CLINICAL REVIEW
of **ORAL**
and **MAXILLOFACIAL**
SURGERY

CLINICAL REVIEW of ORAL and MAXILLOFACIAL SURGERY

A CASE-BASED APPROACH

SHAHROKH C. BAGHERI, DMD, MD, FACS, FICD

Chief, Division of Oral and Maxillofacial Surgery
Department of Surgery, Northside Hospital
Georgia Oral and Facial Surgery, and Eastern Surgical
    Associates and Consultants
Atlanta, Georgia
Clinical Associate Professor
Department of Oral and Maxillofacial Surgery
Georgia Health Sciences University
Augusta, Georgia
Clinical Assistant Professor
Department of Surgery, School of Medicine
Emory University
Atlanta, Georgia
Adjunct Assistant Professor of Surgery
School of Medicine, University of Miami
Miami, Florida

ELSEVIER

SECOND EDITION

3251 Riverport Lane
St. Louis, Missouri 63043

CLINICAL REVIEW OF ORAL AND MAXILLOFACIAL SURGERY: ISBN: 978-0-323-17126-7
A CASE-BASED APPROACH SECOND EDITION

Notices

Knowledge and best practice in this field are constantly changing. As new research and experience broaden our understanding, changes in research methods, professional practices, or medical treatment may become necessary.

Practitioners and researchers must always rely on their own experience and knowledge in evaluating and using any information, methods, compounds, or experiments described herein. In using such information or methods they should be mindful of their own safety and the safety of others, including parties for whom they have a professional responsibility.

With respect to any drug or pharmaceutical products identified, readers are advised to check the most current information provided (i) on procedures featured or (ii) by the manufacturer of each product to be administered, to verify the recommended dose or formula, the method and duration of administration, and contraindications. It is the responsibility of practitioners, relying on their own experience and knowledge of their patients, to make diagnoses, to determine dosages and the best treatment for each individual patient, and to take all appropriate safety precautions.

To the fullest extent of the law, neither the Publisher nor the authors, contributors, or editors, assume any liability for any injury and/or damage to persons or property as a matter of products liability, negligence or otherwise, or from any use or operation of any methods, products, instructions, or ideas contained in the material herein.

Previous edition copyrighted 2008

ISBN: 978-0-323-17126-7

Vice President and Publisher: Linda Duncan
Executive Content Strategist: Kathy Falk
Senior Content Development Specialist: Courtney Sprehe
Publishing Services Manager: Julie Eddy
Senior Project Manager: Richard Barber
Design Direction: Paula Catalano

Printed in China

Last digit is the print number: 9   8   7   6   5   4   3   2

This book is dedicated to...

....all students, residents, and fellows in oral and maxillofacial surgery in all corners of the world, and a tribute to their commitment to improve upon the lives of others despite the many challenges that lie ahead.

....my wife, Nooshin, and to my children, Shaheen and Bijan, whose future is the spark behind this work. My parents, Parviz and Ladan, and my brother, Homayoun, all of whom brighten and bring joy to my day. It is because of them that I was able to complete this project.

....to my prior mentors and friends who have influenced and molded my surgical career. Dr. Robert A. Bays, Dr. Sam E. Farish, Dr. Eric J. Dierks, Dr. Bryce E. Potter, Dr. R. Bryan Bell, Dr. Leon Assael, and Dr. Roger A. Meyer. And to my great friend, Dr. Husain Ali Khan.

Acknowledgments

This book would not have been possible without the support and hard work of the many contributors that gave their time and expertise. It is them who make this book possible.

Special thanks to Dr. Chris Jo, whose help as co-editor and author was instrumental in completion of the first and second editions of this text.

The production of this book would not have been possible without the efficient and enthusiastic team at Elsevier. Special thanks to Ms. Courtney Sprehe, Ms. Kathy Falk, and Mr. Rich Barber.

CHAPTER EDITORS AND CONTRIBUTORS

CHAPTER EDITORS

Deepak Kademani, DMD, MD, FACS
Associate Professor and Fellowship Director
Department of Oral and Maxillofacial Surgery
University of Minnesota
Chief of Oral and Maxillofacial Surgery
North Memorial Medical Center
Minneapolis, Minnesota

Martin B. Steed, DDS
Associate Professor and Residency Program Director
Division of Oral and Maxillofacial Surgery, Department of Surgery
Emory University
Atlanta, Georgia

Husain Ali Khan, DMD, MD
Georgia Oral and Facial Surgery, and Eastern Surgical Associates and Consultants
Attending Surgeon
Division of Oral and Maxillofacial Surgery, Department of Surgery
Northside Hospital
Atlanta, Georgia
Clinical Associate Professor
Department of Oral and Maxillofacial Surgery
Medical College of Georgia
Augusta, Georgia

Roger A. Meyer, MD, DDS, MS, FACS
Director,Maxillofacial Consultations, Ltd.
Greensboro, Georgia
Department of Surgery, Northside Hospital
Atlanta, Georgia
Clinical Assistant Professor
Department of Oral and Maxillofacial Surgery
Georgia Health Science University
Augusta, Georgia
Private Practice, Georgia Oral and Facial Surgery
Marietta, Georgia

CONTRIBUTORS

Nathan G. Adams, DMD, MD
Private Practice, Oral and Facial Reconstructive Surgeons of Utah
Salt Lake City, Utah

Neil Agnihotri, DMD, MD
Private Practice
Virginia Oral and Facial Surgery
Richmond, Virginia

Saif Al-Bustani, MD, DMD
Resident
Division of Plastic and Reconstructive Surgery, School of Medicine
University of North Carolina at Chapel Hill
Chapel Hill, North Carolina

John M. Allen, DMD
Private Practice, Pomona Valley Oral and Maxillofacial Surgery
Pomona, California
Medical Attending Staff, OMS USC University Hospital
Clinical Attending Staff, Los Angeles County/USC Medical Center
Clinical Attending Staff, USC School of Dentistry
Los Angeles, California

Bruce W. Anderson, DDS
Private Practice, South OMS
Peachtree City, Georgia

Leon A. Assael, DMD
Dean, School of Dentistry
University of Minnesota
Minneapolis, Minnesota

Robert S. Attia, DMD
Division of Oral and Maxillofacial Surgery, Department of Surgery
School of Medicine
Emory University
Atlanta, Georgia

Shahid R. Aziz, MD, DMD, FACS
Associate Professor
Department of Oral and Maxillofacial Surgery
New Jersey Dental School
Division of Plastic Surgery, Department of Surgery
New Jersey Medical School
University of Medicine and Dentistry of New Jersey
Newark, New Jersey

Shahrokh C. Bagheri, DMD, MD, FACS, FICD
Chief, Division of Oral and Maxillofacial Surgery
Department of Surgery, Northside Hospital
Georgia Oral and Facial Surgery, and Eastern Surgical
Associates and Consultants
Atlanta, Georgia
Clinical Associate Professor
Department of Oral and Maxillofacial Surgery
Georgia Health Sciences University
Augusta, Georgia
Clinical Assistant Professor
Department of Surgery, School of Medicine
Emory University
Atlanta, Georgia
Adjunct Assistant Professor of Surgery
School of Medicine, University of Miami
Miami, Florida

Michael L. Beckley, DDS
Clinical Assistant Professor
Department of Oral and Maxillofacial Surgery
School of Dentistry
University of the Pacific
San Francisco, California

R. Bryan Bell, MD, DDS, FACS
Medical Director, Oral, Head, and Neck Cancer Program
and Clinic
Providence Cancer Center/Providence Portland Medical
Center
Attending Surgeon, Trauma Service/Oral and Maxillofacial
Surgery Service
Legacy Emanuel Medical Center
Affiliate Professor
Oregon Health and Science University
Head and Neck Surgical Associates
Portland, Oregon

Samuel Bobek, DMD, MD
Private Practice, Head and Neck Surgical Associates
Associate Professor
Oregon Health and Science University
Portland, Oregon

Gary F. Bouloux, MD, DDS, MDSc, FRACDS (OMS)
Associate Professor
Division of Oral and Maxillofacial Surgery, Department of
Surgery
School of Medicine
Emory University
Atlanta, Georgia

Shenan Bradshaw, DDS
Resident, Division of Oral and Maxillofacial Surgery
School of Medicine
Emory University
Atlanta, Georgia

Tuan G. Bui, MD, DMD
Private Practice, Head and Neck Surgical Associates
Attending Surgeon, Oral, Head, and Neck Cancer Program
Providence Cancer Center
Attending Surgeon, Trauma Service/Oral and Maxillofacial
Surgery Service
Legacy Emanuel Medical Center
Affiliate Assistant Professor
Department of Oral and Maxillofacial Surgery
Oregon Health and Science University
Portland, Oregon

Allen Cheng, DDS, MD
Fellow, Head and Neck Oncology and Microvascular
Reconstructive Surgery
Legacy Emanuel Medical Center and Providence Cancer
Center
Portland, Oregon

Sung Hee Cho, MD, DDS
Head and Neck Oncologic Fellow
Department of Otolaryngology
School of Medicine
Emory University
Atlanta, Georgia

Danielle M. Cunningham, DDS
Clinical Attending, St. Joseph's Hospital and Health Center
Syracuse, New York
Private Practice
Camillus, New York

Eric Dierks, MD, DMD
Affiliate Professor
Department of Oral and Maxillofacial Surgery
Oregon Health and Science University
Portland, Oregon

Abdulrahman Doughan, MD, FACC
Atlanta Heart Associates, PC
Stockbridge, Georgia

Fariba Farhidvash, MD, MPH
Neurologist
Atlanta, Georgia

Sam E. Farish, DMD
J. David and Beverly Allen Family Professor of Oral and
Maxillofacial Surgery
Division of Oral and Maxillofacial Surgery, Department of
Surgery
School of Medicine
Emory University
Chief, Department of Oral and Maxillofacial Surgery
VA Medical Center
Atlanta, Georgia

Jaspal Girn, DMD, FRCD(C)
Private Practice, Centrepoint Oral and Facial Surgery
Burnaby, British Columbia
Part-Time Clinical Assistant Professor
Department of Oral Surgery, Faculty of Dentistry
University of British Columbia
Vancouver, British Columbia

Ibrahim M. Haron, DDS
Resident, Division of Oral and Maxillofacial Surgery
School of Medicine
Emory University
Atlanta, Georgia

Eric P. Holmgren, DMD, MD, FACS
Private Practice, Oral and Facial Surgery Associates
Pittsfield, Massachusetts

Bradford Huffman, DMD
Resident, Department of Oral and Maxillofacial Surgery
College of Dental Medicine
Georgia Regents University
Augusta, Georgia

Jason A. Jamali, DDS, MD
Clinical Assistant Professor
Department of Oral and Maxillofacial Surgery
University of Illinois at Chicago
Chicago, Illinois

Damian R. Jimenez, DMD
Chief Resident, Division of Oral and Maxillofacial Surgery
School of Medicine
Emory University
Atlanta, Georgia

Chris Jo, DMD
Atlanta Oral and Facial Surgery, LLC
Atlanta, Georgia

Jenny Jo, MD
Peachtree Women's Clinic
Atlanta Women's Health Group
Atlanta, Georgia

Jeremiah O. Johnson, DDS, MD
Former Chief Resident of Oral and Maxillofacial Surgery
Oregon Health and Science University
Portland, Oregon
Fellow, Royal Melbourne Hospital
Australia

Deepak Kademani, DMD MD FACS
Associate Professor and Fellowship Director
Department of Oral and Maxillofacial Surgery
University of Minnesota
Chief of Oral and Maxillofacial Surgery
North Memorial Medical Center
Minneapolis, Minnesota

Solon Kao, DDS, FICD
Assistant Professor of Oral and Maxillofacial Surgery
Deputy Program Director of OMS Training Program
Department of Oral and Maxillofacial Surgery
School of Dental Medicine
Georgia Regents University
Augusta, Georgia

Husain Ali Khan, DMD, MD, FACS
Georgia Oral and Facial Surgery, and Eastern Surgical
    Associates and Consultants
Attending Surgeon
Division of Oral and Maxillofacial Surgery, Department of
    Surgery
Northside Hospital
Atlanta, Georgia
Clinical Associate Professor
Department of Oral and Maxillofacial Surgery
Medical College of Georgia
Augusta, Georgia

Brian E. Kinard, DMD
Resident, Division of Oral and Maxillofacial Surgery
School of Medicine
Emory University
Atlanta, Georgia

Antonia Kolokythas, DDS, MSc
Department of Oral and Maxillofacial Surgery
University of Illinois at Chicago Cancer Center
Chicago, Illinois

Deepak G. Krishnan, BDS
Assistant Professor of Surgery and Residency Program
    Director
Department of Oral and Maxillofacial Surgery
University of Cincinnati Medical Center
Cincinnati, Ohio

Joyce T. Lee, DDS, MD, FACS
Division of Oral and Maxillofacial Surgery, Department of
    Surgery
School of Medicine
Emory University
Atlanta, Georgia

Patrick J. Louis, DDS, MD
Professor and Residency Program Director
Department of Oral and Maxillofacial Surgery
University of Alabama at Birmingham
Birmingham, Alabama

Michael R. Markiewicz, DDS, MD, MPH
Resident, Division of Oral and Maxillofacial Surgery
School of Medicine
Emory University
Atlanta, Georgia

Robert E. Marx, DDS
Miller School of Medicine
University of Miami
Miami, Florida

Wm. Stuart McKenzie, DMD, MD
Resident, Department of Oral and Maxillofacial Surgery
University of Alabama at Birmingham
Birmingham, Alabama

Mehran Mehrabi, DMD, MD
Private Practice, Advanced Dental Specialists
Glen Dale, Wisconsin

Roger A. Meyer, MD, DDS, MS, FACS
Director, Maxillofacial Consultations, Ltd.
Greensboro, Georgia
Department of Surgery, Northside Hospital
Atlanta, Georgia
Clinical Assistant Professor
Department of Oral and Maxillofacial Surgery
Georgia Health Science University
Augusta, Georgia
Private Practice, Georgia Oral and Facial Surgery
Marietta, Georgia

Michael Miloro, DMD, MD, FACS
Professor and Head
Department of Oral and Maxillofacial Surgery
University of Illinois at Chicago
Chicago, Illinois

Justine Moe, DDS
Resident, Division of Oral and Maxillofacial Surgery
School of Medicine
Emory University
Atlanta, Georgia

Kambiz Mohammadzadeh, MD
Research Fellow
Georgia Oral and Facial Surgery
Atlanta, Georgia

Anthony B.P. Morlandt, MD, DDS
Fellow, Head and Neck Microvascular Reconstruction
Department of Oral and Maxillofacial Surgery, Section of
    Head and Neck Surgery
University of Florida at Jacksonville
Jacksonville, Florida

Timothy M. Osborn, MD, DDS
Assistant Professor
Department of Oral and Maxillofacial Surgery
Henry M. Goldman School of Dental Medicine
Boston University
Boston, Massachusetts

Rebecca Paquin, DMD, BS
Resident, Department of Oral and Maxillofacial Surgery
College of Dental Medicine
Georgia Regents University
Augusta, Georgia

Etern S. Park, MD, DDS
Fellow, Head and Neck Oncologic and Microvascular
    Reconstructive Surgery
Legacy Emanuel Medical Center and Providence Portland
    Cancer Center
Portland, Oregon

Ketan Patel, DDS, PhD
Fellow, Oral/Head and Neck Oncologic Surgery
University of Minnesota
Minneapolis, Minnesota

Kumar J. Patel, BDS, LDSRCS, DMD, MS, FICD
Private Practice
Marietta, Georgia

Mayoor Patel, DDS, MS
Adjunct Clinical Instructor, Craniofacial Pain Center
Tufts University
Boston, Massachusetts
Adjunct Clinical Instructor
Department of Oral Health and Diagnostic Sciences
Georgia Regents University
Augusta, Georgia
Private Practice, Craniofacial Pain Center of Georgia
Atlanta, Georgia

Piyushkumar P. Patel, DDS
Private Practice
Atlanta, Georgia

Sandeep V. Pathak, DMD, MD
Private Practice, Oral and Facial Surgery Associates
Lawrenceville, Georgia

Vincent J. Perciaccante, DDS
Adjunct Associate Professor of Surgery
Division of Oral and Maxillofacial Surgery
School of Medicine
Emory University
Atlanta, Georgia

Ali R. Rahimi, MD, MPH, FACC
Director, Cardiovascular Quality
Kaiser Permanente Georgia/The Southeast Permanente
    Medical Group
Adjunct Assistant Professor
Department of Health Policy and Management
Emory University
Atlanta, Georgia

Kevin L. Rieck, DDS, MD
Assistant Professor of Surgery
Division of Oral and Maxillofacial Surgery, Department of
    Surgery
Mayo Clinic
Rochester, Minnesota

Ma'Ann C. Sabino, DDS, PhD
Parkside Oral and Maxillofacial Surgery Clinic
Hennepin County Medical Center
Minneapolis, Minnesota

Martin Salgueiro, DDS
Department of Oral and Maxillofacial Surgery
Georgia Regents University
Augusta, Georgia

Edward R. Schlissel, DDS, MS
Professor Emeritus of General Dentistry
School of Dental Medicine
Stony Brook University
Stony Brook, New York
Assistant Clinical Professor
Division of Oral and Maxillofacial Surgery, Department of
    Surgery
School of Medicine
Emory University
Atlanta, Georgia

Abtin Shahriari, DMD, MPH
Private Practice, Greater Atlanta Oral Facial Surgery
Cumming, Georgia
Private Practice, Gwinnett Medical Center
Lawrenceville, Georgia
Attending Surgeon, Northside Hospital and Saint Joseph's
    Hospital
Atlanta, Georgia

Jonathan Shum, MD, DDS
Fellow, Head and Neck Oncology and Microvascular
    Reconstructive Surgery
Legacy Emanuel Medical Center and Providence Cancer
    Center
Portland, Oregon
University of Maryland Medical Center
Baltimore, Maryland

Somsak Sittitavornwong, DDS, DMD, MS
Department of Oral and Maxillofacial Surgery
School of Dentistry
University of Alabama at Birmingham
Birmingham, Alabama

A. Michael Sodeifi, DMD, MD, MPH
Private Practice, Silicon Valley Surgical Arts
Cupertino, California
Private Practice, San Francisco Surgical Arts
Adjunct Assistant Professor of Oral and Maxillofacial
    Surgery
University of the Pacific
San Francisco, California

Martin B. Steed, DDS
Associate Professor and Residency Program Director
Division of Oral and Maxillofacial Surgery, Department of
    Surgery
Emory University
Atlanta, Georgia

Brett A. Ueeck, DMD, MD
Assistant Professor
Department of Oral and Maxillofacial Surgery
Oregon Health and Science University
Attending Surgeon, Cleft Lip and Palate Team
Shriners Hospital for Crippled Children
Portland, Oregon

David Verschueren, DMD, MD
Private Practice, Northwest Oral and Facial Surgery
Vancouver, Washington
Clinical Associate and Assistant Professor
Department of Oral and Maxillofacial Surgery
Oregon Health and Sciences University
Portland, Oregon

Lee M. Whitesides, DMD, MMSC
Private Practice
Dunwoody, Georgia

Michael Wilkinson, DMD, MD
Private Practice, Cache Valley Oral and Facial Surgery
Logan, Utah

A Purpose for our Knowledge

Clinical knowledge is like no other. The entire purpose of all the clinical knowledge we retain or access is to help in making a clinical decision. What should I do for this patient? How should I advocate for treatment, select treatment from a variety of options, provide informed consent, sequence patient care, prioritize care, perform it, and evaluate patient care outcomes? All those tasks begin with didactic knowledge. Not didactic knowledge in the abstract, but knowledge that is patient-based (e.g., clinical knowledge). Only knowledge that is applicable to the care of a patient can be deemed clinical knowledge. The traditional surgical textbooks present biomedical knowledge in the abstract. They are a collection of facts and concepts that are left to the reader to determine how to apply in the clinical setting. Although these texts can provide foundational knowledge, their study cannot directly improve patient care.

This text differs fundamentally from that common paradigm in that it strives to impart true clinical knowledge. It is the goal of *Clinical Review of Oral and Maxillofacial Surgery* to bring knowledge directly into the realm of patient care. In this text, Dr. Bagheri and his expert clinician contributors take 103 clinical situations in patient care and apply the appropriate didactic knowledge to making a clinical decision. This text simulates real practice by addressing common clinical situations that for the experienced clinicians will resonate in their daily practice, and for the residents will set the landscape for their eventual clinical decision needs.

Evidence-based medicine is the application of didactic knowledge combined with clinical experience personalized to the needs of an individual patient. Evidence-based medicine is thus the most straightforward, practical, and effective way to practice oral and maxillofacial surgery. Thus, the best evidence-based practice is delivered by experienced clinicians, with a wealth of didactic knowledge, who also access the latest information and who address the needs of their patients through careful listening and knowledge of each patient. How can the tenets of this method be taught to the surgeon who has not yet gained sufficient experience to allow didactics, skill, and patient/doctor communication to flow seamlessly into great care? *Clinical Review of Oral and Maxillofacial Surgery* seeks to do so by simulating the clinical environment by presenting common clinical problems addressed by true experts in each area. The resident in oral and maxillofacial surgery can particularly benefit from this text in that the key elements of the clinical care of each problem are presented. As actual care unfolds, the questions to be asked on rounds, the queries and concerns of the patient, the needs of the health care team, and the verification of one's own clinical thinking are confirmed in the text as each case setting is discussed.

Actual patient care is simulated in the *Clinical Review* by demonstrating common clinical presentation, anamnestic and physical findings, imaging, and laboratory values. These are collated into patient assessment, which is combined with biomedical knowledge to choose the best treatments. Even the best evidence is often controversial. Where the limits of contemporary knowledge and the parameters that define the decision-making environment are not clear, the remaining controversies over treatment are discussed. Finally, key to the success of such an effort, the clinical education presented in *Clinical Review of Oral and Maxillofacial Surgery* details the complications of treatment, such as infection and idiosyncratic drug reactions.

All this can and must be done in an efficient way that uses the precious time of the practicing surgeon wisely. As Shakespeare said, "Brevity is the soul of wit." Clinicians today must make dozens of daily decisions using the tenets of evidence-based medicine. To do so requires knowledge that, as in manufacturing, is accessed "just in time" to care for an individual patient. The large inventory of knowledge that has been traditionally used to make clinical decisions has been supplanted by the rapid increase of new information that must guide clinical decisions. To achieve that goal in a practical way, knowledge must be contemporary, easy to access, easy to read and understand, and of course it must be brief. *Clinical Review of Oral and Maxillofacial Surgery* seeks to allow the reader to find clinically relevant knowledge efficiently.

In the era of a society and specialty that measures the continued competence of surgeons, certification/licensure and credentialing are ongoing processes that must be concurrently achieved and regularly enforced. Although clinical measurements can be obtained by examining clinical outcomes, a continuous monitoring of contemporary knowledge to underlie effective practice is becoming the norm. *Clinical Review of Oral and Maxillofacial Surgery* is particularly suited to this emerging environment of being able to apply contemporary knowledge into clinical practice.

The only purpose of clinical knowledge, as can be read and enjoyed in *Clinical Review of Oral and Maxillofacial Surgery*, is to make a decision that has a positive effect on patient care. The cases presented here resemble an objective-simulated clinical encounter (OSCE). The case-based format allows readers to calibrate their own opinions about a clinical problem in a virtual, live patient setting and to customize it to the needs of their patients in real practice. Using these clinical presentations in real time to evaluate one's own thinking on a clinical problem can result in more effective care influenced by the wealth of clinical evidence underlying the decision as well as the opinion of experts supplied with the latest knowledge. Here in the pages of *Clinical Review of Oral and Maxillofacial Surgery* we can help the sick to be well and achieve our highest purpose.

Dr. Leon Assael, Dean, University of Minnesota

It is clear now, almost 10 decades after the formation of the specialty in 1918, that the demand for and subsequently the scope of oral and maxillofacial surgery have rapidly expanded far beyond what anyone could have envisioned in the beginning. As the world's population ages, and with development of new diagnostic modalities, treatment and surgical procedures to prolong a useful life span even further, there will be a sustained and consistent increase in the need for the services of the modern oral and maxillofacial surgeon.

The traditional array of oral and maxillofacial operations was mostly related to the surgical treatment of conditions such as infections, diseased teeth and associated pathology, or repair of traumatic injuries or developmental deformities limited to the oral region. However, as explained in this textbook, there has been considerable expansion of the recognized scope of the specialty to include the cranium and the neck, and not only to address the eradication of pathology. With the dawn of the twenty-first century, the long-anticipated goal of "expanded scope" of oral and maxillofacial surgery has ceased to be a "buzz word" and has become a reality. Fueled by the energy, imagination, and skill of many young surgeons with post-residency fellowship training, and a realization that mere '"familiarity" about an area of surgical interest does not create true clinical competence that can be transferred to quality surgical care,[1,2] the specialty has moved forward with confidence based on training and documented clinical experience. It has become heavily committed to research, teaching, and patient care in the additional areas of pediatric craniomaxillofacial surgery, oncologic and reconstructive surgery, facial cosmetic surgery, care of nerve injuries, surgery for temporomandibular joint disorders (both open and arthroscopic), endoscopic minimally invasive operations, and dental and craniofacial implantology. None of this would have been possible without the opportunities given to those trainees who wished to expand their knowledge and skills beyond residency by completing fellowship training or seeking further education beyond formal training in one of the areas just mentioned. Not only has the scope of diseases and conditions expanded but also additional efforts have been designed to change the patients' quality of life by improving upon oral and facial anatomic defects that affect both function and aesthetics. In addition to surgical skills, supportive technology in the form of instrumentation, internal fixation and implant systems, and imaging modalities have allowed the evaluation and treatment planning for surgical corrections of complex head and neck pathology, congenital or development craniofacial deformities, loss of teeth and supporting bone, or maxillofacial injuries to be done with increased accuracy and predict-

ability. As the repertoire of procedures increases, so does the risk of unwanted complications of treatment that may require further surgical interventions, and these areas are addressed as well.

Similar to the first edition, the purpose of this edition is to provide its readers with a systematic and comprehensive approach to the management of patients presenting with a wide array of surgical or pathological conditions seen in this specialty. Contrary to traditional textbooks of surgery (which present material in a fashion not directly related to a given patient, but rather list "classical" findings, pathophysiology, and stereotypical treatment modalities), in this publication we emphasize a case-based approach to learning that is suitable for readers of oral and maxillofacial surgery at all levels of training or practice. Case-based learning is a proven and effective method of teaching. Some of the most common (as well as complex) cases are selected to illustrate individual examples of the typical history, physical exam findings, laboratory and imaging studies, analysis of treatment options, complications, and discussion of other relevant information. Learning is enhanced by incorporating teaching around real-patient scenarios. However, each chapter is more than a patient scenario, but rather a carefully written teaching case that outlines essential information pertinent to fundamental aspects of the condition as they present in the practice of oral and maxillofacial surgery. In this manner, the reader is actively engaged in assessing the case, raising the interest, and therefore enhancing the understanding and retention of information.

In the past decades, the specialty of oral and maxillofacial surgery has seen numerous dramatic changes in training, scope, and style of practice. Additional changes in the near future are undoubtedly in the offing. For example, traditional ways of conducting single or small-group private practice in offices may be replaced by a new model,[3] in which groups of subspecialists practice together in a university or large hospital setting and are fully staffed to see patients around the clock. A single area of surgical expertise for a large metropolitan area of several million people may be provided by a group of surgeons practicing together in a large hospital or university medical center setting. These surgeons focus solely on their area of expertise (for example, pediatric craniofacial surgery, maxillofacial trauma, or head and neck oncologic surgery and reconstruction) to the exclusion of other aspects of their specialty. All major surgery with a high demand for technical expertise and experience in patient hospital management is handled in such a fashion. These surgeons may be the new oral and maxillofacial hospitalists of the twenty-first century! Only the more routine procedures or aspects of practice, which comprise the majority of work in today's oral surgery private practices (tooth extractions, biopsies, routine infections, and perhaps dental implants) might continue to be managed by future oral surgeons who choose to practice in an office-based environment. What is contained in this new edition will give the reader a good overview of all areas of the specialty of oral and maxillofacial surgery as it faces the challenges of the twenty-first century.

It is with great excitement and anticipation of the future development of our specialty that we publish this second edition with new cases and updated information. It is hoped that all readers, in all corners of the world, will find within its contents the information and inspiration that helps them improve the care of their patients.

Shahrokh C. Bagheri
Atlanta, Georgia

---

[1]Hupp JR: Surgical training: Is dabbling enough? *J Oral Maxillofac Surg* 69:1535, 2011.
[2]Meyer RA, Bagheri SC: Familiarity does not breed competence, *J Oral Maxillofac Surg* 69:2483, 2011.
[3]Hupp JR: Integrated service-line care—lessons from China, *J Oral Maxillofac Surg* 71:653, 2013.

CONTENTS

CHAPTER 1

Oral and Maxillofacial Radiology

This chapter addresses:
- Multilocular Radiolucent Lesion in the Pericoronal Region (Keratocystic Odontogenic Tumor [Odontogenic Keratocyst])
- Unilocular Radiolucent Lesion of the Mandible
- Multilocular Radiolucent Lesion in the Periapical Region (Ameloblastoma)
- Unilocular Radiolucent Lesion in a Periapical Region (Periapical Cyst)
- Mixed Radiolucent-Radiopaque Lesion (Ossifying Fibroma)
- Cone-Beam Computed Tomography (CBCT)

Interpretation of radiographs is a routine part of the daily practice of oral and maxillofacial surgery. Commonly obtained radiographs at the office include the periapical, occlusal, panoramic, and lateral cephalometric radiographs. Cone beam computed tomography (CBCT) scans are becoming more readily available in many offices. Although this technology is extremely useful, its indications, liabilities, and advantages have to be clearly recognized. As the future unfolds, the advancing technology will improve upon office imaging modalities that will facilitate diagnosis and treatment. Therefore, a knowledge of normal radiographic anatomy and clinical skill in recognizing pathologic conditions become even more essential.

Despite clinicians' ability to read and interpret many different imaging studies, the oral and maxillofacial radiologist will play an increasingly greater role in the practice of oral and maxillofacial surgeons.

This section includes the radiographic presentation of five important and representative pathologic processes, in addition to a new case demonstrating the use of CBCT. Included in each case is the differential diagnosis of associated conditions, to guide further study.

Figure 1-1 shows the most common location of several radiographically detectable maxillofacial pathologic processes.

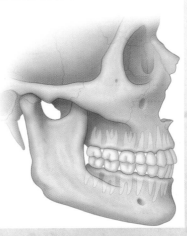

Posterior maxilla
- Pagets disease of bone

Posterior mandible
- Dentigerous cyst
- Keratocytic odontogenic tumor
- Ameloblastoma
- Intraosseous mucoepidermoid carcinoma
- Stafne bone defect (below canal)
- Idiopathic bone marrow defect
- Calcifying epithelial odontogenic tumor (CEOT)

Anterior maxilla
- Adenomatoid odontogenic tumor (AOT)
- Nasopalatine duct cyst
- Lateral periodontal cyst (botryoid type)
- Odontoma
- Paget's disease of bone

Anterior mandible
- Periapical cemento osseous dysplasia
- Central giant cell granuloma
- Odontoma

Figure 1-1 The most common location of several radiographically detectable maxillofacial pathologic processes.

Multilocular Radiolucent Lesion in the Pericoronal Region (Keratocystic Odontogenic Tumor [Odontogenic Keratocyst])

Piyushkumar P. Patel, Chris Jo, and Shahrokh C. Bagheri

CC

A 20-year-old man is referred for evaluation of a swelling on his right mandible.

Keratocystic Odontogenic Tumor (KCOT)

Keratocystic odontogenic tumors (KCOTs) show a slight predilection for males and are predominantly found in individuals of Northern European descent. The peak incidence is seen between 11 and 40 years of age. Patients with larger lesions may present with pain secondary to infection of the cystic cavity. Smaller lesions are usually asymptomatic and are frequently diagnosed during routine radiographic examination.

The World Health Organization (WHO) has recommended the use of the term *keratocystic odontogenic tumor* (KCOT), rather than *odontogenic keratocyst* (OKC), because the former name better reflects the neoplastic behavior of the lesion. Genetically, the lesion shows a repeatable chromosomal abnormality (PTCH gene on chromosome 9q22.3-q31).

HPI

The patient complains of a 2-month history of progressive, nonpainful swelling of his right posterior mandible. (About 65% to 83% of KCOTs occur in the mandible, most often in the posterior body and ramus region. KCOTs account for approximately 3% to 14% of all oral cystic lesions.) The patient denies any history of pain in his right lower jaw, fever, purulence, or trismus. He does not report any neurosensory changes (which are generally not seen with KCOTs).

MHX/PDHX/MEDICATIONS/ALLERGIES/SH/FH

Noncontributory. There is no family history of similar presentations.

Nevoid basal cell carcinoma syndrome (NBCCS) is an autosomal dominant inherited condition with features that can include multiple basal cell carcinomas of the skin, multiple KCOTs, intracranial calcifications, and rib and vertebral anomalies. Many other anomalies have been reported with this syndrome (Box 1-1). The prevalence of NBCCS is estimated to be 1 in 57,000 to 1 in 164,000 persons.

EXAMINATION

Maxillofacial. The patient has slight lower right facial swelling isolated to the lateral border of the mandible and not involving the area below the inferior border. The mass is hard, nonfluctuant, and nontender to palpation (large cysts may rupture and leak keratin into the surrounding tissue, provoking an intense inflammatory reaction that causes pain and swelling). There are no facial or trigeminal nerve deficits (paresthesia of the inferior alveolar nerve would be more indicative of a malignant process). The intercanthal distance is 33 mm (normal), and there is no evidence of frontal bossing. His occipitofrontal circumference is normal (an intercanthal distance [the distance between the two medial canthi of the palpebral fissures] of greater than 36 mm is indicative of hypertelorism, and an occipitofrontal circumference greater than 55 cm is indicative of frontal bossing; both can be seen with NBCCS).

Neck. There are no palpable masses and no cervical or submandibular lymphadenopathy. Positive lymph nodes would be indicative of an infectious or a neoplastic process. A careful neck examination is paramount in the evaluation of any head and neck pathology.

Box 1-1	Diagnostic Criteria for Nevoid Basal Cell Carcinoma Syndrome

A diagnosis can be made when 2 major criteria (or 1 major and 2 minor criteria) are met.

Major Criteria
1. Multiple (>2) basal cell carcinomas, or one in a patient under age 30, or >10 basal cell nevi
2. Any odontogenic keratocyst (confirmed on histology) or polyostotic bone cyst
3. Palmar or plantar pits (3 or more)
4. Ectopic calcification: lamellar or early (< age 20) falx calcification
5. Family history of NBCCS

Minor Criteria
1. Congenital skeletal anomaly: bifid, fused, splayed, or missing rib; or bifid, wedged, or fused vertebra
2. Occipitofrontal circumference (OFC) > 97th percentile, with frontal bossing
3. Cardiac or ovarian fibroma
4. Medulloblastoma
5. Lymphomesenteric cysts
6. Congenital malformation: cleft lip and/or palate, polydactyly, eye anomaly (cataract, coloboma, microphthalmia)

From Evans DG, Ladusans EJ, Rimmer S, et al: Complications of the naevoid basal cell carcinoma syndrome: results of a population based study, *J Med Genet* 30(6):460-464, 1993.

Intraoral. Occlusion is stable and reproducible. The right mandibular third molar appears to be distoangularly impacted (KCOTs do not typically alter the occlusion). The interincisal opening is within normal limits. There is buccal expansion of the right mandible, extending from the right mandibular first molar area posteriorly toward the ascending ramus. Resorption of bone may include the cortex at the inferior border of the mandible, but this is observed at a slower rate than in intermedullary bone, which is less dense. For this reason, KCOTs characteristically extend anteroposteriorly than buccolingually. This pattern of expansion into less-dense bone explains why maxillary KCOTs show more buccal than palatal expansion and often expand into the maxillary sinus. There is no palpable thrill or audible bruit, both of which are seen with arteriovenous malformations. The oral mucosa is normal in appearance with no signs of acute inflammatory processes.

Thorax-abdomen-extremity. The patient has no findings suggestive of NBCCS (e.g., pectus excavatum, rib abnormalities, palmar or plantar pitting, and skin lesions; see Box 1-1).

IMAGING

A panoramic radiograph is the initial screening examination of choice for patients presenting for evaluation of intraosseous mandibular pathology (10% to 20% of KCOTs are incidental radiographic findings). This provides an excellent overview of the bony architecture of the maxilla, mandible, and associated structures. CT scans can be obtained when large lesions are found. CT scans are valuable in that they provide additional information, such as the proximity of adjacent structures (e.g., the mandibular canal), the integrity of cortical plates, and the presence of perforations into adjacent soft tissues. CT scans provide accurate assessment of the size of the lesion and can demonstrate additional anatomic details (or lesions) that do not appear on panoramic radiographs.

A CBCT scan is appropriate for the evaluation of this lesion. Given its higher resolution, lower radiation dose (approximately 20% of the radiation of a conventional [helical] CT), and lower cost, a CBCT can replace helical CT for evaluation and follow up of such a lesion. The CBCT scan can also be used to create a stereolithic model of the area of interest.

It has been demonstrated that T2-weighted magnetic resonance imaging (MRI) can detect KCOTs in 85% of new cases with a readily recognizable pattern. However, the use of MRI for management of suspected OKCs is not routine.

In this patient, the panoramic radiograph reveals a large, multilocular radiolucent lesion with possible displacement of the right mandibular third molar (Figure 1-2). There are also several carious teeth and a retained root tip of the right mandibular second bicuspid (tooth #29). (In a patient with a radiolucent lesion of the mandible presumed to be an odontogenic cystic lesion, a multilocular appearance is associated with a 12-fold increased risk for the diagnosis of KCOT; however, the presence of a unilocular lesion does not exclude the possibility of a KCOT diagnosis.)

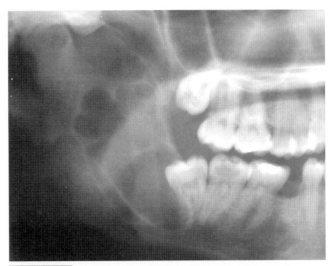

Figure 1-2 Preoperative panoramic radiograph showing a large multilocular radiolucent lesion of the right mandible body and ramus associated with an impacted third molar.

LABS

No laboratory tests are indicated unless dictated by the medical history.

Fine-needle aspiration (FNA) biopsy and cytokeratin-10 immunocytochemical staining have been shown to differentiate KCOTs from dentigerous and other nonkeratinizing cysts. Despite their availability, these techniques are not routinely ordered.

DIFFERENTIAL DIAGNOSIS

The differential diagnosis of multilocular radiolucent lesions can be divided into lesions of cystic pathogenesis, neoplastic (benign or malignant) lesions, and vascular anomalies (least common). The differential diagnosis of multilocular radiolucent lesions is presented in Box 1-2 and can be further narrowed by the clinical presentation. Special consideration should be given to radiolucent lesions with poorly defined or ragged borders, which have a separate differential.

BIOPSY

An incisional or excisional biopsy can be performed, depending on the size of the lesion. A smaller cystic lesion can be completely excised, whereas larger lesions require an incisional biopsy to guide final therapy. It is important to aspirate the lesion before incising into it (entering carefully through the cortical bone) to rule out a vascular lesion. The aspiration of bright red blood alerts the surgeon to the presence of a high-flow vascular lesion, such as an arteriovenous malformation, which could result in uncontrollable hemorrhage. In such a case, the procedure should be aborted to allow for further radiographic and angiographic studies to characterize the vasculature of the area. The aspiration of straw-colored (or clear) fluid is characteristic of a cystic lesion, and the absence of any aspirate may be seen with a solid mass (tumors).

Box 1-2   Differential Diagnosis of Multilocular Radiolucent Lesions

- **Ameloblastoma**—The most frequent location is the posterior mandible, and the tumor's most common radiographic appearance is that of a multilocular radiolucent lesion. This is the most frequently diagnosed odontogenic tumor.
- **Keratocystic odontogenic tumor**—This lesion cannot be differentiated on clinical and radiographic grounds from an ameloblastoma. KCOTs generally do not cause resorption of adjacent teeth. The orthokeratin variant is usually associated with an impacted tooth.
- **Dentigerous cyst**—Large dentigerous cysts can have a multilocular appearance on a radiograph, given the existence of bone trabeculae within the radiolucency. However, they are histologically a unilocular lesion. There is a strong association with impacted mandibular third molars. Painless bony expansion and resorption of adjacent teeth are uncommon but can occur.
- **Ameloblastic fibroma**—The posterior mandible is also the most common site for this lesion. It is predominantly seen in the younger population, and most lesions are diagnosed within the first two decades of life. Large tumors can cause bony expansion. The lesion can manifest as a unilocular or multilocular radiolucent lesion that is often associated with an impacted tooth. Ameloblastic fibro-odontomas are mixed radiopaque-radiolucent lesions.
- **Central giant cell tumor**—Approximately 70% of these lesions occur in the mandible, most commonly in the anterior region. The tumor's radiographic appearance can be unilocular or multilocular. These lesions can contain large vascular spaces that can lead to substantial intraoperative bleeding. The aneurysmal bone cyst has been suggested to be a variant of the central giant cell tumor. The majority of these lesions are discovered before age 30.
- **Odontogenic myxoma**—Although myxomas are seen in all age groups, the majority are discovered in patients 20 to 40 years of age. The posterior mandible is the most common location, and the tumor's radiographic appearance can be unilocular or multilocular. At times, the radiolucent defect may contain thin, wispy trabeculae of residual bone, given its "cobweb" or "soap bubble" trabecular pattern.
- **Aneurysmal bone cyst**—Lacking a true epithelial lining, these cysts most commonly occur in the long bones or the vertebral column. They rarely occur in the jaws, but when they do, it is mostly in young adults. They can present as a unilocular or multilocular radiolucent lesion with marked cortical expansion that usually displaces but does not resorb teeth.
- **Traumatic bone cyst**—This lesion lacks a true epithelial lining and frequently involves the mandibular molar and premolar region in young adults. These cysts can cause expansion and usually show a well-defined unilocular, scalloping radiolucency between the roots without resorption. The lesion always exists above the inferior alveolar canal.
- **Calcifying epithelial odontogenic tumor (CEOT)**—This is an uncommon tumor. The majority are found in the posterior mandible, mostly in patients age 30 to 50 years. A multilocular radiolucent defect is seen more often than a unilocular radiolucency. Although the tumor may be entirely radiolucent, calcified structures of varying sizes and density are usually seen within the defect. CEOTs can also be associated with an impacted tooth.
- **Lateral periodontal cyst (botryoid odontogenic cyst)**—Usually found in older individuals (fifth to seventh decades of life), the botryoid variant often shows a multilocular appearance. It is most commonly seen in the premolar canine areas.
- **Calcifying odontogenic cyst (COC)**—Most commonly found in the incisor canine region, this cyst is usually diagnosed in patients in the mid-30s. Although the unilocular presentation is most common, multilocular lesions have been reported. Radiopaque structures are usually present in approximately one third to one half of the lesions.
- **Intraosseous mucoepidermoid carcinoma**—This is the most common salivary gland tumor arising centrally within the jaws. Most commonly found in the mandible of middle-aged adults, the tumors can appear radiographically as unilocular or multilocular radiolucent lesions. Association with an impacted tooth has been reported.
- **Hyperparathyroidism (brown tumor)**—Parathyroid hormone (PTH) is normally produced by the parathyroid gland in response to decreased serum calcium levels. In primary hyperparathyroidism, uncontrolled production of PTH is due to hyperplasia or carcinoma of the parathyroid glands. Secondary hyperparathyroidism develops in conditions of low serum calcium levels (e.g., renal disease), resulting in a feedback increase in PTH. Patients with hyperparathyroidism usually present with a classic triad of signs and symptoms, described as "stones, bones, and abdominal groans." Patients with primary hyperparathyroidism have a marked tendency to develop renal calculi ("stones"). "Bones" refers to the variety of osseous changes that are seen, including the brown tumor of hyperparathyroidism. These lesions can appear as unilocular or multilocular radiolucent lesions, most commonly affecting the mandible, clavicle, ribs, and pelvis. "Abdominal groans" refers to the tendency of these patients to develop duodenal ulcers and associated pain. When dealing with any giant cell lesions, the clinician must rule out the brown tumor of hyperparathyroidism by evaluating the patient's serum calcium level (it is elevated in hyperparathyroidism). Patients with brown tumor also have elevated levels of PTH (which is confirmed by radioimmunoassay of the circulating parathyroid levels).
- **Cherubism**—In this rare developmental inherited condition, painless bilateral expansion of the posterior mandible produces cherublike facies (plump-cheeked little angels depicted in Renaissance paintings). In addition, involvement of the orbital rims and floor produces the classic "eyes upturned toward heaven." Radiographically, the lesions are usually bilateral multilocular radiolucent lesions. Although rare, unilateral involvement has been reported.
- **Intrabony vascular malformations**—Arteriovenous malformations are most often detected in patients between 10 and 20 years of age and are more commonly found in the mandible. Mobility of teeth, bleeding from the gingival sulks, an audible bruit, or a palpable thrill should alert the clinician. The radiographic appearance is variable, but the malformation most commonly presents as a multilocular radiolucent lesion. The loculations may be small, giving the honeycomb appearance that produces a "soap bubble" radiographic appearance. Aspiration of all undiagnosed intrabony lesions is warranted to rule out the presence of this lesion, because fatal hemorrhage can occur after an incisional biopsy.

ASSESSMENT

Expansile multilocular radiolucent mass of the posterior right mandible associated with an impacted right mandibular third molar (25% to 40% of cases are associated with an unerupted tooth).

With this patient under intravenous anesthesia, an incisional biopsy was performed after aspiration of straw-colored fluid that showed the classic histopathology of the KCOT. Histologic features include a thin squamous cell epithelial lining (eight cells or fewer). Because of the lack of rete ridges, the epithelial–connective tissue interface is flat. The epithelial surface is parakeratinized and often corrugated (wavy). The basal cell layer is hyperchromatic and composed of cuboidal cells, which show prominent palisading, giving a "tombstone" effect. The fibrous wall is usually thin and at times shows a mixed inflammatory response. Keratinization of the lumen is not a pathognomonic finding. The fibrous wall may contain epithelial islands that show central keratinization and cyst formation; these are known as *daughter-satellite cells.*

TREATMENT

Options that have been used to treat KCOTs include the following:
- Decompression by marsupialization
- Marsupialization followed by enucleation (surgical decompression of the cyst, followed by several months of daily irrigation with chlorhexidine via stents secured in the cystic cavity, followed by cystectomy)
- Enucleation with curettage alone
- Enucleation followed by chemoablation or cryotherapy
- Enucleation with peripheral ostectomy
- Enucleation with peripheral ostectomy and chemoablation or cryotherapy
- En bloc resection or mandibular segmental resection

Resection is advocated only if there have been multiple recurrences after enucleation with an adjunctive procedure (e.g., cryotherapy, Carnoy's solution, or peripheral ostectomy) or for a large KCOT exhibiting aggressive behavior, such as destruction of adjacent tissues. Several studies demonstrate that enucleation alone (when the diagnosis of KCOT has been established) has a high recurrence rate; therefore, many surgeons advocate enucleation with a local adjunctive procedure, such as cryotherapy, Carnoy's solution, and/or peripheral ostectomy.

KCOTs do not invade the epineurium; therefore, the inferior alveolar nerve can be separated and preserved. Furthermore, any perforations of the keratinized mucosa should be excised, because they may contain additional epithelial rests, which can lead to recurrences. Aggressive soft tissue excision is not required, because KCOTs do not usually infiltrate adjacent structures. If the cyst is removed in one unit, there is no need for curettage, unless the lining has been shredded or torn.

Some controversy exists regarding the optimal management (extraction versus retention) of teeth involved with an KCOT. It is generally accepted that a KCOT with a scalloped radiographic appearance should have the associated teeth removed, because it is considered impossible to completely remove the thin-walled cystic lining. However, if the KCOT is successfully removed in one unit, the teeth may be spared without compromising recurrence. In most instances there is no need for endodontic therapy, despite surgical denervation. The teeth may not become devitalized due to perfusion of the pulp via accessory canals through the periodontal ligaments.

Some surgeons advocate the application of Carnoy's solution after enucleation and peripheral ostectomy with application of methylene blue. Carnoy's solution is composed of 6 ml of absolute alcohol, 3 ml of ferric chloride, and 1 ml of 100% acetic acid. Chloroform is no longer recommended due to its carcinogenic potential. Carnoy's solution penetrates the bone to a depth of 1.54 mm after a 5-minute application. It is difficult to obtain and needs to be mixed fresh. It does not fixate the inferior alveolar nerve, but some clinicians cover the nerve with sterile petrolatum as a caution.

Synchronous bone grafting is not carried out with this technique. Cryotherapy with liquid nitrogen is an acceptable alternative to the use of Carnoy's solution. Liquid nitrogen is sprayed within the cavity and penetrates to a depth of about 1.5 mm. Suggested protocols include spraying the cavity for 1 minute and then allowing the bone to thaw. This can be repeated two or three times.

Synchronous grafting with cancellous bone can be accomplished after cryotherapy. Patients should be cautioned since liquid nitrogen does weaken the mandible, and this may result in a pathologic fracture. Sensory nerves within the field may show paresthesia; however, the majority recover within 3 to 6 months.

With both techniques, adjacent soft tissue needs to be protected. An alternate technique is used in cases of buccal or lingual plate perforation and with sinus involvement.

This patient was treated under general anesthesia with enucleation of the lesion followed by the application of methylene blue to guide peripheral ostectomy. The patient was placed on a soft diet to reduce the risk of jaw fracture. The postoperative panoramic radiograph confirmed that the inferior border of the mandible remained intact.

The final pathology report confirmed the diagnosis of a KCOT consistent with the initial incisional biopsy specimen. The patient was placed on a strict recall schedule—every 6 months for the first 5 years and then yearly. The recurrence rate for KCOTs has been reported to range from 5% to 60%. It has been reported that most recurrences are seen within 5 years, although they can develop at any time. Recurrences that arise secondary to residual cyst left in the bone may be apparent within 18 months of surgery.

COMPLICATIONS

The KCOT has been described as having clinical features that include potentially aggressive behavior and a high recurrence rate. Because recurrence is a major concern, clinicians vary in their surgical approach. Resection results in the lowest recurrence rate; however, there is considerable morbidity associated with this radical treatment. The primary mechanisms for recurrence have been postulated to be incomplete removal of all the cystic lining; new primary cyst formation from additional activated rests; or the development of a new KCOT in an adjacent area that is interpreted as a recurrence.

KCOTs have been reported to undergo transformation into ameloblastoma and squamous cell carcinoma, although this occurrence is rare. Other common postprocedural complications include inferior alveolar nerve paresthesia, postoperative infection and, with larger lesions, pathologic mandibular fracture (the highest risk is during the first few weeks after enucleation).

DISCUSSION

Ever since the histologic features of the KCOT were established, many investigators have recognized that two major variants exist, based on microscopic findings: a cyst with a parakeratinized epithelial lining and a cyst with an orthokeratinized epithelial lining.

Crowley and colleagues undertook a comparison of the orthokeratin and parakeratinized variants. In their review, they found that the parakeratinized variant occurred more commonly than the orthokeratinized variant (frequency of 86.2% for the parakeratinized variant compared with 12.2% for the orthokeratinized variant); 1.6% of cysts had both orthokeratin and parakeratin features.

These researchers also found that the parakeratinized variant demonstrated a 42% recurrence rate, compared to only 2.2% for the orthokeratinized variant. In addition, the orthokeratinized variant was more frequently associated with impacted teeth. Given the different clinical behaviors of these two entities, many authors designate them as separate pathologic lesions, with the orthokeratinized variant known as an *orthokeratinized odontogenic cyst* (OOC). A lesion with both orthokeratin and parakeratin features should be treated as a parakeratinized KCOT (OKC).

As was mentioned earlier, in 2005 WHO designated the OKC a *keratocystic odontogenic tumor* (KCOT). The lesion was defined as a benign, unicystic or multicystic intraosseous tumor of odontogenic origin with a characteristic lining of parakeratinized, stratified squamous epithelium and the potential for aggressive infiltrative behavior.

Stimulation of residual epithelial cells is a common feature in the development of any cyst. In the case of the KCOT, the epithelial cells implicated are from the rest of Serres or Malassez or from the reduced enamel epithelium. Aberration of a PTCH gene is thought to be a genetic cause for the etiology of the KCOT. Collagenase activity in the cyst's epithelium, with its resorptive properties, appears to regulate the ability of the lesion to grow expansively in bone.

Identification of individuals who may have NBCCS allows the clinician to arrange for appropriate referrals. NBCCS should be suspected when multiple lesions exist. The diagnosis is confirmed upon finding any two of the major criteria, or one major criterion plus two minor criteria (see Box 1-1).

Some abnormalities are pertinent only to the diagnosis and do not require any specific therapy. Other abnormalities may pose further risk to the patient and require the input of other specialists. Spina bifida and central nervous system tumors require referral to a neurosurgeon. In addition, genetic counseling for all patients afflicted with NBCCS is recommended. KCOTs associated with this syndrome are treated in the same manner as an isolated KCOT; however, these lesions have a higher rate of recurrence when associated with NBCCS (which may represent new lesions). KCOTs are often associated with the follicle of a potentially functional tooth and, when possible, marsupialization with orthodontic guidance should be considered.

Bibliography

August M, Caruso PA, Faquin WC: Report of a case: an 18-year-old man with a one-month history of nontender left mandibular swelling, *N Engl J Med* 353:2798-2805, 2005.

August M, Faquin WC, Troulis M, et al: Differentiation of odontogenic keratocysts from nonkeratinizing cysts by use of fine-needle aspiration biopsy and cytokeratin-10 staining, *J Oral Maxillofac Surg* 58:935-940, 2000.

Barnes L, Eveson JW, Reichart P, et al (eds): *Pathology and genetics: head and neck tumours (IARC World Health Organization classification of tumors)*, Lyon, France, 2005, IARC Press.

Buckley P, Seldin E, Dodson T, et al: Multilocularity as a radiographic marker of the keratocystic odontogenic tumor, *J Oral Maxillofac Surg* 70:320, 2012.

Crowley T, Kaugras GE, Gunsolley JC: Odontogenic keratocysts: a clinical and histologic comparison of the parakeratin and orthokeratin variants, *J Oral Maxillofac Surg* 50:22-26, 1992.

Evans DG, Ladusans EJ, Rimmer S, et al: Complications of the naevoid basal cell carcinoma syndrome: results of a population based study, *J Med Genet* 30:460-464, 1993.

Kolokythas A: OKC: to decompress or not to decompress—a comparative study between decompression and enucleation vs resection/peripheral ostectomy, *J Oral Maxillofac Surg* 65(4):640-644, 2007.

Madras J: Keratocystic odontogenic tumor: reclassification of the odontogenic keratocyst from cyst to tumor, *J Can Dent Assoc* 74:2, 2008.

Marx RE, Stern D: *Oral and maxillofacial pathology: a rationale for diagnosis and treatment*, Chicago, 2003, Quintessence.

Pindborg JJ, Hansen J: Studies on odontogenic cyst epithelium: clinical and roentgenographic aspects of odontogenic keratocysts, *Acta Pathol Microbial Scand* 58:283, 1963.

Pogrel MA: Keratocystic odontogenic tumor. In Bagheri S (ed): *Current therapy in oral and maxillofacial surgery*, St Louis, 2012, Mosby.

Pogrel MA, Jordan RC: Marsupialization as a definitive treatment for the odontogenic keratocyst, *J Oral Maxillofac Surg* 62:651-655, 2004.

Pogrel MA, Schmidt BL: The odontogenic keratocyst, *Oral Maxillofacial Surg Clin N Am* 15(3): xi, 2003.

Shear M: Primordial cysts, *J Dent Assoc S Afr* 152:1, 1960.

Tolstunov L, Treasure T: Surgical treatment algorithm for odontogenic keratocyst: combined treatment of odontogenic keratocyst and mandibular defect with marsupialization, enucleation, iliac crest bone graft and dental implants, *J Oral Maxillofac Surg* 66:1025, 2008.

Quereshy F, Barnum G, Demko C, et al: Applications of cone beam computed tomography in the practice of oral and maxillofacial surgery, *J Oral Maxillofac Surg* 66:791, 2008.

Unilocular Radiolucent Lesion of the Mandible

Michael R. Markiewicz, David Verschueren, and Shahrokh C. Bagheri

CC

A 68-year-old Caucasian man is referred for evaluation of "swelling on my right lower jaw."

Dentigerous Cyst

Dentigerous cyst (DC), also known as a *follicular cyst,* has a slight male predilection. It is more common in Caucasians, and it is most frequently seen in the age range of 10 to 30 years.

HPI

Approximately 2 months earlier, the patient noticed a non-painful swelling of the right posterior mandible (dentigerous cysts can cause expansion but are typically nonpainful unless secondarily infected). The most common location of dentigerous cysts is the mandibular third molar region; other frequently involved teeth include the maxillary canines, maxillary third molars, and mandibular second premolars. The patient was seen by the referring general dentist, who discovered a radiolucent lesion on a periapical radiograph. The patient denies any history of pain in his right lower jaw, fever, purulence, or trismus (inability to open the mouth due to contraction of the muscles of mastication, commonly a sign of inflammatory infiltration of the muscles secondary to infection).

PMHX/PDHX/MEDICATIONS/ALLERGIES/SH/FH

Noncontributory. There is no history of similar presentations in his family (there is no familial predisposition).

EXAMINATION

General. The patient is a well-developed and well-nourished anxious man (patients are often anxious because they fear a malignant process).

Maxillofacial. There is noticeable right lower facial swelling isolated to the lateral border of the mandible not involving the area below the inferior border. The mass is hard, nonfluctuant, and nontender to palpation, consistent with a noninflammatory process. There are no facial or trigeminal nerve deficits (paresthesia of the right inferior alveolar nerve would be indicative of a malignant process).

Neck. The patient does not have palpable masses or cervical or submandibular lymphadenopathy. Positive lymph nodes would be indicative of an infectious or neoplastic etiology, so a careful neck examination is paramount in the evaluation of any head and neck pathology.

Intraoral. The occlusion is stable and reproducible. There does not appear to be displacement of the dentition in the involved area (dentigerous cysts do not typically alter the occlusion). Interincisal opening is within normal limits. There is significant buccal expansion of the right mandible, extending from the mental foramen posteriorly and ascending into the ramus (large cysts may be associated with a painless expansion of the bone, but most are asymptomatic and do not cause expansion). The patient does not have a palpable thrill or an audible bruit (both are seen with arteriovenous malformations). The oral mucosa is normal in appearance with no signs of any acute inflammatory processes.

IMAGING

When evaluating large lesions of the mandible, the panoramic radiograph is an excellent initial study for assessment of the bony and dental anatomy. A CT scan is not essential, but it can better delineate the three-dimensional bony and regional architecture, including involvement of the cortices of the mandible (i.e., cortical perforation is seen with some tumors and locally aggressive cysts) and the lesion's position in relation to the inferior alveolar canal.

In this patient, a panoramic radiograph (Figure 1-3, *A*) demonstrates a well-corticated unilocular radiolucent lesion of the right posterior mandible extending from the area of tooth #31 up to the sigmoid notch and coronoid process. The right mandibular third molar (tooth #32) is displaced inferiorly, and the lesion involves the roots of tooth #31, with some resorption and superior displacement of the tooth. After aspiration and incisional biopsy, teeth #31 and teeth #32 were extracted and the cyst was enucleated and curettaged (Figure 1-3, *B* to *E*). Six- and 16-week postoperative orthopantograms demonstrate good progressive bony fill of the defect (Figure 1-3, *F* and *G*).

LABS

No laboratory tests are indicated unless dictated by the medical history. If brown tumor of hyperparathyroidism is in the differential diagnosis, serum calcium levels should be obtained. This tumor is derived from primary hyperparathyroidism, which leads to osseous lesions with abundant hemorrhage and hemosiderin deposition within the tumor (giving it

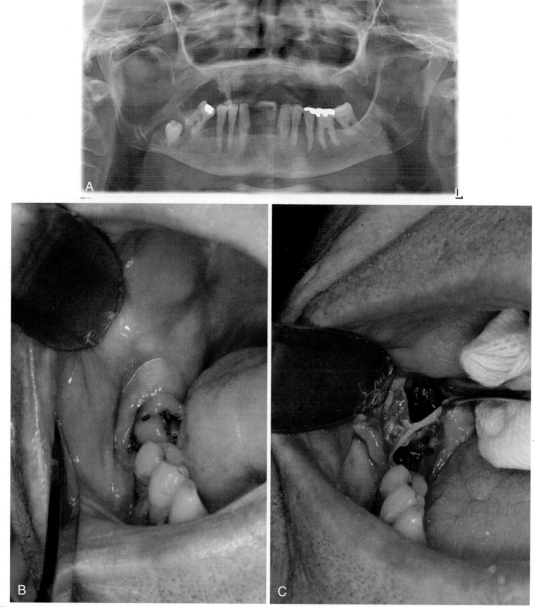

Figure 1-3   **A,** Unilocular radiolucency from posterior mandibular body to sigmoid notch. **B,** Preoperative photograph demonstrating absence of tooth #32. **C,** Initial exposure of the lesion.

a brown color). Removal of the hyperplastic parathyroid tissue is necessary in this condition.

DIFFERENTIAL DIAGNOSIS

The differential diagnosis can be divided into lesions of cystic pathogenesis, neoplastic (benign or malignant) lesions, and vascular anomalies (least common). Well-defined borders and the lack of a multilocular appearance are more suggestive of a cystic process, but this distinction is not predictable. The differentials presented in Box 1-3 should be considered; the first three are the most likely.

BIOPSY

An incisional biopsy would be indicated to guide final therapy for this lesion. This can be done under local, intravenous sedation or general anesthesia, depending on the surgeon's preference and the medical indications. It is important to obtain an aspirate of the mass before perforating the bony cortex. Bright red blood would alert the surgeon to the presence of a high-flow vascular lesion that could result in uncontrollable hemorrhage. In such a case, the procedure should be aborted to allow for further radiographic and angiographic studies to characterize the vasculature of the area.

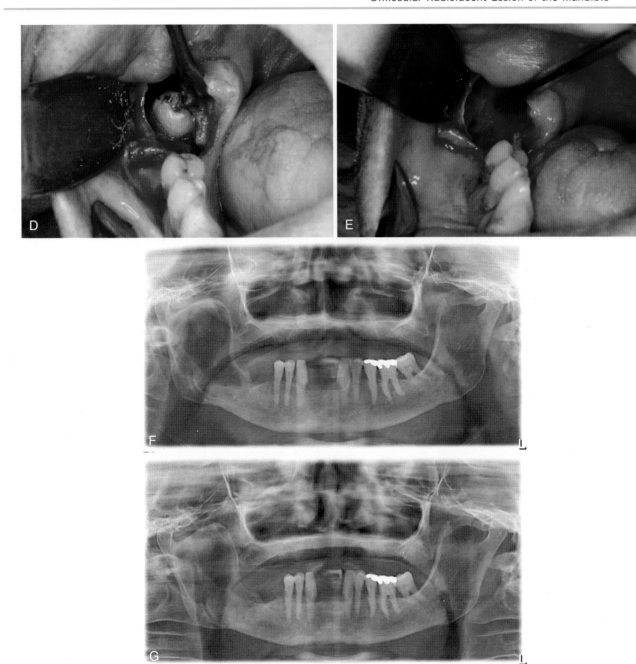

Figure 1-3, cont'd **D,** Unroofing of the lesion and exposure of tooth #32. **E,** Surgical defect after enucleation and curettage of the lesion. **F,** Orthopantogram 6 weeks after enucleation and curettage of the lesion. **G,** Orthopantogram 16 weeks after enucleation and curettage of the lesion.

Straw-colored fluid is characteristic of a cystic lesion, and the absence of any aspirate may be seen with tumors of the jaw.

ASSESSMENT

Expansile radiolucent mass of the posterior mandible associated with impacted right mandibular second and third molars

In this case, under intravenous anesthesia, an incisional biopsy was performed after aspiration (straw-colored fluid),

demonstrating classic dentigerous cyst histopathology (epithelial lining of nonkeratinized, stratified squamous epithelium and a loosely arranged fibrous connective tissue wall; see Figure 1-3, *A* to *D*).

TREATMENT

Complete removal of the cyst by enucleation, along with removal of the unerupted tooth, is the preferred treatment for dentigerous cysts. If eruption of the involved tooth into a functional position is feasible (with or without orthodontic

---

Box 1-3   **Differential Diagnosis of a Unilocular Radiolucency**

- **Dentigerous cyst**—This cyst is considered first on the differential, given the patient's age and the location of the lesion and its radiographic presentation. This cannot be differentiated on clinical and radiographic presentation alone.
- **Calcifying odontogenic cyst**—These cysts have a unilocular radiolucency, and calcifications in the lining sometimes makes them partially radiopaque. Treatment is by enucleation. Show "ghost cells" of histopathologic examination.
- **Keratinizing odontogenic tumor (KCOT)**—Formerly known as an odontogenic keratocyst, this cyst also is most commonly found in the posterior mandible; it can grow to a considerable size and must be distinguished from a dentigerous cyst. Frequently, large unilocular lesions that are thought to be dentigerous cysts prove to be KCOTs. The orthokeratinizing odontogenic cyst can have a similar presentation. These cysts can be treated by decompression or marsupialization, cystectomy with peripheral ostectomy, liquid nitrogen, or Carnoy's solution.
- **Ameloblastoma**—Given the patient's radiographic presentation (most common in the posterior mandible), a unicystic variant is most likely. Ameloblastomas occur equally in males and females and typically cause a painless bony expansion. This would be the most common noncystic pathology for this radiographic and clinical presentation. Histologically it is characterized by benign proliferation of odontogenic epithelium, with stellate reticulum accompanied by a varying composition of solid or cystic features.
- **Odontogenic myxoma**—This lesion arises from the papilla of the primitive dental pulp. Radiographically, it can present as a unilocular or multilocular lesion. Larger lesions tend to be multilocular and have a "soap bubble" appearance. The lesions are treated with resection, and they have a high recurrence rate.

- **Central giant cell granuloma**—This lesion is more common in the anterior mandible. A benign lesion that may be unilocular or multilocular shows a female predilection. In addition to aggressive curettage, treatment alternatives include intralesional steroid injection, systemic calcitonin, and treatment with interferon-alpha.
- **Calcifying epithelial odontogenic tumor (Pindborg tumor)**—This tumor is less likely, given the patient's radiographic presentation. It is a slow-growing mass and usually has a mixed radiolucent-radiopaque appearance, although early lesions may be entirely radiolucent.
- **Ameloblastic fibroma**—This is an uncommon expansile tumor that usually is seen in younger patients (i.e., during the first two decades of life). It may be treated with enucleation and curettage, although larger tumors may require resection.
- **Adenomatoid odontogenic tumor**—This tumor may show calcifications in the lining, much like a calcifying odontogenic cyst. The lesion is most often seen in females, in the anterior maxilla, and in younger patients. However, it cannot be ruled out without a biopsy. Treatment is enucleation.
- **Arteriovenous aneurysm of bone and other vascular bone tumors**—Clinicians should always consider vascular tumors because of the obvious surgical implications. Aspiration before any surgical incision is essential.
- **Carcinoma arising in a dentigerous cyst**—Although this is rare, it is well documented. Radiographically, the borders may be more irregular, with ragged edges.
- **Intraosseous mucoepidermoid carcinoma**—This is also a rare condition, but it should be ruled out, because early diagnosis of malignant neoplasms is essential for improved survival.

---

guidance), enucleation of the cyst can be performed without removal of the tooth. The inferior alveolar neurovascular bundle is commonly displaced by the cyst and should be preserved if possible. Large cysts may be treated with marsupialization when enucleation and curettage would likely result in neurosensory dysfunction or a pathologic fracture of the mandible. Postoperative maxillomandibular fixation may be prudent to allow remodeling of the bone before function, especially in larger lesions.

Marsupialization permits decompression of the lesion and shrinkage of the cyst and bony defect. Definitive removal can be performed at a later date. A disadvantage of marsupialization is the need for greater patient compliance with an open cystic cavity between treatments. In addition, it does not reliably produce a reduction in the size of the cyst.

This patient was taken to the operating room and underwent enucleation and curettage via an intraoral incision. The right mandibular second and third molars were maintained due to the high risk of fracture and inferior alveolar nerve paresthesia; although this may increase the possibility of recurrence, that fact should be weighed against the possible complications of tooth removal.

The patient was placed on a soft diet to reduce the risk of jaw fracture. The postoperative panoramic radiograph

confirmed that the inferior border of the mandible remained intact.

Marsupialization, mentioned earlier, is an alternative treatment; however, the patient must be compliant in serial appointments thereafter and must often undergo final definitive treatment of the shrunken cyst.

The final pathology report confirmed the diagnosis of a dentigerous cyst consistent with the initial incisional biopsy specimen.

COMPLICATIONS

With adequate treatment, the prognosis for a dentigerous cyst is excellent, and recurrence is rare. Left untreated, these cysts may lead to tooth displacement, resorption of adjacent tooth roots, and extensive bone destruction as they increase in size. The most common complications include postoperative infection, inferior alveolar nerve paresthesia and, with larger cysts, mandibular fracture. Neoplastic transformation into an ameloblastoma, a squamous cell carcinoma, and a mucoepidermoid carcinoma has been reported in fewer than 2% of cases. For this reason, a complete histopathologic examination with enucleation may be preferable to marsupialization, which could delay the diagnosis of a neoplastic transformation.

DISCUSSION

A dentigerous cyst is developmental in origin; it forms as a consequence of the buildup of fluid between the dental follicle and the crown of an unerupted tooth. It is the second most common odontogenic cyst after the periapical cyst. Arising from stellate reticulum and forming from the cementoenamel junction, they are the most common type of developmental odontogenic cyst, making up about 20% of all epithelium-lined cysts in the jaws. The pathogenesis is unknown but is possibly related to the accumulation of fluid between the reduced enamel epithelium and the tooth crown. Dentigerous cysts most commonly involve impacted mandibular third molars but may also involve maxillary canine, maxillary third, and mandibular second molars. This cyst is most commonly discovered between the ages of 10 and 30 years. It has a slight male predilection and a higher prevalence for Caucasians than for African Americans.

Dentigerous cysts are commonly asymptomatic on presentation but can grow to a significant size, resulting in painless expansion of the bone in the involved area. Large dentigerous cysts can become secondarily infected, with associated pain and swelling.

Radiographically dentigerous cysts usually show a unilocular radiolucent area that is associated with an unerupted tooth. A large dentigerous cyst may give the impression of a multilocular process because of the bony trabeculations. However, these cysts are grossly and histopathologically a unilocular process.

Bibliography

Angadi PV, Rekha K: Calcifying epithelial odontogenic tumor (Pindborg tumor), *Head Neck Pathol* 5(2):137-139, 2011.

Benn A, Altini M: Dentigerous cysts of inflammatory origin: a clinicopathologic study, *Oral Surg Oral Med Oral Pathol Oral Radiol Endod* 81(2):203-209, 1996.

Boffano P, Gallesio C, Barreca A, et al: Surgical treatment of odontogenic myxoma, *J Craniofac Surg* 22(3):982-987, 2011.

Carneiro JT Jr, Carreira AS, Felix VB, et al: Pathologic fracture of jaw in unicystic ameloblastoma treated with marsupialization, *J Craniofac Surg* 23(6):e537-e539, 2012.

Curran AE, Damm DD, Drummond JF: Pathologically significant pericoronal lesions in adults: histopathologic evaluation, *J Oral Maxillofac Surg* 60(6):613-617; discussion 618; 2002.

de Matos FR, Nonaka CF, Pinto LP, et al: Adenomatoid odontogenic tumor: retrospective study of 15 cases with emphasis on histopathologic features, *Head Neck Pathol* 6(4):430-437, 2012.

Elo JA, Slater LJ, Herford AS, et al: Squamous cell carcinoma radiographically resembling a dentigerous cyst: report of a case, *J Oral Maxillofac Surg* 65(12):2559-2562, 2007.

Gbolahan O, Fatusi O, Owotade F, et al: Clinicopathology of soft tissue lesions associated with extracted teeth, *J Oral Maxillofac Surg* 66(11):2284-2289, 2008.

Gomes CC, Diniz MG, Duarte AP, et al: Molecular review of odontogenic myxoma, *Oral Oncol* 47(5):325-328, 2011.

Koca H, Esin A, Aycan K: Outcome of dentigerous cysts treated with marsupialization, *J Clin Pediatr Dent* 34(2):165-168, 2009.

Marciani RD: Is there pathology associated with asymptomatic third molars? *J Oral Maxillofac Surg* 70(9 Suppl 1):S15-S19, 2012.

Peacock ZS, Jordan RC, Schmidt BL: Giant cell lesions of the jaws: does the level of vascularity and angiogenesis correlate with behavior? *J Oral Maxillofac Surg* 70(8):1860-1866, 2012.

Sandhu SV, Narang RS, Jawanda M, et al: Adenomatoid odontogenic tumor associated with dentigerous cyst of the maxillary antrum: a rare entity, *J Oral Maxillofac Pathol* 14(1):24-28, 2010.

Simiyu BN, Butt F, Dimba EA, et al: Keratocystic odontogenic tumours of the jaws and associated pathologies: a 10-year clinicopathologic audit in a referral teaching hospital in Kenya, *J Craniomaxillofac Surg* 41(3):230-234, 2013.

Smith JL II, Kellman RM: Dentigerous cysts presenting as head and neck infections, *Otolaryngol Head Neck Surg* 133(5):715-717, 2005.

Tabrizi R, Ozkan BT, Dehgani A, et al: Marsupialization as a treatment option for the odontogenic keratocyst, *J Craniofac Surg* 23(5):e459-e461, 2012.

Williams MD, Hanna EY, El-Naggar AK: Anaplastic ameloblastic fibrosarcoma arising from recurrent ameloblastic fibroma: restricted molecular abnormalities of certain genes to the malignant transformation, *Oral Surg Oral Med Oral Pathol Oral Radiol Endod* 104(1):72-75, 2007.

Multilocular Radiolucent Lesion in the Periapical Region
(Ameloblastoma)

Eric P. Holmgren and Shahrokh C. Bagheri

CC

A 34-year-old woman complaining of a painless swelling in the lower jaw (ameloblastomas are often asymptomatic) is referred by her general dentist.

Ameloblastoma

Ameloblastomas are usually diagnosed in the third to fourth decade of life, with no gender or racial predilection; however, unicystic variants tend to occur earlier in life.

HPI

For the past 2 months, the patient has noticed a progressively enlarging "hard mass" in her mandible. There have been no neurosensory changes associated with the swelling (sensory changes are particularly common in malignancies and are not usually seen in benign lesions such as ameloblastomas). On consultation, her general dentist noticed a significant buccal and lingual bony expansion adjacent to normal-appearing first and second molars on the right posterior mandible, in addition to a multilocular radiolucent lesion on the panoramic radiograph (ameloblastomas occur most frequently in the mandible [80% of the time], often in the posterior mandible).

PMHX/PDHX/MEDICATIONS/ALLERGIES/SH/FH

Noncontributory.

EXAMINATION

General. The patient is well developed and well nourished and appears distressed about her possible diagnosis.

Vital Signs. Vital signs are stable, and the patient is afebrile.

Maxillofacial. There is mild right facial enlargement that is most pronounced at the angle of the mandible, with no evidence of trismus. No cervical lymphadenopathy is present. (Ameloblastomas are benign tumors and in general do not cause lymphadenopathy, which may be seen with malignant tumors.) Neurosensory testing reveals normal mandibular nerve (V3) function bilaterally and no other focal neurologic deficits (ameloblastomas generally do not invade the neurovascular bundle).

Intraoral. There is buccal and lingual expansion of the posterior right mandible with mild tenderness but no evidence of fluctuance or purulent secretions. The mesiobuccal tip of the right mandibular third molar is partially visible. The right mandibular second molar is not mobile; however, there are periodontal pocket depths greater than 10 mm on the distal aspect.

IMAGING

The panoramic radiograph is the initial imaging study of choice for evaluation of a mandibular mass. CT scans are particularly useful for outlining the three-dimensional anatomy to demonstrate the amount of expansion and areas of bony perforation implying subsequent soft tissue involvement. Accurate stereolithographic models can be fabricated from the CT scan and can assist in both resection and reconstruction.

In this patient, the panoramic radiograph demonstrates a 5 × 3.5-cm multilocular, cystic-appearing lesion extending from the distal aspect of the impacted right mandibular third molar, involving the entire ramus up to the level of the sigmoid notch. The bone at the inferior border of the mandible has a normal appearance, without loss of continuity (Figure 1-4).

The CT scan shows an expansile lesion of the right posterior mandible, with cortical perforation seen on axial and coronal sections at the anterior border of the ramus. There is no evidence of lymphadenopathy, and no areas of abnormal enhancement are seen (contrast-enhanced imaging provides improved delineation of soft tissue and can aid in determining any associated vascular malformations).

LABS

Baseline hemoglobin and hematocrit levels should be obtained before major maxillofacial surgical interventions. Other laboratory tests are obtained as dictated by the medical history.

DIFFERENTIAL DIAGNOSIS

The differential diagnosis of a multilocular radiolucent lesion of the posterior mandible is best categorized as lesions of cystic, neoplastic, or vascular origin, with the latter being less common. Although the presentation just described is classic for an ameloblastoma (i.e., bony expansion of the posterior mandible with a multilocular or "soap bubble" appearance), this lesion cannot be distinguished on clinical and radiographic parameters. A complete differential diagnosis should be considered (see Differential Diagnosis in the section

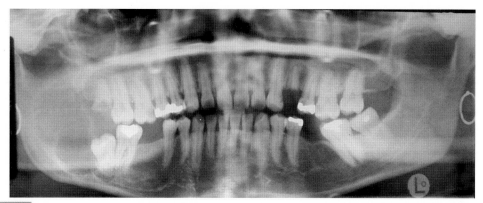

Panoramic radiograph demonstrating a multilocular radiolucent lesion of the right posterior mandible.

Multilocular Radiolucent Lesion in the Pericoronal Region [Odontogenic Keratocyst], earlier in the chapter).

BIOPSY

For diagnosis of this multilocular and expansile lesion, aspiration followed by an incisional biopsy was performed with local anesthesia and intravenous sedation in the clinic. Needle aspiration was negative for blood or any clear fluids and therefore suggestive of a mass lesion. A typical buccal mucoperiosteal third molar incision was reflected (it is important to make the incision where the definitive surgical incision would ultimately be made in order to minimize dehiscence at the time of definitive surgery). No purulence was noted. A cystic lesion with a keratin-like substance was encountered in the large bony concavity. A large sample of the cyst lining was taken from two different locations. The wound was closed with 3-0 chromic interrupted sutures, and a specimen was sent for histopathological examination.

ASSESSMENT

Microscopic evaluation reveals islands of epithelium that resemble enamel organ in a fibrous connective tissue stroma; attached to the basement membrane surrounding the islands are tall columnar cells exhibiting reversed polarity.

This is consistent with the diagnosis of a multicystic, follicular ameloblastoma.

TREATMENT

The treatment of ameloblastomas has raised some controversy. In general, treatment must focus on the ability of the tumor to invade surrounding bone tissue. The average extension into surrounding bone beyond the normal tumor margin is 4.5 mm, with a range of 2 to 8 mm. With this in mind, resection must be at least 10 mm beyond the bony (and radiographic) margin of the tumor for large, multicystic-type ameloblastomas. Resected tumors seldom recur; the cure rate for primary tumors is 95% to 98%. In contrast, there is a high incidence of recurrence (approximately 70%) for treatment with enucleation and curettage alone. Regardless of the

reconstructive measure, close patient follow-up is necessary to monitor for recurrence, especially in patients who do not undergo a resection. Because ameloblastomas can recur within a variable time frame, a cure rate for an ameloblastoma does not necessarily correlate with a 5-year disease-free period, compared with other neoplastic processes. Long-term follow-up is necessary.

For this patient, given the size and extensive, aggressive nature of the lesion, a segmental reconstruction was undertaken via an intraoral approach. Tumor resection was elected because of the close anatomic proximity of the tumor margin at the inferior boarder, in addition to the cortical perforation and involvement of mucosa at the anterior border and near the sigmoid notch. Special attention was paid to the site of perforation, in which a supraperiosteal resection was performed, and the overlying mucosa and periosteum were resected with the specimen. The condyle was retained, and the ramus and angle were reconstructed using a standard reconstruction plate. The inferior alveolar nerve was dissected free and preserved (ameloblastoma cells do not necessarily penetrate the nerve unless there is gross involvement of the inferior alveolar canal, which can theoretically allow the tumor cells to penetrate the perineural tissue).

Other reported treatment alternatives include enucleation, curettage and cryotherapy with or without bone grafting, and excision of the tumor with peripheral ostectomy. Marsupialization of unicystic variants have also been reported. These treatments have not been proved to be curative, are not widely advocated, and have a higher recurrence rate compared with resection.

The mandibular defect in this patient was subsequently reconstructed using an iliac crest cancellous bone graft, performed at 4 months (to allow time for soft tissue healing), via an extraoral approach. A segmental resection with an osteotomized, vascularized fibula free flap and reconstruction plate is a good alternative, especially with recurrences or large, aggressive tumors.

COMPLICATIONS

Complications associated with resection and reconstruction of this tumor include mandibular nerve anesthesia, graft failure, unacceptable facial symmetry, poor bony height and width for implant reconstruction, and donor site morbidity. Plate exposure, plate fracture, and intraoral dehiscence are also possibilities. Recurrence is the most worrisome long-term complication. Recurrence can be due to persistence of the original tumor that was not resected or actual recurrence of new neoplastic cells. Aggressive surgical therapy does not necessarily eliminate the chance of tumor recurrence. In theory, the more aggressive the initial treatment, the lesser the likelihood of tumor recurrence. However, this comes at the expense of a larger residual defect and more complicated reconstructive measures. Surgeons need to determine the extent of the resection and preservation of structures based on the available evidence, tumor biology, patient's preference and availability for follow-up, surgeon experience, and other individual factors.

DISCUSSION

There are seven histologic types of ameloblastomas: follicular, plexiform, acanthomatous, granular cell, desmoplastic, basal cell, and unicystic variant; the first two types are the most common. The desmoplastic variant often presents in the anterior maxilla or mandible and can appear more radiopaque because of the high amount of dense connective tissue. Ameloblastomas can be either solid or multicystic, but they frequently demonstrate both characteristics. The tumor can arise from embryonic remnants of odontogenic cysts, dental lamina, enamel organ, or stratified squamous epithelium of the oral cavity.

Although the majority of the tumors originate from within the maxilla or mandible, they can also be peripheral. The different histological variants do not significantly alter treatment considerations except for the unicystic and the peripheral types, which can typically be treated with enucleation and curettage. Unicystic ameloblastomas represent about 10% to 15% of intraosseous ameloblastomas and can be misdiagnosed as dentigerous cysts. These lesions commonly occur in younger patients and have three distinct variants (luminal, intraluminal, and mural). Luminal and intraluminal types can typically be treated with enucleation and close observation, whereas mural types should be treated more aggressively.

Peripheral ameloblastomas are very uncommon, representing approximately 1% of all ameloblastomas, and are usually successfully treated with local surgical excision because of their nonaggressive behavior. Malignant ameloblastomas are extremely rare and usually metastasize to the lungs (probably from aspiration of oral tumor). The malignant variant has a poor prognosis.

Bibliography

Bianchi B, Ferri A, Ferrari S, et al: Mandibular resection and reconstruction in the management of extensive ameloblastoma, *J Oral Maxillofac Surg* 71:528-537, 2013.

Carlson ER, Marx RE: The ameloblastoma: primary, curative surgical management, *J Oral Maxillofac Surg* 64:484-494, 2006.

Carlson ER, Monteleone K: Analysis of inadvertent perforations of mucosa and skin concurrent with mandibular reconstruction, *J Oral Maxillofac Surg* 62:1103-1107, 2004.

Chapelle K, Stoelinga P, de Wilde P, et al: Rational approach to diagnosis and treatment of ameloblastoma and odontogenic keratocysts, *Br J Oral Maxillofac Surg* 42:381-390, 2004.

Gerzenshtein J, Zhang F, Caplan J, et al: Immediate mandibular reconstruction with microsurgical fibula flap transfer following wide resection for ameloblastoma, *Plast Reconstr Surg* 17:178-182, 2006.

Gold L, Williams TP: Odontogenic tumors: surgical pathology and management. In Fonseca RJ (ed): *Oral and maxillofacial surgery*, ed 2, Philadelphia, 2009, Saunders/Elsevier, pp 466-538.

Laskin DM, Giglio JA, Ferrer-Nuin LF: Multilocular lesion in the body of the mandible: clinicopathologic conference, *J Oral Maxillofac Surg* 60:1045-1048, 2002.

Nakamura N, Mitsuyasu T, Higuchi Y, et al: Growth characteristics of ameloblastoma involving the inferior alveolar nerve: a clinical and histopathologic study, *Oral Surg Oral Med Oral Pathol Oral Radiol Endod* 91:557-562, 2001.

Neville BW, Damm DD, Allen CM, et al: *Oral and maxillofacial pathology*, ed 2, New York, 2002, Saunders.

Sachs SA: Surgical excision with peripheral ostectomy: a definitive, yet conservative, approach to the surgical management of ameloblastoma, *J Oral Maxillofac Surg* 64:476-483, 2006.

Sampson DE, Pogrel MA: Management of mandibular ameloblastoma: the clinical basis for a treatment algorithm, *J Oral Maxillofac Surg* 57:1074-1077, 1999.

Tung-Yiu W, Jehn-Shyun H, Ching-Hung C: Epineural dissection to preserve the inferior alveolar nerve in excision of an ameloblastoma of mandible: case report, *J Oral Maxillofac Surg* 58:1159-1161, 2000.

Unilocular Radiolucent Lesion in a Periapical Region (Periapical Cyst)

Bruce W. Anderson and Shahrokh C. Bagheri

CC

A 37-year-old woman is referred by her general dentist for evaluation of a periapical radiolucency associated with the right mandibular second bicuspid, which was discovered during a new patient examination.

Periapical Cyst

The periapical cyst (also called a *radicular* or *apical periodontal cyst*) is the most common jaw cyst. It develops secondary to the inflammatory process associated with a nonvital tooth and is more common after the third decade of life.

HPI

The patient reports having "a cavity for a long time," with subsequent fracture, approximately 6 months earlier, of a portion of the crown of the right mandibular second bicuspid, which was part of a three-unit bridge. The right mandibular second molar and the right mandibular second bicuspid were treated endodontically 9 years earlier without complications. The patient denies any history of swelling or purulence in the region and is asymptomatic (periapical cysts seldom present with any clinical symptoms, but infected cysts can present with a draining fistula). The patient also denies a history of trauma in the area (periapical cysts are associated with pulpal necrosis secondary to either caries or trauma).

PMHX/PDHX/MEDICATIONS/ALLERGIES/SH/FH

Noncontributory.

EXAMINATION

Maxillofacial. There is no discernible facial asymmetry or swelling (periapical cysts are rarely associated with any cortical expansion).

Neck. No cervical or submandibular lymphadenopathy can be detected (positive node findings could be indicative of an infectious or a neoplastic process).

Intraoral. The right mandibular second bicuspid is grossly carious and fractured at the gingival margin. There is no gingival swelling or palpation tenderness along the buccal or lingual cortices.

IMAGING

A panoramic radiograph is the initial study of choice for any intraosseous lesion, because it provides an excellent overview of the bony anatomy and architecture of the maxilla and mandible and demonstrates the relationship to adjacent anatomic structures. A periapical radiograph can be obtained for small lesions, providing a more detailed outline of the borders and trabecular pattern. More extensive imaging, such as CT scanning, is seldom required for management of a periapical cyst unless the diagnosis is in question.

In this patient, a panoramic radiograph demonstrated a well-circumscribed, radiolucent lesion associated with the right mandibular second bicuspid (Figure 1-5). The lesion is approximately 1 cm in diameter (periapical cysts are generally between 0.5 and 1.5 cm in diameter but may enlarge to fill an entire quadrant). There is no associated root resorption (although root resorption is uncommon in association with a periapical cyst, it can be seen, especially with larger cysts).

LABS

No routine laboratory tests are indicated for the work-up of a periapical cyst unless dictated by the medical history.

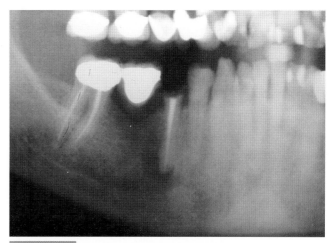

Figure 1-5 Periapical radiolucent lesion associated with endodontic treatment of the right mandibular second bicuspid, seen on a panoramic radiograph. The close association of the lesion with the mental foramen should prompt the clinician to be cautious if performing a biopsy.

DIFFERENTIAL DIAGNOSIS

The differential diagnosis of a periapical radiolucent lesion is greatly influenced by the clinical history and vitality of the associated tooth. If the associated tooth is nonvital and there is radiographic evidence of pulpal pathology, a periapical cyst is the most likely diagnosis. However, a diagnosis based on histopathological examination is warranted, because tumors, developmental cysts, metastatic disease, and early fibro-osseous lesions may also occur in a periapical location. The differential diagnosis is outlined Box 1-4.

BIOPSY

Biopsy and treatment of small periapical cysts are usually synonymous and excisional in nature and vary, depending on the restorative plan for the involved tooth. If extraction is planned, then the cyst can be removed through the extraction socket. If the tooth is to be restored or the lesion is particularly large, a periapical approach through the buccal cortex can be used.

ASSESSMENT

Distinct periapical radiolucent lesion associated with the carious and nonvital right mandibular second bicuspid. The lesion is closely associated with the mental foramen.

In this case, the tooth was extracted and the underlying lesion was carefully removed to avoid injury to the inferior alveolar neurovascular bundle. The specimen was sent for histopathological examination and demonstrated a cystic lining of nonkeratinized, stratified squamous epithelium of varying thickness with numerous curved and round hyaline bodies (Rushton bodies). The wall of the cyst showed dense fibrous connective tissue and significant mixed inflammatory infiltrate of lymphocytes, plasma cells, neutrophils, and histocytes. The central lumen was found to contain proteinaceous fluid and necrotic cellular debris. These clinical and histologic findings are consistent with a periapical cyst.

TREATMENT

Periapical cysts are treated by enucleation and curettage, either through an extraction socket or via a periapical surgical approach when the tooth is restorable or the lesion is greater than 2 cm in diameter. If the tooth is to be preserved, endodontic treatment is necessary, if it has not been done. Some literature supports nonsurgical, conservative endodontic treatment of smaller lesions, ensuring the complete removal of causative organisms, and regular radiographic follow-up to evaluate healing and monitor potential lesion enlargement. Excised cysts should always be sent for histologic evaluation to rule out other possible pathologies. Recurrence is uncommon.

COMPLICATIONS

There are few complications associated with the treatment of a periapical cyst. Extraction of a tooth without removal of the

---

| Box 1-4 | **Differential Diagnosis of Periapical Radiolucent Lesions** |

- **Periapical granuloma**—This lesion is radiographically indistinguishable from a periapical cyst and is treated in the same manner. Differentiation between periapical granulomas and a cyst has no clinical implication (see Residual cyst).
- **Residual cyst**—This is a lesion that remains after the extraction of a tooth or completion of endodontic treatment. It is radiographically and histologically identical to a periapical cyst.
- **Cemento-osseous dysplasias (early)**—The spectrum of these lesions, including focal, periapical, and florid cemento-osseous dysplasias, can be observed in the periapical region. The lesions are most commonly seen in middle-aged women of African descent. With serial observation, these lesions progress to mixed radiolucent-radiopaque lesions and eventually to radiopaque lesions. Associated teeth are asymptomatic and vital.
- **Idiopathic bone cavity (simple bone cyst, traumatic bone cyst)**—Most often seen in the body of the mandible of young adults, this lesion lacks an epithelial lining and has the potential for expansion. Radiographically, it is a well-demarcated, radiolucent lesion that can scallop between teeth without resorption. Associated teeth are asymptomatic and vital.
- **Lingual salivary gland depressions (Stafne defect)**—This well-circumscribed, radiolucent lesion is most commonly seen in males in the posterior mandible inferior to the mandibular canal. It represents a developmental concavity of the lingual cortex containing normal salivary gland tissue. Teeth near this lesion are, of course, asymptomatic and vital, because the radiolucency is in fact superimposed in the periapical location.
- **Other lesions**—Neural lesions (neurilemoma, neurofibroma) could present in a periapical location but are usually associated with the mandibular canal. Other cysts and tumors, including lateral periodontal cysts, ameloblastomas, odontogenic keratocysts, central giant cell tumors, intraosseous mucoepidermoid carcinomas, and metastatic disease, could present in a periapical location and should be investigated. For these lesions, the associated tooth is usually vital unless there has been previous endodontic therapy, or concomitant pathologic processes are present.

---

cyst, or incomplete removal of the cystic lining, can result in a residual cyst. As mentioned previously, residual cysts are histologically identical to periapical cysts and treated with enucleation. Failed conservative endodontic treatment shows a persistent periapical cyst. Endodontic re-treatment may be attempted before a curative surgical apicoectomy and enucleation are performed. When both the buccal and lingual cortices are involved, it is possible for the area to heal with fibrous tissue (periapical scar). No treatment is necessary for periapical scars.

Complications associated with surgical removal of the cyst can be related to the regional anatomy. Neurosensory disturbances secondary to injury to the inferior alveolar nerve or branches of the mental nerve can be seen, especially with larger lesions, but these are usually temporary. Postoperative infection can occur with any surgical intervention.

DISCUSSION

The periapical cyst, or radicular cyst, results from inflammatory stimulation of the rests of Malassez within the periodontal ligament. It is relatively common, accounting for a reported 50% of all oral cysts. Its development is preceded by a periapical granuloma that forms at the tooth apex in response to pulpal bacterial infection and necrosis. A periapical granuloma consists of an outer dense fibrous tissue capsule surrounding a central area of granulation tissue. Expansion of the granuloma leads to central ischemic necrosis and development of a central lumen surrounded by an epithelial membrane. The necrotic cellular debris within the lumen creates an osmotic gradient, drawing in fluid and causing enlargement of the cyst and resorption of surrounding bone secondary to hydrostatic pressure.

There is some debate in the literature as to radiographic distinctions between periapical granulomas and cysts, but the consensus is that they are indistinguishable. It has been shown that there is no significant relationship between preoperative symptoms and lesion type; however, lesions that present with an associated swelling demonstrate worse postoperative bone regeneration. There is a wide range of reported incidences of periapical granulomas versus cysts. The percentage of periapical radiolucent lesions that are attributed to periapical cysts is reported as close to 50%. However, studies with strict histological criteria put the incidence of periapical cysts at about 5% to 22% and that of periapical granulomas at 50% to 85%. Admittedly, this debate might be considered irrelevant, because the eventual treatment of the two lesions is the same. Nonetheless, it has been found that postoperative bone regeneration is diminished in cases involving cysts, compared to granulomas, and that a poorer prognosis is related to larger lesions, which may be a factor in the long-term outcome of endodontic therapy.

Periapical cysts or granulomas are clearly common lesions seen by oral and maxillofacial surgeons. A careful history, the clinical and radiographic presentation and, most important, assessment of the vitality of the associated tooth aid in determining the appropriate diagnosis and management of this common pathologic lesion.

Bibliography

Carrillo C, Penarrocha M, Bagan JV, et al: Relationship between histological diagnosis and evolution of 70 periapical lesions at 12 months, treated by periapical surgery, *J Oral Maxillofac Surg* 66:1606-1609, 2008.

Gallego Romero D, Torres Lagares D, Garcia Calderon M, et al: Differential diagnosis and therapeutic approach to periapical cysts in daily dental practice, *Med Oral* 7:54-58, 2002.

Mass DR, Bhambhani SM: A clinical and histopathological study of radicular cysts associated with primary molars, *J Oral Pathol Med* 24:458-461, 1995.

Nair PN: New perspectives on radicular cysts: do they heal? *Int Endod J* 31:155-160, 1998.

Omoregie OF, Saheeb BDO, Odykoya O, et al: A clinicopathologic correlation in the diagnosis of periradicular lesions of extracted teeth, *J Oral Maxillofac Surg* 67:1387-1391, 2009.

Philipsen HP, Reichart PA, Ogawa I, et al: The inflammatory paradental cyst: a critical review of 342 cases from the literature survey, including 17 new cases from the author's file, *J Oral Pathol Med* 33:147-155, 2004.

Penarrocha M, Carrillo C, Penarrocha M, et al: Symptoms before periapical surgery related to histologic diagnosis and postoperative healing at 12 months for 178 periapical lesions, *J Oral Maxillofac Surg* 69:e31-e37, 2011.

Ramachandran Nair PN, Pajorola G, Schroeder HE: Types and incidence of human periapical lesions obtained with extracted teeth, *Oral Surg Oral Med Oral Pathol Oral Radiol Endod* 81:93-102, 1996.

Regezi JA, Sciubba JJ, Jordan RCK: *Oral pathology: clinical pathologic correlations*, ed 6, St Louis, 2012, Saunders.

Sanchis JM, Penarrocha M, Bagan JV, et al: Incidence of radicular cysts in a series of 125 chronic periapical lesions: histopathologic study, *Rev Stomatol Chir Maxillofac* 98:354-358, 1998.

Spatafore CM, Griffin JA Jr, Keyes GG, et al: Periapical biopsy: an analysis of 10-year period, *J Endod* 16:239-241, 1990.

Stockdale CR, Chandler NP: The nature of the periapical lesion: a review of 1,108 cases, *J Dent* 16:123-129, 1988.

Trope M, Pettigrew J, Petras J, et al: Differentiation of radicular cyst and granulomas using computerized tomography, *Endod Dent Traumatol* 5:69-72, 1989.

Zaiv RB, Roswati N, Ismail K: Radiographic features of periapical cysts and granulomas, *Singapore Dent J* 14:29-32, 1989.

Mixed Radiolucent-Radiopaque Lesion (Ossifying Fibroma)

Danielle Cunningham and Chris Jo

CC

A 32-year-old woman is referred for evaluation of a mandibular lesion. She states, "I have a tumor in my lower jaw."

Ossifying Fibroma

Ossifying fibroma most commonly occurs in the third and fourth decades of life and has a reported female predilection as high as 5:1.

HPI

Approximately 3 years earlier, the patient noticed a painless bony expansion of her anterior mandible (ossifying fibroma is much more common in the mandible than in the maxilla and rarely presents with pain or paresthesia). The patient states that the swelling has been slowly enlarging over the past 3 years and that she was previously scared to seek treatment. Now that the mass is so large and disfiguring, she wants treatment (ossifying fibromas that are left untreated can become very large). She complains of difficulty talking and chewing because of the size of the mass.

PMHX/PDHX/MEDICATIONS/ALLERGIES/SH/FH

Noncontributory.

EXAMINATION

General. The patient is well developed and well nourished and in no apparent distress.

Maxillofacial. There is an obvious enlargement of the anterior mandible. A firm, bony mass is palpable that extends from first premolar to first premolar. The mass has expanded the buccal and inferior cortices ("downward bowing" is common in large ossifying fibromas of the mandible). Sensory examination shows that the mental nerve distributions are intact bilaterally (perineural invasion is not seen with ossifying fibroma).

Neck. No lymphadenopathy is noted (cervical lymphadenopathy is not seen in benign neoplastic processes).

Intraoral. There is a significant amount of bony expansion of the buccal and lingual cortices in the anterior mandible, displacing the tongue posteriorly (Figure 1-6). The left and right mandibular lateral and central incisors are displaced and mobile (larger lesions may cause tooth displacement and root divergence, resorption, or both). The overlying attached

gingiva and mucosa are normal in appearance (mucosal ulcerations can be a sign of a malignant process; however, traumatic ulcerations can occur within large, expansible, benign lesions).

IMAGING

A panoramic radiograph is the initial screening study of choice. It provides an excellent overview of the bony anatomy and architecture of the maxilla and mandible. Osseous lesions are well characterized on a panoramic film, allowing the clinician to make a working differential diagnosis based on the lesion's location, radiodensity, locular or trabecular pattern, border demarcation, size, and effect on adjacent structures (i.e., root resorption, root divergence, scalloping, cortical expansion, cortical erosion, or destruction).

CT is not always essential during the work-up or treatment of a mixed radiopaque-radiolucent lesion that is suspected to be benign. However, when there are radiographic signs of a malignant process (e.g., poorly defined radiolucency, mottled or "moth-eaten" appearance, unilateral widening of the periodontal ligament space, floating teeth, cortical perforation, or "spiked roots"), CT of the mandible and neck is required. CT provides additional information (e.g., lingual or buccal cortex thinning or perforation, location of the inferior alveolar canal) and is especially useful when the lesion is difficult to assess

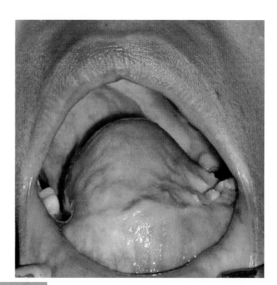

Figure 1-6 Intraoral photograph showing a large, expansile lesion in the anterior mandible, causing posterior and superior displacement of the patient's tongue.

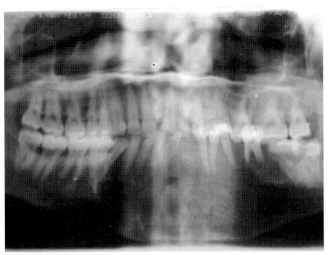

Figure 1-7 Panoramic radiograph showing a large, expansile, mixed radiolucent-radiopaque lesion involving the majority of the dentate segment of the mandible. Note that there is significant root divergence, teeth displacement, root resorption, and cortical expansion.

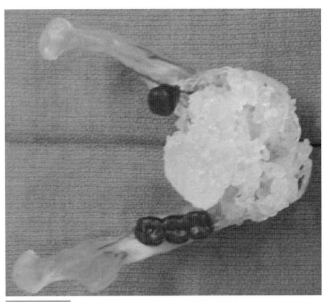

Figure 1-8 Three-dimensional stereolithographic model used to plan the resection and to prebend a reconstruction plate.

on plain films. A three-dimensional stereolithographic model is useful to prebend a reconstruction plate in anticipation of resection.

The radiographic appearance of ossifying fibroma varies, depending on the degree of maturity of the lesion. Early ossifying fibromas are radiolucent, and as they mature, they become mixed radiolucent-radiopaque and may eventually become predominantly radiopaque. Untreated, these tumors are likely to reach large proportions as they continue to grow. Expansion of the lesion is symmetric and has a spherical or egg-shaped appearance on the CT scan.

In this patient, the panoramic radiograph reveals a well-defined, expansile, mixed radiolucent-radiopaque mass in the anterior mandible extending from the right premolar to the left molar regions (Figure 1-7). The borders are smooth and well defined. The anterior mandibular teeth show significant displacement and root resorption. A CT scan reveals a large, circular, expansile mass, in the anterior mandible, of a heterogeneous nature with radiopaque areas (of the same density as bone) within the lesion. There are no air- or fluid-filled spaces noted. The mass is well demarcated from surrounding structures. The stereolithographic model reconstructed from the CT scan illustrates the size of the lesion (Figure 1-8).

LABS

Baseline hemoglobin and hematocrit levels should be obtained before tumor resection. No other laboratory tests are indicated unless dictated by the medical history.

DIFFERENTIAL DIAGNOSIS

The differential diagnosis of a mixed radiolucent-radiopaque mass includes odontogenic cyst, odontogenic

tumor, osteogenic tumor, or a process secondary to infection. Many osseous lesions can change in radiographic characteristics and radiodensity as they mature and progress from a radiolucent to a mixed or radiopaque lesion. The differential diagnosis of a mixed radiolucent-radiopaque lesion can be narrowed when radiographic findings are correlated with clinical findings. Several mixed radiolucent-radiopaque lesions other than an ossifying fibroma are listed in Box 1-5.

BIOPSY

Benign tumors of bone cannot be distinguished on clinical and radiographic information alone and require histological assessment for a definitive diagnosis. In this case, an incisional biopsy would be indicated to guide final therapy. This can be done under local, intravenous sedation or general anesthesia, depending on the surgeon's preference and medical indications. In general, an ossifying fibroma is well demarcated from the surrounding bone but is not encapsulated. During biopsy, it is imperative to preserve the cortical-lesional relationship.

ASSESSMENT

A large, expansile, mixed radiopaque-radiolucent lesion of the mandible.

In this case, the histopathological examination showed a predominance of proliferative fibrous connective tissue with no clear capsule (ossifying fibroma can be seen with a capsule). The stroma appears avascular with some regularly shaped blood vessels (ossifying fibroma can have a mixed vascularity). A mild degree of osteoblastic activity and trabeculae of lamellar bone are also noted. Cementum-like deposits are present in combination with the lamellar bone.

Box 1-5	**Mixed Radiolucent-Radiopaque Lesions**

- **Fibrous dysplasia**—This lesion, which has a higher occurrence in younger patients, presents with a typical "ground glass" appearance on radiographs and a "Chinese script writing" appearance on histologic examination. It can affect one (monostotic) or more (polyostotic) bones in the body. Monostotic fibrous dysplasia is more common, and the jaws are the most common site.
- **Cemento-osseous dysplasias (periapical, focal, and florid)**—These lesions are the most common type of fibro-osseous lesions. They develop in tooth-bearing areas of the jaws and are categorized into three groups (periapical, focal, and florid) based on clinical and radiographic features. Periapical cemento-osseous dysplasia has a 14:1 female predilection and occurs mostly in African Americans between the third and fifth decades of life. Focal cemento-osseous dysplasia also has a high female predilection (4:1) but is seen mostly in Caucasians. Florid cemento-osseous dysplasias occur mostly in African American women. In each case, early lesions appear radiolucent (fibroblastic proliferation stage), and in later stages the lesions become mixed and subsequently radiopaque as bone and cementum-like materials are deposited.
- **Paget's disease of bone (osteitis deformans)**—In general, this disease affects older patients (older than 40 years) and has a 2:1 male predilection. It is characterized by haphazard and abnormal bone resorption and deposition, causing bony expansion and bone pain (most cases are polyostotic). Radiographically, the lesion appears similar to cemento-osseous dysplasia and is described as having a "cotton wool" appearance

(which is also seen in Gardner syndrome and gigantiform cementoma).
- **Osteomyelitis, osteoradionecrosis, and bisphosphonate-induced osteonecrosis of the jaws**—These three pathophysiologically distinct entities can have a mixed radiolucent-radiopaque appearance (see the respective sections for further details).
- **Osteoblastomas**—These are benign tumors of bone that typically present in the second and early third decades of life, causing local expansion. The key feature of this lesion that differentiates it from an ossifying fibroma is the presence of pain. This tumor, which exhibits slow growth, is the result of a genetic alteration during osteoblastic differentiation. Radiographically, the tumor is usually well circumscribed and can be treated by local resection with 5-mm margins. Osteoid osteoma and juvenile active ossifying fibroma may be variants of this lesion.
- **Calcifying odontogenic cyst (Gorlin cyst)**—This lesion is more likely to occur in females than in males (2:1). It initially appears radiolucent but with maturation becomes mixed radiolucent-radiopaque. It is generally asymptomatic and may cause expansion as it enlarges. It has a predilection for the maxilla but can occur in the mandible. Histologic examination shows "ghost cells."
- **Other**—Adenomatoid odontogenic tumor (or cyst), calcifying epithelial odontogenic tumor, ameloblastic fibro-odontoma, odontoma, and cementoblastoma also present as well-demarcated, mixed radiolucent-radiopaque lesions.

Radiographic, clinical, history, and histopathologic findings are consistent with an ossifying fibroma.

TREATMENT

Treatment varies, depending on the size and clinical appearance of the lesion. Small tumors may be treated with enucleation and curettage with 1- to 2-mm margins, as long as they have not lost their encapsulation and the margins remain well demarcated from the surrounding bone. However, resection with 5-mm margins is recommended if:
- Tumors have reached a larger size.
- There is loss of the encapsulation (radiographically or clinically).
- Tumor is within 1 cm of the inferior border of the mandible.
- There is involvement of the maxillary sinus or nasal cavities.

If enucleation and curettage is used, the defect can be left open to heal by secondary intent or closed primarily, using resorbable packs to eliminate the dead space. Packing the defect with materials such as iodoform gauze or various bone regeneration preparations to expedite bone regeneration has not been shown to be effective.

When bony reconstruction is required, various techniques (immediate or secondary cancellous marrow bone graft or immediate vascularized free flap) can be used, depending on

the clinical situation. When cancellous marrow graft is used, secondary bony reconstruction is recommended at least 3 months after the resection to allow for sufficient mucosal healing and tensile strength to prevent mucosal perforation and graft contamination.

In this patient, a partial mandibulectomy with 5-mm margins was performed, with immediate stabilization using a prebent reconstruction plate. Immediate bony reconstruction (cancellous–marrow bone graft) would not be recommended in this case, because the resection involved a dentate segment that would allow oral contaminates to penetrate the graft site. Second-stage bony reconstruction was performed after 3 months of adequate soft tissue healing. Although recurrence is unlikely, the patient should be followed for at least 10 years with serial panoramic radiographs because of the slow-growing nature of this lesion.

COMPLICATIONS

With proper treatment, the prognosis for ossifying fibroma is excellent and recurrence is rare. The potential complications generally reflect the presenting size of the lesion. Smaller lesions often can be treated by enucleation and curettage without complications. Larger lesions requiring resection and reconstruction have the potential for more complex complications (e.g., wound dehiscence, wound infection, hardware failure, graft failure, facial or trigeminal nerve injury, cosmetic deformity). In particular, reconstruction of a continuity defect of the anterior mandible is challenging.

DISCUSSION

Ossifying fibroma (OF) is a slow-growing, benign lesion of bone most commonly associated with the jaws. There have been occurrences in other bones, most commonly the tibia. Many names have been used to describe this lesion (*osteofibroma, fibro-osteoma, cementifying fibroma*) secondary to the tumor's cell of origin. Because it is not possible to determine whether the cell of origin is cementum or bone (both are derived from mesenchymal stem cells), it has become an irrelevant point. Therefore, the name *ossifying fibroma* is used. A variety of chromosomal abnormalities have been described in the small number of OF tumors submitted for cytogenetic analysis.

Multiple studies have shown that OF has a predilection for females (70%) between the second and fourth decades of life. About 58% occur in Caucasians; 23% in African Americans; and 12% in Hispanic individuals. Ossifying fibromas occur predominantly in the mandible (77%), with a greater propensity for the molar regions, followed by the premolar regions.

Juvenile ossifying fibroma is a variant of the ossifying fibroma. It is an uncommon lesion of juveniles and adolescents. It is typically more aggressive than an ossifying fibroma and usually affects the paranasal sinuses and bones around the orbit. *It is further subdivided into two histopathologic variants:* a psammamatous type and a trabecular type. The psammamatous type mainly involves the bones of the orbit and paranasal sinuses, whereas the trabecular type commonly involves the jaws, although there is controversy as to which type has a greater predilection for the maxilla versus the mandible. The psammamatous type occurs in an older and wider age range, compared to the trabecular type, which occurs in children and adolescents.

Frequent clinical features of juvenile ossifying fibroma include proptosis or exophthalmos and nasal symptoms. The lesion may require more aggressive treatment, with larger margins than are needed for the adult counterpart. However, some studies have indicated that smaller lesions may be treated by enucleation and curettage.

Histopathologically, the lesion may contain irregularly mineralized, cellular osteoid strands lined by plump osteoblasts. Juvenile ossifying fibromas have a reported recurrence rate between 38% and 50%.

Bibliography

Abrams AM, Melrose RJ: Fibro-osseous lesion, *J Oral Pathol* 4:158-165, 1975.

Barnes L, Eveson JW, Reichart P, et al (eds): *Pathology and genetics: head and neck tumors (IARC World Health Organization classification of tumors)*, Lyon, France, 2005, p. 319-322, IARC Press.

Brannon RB, Fowler CB: Benign fibro-osseous lesions: a review of current concepts, *Adv Anat Pathol* 8:126-143, 2001.

Eversole LR: Craniofacial fibrous dysplasia and ossifying fibroma, *Oral Maxillofac Surg Clin North Am* 9:625-642, 1997.

Eversole LR, Leider AS, Nelson K: Ossifying fibroma: a clinicopathologic study of sixty-four cases, *Oral Surg Oral Med Oral Pathol* 60:505-511, 1985.

Eversole LR, Merrell PW, Strub D: Radiographic characteristics of central ossifying fibroma, *Oral Surg Oral Med Oral Pathol* 59:522-527, 1985.

Eversole LR, Sabes WR, Rovin S: Fibrous dysplasia: a nosologic problem in the diagnosis of fibro-osseous lesions of the jaws, *J Oral Pathol* 1:189-220, 1972.

Fechner RE: Problematic lesions of the craniofacial bones, *Am J Surg Pathol* 13(Suppl 1):17-30, 1989.

Kramer IRH, Pindborg JJ, Shear M (eds): Histological typing of odontogenic tumors. In *WHO international histological classification of tumors*, ed 2, pp 27-29, Geneva, 1992, WHO.

Marx RE, Stern D: *Oral and maxillofacial pathology: a rationale for diagnosis and treatment*, Chicago, 2003, Quintessence.

Parham DM, Bridge JA, Lukacs JL, et al: Cytogenetic distinction among benign fibro-osseous lesions of bone in children and adolescents: value of karyotypic findings in differential diagnosis, *Pediatr Dev Pathol* 7:148, 2004.

Said AL, Surwillo E: Florid osseous dysplasia of the mandible: report of a case, *Compendium* 20:1017-1030, 1999.

Sciubba JJ, Younai F: Ossifying fibroma of the mandible and maxilla: review of 18 cases, *J Oral Pathol Med* 18:315-321, 1989.

Sissons HA, Steiner GC, Dorfman HD: Calcified spherules in fibro-osseous lesions of bone, *Arch Pathol Lab Med* 117:284-290, 1993.

Su L, Weathers D, Waldron CA: Distinguishing features of focal cemento-osseous dysplasia and cemento-ossifying fibromas. II. A clinical and radiologic spectrum of 316 cases, *Oral Surg Oral Med Oral Pathol Oral Radiol Endod* 84:540-549, 1997.

Su L, Weathers SD, Waldron CA: Distinguishing features of focal cemento-osseous dysplasias and cemento-ossifying fibromas. I. A pathologic spectrum of 316 cases, *Oral Surg Oral Med Oral Pathol Oral Radiol Endod* 84:301-309, 1997.

Summerlin D, Tomich C: Focal cemento-osseous dysplasia: a clinicopathologic study of 221 cases, *Oral Surg Oral Med Oral Pathol* 78:611-620, 1994.

Waldron C: Fibro-osseous lesions of the jaws, *J Oral Maxillofac Surg* 51:828-835, 1993.

Waldron C, Giansanti J: Benign fibro-osseous lesions of the jaws: a clinical-radiologic-histologic review of sixty-five cases. II. Benign fibro-osseous lesions of periodontal ligament origin, *Oral Surg Oral Med Oral Pathol* 35:340-350, 1973.

Wenig B: *Atlas of head and neck pathology*, Philadelphia, 1993, Saunders.

Williams HK, Mangham C, Speight PM: Juvenile ossifying fibroma: an analysis of eight cases and a comparison with other fibro-osseous lesions, *J Oral Pathol Med* 29:13, 2000.

Cone-Beam Computed Tomography (CBCT)

Piyushkumar Patel, DDS and Mayoor Patel, DDS, MS

CC

A 14-year-old girl is referred for exposure and bracketing of her impacted canines.

HPI

The patient's parent states that she had her primary cuspids removed at a younger age, with subsequent failure of her canines to erupt. Her orthodontist has recommended exposure and bracketing of the impacted canines to facilitate correct eruption and to avoid possible root resorption of her adjacent lateral incisors. The patient is otherwise asymptomatic.

PMHX/PDHX/MEDICATIONS/ALLERGIES/SH/FH

Noncontributory.

EXAMINATION

General. The patient is well developed, well nourished, and in no apparent distress.

Intraoral. Teeth #6 and #11 are not visible in the mouth. There is a questionable bulge of the maxillary anterior palate on the left and right sides; however, definitive localization of the impacted canines by palpation is not readily apparent.

Maxillary canines are the second most frequently impacted teeth, after the third molars. The prevalence is 1% to 3% of the population. Approximately 60% to 85% of these impactions are palatal. Impacted canines are seen more commonly in females.

IMAGING

Panoramic imaging revealed that teeth #6 and #11 were impacted and in close association with the adjacent lateral incisors (Figure 1-9). The third molars, also present, were full bone impactions. Given these findings, the risks and benefits of additional imaging were discussed with the patient's parents, who agreed to a CBCT scan to evaluate the maxillary canines (Figure 1-10).

In approximately 38% to 67% of cases, impacted canines can cause varying degrees of resorption of adjacent teeth, especially the lateral incisor. Root resorption can be difficult to diagnose with traditional two-dimensional (2D) radiography, especially when the canine is in a direct palatal or facial position to the lateral incisor roots.

Two-dimensional imaging for surgical or orthodontic planning has several limitations, such as image magnification and distortion, superimposition of structures, and misinterpretation. Three-dimensional (3D) imaging allows the surgeon to determine the best clinical approach and reduces the invasiveness of surgery. Additionally, it allows the orthodontist to determine what orthodontic force vector should be applied to move the canine efficiently, thus reducing involvement of adjacent teeth.

CBCT offers a 3D view that can provide more accurate information about the size, shape, angulation, associated pathology (cysts, tumors, resorption of adjacent teeth), and relationship to adjacent structures (inferior alveolar nerve [IAN] canal, sinus). CBCT software allows anatomic entities in the 3D image to be differentiated by assigning each a color (known as a *mask*). The masks can be turned off, allowing the

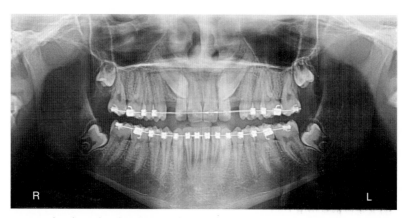

Figure 1-9 Preoperative panoramic view showing impacted teeth #6 and #11. Note the close association with the adjacent lateral incisors.

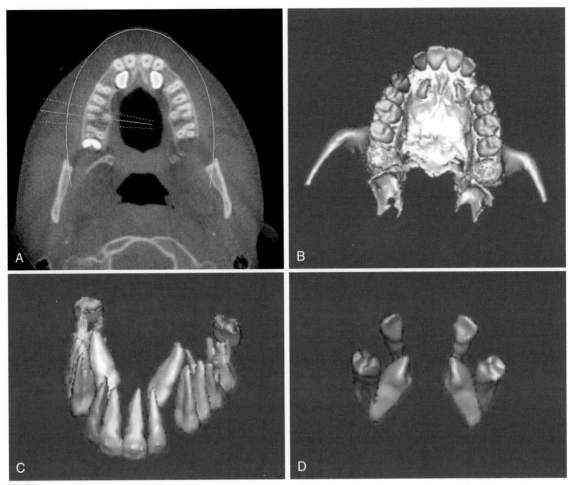

Figure 1-10 Axial view (**A**) and CBCT reconstruction (**B** to **D**) with different-colored masks assigned to the different anatomic structures in the FOV. Segmentation of the adjacent anatomy allows a better appreciation of the region of interest.

clinician a better appreciation of the anatomy. This type of reconstruction can be time-consuming, but it can be referred to third-party companies.

ASSESSMENT

Impacted maxillary canines needing surgically assisted exposure and bracketing for orthodontic correction.

TREATMENT

The precise location of the maxillary canines was determined. No readily apparent resorption of the lateral incisors was noted. (It is possible to underestimate root resorption, owing to inadequate visualization secondary to the limitations of CBCT, such as selecting a large field of view [FOV], which diminishes the resolution of the image.) The 3D reconstruction served two important purposes. It allowed the surgeon to easily appreciate the anatomy, and it also provided a visual aid that enabled the patient to easily understand the anatomic configuration of her problem; this, in turn, facilitated discussion of the procedure and its risks and benefits with the patient and her parents. Subsequently, the impacted canines were

exposed and bracketed without incident in a standard fashion. (See Surgical Exposure of an Impacted Maxillary Canine in Chapter 5, Dentoalveolar Surgery.)

COMPLICATIONS

Clinicians must abide by the "as low as reasonably achievable" (ALARA) principle when ordering an imaging modality for a patient. Exposing the patient to the radiation must provide an image with a diagnostic value that is greater than the detriment the radiation exposure may cause. Not every patient requires CBCT, because the technique does expose the patient to radiation and results in increased cost. The American Dental Association (ADA) Council on Scientific Affairs suggests that CBCT use should be based on professional judgment, and clinicians must optimize technical factors, such as using the smallest FOV possible for diagnostic purposes and using appropriate personal protective shielding.

The radiation dose per U.S. resident has been increasing over the past 30 years. Ionizing radiation is also found in the natural environment in the form of cosmic rays or radon. At doses used in diagnostic and interventional procedures, ionizing radiation may cause DNA damage and increase the risk for future cancer. The probability of effects arising from ionizing radiation (e.g., future cancer, cataracts) is a function of the total radiation dose, although the severity of such effects is also influenced by other factors, such as genetics. The linear no threshold model (LNT) is the most widely used theoretical dose-response model that assumes that any exposure to ionizing radiation can induce future cancer. (Some studies suggest that low doses may not have a detrimental effect.)

The concentration of ionizing radiation in a specific volume of air is a measure of radiation exposure and is expressed in roentgens (R). The amount of radiation absorbed by a specific tissue is measured in grays (Gy) or rads. The effective dose is measured in sieverts (Sv) (1 Sv = 1,000 mSv = 1,000,000 µSv), which provides a quantification of the potential radiobiologic detriment caused by radiation. Calculating the effective dose allows for comparison across different imaging modalities. The International Commission on Radiological Protection (IRCP) estimates a 4% to 5% increased relative risk of fatal cancer after an average person receives a whole-body radiation dose of 1 Sv. Some models predict that 1 in 1,000 persons exposed to 10 mSv (10,000 µSv) will develop cancer as a result of that single exposure.

For comparison purposes, consider the following estimated effective doses:
- Single chest x-ray: 0.02 mSv
- Transcontinental flight: 0.02 mSv
- Annual individual radiation dose from the natural background: 3 mSv
- Intraoral radiograph: 0.005 mSv (5 µSv)
- CT scan of the head: 2 mSv
- CT scan of the neck: 4 mSv
- CT scan of the chest: 8 mSv
- CT pulmonary embolism protocol: 15 mSv

Table 1-1 shows the effective dose estimates for common dental radiographic examinations.

The radiation risk with many newer CBCT machines is lower than that for the most common intraoral full mouth series; therefore, it may be possible, when indicated, to use CBCT with select intraoral images as an option for dental treatment planning in the future.

Currently the results for the use of CBCT for caries detection are mixed. CBCT for this purpose is limited to nonrestored teeth. Because of beam hardening, CBCT for caries detection has a high sensitivity. For periodontics, CBCT promises to be superior to 2D imaging for the visualization of bone topography and lesion architecture (intrabony defects and furcations), but no more accurate than 2D imaging for bone height. Restorations within the dentition can obscure views of the alveolar crest.

CBCT for endodontic purposes is the most promising modality. It has been shown to be useful for detecting apical lesions and root fractures, canal identification, characterizing internal and external resorption, and facilitating apical surgery. In orthodontics, CBCT can be used to evaluate the shape and function of the maxillofacial complex, and it provides a powerful tool for the visualization of root angulations.

Adjacent anatomy outside the region of interest is usually captured with CBCT. Given the volume of tissue that is

Table 1-1	Effective Dose Estimates for Common Dental Radiographic Examinations and Cone-Beam Computed Tomography (CBCT) Imaging*
Imaging Technique	**Effective Dose[†]**
Conventional Radiography	
Four-image posterior bitewings with photostimulable phosphor (PSP)	5.0
Panoramic radiograph with charge-coupled device	3.0-24.3
Cephalometric radiograph, postanterior or lateral with PSP	5.1-5.6
Full Mouth Radiographs	
With PSP storage or F-speed film and rectangular collimation	34.9
With PSP or F-speed film and round collimation	170.7
CBCT[‡]	
Dentoalveolar CBCT (small and medium field of view [FOV])	11-674 (61)
Maxillofacial CBCT (large FOV)	30-1073 (87)

From the American Dental Association Council on Scientific Affairs: The use of cone-beam computed tomography in dentistry, *JADA* 143(8):899-902, 2012.
*Estimates are for adult patients based on data from Paulwels and colleagues, the SEDENTEXCT Project, and Ludlow and colleagues.
[†]Measured in microsieverts.
[‡]Median values for effective dose provided parenthetically.

exposed and readily available for review, there is a moral, ethical, and legal responsibility attached to the interpretation of the volumetric data set. Because of the complexity of the anatomy of the maxillofacial area, review of the images by an appropriately trained radiologist is prudent.

The most common algorithm for reconstructing 3D objects (cone-beam reconstruction) from cone-beam projections is the Feldkemp, Davis, and Kress (FDK) method, which is used by many research groups and commercial vendors. This algorithm has some limitations, such as distortion in the noncentral transverse plane, resolution degradation in the longitudinal direction, and a high computational time required to perform reconstructions. To address these problems, other algorithm and cone-beam geometries are being developed that will likely be incorporated into future machines.

A Web site that provides comparative information on the currently available CBCT machines can be found at *www.conebeam.com/cbctchart*.

DISCUSSION

Dedicated CBCT of the maxillofacial region has created a revolution in all fields of dentistry and has expanded the role of imaging from diagnosis to image guidance for many surgical procedures. CBCT has eliminated some of the inherent limitations of 2D images, such as magnification, distortion, superimposition, and misrepresentation.

CBCT uses a cone-beam–shaped source of ionizing radiation, and the beam is directed through the middle of the area of interest (field of view, or FOV). The beam covers the entire FOV; therefore, only one rotation of the gantry is required. Traditional medical CT uses a fan-shaped beam to acquire individual image slices (each slice requires a separate scan), which are then stacked to obtain a 3D representation. CBCT usually results in a lower dose of radiation than CT, but doses vary widely among different systems and among different imaging protocols (slice thickness, FOV, mAs, kVp, scan time). It is recommended that clinicians use appropriate selection criteria, along with imaging protocols that use the minimal doses that ensure acceptable diagnostic qualities (Table 1-2).

Table 1-2	Summary of Key Advantages and Limitations of CBCT
Advantages	**Disadvantages/Limitations**

Equipment has a smaller physical footprint than conventional CT equipment.	**Artifacts**
	1. X-ray beam artifacts: Beam hardening, which results in two types of artifacts:
	  a. Distortion of metallic structures as a result of differential absorption; this is known as a *cupping artifact*
	  b. Streaks and dark bands that can appear between two dense objects (e.g., a dark band around an amalgam restoration, which can be mistaken for recurrent caries)
	  Limiting the field of view (FOV) and separating the arches are some techniques that can be used to scan regions susceptible to beam hardening.
	2. Patient-related artifacts (e.g., patient motion): These can be minimized by using a head restraint and short scan time. The presence of dental restorations or jewelry can lead to severe streaking artifacts as a result of beam hardening or of photon starvation (insufficient photons reaching the detector).
	3. Scanner-related artifacts: These present as circular artifacts and are usually due to imperfect scanner detection or poor calibration.
	4. Cone-beam–related artifacts: These include partial volume averaging and undersampling.

Considerably cheaper than conventional CT	Image noise: This is due to scattered radiation. The scatter-to-primary ratios are about 0.05 to 0.15 for fan-beam and spiral CT and may be as large as 0.4 to 2 in CBCT (i.e., CBCT appears more grainy).
Rapid scan time: All projection images are acquired in a single rotation.	Poor soft tissue contrast: This is due to the scattered radiation and detector-based artifacts. Newer techniques and devices may improve this.
Collimation limits radiation to the area of interest. In some machines, the FOV can be adjusted to engage only the area of interest, further limiting the dose.	Currently, Hounsfield units cannot be used to assess density information reliably.
Superior image accuracy: Submillimeter isotropic voxel resolution ranges from 0.4 to 0.076 mm.	
Reduced patient radiation dose: Depending on the FOV and CBCT model, the dose can range from 29 to 477 µSv. (The dose for conventional CT for maxillofacial imaging is approximately 2,000 µSv.)	
Interactive display modes, such as cursor-driven measurement algorithms, provide the clinician with on-screen interaction free of distortion and magnification.	
From the volumetric data set, distortion-free additional images can be generated, such as panoramic and cephalometric images.	
Three-dimensional volume rendering can be achieved by either indirect or direct volume rendering methods.	
Multimodal imaging devices are available. These can provide conventional panoramic, cephalometric, and CBCT images.	
Sophisticated third-party software is continuously being developed and updated using data generated by CBCT. The capabilities of such software usually exceed software supplied by CBCT machines. To use this software, the volumetric data is exported from the CBCT manufacturer's software as a digital imaging and communication in medicine (DICOM) data set and imported into the third-party software.	

CBCT image production requires four components.

1. Acquisition configuration
   a. X-ray generation: A pulsed or constant beam of radiation can be used. This is one of the reasons for variation in cone-beam dosimetry between different units.
   b. Field of view: This depends on the detector size and shape, beam projection geometry, and the ability to collimate the beam. CBCT can be categorized by the available FOV, which usually ranges from 4 to 30 cm. The larger the FOV, the poorer the resolution.
   c. Scan factors: During the scan, single exposures (known as *basis, frame,* or *raw images*) are made. (These are similar to the lateral view of PA cephalometric images.) The complete series is known as *projection data.* The number of images comprising a projection data set is determined by the *frame rate* (i.e., the number of images acquired per second; a faster frame rate results in better image quality, but it also exposes the patient to more radiation); the speed of rotation; and the completeness of the trajectory arc. Most CBCT machines scan for a full 360 degrees to acquire projection data. However, some machines limit the scanning arc, thus reducing the time, radiation dose, and mechanical components required. The disadvantages of this approach are greater noise and a higher possibility of artifacts.

2. Image detection
   Current CBCT machines can be divided into two groups based on the detector type: image intensifier tube/charge-coupled device (IIT/CCD) or flat panel imager. The flat panel imager is thought to create less distortion and have fewer artifacts. Flat panel performance limitations are most noticeable at lower and higher exposures.

3. Image reconstruction
   The projection data must be reconstructed to create a usable volumetric data set. This is computationally complex and can involve two computers (an acquisition computer and a processing [workstation] computer). This phase is divided into two stages: the acquisition stage (usually 160 to 600 basis images are collected) and the reconstruction stage (in which algorithms such as the FDK algorithm are used to recombine the data for visualization).

4. Image display
   The data set is presented to the clinician usually in three orthogonal planes (axial, sagittal, and coronal)

CBCT is most widely used for implant planning. Fusion of the CBCT scan data with three-dimensional clinical data (e.g., CBCT of a plaster cast, optical scan of the cast, or optical scan of the oral cavity) facilitates the fabrication of surgical guides (with fiducial markers or, more recently, with corresponding anatomic points). Fusion is necessary to obtain an accurate guide because of the presence of scatter artifact; fusion also allows more accurate visualization of the gingival level.

If CBCT is used for implant planning, the radiographic examination of a potential implant site can include cross-sectional imaging:

- CBCT should be considered as the imaging modality of choice for the preoperative cross-sectional imaging of potential implant sites.
- CBCT is also considered when the initial exam indicates the need for site development (e.g., block grafting, sinus lifting).
- CBCT should be considered for evaluating the results of site development (if bone augmentation procedures were performed before implant placement). In the absence of clinical signs or symptoms, periapical radiographs are appropriate for postoperative assessment.
- CBCT is indicated in the immediate postoperative period if there is altered sensation or implant mobility. CBCT is not indicated for periodic review of asymptomatic implants.
- CBCT can be considered if implant retrieval is anticipated.

In summary, the use of CBCT should be judged based on sound clinical and radiographic parameters. It can provide very valuable information for diagnosis and treatment planning. However, overzealous use of CBCT can result in unnecessary radiation exposure and added cost.

Bibliography

American Dental Association Council on Scientific Affairs: The use of cone-beam computed tomography in dentistry, *JADA* 143(8):899-902, 2012.

Bouwens D, Cevidanes L, Ludlow J, et al: Comparison of mesiodistal root angulation with posttreatment panoramic radiographs and cone-beam computed tomography, *Am J Orthod Dentofacial Orthop* 139:126-132, 2011.

Friedland B, Donoff B, Chenin D: Virtual technologies in dentoalveolar evaluation and surgery, *Atlas Oral Maxillofacial Surg Clin North Am* 20:37-52, 2012.

Kim JW, Cha IH, Kim SJ, et al: Which risk factors are associated with neurosensory deficits of inferior alveolar nerve after mandibular third molar extraction? *J Oral Maxillofac Surg* 70 (11):2508-2514, 2012.

Lee C, Elmore J: Radiation related risks of imaging studies. Available from Wolters Kluwer Health at www.uptodate.com. Accessed January 15, 2013.

Ludlow JB, Davies-Ludlow LE, White SC: Patient risk related to common dental radiographic examinations: the impact of 2007 International Commission on Radiological Protection recommendations regarding dose calculation, *JADA* 139(9):1237, 2008.

Meara DJ: Evaluation of third molars: clinical examination and imaging techniques, *Atlas Oral Maxillofacial Surg Clin North Am* 20:163-168, 2012.

Oberoi S, Knueppel S: Three-dimensional assessment of impacted canines and root resorption using cone beam computed tomography, *Oral Surg Oral Med Oral Pathol Oral Radiol Endod* 113(2):260, 2012.

Okano T, Sur J: Radiation dose and protection in dentistry, *Jpn Dent Sci Rev* 6:112-121, 2010.

Palomo L, Palomo JM: Cone beam CT for diagnosis and treatment planning in trauma cases, *Dent Clin North Am* 53:717-727, 2009.

Pauwels R, Beinsberger J, Collaert B, et al: SEDENTEXCT Project Consortium. Effective dose range for dental cone beam computed tomography scanners, *Eur J Radiol* 81(2):267-272, 2012.

Scarfe W, Farman A: What is cone-beam CT and how does it work? *Dent Clin North Am* 52:707-730, 2008.

The SEDENTEXCT Project. Radiation Protection: Cone Beam CT for Dental and Maxillofacial Radiology: Evidence Based Guidelines 2011 (v2.0 Final). www.sedentexct.eu/files/guidelines_final .pdf. Accessed July 26, 2013.

Tyndall D, Rathore S: Cone-beam CT diagnostic applications: caries, periodontal bone assessment and endodontic applications, *Dent Clin North Am* 52:825-841, 2008.

Tyndall D, Price JB, Tetradis S, et al: Position statement of the American Academy of Oral and Maxillofacial Radiology on selection criteria for the use of radiology in dental implantology with emphasis on cone beam computed tomography, *Oral Surg Oral Med Oral Pathol Oral Radiol* 113:817-826, 2012.

White S, Pharoah MJ: The evolution and application of dental maxillofacial imaging modalities, *Dent Clin North Am* 52:689-705, 2008.

CHAPTER 2

Pharmacology

This chapter addresses:
- Penicillin Allergy/Anaphylaxis
- Antibiotic-Associated Colitis
- Drug-Seeking Behavior
- Acute Acetaminophen Toxicity
- Opioid Side Effects
- Oral Drug-Induced Osteonecrosis of the Jaws
- Intravenous Drug-Induced Osteonecrosis of the Jaws

The use of pharmacotherapy is an important primary or adjunctive modality of treatment in the management of the surgical patient. Antibiotics, anesthetics, and analgesics are the most commonly used medications in oral and maxillofacial surgery. Despite appropriate use of medications, side effects and complications are observed. In this section we present seven cases associated with the use of medications encountered in surgery, along with discussion of related topics. Two cases of drug-induced osteonecrosis of the jaws (DINOJ) are presented—one involving oral and the second involving intravenous bisphosphonates. These two cases are separated since they represent two clinically distinct situations. Cases directly related to anesthesia and anticoagulation therapy are presented separately in the anesthesia and medicine sections.

The undesired effects of medications may result from a single factor or a combination of factors related to the drug: (1) Immunologically mediated reactions ranging from mild cutaneous manifestations to life-threatening anaphylaxis reactions; (2) unwanted systemic or local (side) effects (e.g., antibiotic-associated colitis or bisphosphonate-induced osteonecrosis of the jaws); (3)inappropriate dosing (e.g., acetaminophen overdose); (4) abuse and addictive potential leading to physiologic or social complications (e.g., opioid abuse or addiction); (5) compromised or deficient metabolism and elimination capabilities of the patient leading to toxicities (e.g., renal or hepatic failure); (6) failure of the drug to treat the intended condition, leading to exacerbation of the disease process (e.g., antibiotic resistance); and (7) patient noncompliance compromising treatment (e.g., concomitant alcohol ingestion with opioid or benzodiazepine use).

As the future unfolds, the pharmacological management of oral and maxillofacial surgery patients will become more complex. The greater array of medications on the market will require identification of new unwanted sequelae and interactions of drugs. Integration of technology will allow easier access to information to help ameliorate this emerging phenomenon.

Penicillin Allergy/Anaphylaxis

Piyushkumar P. Patel and Shahrokh C. Bagheri

CC

A 21-year-old woman admitted for treatment of an open mandibular body fracture complains of the sudden appearance of a rash and shortness of breath after receiving her intravenous antibiotics (anaphylaxis is more common with parenteral administration of medications).

HPI

The patient was admitted that day with a diagnosis of an open right mandibular body fracture secondary to assault. The patient did not report any known drug allergies (most frequently, patients do not have a previous history), and the admitting surgeon ordered intravenous penicillin G, morphine sulfate, and nothing-by-mouth (NPO) status in preparation for surgical treatment in the operating room. Upon arrival of the patient on the hospital ward, the nursing staff administered the first dose of intravenous aqueous penicillin G. Approximately 5 to 10 minutes later, the patient developed multiple circumscribed, erythematous, and raised pruritic wheals on her skin (symptoms generally develop within 5 to 60 minutes after exposure; earlier onset is seen with parenteral introduction of the allergen). The patient also reported feeling short of breath and the onset of wheezing (secondary to bronchospasm), nausea, and cramping abdominal pain.

PMHX/PDHX/MEDICATIONS/ALLERGIES/SH/FH

The patient reports no known drug allergies. She has no history of food, environmental, or seasonal allergies. She has no family history of drug allergies. (*Multiple drug allergy syndrome* is a term that may be applied to individuals who have experienced allergic reactions to two or more non-cross-reacting medications. People who are allergic to another drug are likely at increased risk of reacting to penicillin. The reasons are not clear, but genetics may play a role. Genetics may also play a role in the expression of penicillin allergy between family members; however, currently the studies are limited.)

Anaphylaxis is a serious allergic reaction that is rapid in onset and may cause death. Allergic anaphylaxis involves the production of symptoms via an immunologic mechanism. Nonallergic anaphylaxis (previously known as an anaphylactoid reaction) produces a very similar clinical syndrome but is not immune mediated (direct activation of mast cell). Treatment for the two conditions is similar.

EXAMINATION

General. The patient is a well-developed, well-nourished woman in moderate distress who is sitting up and leaning forward in bed.

Vital signs. Her blood pressure is 98/60 mm Hg (hypotension), heart rate 128 bpm (tachycardia), respirations 28 per minute (tachypnea), temperature 36.7°C, and Sao_2 100% on 2 L per nasal cannula.

Neurologic. The patient's Glasgow Coma Scale score is 15; she is alert and oriented × 3 (place, time, and person).

Maxillofacial. Examination is consistent with a mandibular body fracture.

Cardiovascular. She is tachycardic at 128 bpm. The heart rate and rhythm are regular, with no murmurs, gallops, or rubs. Cardiovascular symptoms and signs occur in up to 45% of anaphylactic episodes; they include hypotonia (collapse), syncope, dizziness, tachycardia, and hypotension.

Pulmonary. The patient has bilateral wheezing. Respiratory symptoms and signs occur in up to 70% of anaphylactic episodes; they include nasal congestion and discharge, a change in voice quality, a sensation of throat closure or choking, stridor, shortness of breath, wheezing, and cough.

Abdominal. The abdomen is soft, tender to palpation (secondary to spasm of intestinal smooth muscles), and nondistended with no rebound tenderness and normal bowel sound. Gastrointestinal symptoms and signs occur in up to 46% of anaphylactic episodes; they include nausea, vomiting, diarrhea, and crampy abdominal pain.

Skin. The patient has urticaria (commonly known as "hives," urticaria consists of circumscribed areas of raised erythema and edema of the superficial dermis). Skin symptoms and signs occur in up to 80% to 90% of anaphylactic episodes; they include generalized hives; itching or flushing; swollen lips, tongue, and uvula; periorbital edema; and conjunctival swelling.

The clinical presentation of anaphylaxis is variable and may include any combination of common signs and symptoms. Anaphylaxis is under-recognized and undertreated; the goal is early recognition and treatment with epinephrine. Diagnostic criteria were published by an expert panel in 2006 with the intention of helping clinicians recognize anaphylaxis.

The World Allergy Organization (WAO) has developed a poster that presents the key clinical criteria for both the diagnosis and initial treatment of anaphylaxis (Figure 2-1). These criteria reflect the different clinical presentations;

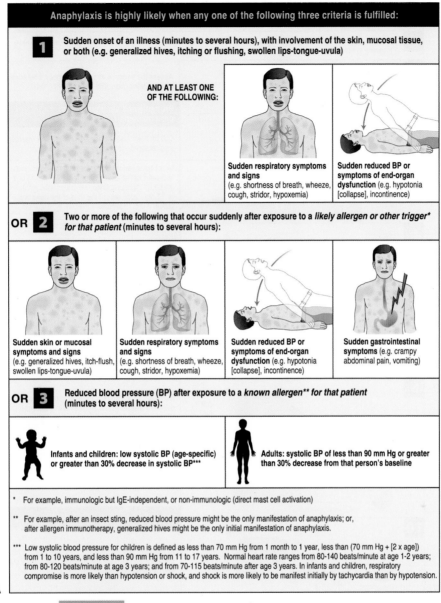

1 Sudden onset of an illness (minutes to several hours), with involvement of the skin, mucosal tissue, or both (e.g. generalized hives, itching or flushing, swollen lips-tongue-uvula)

AND AT LEAST ONE OF THE FOLLOWING:

Sudden respiratory symptoms and signs (e.g. shortness of breath, wheeze, cough, stridor, hypoxemia)

Sudden reduced BP or symptoms of end-organ dysfunction (e.g. hypotonia [collapse], incontinence)

OR **2** Two or more of the following that occur suddenly after exposure to a *likely allergen or other trigger** for that patient* (minutes to several hours):

Sudden skin or mucosal symptoms and signs (e.g. generalized hives, itch-flush, swollen lips-tongue-uvula)

Sudden respiratory symptoms and signs (e.g. shortness of breath, wheeze, cough, stridor, hypoxemia)

Sudden reduced BP or symptoms of end-organ dysfunction (e.g. hypotonia [collapse], incontinence)

Sudden gastrointestinal symptoms (e.g. crampy abdominal pain, vomiting)

OR **3** Reduced blood pressure (BP) after exposure to a *known allergen*** for that patient* (minutes to several hours):

Infants and children: low systolic BP (age-specific) or greater than 30% decrease in systolic BP***

Adults: systolic BP of less than 90 mm Hg or greater than 30% decrease from that person's baseline

* For example, immunologic but IgE-independent, or non-immunologic (direct mast cell activation)

** For example, after an insect sting, reduced blood pressure might be the only manifestation of anaphylaxis; or, after allergen immunotherapy, generalized hives might be the only initial manifestation of anaphylaxis.

*** Low systolic blood pressure for children is defined as less than 70 mm Hg from 1 month to 1 year, less than (70 mm Hg + [2 x age]) from 1 to 10 years, and less than 90 mm Hg from 11 to 17 years. Normal heart rate ranges from 80-140 beats/minute at age 1-2 years; from 80-120 beats/minute at age 3 years; and from 70-115 beats/minute after age 3 years. In infants and children, respiratory compromise is more likely than hypotension or shock, and shock is more likely to be manifest initially by tachycardia than by hypotension.

A

Figure 2-1 **A,** Clinical criteria for the diagnosis of anaphylaxis.

Continued

anaphylaxis is highly likely when any one of the criteria is met. It was acknowledged that no single set of criteria can provide 100% sensitivity and specificity, but it is believed that the WAO's proposed criteria are likely to capture more than 95% of cases of anaphylaxis. The majority of anaphylactic reactions include skin symptoms, which are noted in more than 80% of cases. Thus at least 80% of anaphylactic reactions should be identified by criterion 1, even when the allergic status of the patient and the potential cause of the reaction might be unknown.

IMAGING

In the acute phase of anaphylaxis, no imaging studies are indicated (any unnecessary delay may compromise other life-saving interventions).

LABS

During an acute anaphylactic episode, no laboratory tests are indicated. However, once the patient's condition has been stabilized (or if the diagnosis is in question), in addition to a complete blood cell count (CBC) and comprehensive metabolic panel (CMP), the following tests can be obtained:

Plasma histamine level. This is elevated within 5 to 10 minutes after the onset but remains elevated for only 30 to 60 minutes because of rapid metabolism (histamine is released secondary to IgE-mediated mast cell degranulation).

Urinary N-methyl histamine. A metabolite of histamine, N-methyl histamine remains elevated for several hours. A 24-hour urine sample for N-methyl histamine may be useful.

Serum tryptase. This peaks 60 to 90 minutes after the onset of anaphylaxis and remains elevated for up to 5 hours. Tryptase

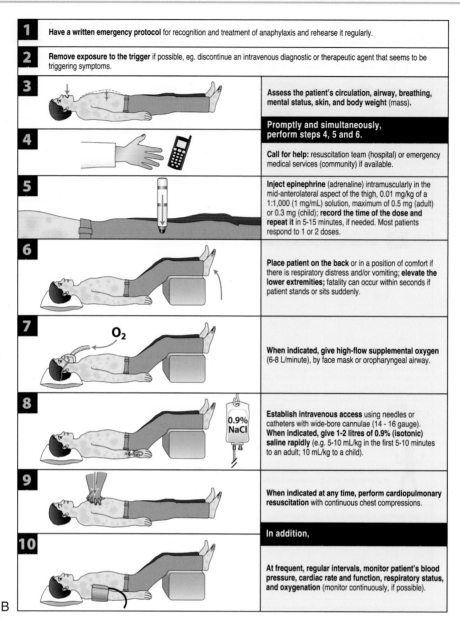

1	**Have a written emergency protocol** for recognition and treatment of anaphylaxis and rehearse it regularly.
2	**Remove exposure to the trigger** if possible, eg. discontinue an intravenous diagnostic or therapeutic agent that seems to be triggering symptoms.
3	**Assess the patient's circulation, airway, breathing, mental status, skin, and body weight** (mass).
	Promptly and simultaneously, perform steps 4, 5 and 6.
4	**Call for help:** resuscitation team (hospital) or emergency medical services (community) if available.
5	**Inject epinephrine** (adrenaline) intramuscularly in the mid-anterolateral aspect of the thigh, 0.01 mg/kg of a 1:1,000 (1 mg/mL) solution, maximum of 0.5 mg (adult) or 0.3 mg (child); **record the time of the dose and repeat it** in 5-15 minutes, if needed. Most patients respond to 1 or 2 doses.
6	**Place patient on the back** or in a position of comfort if there is respiratory distress and/or vomiting; **elevate the lower extremities;** fatality can occur within seconds if patient stands or sits suddenly.
7	**When indicated, give high-flow supplemental oxygen** (6-8 L/minute), by face mask or oropharyngeal airway.
8	**Establish intravenous access** using needles or catheters with wide-bore cannulae (14 - 16 gauge). **When indicated, give 1-2 litres of 0.9% (isotonic) saline rapidly** (e.g. 5-10 mL/kg in the first 5-10 minutes to an adult; 10 mL/kg to a child).
9	**When indicated at any time, perform cardiopulmonary resuscitation** with continuous chest compressions.
	In addition,
10	**At frequent, regular intervals, monitor patient's blood pressure, cardiac rate and function, respiratory status, and oxygenation** (monitor continuously, if possible).

B

Figure 2-1, cont'd   **B,** Initial treatment of anaphylaxis. *(From Simons FER, Ardusso LRF, Bilo MB, et al: World Allergy Organization anaphylaxis guidelines: summary,* J Allergy Clin Immunol *127[3]:587-593, 2011.)*

is a protease specific to mast cells. It is the only protein that is concentrated selectively in the secretory granules of human mast cells. Normal levels of either tryptase or histamine do not rule out the clinical diagnosis of anaphylaxis.

ASSESSMENT

Immediate allergic anaphylactic reaction induced by intravenously administered penicillin G

Box 2-1 outlines the differential diagnosis of anaphylactic shock.

TREATMENT

The initial management of anaphylaxis is to perform a focused examination; discontinue the suspected medication; call for help; administer intramuscular injection of epinephrine; place the patient, if possible, in a Trendelenburg position (to maximize perfusion of vital organs); administer supplemental oxygen; establish a stable airway (with intubation if necessary); obtain venous access (preferably with two large-bore [16-gauge] peripheral intravenous catheters) for volume resuscitation; and continuously monitor the vital signs and level of consciousness.

Immediately upon diagnosis, 0.3 to 0.5 ml of 1 : 1,000 epinephrine (0.3 to 0.5 mg in adults and 0.01 mg/kg in children) should be injected intramuscularly (IM) into the anterolateral thigh (injection at this site has been shown to be more effective than subcutaneous or upper arm [deltoid] injection). The site can be massaged to facilitate absorption. This dose may be repeated every 10 to 15 minutes, up to a total of three doses. The therapeutic effects of epinephrine include:

- **Other forms of shock**—Hemorrhagic/hypovolemic, cariogenic, septic
- **Flush syndromes**—Carcinoid, postmenopausal hot flashes, red man syndrome (vancomycin), oral hypoglycemic agents with alcohol, medullary carcinoma of the thyroid, idiopathic
- **Excess endogenous production of histamine**—Systemic mastocytosis, basophilic leukemia, hydatid cyst
- **Respiratory distress**—Asthma/chronic pulmonary obstructive disease exacerbation, foreign body aspiration, vocal cord dysfunction, pulmonary embolism
- **Nonorganic diseases**—Panic attacks, globus hystericus, Munchausen's stridor
- **Other conditions**—Ingestion of sulfites or monosodium glutamate, hereditary angioedema, neurologic condition (stroke or seizure), drug overdose

- α_1 adrenergic agonist: Increased vasoconstriction, increased peripheral vascular resistance, and decreased mucosal edema (in the upper airway)
- β_1 adrenergic agonist: Increased inotropy and chronotropy
- β_2 adrenergic agonist: Increased bronchodilation and decreased release of mediators from mast cells and basophils

Patients with severe upper airway edema, bronchospasm, or significant hypotension or who do not respond to IM injection (may not be perfusing muscle tissue) and fluid resuscitation should receive 0.5 to 1 ml of 1:10,000 epinephrine intravenously at 5- to 10-minute intervals. Alternatively, a continuous infusion of 1 to 10 μg/min of epinephrine (titrated to effect) may be administered (this is preferred over bolus dosing of epinephrine, because bolus dosing is associated with more adverse effects). Patients receiving intravenous epinephrine require continuous cardiac monitoring because of the potential for arrhythmias and ischemia, which occur most commonly with this route of administration. If intravenous access cannot be established, the epinephrine can be administered via an endotracheal tube (3 to 5 ml of 1:10,000 epinephrine).

It has been recommended that the epinephrine be administered early, because this can prevent progression to severe symptoms. Delayed administration has been implicated in contributing to fatalities.

Nebulized albuterol (β_2 agonist) for respiratory symptoms may be administered, and intravenous aminophylline (bronchodilator) can be considered, although its effectiveness for anaphylaxis is questionable. These are adjunctive treatments to epinephrine. Large volumes of fluids may be required to treat hypotension caused by increased vascular permeability and vasodilatation. Any patients with evidence of intravascular volume depletion (e.g., hypotension, low urine output, low or no response to injected epinephrine) should receive volume replacement. Normal saline is preferred initially. Additional pressors, such as dopamine (5 to 20 μg/kg/min),

norepinephrine (0.5 to 30 μg/kg/min), or phenylephrine (30 to 180 μg/kg/min), may be required.

Antihistamines also are considered adjunctive to epinephrine. The purpose for using antihistamines is to relive itch and hives. A combination of H_1 and H_2 blockers may be superior to either agent alone. Thus, diphenhydramine (H_1-receptor blocker) 25 to 50 mg intravenously/intramuscularly every 4 to 6 hours can be used with cimetidine (H_2-receptor antagonist) 300 mg intravenously every 8 to 12 hours. Alternatively, ranitidine (H_2-receptor antagonist) 1 mg/kg intravenously can be used.

Most authorities also advocate the administration of corticosteroids (methylprednisolone 1 to 2 mg/kg/day); their benefit is not realized for 6 to 12 hours after administration, but they may be helpful in the prevention of biphasic reactions. They can be stopped after 72 hours, because all biphasic reactions reported to date have occurred within 72 hours.

Patients currently taking β-blockers pose a challenge, because these drugs may limit the effectiveness of epinephrine. These patients may develop resistant hypotension, bradycardia, and a prolonged course. Atropine (anticholinergic) may be given for bradycardia. Some clinicians recommend administering glucagon. Glucagon exerts a positive inotropic and chronotropic effect on the heart independent of catecholamines. A 1-mg intravenous bolus followed by 1 to 5 mg every hour may improve hypotension in 1 to 5 minutes, with maximal benefit at 5 to 15 minutes. All patients with anaphylaxis should be monitored for the possibility of recurrent symptoms after initial resolution.

In the current patient, penicillin was immediately discontinued and 0.3 mg of 1:1,000 epinephrine was injected intramuscularly into the right anterolateral thigh. Synchronously a code was called; the patient was placed in a Trendelenburg position; and supplemental oxygen at 10 LPM was administered via a nonrebreather mask. Two 16-gauge peripheral intravenous lines were started at each antecubital fossa, and a bolus of normal saline was given. The patient also received intravenous medications (i.e., 50 mg diphenhydramine, 300 mg cimetidine, 100 mg methylprednisone) and nebulized albuterol. The vital signs were continuously monitored. An additional 0.3 mg of 1:1,000 epinephrine was given intramuscularly after 12 minutes. The patient remained stable, and marked improvement was noted. She was subsequently transferred to the intensive care unit (ICU) for observation.

After an uneventful overnight stay in the ICU, the patient was taken to the operating room the next day, where she underwent open reduction with internal fixation (ORIF) of the mandibular fracture. The anesthesia team was informed of her hospital course (in case the patient experienced a biphasic recurrence, with the signs and symptoms of anaphylaxis occurring during anesthesia). All early symptoms of anaphylaxis usually observed in the awake patient (e.g., malaise, pruritus, dizziness, and dyspnea) are absent in the anesthetized patient. The most commonly reported initial features are pulselessness, difficulty in ventilating, desaturation, and decreased end-tidal CO_2. Also, cutaneous signs may be difficult to notice in a completely draped patient.

Upon discharge, the patient was thoroughly informed of her allergy. She was provided with a medical alert bracelet, and follow-up was arranged with allergy care specialists.

COMPLICATIONS

Complications of anaphylaxis range from full recovery to anoxic brain injury and death despite adequate response and treatment. The factors that determine the course of anaphylaxis are not understood. At the onset of an episode, it is not possible to predict how severe it will become, how rapidly it will progress, or whether it will resolve spontaneously (as a result of endogenous production of compensatory mediators, such as epinephrine) or become biphasic or protracted. The rapidity of onset of symptoms makes this uncommon condition difficult to treat. Early recognition and treatment are essential. It is estimated that anaphylaxis causes approximately 1,400 to 1,500 fatalities per year in the United States. Between 5% and 20% of patients experience biphasic anaphylaxis, with a recurrence of symptoms after apparent initial resolution (typically 1 to 10 hours after initial resolution). Some cases of recurrence have been reported up to 72 hours later. Protracted anaphylaxis also has been reported, with persistence of symptoms for hours, days, or even weeks despite therapy.

Anaphylaxis is known to be difficult to recognize clinically for several reasons, including the broad differential that needs to be considered. Concurrent use of central nervous system (CNS)–active medications, such as sedatives, hypnotics, antidepressants, and first-generation sedating H_1 antihistamines, can interfere with recognition of anaphylaxis triggers and symptoms and with the ability to describe symptoms. In patients with concomitant medical conditions, such as asthma, chronic obstructive pulmonary disease, or congestive heart failure, symptoms and signs of these diseases can also cause confusion in the differential diagnosis of anaphylaxis. Death most commonly results from intractable bronchospasm, asphyxiation from upper airway edema, or cardiovascular collapse.

DISCUSSION

Penicillin allergy is reported by up to 10% of people in the United States. It has also been recognized that 80% to 90% of patients who report a penicillin allergy are not truly allergic to the drug. Of significance is that many people are falsely labeled as being penicillin allergic.

Most clinicians simply accept a diagnosis of penicillin allergy without obtaining a detailed history of the reaction. In their review, Salkind and colleagues stress the importance of a thorough history when faced with a penicillin-allergic patient (Box 2-2). However, it has been shown that patients with a vague history have also been found to have an IgE-mediated allergy. The time elapsed since the last reaction is important, because penicillin-specific IgE antibodies decrease with time (approximately 80% of patients with IgE-mediated penicillin allergy have lost sensitivity after 10 years).

Box 2-2	Taking a Detailed History from a Penicillin-Allergic Patient

Important Questions

What was the patient's age at the time of the reaction?

Does the patient recall the reaction? If not, who informed him or her of it?

How long after beginning penicillin did the reaction start?

What were the characteristics of the reaction?

What was the route of administration?

Why was the patient taking penicillin?

What other medications was the patient taking? Why and when were they prescribed?

What happened when the penicillin was discontinued?

Had the patient taken antibiotics similar to penicillin (e.g., amoxicillin, ampicillin, cephalosporins) before or after the reaction? If yes, what was the result?

From Salkind AR, Cuddy PG, Foxworth JW: The rational clinical examination—is this patient allergic to penicillin?: an evidence-based analysis of the likelihood of penicillin allergy, *JAMA*: 285:2498-2505, 2001.

Nonetheless, it is prudent to refer any patient with a history of IgE-mediated penicillin allergy for testing. Penicillin is the most common cause of drug-induced anaphylaxis. It causes an estimated 40% to 50% of all anaphylactic deaths in the United States.

Allergic drug reactions are one type of adverse drug reaction (ADR). An ADR has been defined by the World Health Organization as any noxious, unintended, and undesired effect of a drug that occurs at doses used for prevention, diagnosis, or treatment. ADRs can be categorized into two types: type A reactions, which account for 85% to 90% of all ADRs and can affect any individual (e.g., diarrhea in response to antibiotics), and type B reactions, which are hypersensitivity reactions that occur in susceptible patients. Although it has been difficult to determine the frequency of drug-induced allergic reactions specifically, it is known that they account for only a small proportion of ADRs, approximately 6% to 10%.

An allergic drug reaction can be classified as immediate (reaction occurs within 1 hour of administration and is usually IgE mediated) or delayed (reaction occurs after 1 hour, at times days or weeks after treatment, and is not IgE mediated). Anaphylaxis is an example of an immediate reaction. Late reactions can range from a rash that develops during treatment with amoxicillin to life-threatening conditions, such as Stevens-Johnson syndrome and toxic epidermal necrolysis (TEN). In rare cases, certain β-lactams can cause interstitial nephritis, hepatitis, or a vasculitis with or without signs of serum sickness.

Allergic reactions can also be classified by the immune mechanism involved, as described by Gell and Coombs. In this classification, type I represents an IgE-mediated response, whereas types II, III, and IV are non–IgE dependent. Type II, type III, and type IV reactions are classified as delayed reactions because they generally occur more than 1 hour after drug administration.

The clinical syndrome of anaphylaxis results from activation and release of mediators from mast cells and basophils (e.g., histamine). The cross-linking of mast cell–bound IgE with antigens causes the release of these mediators, with manifestations that include increases in vascular permeability (causing edema), vasodilatation (causing hypotension), respiratory smooth muscle contraction (causing bronchospasm), stimulation of the autonomic nervous system (causing tachycardia), mucus secretion, platelet aggregation, and recruitment of inflammatory cells.

Middle-aged and elderly patients are at increased risk of severe or fatal anaphylaxis because of known or subclinical cardiovascular diseases and the medications used to treat them. In the healthy human heart, mast cells are present around the coronary arteries and the intramural vessels, between the myocardial fibers, and in the arterial intima. In patients with ischemic heart disease, the number and density of cardiac mast cells is increased in these areas, and mast cells also are present in the atherosclerotic plaques. During anaphylaxis, the mediators released from cardiac mast cells contribute to vasoconstriction and coronary artery spasm.

Foods are the most common trigger for anaphylaxis in children, teens, and young adults (food triggers differ according to local dietary habits). Insect stings and medications (e.g., penicillin, radiocontrast media) are relatively common triggers in middle-aged and elderly adults. Natural rubber latex (NRL) may trigger anaphylaxis in health care settings, where it is found in equipment such as airway masks, endotracheal tubes, blood pressure cuffs, and stethoscope tubing and also in supplies such as disposable gloves, catheters, adhesive tape, tourniquets, and vials with NRL closures. Prompt recognition and treatment are critical in anaphylaxis.

For patients whose history appears to indicate an IgE-mediated response, skin testing to confirm allergy is useful if there is a compelling reason to use penicillin. Penicillin skin testing is performed by three classic methods: prick, intradermal, and patch. Skin testing itself carries a risk of fatal anaphylaxis, and the facility must be prepared to respond should a reaction occur. Studies have shown that among patients who test positive on a penicillin skin test, approximately 2% will react to a cephalosporin.

Patients who are allergic to penicillin and in whom the administration of a penicillin antibiotic is very desirable or even essential can be managed by desensitizing the patient to penicillin. Desensitization is accomplished by administering increasing doses of penicillin over a period of 3 to 5 hours. The mechanism whereby clinical tolerance is achieved is not entirely clear. The most likely hypothesis is that desensitization works by making mast cells unresponsive to the specific antigen. The desensitization procedure should be undertaken in an ICU setting, where continual monitoring is available. Also, the clinician must be at the bedside or readily available.

It has been shown that desensitization is an acceptable, safe approach to therapy in patients who are penicillin allergic but require β-lactams for treatment. Oral desensitization is safer than parenteral desensitization. There are no specific contraindications to desensitization. However, patients who are unable to withstand the consequences of an acute allergic reaction and its management are poor candidates.

Bibliography

Gell POH, Coombe RRA: The classification of allergic mediated underlying disease. In Coombe RRA, Gell POH (eds): *Clinical aspects of immunology*, ed 2, Oxford, 1968, Blackwell Science.

Gomez MB, Torres MJ, Mayorga C, et al: Immediate allergic reactions to beta lactams: facts and controversies, *Curr Opin Allergy Clin Immunol* 4:261, 2004.

Gruchalla R: Drug allergy, *J Allergy Clin Immunol* 111:548, 2003.

Mertes PM, Tajima K, Regnier-Kimmoun MA, et al: Perioperative anaphylaxis, *Med Clin North Am* 94:761, 2010.

Miller EL: The penicillins: a review and update, *J Midwifery Womens Health* 47:426, 2002.

Park MA, Li JT: Diagnosis and management of penicillin allergy, *Mayo Clin Proc* 80:405, 2005.

Riedl M, Casalias A: Adverse drug reactions: types and treatment options, *Am Fam Physician* 68:1781, 2003.

Romano A, Blanca M, Torres MJ, et al: Diagnosis of nonimmediate reactions to β-lactam antibiotics, *Allergy* 59:1153, 2004.

Salkind AR, Cuddy PG, Foxworth JW: The rational clinical examination—is this patient allergic to penicillin?: an evidence- based analysis of the likelihood of penicillin allergy, *JAMA* 285:2498, 2001.

Sampson H, Muñoz-Furlong A, Campbell RL, et al: Second symposium on the definition and management of anaphylaxis: Summary report: Second National Institute of Allergy and Infectious Disease/Food Allergy and Anaphylaxis Network Symposium, *J Allergy Clin Immunol* 117(2):391, 2006.

Simons F, Estelle R, Ardusso Ledit RF, et al: World Allergy Organization guidelines for the assessment and management of anaphylaxis, *World Allergy Organ J* 4(2):13-37, 2011.

Tang AW: A practical guide to anaphylaxis, *Am Fam Physician* 68:1325, 2003.

Torres MJ, Blanca M, Fernandez J, et al: Diagnosis of immediate allergic reactions to beta-lactam antibiotics, *Allergy* 58:961, 2003.

Wendel GD, Stark BJ, Jamison RB, et al: Penicillin allergy and desensitization in serious infections during pregnancy, *N Engl J Med* 312:1229, 1985.

Antibiotic-Associated Colitis

Piyushkumar P. Patel and Shahrokh C. Bagheri

CC

A 65-year-old man, status post incision and drainage (I & D) of a severe facial infection, who was previously admitted to the hospital for treatment of an odontogenic infection, complains of the new onset of severe "watery diarrhea."

HPI

The patient was admitted 6 days earlier and was taken to the operating room on that day, where I & D of the right submandibular/medial masticator and submental spaces, with extraction of a grossly carious right mandibular first molar, was performed. He remained intubated for 3 days and was maintained on intravenous clindamycin (900 mg every 8 hours). A previously placed nasogastric tube was also removed. The patient continued to do well and was transferred to the ward from the ICU on the fourth postoperative day, with continuation of the intravenous clindamycin therapy.

On hospital day 6, the patient reported lower abdominal pain and cramping of over 12 hours' duration. He also reported experiencing nausea, malaise, fever, and chills. He had several episodes of profuse, watery diarrhea, which were documented by the nursing staff. There was no evidence of blood in his stool, but he has had minimal oral intake since the symptoms began.

PMHX/PDHX/MEDICATIONS/ALLERGIES/SH/FH

Allergies. The patient has a penicillin allergy (history of rash).

Current medications. He is receiving clindamycin 900 mg intravenously every 8 hours and morphine sulfate 2 mg every 4 hours as needed for pain.

EXAMINATION

General. The patient is an obese man in mild distress who is resting in bed.

Vital signs. His blood pressure is 110/68 mm Hg, heart rate 118 bpm (tachycardia secondary to elevated temperature and gastrointestinal fluid losses), respirations 18 per minute, and temperature 38.8°C (fever secondary to release of inflammatory mediators in the gastrointestinal tract).

Maxillofacial. With decreasing facial edema, drains in the submandibular and submental spaces are nonproductive; removal is pending.

Abdominal. The abdomen is soft, nontender, and nondistended, with hyperactive bowel sounds in all four quadrants. There is no guarding or rebound tenderness (these would be indicative of peritonitis).

IMAGING

Plain radiographic imaging studies of the abdomen (e.g., kidney-ureter-bladder [KUB]) can be used to assist in the diagnosis of *Clostridium difficile*–associated diarrhea. Plain radiographs may reveal a dilated colon suggestive of ileus. (Patients with severe disease may develop colonic ileus or toxic dilatation with abdominal pain and distension with minimal or no diarrhea). A diffusely thickened or edematous colonic mucosa is often better visualized on an abdominal computed tomography (CT) scan. Thickening can sometimes be seen on abdominal plain films.

Colonoscopy or sigmoidoscopy is a more invasive diagnostic modality that is reserved for cases in which rapid diagnosis is necessary or stool samples cannot be obtained secondary to ileus. The finding of pseudomembranes is pathognomonic for *C. difficile* colitis. Because of the increased risk for intestinal perforation, endoscopy should be used sparingly in patients with suspected *C. difficile*–associated diarrhea.

Because this patient is relatively stable, abdominal imaging and/or endoscopy is not indicated.

LABS

A basic metabolic panel (BMP) demonstrated an elevated sodium level (148 mEq/L) and elevated BUN and creatinine (secondary to dehydration). Serial CBCs demonstrated elevation of the white blood cell (WBC) count, from 12,000 to 20,000 cells/µl, with bandemia.

The patient's stool guaiac test was negative for blood. Enzyme-linked immunosorbent assay (ELISA) for *C. difficile* toxin was positive.

The gold standard test for diagnosis of *C. difficile*–mediated disease is a cytotoxin assay. Although this test is highly sensitive and specific, it is difficult to perform, and the results are not available for 24 to 48 hours. In addition, the testing facility must be equipped with tissue culture capabilities. ELISA can be used to detect *C. difficile* toxin (A and/or B) in stool. This test has a sensitivity of 63% to 99% and a specificity of 93% to 100%. ELISA can be quickly performed (2 to 6 hours) and is the laboratory test most frequently used to diagnose *C. difficile* infection.

The average range for peripheral WBCs in patients with *C. difficile*–associated diarrhea is 12,000 and 20,000 cells/µl, but occasionally the count is higher. An important indicator of impending fulminant colitis is a sudden rise in peripheral WBCs to 30,000 to 50,000 cells/µl. Because progression to shock can occur even in patients who have had benign symptoms for weeks, early warning signs, such as the leukocytosis, can be invaluable.

ASSESSMENT

Resolving odontogenic infection now complicated by C. difficile*–associated diarrhea.*

TREATMENT

In otherwise healthy adults, the first step is to discontinue the precipitating antibiotic and to administer fluids and electrolytes to maintain hydration. For many patients, antibiotic-associated diarrhea is a mild and self-limited illness that responds to the discontinuation of antibiotics, supportive care, and fluid and electrolyte replacement. Specific pharmacotherapy for *C. difficile*–associated diarrhea should be initiated once the diagnosis of *C. difficile* has been confirmed or in highly suggestive cases of severely ill patients (Box 2-3). The use of opiates and antidiarrheal medications has previously been discouraged; however, some studies have shown that evidence supporting this hypothesis is lacking. Additionally, antimotility agents may be beneficial in providing symptomatic relief and reducing environmental contamination with infectious stool.

Box 2-3	**Guidelines for the Treatment of *Clostridium Difficile* Colitis**

- Discontinue antibiotics.
- Initiate supportive therapy. Prophylactic antibiotic therapy should not be given routinely. Once the diagnosis of *C. difficile* diarrhea has been confirmed and specific therapy is indicated, metronidazole given orally is preferred. If the diagnosis is highly likely and the patient is seriously ill, metronidazole may be given empirically before the diagnosis is established.
- Vancomycin given orally is reserved for the following conditions:
  - The patient has failed therapy with metronidazole.
  - The causative organism is resistant to metronidazole.
  - The patient is allergic to or cannot tolerate metronidazole or is being treated with ethanol-containing solutions.
  - The patient is pregnant.
  - The patient is a child under 10 years of age.
  - The patient is critically ill because of *C. difficile*–associated diarrhea or colitis.
  - There is evidence suggesting that the diarrhea is caused by *Staphylococcus aureus*.

From Pimental R, Choure A: Antibiotic associated diarrhea and *Clostridium difficile.* In Carey WD (ed): *Cleveland Clinic: current clinical medicine: expert consult premium edition,* ed 2, St Louis, 2010, Saunders.

For persisting symptoms, first-line therapy consists of metronidazole 500 mg orally three times daily for 10 to 14 days. Vancomycin is also an effective treatment, with a response rate greater than 95%. If the patient is pregnant or does not respond to or cannot tolerate metronidazole, then vancomycin should be initiated at 125 mg orally four times daily for 10 to 14 days. Response to therapy can be assessed by the resolution of fever, usually within the first 2 days. Diarrhea should resolve within 2 to 4 days; however, treatment is continued for 10 to 14 days. Therapeutic failure is not determined until treatment has been given for at least 5 days.

The best treatment is prevention. This includes the judicious use of antibiotics; hand washing between patient contacts (hand washing with soap and water may be more effective than the use of alcohol-based hand sanitizers, because *C. difficile* spores are resistant to killing by alcohol); rapid detection of *C. difficile* by immunoassays for toxins A and B; and isolation of patients who have *C. difficile*–associated diarrhea.

In the current case, the patient was placed on contact precautions. Current guidelines from the Centers for Disease Control and Prevention (CDC) indicate that patients should be placed under contact precautions and in isolation until the diarrhea has resolved. This patient was given a bolus of normal saline (NS) and started on maintenance fluids of D5½NS at 110 ml/hr. Clindamycin was discontinued, and the patient was started on metronidazole 500 mg orally three times daily. His diarrhea resolved in 2 days, and he was subsequently discharged. He was given a nonopiate pain medication during his hospital stay and upon discharge. The patient was educated about his diagnosis, and it was recommended that he inform other practitioners of it before initiation of antibiotic therapy.

COMPLICATIONS

Recurrence can develop and is usually due to the germination of persistent *C. difficile* spores in the colon after treatment or secondary to reinfection by the pathogen. Relapse is reported to occur in 15% to 20% of cases regardless of the initial treatment used. Some conditions identified as potential markers for relapse include previous relapses, chronic renal failure, marked leukocytes, and continued antibiotic use. In patients who have had more than one relapse, the recurrence rate can be as high as 65%; in such cases, avoidance of unnecessary antibiotics is strongly advised. Different agents, regimens, doses, and even unusual forms of therapy, such as fecal enemas, have been tried in these cases, with varying success.

Approximately 3% of patients develop severe *C. difficile*–associated diarrhea. The mortality rate in these patients ranges from 30% to 85%. Treatment of severe cases must be aggressive, with intravenous metronidazole and oral vancomycin used in combination. If ileus occurs, vancomycin can be administered by nasogastric tube with intermittent clamping, retention enemas, or both. If medical therapy fails or perforation or toxic megacolon develops, surgical intervention with colectomy and ileostomy is indicated but carries a high mortality rate.

Of concern is the fact that recent studies indicate the emergence of a new, more virulent strain of *C. difficile* that is associated with more severe disease (higher rates of toxic megacolon, leukemoid reaction, shock, need for colectomy, and death). This new strain is commonly designated as NAP1/BI/027 (the designation denotes the following: NAP1—a North American Pulse Field type 1 pattern on gel electrophoresis; BI—a BI pattern on restriction endonuclease analysis; 027—type 27 on ribotyping). Deletion of a gene in this new strain may be responsible for its greater pathogenicity. This deletion is thought to be responsible for production of 16 to 23 times more toxin A and B. The emergence of this virulent strain underscores the importance of judicious use of antibiotics (especially cephalosporins, clindamycin, and fluoroquinolones). Strict infection control measures, including contact isolation and enhanced environmental cleaning, are mandatory. Recent outbreaks of the more virulent strain in hospitals in the United States and Canada, which have been reported in the popular press, have increased public awareness of this disease process.

DISCUSSION

C. difficile is a gram-positive, spore-forming rod that is responsible for 20% to 30% of antibiotic-related cases of diarrhea. *C. difficile* infection results in more than 300,000 cases of diarrhea in the United States and is the most common cause of nosocomial diarrhea. The case mortality rate is approximately 1% to 2.5%.

Acquisition of *C. difficile* occurs primarily in the hospital setting or long-term care facilities, where the organism has been cultured from bed rails, floors, windowsills, and toilets, in addition to the hands of hospital workers who provide care for patients with *C. difficile* infection. The rate of *C. difficile* acquisition is estimated to be 13% to 20% in patients with hospital stays up to 2 weeks and 50% in those with hospital stays longer than 4 weeks.

The risk factors for the development of symptomatic *C. difficile*–associated diarrhea are summarized in Box 2-4. The most important modifiable risk factor for the development of *C. difficile* infection is exposure to antimicrobial agents. Even very limited exposure, such as single-dose surgical antibiotic prophylaxis, increases a patient's risk of both *C. difficile* colonization and symptomatic disease. The initiating event for *C. difficile* colitis is disruption of colonic flora, with subsequent colonization. Depending on host factors, a carrier state or disease results. The disruption is usually caused by broad-spectrum antibiotics. Clindamycin and broad-spectrum penicillins and cephalosporins are most commonly implicated. *C. difficile* colitis can occur up to 8 weeks after discontinuation of antibiotics.

C. difficile produces two toxins that are responsible for its pathogenesis, toxin A and B. Both toxins play a role in the pathogenesis of *C. difficile*–associated diarrhea. Toxin B is approximately 10 times more potent than toxin A. The toxins

---

Box 2-4	Risk Factors for *Clostridium Difficile*–Associated Diarrhea

Admission to the ICU
Advanced age
Antibiotic therapy
Immunosuppressive therapy
Multiple and severe underlying diseases
Placement of a nasogastric tube
Prolonged hospital stay
Recent surgical procedure
Residing in a nursing home
Sharing a hospital room with a *C. difficile*–infected patient
Antacid use

---

bind to intestinal receptors, leading to disruption of the cellular skeleton and intracellular junctions. Protein synthesis and cell division are inhibited. Inflammatory mediators attract neutrophils and monocytes, increasing capillary permeability, tissue necrosis, hemorrhage, and edema. As colitis worsens, focal ulcerations occur, and the accumulation of purulent and necrotic debris forms the typical pseudomembranes.

The diagnosis of *C. difficile* colitis requires a detailed history, including use of any antibiotics over the past 3 months. A detailed description of the type, frequency, and consistency of diarrhea is important. The enzyme immunoassay that detects toxins A and B is the laboratory test most commonly used to diagnose *C. difficile*–mediated disease.

Fidaxomicin is a macrocyclic antibiotic that is bactericidal against *C. difficile*. It was approved by the U.S. Food and Drug Administration (FDA) in 2011. Trials have shown that fidaxomicin 200 mg twice daily has clinical cure rates similar to those of vancomycin; also, the recurrence rates with fidaxomicin are lower with non-NAP1 strains, but not with the NAP1 strain. Fidaxomicin may be appropriate in patients with relapsing C- difficile. Parameters for its most appropriate use are still being developed.

Probiotics, a group of agents designed to resist colonization and restore normal flora, have been tried in antibiotic-associated diarrhea. The most promising probiotic agent is *Saccharomyces boulardii*, a live, nonpathogenic yeast. Some studies have shown that when *S. boulardii* was given prophylactically to patients receiving antibiotics, it was safe and beneficial in reducing the incidence of *C. difficile* colitis. *Lactobacillus GG*, another popular probiotic, has been shown to improve intestinal immunity by increasing IgG and IgA levels at the intestinal mucosal level. However, despite some positive findings, conclusive studies are still lacking to recommend the use of probiotics for routine prevention of antibiotic-associated diarrhea. Although usually considered harmless, both *S. boulardii* and *Lactobacillus* therapy are capable of inducing fungemia and bacteremia, respectively.

Other types of diarrhea should be considered and ruled out based on the history and physical examination. These include infectious enteritis or colitis, bacterial gastroenteritis, viral gastroenteritis, amebic dysentery, inflammatory bowel disease (e.g., Crohn's disease), ulcerative colitis, and ischemic colitis.

Antibiotic intolerance manifested as diarrhea in which there is no evidence of colitis usually resolves upon antibiotic withdrawal.

Bibliography

Bartlett JG: Antibiotic-associated diarrhea, *N Engl J Med* 346:334, 2002.

Bartlett JG, Perl TM: The new *Clostridium difficile*: What does it mean? *N Engl J Med* 353:2503-2505, 2005.

Cohen S, Gerding DN, Johnson S, et al: Clinical practice guidelines for *Clostridium difficile* infection in adults—2010: update by the Society for Healthcare Epidemiology of America (SHEA) and the Infectious Diseases Society of America (IDSA), *Infect Control Hosp Epidemiol* 31(5):431-455, 2010.

Efron P, Mazuski J: *Clostridium difficile* colitis, *Surg Clin North Am* 89(2):483-500, 2009.

Koo HL, Koo DC, Musher DM, et al: Antimotility agents for the treatment of *Clostridium difficile* diarrhea and colitis, *Clin Infect Dis* 48(5):598, 2009.

Loo VG, Poirier L, Miller MA, et al: A predominantly clonal multi-institutional outbreak of *Clostridium difficile*–associated diarrhea with high morbidity and mortality, *N Engl J Med* 353(23):2442-2449, 2005.

Louie TJ, Miller MA, et al: Fidaxomicin versus vancomycin for *Clostridium difficile* toxins, *N Engl J Med* 364:422, 2011.

McDonald LC, Killgore GE, Thompson A, et al: An epidemic, toxin gene-variant strain of *Clostridium difficile*, *N Engl J Med* 353(23):2433-2441, 2005.

Mylonakis E, Ryan E, Calderwood S: *Clostridium difficile*–associated diarrhea: a review, *Arch Intern Med* 161:525, 2001.

Pimental R, Choure A: Antibiotic associated diarrhea and *Clostridium difficile*. In Carey WD (ed): *Cleveland Clinic: current clinical medicine: expert consult premium edition*, ed 2, St Louis, 2010, Saunders.

Savola KL, Baron EJ, Tompkins LS, et al: Fecal leukocyte stain has diagnostic value for outpatients but not inpatients, *J Clin Micriobiol* 39:266, 2001.

Schroeder M: *Clostridium difficile*–associated diarrhea, *Am Fam Physician* 71(5):921, 2005.

Thomas RV: Nosocomial diarrhea due to *Clostridium difficile*, *Curr Opin Infect Dis* 17:323, 2004.

Drug-Seeking Behavior

Fariba Farhidvash, Chris Jo, and Shahrokh C. Bagheri

CC

A 40-year-old man presents to your office, stating, "My tooth is killing me, and I ran out of my pain meds."

HPI

The patient complains of a 3-day history of exquisite tooth pain. When interviewed, the patient immediately emphasizes that he has tried everything and that only "Percocet" helps with the pain. He states that he is unable to tolerate all non-steroidal antiinflammatory drugs (NSAIDs) because of gastric upset, and he also states that he has a "very high tolerance" for pain medications because of a history of chronic pain associated with a herniated lumbar disc. The patient is given a prescription for 20 oxycodone/acetaminophen (325/5 mg) tablets, to take as needed, and he is scheduled for surgery the next morning. On the morning of surgery, he calls to cancel his appointment for "financial reasons" and requests more pain medication to last him through the weekend. You call his referring dentist to obtain a more detailed history and find out that this patient has called several times in the past requesting opioid pain medications without compliance with the proposed treatment plans (restoration versus extraction).

PMHX/PDHX/MEDICATIONS/ALLERGIES/SH/FH

The patient has a history of back pain caused by lumbar disc herniation, which resulted from a fall at work (a previous history of chronic pain and narcotic analgesic use would likely indicate tolerance). He also has a history of depression (this may be a consequence of chronic pain, but patients with depression and/or anxiety also are more likely to exhibit dependence or addiction).

EXAMINATION

General. The patient is a well-developed and well-nourished man who appears mildly agitated. He reports a pain level of 10/10 on the visual analog scale (VAS), although his behavior (and examination findings) do not correlate with his reported level of pain (although this is a subjective observation and its value is questionable, clinicians need to correlate subjective complaints of pain with objective clinical findings).

Intraoral. The dentition is in good general repair. The right maxillary first molar (tooth #3) has a small occlusal carious lesion. The patient has a dramatic painful reaction upon palpation and percussion of the tooth. No vestibular swelling, erythema, or any other signs of acute infection are noted.

Pain perception is a physical sensation interpreted in the light of experience. It is influenced by a great number of interacting physical, mental, biologic, physiologic, psychological, social, cultural, and emotional factors. Each individual learns the application of the word "pain" through experiences related to injury early in life. The response to pain is very variable subjectively, behaviorally (crying, yelling, teeth clenching, wincing), and physiologically through various individual ranges of sympathetic nervous system manifestations (hypertension, tachycardia, nausea, pupillary dilatation, pallor, perspiration). A remarkable aspect of pain perception is the extreme variability of reactions that it evokes. Many factors affect the perception of pain; therefore, clinicians need to exercise caution when interpreting a patient's perception of pain.

IMAGING

A panoramic radiograph is an excellent screening tool for evaluating odontogenic sources of pain. A bitewing and periapical radiographs provide better resolution for detection of caries.

The panoramic radiograph for the current patient showed a carious lesion on the right maxillary first molar that does not appear to involve the pulp. There is no periapical radiolucent lesion or widening of the periodontal ligament space.

LABS

No laboratory tests are needed in the work-up of acute odontogenic pain unless dictated by the patient's medical history. For patients being admitted to the hospital for maxillofacial injuries or pathology, a urine drug screen (UDS) or blood alcohol level (BAL) can be obtained to detect recent use of illicit drugs that may influence treatment interventions. However, this may not be feasible for the patient presenting to the office.

ASSESSMENT

Carious right maxillary first molar, with subjective report of refractory odontogenic pain in the setting of other chronic pain syndromes and a history of substance abuse; patient demands to be treated for his acute dental pain with opioid medications, displaying signs of drug-seeking behavior.

A patient who presents to your clinic for acute or chronic pain that is refractory to multiple pain medications, who has made multiple visits to other medical facilities to obtain medications, and who is demanding or aggressive in his attempt to receive narcotic medications raises concerns about drug-seeking behavior. "Drug-seeking behavior" is a common term used among physicians; it may be defined as "a patient's manipulative, demanding behavior to obtain medication." Although there is no definition of drug-seeking behavior in the *Diagnostic and Statistical Manual of Mental Disorders–Fourth Edition* (DSM-IV), the condition is related to, but not synonymous with, drug abuse, dependence, and addiction.

DSM-IV criteria for abuse include the presence of the following symptoms within a 12-month period:

- Recurrent use resulting in a failure to fulfill major obligations at work, school, or home
- Recurrent use in situations that are physically hazardous (e.g., driving while intoxicated)
- Legal problems resulting from recurrent use
- Continued use despite significant social or interpersonal problems caused by the substance use

DSM-IV criteria for dependence include the following:

- Excessive amount of time spent to obtain or use the substance
- Continuation of use despite related problems
- Increase in tolerance (more of the drug is needed to achieve the same effect)
- Withdrawal symptoms

Although addiction is not included in the DSM-IV, it is characterized by preoccupation with and seeking of the drug and with continued use of the drug, leading to tolerance, physical dependence, and other adaptive changes in the brain.

TREATMENT

It is important for physicians to treat pain effectively and without fear of addiction or dependence. There are steps to effectively treat the patient's pain and curb the physician's concern. First and foremost, it is important to become familiar with the patient's medical history, especially any other pain syndromes or psychological comorbidities. It is also essential to become familiar with the different schedules of medications, dosing, adverse effects, and general pharmacokinetics. Dosing schedules and any recent changes, along with any side effects the patient may experience, should be followed closely. An interdisciplinary approach to pain and other alternatives to treatment, such as various injections or blocks or even nonmedication routes, such as psychotherapy, should not be excluded. Pain should not be treated in isolation but as part of the patient's overall medical picture.

Treating acute or chronic pain should be approached in a stepwise manner. Pain management should be individualized and applied in the appropriate clinical situation. The World Health Organization (WHO) guidelines for the management of chronic facial pain have established a three-step ladder approach. Step 1 involves the use of nonopioids, including acetaminophen (the drug of choice for patients with bleeding disorders, renal disease, or peptic ulcer disease), NSAIDs, aspirin, and propoxyphene napsylate. Step 2 involves the use of acetaminophen combined with various narcotic medications (codeine, hydrocodone, and oxycodone). Step 3 involves the use of opioid medications for moderate to severe pain plus a nonopioid medication. In the case of facial pain, nonopioid choices include anticonvulsants and tricyclic antidepressants (gabapentin, amitriptyline, carbamazepine, clonazepam, imipramine), which are reserved for chronic or neuropathic pain states.

In the setting of mild to moderate acute odontogenic or postoperative pain, nonopioid analgesics (NSAIDs and acetaminophen) should be initiated. A short course of scheduled dosing of an NSAID (e.g., ibuprofen 800 mg every 8 hours for 3 days, in the absence of contraindications), along with narcotic pain medication (e.g., hydrocodone, oxycodone, meperidine, with or without acetaminophen) may be prescribed for moderate to severe breakthrough pain. However, drug seekers commonly preclude the use of NSAIDs in their pain management by stating that they are allergic to or intolerant of them. If the patient has more moderate to severe pain, then higher doses of opioids with the nonopioid analgesics are used. Each medication can be increased in dose, or the dosing frequency can be adjusted according to the patient's needs. In conjunction with analgesics, antibiotic therapy should be initiated when indicated. Although chronic opioid treatment has been successful and is recommended for cancer patients, controversy exists regarding the use of opioid versus nonopioid drugs in the management of chronic nonmalignant orofacial pain.

If the chronic pain is characterized as neuropathic, tricycle antidepressants or selected antiepileptics (Neurontin, Tegretol, or Lyrica) can be very effective. Other options for pain management, such as regional sympathetic blockade, steroid injections, neuroablative procedures, and the like, may have longer lasting effects without the fear of abuse. It should be noted that pain is characteristically a manifestation of an underlying problem and associated comorbidities that may include organic or psychiatric conditions that influence the perception of pain. Treatment of underlying mood or other psychiatric disorders can help relieve the subjective experience of pain.

If drug-seeking behavior is observed or if there is suspicion of dependence or abuse of prescription medication, medical intervention may be warranted. This is usually out of the realm of most specialties and is best handled by primary care physicians or psychiatrists. Various methods include pharmacologic detoxification (e.g., supervised use of methadone) and various behavioral therapies, such as biofeedback and relaxation techniques and psychotherapy—all addressing the multiple facets of addiction and dependence.

With the current patient, he continues to focus on the tooth pain and the need for narcotic medications. He becomes more agitated, raising his voice as he explains that "nothing else has worked so far." You emphasize that there are other, non-narcotic alternatives and that further narcotic use will cause increased tolerance. Despite continued disagreement, the patient is emphatically informed that you will work closely with him to monitor the pain and modify treatment accordingly but will not prescribe further narcotic medication. The patient is hesitant but finally agrees to follow the strict but thorough plan for pain management.

COMPLICATIONS

Overuse of opioid analgesics, sedative-hypnotics, and stimulants is typically implicated in drug tolerance and dependence. If this problem is further escalated, it can lead to abuse, physical dependence with disruption of daily activities and functioning, and even death in the event of overdose. Beyond these effects, there are the individual adverse effects associated with each medication. The most common side effects related to narcotic or opioid drugs include nausea and vomiting, constipation, anorexia, sedation or decreased cognitive functioning, euphoria, and respiratory depression and hypotension. Although uncommon, overdose with any of the medications can cause death. These side effects may be magnified if the drug is used in combination with other analgesic or nonanalgesic medications. Drug interactions may result in changes in absorption, metabolism, or excretion of either medication.

DISCUSSION

With the increased availability of narcotic and opioid medications, the use and abuse of these drugs have significantly increased in the past few decades. Emergency department visits for narcotic medications rose at least 75% or more for all age groups between 2004 and 2009. In addition, deaths involving opioid analgesics increased by 142% between 1999 and 2004. Multiple factors contribute to this epidemic, including inappropriate and incorrect prescribing, lack of physician education, slow governmental response, marketing by pharmaceutical companies, and variable sources for the medications, including multiple physicians, friends and family, and the Internet.

Addiction disorders can be seen in up to 15% to 30% of patients in the primary care setting and in 20% to 50% of hospitalized patients. Opioid analgesics, sedative-hypnotics, and stimulants are the most commonly abused medications. Patients with acute or chronic pain, anxiety disorders, a history of substance abuse, or attention deficit/hyperactivity disorder are at increased risk for addiction. Identifying patients at risk is important, so obtaining the past medical, psychiatric, and substance abuse histories, in addition to histories of other pain disorders and psychosocial stressors, is paramount.

Recognizing drug-seeking behavior can help the clinician identify patients who need close follow-up. Patients may increase the use of analgesics over time as a result of increased tolerance to the drug. Patients typically focus excessively on their pain and emphasize the need for a particular drug with abuse potential. They frequently present with multiple claims that non-narcotic medications are not effective and that they have several "allergies." Commonly, if one doctor does not "meet their needs" or if they wish to avoid suspicion, they "doctor shop," a pattern difficult to identify, because physicians do not have access to other physicians' or hospitals' medical records. Also, patients may be involved in scams to obtain brand names or stronger medications, especially for sale on the street.

With this increasing problem, steps can be taken to protect both physician and patient. Physician education regarding appropriate medication selection and use is paramount. Physicians should also be aware of the regulations set forth by their state boards regarding controlled substances. If controlled substances are to be prescribed, an agreement can be signed between the patient and the physician in which the patient is informed of the risks of opioid medications and agrees to monitoring of his or her narcotic use (e.g., a pill count or random urine drug screens). Following the stepwise approach to pain control may help prevent inappropriate opioid use.

Bibliography

Bagheri SC, Perciaccante VJ, Bays RA: Comparison of patient and surgeon assessments of pain in oral and maxillofacial surgery, *J Calif Dent Assoc* 36(1):43-50, 2008.

Longo LP, Johnson B: Addiction. II. Identification and management of the drug-seeking patient, *Am Fam Physician* 61:2121-2128, 2000.

Manubay JM, Muchow C, Sullivan MA: Prescription drug abuse: epidemiology, regulatory issues, chronic pain management with narcotic analgesics, *Prim Care* 38:71-vi, 2011.

Maxwell JC: The prescription drug epidemic in the United States: a perfect storm, *Drug Alcohol Rev* 30:264-270, 2011.

Mersky H, Bogduk N: Classification of chronic pain. In Merskey H, Bogduk N (eds): *Task Force on Taxonomy*, pp 209-214, Seattle, 1994, International Association for the Study of Pain.

Swift JQ: Nonsteroidal anti-inflammatory drugs and opioids: safety and usage concerns in the differential treatment of postoperative orofacial pain, *J Oral Maxillofac Surg* 58(Suppl 2):8-11, 2000.

Swift JQ, Roszkowski MT: The use of opioid drugs in management of chronic orofacial pain, *J Oral Maxillofac Surg* 56:1081-1085, 1998.

Vukmir RB: Drug-seeking behavior, *Am J Drug Alcohol Abuse* 3:551-571, 2004.

Zuniga JR: The use of nonopioid drugs in management of chronic orofacial pain, *J Oral Maxillofac Surg* 56:1075-1080, 1998.

Acute Acetaminophen Toxicity

Bruce W. Anderson and Shahrokh C. Bagheri

CC

A 53-year-old man is referred to your clinic with a chief complaint of severe pain associated with the left mandibular second molar. The patient also complains of generalized malaise and right upper quadrant abdominal pain.

HPI

The patient reports a 3-month history of diffuse intermittent pain of the right posterior mandible that he has treated with several over-the-counter analgesics. In the past 4 days, the pain has become constant and has progressively exacerbated. It has localized to the left mandibular second molar, causing him to repeatedly wake up during the night. Two days prior to presentation, he was seen at a walk-in dental clinic, where he was prescribed penicillin and oxycodone/acetaminophen (5/325 mg) and referred to your clinic for evaluation and extraction. Careful questioning reveals that during the past 48 hours, he has ingested the 30 prescribed tablets of oxycodone/acetaminophen and, due to continued pain, also ingested 12 additional 500-mg tablets of acetaminophen that he purchased over the counter from the local pharmacy (total ingested dose of acetaminophen in 48 hours is estimated at 15,750 mg). During the last 6 hours, he reports the onset of right upper quadrant abdominal pain and nausea.

Abdominal pain and a history of excessive acetaminophen ingestion should alert the clinician to possible hepatotoxicity and warrant immediate referral to an emergency department.

PMHX/PDHX/MEDICATIONS/ALLERGIES/SH/FH

His past medical history is significant for chronic alcohol abuse. He admits to drinking at least six cans of beer per day (suggestive of preexisting compromised liver function).

Patients with compromised liver function, as in chronic alcoholism, have a decreased ability to clear acetaminophen and are more prone to toxic injury. Conversely, acute alcohol ingestion in an otherwise healthy individual will induce the hepatic microsomal oxidase system and increase the removal of acetaminophen from plasma.

EXAMINATION

General. The patient is in mild distress (secondary to pain) but is cooperative. He is alert and oriented (altered mental status can be seen several days after ingestion of toxic doses of acetaminophen due to severe hepatotoxicity). He appears mildly cachectic (suggestive of malnutrition), slightly lethargic, and pale.

Weight. 70 kg

Vital signs. Blood pressure is 127/83 mm Hg, heart rate 112 bpm (tachycardia due to pain), respirations 17 per minute, and temperature 37.4°C.

Intraoral. The examination is consistent with acute pulpitis of the left mandibular second molar.

Abdominal. Palpation of the right upper quadrant elicits mild pain. The liver is palpated at 6 cm inferior to the costal margin and measures over 17 cm using percussion (hepatomegaly). (A normal liver margin is generally not palpable or is palpated just superior to the costal margin upon inspiration).

There are no signs of progressive hepatic encephalopathy (disturbances in consciousness, hyperreflexia, asterixis or, rarely, seizures).

IMAGING

No immediate imaging studies are indicated in patients suspected of acute acetaminophen toxicity. The patient should be immediately transported to a local emergency department for treatment. Referral to an emergency department should not be delayed by dental radiographs or nonurgent surgical procedures.

In this case, a periapical and a panoramic radiograph had been obtained at the walk-in dental clinic 2 days prior for evaluation of the odontogenic pathology, demonstrating pulpal caries and a fractured left mandibular second molar with a corresponding periapical radiolucency.

LABS

Several laboratory studies are obtained in the emergency department to evaluate the extent of hepatic injury. A serum acetaminophen concentration should be immediately obtained, because its result will be helpful to guide treatment and to predict the outcome of hepatotoxicity. Liver function tests (LFTs) should be performed, including aspartate aminotransferase (AST), which is the best early indicator of hepatic injury. Patients with marked elevations in AST who demonstrate clinical manifestations of hepatotoxicity or failure should have expanded laboratory monitoring, including alanine aminotransferase (ALT), lactate dehydrogenase

(LDH), total bilirubin, coagulation studies (prothrombin time [PT], partial thromboplastin time [PTT], and international normalized ratio [INR]), pH, and blood glucose. Serial laboratory testing is used to monitor the progression of hepatic injury or recovery. A complete metabolic panel can also be obtained to monitor electrolyte disturbances, especially with concomitant alcohol ingestion. A blood alcohol level (BAL) may be obtained as indicated by the history.

For the current patient, the initial AST was 1,320 U/L (normal range, 5 to 40 U/L).

ASSESSMENT

Acetaminophen toxicity (stage II) secondary to pain caused by irreversible pulpitis of the left mandibular second molar and excessive self-administration of acetaminophen containing analgesics.

TREATMENT

Recognition of acetaminophen toxicity requires immediate transfer of the patient to a hospital emergency department for work-up and treatment.

Management of acetaminophen toxicity requires an understanding of its pharmacokinetics and pathophysiology. Acetaminophen (N-acetyl-p-aminophenol, or APAP) is an analgesic and antipyretic agent that is rapidly absorbed from the gastrointestinal tract, achieving peak serum concentrations between 45 minutes and 2 hours after ingestion. Peak serum concentrations after acute toxic ingestion are observed at approximately 4 hours. The elimination half-life is between 2 and 4 hours. Therapeutic doses of acetaminophen are 10 to 15 mg/kg per dose, with a daily maximum of 80 mg/kg in children and 4 g in adults. Therapeutic serum concentrations are reported at 10 to 30 µg/ml. Toxicity is probable with single doses greater than 250 mg/kg or a daily ingestion greater than 12 g and is certain with single doses greater than 350 mg/kg.

Approximately 5% of acetaminophen is excreted unchanged in the urine. Another 75% to 90% is metabolized by the hepatic glucuronic acid pathway prior to excretion. The remaining portion is metabolized by the hepatic P450 microsomal oxidase pathway into N-acetyl-p-benzoquinoneimine (NAPQI), a toxic metabolite. At therapeutic doses, NAPQI is rapidly conjugated by hepatic glutathione and excreted; at toxic doses, glutathione stores are depleted, with subsequent accumulation of NAPQI, resulting in oxidative damage and hepatocellular necrosis (Figure 2-2).

Considerations for the management of acute acetaminophen toxicity include a detailed dosing history, time of presentation, indicated laboratory studies, the presence of comorbid conditions, and clinical manifestations. The current methods of treatment include induced emesis (if diagnosed early), gastric lavage, gastrointestinal decontamination with activated charcoal (AC), and administration of N-acetylcysteine (NAC). Activated charcoal acts by readily absorbing acetaminophen, resulting in a reduction of gastrointestinal absorption of 50% to 90%. AC is administered as a single dose of

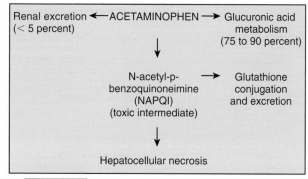

Figure 2-2   Overview of acetaminophen metabolism.

1 g/kg and is only indicated within the first 4 hours after ingestion, because gastrointestinal absorption is complete beyond this time. NAC is a precursor of glutathione and acts to increase glutathione stores, in addition to combining with NAPQI directly. NAC has other beneficial effects, including acting as an antiinflammatory, antioxidant, and vasodilator, thereby aiding in the preservation of multiorgan function.

The standard adult oral regimen of NAC is a loading dose of 140 mg/kg, followed by 17 doses of 70 mg/kg every 4 hours for a total of 72 hours. NAC is supplied as either a 10% or 20% oral solution (generic acetylcysteine). It is also available in an intravenous (IV) formulation (Acetadote), for which the adult regimen is 150 mg/kg IV over 60 minutes, followed by 50 mg/kg IV over 4 hours, and 100 mg/kg IV over 16 hours. Patients developing hepatic failure require a longer course of NAC therapy, until clinical improvement is demonstrated and the INR falls below 2.0. The efficacy of NAC treatment is significantly decreased if the drug is not administered within 8 to 10 hours of acetaminophen ingestion, because cell injury may have already begun. Severe hepatotoxicity and death are rare when NAC therapy is initiated early (within 8 hours), regardless of the initial serum acetaminophen concentrations. Early discontinuation of NAC therapy may be considered if the patient has become asymptomatic, has an acetaminophen concentration of less than 10 µg/ml, and has normal AST levels 36 hours after ingestion. These markers demonstrate completion of acetaminophen metabolism and safely determine that no subsequent hepatic injury will occur. The indications for initiation of NAC therapy, paired with expanded laboratory testing, are variable between acute and chronic toxic ingestions and are addressed later.

The current patient was treated in the emergency department with NAC therapy. He was admitted to a medical service, and his LFTs were normalized over 30 days. The left mandibular second molar was extracted the day after initiation of therapy to aid in pain control. Prior to discharge, he was referred to an alcohol cessation program, and he was to be followed by a primary care provider.

COMPLICATIONS

The most feared complication associated with acute acetaminophen toxicity is severe hepatotoxicity leading to fulminant hepatic failure, hepatic encephalopathy, multiorgan failure, and death. Acute renal failure occurs in 25% and 50% of patients with significant hepatotoxicity and hepatic failure, respectively; this is primarily due to acute tubular necrosis. Hypoglycemia, lactic acidosis, hemorrhage, acute respiratory distress syndrome (ARDS), and sepsis may also occur in severe cases. Liver transplantation is indicated in patients who show a pH lower than 7.30 after hemodynamic resuscitation, a PT greater than 1.8 times the control, a creatinine level greater than 3.3 mg/dl, and grade III or IV encephalopathy. Death usually occurs as a result of multiorgan failure.

The existence of comorbid conditions, including chronic alcoholism, malnutrition, and the use of drugs that influence the mixed-function oxidase pathway, may increase the risk of toxicity in some patients. Chronic alcohol abuse both depletes glutathione stores and increases P450 activity, resulting in higher production of NAPQI. Chronic alcoholics are reported to be at higher risk for toxicity after multiple doses of acetaminophen, although they do not appear to be at higher risk after single acute toxic ingestions. Malnutrition or fasting also depletes glutathione stores, in addition to adversely affecting the carbohydrate-dependent glucuronide conjugation pathway. Examples of drugs that increase P450 activity and subsequent NAPQI production include barbiturates, anticonvulsants, and antituberculotic medications.

The inability of some patients to tolerate oral NAC therapy is noteworthy and is usually successfully managed by aggressive antiemetic treatment. If this fails, intravenous administration of NAC should be considered to ensure delivery within 8 to 10 hours after ingestion. Although intravenous NAC therapy provides advantages of equivalent efficacy, a shorter duration of treatment, and improved ease of administration and patient acceptance, it is also associated with an increased risk of complications, including anaphylactoid reactions, bronchospasm, hypotension, nausea and vomiting, status epilepticus, and cerebral edema. Other indications for intravenous NAC include patients who have medical conditions that contraindicate oral delivery of NAC (e.g., active gastrointestinal bleeding, gastrointestinal obstruction), pregnant patients (theoretical improved transplacental delivery secondary to higher serum concentrations), and patients with established fulminant hepatic failure (demonstrate little benefit from oral NAC).

DISCUSSION

Acetaminophen, which was introduced clinically in 1950, is a widely used over-the-counter analgesic that is extremely safe when used at appropriate therapeutic doses. It is present in numerous individual and combination (usually with an opioid) pharmaceuticals and is most commonly used for the treatment of pain and fever. It is also found in many over-the-counter medications in combination with sedatives, decongestants, and antihistamines. It may be this wide availability, coupled with the general public's lack of knowledge of potential toxicity, that has resulted in acetaminophen being responsible for the most overdoses and overdose-associated deaths

yearly in the United States, as reported by the American Association of Poison Control Centers. In 2011, 67 deaths were attributed to overdose of acetaminophen alone, and 39 deaths were attributed to overdose of acetaminophen combination drugs. Other sources combining data from hospitals, emergency facilities, and poisoning databases estimate that more than 400 deaths occur per year as a result of acetaminophen overdose in the United States, and reported toxic exposures for acetaminophen exceed 140,000 cases annually.

In 2011 the U.S. Food and Drug Administration (FDA) required changes in the manufacture of prescription combination products to limit the amount of acetaminophen to 325 mg per dose; also, packaging was updated to include a warning of the potential risks of severe liver injury. The first reported case of acetaminophen-related hepatic necrosis appeared in 1966; subsequently, the pharmacokinetics, risk stratification, and management of acetaminophen toxicity have been and continue to be well studied and documented.

Prompt recognition of potential toxicity is vital in reducing morbidity and mortality. A detailed dosing history, including the time of last ingestion, is important. The diagnosis may be difficult to establish in cases of chronic overdose, because the patient often presents with only mild symptoms or no symptoms at all. The clinical sequence of acetaminophen toxicity can be divided into four stages.

- **Stage I (0 to 24 hours).** Hepatic injury has not yet occurred, and patients are often clinically asymptomatic, giving a false sense of well-being. Some vague symptoms may be present, including nausea and vomiting, pallor, lethargy, malaise, and diaphoresis. AST levels are usually normal during this stage but may start to rise at 8 to 12 hours in severe cases.
- **Stage II (24 to 72 hours).** It is during stage II that hepatic injury begins, along with its associated signs and symptoms. Patients develop abdominal right upper quadrant pain and liver enlargement but are likely to demonstrate resolution of previous symptoms evident in stage I. Laboratory markers of liver dysfunction also become evident during this stage. AST elevation is present in all patients with hepatotoxicity by 36 hours and is the most sensitive value in predicting progressive hepatic injury.
- **Stage III (72 to 96 hours).** This is the stage of maximum hepatotoxicity, and resulting signs and symptoms vary, depending on the severity of hepatic injury. Patients demonstrate nausea and vomiting, diaphoresis, jaundice, lethargy, and malaise and may progress to develop fulminant hepatic failure, acute renal failure, lactic acidosis, hepatic encephalopathy, exsanguinating hemorrhage, ARDS, sepsis, and death. Pertinent laboratory findings include marked elevation of AST and ALT, elevated total bilirubin, hypoglycemia, decreased pH, and elevated PT/INR.
- **Stage IV (4 to 7 days).** This is the recovery stage for survivors of stage III. Laboratory abnormalities normalize, and symptoms resolve, but this may take weeks in severely ill patients. Histologic repair of hepatic necrosis may take up to 3 months to complete, but chronic hepatic injury has not been reported in cases of acetaminophen toxicity.

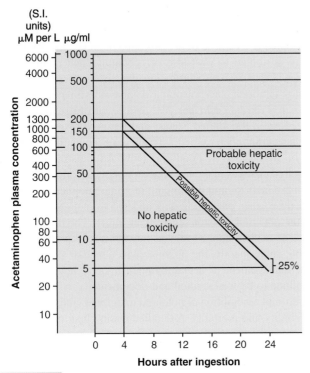

(S.I. units)
μM per L   μg/ml

Acetaminophen plasma concentration

Probable hepatic toxicity

Possible hepatic toxicity

No hepatic toxicity

25%

Hours after ingestion

Figure 2-3   Rumack-Matthew nomogram. *(Modified from Rumack BH, Matthew H:* Acetaminophen poisoning and toxicity, Pediatrics *55:871, 1975).*

Diagnosis and risk stratification of acetaminophen toxicity need to be assessed in a timely fashion. Patients presenting with suspicion of toxicity are usually categorized as having either an acute or a chronic overdose, and there are slight differences in the treatment protocols. In both groups, the history and timing of ingestion, in addition to the existence of any comorbid conditions, must be determined.

Patients with a single acute overdose are normally evaluated based on the Rumack-Matthew nomogram, which relates the serum acetaminophen concentration to the time from ingestion as a predictor of hepatotoxicity. Blood for serum acetaminophen measurement should be drawn at 4 hours after ingestion or immediately if the time of ingestion is unknown. NAC therapy is the standard of care for any patient whose serum concentration is above the line in the nomogram, indicating a possible risk of hepatic toxicity (Figure 2-3).

Chronic overdose patients often present to emergency departments at a later stage of toxicity because of the absence of early symptoms. These patients are at high risk for hepatotoxicity if they have ingested greater than 7.5 to 10 g within 24 hours or greater than 4 g within 24 hours in the presence of comorbid conditions.

Indications for the initiation of NAC therapy include acute overdose patients with a serum acetaminophen concentration above the possible risk line of the Rumack-Matthew nomogram; single ingestions greater than 7.5 g; unknown dose or time of ingestion with a serum acetaminophen concentration greater than 10 μg/ml; repeated supratherapeutic doses in the presence of comorbid conditions; and any patient with elevated AST levels or right upper quadrant abdominal pain.

Most patients with toxicity recover after the standard 72-hour protocol of NAC therapy; however, in severe cases of hepatic failure, NAC therapy should continue until the INR falls below 2.0, other laboratory values normalize, and clinical symptoms resolve.

Low-risk patients are defined as those who are asymptomatic with acetaminophen concentrations less than 10 μg/ml at 4 hours and normal AST levels. Low-risk patients do not require NAC therapy and can be discharged with detailed instructions and scheduled 24-hour follow-up.

Health care providers, particularly oral and maxillofacial surgeons and other clinicians who frequently prescribe acetaminophen-containing analgesic medications, should be aware of symptoms of acute and chronic acetaminophen toxicity. Patients should be carefully instructed to avoid other medications containing acetaminophen in conjunction with prescribed medications and should be made aware of the risks of toxicity. Practitioners should be aware of the surgical patient presenting with a history of pain who has been self-medicating. Detailed questions to determine all ingested medications, in addition to the possible existence of any comorbid conditions, are necessary. A working knowledge of the risks and symptoms of acetaminophen toxicity is vital to early recognition and subsequent treatment of this potentially fatal condition.

Bibliography

Bagheri SC, Beckley ML, Farish SE: Acute acetaminophen toxicity: report of a case, *J Calif Dent Assoc* 29:687, 2001.

Bessems JG, Vermeulen NP: Paracetamol (acetaminophen)–induced toxicity: molecular and biochemical mechanisms, analogues and protective approaches, *Crit Rev Toxicol* 31:55, 2001.

Bronstein AC, et al: 2010 Annual report of the American Association of Poison Control Centers National Poison Data System (NPDS): twenty-eighth annual report, *Clin Toxicol* 49:911, 2011.

Bronstein AC, Spyker DA, Cantilena LR, et al: 2011 Annual report of the American Association of Poison Control Centers National Poison Data System (NPDS): twenty-ninth annual report, *Clin Toxicol* 50:911, 2012.

Davidson DG, Eastham WN: Acute liver necrosis following overdose of paracetamol, *Br Med J* 5512:497, 1966.

Heard KJ: Acetylcysteine for acetaminophen poisoning, *N Engl J Med* 359(3):285, 2008.

Holdiness MR: Clinical pharmacokinetics of N-acetylcysteine, *Clin Pharmacokinet* 20:123, 1991.

Keays R, Harrison PM, Wendon JA, et al: Intravenous acetylcysteine in paracetamol induced fulminant hepatic failure: a prospective controlled study, *Br Med J* 303:1026, 1991.

Litovitz TL, Klein-Schwartz W, Dyer KS, et al: 1997 Annual report of the American Association of Poison Control Centers Toxic Exposure Surveillance System, *Am J Emerg Med* 16:443, 1998.

Makin AJ, Wendon J, Williams R: A 7-year experience of severe acetaminophen-induced hepatotoxicity (1987-1993), *Gastroenterology* 109:1907, 1995.

Makin AJ, Williams R: The current management of paracetamol overdosage, *Br J Clin Pract* 48:144, 1994.

Nourjah P, Ahmad SR, Karwoski C, et al: Estimates of acetaminophen (paracetamol)–associated overdoses in the United States, *Pharmacoepidemiol Drug Saf* 15:398, 2006.

Novak D, Lewis JH: Drug-induced liver disease, *Curr Opin Gastroenterol* 19(3):203-215, 2003.

O'Grady JG, Alexander GJ, Hayllar KM, et al: Early indicators of prognosis in fulminant hepatic failure, *Gastroenterology* 97:439, 1989.

Prescott LF: Paracetamol overdosage: pharmacological considerations and clinical management, *Drugs* 25:290, 1983.

Prescott LF, Critchley JAJH: The treatment of acetaminophen poisoning, *Annu Rev Pharmacol Toxicol* 23:87, 1983.

Prescott LF, Proudfoot AT, Cregeen RJ: Paracetamol-induced acute renal failure in the absence of fulminant liver damage, *Br Med J* 284:421, 1982.

Rose SR, Gorman RL, Oderda GM, et al: Simulated acetaminophen overdose: pharmacokinetics and effectiveness of activated charcoal, *Ann Emerg Med* 20:1064, 1991.

Rumack BH, Bateman DN: Acetaminophen and acetylcysteine dose and duration: past, present and future, *Clin Toxicol* 50:91, 2012.

Rumack BH: Acetaminophen hepatotoxicity: the first 35 years, *J Toxicol Clin Toxicol* 40:3, 2002.

Rumack BH, Matthew H: Acetaminophen poisoning and toxicity, *Pediatrics* 55:871, 1975.

Sandilands EA, Bateman DN: Adverse reactions associated with acetylcysteine, *Clin Toxicol* 47:81, 2009.

Schiødt FV, Lee WM, Bondesen S, et al: Influence of acute and chronic alcohol intake on the clinical course and outcome in acetaminophen overdose, *Aliment Pharmacol Ther* 16:707, 2002.

Singer AJ, Carracio TR, Mofenson HC: The temporal profile of increased transaminase levels in patients with acetaminophen-induced liver dysfunction, *Ann Emerg Med* 26:49, 1995.

Smilkstein MJ, Knapp GL, Kulig KW, et al: Efficacy of oral N-acetylcysteine in the treatment of acetaminophen poisoning, *N Engl J Med* 319:1557, 1988.

Smilkstein MJ: Techniques used to prevent absorption of toxic compounds. In Goldfrank LR, et al (eds): *Goldfrank's toxicologic emergencies*, p 541, Stamford, Conn, 1998, Appleton & Lange,.

Smilkstein MJ: Chronic ethanol use and acute acetaminophen overdose toxicity, *J Toxicol Clin Toxicol* 36:476, 1998.

Watson WA, Litovitz TL, Klein-Schwartz W, et al: 2003 Annual report of the American Association of Poison Control Centers Toxic Exposure Surveillance System, *Am J Emerg Med* 22:335, 2004.

Opioid Side Effects

Piyushkumar P. Patel and Shahrokh C. Bagheri

CC

A 30-year-old woman presents to the office complaining that "the pain medication is making me feel nauseous." (Nausea is one of the most commonly seen adverse effect of orally administered opioids. In a large retrospective review, it was found that women have a 60% higher risk of nausea and vomiting than men when administered opioids.)

HPI

The patient had several mandibular teeth extracted with no intraoperative complications 2 days before presentation. She was given a prescription for a combination analgesic containing hydrocodone (an opioid) and acetaminophen. She reports poor oral intake since her procedure and has been feeling nauseated, with one episode of vomiting since taking the medication (opioids have a greater tendency to cause nausea and vomiting when taken on an empty stomach). She has not had any relief from pain and explains that she is now worse because she has both pain and nausea.

A detailed history of symptoms can provide clues to rule out other causes for this acute nausea episode. Abrupt onset of nausea and vomiting is suggestive of cholecystitis, food poisoning, gastroenteritis, pancreatitis, or drug-related etiologies. If a patient has pain, obstructive etiologies must be considered.

Postoperative nausea and vomiting (PONV), defined as nausea and vomiting occurring in the 0- to 24-hour postoperative period, is one of the most common complaints after surgery. It has a multifactorial etiology, and risk factors for the development of PONV have been identified (Table 2-1). A simplified scoring system by Apfel and colleagues is one of the most popular and widely used scoring systems. They identified four highly predictive risk factors for PONV: female gender, history of motion sickness or PONV, nonsmoker, and use of perioperative opioids. The presence of 0, 1, 2, 3, or 4 of these factors corresponded to a PONV incidence of 10%, 21%, 39%, 61%, and 79%, respectively.

Risk factors for post discharge nausea and vomiting (PDNV), in which symptoms occur late (24 to 72 hours) appear to be similar to the typical risk factors for PONV and are also likely related to, among other factors, emetic symptoms before discharge, increased pain at home, and the use of postoperative opioids.

The term *opioid* is used to refer to all the agonists and antagonists of the morphinelike family of compounds. This term is preferred to older terms, such as opiate or narcotic. *Narcotic* refers to any drug that can cause dependence; the term is not specific for opioids (i.e., not all narcotics are opioids).

PMHX/PDHX/MEDICATIONS/ALLERGIES/SH/FH

The patient has no known history of narcotic abuse (a risk factor for drug-seeking behavior). Current medications include hydrocodone/acetaminophen (5/325 mg tablets). She admits to having ingested four tablets in the past 6 hours, with minimal oral intake.

EXAMINATION

General. The patient is a well-developed and well-nourished woman who appears her stated age and is in mild discomfort secondary to nausea. (The physical examination of this patient should focus initially on signs of dehydration, evaluating skin turgor and mucous membranes, and observing for hypotension or orthostatic changes.) She is alert and oriented to time, place, and person (it is important to assess mental status in cases of acute opioid toxicity).

Vital signs. Her vital signs are stable, and she is afebrile (AF), except for slight tachycardia at 110 bpm (caused by dehydration second to decreased oral intake).

Table 2-1	Risk Factors for PONV and PDNV	
Patient Factors	**Anesthetic Factors**	**Surgical Factors**
Female	Use of perioperative opioids	Duration of surgery
		Type of surgery
		Abdominal
Nonsmoker	Use of volatile anesthetics	Ear, nose, and throat
History of motion sickness or PONV	Nitrous oxide ___	Gynecologic
		Laparoscopic
Family history of motion sickness or PONV (pediatric)		Ophthalmologic
		Orthopedic
		Plastic
Age ≥ 3 yr (pediatric)		Strabismus (pediatric)

From Le T, Gan T: Update on the management of postoperative nausea and vomiting and post discharge nausea and vomiting in ambulatory surgery, *Anesthesiol Clin* 28:225-249, 2010.
PDNV, Post discharge nausea and vomiting; *PONV,* postoperative nausea and vomiting.

Maxillofacial. Pupils are 3 mm, equal, round, and bilaterally reactive (pupillary constriction, or *miosis,* would be a sign of excessive opioid intake and is not affected by tolerance).

Intraoral. The examination is consistent with healing extraction sockets with no evidence of alveolar osteitis or acute infection. Mucous membranes are moist and within normal limits (WNL).

Abdominal. The abdomen is soft, nontender, and nondistended; bowel sounds are present but hypoactive in all four quadrants. (Abdominal examination may not be routine in this situation, but it may demonstrate decreased bowel sounds secondary to the effect of opioids on gastrointestinal motility or distention with tenderness suggestive of a bowel obstruction. Pain in the right upper quadrant is more consistent with cholecystitis or biliary tract disease.)

IMAGING

No imaging studies are indicated unless the situation is compounded by other medical conditions. For patients with a suspicion of aspiration, such as those with concomitant alcohol consumption or decreased mental status secondary to excessive opioid intake, a chest radiograph may be indicated.

LABS

No laboratory studies are indicated unless dictated by preexisting medical conditions, such as uncontrolled diabetes. In patients with prolonged vomiting, metabolic alkalosis and other electrolyte abnormalities may ensue. Appropriate laboratory studies should be ordered as needed.

ASSESSMENT

Acute nausea and vomiting associated with postoperative opioid analgesia, status post dentoalveolar surgery; subjective report of moderate pain that is nonresponsive to the current pharmacologic regimen.

It is important to distinguish acute pain, which is of recent onset and limited duration, from chronic pain, which is described as lasting for an undefined period, beyond that expected for the injury to heal. This distinction has both diagnostic and treatment implications. Caution should be exercised when treating chronic pain with opioids because of the development of dependence.

TREATMENT

Several different approaches can be used, either alone or in combination, for the management of the adverse effects of opioids; these include:
- Dose reduction of the systemic opioid
- Symptomatic management of the adverse effect
- Opioid rotation (or switching)
- Alternate routes of systemic administration

Reducing the dose of the administered opioid can result in a reduction of dose-related adverse effects. To compensate for the loss of pain control, adjunctive strategies can be used to maintain control while reducing the dose or eliminating the opioid. Common strategies include addition of a nonopioid coanalgesic or an adjuvant analgesic that is appropriate to the pain syndrome and mechanism (e.g., addition of Neurontin for the treatment of neuropathic pain). In addition, therapy targeting the cause of the pain (e.g., placement of packing material into a dry socket wound), application of a regional anesthetic, or a neuroablative intervention may be used.

Symptomatic management of the adverse effect is usually based on cumulative anecdotal experiences. In general, this involves the addition of one or more new medications. However, polypharmacy adds to medication burden, and the possibility of drug interactions needs to be considered.

Opioid rotation (also called *opioid switching* or *substitution*) requires familiarity with a range of opioid agonists and with the use of opioid dose conversion tables to find equianalgesic dosages. The objective of switching one opioid with another is to reduce the adverse effects. Alternatively, switching the route of systemic administration, such as changing from the intravenous to the oral route, has been shown to ameliorate symptoms of nausea, constipation, and drowsiness. In many acute situations, nonsteroidal antiinflammatory drugs (NSAIDs) provide analgesia equal to the starting doses of opioids. However, unlike opioids that lack a ceiling dose, NSAIDs have a maximum dose above which no additional analgesic effect is obtained.

The current patient was treated with a single dose of oral promethazine (Phenergan) 12.5 mg. (Studies have shown that 12.5 mg of oral Phenergan is as effective in reducing symptoms of nausea as 25 mg of oral Phenergan and may result in fewer adverse effects.) The patient's medication was switched to a nonopioid analgesic (ibuprofen 400 mg orally every 6 hours). She was also instructed to increase her oral intake, preferably with isotonic drinks. She responded well to this regimen, with resolution of her nausea and reduction of pain to an acceptable level. Should the initial antiemetic agent fail, a rescue antiemetic from a different treatment class can be considered.

COMPLICATIONS

Although opioids are well recognized as being effective for moderate to severe pain, they are frequently associated with an array of troublesome side effects (Table 2-2). Genuine allergy to opioids is rare. In most cases, patients report having an opioid allergy when they actually have had an opioid-related adverse effect.

The following are some of the complications that can arise with opioid therapy.

Nausea and vomiting. More than 30% of patients using opioids report experiencing nausea or vomiting. It is a common and unpleasant adverse effect of opioids. Opioid receptors play an important role in the control of emesis (vomiting). They directly stimulate the chemoreceptor trigger zone (CTZ), depressing the vomiting center and slowing gastrointestinal motility. Signaling between the CTZ and the vomiting center

Table 2-2	Common Opiate-Induced Adverse Effects
Body System	**Adverse Effects**
Gastrointestinal	Nausea
	Vomiting
	Constipation
Autonomic	Xerostomia
	Urinary retention
	Postural hypotension
CNS	Drowsiness
	Cognitive impairment
	Hallucinations
	Delirium
	Respiratory depression
	Myoclonus
	Seizure disorder
	Hyperalgesia
Cutaneous	Itch
	Sweating

Table 2-3	Antiemetic Drugs	
Pharmacologic Group	**Common Generic Name**	**Common Trade Names**
Anticholinergic	Scopolamine	Scopace, Transderm Scop
Antihistamine	Cyclizine	Merezine, Migril
	Dimenhydrinate	Dimentabls, Dramamine
	Diphenhydramine	Benadryl
	Promethazine	Phenergan
Antiserotonins	Dolasetron	Anzemet
	Granisetron	Zofran
	Ondansetron	Zotran
Benzamides	Metoclopramide	Reglan, Octamide
Butyrophenones	Droperidol	Droleptan, Inapsine
	Haloperidol	Haldol
Phenothiazines	Chlorpromazine	Thorazine
Steroids	Betamethasone	Celestone
	Dexamethasone	Decadron

is mediated through a variety of neurotransmitter receptor systems, including the serotonergic, dopaminergic, histaminergic, cholinergic, and neurokininergic receptors. The available antiemetics block one or more of the associated receptors (Table 2-3). There is no "universal" antiemetic, and no current single antiemetic is 100% effective for all patients. The variability of clinical studies makes it difficult to recommend one of these medications over another. The 5-hydroxytryptamine-3 receptor antagonists (5-HT3 RAs), which include ondansetron (Zofran), granisetron droxytr (Kytril), dolasetron (Anzemet), and palonosetron (Aloxi), act by inhibiting the action of serotonin in 5-HT3 receptor–rich areas of the brain. These agents have been shown to be effective antiemetic agents; their differing chemical structures may explain slight differences in receptor binding affinity, dose response, and

duration of action. Palonosetron has a longer duration of action and may be beneficial in preventing nausea for up to 72 hours after discharge.

The phenothiazines, including promethazine (Phenergan), are some of the most commonly used antiemetics in the world. However, their use has fallen out of favor because of their high incidence of adverse effects, such as sedation, restlessness, diarrhea, agitation, central nervous system depression and, more rarely, extrapyramidal effects, hypotension, neuroleptic syndrome, and supraventricular tachycardia. In 2009 the U.S. Food and Drug Administration (FDA) issued a black box warning for promethazine, advising practitioners of possible severe tissue injury, including gangrene, from injection into an artery, under the skin, or even after intravenous administration.

Nausea or vomiting has been shown to occur despite the use of pre-emptive antiemetics. Switching to an alternative opioid can reduce the severity of nausea and vomiting. In addition, it has been shown that patients who receive opioids intravenously (primarily through patient-controlled analgesia pumps) exhibit more nausea and vomiting. It should also be remembered that independent of other factors, pain could be the cause of nausea or vomiting.

Constipation. This is another common adverse effect of opioids, one that is more problematic for patients on chronic opioid therapy. Constipation may also contribute to nausea and vomiting. It is defined by the four "too's": stools that are too hard, too small, too difficult to expel, or too infrequent. Opioids cause constipation by binding to receptors in the gastrointestinal tract, thereby slowing peristalsis and increasing transit time. Consequently, sodium and water are reabsorbed, resulting in dry, hardened stools. Patients on long-term therapy seldom develop tolerance to this side effect and should be advised to increase their fluid intake and dietary fiber to compensate for the constipation. It has been suggested that a stool softener and a large bowel stimulant (e.g., docusate sodium) be used for chronic opioid therapy. A stool softener alone should not be prescribed, because opioids slow normal peristalsis and may result in an uncomfortable patient who is unable to evacuate his or her bowel. Thus, a stimulant laxative may also be prescribed. In the absence of a bowel movement for 3 to 4 days, more invasive measures may be necessary, such as stool disimpaction or rectally administered bowel evacuants (e.g., Fleet enema). A single dose of an opioid can affect gastrointestinal tract motility. In addition, opioids are thought to have a role in the development of postoperative ileus (a multifactorial phenomenon).

Respiratory depression. This is the most serious and most feared adverse effect of opioid therapy. Respiratory depression to the point of apnea is dose dependent and caused by opioids acting directly on respiratory centers within the brainstem. This is characterized by a reduction in tidal volume, minute volume, respiratory rate, and the response to hypoxia and hypercapnia. Careful monitoring of the patient can prevent this adverse outcome. Equianalgesic dosages of other opioids produce the same degree of respiratory depression. Patients with impaired respiratory function or bronchial asthma are at greater risk of experiencing clinically significant respiratory depression in response to the usual doses of these drugs. If respiratory depression does occur, it is often in an opioid-naïve patient; other signs and symptoms, such as sedation and mental clouding, can also be seen. Tolerance to this effect occurs with repeated use of opioids, allowing the management of chronic pain without significant risk of respiratory depression. Naloxone (Narcan) can be used to reverse opioid-induced respiratory depression. To avoid an abrupt reversal of analgesia (which may produce a catecholamine surge, resulting in tachycardia, hypertension, pulmonary edema, and arrhythmias), naloxone is administered in doses of 40 µg repeated every few minutes as necessary.

Sedation. Opioid analgesics produce sedation and drowsiness. These properties are useful in certain situations (e.g., preoperatively), but they are not desirable in ambulatory patients. The central nervous system (CNS)–depressant actions, in addition to respiratory depressant effects, are synergistic with alcohol, barbiturates, and benzodiazepines. Concurrent administration of dextromethamphetamine (2.5 to 5 mg orally twice daily) has been reported to reduce the sedative effects of opioids. However, it has also been reported that using dextromethamphetamine and similar agents can, in certain individuals, produce adverse effects such as hallucinations, delirium, psychosis, decreased appetite, tremor, and tachycardia; therefore, these drugs are contraindicated in those with psychiatric disorders and are relatively contraindicated given a history of paroxysmal tachyarrhythmia. Opioid rotation or switching the route of administration can reduce the severity of opioid sedation. Tolerance to sedative effects of opioids develops within the first several days of long-term administration. Mild cognitive impairment, delirium, and agitated confusion have also been reported in patients taking opioids. CNS effects appear to be idiosyncratic, not dose related. Meperidine is the opioid most commonly associated with adverse CNS events. (Meperidine is currently considered for brief use as a second-line agent for the treatment of acute pain.) After gastrointestinal effects (nausea, vomiting, and constipation), the combined CNS effects account for the second highest percentage of adverse drug events.

Pruritus. The mechanism by which opioids cause itching is not fully known, although opioid-mediated direct release of histamine from mast cells is thought to contribute to this effect (most notably with meperidine). Some opioids, such as fentanyl and alfentanil, do not cause histamine release but can cause mild pruritus; the mechanism of this is not clear. (Morphine, codeine, and meperidine stimulate histamine release; fentanyl, sufentanil, and alfentanil do not.) If pruritus is accompanied by a rash, allergic reactions cannot be ruled out. In such patients, an opioid from a different chemical class may be used. Options for managing itching include the use of histamine-blocking agents (e.g., diphenhydramine), administration of naloxone, or changing the opioid.

Urinary retention. Although urinary retention is a known side effect of opioid administration, it is uncommon when the drug is administered for a short period. Opioids increase smooth muscle tone, cause bladder spasm, and increase sphincter tone, resulting in urinary retention, which occurs more frequently in the elderly. Catheterization may be required.

Cough suppression. Suppression of the cough reflex is a well-known effect of opioids. In particular, codeine and derivatives are extensively used in antitussive preparations. Dextromethorphan is an over-the-counter antitussive agent that acts centrally at therapeutic doses by binding to opioid receptors. The drug is about equal to codeine in depressing the cough reflex.

Miosis. Constriction of the pupils is seen with all opioids. It is an action to which little or no tolerance develops even in chronic users. This is a valuable sign in the diagnosis of opioid overdose and toxicity (and one commonly used by law enforcement agents).

Truncal rigidity. An increase in the tone of large trunk muscles (stiff chest) has been seen with administration of large doses of primarily highly lipophilic opioids (e.g., fentanyl, sufentanil, alfentanil) that are administered rapidly (bolus administration). In the setting of acute respiratory distress, a rapidly acting neuromuscular agent, such as succinylcholine, can be administered to paralyze the muscles and allow ventilation. Alternatively, an opioid antagonist can be used, but this will also antagonize the analgesic effects.

Tolerance. Tolerance is a physiologic adaptation to a drug. As a person becomes tolerant to the pharmacologic effects, increasing doses are required to produce the same effect. Patients may develop tolerance to some but not all the effects of the opioid. In general, tolerance develops rapidly to the sedative, analgesic, and respiratory effects but is not commonly seen with the constipating effects or the development of miosis. The hallmark of the development of tolerance is a decrease in the duration of effective analgesia. The rate of development of tolerance varies greatly among individuals. However, a sudden increase in opioid requirement may also represent progression of the disease. Opioid rotation may be of value for patients requiring long-term treatment. In addition, combining the opioid with a nonopioid not only provides additive analgesia, but also delays the development of tolerance.

Dependence. An individual is physically dependent on a drug when cessation of the drug or a rapid dose reduction initiates symptoms of withdrawal. This generally includes autonomic signs, including diarrhea, rhinorrhea, piloerection, sweating, and indicators of central arousal, such as sleeplessness, irritability, and psychomotor agitation. Dependence is an expected physiologic phenomenon when certain drugs are used for sufficiently long periods; it is neither a necessary nor a defining characteristic of addiction. Withdrawal can be avoided by slowly tapering the dosage.

Addiction. According to the American Society of Addiction Medicine, addiction is a primary chronic neurobiologic disease that is influenced by genetic, psychosocial, and environmental factors. Characteristics of addiction include impaired control over drug use, and/or continued use despite harm, and cravings. It has been shown that among persons without a history of substance abuse who are being treated for

Table 2-4	Major Opioid Receptors

Receptor	Effects
Mu (μ)	
Mu 1	Analgesia
Mu 2	Respiratory depression, bradycardia, physical dependence, euphoria, ileus
Delta (δ)	Analgesia; modulates activity at the mu receptor. It is thought that mu and delta receptors coexist
Kappa (κ)	Analgesia, sedation, dysphoria, psychomimetic effects

acute pain, the risk of true iatrogenic addiction is extremely low, and concern over the development of addiction should be a minor factor in therapeutic decision making.

Pseudoaddiction. Pseudoaddiction is an iatrogenic syndrome that mimics substance abuse. It resembles addiction but is a direct result of inadequate treatment of pain. In the treatment of acute pain (e.g., postsurgical pain), clinicians should attempt to provide an adequate regimen of analgesics to prevent this phenomenon.

DISCUSSION

There are three major classes of opioid receptors in the CNS, designated by the Greek letters mu (μ), kappa (κ), and delta (δ) (Table 2-4). Most of the opioids used work clinically by binding with relative selectivity to the mu receptors. Peripheral opioid receptors also exist and are thought to be responsible for some of the adverse events. Mu receptor agonists have no therapeutic ceiling effect. Therefore, unlike nonopioid analgesics, the dose of these drugs can be adjusted until satisfactory pain control is achieved.

Most members of the opioid family are chemically similar to morphine, with minor chemical modifications that change the pharmacokinetics and pharmacodynamics. *Pharmacodynamics* refers to the biochemical effects of drugs and their mechanism of action. *Pharmacokinetics* refers to the factors (absorption, distribution, biotransformation, and excretion) that determine the concentration of drug at its sites of action. Pharmacodynamics can be thought of as "what the drug does to the body," and pharmacokinetics can be thought of as "what the body does to the drug."

Individual patients could also be genetically predisposed to poor analgesia. Codeine has very little affinity for the mu receptor and may be considered a prodrug, because 10% of the parent drug is converted to morphine by cytochrome P450 (CYP) 2D6. Hydrocodone and oxycodone require demethylation to hydromorphone and oxymorphone, respectively. Approximately 7% to 10% of the Caucasian population metabolizes codeine, oxycodone, and hydrocodone poorly because of inherited deficiencies of CYP2D6; therefore, analgesia from these drugs will be less than expected.

Pre-emptive analgesia, the administration of analgesics before the onset of a noxious stimuli, has been shown to reduce postoperative opioid use and thus opioid side effects. Pre-emptive analgesia can be achieved with the use of agents to modify both peripheral CNS processing of noxious stimuli (e.g., use of a long-acting local anesthetic) and also central CNS processing of these stimuli (e.g., preoperative ibuprofen 800 mg orally or ketorolac 30 mg intravenously).

A large number of analgesics have both nonopioid and opioid ingredients. Combinations allow a lower dosage of the opioid being used (an "opioid-sparing effect") with a decrease in opioid-related adverse effects. When prescribing these agents, clinicians must be sure to be aware of the toxic dose of the nonopioid agent.

Bibliography

Apfel CC, Laara E, Koivuranta M, et al: A simplified risk score for predicting postoperative nausea and vomiting: conclusions from cross-validations between two centers, *Anesthesiology* 91(3):693-700, 1999.

Barrett TW, DiPersio DM, Jenkins CA, et al: A randomized placebo controlled trial of ondansetron, metoclopramide and promethazine in adults, *Am J Emerg Med* 29:3, 2011.

Bates JJ, Foss JF, Murphy DB, et al: Are peripheral opioid antagonists the solution to opioid side effects? *Anesth Analg* 98:116-122, 2004.

Cherny N, Ripamonti C, Pereira J, et al: Strategies to manage the adverse effects of oral morphine: an evidence based report, *J Clin Oncol* 19:2542-2554, 2001.

Cepeda MS: Side effects of opioids during short term administration: effect of age gender and race, *Clin Pharmacol Ther* 74:102-112, 2003.

Fletcher M, Spera J: Management of acute postoperative pain after oral surgery, *Dent Clin North Am* 56:95-111, 2012.

Inturrisi CE: Clinical pharmacology of opioids for pain, *Clin J Pain* 18:S3-S13, 2002.

Katzung BG (ed): *Basic and clinical pharmacology*, ed 9, New York, 2004, Lang/McGraw-Hill.

Le T, Gan T: Update on the management of postoperative nausea and vomiting and post discharge nausea and vomiting in ambulatory surgery, *Anesthesiol Clin* 28:225-249, 2010.

Phero JC, Becker DE, Dionne RA, et al: Contemporary trends in acute pain management, *Curr Opin Otolaryngol Head Neck Surg* 12:209-216, 2004.

Plaisance L: Opioid induced constipation, *Am J Nurs* 102:72, 2002.

Sachs CJ: Oral analgesics for acute nonspecific pain, *Am Fam Physician* 71:913-918, 2005.

Scorza K: Evaluation of nausea and vomiting, *Am Fam Physcian* 76(1):76-84, 2007.

Scuderi PE: Pharmacology of antiemetics, *Int Anesthesiol Clin* 41:41-66, 2003.

Strassels SA: Postoperative pain management: a practical review. Part 1, *Am J Health Syst Pharm* 62:1904-1916, 2005.

Strassels SA: Postoperative pain management: a practical review. Part 2, *Am J Health Syst Pharm* 62:2019-2025, 2005.

Swift JQ: Nonsteroidal anti-inflammatory drugs and opioids: safety and usage concerns in the differential treatment of postoperative orofacial pain, *J Oral Maxillofac Surg* 58:8-11, 2000.

Wheeler M, Oderda GM, Ashburn MA, et al: Adverse events associated with postoperative opioid analgesia: a systematic review, *J Pain* 3:159-180, 2002.

Oral Drug–Induced Osteonecrosis of the Jaws

Robert E. Marx

CC

A 65-year-old woman is referred for evaluation because "the right side of my face aches, and I feel it is swollen."

Oral Drug–Induced Osteonecrosis of the Jaws

Patients who take oral bisphosphonates must be treated differently from other patients and must also be treated differently from patients receiving intravenous bisphosphonates. Although drug-induced osteonecrosis of the jaws (DIONJ) caused by oral bisphosphonates can result in a severe and extensive exposure of bone and also may require extensive surgery, it generally is less common, less severe, and more amenable to office-based debridement surgeries than intravenous DIONJ.

HPI

The patient is a 65-year-old woman who was referred by her periodontist after she developed exposed bone as a complication of periodontal surgery to graft vertical defects in the #3 and #4 areas. The referring periodontist did not realize that this woman had been taking alendronate (Fosamax) 70 mg/week for the past 7 years. The bone exposure apparently developed soon after the surgery, about 10 months ago. The patient states that the initial area of exposed bone has increased in size since that time, despite attempts to advance local tissue to cover the bone, various courses of antibiotics, and even hyperbaric oxygen treatment. She reports episodes of increased pain accompanied by swelling of her cheek and some drainage. She also complains that her nose "feels stuffy."

PMHX/PDHX/MEDICATIONS/ALLERGIES/SH/FH

This woman has a history of hypertension and age-related hypothyroidism, in addition to the osteopenia, for which she was started on Fosamax to "prevent osteoporosis." However, she relates that her DEXA scan–generated T scores last year went beyond the −2.5 benchmark for osteoporosis. She currently takes Norvasc and HCTZ for her hypertension and Synthroid for her hypothyroidism. She stopped taking Fosamax 6 months ago. She relates an allergy to penicillin, manifested as a rash. She is currently taking clindamycin 300 mg three time daily for her facial swelling and pain.

EXAMINATION

The right side of the face is mildly edematous and tender to the touch. Vital signs indicate that her hypertension is under control (126/76 mm Hg), heart rate 80 bpm, and respirations 14 per minute.

Maxillofacial. The oral examination identified exposed necrotic bone and loss of gingiva and oral mucosa on the facial aspect of the bicuspid and molar teeth in the right side of the maxilla (Figure 2-4). There is a slight suppurative exudate, and the edge of the retracted mucosa is mildly inflamed. The roots of the teeth within the exposed bone are discolored, and the teeth have 1+ to 2+ mobility.

IMAGING

A cone-beam CT scan shows a disrupted and irregular trabecular bone pattern in the alveolar bone in the right side of the maxilla. The right maxillary sinus has a complete opacification with what appears to be a swollen sinus mucous membrane (Figure 2-5).

LABS

The routine laboratory studies of a CBC and basic metabolic panel (BMP) were within normal ranges. In particular, the

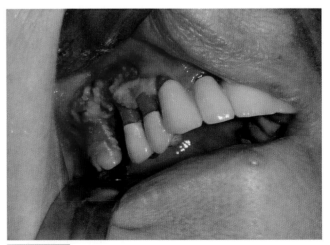

Figure 2-4 Exposed bone and tooth roots in the right maxillary alveolus.

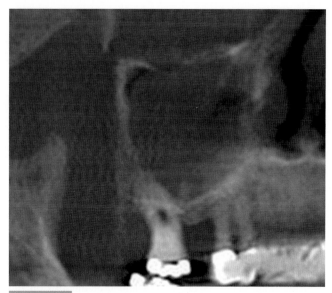

Figure 2-5   Cone-beam CT scan shows complete opacification of the right maxillary sinus, indicative of secondary sinus inflammation from the necrotic bony sinus floor.

white blood cell count was normal at 5,000/µl with a normal differential. A morning fasting C-terminal telopeptide (CTX) test was returned as a 101 pg/ml.

ASSESSMENT

Stage III drug-induced osteonecrosis of the maxilla secondary to alendronate therapy.

What was once referred to as bisphosphonate-induced, related, or associated osteonecrosis of the jaws has now been clearly defined as drug-induced osteonecrosis of the jaws. This is because denosumab, which also works by an antiresorptive affect via osteoclast impairment and death but is not a bisphosphonate, also causes osteonecrosis of the jaws. The misleading and ill-defined terms "associated" and "related" have been dropped by the American Medical Association; this is reflected in the 2010, 2011, and 2012 versions of the ICD-9-CM coding manual, which lists drug-induced osteonecrosis of the jaws, 733.45.

In the current patient, the stage III designation follows the simplified staging system by Marx. That is, extension into the maxillary sinus indicates an advanced presentation and, therefore, stage III disease. The failure of other staging systems is their reliance on pain. Because the dead bone is not painful by itself and only becomes painful if colonized or infected by microorganisms, pain does not relate to the extensiveness or severity of the disease. Additionally, the use of antibiotics or analgesics changes the pain (but not the severity or extension of the disease) and therefore also changes the stage.

TREATMENT

This patient was placed on doxycycline 100 mg daily to palliate the secondary infection and pain. She was told to take the doxycycline without milk products or yogurt, which are known to bind doxycycline and reduce its absorption. Doxycycline is the best choice, after phenoxymethyl penicillin, for long-term use in patients with DIONJ. Clindamycin, which this patient was taking at the time of presentation, is not a good choice. In DIONJ, most exposed bone is colonized by *Actinomyces* species, which are not very sensitive to clindamycin. The patient was also placed on a drug holiday, with the approval of her prescribing physician. In addition, the prescribing physician was advised to obtain radiographs of the patient's femur and was informed of the increased reports of spontaneous subtrochanteric femur fractures in women taking alendronate for 6 years or longer.

After an additional 3-month drug holiday, a repeat morning fasting serum CTX test was obtained, and its results were 180 pg/ml. This value was 30 pg/ml above the benchmark where debridement surgery can be accomplished in an otherwise normal postmenopausal woman without cancer so that normal healing can be anticipated.

The patient was subsequently treated in the operating room, where the necrotic bone was removed; this amounted to the entire floor of the right maxillary sinus and the teeth within the alveolar bone (Figure 2-6, *A*). The sinus was entered, and multiple mucoceles (often also called *sinus polyps*) and the entire edematous sinus membrane were removed with vigorous curettage (Figure 2-6, *B*). An incision was then made through the periosteum in the posterior superior area of the vestibule to expose the buccal fat pad. A pericapsular dissection around the buccal fat pad and gentle traction were used to bring the vascular buccal fat pad forward to completely fill the floor of the sinus (Figure 2-6, *C*). The fat pad was sutured to bur holes placed into the buccal cortex of the remaining sinus wall and to the periosteum of the palatal soft tissue (Figure 2-6, *D*). The buccal mucosa was then undermined so as to advance it sufficiently to gain a primary closure by suturing it to the palatal soft tissue (Figure 2-6, *E*).

OUTCOME

The closure healed and matured without further exposure of bone (Figure 2-7). The patient's physician discontinued the alendronate. After 3 years, her osteoporosis-related T scores have not changed, and no osteoporosis-related fractures have occurred.

DISCUSSION

Any drug that impairs or eliminates the normal function of an osteoclast or kills it has the potential to cause DIONJ and/or subtrochanteric fractures of the femur. Alendronate (Fosamax) has caused more than 96% of all cases of oral bisphosphonate–induced osteonecrosis, simply because it is marketed at twice the dose of its competitors, even though all these drugs have the same mechanism of action, are equally potent, are absorbed in the same amount, and have the same 11-year half-life in bone. Denosumab, a newer and different type of drug, recently has become available. Denosumab is a RANK ligand (reactor activator of nuclear kappa-B ligand) inhibitor and currently is

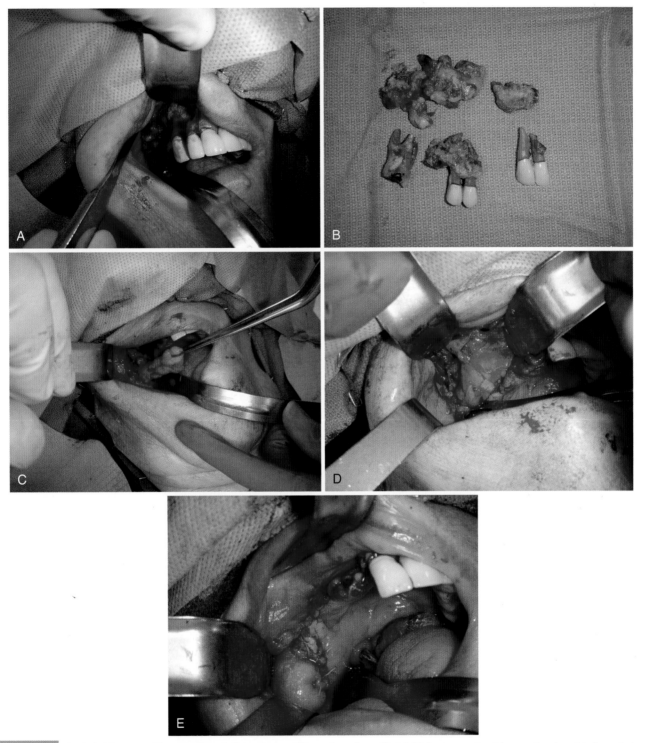

Figure 2-6 **A,** Debridement of bone and teeth from the maxillary sinus floor. **B,** Multiple mucoceles (sinus polyps) and inflamed sinus membrane are removed from the sinus. **C,** Buccal fat pad is advanced forward after a pericapsular dissection. **D,** Buccal fat pad is sutured to the lateral sinus wall and palatal mucosa to stabilize it in the sinus. **E,** Primary mucosal closure over the buccal fat pad is achieved after extensive undermining.

marketed as Prolia (60 mg given by injection every 6 months) and as Xgeva (120 mg given by injection every month). Denosumab, in both forms, already has produced cases of osteonecrosis of the jaws. Hence, the name change from bisphosphonate-induced osteonecrosis of the jaws to drug-induced osteonecrosis of the jaws.

Although alendronate caused osteonecrosis of the jaws (ONJ) as early as 1999, the focus of ONJ publications centered on the more common and more severe cases attributed to pamidronate (Aredia, Novartis Pharmaceutical) and zoledronate (Zometa, Novartis Pharmaceutical). It was not until Marx published his textbook, *Oral and Intravenous*

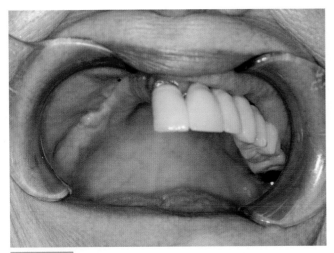

Figure 2-7   Healed oral mucosa and resolved ONJ.

Bisphosphonate-Induced Osteonecrosis of the Jaws, in 2005, and followed it with a publication in 2007, that the profession was alerted to the fact that oral bisphosphonates can cause ONJ and to the management of this problem. Since then, numerous publications, most identifying alendronate (Fosamax) as the cause of ONJ, have left little doubt that oral bisphosphonates can and do cause ONJ. However, by 2008 several publications had identified an unusual location of fractures in the femur unassociated with trauma. These were linked to alendronate taken as the commercial drug Fosamax and became known as *subtrochanteric fractures of the femur.* The number of publications on these fractures and on ONJ has increased yearly as cases of both have mounted.

The prevention and treatment guidelines for patients on oral bisphosphonates have been published by several associations, in addition to several publications and textbooks. Although they may differ slightly, there is mostly a consistency between them.

For the restorative dentist, it is well to remember that the teeth themselves do not take up bisphosphonates but that the alveolar bone does and is the target and initiation point for ONJ. Therefore, before, during, and after treatment with any bisphosphonate or denosumab, dentistry that does not invade the alveolar bone is safe. Restorative dentistry, crown and bridge work, dentures, root canals, and even scaling of the teeth that does not contact alveolar bone is safe. In fact, many cases of DIONJ caused by oral bisphosphonates can be prevented by restoring teeth and by eradicating periodontal inflammation before or in the early time course of treatment.

About 50% of cases of DIONJ caused by an oral bisphosphonate occur spontaneously. However, many of them are actually initiated by traumatic injury or by heavy occlusion. This is particularly noted in spontaneous cases in which the lingual cortex in the mandibular molar region is the first area to exhibit exposed bone (Figure 2-8, *A*). This, in turn, is due to the wide occlusal table of molar teeth and its closer proximity to the hinge effect of the temporomandibular joint. This greater force on the molar teeth is transmitted to the underlying bone which, if sufficiently loaded with a bisphosphonate, cannot remodel to adjust and compensate for this loading and becomes necrotic and exposed (Figure 2-8, *B*). It is further seen that the axial loading on molar teeth is not on the inferior border, as it is in other mandibular teeth, but on the lingual cortex instead (Figure 2-8, *C*). The clinical importance of this is that a balanced occlusion reduces the risk of developing DIONJ as much as anything else.

The remaining 50% of DIONJ cases caused by an oral bisphosphonate are initiated by a surgical procedure on the alveolar bone, mostly tooth extractions. All surgical procedures on the alveolar bone require bone remodeling and renewal to heal. Once again, if the alveolar bone is sufficiently loaded with a bisphosphonate, it cannot meet this enhanced healing requirement and may become necrotic. The clinical importance of this is that by preventing the need to extract teeth or by reducing periodontal inflammation, which also increases the requirement for bone remodeling, the risk of developing DIONJ can be reduced.

Today, many clinicians are faced with the need to perform some invasive surgery on a patient taking an oral bisphosphonate. Because of the minimal absorption of oral bisphosphonates, their accumulation in bone is delayed, compared with IV forms, and their impact on the bone marrow precursors of osteoclasts in less and also delayed. Therefore, the risk of developing DIONJ after an oral surgical procedure begins at around 2 years of steady weekly or monthly dosing and first becomes significant at 3 years. During this time and later, the author uses and recommends the morning fasting serum CTX test. This is the most accurate blood marker for the suppression of bone turnover and was used in most bisphosphonate research studies. It measures an eight amino acid split product of collagen released by the osteoclast during bone resorption. Therefore, it is an index of osteoclast function. Although the usefulness of the CTX is limited to women with uncomplicated osteopenia or osteoporosis, and it is not included in the major dental and medical association position papers, it can be a useful technique for assessing the risk for DIONJ related to surgery in a patient taking oral bisphosphonates. The usefulness of the CTX test has been documented by several independent studies. A CTX value above 150 pg/ml (as seen in the current patient's repeat test) is associated with alveolar bone healing and remodeling. Values lower than 150 pg/ml indicate a risk for DIONJ.

The limitations of the CTX test are that it is inaccurate in cancer patients and therefore cannot correlate with the effects of Aredia and Zometa on these patients. This is due to the fact that the cancer's invasion into bone and soft tissues also creates collagen split products. These cross-react with the CTX test to register higher values. Another limitation of the CTX text is seen in patients taking or who have taken significant amounts of steroids or methotrexate. Both suppress collagen synthesis and register lower values on the CTX test. The clinical experience with these patients and others has been that a 9-month to 1-year drug holiday from an oral bisphosphonate allowed alveolar bone surgery without the development of DIONJ. Therefore, either a CTX test result

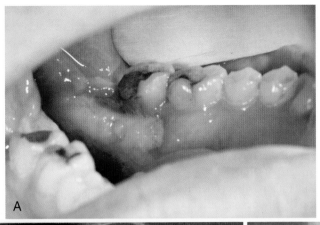

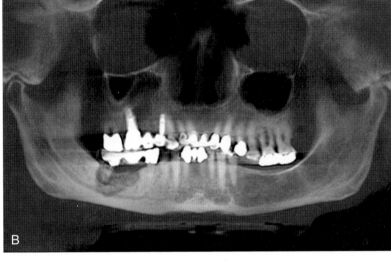

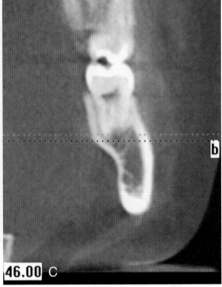

Figure 2-8   **A,** The mandibular lingual cortex is a site of predilection for spontaneous oral bisphosphonate–induced osteonecrosis. **B,** Osteolysis of DIONJ caused by an oral bisphosphonate but initiated by hyperocclusion. **C,** Cone-beam CT scan identifies the lingual cortex of the mandible as the point of axial loading of its molar teeth.

of 150 pg/ml or greater or a drug holiday of 9 months or longer is recommended in these cases.

TREATMENT OF ORAL BISPHOSPHONATE DIONJ

The general principles of treating oral bisphosphonate–induced osteonecrosis of the jaws were illustrated in the current patient's case. Once the exposed bone develops, it is best to consult the prescribing physician to confirm the dose and the length of time the patient has been taking the drug. The higher the dose (Fosamax is prescribed at 70 mg/week; Actonel at 35 mg/week; and Boniva at 150 mg/month, averaging 35 mg/week) and the greater the number of doses, the greater the severity of the ONJ. The clinician should request a drug holiday from the bisphosphonate for 9 months to 1 year. Should the prescribing physician be reluctant to discontinue the oral bisphosphonate, he or she should be encouraged to read the *JAMA* article by Black, Schwartz, Ensrud, et al. and the FDA's 2011 publication on drug safety (see the Bibliography for information on both citations). Both of these

publications concluded that the therapeutic benefit of alendronate (Fosamax) does not extend beyond 3 years of taking the drug and that the risk of complications overtakes the benefit at 5 years. Most prescribing physicians are very compliant with a drug holiday and often use no alternative therapy or use only calcium and vitamin D, or raloxifene (Evista), or recombinant human parathyroid hormone 1-34 (Forteo) as an alternative treatment.

The author obtains a morning fasting serum CTX value as a base line and repeats it at 6 months. When the CTX value exceeds 150 pg/ml, about 50% of cases will have sloughed the exposed bone and healed over the area with normal-appearing mucosa. The remaining 50% at that time can undergo debridement with the expectation of normal bone and wound healing. Only 10% of oral bisphosphonate DIONJ cases are sufficiently severe to need a mandibular continuity resection or a radical sinusotomy (as was required in the current patient's case). In cases in which a CTX value cannot be obtained for any reason, an arbitrary 9-month to 1-year drug holiday has been associated with normal bone and soft tissue healing.

In patients whose oral bisphosphonate DIONJ has resolved, reconstruction of the alveolar bone with the clinician's preferred bone grafting materials and/or dental implant placements can be accomplished with the same success rate as that for any similar patient who has not taken a bisphosphonate— as long as a bisphosphonate or denosumab has not been reinitiated.

Although hyperbaric oxygen is the standard of care for treating osteoradionecrosis, it is of no use in DIONJ. This is due to the fact that radiation injury creates an oxygen gradient deficit, which hyperbaric oxygen corrects; in DIONJ, however, there is no oxygen gradient deficit, but rather a direct chemical toxicity to bone, which hyperbaric oxygen does not affect.

Bibliography

Advisory Task Force on Bisphosphonate-Related Osteonecrosis of the Jaws: American Association of Oral and Maxillofacial Surgeons position paper on bisphosphonate-related osteonecrosis of the jaws, *J Oral Maxillofac Surg* 65:369-376, 2007.

Aghaloo TL, Felsenfeld AL, Etradis S: Osteonecrosis of the jaw in a patient on denosumab, *J Oral Maxillofac Surg* 68(5):959-963, 2010.

Black DM, Thompson DE, Bauer DC, et al: Fracture risk reduction with alendronate in women with osteoporosis: the Fracture Intervention Trial, *J Clin Endocrinol Metab* 85:4118-4124, 2000.

Black DM, Schwartz AV, Ensrud KE, et al: Effects of continuing or stopping alendronate after five years of treatment: the Fracture Intervention Trial Long-Term Extension (FLEX)—a randomized trial, *JAMA* 296:2927-2938, 2006.

Das De S, Setiobudi T, Shen L, et al: A rationale approach to management of alendronate-related subtrochanteric fractures, *J Bone Joint Surg* 92-b:679-686, 2010.

Edwards NH, McCrae FC, Young-Min SA: Alendronate-related femoral diaphysis fracture: What should be done to predict and prevent subsequent fracture of the contralateral side? *Osteoporosis Int* 4:701-703, 2010 (EPUB: June 27, 2009).

Ingenix *ICD-9-CM for physicians,* vol 1, Eden Prairie, MN, 2012, Ingenix, Inc.

Kunchur R, Need A, Hughes T, et al: Clinical investigation of C-terminal cross linking telopeptide test in prevention and management of bisphosphonate-associated osteonecrosis of the jaws, *J Oral Maxillofac Surg* 67:1167-1173, 2009.

Kwon YD, Ohe JY, Lim DY, et al: Retrospective study of two biochemical markers for the risk assessment of oral bisphosphonate related osteonecrosis of the jaws: Can they be utilized as risk markers? *Clin Oral Implants Res* 22:100-105, 2011.

Lasseter KC, Porras AG, Denker A, et al: Pharmacokinetic considerations in determining the terminal elimination half-lives of bisphosphonates, *Clin Drug Invest* 25:107-114, 2005.

Marx RE (ed): *Oral and intravenous bisphosphonate-induced osteonecrosis of the jaws: history, etiology, prevention, and treatment,* ed 2, Hanover Park, Ill, 2010, Quintessence.

Marx RE, Cillo JE Jr, Ulloa JJ: Oral bisphosphonate–induced osteonecrosis: risk factors, prediction of risk using serum CTX testing, prevention, and treatment, *J Oral Maxillofac Surg* 65(12):2397-2410, 2007.

Neviaser AS, Lane JM, Lenart BA, et al: Low energy femoral shaft fractures associated with alendronate use, *J Orthop Trauma* 22:346-350, 2008.

Park-Wyllie LY, Mamdani MM, Juirlink DN, et al: Bisphosphonate use and atypical fractures of the femoral shaft, *N Engl J Med* 36:1728-1737, 2011.

Rosen HN, Moses AC, Garber J, et al: Serum CTX: a new marker of bone resorption that shows treatment effect more often than other markers because of low coefficient of variability and large changes with bisphosphonate therapy, *Calcif Tissue Int* 66:100-103, 2000.

Taylor KH, Middlefell LS, Mizen KD: Osteonecrosis of the jaws induced by anti-RANK Ligand therapy, *Br J Oral Maxillofac Surg* 48:221-223, 2010.

US Food and Drug Administration: Background document for meeting of Advisory Committee for Reproductive Health Drugs and Drug Safety and Risk Management Advisory Committee. September 9, 2011. Available at: http:11wwwfda.gov/downloads/advisorycommittees/committees meeting materials/drugs/drug safety and risk management advisory committee/UCM 270958.

Intravenous Drug–Induced Osteonecrosis of the Jaws

Robert E. Marx

CC

A 71-year-old woman with a history of multiple myeloma of the past 5 years is referred by her oncologist because of "exposed bone" and a draining fistula (Figure 2-9).

Intravenous Drug–Induced Osteonecrosis of the Jaws

Two classes of drugs have been directly linked to osteonecrosis of the jaws: bisphosphonates and reactor activator of nuclear kappa-B (RANK) ligand inhibitors. Therefore, what was once referred to as bisphosphonate–induced osteonecrosis of the jaws (BIONJ) now is best called *drug-induced osteonecrosis of the jaws* (DIONJ).

The clinically important distinction is the route of administration, intravenous versus oral, across both classes of drugs. Therefore, a sample case of an oral bisphosphonate ONJ was presented in the preceding section, and a sample case of an intravenous bisphosphonate ONJ is presented here.

HPI

The current patient's multiple myeloma is stated to be in remission as a result of stem cell transplantation and Velcade treatment in the past. She now takes only Revlimid, but she took zoledronic acid (Zometa) in the recent past. She took Zometa 4 mg monthly for 2 years; this treatment was discontinued 9 months ago when exposed bone and pain developed spontaneously. Since then, the exposed bone has failed to heal. The patient was initially treated with clindamycin 300 mg three times daily, but without relief of pain. Pain relief was obtained when she was placed on phenoxymethyl penicillin (penicillin VK) 500 mg four times daily, along with 0.12% chlorhexidine oral rinses three times daily. Despite initial pain control, the area of exposed bone increased, and two draining cutaneous fistulas developed, along with a return of pain.

PMHX/PDHX/MEDICATIONS/ALLERGIES/SH/FH

Other than multiple myeloma and its related treatments, the patient has had a left total knee replacement for degenerative arthritis (8 years ago) and placement of a coronary artery stent (6 years ago). She is a past smoker of one pack per day but quit 10 years ago. She takes no medications other than Zometa and Revlimid.

EXAMINATION

Exposed bone is noted in the lingual alveolar bone in the right mandibular molar area (see Figure 2-9, *A*). There is a draining fistula at the level of the inferior border of the mandible (see Figure 2-9, *B*). Although there is no exposed bone seen on the buccal, there is prominent exposed bone seen on the lingual, which is jagged. There are also several fistulas arising from

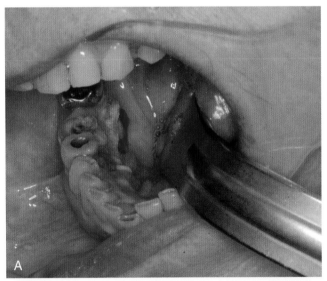

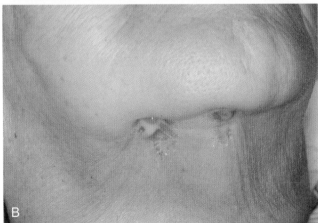

Figure 2-9 **A,** Exposed bone with ragged edges on the lingual mandibular cortex in the molar region. **B,** Draining cutaneous fistula.

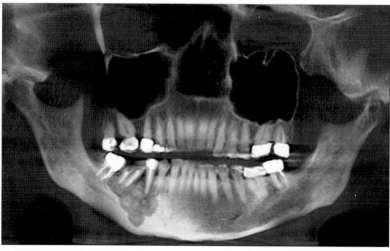

Figure 2-10 Osteolysis extending into the inferior border. Note the surrounding sclerotic bone and the beginning sequestra with the radiolucency.

the adjacent lingual mucosa, which suggests that the nonvital bone extends beyond the clinically exposed bone.

IMAGING

A cone-beam CT scan shows significant osteolysis in the right midbody area of the mandible and a diffuse surrounding sclerosis (Figure 2-10). Compared with a cone-beam CT scan taken 6 months earlier, a greater amount of osteolysis and osteosclerosis is noted.

LABS

Routine laboratory testing is required to particularly assess for anemia and blood chemistry changes. This patient showed a clinically insignificant anemia, with an Hb of 11.3 g/dl and an HCT of 34%. She also exhibited slightly elevated myeloma proteins (IgG 160.8 mg/ml; normal range, 3 to 19.4 mg/ml. This IgG value is still not a contraindication to nonsurgical or even surgical management of the exposed bone.

ASSESSMENT

Stage III drug-induced osteonecrosis of the jaws (DIONJ), by virtue of its osteolysis to the inferior border threatening a pathologic fracture.

TREATMENT

The treatment choices discussed with the patient included palliative nonsurgical management using intermittent or ongoing antibiotic therapy, along with oral rinses of 0.12% chlorhexidine three times daily, and adaptation to long-term and probably permanent exposed bone, or surgical resection to achieve resolution and a cure. Because this patient had endured the pain, odor, and foul taste of the exposed bone for 9 months already, and because the bone deterioration was advancing, she chose to undergo surgical resection.

Surgical resection was performed after consultation with and clearance from her medical oncologist and her internist. The surgical access was made through a convenient neck crease to expose the right hemimandible (Figure 2-11, *A*). A 2.9-mm titanium reconstruction plate (the strongest made) then was placed and fixated onto the intact mandible with locking screws so as to index the position of the condyle and the remaining occlusion (Figure 2-11, *B*). The plate was subsequently removed, with each screw marked to correlate with the appropriate screw hole. The mandible was then resected from the right canine area to the right midramus, with the surgeon observing for residual viable marrow space as the best assessment for an adequate resection margin (Figure 2-11, *C* and *D*). The titanium plate was replaced and fixated in its preoperative position after the resection edges have been rounded off (Figure 2-11, *E*). The mucosa and skin were closed primarily over the reconstruction plate.

OUTCOME

The patient has been followed for the past 3 years. Her multiple myeloma remains under control, and her DIONJ remains resolved, with no further exposed bone; the secondary infection, foul order, and taste also have resolved, and there are no fistulas (Figure 2-12). The patient eats in a near-normal fashion with her residual dentition in the anterior region and left side. She has not been restarted on zoledronic acid but continues to be on maintenance chemotherapy.

PATHOLOGY

The specimen microscopically showed the features characteristic of DIONJ. Specifically, one section showed nonvital bone with scalloped edges representing empty resorption pits (Figure 2-13, *A*). These were generated by osteoclasts that began resorbing the dead bone but died as they ingested the metabolic poison of the bisphosphonate, leaving an incompletely resorbed portion of dead bone with scalloped edges.

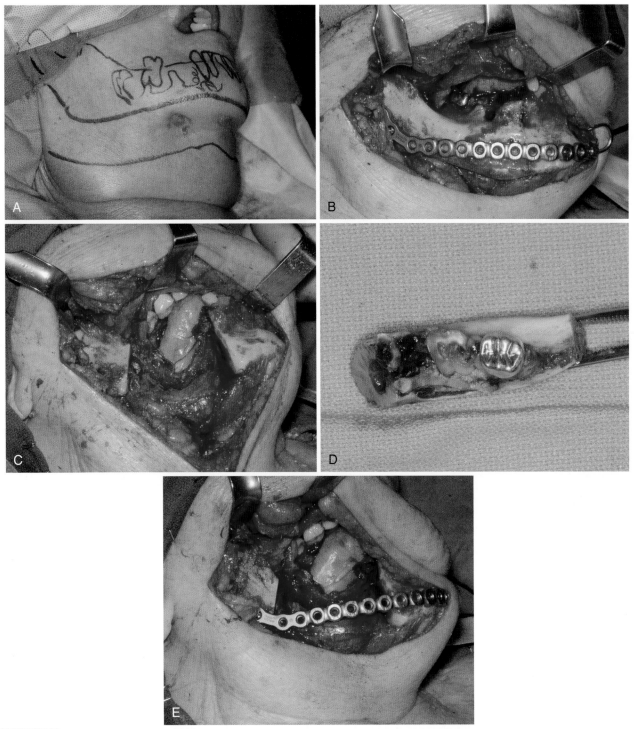

Figure 2-11 **A,** Outline of the mandible and area of necrotic bone with planned incision placement for maximum cosmetic outcome. **B,** A 2.9-mm titanium reconstruction plate fixated to the intact mandible with intended resection margins. **C,** Defect of the mandible after resection of necrotic bone. Note the bleeding marrow space and residual cancellous marrow at the distal resection margin. This is currently the best indicator of an adequate margin. **D,** Resection specimen with discolored necrotic bone. **E,** Reconstruction plate returned after the resection, positioning the occlusion and the condyle in their preresection positions.

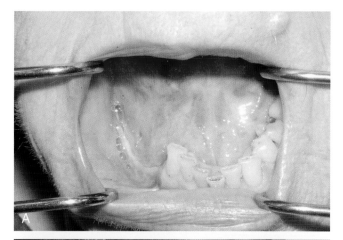

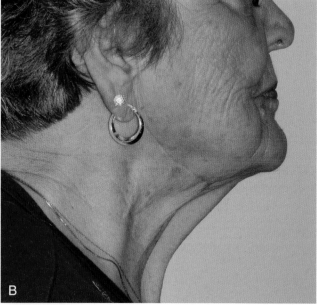

Figure 2-12   **A,** Healed mucosa and resolution of DIONJ after resection surgery. **B,** Profile facial view identifies resolution of the cutaneous fistula and a well-hidden incision scar in the neck.

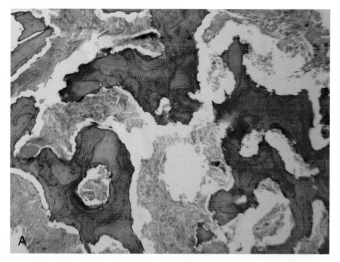

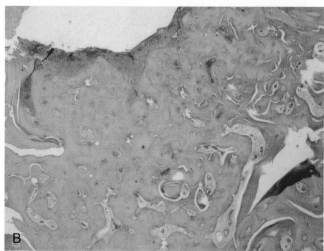

Figure 2-13   **A,** Resection specimen showed necrotic bone with scalloped edges representing empty resorption lacunae for osteoblastic death. Colonies of *Actinomyces* organisms also are seen, but no residual bone marrow cells. **B,** Surface inflammation with no marrow inflammation ruled out a primary osteomyelitis in this case. Note the thick trabecular bone, which accounts for the sclerosis seen on the cone-beam CT scan.

Between the necrotic bone trabeculae were dense colonies of *Actinomyces* organisms, the most common microorganisms to colonize DIONJ-exposed bone (Figure 2-13, *A*). Another section at the resection edge showed surface inflammation but normal marrow spaces without inflammation, which distinguished the condition from a primary osteomyelitis. A thick, bony trabecular network also was noted, which is the result of the antiresorptive effect of bisphosphonates and is related to the osteosclerosis seen on imaging (Figure 2-13, *B*).

DISCUSSION

DIONJ was first recognized in 2003 as bisphosphonate-induced osteonecrosis of the jaws. Since then researchers have noted that denosumab, a RANK ligand inhibitor (marketed as Prolia, given orally, and Xgeva, given by injection), causes the same type of osteonecrosis of the jaws. For this reason, the American Medical Association has settled on DIONJ as the correct term. In just under one decade, more

than 1,300 scientific articles, reporting more than 10,000 cases, have underscored the clinical epidemic predicted by the first article.

The takeaway lessons from the case presented here are many. One is that about 25% of cases occur spontaneously because of the dose, potency of the drug, and duration of drug exposure. The current patient took zoledronic acid, the most potent bisphosphonate, for approximately 24 doses, which was the cause of her DIONJ. The fact that she persisted with exposed bone for longer than 9 months and actually experienced a worsening of her DIONJ is due to the 11-year half-life of these drugs. Although a drug holiday of 9 months is effective in cases of oral bisphosphonate DIONJ, drug holidays are not effective with intravenous bisphosphonate DIONJ, even if they last several years. This is due to the IV route itself, which loads the bone 140 times faster and more completely than an oral bisphosphonate, which is poorly absorbed into

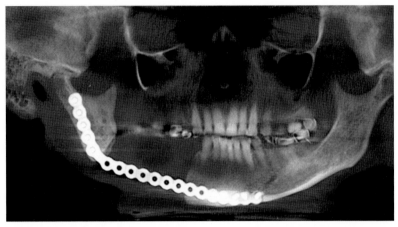

Figure 2-14   The continuity defect of the mandible was reconstructed with only the titanium plate and has been stable for 2 years.

the systemic circulation (0.64% of an oral bisphosphonate is absorbed into the systemic circulation). It is also due to this greater drug load on the bone marrow osteoclast precursors, which do not quickly recover to replenish functioning osteoclasts when an IV bisphosphonate is discontinued. The clinical value of discontinuing Zometa in this case, and in others like it, is more to reduce the probability of DIONJ developing in other sites in the jaws.

As a result of the influence of the drug companies, the medical and dental associations have each put forth a confusing and overcomplicated staging system. This is because pain is incorporated as part of these staging systems; however, pain is unrelated to the extent or the severity of DIONJ. Pain is related only to secondary infection, and it changes with the use of antibiotics; therefore, a patient's disease may jump from stage Ia to stage Ib or to stage IIb, or back and forth, as a function of secondary infection or of the patient's use of analgesics. The following is a more straightforward staging system:

- Stage I: Exposed bone limited to one quadrant
- Stage II: Exposed bone involving two quadrants
- Stage III: Exposed bone involving three or four quadrants, or osteolysis to the inferior border, or a pathologic fracture, or extension into the maxillary sinus if in the maxilla

The importance of a stage III presentation is that it brings surgery to the forefront, as it did in this case. The value of nonsurgical management is that it avoids the risks of general anesthesia and surgery. In some patients with metastatic cancer, debilitation and systemic compromise may not allow a safe anesthesia or surgery. These patients and patients who decide against surgery must accept the continuation of exposed bone, the expectation of episodes of pain, and ongoing courses of antibiotics. In such cases, penicillin VK 500 mg four times daily is the drug of choice. As an alternative in refractory cases or in a patient who is allergic to penicillin, doxycycline 100 mg daily is a good choice. In patients whose DIONJ is refractory to either of those drugs, the addition of metronidazole 500 mg three times daily for a 10-day course is usually effective. Patients whose condition remains refractory despite

all these medications usually choose the surgical option. In accepting a palliative course, with continued exposed bone with colonization and episodes of bacterial infection, the clinician should take into account the potential for bacterial feeding on implanted devices, such as prosthetic heart valves, knee or hip replacements, and cardiac stents.

The surgical option is mostly a continuity resection of the mandible or, if the disease is in the maxilla, local resection of the maxilla with sinus debridement. Limited office-based debridements have usually been unsuccessful and have actually eventuated into a greater amount of exposed bone. However, with a resection (such as was performed with the patient in the example case), bony reconstruction of the defect is problematic and usually is not accomplished. This is because disease-free donor bone is not available because of the presence of malignant cells in the donor bone, and rhBMP-2/ACS is contraindicated in patients with active cancers. Therefore, a titanium plate, used as an "artificial jaw" to establish and maintain continuity, becomes the permanent reconstruction in the mandible (Figure 2-14), and a closed mucosa with no underlying bone is the permanent outcome in the maxilla.

Bibliography

Aghaloo TL, Felsenfeld AL, Tetradis S: Osteonecrosis, *J Oral Maxillofac Surg* 68(5):959-963, 2010.

Buck CJ: *American Medical Association ICD-9-CM for physicians,* St Louis, 2011, p 962, Saunders.

Khosla S, Burr D, Cauley J, et al: Bisphosphonate-associated osteonecrosis of the jaw: report of a task force of the American Society for Bone and Mineral Research, *J Bone Miner Res* 22(10):1479-1491, 2007.

Lasseter KC, Porros AG, Denker A, et al: Pharmacokinetic considerations in determining the terminal elimination half lives of bisphosphonates, *Clin Drug Invest* 25(2):107-114, 2005.

Marx RE: Pamidronate (Aredia) and zolendronate (Zometa) induced avascular necrosis of the jaws: a growing epidemic, *J Oral Maxillofac Surg* 61:1115-1157, 2003.

Marx RE, Sawatari Y, Fortin M, et al: Bisphosphonate induced exposed bone (osteonecrosis/osteopetrosis) of the jaws: risk factors, recognition, prevention, and treatment, *J Oral Maxillofac Surg* 63:1567-1575, 2005.

Marx RE, Cillo JE Jr, Ulloa JJ: Oral bisphosphonate-induced osteo-necrosis: risk factors, prediction of risk using serum CTX testing, prevention, and treatment, *J Oral Maxillofac Surg* 65(12):2397-2410, 2007.

Merck & Co: Fosamax (alendronate sodium) tablets and oral solution. Product information sheet, 2012. Available at www.merck.com/product/usa/pi_circulars/f/fosamax/fosamax_pi.pdf. Accessed April 2, 2013.

Ruggiero SL, Dodson TB, Assael LA, et al: American Association of Oral and Maxillofacial Surgeons position paper on bisphosphonate-related osteonecrosis of the jaws: 2009 update, *J Oral Maxillofac Surg* 67(5 Suppl):2-12, 2009.

Taylor KH, Middlefell LS, Mizen KD: Osteonecrosis of the jaws induced by anti-RANK ligand therapy, *Br J Oral Maxillofac Surg* 48:221-223, 2010.

CHAPTER 3

Anesthesia

This chapter addresses:
- Laryngospasm
- Perioperative Considerations of the Pregnant Patient
- Respiratory Depression Secondary to Oversedation
- Inadequate Local Anesthesia
- Trigeminal Neuralgia
- Malignant Hyperthermia
- Emergent Surgical Airway

Administration of anesthesia remains an important part of office-based oral and maxillofacial surgery. The most important step in delivering safe and effective anesthesia is preparation. Preparation begins with a thorough knowledge and understanding of the anatomy, physiology, and pharmacology relevant to anesthesia. From this point, safe anesthetic techniques are developed and used based on the preoperative patient evaluation, practitioner's preference, and individual clinical situations. Preparation also includes measures to prevent and manage emergencies. Despite a thorough preoperative patient evaluation, use of safe and proven anesthetic techniques, and vigilant monitoring, emergency situations may arise. For these reasons, it is essential that all practitioners continually hone their skills in the recognition and management of life-threatening emergencies in the office or operating room. Our excellent safety record is evidence of oral and maxillofacial surgeons' training and preparation in the delivery of safe anesthesia.

Each of the following teaching cases deals with the management of specific clinical scenarios. We also include a new case discussing trigeminal neuralgia/facial pain. The sections are structured to emphasize the key points in the preoperative evaluation and recognition of impending emergencies. Strategies for reducing the risk of emergent situations—and for their management when they do arise—are discussed. The highlighted clinical pearls in the preoperative patient evaluation should be incorporated into all practitioners' routine preoperative assessment.

The intent of this section is to familiarize readers with the risk factors and clinical signs associated with disastrous outcomes involving anesthesia (local, sedation, or general).

Laryngospasm

Michael L. Beckley and Shahrokh C. Bagheri

CC

A 12-year-old female is scheduled for extraction of four bicuspids under intravenous general anesthesia. (Laryngospasm may occur more often in children because of the frequency of upper respiratory tract infections in this patient population.)

HPI

Preoperative evaluation of the patient revealed no recent respiratory tract infections. The lungs were clear to auscultation. After ECG, blood pressure, pulse oximeter, and capnography monitors were applied, the patient was administered 4 L of oxygen and 2 L of nitrous oxide via nasal hood. Sedation was achieved using 4 mg of midazolam and 50 µg of fentanyl titrated to effect. Prior to administration of local anesthesia, 40 mg of propofol was infused. During the first extraction, respiratory stridor (a high-pitched, inspiratory "crowing" sound) was noted. A noisy, harsh sound was heard on inspiration through the precordial stethoscope, and the patient's oxygen saturation decreased from 99% to 65%. Capnography indicated no ventilation. At this point, the respiratory noises ceased. Tracheal tug and paradoxical chest wall motion were observed (signs of upper airway obstruction), and the patient began to appear cyanotic.

PMHX/PDHX/MEDICATIONS/ALLERGIES/SH/FH

Noncontributory. A recent history of upper respiratory tract infection (URI) may indicate an increased risk of perioperative respiratory complications, especially laryngospasm. In the event of a recent URI, it may be prudent to reschedule surgery after a 2-week symptom-free period. Patients with reactive airway disease may be more prone to experience laryngospasm.

EXAMINATION

General. A harsh inspiratory noise, or crowing, is audible on inspiration, which is best heard through the precordial stethoscope. The patient's skin color is assessed for signs of cyanosis, which is seen with severe hypoxemia. In pediatric patients, hypoxemia is often a late finding of decreased ventilation or apnea. End tidal CO_2 monitoring and use of the precordial stethoscope indicate hypoventilation or apnea prior to changes in pulse oximetry.

Oropharynx. The throat pack is removed, and there is no evidence of foreign bodies. Copious amounts of mucous secretions are observed. (Blood and mucus are common stimuli for airway irritation.)

Neck and chest. There is evidence of tracheal tug and paradoxical chest wall motion (despite chin-lift and jaw-thrust maneuvers). This phenomenon is the result of forced inspiration against a closed glottis.

Vital signs. The patient's heart rate is 160 bpm, blood pressure 145/78 mm Hg, $EtCO_2$ 0, and respirations 0 breaths per minute.

Oxygen saturation. Oxygen saturation decreased from 99% to 65% with the onset of laryngospasm. (Continued decline in the oxygen saturation can result in respiratory acidosis.)

ECG. The patient is in sinus tachycardia. (This is a common finding, but hypoxia can trigger more life-threatening cardiac arrhythmias. Hypoxemia in children may result in bradycardia.)

IMAGING

Imaging is not relevant in the acute management of laryngospasm. This is an anesthetic emergency and is diagnosed based on the clinical presentation. Chest films can be ordered if there is suspicion of foreign body aspiration or to aid in the diagnosis of negative pressure/post obstructive pulmonary edema after the acute management of the airway.

LABS

None are indicated in the acute setting.

ASSESSMENT

Intraoperative laryngospasm during odontectomy under general anesthesia

TREATMENT

Prompt recognition and treatment of laryngospasm usually result in a good outcome. Upon diagnosis, the airway should be suctioned clear of noxious stimuli and the surgical site should be packed. Any foreign bodies are removed from the oral cavity and 100% oxygen is administered. Positive pressure ventilation should be attempted, ideally with a two-person technique and jaw-thrust maneuver; this often "breaks" the laryngospasm (jaw thrust and pressure at the angle of the mandible may also assist in breaking laryngospasms).

A technique described by Dr. N.P. Guadagni also has been found to effective at "breaking" laryngospasm. This involves placing the middle finger of each hand anterior to the mastoid and posterior to the condyle. The fingers then press inward while at the same time positioning the mandible forward. If the patient cannot be ventilated, the plane of anesthesia may be deepened with a short-acting intravenous general anesthetic; this often obviates the need for a skeletal muscle relaxant.

In rare situations these methods are unsuccessful, and it is necessary to administer succinylcholine, a short- and fast-acting depolarizing neuromuscular blocking agent. If intravenous access is not available, succinylcholine may be administered intramuscularly at a dose of 4 mg/kg. A dose of 20 mg intravenously is usually sufficient to break the spasm (pediatric dose, 0.25 mg/kg). However, up to 60 mg can be administered if laryngospasm persists. Rapacurium, rocuronium, and mivacurium can be used for patients in whom succinylcholine is contraindicated. The longer half-life of these nondepolarizing muscle relaxants may require continuous bag-mask ventilation until spontaneous respiration resumes.

Bradycardia is not uncommon after administration of succinylcholine. This usually occurs in children and in adults after repeated doses. Atropine may be administered in an effort to prevent this. Intravenous lidocaine 2 mg/kg administered before extubation was found to be effective in preventing postextubation laryngospasm in patients undergoing tonsillectomy. Other studies have found the prophylactic use of intravenous lidocaine to be ineffective.

COMPLICATIONS

Laryngospasm may produce partial or complete respiratory obstruction. Fortunately, early recognition and management allow for rapid resolution and minimal morbidity. However, with prolonged hypoxemia, the complications can be devastating. Laryngospasm may result in an acid-base disturbance, such as respiratory acidosis. Rare complications of laryngospasm include cardiac arrhythmias, anoxic brain injury, negative pressure pulmonary edema, and death.

If succinylcholine is administered, the patient may complain of general postoperative myalgia secondary to the rapid muscle depolarization. Other potential complications of succinylcholine include masticator muscle rigidity, malignant hyperthermia, and hyperkalemic cardiac arrest (secondary to the transient hyperkalemia), which can be seen in patients with undiagnosed myopathies (e.g., Duchenne's and Becker's muscular dystrophies).

DISCUSSION

Laryngospasm results in tight approximation of the true vocal cords (Figure 3-1). It is a protective reflex that is most commonly caused by a noxious stimulus to the airway during a light plane of anesthesia. The structural and functional bases

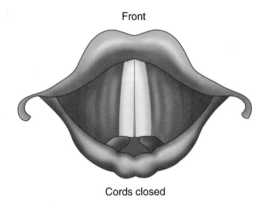

Front

Cords closed

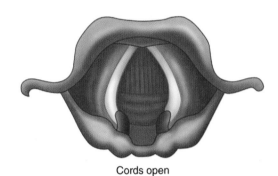

Cords open

Figure 3-1   Tight approximation of the true vocal cords as seen during laryngospasm. *(From Malamed SF: Sedation: a guide to patient management, ed 5, St Louis, 2010, Mosby.)*

of the laryngospasm reflex were described by Rex. Secretions, vomitus, blood, pungent volatile anesthetics, painful stimuli, and oral and nasal airways may elicit this protective reflex. Mediated by the vagus nerve, this reflex is designed to prevent foreign materials from entering the tracheobronchial tree. During laryngospasm, the false vocal cords and supraglottic tissues act as a ball valve and obstruct the laryngeal inlet during inspiration. Laryngospasm has a reported occurrence of 8.7 per 1,000 patients receiving general anesthesia. It is 19 times more frequent than bronchospasm.

Laryngospasm accounts for more than 50% of the cases of negative pressure/post obstructive pulmonary edema. With the use of general endotracheal intubation, laryngospasm classically occurs during extubation in a light plane of anesthesia (stage II). Children and patients who have had a recent upper respiratory tract infection are predisposed to developing laryngospasm during anesthesia.

Efforts to prevent laryngospasm include postponing surgery in patients who have had recent upper respiratory infections, maintaining a dry surgical field, and using anticholinergics and avoiding extubation during stage II of anesthesia. Laryngospasm is not uncommon in outpatient and inpatient oral and maxillofacial surgery. Recognition and early intervention are essential in preventing morbidity and mortality.

Bibliography

Baraka A: Intravenous lidocaine controls extubation laryngospasm in children, *Anesth Analg* 57:506-507, 1978.

Ciavarro C, Kelly JP: Postobstructive pulmonary edema in an obese child after an oral surgery procedure under general anesthesia: a case report, *J Oral Maxillofac Surg* 60(12):1503-1505, 2002.

Hartley M, Vaughan RS: Problems associated with tracheal extubation, *Br J Anaesth* 71:561-568, 1993.

Hurford WE, Bailin MT, Davison JK, et al: *Clinical procedures of the Massachusetts General Hospital*, ed 5, pp 299-300, 514, 609, Philadelphia, 1998, Lippincott-Raven.

Larson CP: Laryngospasm–the best treatment, *Journal of the American Society of Anesthesiologists*, 89(5): 1293-1294, 1998.

Leicht P, Wisborg T, Chraemmer-Joorgensen B: Does intravenous lidocaine prevent laryngospasm after extubation in children? *Anesth Analg* 64:1193-1196, 1985.

Louis PJ, Fernandes R: Negative pressure pulmonary edema, *Oral Surg Oral Med Oral Pathol Oral Radiol Endod* 93(1):4-6, 2002.

Rex MAE: A review of the structural and functional basis of laryngospasm and a discussion of the nerve pathways involved in the reflex and its clinical significance in man and animals, *Br J Anaesth* 42:891-898, 1970.

Stoelting RK, Miller RD: *Basics of anesthesia*, ed 3, pp 85-90, 161, New York, 1994, Churchill Livingstone.

Perioperative Considerations for the Pregnant Patient

Chris Jo and Jenny Jo

CC

A 29-year-old primigravida (first pregnancy) with twins at 25 weeks of gestation presents to your office for evaluation and management of an odontogenic abscess.

HPI

The patient presents complaining of a 2-week history of dental pain in the right mandible and a 2-day history of progressive swelling of her right face. She is being followed by her obstetrician, and she states that her pregnancy is progressing without complications. Recently she has noted good fetal movements. She denies having any vaginal bleeding or leakage of vaginal fluid (a sign that amniotic fluid may be leaking from ruptured membranes). She started having pelvic cramping just recently (cramping described by pregnant patients may actually be contractions). She has been taking acetaminophen (the analgesic of choice during pregnancy) for pain and has not been able to eat adequately for the past 3 days (pregnant patients have a higher nutritional and fluid requirement). There is no history of dysphagia (difficulty swallowing), odynophagia (painful swallowing), dyspnea (difficulty breathing), or subjective fevers.

PMHX/PDHX/MEDICATIONS/ALLERGIES/SH/FH

Noncontributory.

POBHx. This is the patient's first pregnancy. Her only high-risk diagnosis is carrying twins. They are diamniotic/dichorionic (two separate sacs). The twins have had concordant growth on serial ultrasounds, and her cervical length was 4 cm (good length) at 24 weeks. (A normal cervical length indicates a reduced risk for an incompetent cervix and preterm labor and delivery. Twins are at higher risk compared to singleton pregnancies).

EXAMINATION

Vital signs. The patient's blood pressure was 110/55 mm Hg, heart rate 110 to 140 bpm (tachycardic), respirations 20 per minute, and temperature 39°C (febrile).

General. She is well developed and well nourished and in no apparent distress.

Maxillofacial. There is a large right-sided facial swelling. The swelling is above the inferior border of the mandible (rules out submandibular space involvement) and below the zygomatic arch (buccal space abscess). It extends from the masseter (submasseteric space involvement) to the oral commissure. The swelling is tense, erythematous, warm, and tender to palpation. The submandibular and submental regions are normal. She has limited opening (trismus due to involvement of the lateral masticator space) secondary to pain, which limits the intraoral examination. The right mandibular first molar is grossly decayed, with adjacent vestibular swelling and purulence extravasating from the gingival sulcus. The oropharynx is not completely visible due to limited mouth opening. The floor of the mouth is nonelevated (rules out sublingual space involvement). She is in no respiratory distress and is tolerating her secretions well.

Cardiovascular. The patient is tachycardic with an II/VI systolic ejection murmur. (Early systolic ejection murmur is very common in pregnant women due to the high volume of flow; it is accentuated by acute tachycardia secondary to the elevated temperature.)

Abdominal. Examination reveals a gravid uterus (pregnant uterus) appearing larger than the stated gestational age (due to twins), nontender abdomen, and fetal heart rates of 190s for twin A (the lower presenting fetus in the uterus) and 180s for twin B (the heart rates are elevated above normal due to maternal temperature).

Extremities. The extremities are nontender with 1+ pitting edema at the ankles bilaterally (common during pregnancy), no cords, and 2+ equal pulses. She has a negative Homans sign (calf pain upon dorsiflexion of the foot, suggestive of deep vein thrombosis [DVT]).

IMAGING

A panoramic radiograph is the initial diagnostic study of choice. When the oropharynx cannot be adequately visualized due to trismus or when a deep neck space abscess is suspected, computed tomography (CT) scanning of the head and neck is necessary to rule out involvement of the parapharyngeal spaces (lateral pharyngeal and retropharyngeal spaces). The use of CT with intravenous contrast material is generally considered safe during pregnancy; however, special attention must be paid to the gestational age of the fetus and the amount of ionizing radiation that would be absorbed. In this particular case, the approximate exposure rate is less than 0.05 rad per examination, which is significantly less than the 5 rad cumulative upper limit for exposure during pregnancy (Dollard). The use of iodinated IV contrast does not produce any radiation exposure. The benefit of using IV contrast outweighs any theoretical risk of transient neonatal thyroid suppression; therefore, it can be used as needed, as long as there is no other contraindication to using the contrast material.

Despite the potential theoretical effects of radiation exposure to the fetus, all necessary plain film and CT studies for diagnosing and managing head and neck infections can be safely performed as needed. The radiation exposure to the developing fetus is minimal, especially when imaging the head and neck, and is further reduced by using shielding devices. Furthermore, the benefits outweigh the risks of exposure when dealing with acute head and neck infections. Nonionization techniques, such as ultrasound scans and magnetic resonance imaging (MRI) of the head and neck, are also considered safe during pregnancy and can aid in imaging soft tissue pathology. The use of gadolinium contrast with an MRI is currently not recommended during pregnancy, although there have not been any reported adverse fetal outcomes. Gadolinium does cross the placenta and can accumulate in the amniotic fluid of the fetus. The risk of nephrogenic systemic fibrosis with gadolinium is rare but warrants special attention in patients with renal insufficiency.

In this particular patient, the panoramic radiograph showed a grossly decayed right mandibular first molar with a large periradicular radiolucent lesion. CT was not indicated, because the clinical suspicion of parapharyngeal space involvement was low.

LABS

A complete blood count (CBC) with platelets and differential is the baseline study.

This patient's hemoglobin and hematocrit were 11 g/dl and 32.6%, respectively. (Anemia is commonly seen during pregnancy secondary to hemodilution, because the increase in plasma volume is relatively larger than the increase in red blood cells; however, pregnant patients are also at risk for iron deficiency anemia.) The patient's white blood cell (WBC) count was $18,000/mm^3$ with a 15% bandemia. (Although a slight, nonspecific elevation in the WBC count can be seen during pregnancy, this patient's elevated WBC count, in conjunction with bandemia and fever, is indicative of an acute infection until proven otherwise.)

ASSESSMENT

A 29-year-old primigravida with twins at 25 weeks of gestation with a large right-sided buccal and submasseteric space abscess secondary to a necrotic right mandibular first molar, complicated by dehydration and potential early onset of sepsis.

TREATMENT

The ideal time to perform elective or semielective oral and maxillofacial surgical procedures is postpartum; otherwise, the second trimester is considered the safest period for performing nonelective surgery. However, urgent or emergent surgery should not be delayed at any gestation of pregnancy, especially if procedures can be carried out under local anesthesia. Local anesthesia is the preferred method for simple procedures that can be performed in an office setting (there are no contraindications to vasoconstrictors, but aspiration to avoid intravascular injection is important). If the need arises, intravenous sedation and general anesthesia (in a hospital setting, when appropriate) can be safely performed without significant risk to the mother or fetus in an uncomplicated pregnancy (this is discussed later in the chapter).

There should be a lower threshold for hospital admission in the pregnant patient with a maxillofacial infection. Fever, dehydration, inability to tolerate oral intake, and potential airway compromise are all indications for hospital admission and initiation of supportive measures. (The risk of airway and pharyngeal edema is higher during pregnancy, especially when parapharyngeal spaces are involved.) Other obstetric concerns include risk factors for preterm contractions and preterm labor (onset of labor before 37 weeks of gestation): twins, dehydration, infection, and potential early sepsis.

When a pregnant woman is hospitalized, an obstetric consultation should be obtained. Fluid resuscitation, intravenous antibiotics, fetal monitoring, and nutritional support are extremely important. Caution should be exercised to avoid excessive fluid overload that can lead to pulmonary edema, because pregnancy and sepsis both can lead to third spacing due to increased capillary permeability. Usually, a 500-ml crystalloid bolus, followed by a maintenance level of 100 to 150 ml/hr until the patient is tolerating liquids, is appropriate for the average patient. Intravenous antibiotics should also be initiated (the penicillin and cephalosporin families are considered safe first-line antibiotics during pregnancy). Oral and maxillofacial infections should be aggressively treated, because untreated infections and abscesses have been associated with preterm labor and maternal sepsis.

If a pregnant woman is admitted to the hospital, she and the fetus should be monitored for contractions and fetal well-being. Pain management with a patient-controlled analgesia pump until the patient is tolerating oral medications is appropriate. Intravenous morphine, meperidine (Demerol), and fentanyl or orally administered hydrocodone, oxycodone, or codeine with acetaminophen combinations are all considered safe during pregnancy for necessary pain control. Routine use of nonsteroidal antiinflammatory drugs (NSAIDs), such as ibuprofen and aspirin, for postoperative pain control during pregnancy is generally not recommended; however, these drugs can be used short term in the second trimester only.

The current patient was admitted to the hospital, and an obstetric consultation was obtained. Intravenous fluids and piperacillin/tazobactam 3.375 g every 6 hours were administered. The twins were evaluated for heart tones and contractions. No significant abnormalities were noted. The fetal heart rates were slightly higher than normal due to the maternal temperature but were otherwise reassuring. There were no contractions noted. The pelvic examination was unremarkable, with no evidence of cervical effacement (thinning and shortening of the cervix associated with labor) or of cervical dilatation (also a sign of labor).

The patient was taken to the operating room for incision and drainage of the submasseteric and buccal space abscess and extraction of the right mandibular first molar. Ideally, pregnant patients should be NPO (nothing to eat or drink, including chewing gum) for at least 8 hours before surgery. In addition to the slower gastric emptying time and the enlarged uterus (which takes up more abdominal space, thus leaving less room for the gastrointestinal organs), pregnancy causes relaxation of the esophageal sphincter. The combination of these conditions increases the risk of aspiration associated with general anesthesia. Therefore, preoperatively, this patient received an oral antacid (to increase the pH of gastric contents), an H_2 antagonist (to decrease gastric acid production), and metoclopramide (to accelerate gastric emptying). Due to the gestational age of the patient, the uterus was enlarged (especially with twins). Therefore, a roll was placed under her right back and hip, and she was slightly tilted to the left. (A left lateral tilt of 15 to 30 degrees displaces the uterus off the aorta and inferior vena cava and prevents supine hypotensive syndrome, which is due to prolonged compression of the great vessels, leading to decreased venous return and cardiac output.)

After the patient had been positioned, she was intubated via an awake nasal fiberoptic intubation, due to her trismus (pregnant patients have edematous nasal mucosa and a potential for epistaxis, especially during a traumatic nasal intubation). The procedure was completed without complications. A thorough intraoperative examination of the oropharynx revealed no parapharyngeal involvement or edema. Her mouth opening increased to normal range after decompression of the lateral masticator (submasseteric) space. Her airway was deemed stable, without risk for postoperative upper airway obstruction, and she was successfully extubated. She remained in the hospital for a total of 4 days. She received daily antenatal testing to check for fetal well-being and contractions.

The patient was discharged home on postoperative day 4 after she had been afebrile for longer than 48 hours and was tolerating full liquids and a regular diet. She received intravenous antibiotics postoperatively until she was able to tolerate medications by mouth; she was then switched to oral antibiotics. Upon discharge, the patient's facial swelling had decreased significantly, there was no oral purulent discharge, the WBC count had normalized and there was no bandemia, and pain control was adequate with opioid analgesics.

COMPLICATIONS

Complications associated with surgery under general anesthesia during pregnancy include the risk of DVT, pulmonary embolism (PE), aspiration (decreased esophageal sphincter tone, decreased gastric emptying, increased gastric pressures, and hyperemesis increase the risk of regurgitation and aspiration), pulmonary edema, acute respiratory distress syndrome (ARDS), spontaneous abortion during the first trimester, and

preterm labor. These are weighed against the risks of an untreated oral or maxillofacial infection, which pose a greater direct danger to both the fetus and the mother; these risks include preterm labor and delivery with complications of a premature neonate, fetal death, maternal sepsis, and septic shock. All elective surgical procedures should be avoided during pregnancy, but necessary surgical interventions should not be delayed.

For the pregnant female undergoing general anesthesia, surgery should be performed in a setting where an obstetrician is available for consultation and where anesthesiologists are familiar with the physiologic changes associated with pregnancy. Teratogenic and abortive agents should be avoided (this is most important during the first trimester). Specific modifications may be needed as the gestational age of the fetus advances (discussed previously). A collaborative, multidisciplinary approach involving obstetricians, anesthesiologists, and oral and maxillofacial surgeons provides the most appropriate management and treatment plan for the pregnant patient.

A potential complication risk that is increased in pregnancy is the risk of deep vein thrombosis and pulmonary embolism due to the prothrombotic state of a pregnant woman. Physiologic changes that occur during pregnancy, such as increased clotting factors, increased plasma volume, increased venous stasis, decreased blood flow velocity, and decreased fibrinolytic activity, increase the risk of DVT (signs include leg pain, tenderness, edema, discoloration, palpable cord, and positive Homans sign) and subsequent PE (signs include shortness of breath, tachypnea, hypoxemia, and respiratory distress) by twofold to fourfold during pregnancy and early postpartum (Cromwell). Other exogenous factors, such as tobacco use, obesity, and immobility, add even further risks. Venous thromboembolic events are still a leading cause of maternal morbidity and mortality. Early detection of DVT (using duplex Doppler ultrasound) and initiation of heparin therapy have significantly reduced maternal mortality. Chest CT or a V/Q scan are options for evaluation if a pulmonary embolus is suspected. DVT/PE prophylaxis should be initiated upon the patient's admission, with the use of support stockings, compression devices, and/or subcutaneous heparin.

DISCUSSION

Several other anesthetic considerations in pregnancy are noteworthy. Propofol, thiopental, etomidate, and ketamine are examples of generally safe induction agents for the pregnant patient. The use of a 50:50 mixture of nitrous oxide and oxygen, and of halogenated agents (desflurane, isoflurane, sevoflurane) in low concentrations, is also considered safe. Careful examination of the patient's oropharyngeal and neck structures, noting range of movement and any obstructing lesions, is critical. Preoxygenation, intravenous fluid resuscitation, and left lateral tilt are all important steps in preventing hypoperfusion in both the mother and the fetus. Opiates, including fentanyl and morphine, are also considered safe to administer.

The use of local anesthesia is safe during pregnancy and is well tolerated by most pregnant patients undergoing minor oral surgical procedures. Although there is a theoretical concern that epinephrine-induced vasoconstriction could lead to decreased placental blood flow, epinephrine in local anesthetics is generally considered safe. Local anesthesia without epinephrine is an alternative. Despite concerns about potential teratogenic effects of benzodiazepines in the first trimester, they can be safely administered when the usual and appropriate doses are used.

For nursing mothers, it has been historically recommended that the patient "pump and dump" after receiving a general anesthetic. With current medications, nursing mothers can pump and discard breast milk for 8 to 24 hours after receiving an intravenous sedative or general anesthetic, to err on the side of caution. However, most agents have a very short half-life and very minimal crossover into breast milk that would affect the baby. Postoperative analgesics (hydrocodone, oxycodone, morphine, ketorolac [Toradol], NSAIDs) are safe to use without pumping and discarding breast milk. Perioperative intravenous steroids to help reduce postoperative swelling can be used in pregnancy and in breast-feeding mothers if necessary. Antinausea medications, as needed, also are generally safe to use.

Bibliography

Briggs GG, Freeman RK, Yaffe SJ: *Drugs in pregnancy and lactation*, ed 5, Philadelphia, 2005, Williams & Wilkins.

Cromwell C: Hematologic changes in pregnancy. In Hoffman R, Benz EJ Jr, Silberstein L, et al (eds): *Hoffman hematology: basic principles and practice*, ed 6, St Louis, 2012, Saunders.

Cumminham FG, Leveno KJ, Bloom SL, et al: *Williams obstetrics*, ed 21, New York, 2005, McGraw-Hill Professional.

Dollard DF: Radiation in pregnancy and clinical issues of radiocontrast agents. In Roberts JR, Hedges JR (eds): *Clinical procedures in emergency medicine*, ed 5, St Louis, 2009, Saunders.

Hawkins JL, Bucklin BA: Obstetrical anesthesia. In Gabbe SG, Niebyl JR, Galan HL, et al (eds): *Obstetrics: Normal and problem pregnancies*, ed 6, St Louis, 2012, Saunders.

Lawrenz DR, Whitley BD, Helfrick JF: Considerations in the management of maxillofacial infections in the pregnant patient, *J Oral Maxillofac Surg* 54:474-485, 1996.

Mozurkewich EL, Pearlman MD: Trauma and related surgery in pregnancy. In Gabbe SG, Niebyl JR, Galan HL, et al (eds): *Obstetrics: Normal and problem pregnancies*, ed 6, St Louis, 2012, Saunders.

Schwartz N, Adamczak J, Ludmir J: Surgery during pregnancy. In Gabbe SG, Niebyl JR, Galan HL, et al (eds): *Obstetrics: Normal and problem pregnancies*, ed 6, St Louis, 2012, Saunders.

Turner M, Aziz SR: Management of the pregnant oral and maxillofacial surgery patient, *J Oral Maxillofac Surg* 60:1470-1488, 2002.

Respiratory Depression Secondary to Oversedation

Piyushkumar P. Patel, Chris Jo, and Shahrokh C. Bagheri

CC

A 45-year-old woman presents to your office for cosmetic eyelid surgery (blepharoplasty).

HPI

The patient is an otherwise healthy woman for whom treatment was planned for bilateral upper and lower eyelid blepharoplasties with intravenous sedation. After the incision lines had been marked in the usual manner, ECG, blood pressure, pulse oximeter and a sidestream capnograph monitors were applied. The patient was administered 4 L of oxygen and 2 L of nitrous oxide via nasal hood (nitrous oxide decreases the amount of intravenous sedatives needed). Sedation was achieved using 5 mg of midazolam, 100 µg of fentanyl, and a propofol drip titrated to effect. Verrill's sign (50% upper eyelid ptosis, indicating adequate sedation) was observed. Prior to administration of local anesthesia, 40 mg of propofol was administered as a bolus (propofol may cause a 20% to 25% drop in systolic blood pressure when given as a bolus). Upon administration of local anesthesia, loss of the capnogram, with no chest wall movement, was observed. (This indicates the presence of central apnea. Capnography is considered to be more sensitive than clinical assessment of ventilation in the detection of apnea. In a study by Soto and colleagues (2004), 10 of 39 patients (26%) experienced 20-second periods of apnea during procedural sedation and analgesia. All 10 episodes of apnea were detected by capnography but not by the anesthesia providers.) The apnea was attributed to the propofol bolus (combined with the respiratory depressant effects of fentanyl), which was anticipated to resolve shortly. However, the patient continued to be apneic, and her oxygen saturation decreased from 99% to 80% (pulse oximeter readings are about 30 seconds behind the real-time oxygen saturation). Tracheal tug and paradoxical chest wall motion were not observed (these would be signs of upper airway obstruction and inspiratory efforts). The patient began to appear cyanotic (bluish hue to facial skin and lips due to prolonged hypoxemia).

PMHX/PDHX/MEDICATIONS/ALLERGIES/SH/FH

A thorough medical history is important during the preoperative evaluation of any patient undergoing intravenous sedation or general anesthesia to identify potential risk factors of intraoperative or postoperative anesthetic complications.

The past medical and surgical histories are noncontributory. This patient is categorized as American Society of Anesthesiologist (ASA) Class I (Table 3-1). She does not use any medications and has no known drug allergies. She denies previous problems with local anesthetics (e.g., methemoglobinemia), intravenous sedation, or general anesthetics (problems with previous anesthesia or adverse drug reactions should alert clinicians to possible complications that may require modification of anesthetic techniques). There is no family history of complications with general anesthetics (e.g., malignant hyperthermia). She denies a history of drug or alcohol use (patients with a previous drug history or alcohol abuse may require higher doses of sedative-hypnotic drugs), and she does not smoke (smoking decreases oxyhemoglobin concentrations and increases pulmonary secretions).

Table 3-1	American Society of Anesthesiologists (ASA) Classification System for Stratifying Patients Preoperatively by Risk			
ASA Category	**Patient's Health**	**Status of Underlying Disease**	**Limitations on Activities**	**Risk of Adverse Effects**
I	Excellent; no systemic disease; excludes persons at extremes of age	None	None	Minimal
II	Disease of one body system	Well controlled	None	Minimal
III	Disease of more than one body system or one major system	Controlled	Present but not incapacitated	No immediate danger
IV	Poor with at least one severe disease	Poorly controlled or end stage	Incapacitated	Possible
V	Very poor, moribund		Incapacitated	Imminent

Modified from the American Society of Anesthesiologists: *Relative value guide,* 2003, Park Ridge, Ill, the American Society of Anesthesiologists.

ABCs

- **A (airway):** The upper airway is rapidly evaluated and found to be clear of any obstruction. The patient's oropharynx is clear (secretions are suctioned with a tonsillar suction), and no inspiratory or expiratory noises are heard (stridor or gurgling noises may indicate upper airway obstruction). No tracheal tug is present. Chin tilt/jaw thrust maneuvers are applied.
- **B (breathing):** There are no inspiratory efforts, and no chest wall or abdominal motion (apnea) is seen. Breath sounds are not heard with the precordial stethoscope (placed above the suprasternal notch), and the reservoir bag is motionless. The pulse oximetry (SpO_2) reading has been steadily falling from 99% to 80%. (An SpO_2 of 90% correlates with a PaO_2 of 60 mm Hg; values below this correspond to the steep portion of the oxygen-hemoglobin dissociation curve.)
- **C (circulation):** Blood pressure and heart rate are stable (bradycardia and hypotension resulting from an extended period of hypoxemia are ominous signs of impending circulatory collapse). The electrocardiogram shows normal sinus rhythm without any ST changes. (Leads II and V_5 are most sensitive in detecting myocardial hypoxia.)

EXAMINATION

Preoperative. A thorough preoperative evaluation is important to identify potential risk factors for negative anesthetic outcomes, with an emphasis on airway anatomy.

General. The patient is a well-developed and well-nourished woman in no apparent distress who weighs 60 kg.

Airway. Maximal interincisal opening (MIO) is within normal limits (difficult intubation occurs with decreased MIO). Her oropharynx is Mallampati class I (soft palate, tonsillar pillars, and uvula completely visualized), and the thyromental distance (TMD) is three finger-breadths (intubation is more difficult with retrognathia, a short TMD, and/or a higher Mallampati classification). The cervical spine has a full range of motion.

Cardiovascular. Heart is regular rate and rhythm without murmurs, rubs, or gallops.

Pulmonary. Lung fields are clear to auscultation bilaterally (preoperative wheezing may increase the risk of intraoperative bronchospasm).

Intraoperative. During the course of intravenous sedation (conscious sedation, deep sedation, or general anesthesia), it is important to continuously monitor the patient's level of sedation and anesthesia (to prevent oversedation and respiratory depression) and to survey the ABCs (airway, breathing, and circulation [Box 3-1]).

General. The patient is sedated/unconscious and unresponsive to painful stimulus (a state of general anesthesia).

IMAGING

Preoperative and serial postoperative photoimaging is mandatory for cosmetic procedures. A preoperative chest radiograph has a limited role in healthy individuals and is not warranted unless dictated by other medical factors.

LABS

Routine laboratory tests are not indicated in healthy patients undergoing cosmetic blepharoplasty with intravenous sedation. Females of childbearing age who are sexually active and/or have missed their last menstrual period may require a urine pregnancy test (UPT).

ASSESSMENT

Central apnea secondary to oversedation during intravenous sedation for cosmetic upper and lower eyelid blepharoplasties.

TREATMENT

Before the diagnosis of respiratory depression (apnea or hypopnea) as the cause of hypoxemia, possible causes of upper airway obstruction need to be rapidly ruled out by evaluating the airway, jaw position, and possibility of foreign body aspiration. Subsequently, the procedure should be stopped, any open or bleeding wounds packed, and necessary assistance should be elicited. Attempts to arouse the patient with verbal command and painful stimulus should be made. Unresponsiveness to painful stimulus is considered to be a state of general anesthesia.

Respiratory depression secondary to oversedation is a self-limiting process that requires adequate supportive measures or pharmacologic interventions until spontaneous respirations resume. Respiratory depression causes a reduction in alveolar ventilation through a decrease in the respiratory rate or tidal volume, which in turn is caused by a decrease in respiratory drive. All sedatives, opioids, and potent inhalation general anesthesia agents have the potential to depress central hypercapnic and/or peripheral hypoxemic drives. Opioids primarily depress the central chemosensitive area (i.e., hypercapnic drive), whereas inhalation anesthetics and benzodiazepines exert greater influence on the chemoreceptors in the carotid and aortic bodies (i.e., hypoxemic drive). At high doses, all classes can depress both these mechanisms

Nitrous oxide is not a respiratory depressant; however, when it is combined with sedatives or opioids that depress ventilation, a more pronounced and clinically important depression may result. Therefore, it should be discontinued to allow more rapid arousal from anesthesia and delivery of 100% oxygen, with subsequent resolution of spontaneous respirations. Any anesthetic intravenous drips should be discontinued immediately. Jaw-thrust maneuvers and/or tugging on the tongue anteriorly will improve the opening of the airway for more effective oxygen delivery. The anesthesia circuit should be flushed to evacuate residual nitrous oxide and to deliver a higher flow of oxygen. If these measures fail, the patient's breathing can be assisted with positive pressure ventilation (PPV), at one breath every 5 seconds (coordinated with any apparent shallow breathing). If oxygenation proves to be successful with PPV, continued ventilatory support is maintained until the sedation lightens and respiratory depression resolves. However, if ventilation is not achieved, rapid re-evaluation for other etiologies (laryngospasm, bronchospasm, foreign body aspiration, chest wall rigidity) should be considered. The airway is reassessed, and chin lift/jaw thrust maneuvers should be optimized. Oral and/or nasal airways can be inserted if there is continued difficulty with PPV. If laryngospasm or bronchospasm is diagnosed, it should be treated promptly (see Laryngospasm earlier in this chapter). If these measures fail to re-establish ventilation, more advanced airway interventions may be necessary. These include the use of a laryngeal mask airway, endotracheal intubation, or establishment of a surgical airway (cricothyrotomy). Despite the infrequency of the latter scenario, the clinician should be prepared to establish an airway as soon as possible (see Emergent Surgical Airway later in this chapter). Once the oxygen saturation returns above 95%, the clinician can decide whether to cautiously continue with the procedure and intermittently apply PPV as needed or to abort the procedure for further evaluation.

If prolonged respiratory depression occurs, the sedative effects of some agents can be pharmacologically reversed. Flumazenil (Romazicon) reverses the sedative effects of benzodiazepines. It is given at 0.2 mg intravenously (or 0.01 to 0.02 mg/kg in small children) every minute up to five doses (maximum total dose of 1 mg) until reversal of sedation is accomplished. It may be repeated every 20 minutes for resedation. Naloxone (Narcan) is an opioid antagonist that reverses the sedative, respiratory depressant, and analgesic effects of opiates. Low doses are recommended (to prevent adverse effects of reversal) at 0.04 mg intravenously (or 0.001 mg/kg) every 2 to 3 minutes until reversal is accomplished (a higher dosing schedule is used in narcotic overdose). Once sedation has been reversed, the patient needs to be monitored for resedation, because the half-lives of naloxone and flumazenil are shorter than those of their sedative counterparts, potentially requiring redosing of the reversal agent(s). There are no reversal agents for barbiturates or propofol. Reversal of sedation from these agents relies on rapid redistribution of the drugs. It is important to remember that hypoxemia and hypercarbia can further contribute to central nervous system (CNS) depression.

In the current patient, supportive measures included 100% oxygen delivered via PPV with a bag-valve-mask device. PPV was easily accomplished, and the patient's oxygen saturation steadily increased to 99%. After sufficient ventilation and oxygenation, the surgery was resumed. The propofol intravenous drip was discontinued during the apnea/hypopnea episode and was subsequently titrated down as the procedure was completed. The patient began to have spontaneous respirations and maintained a normal capnogram and an adequate oxygen saturation, and she arose from sedation shortly after completion of the procedure. Reversal agents were not required.

COMPLICATIONS

Oversedation and respiratory depression can have devastating outcomes if not promptly treated as outlined here. In most circumstances, the patient's airway and breathing can be easily supported. However, it is important to identify those patients at higher risk of difficult mask ventilation and endotracheal intubation (see Emergent Surgical Airway later in this chapter) before administering deep sedation. The loss of the patient's airway (cannot intubate and cannot ventilate scenario) can lead to prolonged hypoxemia, which can in turn lead to cardiovascular collapse, cerebral anoxia, and death if not managed promptly.

Precipitous reversal of sedation and respiratory depression with opioid antagonists is not without adverse side effects. Naloxone (Narcan) may cause cardiac arrhythmias, pulmonary edema, severe hypotension, and cardiac arrest when given at higher doses. The analgesic effects are also reversed, which may cause the patient to experience profound surgical pain, accompanied by hypertension and tachycardia. Patients with acute or chronic opioid dependence can experience acute withdrawal symptoms. Naloxone and flumazenil have short half-lives and may require redosing every 20 to 30 minutes if resedation occurs; therefore, close patient observation is paramount.

DISCUSSION

Various levels of intravenous sedation can be administered by oral and maxillofacial surgeons. Conscious sedation is defined as "a controlled, pharmacologically induced, minimally depressed level of consciousness that retains the patient's ability to maintain a patent airway independently and continuously, with the ability to respond appropriately to physical stimulation and/or verbal command." Deep sedation is defined as "a controlled, pharmacologically induced state of depressed consciousness from which the patient is not easily aroused, and which may be accompanied by a partial loss of protective reflexes, including the ability to maintain a patent airway independently and/or respond purposefully to physical stimulation or verbal command." General anesthesia is defined as "an induced state of unconsciousness accompanied by partial or complete loss of protective reflexes, including the ability to independently maintain an airway and respond purposefully to physical stimulation or verbal command."

Respiratory depression from oversedation can occur during the course of a procedure or in the recovery period; however, it is relatively uncommon when sedation is administered by an experienced oral and maxillofacial surgeon (short half-lives and lack of active metabolites are ideal properties of intravenous anesthetic agents). The short duration of action of modern intravenous anesthetics relies on rapid redistribution (alpha half-life) and/or rapid metabolism. However, repeated doses of opioids, benzodiazepines, or barbiturates for longer procedures may cause accumulation in inactive tissues (especially adipose tissue), which is later released into circulation to cause delayed emergence (beta half-life), thereby on occasion requiring a reversal agent. Naloxone is an opioid antagonist that competitively binds to mu receptors, effectively reversing the sedative, analgesic, and respiratory-depressant effects of any given opioid (e.g., fentanyl, morphine, sufentanil, alfentanil, remifentanil, meperidine). Flumazenil is a competitive antagonist to benzodiazepines (e.g., midazolam, lorazepam, diazepam) at the central benzodiazepine receptor (alpha subunits of the GABA receptor), and it reverses all effects of benzodiazepines (e.g., sedation, respiratory depression, anxiolysis). The respiratory-depressant effects of midazolam (Versed, the most commonly used benzodiazepine) are minimal compared to those of propofol and narcotics.

Inadequate local anesthesia or insufficient time allocation for its onset may make the sedated patient appear uncooperative or undersedated. The clinician may decide to deepen the sedation to control the uncooperative patient and overcome the effects of inadequate local anesthesia. Once the painful stimulus is gone or the local anesthesia has set in, the patient may return to a deeper level of sedation or may become oversedated with respiratory depression. Risk of oversedation and respiratory depression can be minimized by using local anesthesia effectively.

Some additional precautions should be noted when administering anesthesia to pediatric and elderly patients. Small doses of benzodiazepines and opioids can cause significant respiratory depression in the elderly patient. The changes in physiology and medical comorbidities associated with aging are beyond the scope of this section, but a general precaution used by clinicians is "go low and go slow." It is important to remember that children have a lower functional residual capacity (FRC) and do not tolerate hypoventilation and hypoxemia well, which is evidenced by a more rapid drop in oxygen saturation. Differences in the pediatric airway (larger tongue, lymphoid hypertrophy, more rostrally positioned larynx, long and floppy epiglottis, narrowest at cricoid cartilage, more compliant tracheal walls, more caudal anterior cord attachment, underdeveloped accessory muscles) are important to recognize.

Capnography is the noninvasive measurement of the partial pressure of CO_2 in the exhaled breath. The relationship of CO_2 concentration to time is graphically represented by the CO_2 waveform or capnogram (Figure 3-2). (Time capnograms are more commonly used than volume capnograms, on which CO_2 is plotted against expired volume.) Pulse oximetry provides real-time information about arterial oxygenation, whereas capnography provides breath-to-breath information about ventilation (how effectively CO_2 is being eliminated by the pulmonary system), perfusion (how effectively CO_2 is being transported through the vascular system), and metabolism (how effectively CO_2 is being produced).

Capnography refers to monitors that display a continuous waveform reflecting inspiration and expiration. Although capnometers and capnographs both display numeric values for the end-tidal carbon dioxide ($Etco_2$) level and respiratory rate, capnography is preferred because visualization of the waveform allows continuous assessment of the depth and frequency of each ventilatory cycle (see Figure 3-2).

CO_2 monitors measure the gas concentration, or partial pressure, using one of two configurations, depending on the location of the sensor: mainstream or sidestream. Mainstream

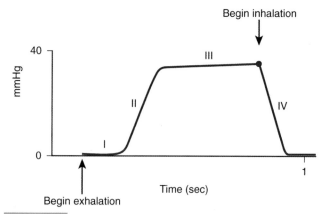

Figure 3-2 The relationship of CO_2 concentration to time, represented by a capnograph. *(From Krauss B, Hess DR: Capnography for procedural sedation and analgesia in the emergency department, Ann Emerg Med 50:172, 2007.)*

devices measure CO_2 directly from the airway, with the sensor located directly on the endotracheal tube. Sidestream devices measure CO_2 by sampling from the exhaled breath and analyzing via a sensor located inside the monitor.

The capnogram, corresponding to a single tidal breath (see Figure 3-2), consists of four phases. Phase I represents the beginning of exhalation. Phase II (ascending phase) represents the increase in CO_2 concentration in the breath stream as the CO_2 reaches the upper airway. Phase III (alveolar plateau) represents the CO_2 concentration reaching a uniform level in the entire breath stream (from alveolus to nose) and the point of maximum CO_2 concentration ($EtCo_2$); this is the value displayed on the monitor. Phase IV represents the inspiratory cycle, in which the CO_2 concentration drops to zero.

In a normal capnogram, for patients of all ages, the CO_2 concentration starts at zero and returns to zero (there is no rebreathing of CO_2); a maximum CO_2 concentration is reached with each breath ($Etco_2$); the amplitude is determined by the $Etco_2$ concentration; the width is determined by the expiratory time; and a characteristic shape is seen for normal lung function.

Capnography has been shown to be one of the earliest indicators of airway or respiratory compromise; it registers changes well before pulse oximetry registers a decreasing oxyhemoglobin saturation, especially in individuals receiving supplemental oxygen.

Both central and obstructive apnea can readily be detected by capnography (Table 3-2). Central apnea is confirmed with the loss of the capnogram, in conjunction with no chest wall movement and no breath sounds on auscultation. Obstructive apnea is characterized by loss of the capnogram, chest wall movement, and absent breath sounds. Two types of drug-induced hypoventilation occur during procedural sedation and analgesia (see Table 3-2): bradypneic hypoventilation (type 1), which is commonly seen with opioids, and hypopneic hypoventilation (type 2), which is commonly seen with sedative-hypnotic drugs.

The $Etco_2$ may initially be high (bradypneic hypoventilation) or low (hypopneic hypoventilation) without significant

Table 3-2 Capnographic Airway Assessment for Procedural Sedation and Analgesia

Diagnosis	Waveform	Features		Intervention
Normal		SpO_2	Normal	No intervention required
		$EtCO_2$	Normal	Continue sedation
		Waveform	Normal	
		RR	Normal	
Hyperventilation		SpO_2	Normal	No intervention required
		$EtCO_2$	↓	Continue sedation
		Waveform	Decreased amplitude and width	
		RR	↑	
Bradypneic hypoventilation (type 1)		SpO_2	Normal	Reassess patient
		$EtCO_2$	↑	Continue sedation
		Waveform	Increased amplitude and width	
		RR	↓ ↓ ↓	
OR		SpO_2	↓	Reassess patient
		$EtCO_2$	↑	Assess for airway obstruction
		Waveform	Increased amplitude and width	Provide supplemental oxygen
		RR	↓ ↓ ↓	Stop medication or reduce dosing
Hypopneic hypoventilation (type 2)		SpO_2	↓	Reassess patient
		$EtCO_2$	↓	Continue sedation
		Waveform	Decreased amplitude	
		RR	↓	
OR		SpO_2	↓	Reassess patient
		$EtCO_2$	↓	Assess for airway obstruction
		Waveform	Decreased amplitude	Provide supplemental oxygen
		RR	↓	Stop medication or reduce dosing
Hypopneic hypoventilation with periodic breathing		SpO_2	Normal or ↓	Reassess patient
		$EtCO_2$	↓	Assess for airway obstruction
		Waveform	Decreased amplitude	Provide supplemental oxygen
		RR	↓	Stop medication or reduce dosing
		Other	Apneic pauses	
Physiologic variability		SpO_2	Normal	No intervention required
		$EtCO_2$	Normal	Continue sedation
		Waveform	Amplitude and width vary	
		RR	Normal	
Bronchospasm		SpO_2	Normal or ↓	Reassess patient
		$EtCO_2$	Normal, ↑, or ↓*	Bronchodilator therapy
		Waveform	Curved	Stop medication
		RR	Normal, ↑, or ↓*	
		Other	Wheezing	
Partial airway obstruction / Partial laryngospasm		SpO_2	Normal or ↓	Reassess patient
		$EtCO_2$	Normal	Stimulation
		Waveform	Normal	Bag-mask ventilation
		RR	Variable	Reversal agents (where appropriate)
		Other	Noisy breathing and/or inspiratory stridor	Stop medication
Apnea		SpO_2	Normal or ↓*	Reassess patient
		$EtCO_2$	0	Stimulation
		Waveform	Absent	Bag-mask ventilation
		RR	0	Reversal agents (where appropriate)
		Other	No chest wall movement or breath sounds	Stop medication
Complete airway obstruction		SpO_2	Normal or ↓*	Airway patency restored with airway alignment
		$EtCO_2$	0	Waveform present
Complete laryngospasm		Waveform	Absent	Airway not patent with airway alignment
		RR	0	No waveform
		Other	No chest wall movement or breath sounds	Positive pressure ventilation

From Krauss B, Hess DR: Capnography for procedural sedation and analgesia in the emergency department, *Ann Emerg Med* 50:172, 2007.
*Depending on duration and severity of bronchospasm.
EtCO₂, End-tidal carbon dioxide; *RR,* respiratory rate; *SpO₂,* oxygen saturation; ↓ decreased; ↑ increased; ↓ ↓ ↓.

changes in oxygenation, especially with the use of supplemental oxygen. Therefore, drug-induced changes in the $EtCO_2$ do not necessarily lead to oxygen desaturation and thus may not require intervention.

Hypopneic hypoventilation can remain stable, with low tidal volume breathing resolving over time as CNS drug levels decrease with redistribution; or, it may lead to periodic breathing, with intermittent apneic pauses (which may resolve spontaneously or progress to central apnea) or progress directly to central apnea.

Capnography to monitor ventilation has been shown to provide the earliest indicator of airway or respiratory compromise. It is the only single monitoring modality that provides airway, breathing, and circulation assessment. The presence of a normal waveform denotes that the airway is patent and that the patient is breathing. A normal $EtCO_2$ value (35 to 45 mm Hg), in the absence of obstructive lung disease, reflects adequate perfusion. Unlike pulse oximetry, the capnogram remains stable during patient motion and is reliable in low-perfusion states. Capnography has been shown to trigger early intervention and decrease the incidence of oxygen desaturation. Capnography can forewarn of impending hypoxia by about 5 to 240 seconds. Administration of supplemental oxygen delays the onset of desaturation after apnea; therefore, relying on pulse oximetry alone delays that intervention. Starting in January, 2014, capnography will be required by law for procedural sedation in oral surgery offices.

Bibliography

Becker DE, Haas DA: Recognition and management of complications during moderate and deep sedation. Part 1. Respiratory considerations, *Anesth Prog* 58(2):82-92, 2011.

Becker DE, Rosenberg M: Nitrous oxide and the inhalation anesthetics, *Anesth Prog* 55(4):124-131, 2008.

Bennet J: Intravenous anesthesia for oral and maxillofacial office practice, *Oral Maxillofac Surg Clin North Am* 11(4):601-610, 1999.

Burton JH, Harrah JD, Germann CA, et al: Does end-tidal carbon dioxide monitoring detect respiratory events prior to current sedation monitoring practices? *Acad Emerg Med* 13:500-504, 2006.

D'Eramo EM, Bookless SJ, Howard JB: Adverse events with outpatient anesthesia in Massachusetts, *J Oral Maxillofac Surg* 61:793-800, 2003.

Dripps RD, Eckenhoff JE, Vandam LD (eds): *Introduction to anesthesia: the principles of safe practice*, ed 7, Philadelphia, 1988, Saunders.

Krauss B, Hess DR: Capnography for procedural sedation and analgesia in the emergency department, *Ann Emerg Med* 50:172, 2007.

Perrott DH, Yuen JP, Andresen RV, et al: Office-based ambulatory anesthesia: outcomes of clinical practice of oral and maxillofacial surgeons, *J Oral Maxillofac Surg* 61:983-995, 2003.

Roberts JR, Hedges JR: *Clinical procedures in emergency medicine*, ed 5, St Louis, 2010, Saunders.

Rodgers SF: Safety of intravenous sedation administered by the operating oral surgeon: the first 7 years of office practice, *J Oral Maxillofac Surg* 63:1478-1483, 2005.

Soto RG, Fues ES, Miguel RV: Capnography accurately detects apnea during monitored anesthesia care, *Anesth Analg* 99(2):379-382, 2004.

Vezeau PJ: Anesthetic and medical management of the elderly oral and maxillofacial surgery patient, *Oral Maxillofac Surg Clin North Am* 11(4):549-559, 1999.

Winikoff SI, Rosenblum M: Anesthetic management of the pediatric patient for ambulatory surgery, *Oral Maxillofac Surg Clin North Am* 11(4):505-517, 1999.

Inadequate Local Anesthesia

Gary F. Bouloux, Shenan Bradshaw, and Shahrokh C. Bagheri

CC

A 38-year-old man presents with left facial swelling and pain secondary to a carious left maxillary cuspid (acute infection decreases the efficacy of local anesthetics).

HPI

The patient reports a 2-month period of a toothache localized to the upper left quadrant. Two days ago, he experienced an acute exacerbation of his pain along with the development of progressively enlarging left facial swelling. He was subsequently seen by his general dental practitioner, who attempted to extract the tooth but was unsuccessful due to persistent pain despite several local anesthetic injections.

PMHX/PDHX/MEDICATIONS/ALLERGIES/SH/FH

Noncontributory. The patient has had multiple dental restorations under local anesthesia without any complications. He has no known drug allergies.

Although occasionally patients report an "allergy" to epinephrine, this is a naturally occurring catecholamine present in all individuals that plays a critical role in homeostasis and is not a source of allergic reactions. The transient tachycardia that may be seen with local anesthetic injections that contain epinephrine (especially with intravascular injection) is simply an adrenergic response to the epinephrine.

EXAMINATION

Maxillofacial. There is a fluctuant and tender swelling extending from the midline of the upper lip to the left cheek, consistent with left canine space abscess.

IMAGING

Panoramic radiograph reveals a carious left maxillary cuspid with an associated 1.5-cm periapical radiolucent lesion.

LABS

No routine laboratory tests are indicated unless dictated by the medical history. A WBC count may be obtained to evaluate the degree of leukocytosis during an infection.

ASSESSMENT

Left canine space infection complicated by failure to extract the left maxillary cuspid secondary to inadequate local anesthesia.

TREATMENT

Management of failure to achieve adequate local anesthesia should involve a thorough examination for the cause of the failure. Anatomic variation, accessory innervation, poor technique, inadequate volume or concentration of local anesthetic, the presence of infection, or an excessively anxious patient may all contribute to the failure to achieve adequate local anesthesia. Upon identification of potential causes, the clinician should develop a stepwise plan to address the problem. A reasonable approach may use supplemental anesthetic injections, regional block anesthesia (rather than infiltration), intraligamentary injections, intraosseous injections, intrapulpal injections, or addition of other medications, such as nitrous oxide, for anxiolysis and analgesia. With failure of all the above measures, consideration must be given to either deep sedation or general anesthesia.

In the current patient, the infraorbital rim (the infraorbital foramen is approximately 8 mm inferior to the rim) was palpated, and the overlying tissues was cleansed with an alcohol wipe. A total of 5 ml of 2% lidocaine with 1 : 100,000 epinephrine was injected after the tip of the hypodermic needle was placed through the skin against the foramen. The tissue was gently massaged to facilitate diffusion of the local anesthetic into the foramen to anesthetize the infraorbital and anterior superior alveolar nerves. The nasopalatine and greater palatine nerves were anesthetized in the usual manner. After 10 minutes, the left maxillary cuspid was extracted without any subjective pain. No purulent drainage was obtained through the socket; therefore, a horizontal vestibular incision was made, allowing the release of approximately 10 ml of purulent drainage. A sample of the pus was sent for Gram stain, aerobic and anaerobic cultures, and antibiotic sensitivity. A drain was placed, and the wound was left open to facilitate continued drainage. The patient was prescribed a 10-day course of penicillin and instructed to rinse with warm saltwater five times a day. An opioid with acetaminophen was prescribed for postoperative pain control. The patient was seen at 2 and 7 days for drain removal and follow-up, with subsequent resolution of the infection.

COMPLICATIONS

Complications related to failure to achieve local anesthesia are related to the psychological impact on and frustration of the patient and clinician, the added cost and time to complete a necessary procedure using a different modality, and possible toxic effects of local anesthetic due to repeat injections. The negative impact on a patient's perception of the dental profession should not be underestimated.

Complications may also be related to progression of the disease process (e.g., the spread of infection) that could not be treated due to the inadequacy of local anesthesia to permit extraction. Infection must be treated as soon as possible to reduce the likelihood of the patient becoming septic (disseminated infection). Furthermore, infections in close proximity to vital structures (e.g., the eye) may rapidly spread, resulting in dissemination of the infection into distant areas. This includes spread of infection into the orbit or, via communicating veins, into the cavernous sinus, with the development of cavernous sinus thrombosis. The presence of significant infraorbital swelling and tenderness is a relative contraindication to the use of the extraoral infraorbital anesthetic block due to concern for the development of cavernous sinus thrombosis.

There are several strategies to overcome the inadequacy of local anesthesia in the presence of infection. A larger volume or a higher concentration of the local anesthetic solution may be used. However, care must be taken to avoid toxicity from an excessive volume of local anesthetic. Toxicity initially presents as central nervous system (CNS) excitation, but with increasing doses, CNS depression (including respiratory depression) can be seen. Epinephrine substantially reduces toxicity by decreasing tissue absorption. However, epinephrine can result in tachyarrhythmias and increased blood pressure, particularly with inadvertent intravascular injection. Also, attention must be paid to the concentration of local anesthetic used, because anesthetics with higher concentration, such as 4% articaine and 4% prilocaine, have been found to be associated with an increased incidence of neurotoxicity. For this reason, it may be wise to limit the use of these anesthetics to local infiltrations rather than direct nerve blocks.

Care must be taken when infiltrating the area of the mandibular premolars with these anesthetics, because the mental nerve is in close proximity and could be affected by the higher concentration anesthetics.

The initial excitement and agitation seen with local anesthetic toxicity are due to suppression of the inhibitory cortical neurons, whereas the more common somnolence and decreased consciousness are secondary to inhibition of excitatory cortical neurons. Treatment is purely supportive, with attention to the airway, breathing, and circulation (ABCs) (see Box 3-1). An increase in heart rate (β_1-receptor stimulation) and blood pressure (α_1-receptor stimulation) may also follow inadvertent intravascular administration of a local anesthetic containing epinephrine. This should be considered carefully when patients with cardiac conditions are treated, although local anesthetics containing epinephrine are more efficacious due to the localized vasoconstriction that reduces systemic absorption of the catecholamine. However, the pain and anxiety generated with inadequate local anesthesia may be more harmful than the administration of a local anesthetic containing epinephrine due to the release of endogenous catecholamines. Aspiration after placement of the local anesthetic needle in the tissues and prior to injection should always be performed to reduce the likelihood of intravascular injection. The maximum doses of the most commonly used anesthetics are listed in Table 3-3.

DISCUSSION

Failure to achieve local anesthesia can be due to multiple factors, including the technique, anatomy, infection, and patient selection. The latter can often be predicted from the initial patient consultation and can potentially be avoided by alternate or modified surgical planning (sedation, regional block, preoperative anxiolytics). The appropriate choice of local anesthetic agent and adequate volume, and of infiltration versus regional block anesthesia, must be considered carefully. Anatomic variations may result in unusual neural innervation of mandibular and maxillary structures. A stepwise progression from more distal infiltration to more proximal regional block anesthesia often overcomes this difficulty. Anesthesia of maxillary structures may necessitate extraoral infraorbital anesthesia (as in the current case) or a maxillary

Table 3-3	Commonly Used Local Anesthetics in Oral and Maxillofacial Surgery			
Local Anesthesia	**Onset (min)**	**Duration of Action (min)**	**pKa**	**Maximum Dose**
Lidocaine	3-5	60-90	7.9	7 mg/kg (with epinephrine) 4 mg/kg (no epinephrine)
Bupivacaine	5-10	90-180	8.1	2 mg/kg*
Mepivacaine	3-5	45-90	7.8	5 mg/kg*
Articaine	3-5	60-180	7.8	7 mg/kg*
Etidocaine	5-10	90-180		8 mg/kg (with epinephrine) 4 mg/kg (no epinephrine)

*With or without epinephrine.
pKa, Dissociation constant.

(V2) block anesthesia via the greater palatine foramen or pterygomaxillary fissure. Anesthesia of the mandibular structures may necessitate consideration of accessory neural pathways, such as the nerve to the mylohyoid. The use of the closed mouth (Akinosi) technique for patients with trismus should be considered. The Gow-Gates technique may also be helpful when anesthesia of the mandibular trunk is desired or in cases of failed attempts at inferior alveolar nerve block using standard technique.

The presence of infection is generally considered to reduce the effectiveness of local anesthetics due to several mechanisms. The primary mechanism is due to the altered pH of the tissue. Different local anesthetics have different dissociation constants (pKa), which define the concentration of ionized and nonionized local anesthetic at a given pH. The nonionized form of the local anesthetic is responsible for penetrating nerve membranes and subsequently dissociating to give the ionized form, which blocks sodium channels. In the presence of infection (and hence a lower tissue pH), lidocaine, with a pKa of 7.9, exists predominantly in the ionized form, which is unable to diffuse through membranes. Although giving additional anesthetic is reasonable, a better choice would be to increase the concentration (percent) of the agent or to use a different agent with a lower pKa so that more of the nonionized form is available. Articaine is an amide local anesthetic with a lower pKa of 7.8 (more rapid onset), which when combined with high lipid solubility (depth of anesthesia) may be of benefit when infection is present.

Additionally, the increased tissue perfusion secondary to inflammation may increase removal of the local anesthetic from the site of administration, although this plays a minor role. A more proximal regional block anesthetic injection may also suffice in the presence of infection, because the local anesthetic is delivered into the uninfected tissue, and therefore problems related to a decreased tissue pH are avoided. It should be remembered, however, that chronic pain may result in both peripheral and CNS sensitization, which may reduce the efficacy of the local anesthetic, even when it is given as a regional block away from the source of infection or pain.

In the management of postoperative pain and discomfort, long-acting local anesthetics are often used when significant pain is expected, such as after multiple or third molar extractions. Bupivacaine and etidocaine are long-acting anesthetics with a duration of action approximately two to three times that of lidocaine or mepivacaine. The effectiveness of bupivacaine in obtaining profound anesthesia has been shown to be comparable to that of lidocaine, although the former drug has been shown to have a slower onset of action. Etidocaine has a slightly faster onset than bupivacaine and provides equally profound mandibular anesthesia when given as a regional block. However, the depth of anesthesia obtained when it is given as maxillary infiltrates has been shown to be somewhat less. A long-acting anesthetic is typically used in conjunction with another, shorter acting anesthetic for profound anesthesia during the procedure and extended pain control postoperatively. The benefit of prolonged anesthesia must be weighed against the risks, such as self-inflicted trauma and patient concern over prolonged numbness. If the decision is made to use a long-acting anesthetic, the postoperative expectations should be discussed thoroughly with the patient; delay in recovery of sensation beyond 10 hours is not uncommon.

Bibliography

Bouloux GF, Punnia-Moorthy A: Bupivacaine versus lignocaine for third molar surgery: a double blind randomized crossover study, *J Oral Maxillofac Surg* 57:510-514, 1999.

Feldman H: Toxicology of local anesthetic agents. In Rice S, Fish K (eds): *Anesthetic toxicity*, pp 107-133, New York, 1994, Raven Press.

Gaffen AS, Haas DA: Retrospective review of voluntary reports of nonsurgical paresthesia in dentistry, *J Can Dent Assoc* 75(8):579, 2009.

Garisto GA, Gaffen GA, Lawrence HP, et al: Occurrence of paresthesia after dental local anesthetic administration in the United States, *J Am Dent Assoc* 141(7):836-844, 2010.

Hawkins JM, Moore PA: Local anesthesia: advances in agents and techniques, *Dent Clin North Am* 46(4):719-732, 2002.

Tofoli GR, Ramacciato JC, De Oliveira PC, et al: Comparison of effectiveness of 4% articaine associated with 1:100,000 or 1:200,000 epinephrine in inferior alveolar nerve block, *Anesth Prog* 50:164-168, 2003.

Trigeminal Neuralgia

Mayoor Patel and Piyushkumar P. Patel

CC

A 52-year-old Caucasian female is referred by her physician for evaluation of an 11-month history of intermittent severe, stabbing pain and dull throbbing pain in the right maxillary zygomatic buttress area. (Trigeminal neuralgia [TN] is more common in women than in men by a ratio of 3:2. The condition usually affects the middle aged or older; however, young adults and children can also be affected.)

HPI

The patient reports the pain over her right check area as stabbing and at times shocklike, superimposed on a dull background pain of varying duration (95% of the time TN is located in the lower face and/or malar region). She rates her pain severity as a 9 on a 0 to 10 visual analog scale (most patients with TN rate their pain as 9 or 10 on a VAS). These episodes last about 10 to 35 seconds and are triggered by chewing, washing her face, or brushing her teeth. (Triggering stimuli may include talking [76%], chewing [74%], touch [65%], cold temperature [48%], wind, applying makeup and shaving. Intraoral TN triggers are associated with the gingiva). Between attacks the individual has periods of temporary remission, called *refractory periods,* during which it is impossible or extremely difficult to trigger pain (trigger zones characteristic of TN are not clinically identifiable in 40% to 50% of cases). The pain does not awake her from sleep unless she has slept on her right side (pain occurs on the right side over the left by a ratio of 3:2; it is typically unilateral, with bilateral pain reported in 1% to 4% of cases).

PMHX/PDHX/MEDICATIONS/ALLERGIES/SH/FH

The patient's medical history is unremarkable (the presence of hypertension increases the risk of TN 2.1 times in females and 1.5 times in males; multiple sclerosis increases the risk by a factor of 20). Her dental history indicates that she saw a dentist shortly after her symptoms began. She had received two root canals on her upper right first and second molars. Her symptoms did not resolve, and both teeth were subsequently extracted (due to its location and paroxysmal nature, TN has often been confused with dental pathology, leading to unnecessary dental treatment in 33% to 65% of cases). She still experiences bouts of pain that are triggered by eating, and she was treated for a temporomandibular disorder (pain with chewing is consistent with TMD) with oral appliance therapy.

She is anxious, depressed, and fearful of recurring attacks (quality of life is severely impaired with TN; depression is common, and suicides have been reported). She is married and has two young children. Presently she does not work because of her symptoms (talking provokes attacks in 74% of patients).

EXAMINATION

The patient is anxious; she appears well developed and well nourished. (Some patients limit their diet and thus exhibit signs of undernourishment.) There is no extraoral swelling or asymmetry. On palpation there is tenderness of the temporalis and masseter on her right side. She is very resistant to any palpation over her zygomatic area and to opening her mouth, for fear of eliciting sharp, shooting pain. Her opening is 42 mm with lateral excursions of 11 mm bilaterally and protrusive movement of 6 mm. Cranial nerve examination is noncontributory, and sensory testing is normal (this potentially differentiates between symptomatic and idiopathic TN). Oral hygiene is poor, with significant plaque buildup on the buccal surfaces of her right premolar area. No evidence of dental caries noted. Percussion and palpation over her premolars were negative. Gingival tissue is inflamed, primarily due to plaque buildup.

The physical examination in patients with TN is generally normal. Diagnosis of trigeminal neuralgia is largely based on an accurate clinical history (sudden onset of severe, unilateral facial pain lasting seconds) and necessary imaging (MRI with contrast or CT scan) to differentiate between symptomatic and idiopathic TN, regardless of age. Ruling out ear, mucosal, sinus, teeth, and temporomandibular joint (TMJ) pathologies is necessary, because problems in these areas may cause facial pain (see Table 3-6 for differential diagnoses).

IMAGING

Obtaining a panoramic radiograph (and, when indicated, periapical radiographs) is prudent to rule out the presence of dental pathology.

Radiologic investigations are important to distinguish between symptomatic and idiopathic TN. An MRI scan with gadolinium enhancement can demonstrate arterial compression of the nerve or rule out tumor or demyelination, as is seen in multiple sclerosis. (Compression lesions, such as vestibular schwannomas, meningiomas, epidermoid cysts, and other tumors, can cause symptomatic TN.) Magnetic resonance angiography (MRA) is useful diagnostically and can aid surgical treatment of the offending blood vessel. (Compression of the fifth or the ninth nerve root by a blood vessel, usually a tortuous artery at the root entry zone into the brainstem, is the most common source of neuropathic pain in idiopathic TN). If neither MRI nor MRA is available, contrast-enhanced CT scanning is effective in ruling out neoplastic causes.

In the current patient, the panoramic radiograph revealed multiple missing teeth. No osseous pathology was noted, and the results were otherwise unremarkable. The MRI scan of the head was within normal limits (WNL).

LABS

There are no specific laboratory tests required for diagnosis of TN. However, because TN is a diagnosis of exclusion, specific tests can be ordered to rule out other infectious or inflammatory conditions.

ASSESSMENT

Idiopathic TN predominantly involving the second division of the right trigeminal nerve (V2).

TREATMENT

For newly diagnosed TN, medical management is the first-line therapy (it reduces or eliminates pain in approximately 75% of patients). Medications used in the medical management of TN can be divided into antiepileptic drugs (AEDs) and non-AEDs (Tables 3-4 and 3-5).

Patients with TN do not respond to conventional analgesic drugs. However, almost all these patients (80% to 90%) respond to carbamazepine (Tegretol), and some clinicians use this response as a diagnostic criterion. Although the initial response is good, the long-term response is not as favorable, and a significant number of patients may become refractory as the symptoms increase. The dose of carbamazepine should be slowly increased until the pain disappears or the patient experiences side effects. After the pain has been adequately controlled for 6 to 8 weeks, it is advisable to titrate the dosage of carbamazepine to the lowest level that controls the pain. To avoid the side effects of carbamazepine, oxcarbazepine (Trileptal, a keto analogue of carbamazepine) can be used instead. Oxcarbazepine appears to achieve similar levels of pain control with a less distressing side effect profile and without the need for monitoring of hematologic profiles.

Over time many patients with TN on carbamazepine experience "breakthrough" pain attacks and require increased dosages for pain control. This is also true for other AEDs and may reflect progression of the disease process (see Table 3-4 for AED medications and dosing).

Other strategies worth considering for acute management of TN pain attacks are peripheral local anesthetic block (injecting the trigger zone), intravenous lidocaine (100 mg infused at 20 mg/min) and intravenous AED administration. Several case studies have reported on the use of botulinum toxin A (50 U), which is injected into trigger zones, in patients who are drug refractory. This approach was shown to improve the pain threshold, and a stronger stimuli was necessary to provoke pain. In one open label trial, topical capsaicin (Zostrix), applied locally to the trigger zone, was helpful for TN pain.

Surgical treatment options are divided into procedures that directly decompress the trigeminal nerve (involving a posterior fossa craniectomy and translocation of the offending structures); procedures that partially injure the nerve (percutaneous thermal radiofrequency ablation, percutaneous glycerol rhizotomy, mechanical balloon compression, trigeminal rhizotomy, and stereotactic radiosurgery); and palliative procedures (deep pain stimulation). Factors such as the patient's age, the location of the pain, and any associated comorbidities all are considered before a decision is made on which procedure to perform.

The current patient was started on carbamazepine 200 mg two times a day, which relieved her attacks for a month only. For her recurrent episodes, the carbamazepine dosage was increased to 1,000 mg a day. The patient's liver function test (LFT) results and CBC were monitored prior to medication initiation and at 3 months, with no significant changes seen while the patient was taking the medication. After 3 months the patient was experiencing some attacks, although not as frequently as before. Baclofen 10 mg three times a day was added to her regimen, which helped control her pain. After she had been pain free for 3 months, her medications were tapered over a 1-month period (if mild pain remains, maintenance at a low dose of an effective drug is preferable).

COMPLICATIONS

Medication management comes with its own risks and benefits. Carbamazepine, although an effective drug, produces several adverse effects that need to be considered and monitored. Carbamazepine is metabolized by the liver cytochrome P450 enzyme 3A4; in addition, it induces the several cytochrome P450 enzyme systems, thus altering the circulation levels of other medications. It is necessary to conduct serologic assessments of the patient's liver function and hematologic status; also, to determine whether the drug is in the suggested therapeutic range, the patient must have regular blood tests (these are repeated monthly for 3 months and then once every 3 to 6 months). The administration of carbamazepine during pregnancy has been associated with various birth defects, ranging from neural tube defects to congenital heart disease. (See Table 3-4 for additional information.)

Surgical procedures that produce destructive lesions in the trigeminal system usually provide effective pain control. However, these procedures do not treat the cause of the TN, which leads to the recurrence of pain over time. In addition, these procedures are more likely to produce other sensory disturbances involving the trigeminal nerve; these can vary

Table 3-4	Antiepileptic Drugs Most Commonly Used for Trigeminal Neuralgia				
Generic	**Brand**	**Classification/ Mechanism of Action**	**Dosing Guidelines**	**Side Effects**	**Comments**
Carbamazepine (CBZ)	Tegretol	Anticonvulsant/sodium (Na$^+$) channel blockade	Start at 200 mg bid; increase to 600-1,200 mg/day	Dizziness; rash; vertigo; drowsiness; fatigue; can increase liver enzyme levels; can cause marrow depression; aplastic anemia, causing irreversible cardiac or hepatic damage; reversible leukopenia; Stevens-Johnson syndrome (in patients with genetic predisposition)	Serologic assessments of liver function and hematologic status required; regular blood tests to ensure drug is in suggested therapeutic range; hyponatremia may occur (at higher doses)
Oxcarbazepine	Trileptal	Anticonvulsant/sodium (Na$^+$) channel blockade	Start at 150 mg bid; increase to 1,800-2,400 mg/day	Hyponatremia (at high dose), vertigo, fatigue, nausea, Stevens-Johnson syndrome (in genetically predisposed patients)	Serologic assessments not required; drinking milk daily can prevent hyponatremia
Gabapentin	Neurontin	Anticonvulsant/ unknown	Start at 100-300 mg hs; increase by 300 mg every third day to maximum of 3,600 mg	Somnolence, dizziness, ataxia, fatigue, nervousness, weight gain, nausea, headache	No drug-drug interaction, considered in patients with altered liver function, better tolerated than CBZ
Pregabalin	Lyrica	Anticonvulsant/ unknown	Start at 25 mg tid; increase to 100-200 mg tid	Dizziness, somnolence, peripheral edema, weight gain, nausea, headache	No drug-drug interaction, considered in patients with altered liver function, rapid escalation possible
Lamotrigine	Lamictal	Anticonvulsant/mixed	Start at 25 mg/day; increase to maximum of 100-400 mg/day	Dizziness, sedation, ataxia, nystagmus, irritability, diplopia, skin rash (rapid dose escalation), insomnia	Slower titration, recommended in combination with another anticonvulsant for refractory pain
Topiramate	Topamax	Anticonvulsant/mixed	Start at 15-25 mg hs; increase to maximum of 600 mg/day in divided doses	Abnormal delusional, psychotic thinking, impairment of word finding, renal stones	No drug-drug interaction
Divalproex sodium	Depakote	Anticonvulsant/GABA agonist	Start at 15 mg/kg/day; increase to maximum of 60 mg/kg/day	Nausea, vomiting, anorexia, ataxia, sedation, tremor	Second-line drug for patients who have not responded to other anticonvulsants or have developed significant side effects from them
Dilantin	Phenytoin	Anticonvulsant/sodium (Na$^+$) channel blockade	Start at 200 mg; increase to 300-500 mg bid	Nausea, vomiting, constipation, epigastric pain, dysphagia, loss of taste, anorexia, weight loss, headache, behavioral changes, folate deficiency (prolonged use)	Structurally similar to CBZ; gingival hyperplasia may develop

Table 3-5		Non-Antiepileptic Drugs Most Commonly Used for Trigeminal Neuralgia			
Generic Name	Brand Name	Classification/ Mechanism of Action	Dosing Guidelines	Side Effects	Comments
Clonazepam	Klonopin	Anticonvulsant/GABA agonist	Start at 0.5 mg tid; increase to 15 mg/day	Can elevate liver function values; drowsiness, ataxia, respiratory depression	Indicated when carbamazepine (CBZ) is ineffective or cannot be tolerated
Baclofen	Lioresal	Skeletal muscle relaxant/GABA agonist	Start at 5 mg tid; increase 5-10 mg every 2-3 days to 80 mg/day tid	Drowsiness, dizziness, muscle weakness, constipation, headache, itching, hypotension, nausea	Can be used as a substitute for CBZ in nonresponding patients on CBZ, prescribed in combination with CBZ or gabapentin if effectiveness of those medications decreases

Modified from Reisner L, Pettengill CA: The use of anticonvulsants in orofacial pain, *Oral Surg Oral Med Oral Pathol Oral Radiol Endod* 91:2-7, 2001.

from minor dysesthesias to more severe symptoms, such as analgesia dolorosa or anesthesia dolorosa.

DISCUSSION

Patients with TN report that they have severe head pain that lasts for hours to days; however, they may not specify that the individual unit of pain is brief (lasting seconds to 1 to 2 minutes) but occurs repetitively over the duration of the attack. Generally the first attack is totally unexpected, and most patients describe it as by far the worst pain they have ever experienced. The details of the first attack generally are remembered forever. The pain is described as lancinating, resembling an electric shock, feeling as if glass is grinding into the face, or much worse (Table 3-6). Patients may comment that attacks can be precipitated by various stimuli to the face. No neurologic deficits are present except when a tumor exists. Pain is confined to the distribution of the trigeminal nerve and is almost always unilateral. It is estimated that in 5% to 8% of cases, TN is precipitated by trauma, most commonly an acute flexion-extension injury. The pain is more commonly located in the V3>V2>V1 nerve distribution.

In deciding on the treatment options for a patient with TN, the clinician must take into account various clinical factors. The International Headache Society has classified TN into two categories: classic (idiopathic) and secondary (symptomatic). The two categories present with similar symptoms, but they differ with respect to causality. Classic TN includes neuralgia that is idiopathic or caused by compression of the trigeminal nerve by a nearby blood vessel (arterial loop of the basilar artery, most commonly anterior inferior cerebellar or

superior cerebellar), and it is by far more common (90%) than the secondary type. Secondary TN accounts for cases triggered by structural abnormalities (tumors, vascular malformation or demyelinating diseases). Rarely TN results from bony compression of the nerve (e.g., due to an osteoma or deformity resulting from osteogenesis imperfecta).

TN rarely occurs bilaterally; when it does, it is usually secondary to multiple sclerosis. TN never crosses the midline but on rare occasions may switch to the opposite side in different attack periods. Typically the time pattern of the pain is episodic, and the pain lasts for a few weeks to approximately a month. This can be followed by a remission period of several weeks, months, or years. Over time, there is a tendency to exacerbations and remissions, with an overall progressive increase in the frequency, duration, and severity of the attacks until the symptoms become continuous without remission. The character of the pain may also change, with an aching or burning sensation accompanying the shooting pains.

TN was originally called *tic douloureux* (painful tic), because the patient, when experiencing the pain, grimaces, especially on the ipsilateral side. Before the onset of TN, some patients have a prodrome of discomfort or moderate pain in the tooth, face, or jaw. In some cases this may precede an actual TN attack by weeks to months. During this period, patients usually present to a dentist and in many cases have teeth extracted, root canal procedures, and sometimes oral appliance therapy. A timely, accurate diagnosis of TN is particularly important, because a variety of specific treatments can greatly reduce or eliminate TN pain symptoms in many patients.

Table 3-6	Types of Facial Pain					
Diagnosis	**Location**	**Quality**	**Intensity**	**Duration**	**Triggers**	**Other Characteristics**
Trigeminal neuralgia	Second and third divisions of trigeminal nerve; unilateral Rarely, first division	Stabbing, sharp, shooting; electric shock like	Severe	Seconds	Touching or washing the face, eating, chewing, smiling, talking, brushing teeth, shaving	No sensory or motor paralysis in idiopathic cases
Postherpetic neuralgia	Usually ophthalmic or maxillary branch of fifth cranial nerve; unilateral	Burning, tingling, shooting	Severe	Continuous	Touch, movement	Allodynia, hyperalgesia, altered sensation
Glossopharyngeal neuralgia	Ear, tonsils, neck, posterior tongue	Sharp, shooting, stabbing	Severe	Seconds	Swallowing, chewing, yawning, coughing, touch	Unilateral Rule out eagle syndrome due to similar pain associations
Atypical facial pain	One side of face, nasolabial fold or side, chin, jaw, neck; poorly localized	Aching, burning, often stabbing	Mild to severe	Constant		Depressive and anxiety states
TMD	Jaw, mandible, preauricular region, masticatory muscles	Dull, aching, throbbing, sharp, stabbing	Mild to moderate	Minutes to hours	Prolonged chewing, talking, opening wide	Clicking, crepitus, limited opening, deviation of mandible on opening, ear pain and/or fullness, tinnitus
Tolosa-Hunt syndrome	Mainly retro-orbital; unilateral	Aching	Severe	Constant		Ophthalmoplegia, sensory loss over forehead, ptosis
Carotidynia	Face, ear, jaws, teeth, upper neck; unilateral	Throbbing	Moderate	Constant	Compression of common carotid artery	Compression of common carotid at or below bifurcation reproduces pain in some
Temporal arteritis	Temporal region; unilateral/ bilateral	Throbbing, dull, aching, tender	Moderate to severe	Constant	Pressure over temporal artery	Jaw claudication Usually seen in elderly Elevated ESR and C-reactive protein Temporal artery biopsy (4- to 6-cm segment) to confirm diagnosis

	Location	Quality	Severity	Duration	Triggers	Associated features
Alveolar osteitis (dry socket)	Affected bone	Sharp, aching, throbbing	Moderate to severe	Continuous 4-5 days postextraction	Open socket	Loss of clot, exposed bone, halitosis
Mucosal pathology	Affected mucosa	Sharp, burning, tingling	Mild to severe	Intermittent	Touch	Erosive or ulcerative lesions, redness
Pulpitis	Teeth	Intermittent, throbbing	Mild to severe	Minutes to hours	Mechanical, cold, heat, lying supine	Deep caries, extensive restoration
Maxillary sinusitis	Over affected sinus; unilateral or bilateral	Dull, aching	Mild to moderate	Constant	Touch, bending	History of URTI, nasal discharge, fullness over cheek with or without erythema over cheek
Burning mouth syndrome (BMS)	Tongue, palate, lips, pharynx	Burning, tingling, tender	Mild to moderate	Constant	Stress; spicy, acidic foods; vitamin and iron deficiency; candidiasis	Altered taste, xerostomia
Cluster headache	Orbital, suborbital, and/or temporal; unilateral	Boring, throbbing	Severe	Minutes to hours	Alcohol, smoking, stress, heat, cold, REM sleep	Autonomic symptoms
Tension-type headache	Frontotemporal and/or parietal; bilateral	Pressure, tight	Mild to moderate	Minutes to days	Stress	Not aggravated by routine physical activity
Migraine	Frontotemporal, orbital; usually unilateral	Pulsating, throbbing	Moderate to severe	Hours	Physical activity, stress, foods, odors, estrogen, alcohol, lack of sleep, barometric pressure	Aura (in migraine with aura) Nausea or vomiting, photophobia or phonophobia
Paroxysmal hemicrania	Periorbital, temple; unilateral	Boring	Moderate to severe	Paroxysmal: 1-40 attacks/day lasting 2-30 min	Neck movement	Autonomic features
SUNCT/SUNA	First and second divisions of trigeminal nerve; unilateral	Stabbing	Moderate to severe	Recurring: 1-200 attacks/day, 10-250 seconds each	Cutaneous triggers	Tearing, conjunctival injection
Orofacial tumors	Variable	Variable (atypical)	Severe		Jaw movement	Frequently neurologic signs, WBC abnormalities

Modified from Agostoni E, Frigerio R, Santoro P: Atypical facial pain: clinical considerations and differential diagnosis, *Neurol Sci* 26:s71-s74, 2005.

ESR, Erythrocyte sedimentation rate; *SUNA*, short-lasting unilateral autonomic headaches; *SUNCT*, severe unilateral neuralgiform headache with conjunctival injection and tearing; *TMD*, temporomandibular disorder; *URTI*, upper respiratory tract infection.

Bibliography

Bagheri SC, Farhidvash F, Perciaccante VJ: Recognition and management of trigeminal neuralgia, *J Am Dent Assoc* 135:1713-1717, 2004.

Bohluli B, Motamedi MHK, Bagheri SC, et al: Use of botulinum toxin A for drug refractory trigeminal neuralgia: preliminary report, *Oral Surg Oral Med Oral Pathol Oral Radiol Endod* 111:47-50, 2011.

Clark GT, Teruel A: Anticonvulsant agents used for neuropathic pain including trigeminal neuralgia. In Clark GT, Dionne RA (eds): *Orofacial pain: a guide to medications and management*, pp 95-114, West Sussex, UK, 2012, Wiley-Blackwell.

Cohen J: Current medical therapy. In Jannetta PJ (ed): *Trigeminal neuralgia*, pp 56-73, New York, 2011, Oxford University Press,

Elias WJ, Burchiel KJ: Trigeminal neuralgia and other neuropathic pain syndromes of the head and face, *Curr Pain Headache Rep* 6:115-124, 2002.

International Headache Society, Headache Classification subcommittee: The international classification of headache disorders, second edition, *Cephalgia* 24(Suppl 1): 2004.

Jannetta PJ: Typical and atypical symptoms. In Jannetta PJ (ed): *Trigeminal neuralgia*, pp 41-45, New York, 2011, Oxford University Press.

Jannetta PJ, Hadeed GJ: Medical therapy: the dentist's perspective. In Jannetta PJ (ed): *Trigeminal neuralgia*, pp 46-50, New York, 2011, Oxford University Press.

Krafft RM: Trigeminal neuralgia, *Am Fam Physician* 77(9):1291-1296, 2008.

Linskey ME, Jannetta PJ: Differential diagnosis: look-alike diseases, atypical trigeminal neuralgia. In Jannetta PJ (ed): *Trigeminal neuralgia*, pp 74-86, New York, 2011, Oxford University Press.

Love S, Coakham HB: Trigeminal neuralgia: pathology and pathogenesis, *Brain* 24:2347-2360, 2001.

Pawl RP: Trigeminal neuralgia and atypical facial pain, *Curr Pain Headache Rep* 1:175-181, 1997.

Reisner L, Pettengill CA: The use of anticonvulsants in orofacial pain, *Oral Surg Oral Med Oral Pathol Oral Radiol Endod* 91:2-7, 2001.

Scrivani SJ, Mathews ES, Maciewicz RJ: Trigeminal neuralgia, *Oral Surg Oral Med Oral Pathol Oral Radiol Endod* 100:527-538, 2005.

Scrivani SJ, Keith DA, Bassiur JP, et al: Nonsurgical management of facial pain. In Bagheri SC, Bell RB, Khan HA (eds): *Current therapy in oral and maxillofacial surgery*, pp 247-264, Philadelphia, 2011, Elsevier/Mosby.

Scrivani SJ, Keith DA, Mathews ES, Kaban LB: Percutaneous stereotactic differential radiofrequency thermal rhizotomy for the treatment of trigeminal neuralgia, *J Oral Maxillofac Surg* 57(2):104-111; discussion, 111-112; 1999.

Zakrzewska JM, Linksey ME: Trigeminal neuralgia. In Zakrzewska JM: *Orofacial pain*, pp 119-133, New York, 2009, Oxford University Press.

Zakrzewska JM, McMillan R: Trigeminal neuralgia: the diagnosis and management of this excruciating and poorly understood facial pain, *Postgrad Med J* 87:410-416, 2011.

Malignant Hyperthermia

Vincent J. Perciaccante and Shahrokh C. Bagheri

CC

A 15-year-old boy (incidence of malignant hyperthermia [MH] is highest in children and 75% in males) is undergoing an open reduction with internal fixation (ORIF) of a left mandibular angle fracture in the operating room. He had presented to the emergency department complaining of pain, swelling, and malocclusion. He has previously had ear tubes and a tonsillectomy under general anesthesia without anesthesia complication.

HPI

While playing ball, the patient sustained an accidental blow to the left side of the jaw from an opponent's elbow. He was diagnosed with a fractured mandible and subsequently was admitted to the hospital for treatment of his injury under general anesthesia. The patient was induced with propofol, given succinylcholine, and nasotracheally intubated without difficulty. He was maintained on sevoflurane (halogenated inhaled anesthetic) and intravenous agents. The patient had a smooth anesthetic course for the first 20 minutes of the procedure before the onset of unexplained tachycardia and elevation in his end-tidal CO_2 (earliest signs of MH). The diagnosis of MH was considered.

PMHX/PDHX/MEDICATIONS/ALLERGIES/SH/FH

The patient underwent tonsillectomy and adenoidectomy at age 6 under general anesthesia without any surgical or anesthetic complications (50% of MH cases occur in patients with two or more prior uneventful experiences with anesthetics). His family history is negative for MH. (MH is an autosomal dominant inherited disorder. However, many patients present with MH without any prior documented family history.)

EXAMINATION

MH is a life-threatening, pharmacogenetic hypermetabolic state that can be recognized by a variety of signs and symptoms, most commonly while the patient is under general anesthesia.

General. Muscle rigidity (commonly seen in the masseter, including masseter spasm) and skin mottling are present.

Vital signs. Heart rate is 130 bpm (unexplained tachycardia is one of the early signs), temperature 39.2°C (hyperthermia is regarded as a hallmark, but it may be a late finding, and the likelihood of complication increases 2.9 times per 2°C increase in maximum temperature), and respirations 34 per minute (tachypnea).

Adjunctive monitors. End-tidal CO_2 is 57 mm Hg and rising (hypercapnia). (The end-tidal CO_2 can rise to two to three times normal at a constant minute ventilation.)

ECG. Sinus tachycardia at 130 bpm (supraventricular and ventricular arrhythmias, including cardiac arrest, can be observed).

IMAGING

No imaging studies are indicated in the acute management of MH. A chest radiograph is obtained after the initial treatment to evaluate the position of the endotracheal tube if the patient remains intubated and for evaluation of the lung fields.

LABS

Upon diagnosis of MH, a full set of serum electrolytes, liver function tests, urinalysis, and arterial blood gases should be ordered to aid in the correction and diagnosis of electrolyte and acid-base disturbances.

The laboratory findings would characteristically reflect the following metabolic conditions:

- Acidemia (elevated P_{CO_2} and metabolic acidosis) (of cases seen between 1987 and 2006, 78.6% presented with both muscular abnormalities and respiratory acidosis; only 26% had metabolic acidosis).
- Hyperkalemia (secondary to acidosis)
- Hypercalcemia (secondary to reduced uptake of calcium from the sarcoplasmic reticulum of skeletal muscles)
- Elevated serum transaminases and creatinine kinase (CK) and subsequent rhabdomyolysis, causing myoglobinuria (secondary to hypermetabolic skeletal muscle activity)

The standard for diagnostic testing for suspected susceptibility to malignant hyperthermia is the caffeine-halothane contracture test (CHCT), which is performed on muscle biopsy specimens at specialized centers.

ECG changes and dysrhythmias can occur; these are late findings. They are due to elevated potassium levels from muscle breakdown. They can occur more rapidly in muscular patients.

The presence of premature ventricular contractions may indicate a life-threatening hyperkalemia and is an ominous sign, because this condition may degrade into ventricular tachycardia or ventricular fibrillation.

| Box 3-2 | **Steps for Treating Malignant Hyperthermia** |

1. Activate EMS if not in a hospital.
2. Discontinue the surgical procedure as quickly as possible.
3. Discontinue the triggering agents.
4. Hyperventilate with 100% O_2 at 3 to 4 times the normal minute ventilation.
5. Give dantrolene sodium 2.5 mg/kg intravenously, repeated every 5 to 10 minutes based on ongoing signs of MH.
   - 36 vials should be on hand (20 mg/vial)
   - Add 60 ml of sterile water without bacteriostatic agent to each vial of dantrolene to reconstitute the drug
   - Shake vigorously to reconstitute (until clear)
   - Use IV spike transfer pins to reconstitute
   - Once mixed, protect from direct light
   - 2.5 mg/kg body weight given initially, repeated every 5 to 10 minutes
   - Continue administration until signs of malignant hyperthermia (MH) abate
6. Obtain ABGs, treat hyperkalemia (glucose, insulin, and calcium) and acidosis (bicarbonate 1 to 2 mEq/kg).
7. In case of hyperthermia: Cooling measures should be instituted, with cold IV fluids (normal saline), external ice packs to the groin and axilla, and gastric lavage with cold solutions.
8. Call the MH hotline for immediate consultation in the United States and Canada at 1-800-644-9737.

ASSESSMENT

Acute onset of malignant hyperthermia during ORIF of a mandibular fracture.

TREATMENT

Successful treatment of MH consists of early administration of dantrolene (the likelihood of complication increases 1.6 times per 30-minute delay in dantrolene administration) and removal of the triggering agent. Box 3-2 details the steps that should be followed in treating MH.

Arrhythmias usually respond to correction of acidosis and hyperkalemia. Antiarrhythmic agents, excluding calcium channel blockers, may be used for arrhythmias that do not respond to correction of acidosis and hyperkalemia.

COMPLICATIONS

The mortality rate for untreated MH has been reported to be as high as nearly 70%. Approximately 25% of patients who experience MH relapse within the first 24 hours (recrudescence). After an MH episode, the patient should be transferred to an intensive care unit until all vital signs have returned to normal. Dantrolene treatment should be continued during this period; the usual dose is 1 mg/kg intravenously every 4 to 6 hours.

DISCUSSION

The incidence of MH in children may be as high as 1 in 5,000 to 1 in 65,000. In a genetically predisposed patient, triggering agents, such as succinylcholine and volatile anesthetic agents, release calcium from the sarcoplasmic reticulum, leading to elevated concentrations of calcium in the muscle cells. This increased metabolism causes the muscles to contract and become rigid. The increased metabolism leads to the elevated end-tidal CO_2 and acidosis. Rhabdomyolysis leads to hyperkalemia and potential arrhythmias, in addition to myoglobinuria and potential renal failure.

The routine use of succinylcholine has fallen out of favor. Many anesthesiologists use nondepolarizing agents, such as rapacuronium or rocuronium, when possible. However, none of these drugs have replaced succinylcholine for rapid sequence intubation or the reversal of laryngospasm. Dantrolene sodium should be available in all facilities at which any triggering agents are routinely used.

In preparation for an anesthetic procedure on a known MH-susceptible patient, anesthetic vaporizers are removed or taped in the OFF position. The carbon dioxide absorbent (soda lime or baralyme) is changed. Oxygen at 10 L/min is flushed through the circuit via the ventilator for at least 20 minutes. During this time, a disposable, unused breathing bag should be attached to the Y-piece of the circle system and the ventilator set to inflate the bag periodically. The use of a new or disposable breathing circuit is recommended.

Bibliography

Allen GC, Larach MG, Kunselman AR: The sensitivity and specificity of the caffeine-halothane contracture test: a report from the North American Malignant Hyperthermia Registry, *Anesthesiology* 88:579-588, 1998.

Ball SP, Johnson KJ: The genetics of malignant hyperthermia, *J Med Genet* 30:89, 1993.

Collins CP, Beirne OR: Concepts in the prevention and management of malignant hyperthermia, *J Oral Maxillofac Surg* 61(11):1340-1345, 2010.

Davison JK, Eckhardt WF, Perese DA: *Clinical anesthesia procedures of the Massachusetts General Hospital*, Boston, 2003, Little, Brown.

Larach MG, Gronert GA, Allen GC, et al: MH presentation, treatment, and complications, 1987-2006, *Anesth Analg* 110(2): 498-507, 2010.

Malignant Hyperthermia Association of the United States Web site. Available at: www.mhaus.org. Accessed February 6, 2013.

Patil PM: Malignant hyperthermia in the oral and maxillofacial surgery patient: an update, *Oral Surg Oral Med Oral Pathol Oral Radiol Endod* 112:e1-e7, 2011.

Rosenberg H, Fletcher JE: An update on the malignant hyperthermia syndrome, *Ann Acad Med Singapore* 23:84, 1994.

Emergent Surgical Airway

John M. Allen and Chris Jo

CC

A 48-year-old male presents to the emergency department (ED) complaining of difficulty breathing and the inability to swallow.

HPI

The patient has a 2-month history of intermittent swelling of his right mandible associated with caries affecting tooth #30. For the past 3 days he has developed rapidly increasing swelling of the right floor of the mouth (sublingual space) and submandibular triangle (submandibular space) that has spread to the contralateral side, consistent with Ludwig's angina (see Ludwig's angina in Chapter 4). For the past 24 hours, he has been sitting upright in the sniffing position (unable to lie supine because of a choking sensation), unable to control his secretions, having difficulty swallowing (dysphagia), and unable to open his mouth (trismus). His tongue protrudes (glossoptosis), and he experiences difficulty talking (dysphonia). His level of anxiety has increased with the onset of progressive dyspnea (difficulty breathing), and he is now unable to clear his airway. He makes gurgling noises with a faint, high-pitched, crowing sound (stridor); these are signs of upper airway obstruction.

PMHX/PDHX/MEDICATIONS/ALLERGIES/SH/FH

The patient's past medical history includes type II diabetes (well controlled) and morbid obesity.

EXAMINATION

General. Well-developed, moderately obese male in severe respiratory distress (obesity increases the difficulty of endotracheal intubation).

Vitals signs. Blood pressure is 168/94 mm Hg (hypertension), heart rate 120 bpm (tachycardia), respirations 25 per minute (tachypnea), temperature 39.4°C, and oxygen saturation 96% on 5 L oxygen via nasal cannula.

Maxillofacial exam. Bilateral submandibular and submental brawny cellulitis that is tender to palpation, warm to the touch, and erythematous. The neck is of moderate size; however, the trachea and larynx are easily palpable. The trachea is midline (a deviated trachea increases the difficulty of intubation). The cervical spine has full range of motion (neck extension facilitates intubation or securing a surgical airway).

Intraoral exam. Oral exam is limited due to decreased mouth opening. The patient is unable to control his secretions (dysphagia, evidenced by drooling of saliva). The floor of the mouth (FOM) is elevated, tender, and edematous. The tongue is large and protruding. The uvula and soft palate are not visible (Mallampati class IV). Tooth #30 is grossly carious. Further airway evaluation can be performed with fiberoptic nasopharyngoscopy (visualizing the hypopharynx, base of the tongue, pharyngeal walls, epiglottis, and vocal cords) to determine airway patency and the extent of airway edema. Figure 3-3 shows the surgical landmarks related to the airway; these are the thyroid notch, cricothyroid membrane, cricoid cartilage, and suprasternal notch.

IMAGING

In the setting of impending airway embarrassment, any attempt to obtain imaging studies should be delayed until a secure airway has been established. Loss of an airway in the radiology suite, where adequately trained personnel are not immediately available, can be devastating. For this reason, upon evaluation of the patient, the surgeon must quickly decide either to proceed to the operating room (OR), where optimal personnel and equipment for advanced airway intervention are available or, in a sudden emergency, proceed with immediate placement of a surgical airway in the ED. Immediate intervention should be considered only when the circumstances allow for other options.

If the patient is deemed stable, with no immediate threat to airway obstruction, a panoramic radiograph (to evaluate possible odontogenic sources of infection), and a computed tomography (CT) scan with contrast (to localize loculated areas of abscess formation and to assist in airway evaluation) can be obtained. A lateral cephalometric radiograph provides a reliable study that can be obtained at bedside. It can provide important information regarding the posterior airway space (prevertebral soft tissue should be less than 7 mm at the level of C3 and 20 mm at the level of C7). However, with the recent advent of fiberoptic nasopharyngoscopy and the use of CT, lateral cephalographs are rarely used today.

In the current patient, no radiographic studies were ordered due to airway instability; the patient was taken directly to the operating room.

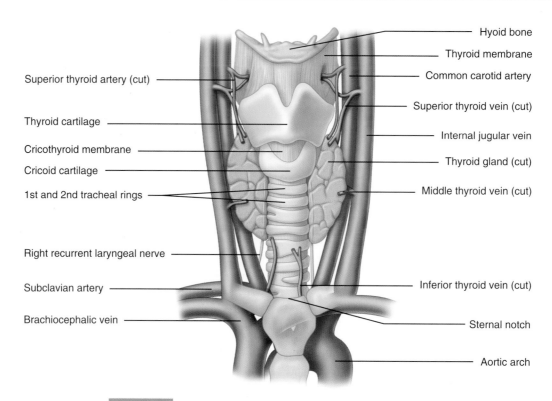

Superior thyroid artery (cut)

Thyroid cartilage

Cricothyroid membrane

Cricoid cartilage

1st and 2nd tracheal rings

Right recurrent laryngeal nerve

Subclavian artery

Brachiocephalic vein

Hyoid bone

Thyroid membrane

Common carotid artery

Superior thyroid vein (cut)

Internal jugular vein

Thyroid gland (cut)

Middle thyroid vein (cut)

Inferior thyroid vein (cut)

Sternal notch

Aortic arch

Figure 3-3   Surgical landmarks of the neck in relation to the airway.

LABS

Laboratory studies should not delay the establishment of a secure airway. When possible, a complete blood count (CBC) with differential and a basic metabolic panel (BMP) are indicated for evaluation of the systemic response and metabolic derangements associated with severe odontogenic fascial space infections. Arterial blood gas analysis can be used to determine the adequacy of ventilation. Other laboratory values are ordered based on pertinent medical information.

In the current patient, a STAT laboratory study obtained by the ED physician demonstrated a white blood cell (WBC) count of 18,000 cells/mm³ and a blood glucose level of 310 mg/dl.

ASSESSMENT

A 46-year-old male with Ludwig's angina, now complicated by an impending loss of airway.

TREATMENT

Upon suspicion or diagnosis of impending airway embarrassment, the anesthesia team and OR/ED staff must be notified immediately. The surgeon and anesthesiologist (if available) must decide upon the safest means of rapidly obtaining a secure airway. Risk factors that predispose patients to difficult mask ventilation and intubation should be identified in anticipation of using advanced airway intervention techniques. Such risk factors include obesity, a short neck, a rigid neck, a small mouth opening, retrognathia, Mallampati class III or

IV, and prominent upper incisors. An awareness of these factors by the surgeon contributes greatly to successful management of a compromised airway.

Patients deemed difficult to intubate are potential candidates for awake fiberoptic nasal intubation or an elective awake tracheotomy in a controlled OR setting. However, it is possible for a "routine" intubation procedure to develop into a difficult airway scenario. During the course of a difficult laryngoscopy, the anesthetist or anesthesiologist may not be able to intubate or adequately ventilate the patient, requiring an emergent surgical airway (fortunately, this is uncommon).

For emergent intervention for a comprised airway in the adult patient, a cricothyroidotomy is the procedure of choice. Tracheostomy is used for emergency surgical airways in pediatric patients younger than 10 to 12 years. The small size of the cricothyroid membrane (3 mm) and the poorly defined anatomic landmarks make performing a cricothyroidotomy extremely difficult in children. There is also an increased risk of laryngeal and vocal cord injury with cricothyroidotomy in this age group.

Needle cricothyroidotomy with jet insufflation can also be performed by skilled anesthesia personnel (providing temporary oxygenation, but not ventilation). The patient can be oxygenated while the surgeon establishes a definitive surgical airway (tracheotomy or cricothyroidotomy). If a surgical cricothyroidotomy is performed, conversion into a formal tracheotomy should be considered, primarily depending on the anticipated duration of the surgical airway (patients requiring prolonged ventilatory support should be converted to a tracheotomy).

Needle cricothyroidotomy with jet insufflation. Ideally the patient should be supine or semisupine with a shoulder bolster to hyperextend the neck. The cricothyroid membrane (the slight depression between the thyroid cartilage and cricoid cartilage) is palpated, and the larynx is stabilized using the thumb and forefinger. In a thin neck with prominent landmarks, an incision is not usually needed, and direct puncture through the skin and cricothyroid membrane can be accomplished. Otherwise, it may be necessary to make a small incision through the skin over the identified region of the cricothyroid membrane. A 3-cc syringe is then attached to a 14-gauge angiocatheter, and the catheter and needle are inserted through the cricothyroid membrane at a 45-degree angle caudally. Negative pressure is applied by withdrawing the plunger of the syringe while the needle is advanced (aspiration of air indicates entry into the tracheal lumen). The 14-gauge needle is removed from the angiocatheter, leaving the angiocatheter in the trachea. Once in place, the catheter can be insufflated with oxygen to provide aeration of the lungs. The intent is to provide oxygen to the lungs and also to allow passive exhalation. Various "kits" are commercially available that accomplish this; however, the effect can be obtained by cutting a small hole in the oxygen tubing near the attachment to the 3-cc syringe (can also be attached to a 7.5 endotracheal tube connector). The hole is occluded for 1 second and left open for 4 seconds, forcing oxygen into the trachea and allowing for some passive exhalation (if any). Adequate oxygenation can be maintained for 30 to 45 minutes, but hypercarbia results from inadequate ventilation. Therefore, preparations should be made to convert the airway to a tracheotomy to secure a patent, reliable airway.

Surgical cricothyroidotomy. The nondominant hand is used to stabilize the laryngeal cartilage, and a vertical skin incision is made using a #15 or #11 scalpel blade over the cricothyroid membrane (this provides the option of superior-inferior extension of the incision, if needed). The incision is carried through the skin and superficial fat layer, immediately over the cricothyroid membrane, which is also vertically incised with the blade. The scalpel handle is inserted into the incision site and rotated 90 degrees to provide access into the tracheal lumen. The lumen is further dilated with finger dissection or with the use of a Trousseau dilator. A small, cuffed endotracheal tube or a tracheotomy tube is inserted, and the patient is ventilated. A positive return of carbon dioxide is the best means of confirming correct tube placement. The tube is secured, and the chest is auscultated for bilateral breath sounds.

In the current patient, an emergent surgical cricothyroidotomy was performed after the airway was lost during an unsuccessful attempt at an awake fiberoptic nasal intubation. Due to the severity of the infection, the difficult airway, and the anticipation of prolonged cannulation, the cricothyroidotomy was subsequently converted to a formal tracheotomy.

COMPLICATIONS

The most feared complication of a needle cricothyroidotomy procedure is inadequate oxygenation and ventilation, leading to anoxic brain injury and cardiovascular collapse. Proper placement of the insufflating needle is paramount for a successful outcome. Placement and manipulation of the 14-gauge needle under emergency circumstances is also a grave concern. Laceration of adjacent structures, including the thyroid, posterior tracheal wall, and the esophagus, can occur, leading to severe hemorrhage that can cause embarrassment of the already compromised airway. Hematoma formation and aspiration of blood can contribute to a negative outcome. Improper placement of the needle can also result in subcutaneous or mediastinal emphysema.

Complications associated with surgical cricothyroidotomy include all the acute events discussed previously with the needle cricothyroidotomy procedure, in addition to chronic complications associated with the surgical intervention. Creation of a false passage into the surrounding connective tissue and damage to the larynx and vocal cords can result from improper or forced introduction of the endotracheal tube. Subsequent laryngeal stenosis or vocal cord paralysis may occur, resulting in permanent damage.

DISCUSSION

The possible etiologies of airway embarrassment (loss of airway) secondary to upper airway obstruction include severe maxillofacial trauma, infection, tumors, congenital or developmental deformities, laryngospasm, foreign body obstruction, and edema. Determination of the exact cause of airway embarrassment is based on physical and radiographic findings, in addition to the chronologic progression. A true loss of the airway is defined as the inability to ventilate (with a bag-valve-mask airway, a laryngeal mask airway, or a Combitube) and the inability to intubate. Although airway loss is usually progressive, it may have a sudden onset and occur prior to arrival in the operating room, during attempted intubation, after extubation, or during intravenous sedation.

It is important to differentiate loss of the airway from loss of protective airway reflexes, in which the patient has an upper airway obstruction that can be alleviated with chin lift/jaw thrust maneuvers, placement of an oral or a nasal airway, or positive pressure mask ventilation (see respiratory Depression Secondary to Oversedation early in this chapter).

There are numerous situations in which an oral and maxillofacial surgeon may encounter patients with difficult airways and/or acute airway embarrassment. The surgeon and anesthesia team should communicate to anticipate the likelihood of a difficult intubation (requiring awake fiberoptic nasal intubation) or possible loss of the airway (requiring emergent surgical intervention). The surgeon should take charge once the airway has been lost (cannot intubate, cannot ventilate scenario) and rapidly secure a surgical airway, as described previously. The operating room staff should be prepared to assist in an emergent cricothyroidotomy (in adults) or a tracheotomy (in pediatric patients).

Recognition of a compromised airway is the most difficult and crucial step in airway management. A compromised airway may be classified as sudden and complete, insidious and partial, or progressive. Assessment and frequent reassessment of airway patency and adequacy of ventilation are crucial. A patient's refusal to lie down may indicate that the patient is unable to maintain the airway or handle the secretions. Tachypnea is generally related to pain and anxiety, but it may also be an early indicator of airway or ventilatory collapse. Compromised ventilatory efforts may occur in unconscious patients suffering from alcohol and drug abuse, neck or thoracic injury, or intracranial damage. These patients often require endotracheal intubation to establish and maintain a definitive airway and to protect against pulmonary aspiration.

Objective signs of airway obstruction may be revealed with visual assessment to determine whether the patient is agitated or obtunded. Agitation may suggest hypoxia, whereas an obtunded patient may have hypercarbia. The abusive patient may be hypoxic and should not be presumed to be intoxicated. Cyanosis related to hypoxemia is manifested by the presence of a blue hue in the perioral tissues and nail beds. Visualization of chest retractions and the use of accessory muscles provides further evidence of airway compromise. The chest should be evaluated by auscultation. Noisy breath sounds, snoring, gurgling, and crowing sounds (stridor) may be associated with partial upper airway obstruction. Hoarseness (dysphonia) may indicate laryngeal obstruction or edema. The trachea should be palpated to determine its position.

A definitive airway comprises an endotracheal tube, connected to an oxygen source, that is positioned in the trachea. The three forms of definitive airways are (1) an orotracheal tube, (2) a nasotracheal tube, and (3) a surgical airway (cricothyroidotomy or tracheotomy).

Initial attempts should be directed toward placement of an orotracheal or a nasotracheal tube. If edema or severe oropharyngeal hemorrhage obstructs the airway, preventing endotracheal tube placement, then a surgical airway must be created. Depending on the experience of the surgeon, a surgical cricothyroidotomy is preferred to a tracheotomy in the emergent setting, because it is easier to perform; it is associated with less bleeding; and it requires less time. An awake tracheotomy is more appropriate in the difficult airway without acute loss of the airway.

Bibliography

Altman KW, Waltonen JD, Kern RC: Urgent airway intervention: a 3-year county hospital experience, *Laryngoscope* 115:2101-2104, 2005.

American College of Surgeons Committee on Trauma: Advanced Trauma Life Support for Doctors, 2004.

Bernard AC, Kenady DE: Conventional surgical tracheostomy as the preferred method of airway management, *J Oral Maxillofac Surg* 57(3):310-315, 1999.

Bobek S, Bell RB, Dierks EJ, et al: Tracheotomy in the unprotected airway, *J Oral Maxillofacial Surg* 69:2198-2203, 2011.

Dierks EJ: Tracheotomy: elective and emergent, *Oral Maxillofacial Surg Clin North Am* 20:513-520, 2008.

Haspel AC, Coviello VF, Stevens M: Retrospective study of tracheostomy indications and perioperative complications on oral and maxillofacial surgery service, *J Oral Maxillofac Surg* 70:890-895, 2012.

Lewis RJ: Tracheostomies: indications, timing and complications, *Clin Chest Med* 13(1):137-149, 1992.

Paw HG, Sharma S: Cricothyroidotomy: a short-term measure for elective ventilation in a patient with challenging neck anatomy, *Anaesth Intensive Care* 34(3):384-387, 2006.

Salvino CK, Dries D, Gamelli R, et al: Emergency cricothyroidotomy in trauma victims, *J Trauma* 34(4):503-505, 1993.

Spitalnic SJ, Sucov A: Ludwig's angina: a case report and review, *J Emerg Med* 13:499, 1995.

Standley TD, Smith HL: Emergency tracheal catheterization for jet ventilation: a role for the ENT surgeon, *J Laryngotology Otol* 119(3):235-236, 2005.

Stauffer JL, Olsen DE, Petty TL: Complications and consequences of endotracheal intubation and tracheostomy, *Am J Med* 70:65, 1981.

Stock CR: What is past is prologue: a short history of the development of tracheostomy, *Throat* 66(4):166-169, 1987.

Taicher S, Givol N, Peleg M, et al: Changing indications for tracheostomy in maxillofacial trauma, *J Oral Maxillofac Surg* 54(3):292-295, 1996.

Walts PA, Murphy SC, DeCamp NM: Techniques of surgical tracheostomy, *Clin Chest Med* 24(3):413-427, 2003.

Wood DE: Tracheostomy, *Chest Surg Clin North Am* 6(4):749-764, 1996.

CHAPTER 4

Oral and Maxillofacial Infections

This chapter addresses:
- Ludwig's Angina
- Buccal and Vestibular Space Abscess
- Lateral Pharyngeal and Masticator Space Infection
- Osteomyelitis

Odontogenic and nonodontogenic maxillofacial infections are among the oldest disease processes treated by oral and maxillofacial surgeons. They commonly present to the office, or in severe cases to the hospital emergency department. Although the majority of infections can be treated in a nonemergent fashion, early recognition and correct management of severe infections can be lifesaving. Knowledge of the surgical anatomy and path of spread of infections in the head and neck is fundamental to correct diagnosis and treatment. Severe infections of the sublingual, submandibular, and parapharyngeal spaces can cause airway compromise, cavernous sinus thrombosis, and possibly mediastinal spread of infection, resulting in significant mortality and morbidity, especially in the medically compromised patient who presents late in the disease process.

Despite the availability of a wide spectrum of antimicrobial agents and increasing knowledge of microbiology, the treatment of odontogenic infections remains primarily surgical. Removal of the source of infection and establishment of adequate drainage for elimination of the purulent material is the mainstay treatment. However, adequate antibiotic coverage is important and should not be overlooked.

The response to treatment can be monitored by several clinical (swelling, erythema, pain, interincisal opening) and laboratory (white blood cell [WBC] count, C-reactive protein) parameters. The measurement of temperature is an ancient method of monitoring the response to an infectious process. Fever occurs secondary to the production of endogenous pyrogens (cytokines, interleukins, tumor necrosis factor), which affect the hypothalamus and medulla to increase the temperature set point. The definition of fever is arbitrary, and there is considerable variability in "normal temperature" for a population of healthy adults. A range of definitions is acceptable (37.5° to 38.5°C), depending on how sensitive an indicator the surgeon wants to use. The lower the temperature used to define fever, the more sensitive the indicator is for detecting an infectious process, but the less specific it will be. Normal body temperature is generally considered to be 37°C and varies according to circadian rhythm and menstrual cycle. Many different variables can influence temperature such as exercise and environmental factors.

Chills occur in response to the elevation in temperature set point during the initiation of fever. This is often accompanied by the need for increased insulation and decreased exposure of skin. Shivering is also seen, contributing to the increase in temperature.

The differential is a ratio of the different types of white blood cells present (polymorphonuclear neutrophils [PMNs], lymphocytes, monocytes, eosinophils, and basophils). With a rise in the WBC count, as is seen during an acute infection, the predominant increase occurs in the PMNs. Chemotactic factors contribute to the recruitment of PMNs to the site of infection (or injury), with a subsequent increase in production of neutrophils by the bone marrow. Production of the precursor forms of the PMN (myelocytes and promyelocytes) increases, and these cells are released into the circulating blood. The movement toward circulation of immature forms is termed a *shift to the left* and is usually seen during acute infections.

In this chapter we present four teaching cases of infections that have an odontogenic etiology. We also present a case of osteomyelitis of the mandible.

Ludwig's Angina

*Solon Kao, Jaspal Girn, Chris Jo, and Shahrokh C. Bagheri**

CC

A 34-year-old, otherwise healthy man presents to the emergency department, stating, "My neck and tongue are swollen, and it all started with a toothache." (Ludwig's angina is predominantly seen in young adults, with as much as a 3 : 1 male predilection.)

HPI

The patient presented to the emergency department with a 3-day history of progressive swelling and pain in his neck. He reports a 3-week history of severe, intermittent pain in his lower right third molar. Ten days ago, his general dentist prescribed him amoxicillin for a periapical abscess and pericoronitis associated with his right mandibular third molar, which was partially impacted and decayed. Despite compliance with antibiotics, he progressively developed persistent swelling and a foul-tasting drainage around the tooth. He began to have swelling under the right side of his tongue (right sublingual space), which spread to the contralateral side (there is no anatomic barrier between the right and left sublingual spaces). Simultaneous with the floor of the mouth swelling, the neck began to swell on the right side, and the swelling spread to the other side. The patient reports having subjective fevers and chills (signs of systemic inflammatory involvement), in addition to dysphagia (difficulty swallowing) and odynophagia (painful swallowing). He states that he has not been able to eat or drink in the past 48 hours (causing dehydration). He denies dysphonia (difficulty speaking, seen with edema of the vocal cords and upper airway) or any chest discomfort (seen with advanced mediastinal involvement).

PMHX/PDHX/MEDICATIONS/ALLERGIES/SH/FH

This patient is otherwise healthy. (Diabetes mellitus and other immunocompromised states are risk factors for poor outcome and death [see Complications]).

EXAMINATION

General. The patient is sitting upright, appears very restless, and is unable to tolerate his oral secretions (evidenced by constant use of a Yankauer suction and drooling of saliva). He appears to be in mild respiratory distress, but there is no evidence of stridor (a high-pitched, crowing noise due to partial upper airway obstruction).

Airway. The airway is stable on examination. The trachea is difficult to palpate due to edema but appears to be in the midline. Fiberoptic nasopharyngoscopy can be performed to further evaluate the patency of the upper airway and the amount of edema of the surrounding soft tissue (see Emergent Surgical Airway in Chapter 3). Alternatively, computed tomography (CT) scans of the neck can delineate neck and airway swelling.

Vital signs. The patient's blood pressure is 138/89 mm Hg, heart rate 110 bpm (tachycardia), respirations 28 per minute (tachypnea), temperature 40°C (febrile), and oxygen saturation 96% on room air.

Maxillofacial. There is obvious moderate to severe facial swelling over the lower third of the face. Brawny and painful induration of the submandibular and submental spaces is noted bilaterally (Figure 4-1). There is erythema over the anterior neck extending down to the clavicles. However, subcutaneous crepitus (indicative of subcutaneous air from gas-producing organisms) is not present. No cervical lymphadenopathy or fluctuance was palpated (lymphadenopathy would be difficult to assess in the presence of neck edema or induration).

Intraoral. The patient's mouth opening is limited, with a maximal interincisal opening of 20 mm (trismus indicates

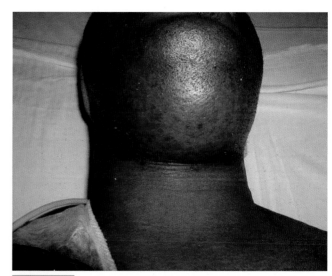

Figure 4-1 Brawny cellulitis and erythema of the bilateral submandibular and submental spaces.

*The authors and publisher wish to acknowledge Jaspal Girn, DMD, for his contributions to previous editions on this topic.

masticator space involvement or guarding secondary to pain). The floor of the mouth and tongue are elevated and edematous (sublingual space). The oropharynx is not clearly visualized due to the limited mouth opening and elevated tongue (positive predictors of difficult laryngoscopy and endotracheal intubation).

Cardiovascular. The patient is tachycardic, without rubs, murmurs, or gallops (tachycardia and friction rubs can be indicative of mediastinitis). He is negative for Homan's sign (crepitus heard with a stethoscope during systole, indicative of mediastinitis).

Pulmonary. Lung fields are clear to auscultation bilaterally, without rales, bronchi, or wheezes (aspiration of saliva or exudates can be seen with advanced cases).

IMAGING

Before obtaining any imaging studies, the surgeon needs to decide on the urgency of the infectious process compromising the airway. If the airway is deemed stable, imaging studies should be obtained to guide surgical treatment. However, any possibility of acute airway embarrassment should not delay direct transfer to the operating room for advanced airway interventions. Once the airway is stabilized, imaging studies can be safely obtained.

A panoramic radiograph is the initial screening study of choice. It provides an excellent overview of the dentition, identifying any odontogenic sources of the infection. CT scans of the neck with contrast material are indicated when dealing with deep neck space infections (chest CT should be included if there is a suspicion of descending mediastinitis). This study can help determine the anatomic spaces involved, localize any fluid collections (loculations of purulence), and determine whether the airway is deviated or compromised. CT is also helpful in surgical planning for incision and drainage. When a chest CT is deemed unnecessary, chest radiographs (posteroanterior and lateral views) can be an important screening tool to detect a widened mediastinum, which may be indicative of descending mediastinitis.

In the current patient, the panoramic radiograph revealed a carious right mandibular third molar with a large periapical radiolucent lesion. The CT scan of the patient's neck revealed a rim-enhancing fluid collection involving the bilateral submandibular, submental, and right sublingual spaces (Figure 4-2). In addition, there was diffuse soft tissue edema consistent with cellulitis in the involved spaces. No subcutaneous emphysema was seen in the cervical tissues (subcutaneous gas collection is considered a hallmark of cervical necrotizing fasciitis and is seen in up to 46% to 67% of cases). The patient's airway was patent and midline. A chest CT was ordered due to the erythema tracking down the anterior neck. No mediastinal involvement was observed.

LABS

A complete blood count (CBC) and complete metabolic panel (CMP) are indicated during the work-up of severe odontogenic infections. The presenting WBC count is a marker of the severity of infection, and this value should be followed during the course of treatment. C-reactive protein (CRP) is an acute-phase reactant that is released in response to inflammation, and it can be used to monitor the response to therapy. Studies have also suggested that a very high CRP level at the time of admission is a predictor of a complicated hospital course. Electrolyte disturbances (sodium, potassium, magnesium, calcium) are common among patients with severe head and neck infections, especially when the patient is not able to tolerate oral intake due to swelling or pain. Blood urea nitrogen (BUN) and creatinine levels are useful for evaluating for prerenal azotemia due to hypovolemia. Blood cultures are indicated in the patient with persistent fever. An electrocardiogram (ECG) should be obtained with suspicion of mediastinitis. Arterial blood gas (ABG) measurement is warranted in the critically ill patient presenting with septic shock.

The current patient presented with these lab values: WBC count 21,000 cells/mm^3 with a 35% bandemia, BUN 30 mg/dl (normal range, 7 to 18 mg/dl), and creatinine 1.2 mg/dl (normal range, 0.6 to 1.2 mg/dl). The BUN/creatinine ratio was 25 (a ratio greater than 20 is indicative of prerenal azotemia). The remainder of his electrolyte values were within normal limits.

ASSESSMENT

Ludwig's angina secondary to carious right mandibular third molar (odontogenic source of infection accounts for 70% to 90% of cases, the vast majority arising from second or third molars).

Ludwig's angina was first described by Karl Friedrich Wilhelm von Ludwig in 1836 as a rapidly progressing, gangrenous cellulitis originating in the region of the submandibular area that extends without any tendency to form abscesses. Ludwig's angina is now known as an aggressively spreading cellulitis that simultaneously affects the bilateral submandibular, sublingual, and submental spaces. Although Ludwig's angina is classically described as a cellulitis, progression to abscess formation within the involved spaces is most often the case, and to this date, clinicians still use the term "Ludwig's angina" when describing a bilateral submandibular, sublingual, and submental space infection. Grodinsky and Holyoke's criteria for Ludwig's angina may no longer have any useful clinical application. The term "angina" is a misleading term, because any chest discomfort seen with this is from descending mediastinitis and is not related to ischemic heart disease.

TREATMENT

Treatment begins with evaluation of the patient's airway and appropriate management to prevent acute airway embarrassment (see Emergent Surgical Airway in Chapter 3). The airway is first evaluated by the general appearance of the patient (a distressed patient with stridorous respirations is assumed to have an airway compromise until proved

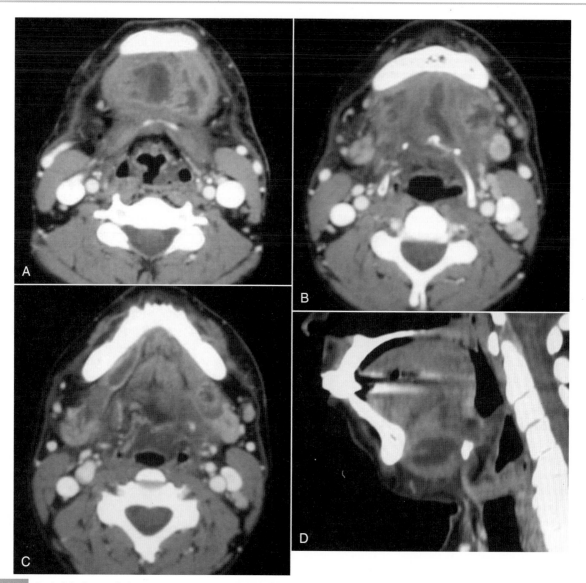

Figure 4-2   **A,** Axial view, soft tissue CT neck scan with contrast, showing an enhancing fluid collection in the submental space. **B,** Axial view, soft tissue CT neck scan with contrast, showing enhancing fluid collections in the submental and bilateral submandibular spaces. **C,** Axial view, soft tissue CT neck scan with contrast, showing an enhancing fluid collection in the right sublingual space. Note that Wharton's duct, seen on this view, confirms that this abscess is above the mylohyoid muscle. **D,** Sagittal reconstruction, soft tissue CT neck scan with contrast, showing a large submandibular space abscess extending from the inferior border of the anterior mandible to the hyoid bone.

otherwise). The oral cavity should be examined to evaluate the amount of tongue, floor of the mouth, soft palate, and pharyngeal wall edema (many times an oral examination is very limited due to the patient's inability to open). A fiberoptic nasopharyngoscopy can be performed in the emergency department to further assess the airway, including the vocal cords. Intravenous dexamethasone can be given to reduce the airway edema in patients with impending upper respiratory obstruction. An emergent cricothyroidotomy should be performed if the patient loses the airway before arrival in the operating room. An awake tracheotomy or an awake fiberoptic nasal intubation can be performed in the operating room if the situation is less acute (oral intubation by direct laryngoscopy may also be possible in less severe cases). There is support in the current literature for the assumption that a

tracheotomy may be indicated in patients with Ludwig's angina (see Complications).

Supportive measures should be initiated while arrangements are made with the operating room. This should include fluid resuscitation and initiation of broad-spectrum empiric antibiotic therapy. Fluid resuscitation is commonly needed because patients present with hypovolemia due to lack of oral intake (insensible losses are accelerated by fever) and/or some degree of sepsis or septic shock. Adequacy of fluid resuscitation should be continuously monitored (heart rate, blood pressure, urine output, and BUN/creatinine). Vasopressive therapy may be indicated in patients presenting with septic shock. Tight glycemic control (blood glucose 90 to 110 mg/dl) is desirable, especially in the critically ill patient.

Empiric antimicrobial therapy should be promptly initiated to cover the mixed aerobic-anaerobic polymicrobial organisms (gram positive, gram negative, aerobic, and anaerobic) commonly involved in these infections. Penicillin G at an adult dose of 4 million to 30 million units per day, divided and given every 4 to 6 hours, in combination with metronidazole, is an appropriate regimen. Other recommendations include clindamycin 900 mg given intravenously every 8 hours; ticarcillin clavulanate 3.1 g given intravenously every 6 hours; ampicillin sulbactam 3 g given intravenously every 6 hours; and piperacillin tazobactam 3.375 g given intravenously every 6 hours. Chow in 1992 recommended high-dose intravenous penicillin G combined with clindamycin, metronidazole, or cefoxitin. When available, the antibiotic regimen should be guided by cultures and sensitivity studies. The CRP has been shown to be an excellent marker for the severity of the infection and the patient's response to surgical and antibiotic therapy.

Aggressive surgical drainage and debridement, along with elimination of the source of infection, are necessary for definitive treatment. Delay in taking the patient to the operating room for surgical treatment is associated with a worse outcome. Cultures should be taken either via aspiration techniques or with a culturette swab. Most cases of Ludwig's angina can be managed using small incisions in the submandibular and submental regions (larger cervical hockey-stick or apron incisions may be indicated when the condition is complicated by necrotizing fasciitis). Blunt dissection is carried out to explore all the involved spaces. Subperiosteal dissection and debridement are important in the area around the source of infection, and any offending teeth should be extracted. The intraoral and extraoral dissections can be dissected to freely communicate, allowing for dependent extraoral drainage. Therefore the abscess is decompressed, the necrotic debris is debrided, and the wounds are copiously irrigated. Red rubber catheters and/or Penrose drains can be used to facilitate postoperative wound irrigation and to allow dependent drainage. Drains can be slowly advanced out of the wound postoperatively or removed when purulent drainage ceases. Repeat drainage and lavage procedures in the operating room should be considered, especially in more severe infections that are refractory to treatment. Bouloux and associates evaluated the efficacy of irrigating surgical drains on postoperative odontogenic infections. They found that nonirrigating drains (Penrose drains) appear to be equally efficacious as irrigating drains (red rubber catheter).

The current patient was given 16 mg of dexamethasone intravenously in the emergency department; intravenous fluid resuscitation was initiated; and empiric intravenous antibiotics were administered. Antibiotic therapy consisted of ampicillin-sulbactam (Unasyn) 3 g every 6 hours and clindamycin 900 mg every 8 hours. The patient was urgently taken to the operating room for incision and drainage of the involved anatomic spaces of the neck and extraction of the right mandibular third molar. The patient was intubated successfully via an awake nasal fiberoptic endotracheal intubation. An 18-gauge needle was used to aspirate purulent exudate from the submandibular space, which was sent for Gram stain, aerobic and anaerobic cultures, and antibiotic sensitivity studies. The surgical drainage consisted of three incisions of 1.5 to 2 cm in length, 2 cm below the inferior border at the angle of the mandible bilaterally and anteriorly in the submental area. Consideration should be given to placement of the incisions to allow dependent drainage. Blunt dissection with a hemostat and a Kelly clamp was carried out to explore all involved spaces. Copious amounts of purulence and necrotic tissue were expressed from the surgical sites. The right mandibular third molar was elevated and extracted. The gingival cuff was elevated, and subperiosteal dissection was carried out along the lingual plate to enter the sublingual and submandibular spaces. All the incisions were connected to each other in the subplatysmal and subperiosteal planes. Irrigation drains were placed in the submandibular, sublingual, and submental spaces. All drains were irrigated with copious amounts of antibiotic irrigation and/or normal saline irrigation. The patient was left intubated for 3 days postoperatively due to surgical and airway edema. After significant resolution of the infection and edema, he had a positive cuff leak test and was extubated over an Eschmann tube, which was left in place for several hours. He did not experience any postextubation airway compromise and was transferred to the ward the following day.

COMPLICATIONS

The most feared complication associated with Ludwig's angina is death due to airway compromise. Loss of airway from upper airway obstruction can occur at any time during the perioperative period, before arrival at the operating room, during an attempted intubation, after an accidental or self-extubation in the intensive care unit (ICU), or after a planned extubation (see Emergent Surgical Airway in Chapter 3). Potter and colleagues in 2002 reported a 3% incidence of loss of airway for patients who received a tracheotomy versus 6% for patients maintained with endotracheal intubation. They reported two deaths (4% mortality rate) secondary to loss of airway, and both deaths occurred in the endotracheal intubation group (one occurred after a planned extubation and the other occurred after an unplanned extubation). The tracheotomy group had shorter ICU stay (1.1 versus 3.1 days) and shorter overall hospital stay (4.9 versus 5.9 days). Patients with Ludwig's angina or a retropharyngeal space abscess have a significant need for tracheotomy. Har-El et al's review of 110 patients showed that 4 of 8 patients meeting their criteria for severe infection who did not receive a tracheostomy developed upper airway obstruction necessitating an emergent surgical airway (50% incidence of airway loss in the endotracheal intubation group). They concluded that tracheotomy is indicated in patients with Ludwig's angina. In 1985, Loughnan and Allen reported successful endotracheal intubation in 9 of 10 patients with Ludwig's angina using an inhalational induction technique and direct laryngoscopy, but they did not report on the postoperative morbidity and mortality. If postoperative endotracheal intubation

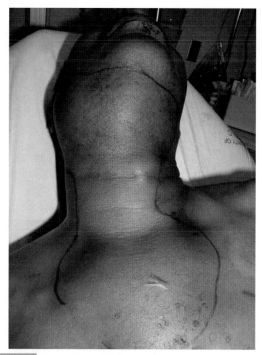

Figure 4-3   A patient with Ludwig's angina and descending mediastinitis via the anterior paratracheal spaces and bilateral carotid spaces. Note the soft tissue edema and erythema of the anterior neck tracking down to the sternum.

is planned, adequate sedation, four-point restraints, and a secured tube (taped around the head or wired to the teeth) are paramount to prevent unanticipated self or iatrogenic extubation. Upon extubation, a cuff leak test should be performed and an Eschmann tube should be left in place to facilitate reintubation if needed (postextubation laryngeal edema may cause loss of airway despite having a good cuff leak test result).

Before the advent of antibiotics, the mortality rate from Ludwig's angina was greater than 50%. Fortunately, the prevalence and mortality rates have significantly decreased due to better access to dental care and antibiotic therapy. When the condition is complicated by descending mediastinitis and thoracic empyema, the mortality rate remains as high as 38% to 60% despite antibiotic therapy (Figure 4-3). When the condition in complicated by cervical necrotizing fasciitis, the more recent reported mortality rate is 18% to 22% (any delay in surgical treatment increases mortality). Tung-Yiu and colleagues reported that an immunocompromised state (e.g., diabetes mellitus) increases the risk of an odontogenic infection developing into cervical necrotizing fasciitis. Of their series of 11 cases, seven patients were immunocompromised (four with diabetes mellitus), which accounted for all major complications, including two deaths. Others have reported a mortality rate as high as 67% with severe odontogenic infections associated with diabetes mellitus. Currently there is no evidence to suggest that HIV/AIDS status increases the risk of developing Ludwig's angina and its associated complications.

Other potential complications include aspiration, ventilator-acquired pneumonia, septic shock, and acute renal failure.

DISCUSSION

Ludwig's angina is defined by the involvement of specific anatomic spaces (bilateral submandibular, sublingual, and submental spaces). The sublingual spaces are bounded anteriorly and laterally by the mandible, superiorly by the floor of the mouth and tongue, and inferiorly by the mylohyoid muscle. There is no anatomic barrier between the left and right sublingual spaces. The submandibular space is separated from the sublingual space by the mylohyoid muscle, thus forming the roof of the submandibular space. The hyoglossus and styloglossus muscles form the medial border, and the body of the mandible forms the lateral border. The skin, superficial fascia, platysma, and superficial layer of the deep cervical fascia form the superficial boundary. The anterior bellies of the digastric muscles form the lateral borders of the submental space. The roof is formed by the mylohyoid muscle. The symphysis of the mandible and the hyoid bone form its anterior and posterior borders, respectively. The sublingual and submandibular spaces posteriorly communicate freely with each other and with the medial masticator and lateral pharyngeal spaces, which in turn is contiguous with the retropharyngeal space. Extension of the infection along the carotid sheath (contained within the posterior compartment of the lateral pharyngeal space [LPS]) or retropharyngeal space can lead to descent into the superior mediastinum. The alar fascia separates the retropharyngeal space from the "danger space" (space 4 of Grodinksy and Holyoke), which extends to the diaphragm and the posterior mediastinum. The anterior paratracheal spaces provide anterior access to the superior mediastinum (Figure 4-4).

Ludwig's angina most commonly has an odontogenic etiology (70% to 90%). A periapical abscess from the second or third mandibular molars is the most common cause. The roots of these teeth are commonly below the attachment level of the mylohyoid muscle to the internal oblique ridge. The periapical abscess perforates the lingual cortex, with spread into the sublingual (if the root is above the mylohyoid attachment) or submandibular (if the root is below the mylohyoid attachment) space. The infection can then rapidly spread to adjacent continuous or contiguous spaces. Other causes include peritonsillar or parapharyngeal abscesses, oral lacerations, mandibular fractures, and submandibular sialadenitis.

The bacteriologic profile of Ludwig's angina is usually polymicrobial and includes aerobes and anaerobes. The most common organisms are *Streptococcus viridans,* β-hemolytic streptococci, staphylococci, *Klebsiella pneumoniae,* anaerobic *Bacteroides* organisms, and *Peptostreptococcus* organisms. *S. viridans* is one of the most commonly isolated organisms. This is consistent with previous reports associating this organism with odontogenic infections. *K. pneumoniae* is another commonly isolated organism that has a higher incidence in patients with diabetes mellitus.

Sagittal section through neck

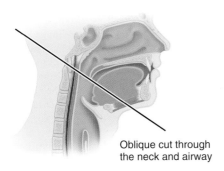

Oblique cut through
the neck and airway

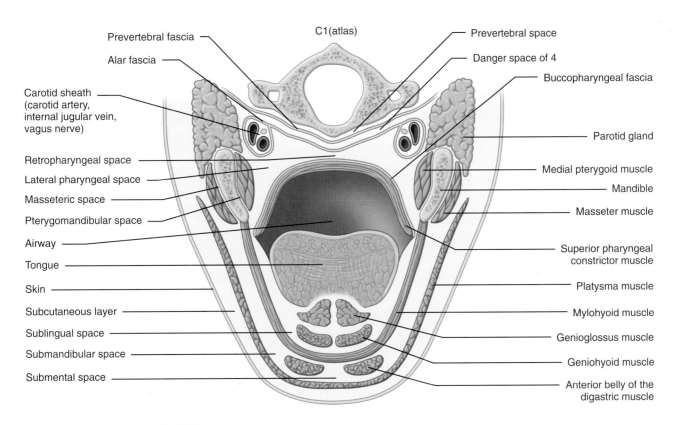

Prevertebral fascia

Alar fascia

Carotid sheath
(carotid artery,
internal jugular vein,
vagus nerve)

Retropharyngeal space

Lateral pharyngeal space

Masseteric space

Pterygomandibular space

Airway

Tongue

Skin

Subcutaneous layer

Sublingual space

Submandibular space

Submental space

C1(atlas)

Prevertebral space

Danger space of 4

Buccopharyngeal fascia

Parotid gland

Medial pterygoid muscle

Mandible

Masseter muscle

Superior pharyngeal
constrictor muscle

Platysma muscle

Mylohyoid muscle

Genioglossus muscle

Geniohyoid muscle

Anterior belly of the
digastric muscle

Figure 4-4 The fascial spaces seen as a transverse section cut at an oblique angle.

Bibliography

Allen D, Loughnan TE, Ord RA: A re-evaluation of the role of tracheostomy in Ludwig's angina, *J Oral Maxillofac Surg* 43:436-439, 1985.

Barsamian JG, Scheffer RB: Spontaneous pneumothorax: an unusual occurrence in a patient with Ludwig's angina, *J Oral Maxillofac Surg* 45:161-168, 1987.

Bouloux GF, Wallace J, Xue W: Irrigating drains for severe odontogenic infections do not improve outcome, *J Oral Maxillofac Surg* 71:42-46, 2013.

Chidzonga MM: Necrotizing fasciitis of the cervical region in an AIDS patient: report of a case, *J Oral Maxillofac Surg* 63:855-859, 2005.

Chow AW: Life-threatening infections of the head and neck, *Clin Infect Dis* 14:991, 1992.

Dugan MJ, Lazow SK, Berger JR: Thoracic empyema resulting from direct extension of Ludwig's angina: a case report, *J Oral Maxillofac Surg* 56:968-971, 1998.

Fischmann GE, Graham BS: Ludwig's angina resulting from infection of an oral malignancy, *J Oral Maxillofac Surg* 43:795-796, 1985.

Har-El G, Aroesty JH, Shana A, et al: A retrospective study of 110 patients, *Oral Surg Oral Med Oral Pathol* 77(5):446-450, 1994.

Loughnan TE, Allen DE: Ludwig's angina: the anaesthetic management of nine cases, *Anaesthesia* 40:295-297, 1985.

Mihos P, Potaris K, Gakidis I, et al: Management of descending necrotizing mediastinitis, *J Oral Maxillofac Surg* 62:966-972, 2004.

Potter JK, Herford AS, Ellis E: Tracheotomy versus endotracheal intubation for airway management in deep neck space infections, *J Oral Maxillofac Surg* 60:349-354, 2002.

Steiner M, Gau MJ, Wilson DL, et al: Odontogenic infection leading to cervical emphysema and fatal mediastinitis, *J Oral Maxillofac Surg* 40:600-604, 1982.

Sugata T, Fujita Y, Myoken Y, et al: Cervical cellulitis with mediastinitis from an odontogenic infection complicated by diabetes mellitus: report of a case, *J Oral Maxillofac Surg* 55:864-869, 1997.

Tsuji T, Shimono M, Yamane G, et al: Ludwig's angina as a complication of ameloblastoma of the mandible, *J Oral Maxillofac Surg* 42:815-819, 1984.

Tsunoda R, Suda S, Fukaya T, et al: Descending necrotizing mediastinitis caused by an odontogenic infection: a case report, *J Oral Maxillofac Surg* 58:240-242, 2000.

Tung-Yiu W, Jehn-Shyun H, Ching-Hung C, et al: Cervical necrotizing fasciitis of odontogenic origin: a report of 11 cases, *J Oral Maxillofac Surg* 58:1347-1352, 2000.

Ylijoki S, Suuronen R, Jousimies-Somer H, et al: Differences between patients with or without the need for intensive care due to severe odontogenic infections, *J Oral Maxillofac Surg* 59:867-872, 2001.

Zachariades N, Mezitis M, Stavrinidis P, et al: Mediastinitis, thoracic empyema, and pericarditis as complications of a dental abscess: report of a case, *J Oral Maxillofac Surg* 46:493-495, 1988.

Buccal and Vestibular Space Abscess

Abtin Shahriari, Piyushkumar P. Patel, and Shahrokh C. Bagheri

CC

A 34-year-old woman presents to the urgent care clinic complaining of pain and progressively enlarging swelling of her right cheek within the past 4 days.

HPI

The patient has not received any dental care for the past several years (risk factor for odontogenic infections). Two weeks earlier, she noticed that a segment of a restoration broke off the right maxillary second molar. At the time, there was an acute, localized pain in the right posterior maxillary molar with subsequent development of swelling in the right buccal vestibule (buccal vestibular space infection). The patient decided to take over-the-counter medications, and her pain subsided but the swelling persisted. Two days before presentation, she developed acute onset of right-side swelling of the cheek associated with mild pain and discomfort that have progressively exacerbated. There is no history of trismus, visual changes, dysphagia, swelling of the floor of the mouth, or difficulty breathing (all of which are signs of more severe facial space involvement, such as masticator space infection, periorbital extension, and parapharyngeal or sublingual infections; these signs are not seen with pure buccal and vestibular space involvement).

PMHX/PDHX/MEDICATIONS/ALLERGIES/SH/FH

Noncontributory. Severe odontogenic infections are most commonly seen in patients with a history of dental neglect, although they are not exclusive to any group. When infections are seen in patients with compromised immunity (AIDS, diabetes, chemotherapy), the infectious process may prove more resistant to treatment.

EXAMINATION

General. The patient was a well-developed and well-nourished woman in mild distress (patients with buccal space infections are frequently very concerned due to the extent of swelling and pain).

Vital signs. Stable and WNL. Temperature of 98.8°F (an elevated temperature is not always seen, especially in well-localized infections, unless there is surrounding cellulitis or systemic dissemination of the infection).

Maxillofacial. Significant right-side facial edema extending from the inferior border of the mandible superiorly to the level of the zygoma (Figure 4-5). The swelling is soft and fluctuant and with no apparent intraoral or extraoral drainage (untreated buccal space infections may spontaneously drain, providing some relief or spread into other fascial spaces). There is tender right submandibular lymphadenopathy (due to active infection).

Intraoral. The maximal interincisal opening is 35 mm (trismus is not seen with vestibular space or buccal space infections, because it does not involve the muscles of mastication, unless the infection has spread from buccal space to the submasseteric space posteriorly, pterygomandibular space inferiorly, and infratemporal space superiorly). Bimanual examination of the right posterior buccal vestibule and right cheek reveals fluctuance within the right maxillary vestibule extending to the depth of the mandibular vestibule. The right maxillary second molar (tooth #2) is grossly carious. The floor of the mouth is soft and not elevated (it is important to assess the airway for patency), the oropharynx is clear, and the uvula is midline (deviation is seen with lateral pharyngeal space [LPS] infections).

A key clinical finding of buccal space infections is the general lack of extension of swelling below the inferior border of the mandible. Infections can spread in a subcutaneous plane to the neck or the periorbital tissue, but extension beyond the buccal area implies tissue involvement beyond this space. The buccal space does not compromise the airway.

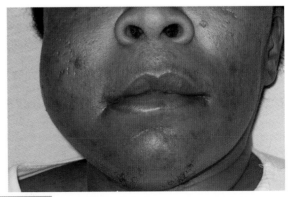

Figure 4-5 Swelling of the right face secondary to a buccal space abscess.

IMAGING

The panoramic radiograph is the imaging study of choice for the evaluation of the odontogenic etiology of suspected vestibular and buccal space infections and is frequently the only imaging study that is necessary. It allows a general screening of the bony anatomy of the maxillofacial region, in addition to identification of potential odontogenic sources of infection (most commonly, the maxillary or mandibular first or second molars). A CT scan with intravenous contrast material can be obtained if there is clinical suspicion of orbital, parapharyngeal, or submandibular space involvement.

For the current patient, the panoramic radiograph demonstrated a severely carious right maxillary second molar with a well-demarcated periapical radiolucent lesion.

LABS

No routine laboratory tests are indicated for the evaluation and treatment of buccal space infections. A CBC can be obtained to assess for leukocytosis (elevated WBC count). The results of this test may be valuable in cases that are refractory to treatment or in the presence of other medical comorbidities. The WBC count may not be elevated with isolated vestibular or buccal space infections.

Routine use of culture and sensitivity studies for all vestibular and buccal space infections is not indicated. However, in patients with multiple comorbidities or infections that are resistant to conventional therapy, culture and sensitivity studies may be useful to guide antimicrobial therapy.

ASSESSMENT

Right vestibular space infection and subsequent spread to buccal space secondary to carious right maxillary second molar.

TREATMENT

Surgical establishment of drainage, along with removal of the source of infection, is the most important treatment for vestibular and buccal space infections. Antibiotic therapy is considered beneficial and should be initiated to aid resolution of the infection.

In cases of odontogenic etiology, tooth extraction or endodontic therapy eliminates the source of infection. Extraction, when possible, is more effective, because it also allows spontaneous drainage of the infection. Drainage allows removal of purulent material, increases tissue perfusion, and therefore enhances the delivery of both oxygen and antibiotics. Incision and drainage is one of the oldest and most effective surgical procedures. Ideally, abscesses should be drained when fluctuant, before spontaneous rupture and drainage.

Several basic principles should be applied when draining an infection:

- The incision is best placed in healthy mucosa or skin when possible.

- Camouflage of the incision can be achieved by placing the incision in an aesthetic area, such as inside the mouth or in the crease of the neck (for a buccal space infection).
- Anatomic placement of an incision allows drainage by gravity. Careful attention is given to the position of the mental nerve.
- A drain should be placed for open communication, with subsequent removal once drainage has ceased.

The incision is frequently placed intraorally through the mucosa in a transverse orientation (although transcutaneous incisions may be necessary in select cases). For a buccal space infection, the buccinator muscle is bluntly penetrated using a hemostat, entering the buccal space. Culture and sensitivity studies should be obtained when indicated (see earlier discussion). Frequent irrigation of the wound can be helpful. Other supportive measures, such as intravenous fluid therapy (hydration), good oral hygiene, and nutritional support, are prescribed as necessary.

In the current case, with the patient under intravenous sedation anesthesia, needle aspiration of the buccal space was accomplished, collecting 5 ml of brown, purulent material that was sent for culture and sensitivity studies. Subsequently, the second molar was extracted and the apex was curetted. Blunt dissection was carried to the buccal maxillary cortex, and an area of perforation adjacent to the tooth was identified. Next, a small transverse incision was placed intraorally about 1 cm superior to the depth of the mandibular vestibule, allowing drainage of another 8 ml of pus.

The vestibular and buccal spaces and the extraction socket were copiously irrigated, and a Penrose drain was placed in the buccal space and secured with a 2-0 silk suture. The patient was prescribed a 10-day course of penicillin (penicillin remains the empiric antibiotic of choice for outpatient odontogenic infections). The patient was seen in the office the next day and then 3 days later for removal of the drain because of progressive resolution of the infection.

COMPLICATIONS

Complications of vestibular and buccal space infections are related to:
- Delay in the diagnosis, leading to systemic or local spread of the infection (sepsis)
- Surgical interventions that result in inadequate drainage
- Compromised host immunity, leading to failure of therapy
- Antibiotic-resistant organisms or inadequate pharmacotherapy
- Damage to vital structures due to surgical interventions

Rapid recognition of these complications can improve the outcome.

The vestibular space primarily contains areolar connective tissue, but it is crossed by the parotid duct and the long buccal and mental nerves. Incisions should be made to avoid Stensen's duct in the posterior maxillary vestibule, the mental nerve in the apical region of the mandibular premolars, the infraorbital nerve in the apical region of the maxillary cuspids, and the greater palatine neurovascular bundle in cases of palatal infections. Vestibular infections can pass around the levator anguli oris muscle to enter the infraorbital space or between the buccinator and depressor anguli oris to enter the subcutaneous or buccal space.

Once in the buccal space, the infection can spread to the cavernous sinus via the transverse facial vein (uncommon), periorbital space through the subcutaneous plane, superficial to the submandibular space via inferior or posterior extensions, submasseteric space and pterygomandibular space superficially and inferiorly respectively and superficial temporal and infratemporal spaces via the buccal fat pad. Injury to adjacent structures is usually avoided by careful attention to the regional anatomy. The buccal fat pad, Stensen's (parotid) duct, and facial artery should be avoided. However, altered anatomy due to regional edema may alter the surgical anatomy.

In infections that do not appropriately respond to treatment, consideration should be given to inadequate drainage or resistant bacterial strains. Culture and sensitivity studies should then be obtained to guide antimicrobial therapy. By far the most common etiology of vestibular and buccal space infections is odontogenic. However, recurrent buccal space infections can be seen in patients with Crohn's disease (a chronic, granulomatous inflammatory bowel disorder of unknown etiology that can affect any part of the gastrointestinal tract with "skip lesions"). According to Mills, the recurrent buccal space infections in patients with Crohn's disease is due to soft tissue development of secondary infections within the deep mucosal fissures. Treatment of buccal space infections of odontogenic etiology in a patient with Crohn's disease or other granulomatous disease may prove to be more challenging.

DISCUSSION

Carious exposure and subsequent bacterial invasion of the pulp lead to necrosis of the pulpal tissues. The inflammatory process then spreads to the surrounding periodontal ligament and bone. The first pathologic change in the area is apical periodontitis. This results in an inflammatory and immunologically mediated process that causes bone resorption and results in a localized abscess. Certain bacteria that produce enzymes that aid in the destruction of tissue (e.g., hyaluronidases produced by streptococci and collagenases produced by *Bacteroides* organisms) are more virulent (the relative pathogenicity or the relative ability to do damage to the host). Such bacteria more easily invade the potential spaces.

If allowed to continue, the inflammatory process spreads peripherally until cortical bone is destroyed and a subperiosteal abscess is formed. Eventually the periosteum is perforated as the infection spreads via the "path of least resistance." The severity of the abscess depends on factors such as the virulence of the microorganism and the anatomic arrangement of adjacent muscles and fascia. Dense sheets of connective tissue, called *fascia,* encompass muscles, glands, and vascular and neural structures, facilitating movement during function. Bacterial infections that penetrate the fascial spaces can therefore spread via the anatomic confines of these "potential" spaces. Bacterial infections spread via hydrostatic pressure and follow the path of least resistance, which is the loose, areolar connective tissue that surrounds the muscles enclosed by the fascial layers.

The vestibular space is the potential space between the vestibular mucosa and the underlying muscles of facial expression. The posterior boundary is bounded by the buccinator in either jaw, and the anterior boundary is made up by the intrinsic muscles of the lips and the orbicularis oris. In the anterior mandible, the abscess is confined to the vestibular space by the attachment of the mentalis muscle.

Vestibular space infections (Figure 4-6) are caused by perforation of the abscess through the buccal cortex superior to the attachment of the buccinator muscle in the mandible and inferior to the attachment of the buccinator muscle in the maxillary posterior region. The vestibular abscess is far more common than a palatal infection due to the thicker bone of the palate.

The buccal space (included in the primary fascial spaces) is confined anatomically by the subcutaneous skin layer superficially and medially by the buccinator muscle. Anteriorly, it ends at the modiolus (aponeurotic junction of the buccinator and orbicularis oris muscles just posterior to the oral commissure; Figure 4-7). Posteriorly and just medial to the ascending ramus, the buccinator muscle is attached to the superior pharyngeal constrictor muscle at the pterygomandibular raphe. This formation leads to important anatomic pathways for the spread of infection into other spaces. Laterally, it creates a communication with the masseteric space (the space between the masseter muscle and the lateral body of the ramus). Posteriorly and medially, the space communicates with the pterygomandibular, lateral pharyngeal, and infratemporal spaces superiorly. Extension of the buccal fat pad can allow buccal space infections to enter the superficial temporal space, extending via the transverse facial vein and pterygoid plexus into the infratemporal space. Rarely, it can erode into the transverse facial vein or pterygoid plexus and follow a posterior route to the cavernous sinus (the earliest sign of cavernous sinus thrombosis is congestion of the retinal veins of the eye and limitation in lateral movement of the eye due to pressure on the abducens nerve [CN VI]).

Infections that spread to the subcutaneous plane have no superficial anatomic barriers and can therefore spread to adjacent anatomic areas along this plane. Clinical inspection of the overlying skin can frequently aid in identification of subcutaneous spread of the infection. Demarcation of the areas of erythema with a skin-marking pen can be used to monitor the progression of the infectious process.

Odontogenic infections (e.g., buccal space infections) are mixed infections. A large proportion (more than half) are composed of anaerobes, mostly gram-negative rods (*Fusobacterium, Bacteroides* spp.). Gram-positive cocci

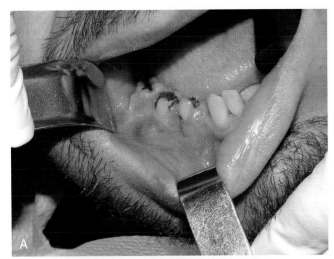

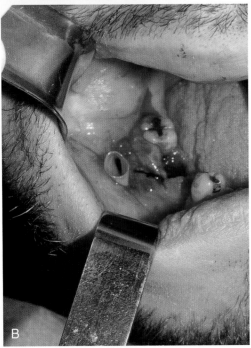

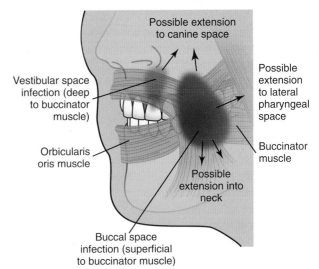

Figure 4-7   The distinction between buccal and vestibular space infections.

Figure 4-6   **A,** Right vestibular abscess secondary to carious right mandibular first molar. **B,** Extracted right mandibular first molar with placement of a Penrose drain in the right vestibule.

This finding suggests a correlation between the severity of an infection and penicillin resistance and is the basis for the recommendation of clindamycin or a β-lactam/β-lactamase inhibitor combination as the empiric antibiotic of choice in odontogenic infections serious enough to require hospitalization. For outpatient treatment, penicillin resistance has not been shown to be a significant problem; therefore, penicillin remains an acceptable antibiotic for the treatment of outpatient odontogenic infections. It has also been shown that amoxicillin may provide more rapid improvement in pain and swelling and that compliance with amoxicillin is better because of its longer dosage interval; therefore, the use of amoxicillin is gaining popularity as the antibiotic of choice for outpatient management of odontogenic infections. Additionally, in patients with orofacial odontogenic infections who received appropriate surgical treatment and/or extraction or endodontic therapy, studies have found no difference in the number of patients cured when patients were prescribed antibiotics for 3 to 4 or 7 days. Therefore, a 3- to 4-day regimen is usually adequate in otherwise healthy patients.

Bibliography

Flynn RT, Halpern RL: Antibiotic selection in head and neck infections, *Oral Maxillofacial Surg Clin North Am* 15:17, 2003.

Flynn RT, Shanti MR, Levi HM, et al: Severe odontogenic infections. Part 1. Prospective report, *J Oral Maxillofac Surg* 64:1093, 2006.

Flynn TR: Surgical management of orofacial infection, *Atlas Oral Maxillofac Surg Clin* 8:77-99, 2000.

Flynn TR: What are the antibiotics of choice for odontogenic infections, and how long should the treatment course last? *Oral Maxillofacial Surg Clin North Am* 23:519-536, 2011.

Grodinsky M, Holyoke EA: The fasciae and fascial spaces of the head, neck, and adjacent regions, *Am J Anat* 63:367, 1938.

Hollinshead WH: *Anatomy for surgeons: the head and neck*, ed 2, Hagerstown, Md, 1968, Harper & Row.

(streptococci and peptostreptococci) are also seen in large numbers (more than 25%).

Noncomplicated buccal space infections frequently can be treated in the office using intravenous sedation and close outpatient follow-up. However, systemic involvement (fever, sepsis, leukocytosis), dehydration, medical comorbidities, noncompliant patients, compromised immune status (diabetes, AIDS, chemotherapy, malnutrition), or infections that involve other deep fascial spaces may warrant hospital admission for intravenous antibiotics and medical evaluation.

In 2006, Flynn and associates conducted a prospective study to predict the length of hospital stay and the failure to respond to penicillin in severe odontogenic infections. They reported a failure rate exceeding 20% with penicillin therapy.

Jones JL, Candelaria LM: Head and neck infections. In Fonscea RJ (ed): *Oral and maxillofacial surgery*, vol 5, Philadelphia, 2000, Saunders.

Laskin DM: Anatomic considerations in diagnosis and treatment of odontogenic infections, *J Am Dent Assoc* 69:308, 1964.

Matthews DC, Sutherland S, Basrani B, et al: Emergency management of acute apical abscesses in the permanent dentition: a systematic review of the literature, *J Can Dent Assoc* 69:660, 2003.

Mills CC, Amin M, Manisali M: Salivary duct fistula and recurrent buccal space infection: a complication of Crohn's disease, *J Oral Maxillofac Surg* 61:1085, 2003.

Mittal N, Gupta P: Management of extra oral sinus cases: a clinical dilemma, *J Endod* 30:541-547, 2004.

Topazian RG, Goldberg MH, Hupp JR: *Oral and maxillofacial infections*, ed 4, Philadelphia, 2002, Saunders.

Lateral Pharyngeal and Masticator Space Infection

Piyushkumar P. Patel and Shahrokh C. Bagheri

CC

A 25-year-old man presents to the emergency department with the complaint that "my throat is swollen, and I cannot swallow."

HPI

Approximately 1 week earlier, the patient began to experience acute pain localized to the posterior mandibular molars, with subsequent development of edema in his left posterior oropharynx 3 days later. He reports the onset of limited mouth opening, progressively worsening dysphagia (difficulty swallowing), and globus (sensation of a lump in the throat) that eventually prompted him to seek care. (Trismus and dysphagia have been shown to be significant indicators of severe odontogenic infection.) He has difficulty swallowing his secretions, either drooling or spitting them out (this is an important clinical note, because it denotes life-threatening oropharyngeal edema). He explains that he has had minimal oral intake with the onset of fever and chills. At this time he does not report any difficulty with breathing, but he feels more comfortable when sitting up (an important clinical sign of dangerous oropharyngeal edema). The patient has a muffled, "hot potato" voice (secondary to supraglottic edema).

Dental infections have become the most common etiology of deep neck infections in the Western world, involving the masticator, parapharyngeal, and submandibular spaces. More than 50% of patients presenting with infection involving these spaces have an odontogenic etiology, making oral and maxillofacial surgeons a preferred provider of surgical care for this group.

PMHX/PDHX/MEDICATIONS/ALLERGIES/SH/FH

The past medical and dental histories are unremarkable. The patient lives in a shelter and does not currently hold a job (although masticator space infections can be seen in individuals of all socioeconomic strata, the condition is far more predominant in the population with less access to health care, including frequent dental examinations).

Despite the lack of coexisting medical diseases in this patient, it is important to consider any conditions that impair the immune system, such as AIDS, diabetes mellitus, chronic corticosteroid therapy, or chemotherapy. Patients should be questioned about risk factors for HIV infection and appropriately tested as needed. Masticator space infections can have very aggressive behavior in the face of immunosuppression.

EXAMINATION

General. The patient is a thin and unkempt-appearing man with a noticeable pungent odor (indicative of neglect to health and hygiene). The patient is not in respiratory distress (it is important to assess the need for advanced airway intervention immediately upon examination). He appears anxious, sitting up holding an emesis basin to catch his secretions as they drool from his mouth (difficulty maintaining secretions).

Vital signs. His blood pressure is 104/68 mm Hg (hypotension secondary to dehydration), heart rate 116 bpm (tachycardia secondary to hypotension and fever), respirations 20 per minute, and temperature 39.2°C (febrile), with an oxygen saturation of 98% on room air.

Maxillofacial. There is significant swelling and induration of the left side extending from the level of the hyoid bone anterior to the sternocleidomastoid to the zygomatic arch. Cranial nerves II through XII are grossly intact. The pupils are equal, round, and reactive to light and accommodation (PERRLA), with no proptosis or ptosis of the eyelid (these would be suggestive of cavernous sinus involvement).

Intraoral. Maximal interincisal opening is 17 mm (trismus) (Figure 4-8, *A*). The floor of the mouth is soft (sublingual space not involved). The patient is able to protrude his tongue past the vermillion-cutaneous border of the upper lip (the ability to protrude the tongue past the vermilion border of the upper lip is a reliable sign that the sublingual space is not severely involved). There is significant fluctuant swelling of the left oropharynx toward the right tonsillar area, with the tip of the uvula touching the right pharyngeal wall (Figure 4-8, *B*). The operculum overlying the partially bony impacted left mandibular third molar is edematous, erythematous, and tender to palpation, with no obvious purulent discharge (mandibular third molars are a common cause of lateral pharyngeal infections). Mucous membranes of the buccal mucosa are dry (secondary to dehydration).

IMAGING

Before any further diagnostic imaging, the treating surgeon must decide whether the patient (and the airway) is stable enough for obtaining further studies, or arrangements should be made to proceed directly to the operating room

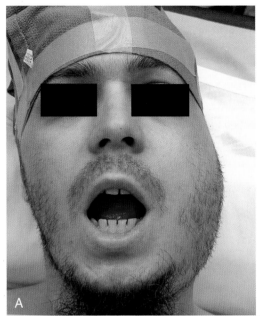

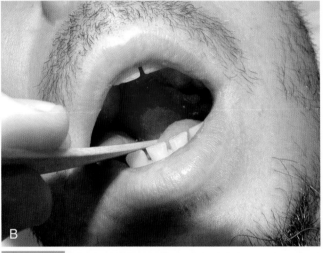

Figure 4-8   **A,** Significant swelling of the left face and maximal interincisal opening of 17 mm. **B,** Large, fluctuant swelling of the posterior oropharynx partially obstructing the airway.

and establish a secure airway (endotracheal or nasotracheal intubation, tracheostomy, cricothyrotomy). Any possibility of acute respiratory obstruction should prompt the surgeon to proceed directly to the operating room. Imaging studies can be safely obtained to guide further treatment at a later time.

When available, a panoramic radiograph is an important imaging study for evaluation of suspected odontogenic infections. It provides an excellent overview of the mandible and maxilla and serves as a screening tool for evaluation of the dentition. Also, in patients with trismus, other dental radiographs may be difficult to obtain. Because mandibular third molars are the most common odontogenic cause of parapharyngeal space infections, this radiograph becomes necessary to evaluate the third molars. In addition, it delineates the relationship to adjacent structures, such as the inferior alveolar canal, and other possible bony pathology.

The combination of contrast-enhanced CT scans and clinical examination has the highest sensitivity and specificity in the diagnosis of deep neck infections. The use of contrast improves the ability to identify the hyperemic capsule of a longstanding abscess (abscesses are seen as discrete, hypodense areas that show an enhancing peripheral rim with use of intravenous contrast material). In general, most radiologists interpret hypodense areas without ring enhancement to represent cellulitis or edema. However, studies have shown that, when drained, approximately 45% of hypodense areas without ring enhancement yield pus. In a study by Miller and associates, a hypodense area of greater than 2 ml without ring enhancement yielded purulence at the time of surgery. In the same study, CT scans were able to correctly differentiate cellulitis from an abscess in 85% of deep neck space (lateral and retropharyngeal) infections.

CT also provides important information regarding the details of adjacent anatomic structures, such as the integrity of the airway, tracheal deviation, and the proximity of vascular structures (the carotid sheath). Airway deviation and the risk of rupture of the pharyngeal abscess during intubation are important factors in determining the choice of technique to secure the airway.

Magnetic resonance imaging (MRI) is also a useful imaging modality for soft tissue evaluation. Compared with CT, advantages of MRI include superior anatomic multiplanar display, high soft tissue contrast, fewer artifacts from dental amalgam, and lack of ionizing radiation. However, MRI is difficult and slower to perform on an emergency basis and is more costly, and claustrophobia may preclude examination in some patients. MRI, when possible, has been shown to be superior in the assessment of deep neck infections.

Ultrasonography has shown some benefit in differentiating cellulitis from an abscess in superficial locations, but the use of this modality as a sole imaging technique for deep neck infection is in its infancy. The ultrasound probe can be placed intraorally, although in the setting of an acute infection and trismus, this can be difficult. An abscess is seen as an echo-free cavity with an irregular, well-defined circumference.

In the current patient, the airway appeared clinically stable, and a panoramic radiograph demonstrated a carious and partially bony impacted left mandibular third molar. A CT scan with contrast demonstrated significant swelling of the lateral pharyngeal area and deviation of the airway (Figure 4-9). Large rim-enhancing hypodense areas consistent with pus are seen on the left lateral masticator and lateral pharyngeal (anterior compartment) spaces.

LABS

A CBC and a basic metabolic panel should be obtained during the initial evaluation of deep neck space infections. The WBC count is an indicator of the severity of the systemic response to the infection and can be obtained periodically to monitor the progression of infection (caution should be exercised in interpretation of this value in a patient who is at high risk for undiagnosed AIDS, because the WBC count may appear

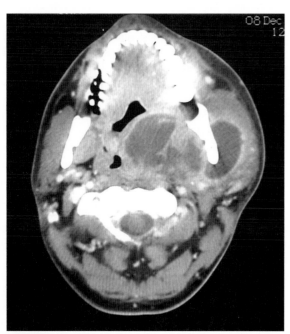

Figure 4-9 Axial cut, contrast-enhanced CT scan, demonstrating large areas of rim-enhanced hypodensities (loculations) both medial and lateral to the left mandible with significant deviation of the airway.

Box 4-1	Risk Factors for Contrast-Associated Nephropathy

- Preexisting renal disease
- Diabetes
- Volume of contrast dye used
- Dehydration
- Congestive heart failure
- Advanced age
- Presence of nephrotoxic drugs (NSAIDs, ACE-Is)

From Soma VR: Contrast-associated nephropathy, *Heart Dis* 4:372-379, 2002. *ACE-Is,* Angiotensin-converting enzyme inhibitors; *NSAIDs,* nonsteroidal antiinflammatory drugs.

within the normal range secondary to the inability to mount an adequate immune response).

The serum creatinine and BUN levels should be obtained before contrast material is used for imaging. Contrast material has been known to cause contrast-associated nephropathy. The condition is defined as an increase in serum creatinine greater than 25% from baseline or a rise greater than 0.5 mg/dl within 48 hours of contrast exposure, in the absence of other causes. Risk factors for the development of contrast-associated nephropathy are summarized in Box 4-1. In the presence of risk factors, renal function should be carefully monitored, and a baseline serum creatinine obtained before and within 48 to 72 hours after the procedure.

The WBC count for the current patient was 18,500 cells/mm³; the differential included 80% polymorphonucleocytes with a shift to the left (indicative of an acute inflammatory process).

Serum chemistries showed a sodium level of 150 mEq/dl (hypovolemic hypernatremia due to dehydration), BUN of 48 mg/dl, and creatinine of 1.1 mg/dl (prerenal azotemia consistent with dehydration).

ASSESSMENT

Deep neck infection involving the anterior compartment of the left LPS with significant upper airway deviation and edema, and left medial and lateral masticator space infections secondary to an impacted mandibular third molar, complicated by dehydration and potential onset of sepsis.

TREATMENT

Successful treatment of fascial space infections should include the following:
- Surgical drainage of an abscess or, in select cases, drainage of cellulitis
- Identification and removal of the source of infection (the tooth, in cases of odontogenic etiology)
- Administration of antibiotics (guided by culture and sensitivity when possible)
- Optimization of host nutritional and immune status

Antimicrobial therapy can abort abscess formation if administered at an early stage of infection. However, once an abscess has formed, antimicrobial therapy is more effective in conjunction with adequate surgical drainage.

Impending airway obstruction may require immediate airway management (see Ludwig's Angina, earlier in this chapter, and Emergent Surgical Airway in Chapter 3). Maintaining spontaneous ventilation and airway patency is critical in patients with a compromised airway. Even a small dose of a respiratory depressant may change an apparently controlled situation into an emergent one, especially in the presence of a fatiguing patient. Morbidity or death due to the loss of an airway is still reported. Available options include endotracheal intubation versus establishment of a surgical airway. The advantages and disadvantages of these methods are summarized in Table 4-1. Consideration should be given to endotracheal intubation using an awake fiberoptic technique. This requires a skilled anesthesiologist and patient cooperation and can be time-consuming.

Regardless of the airway technique used, caution should be exercised to prevent rupture of the abscess during intubation, which can result in aspiration of purulent material and is associated with significant morbidity (aspiration pneumonitis, pneumonia, lung abscess, acute respiratory distress syndrome) and mortality. One useful technique is to aspirate the LPS before any intubation attempts. This can be done in the operating room under local anesthesia. The abscess can be decompressed significantly, thereby reducing the risk of aspiration during intubation.

The anterior compartment can be approached intraorally via an incision over the pterygomandibular raphe, with blunt dissection around the medial side to enter the LPS. The extraoral approach is accomplished by making a 1- to 2-cm

Table 4-1	Intubation Versus Surgical Airway	
Procedure	**Advantages**	**Disadvantages**
Intubation	Potentially fast method	Nonsecured airway
	Nonsurgical procedure	Patient discomfort is required for extended periods
		Difficult to perform with upper airway edema
		Risk of rupture of abscess, with subsequent aspiration
		Requires mechanical ventilation during period of intubation
		Laryngotracheal stenosis
Tracheotomy	Airway security	Surgical procedure
	Patient comfort	Bleeding
	Less need for ventilation and sedation	Scarring
		Pneumothorax
	Earlier transfer from unit to floor	

From Potter JK: Tracheotomy versus endotracheal intubation for airway management in deep neck space infections, *J Oral Maxillofac Surg* 60:349-354, 2002.

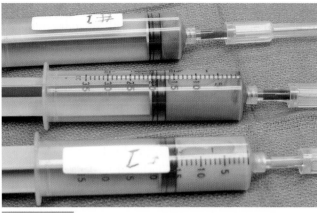

Figure 4-10 Samples of the aspirate to be sent for Gram stain and aerobic and anaerobic culture and sensitivity studies.

incision approximately two finger-breadths inferior to the mandible; dissection is then carried through the platysma to the superficial layer of the deep cervical fascia. Sufficient fascia is exposed to identify the submandibular gland and the posterior belly of the digastric muscle. Dissection is then carried just posterior to the posterior belly of the digastric muscle in a superior, medial, and posterior direction into the LPS. If finger dissection is also used, the surgeon will be able to palpate the endotracheal tube medially and the carotid sheath posterolaterally. Through-and-through intraoral-extraoral drainage can be obtained by combining the intraoral approach with the extraoral approach. If old clots are found or if any signs of carotid sheath involvement are present, then vertical extension of the incision can be made along the anterior border of the sternocleidomastoid muscle. This extension allows the carotid artery to be pulled anteriorly and controlled as necessary.

The extraoral incision should parallel the lines of relaxed skin tension and lie in a cosmetically acceptable site whenever possible. The incision should also be supported by healthy underlying dermis and subcutaneous tissue. Placement of drains should allow for gravity-dependent drainage. A rigid drain should not be placed into the LPS because of the potential for erosion into the carotid sheath.

Supportive care to ensure adequate hydration, caloric intake, and analgesia is also important. It is reported that minimum daily fluid requirements increase by 300 ml per degree of fever (1°C) per day. Caloric requirements also increase by approximately 5% to 8% per degree of fever per day.

Studies have shown that gram-positive cocci and gram-negative rods have the greatest growth percentage in cultures from deep neck space infections of odontogenic origin. It should be noted that some microbiologists estimate that only 50% of the bacteria that comprise oral flora can be cultured in the laboratory. Additionally, it is believed that the majority of human infections are caused by bacteria in biofilms (a complex, usually multispecies, highly communicative community of bacteria that is surrounded by a polymer matrix). Bacteria present in biofilms are difficult to culture with traditional methods. Future trends indicate that rather than relying on traditional culture and sensitivity testing, DNA analysis may be used for identification. Until strategies for the prevention of biofilm formation and disruption of existing biofilms are developed, surgical therapy is still necessary. Due to the rising incidence of penicillin resistance and failure of penicillin therapy, many clinicians advocate the empiric use of clindamycin (in a penicillin-allergic patient) or a combination of a β-lactam with penicillinase inhibitor (e.g., ampicillin/sulbactam) for deep neck space infections of odontogenic origin until an antibiogram is obtained. Clindamycin has the disadvantage of not covering *Eikenella corrodens*. If *E. corrodens* has been cultured, moxifloxacin is an excellent choice.

The current patient was given a bolus of normal saline and was taken urgently to the operating room. The anesthesiologist was informed about the parapharyngeal space involvement, and the anesthesiologist and surgeon agreed on a plan for airway management. Before any attempts at intubation, 6 ml of lidocaine was injected on the mucosa of the oropharynx superficially; subsequently, 35 ml of purulent material was evacuated, allowing decompression of the swelling (Figure 4-10). Subsequently, the patient was placed in the supine position, and anatomic landmarks were marked on the neck for a tracheotomy or cricothyroidotomy. The surgeon and operating room personnel were positioned and prepared for an emergent surgical airway, should the need arise. The anesthesiologist successfully intubated the patient using an awake fiberoptic nasal intubation technique. With a large-bore needle, the LPS was further aspirated and the material was sent for culture and sensitivity. The left mandibular third molar was extracted. The left medial and lateral masticator and the LPS were explored and drained via an intraoral and extraoral approach. A red rubber catheter was secured into the medial and lateral masticator spaces, and a Penrose drain was secured in the LPS. The patient was started on ampicillin/sulbactam 3 g intravenously every 6 hours. He remained intubated postoperatively and was transferred to the ICU. On the night of his surgery, he was weaned to minimal ventilator settings. He was awake and alert and in no apparent distress, with a Glasgow Coma Scale score of 11T.

The wound care regimen included meticulous irrigation of the drains. On postoperative day 1, the patient's WBC count decreased to 13,000 cells/mm^3 (it is not uncommon for the WBC count to increase immediately after surgery due to demargination), and there was a notable decrease in pharyngeal and facial edema (it is not uncommon for surgical edema and fluid resuscitation to worsen the preexisting edema). A Gram stain revealed the presence of gram-positive cocci in pairs and chains (*Streptococcus* species) and gram-negative rods (mixed infection). On the second postoperative day, the WBC count decreased to 10,200 cells/mm^3 with a significant decrease in edema and return of the uvula to midline. All sedative medications were discontinued, and the patient was extubated after passing a cuff leak test. He was subsequently transferred to the ward and discharged to home care with oral antibiotics after 5 days of wound care and intravenous medications. At discharge there was no significant drainage, and all drains were removed. He was given instructions for jaw range-of-motion exercises and a follow-up appointment.

COMPLICATIONS

Complications of masticator space infections are partially dependent on the severity of the presenting infection, the status of the host immune system, the virulence and resistance patterns of the infecting bacteria, and the time of presentation. Complications can be major, ranging from unsightly scars from incisions for drainage or tracheostomy to death from airway embarrassment.

Infections that have gained entry into the LPS may erode into the carotid sheath or impair any of the nerves found in the posterior compartment. Signs that indicate possible carotid sheath involvement include the following:
- Ipsilateral Horner's syndrome (ptosis, miosis, anhidrosis)
- Unexplained palsies of cranial nerves IX through XII
- Recurrent small hemorrhages from the nose, mouth, or ear (herald bleeds)
- Hematoma in the surrounding tissue
- Persistent peritonsillar swelling despite adequate drainage
- Protracted clinical course
- Onset of shock

Any signs of carotid sheath involvement warrant immediate radiologic evaluation, CT, or CT angiography. Surgical exploration and control of the great vessels may be required.

Table 4-2	Boundaries of the Lateral Pharyngeal Space
Space	**Boundary**
Anterior	Pterygomandibular raphe (junction of buccinators and superior constrictor muscles)
Posterior	Prevertebral fascia that communicates with the retropharyngeal space
Medial	Buccopharyngeal fascia on lateral surface of the superior constrictor muscle
Lateral	Fascia over the medial masticator, the parotid gland, and mandible

Involvement of the cranial nerves (vagus and glossopharyngeal nerves) can result in sudden death from bradycardia, asystole, and cardiac arrhythmia. Involvement of the retropharyngeal space can lead to descending infection involving the mediastinum. Erythema over the upper chest is suggestive of descending infection and may require cardiothoracic consultation.

Of particular concern are infections that do not appropriately respond to treatment. Consideration should be given to inadequate drainage or resistant bacterial strains. Culture and sensitivity studies can be obtained on purulent aspirates to guide antimicrobial therapy.

DISCUSSION

The LPS has the shape of an inverted pyramid or cone, the base of which is the sphenoid and the apex is the hyoid bone. The boundaries of this space are summarized in Table 4-2.

The LPS is divided by the styloid process and its muscles into an anterior and a posterior compartment. The anterior compartment contains only fat, muscle, connective tissue, and lymph nodes. The posterior compartment contains the glossopharyngeal, spinal accessory, and hypoglossal nerves. It also contains the carotid sheath (the carotid artery, internal jugular vein, and vagus nerve; the cervical sympathetic trunk lies posterior and medial to the carotid sheath). A strong fascial plane, the stylopharyngeal aponeurosis of Zuckerkandl and Testut, separates the anterior and posterior compartments. It is a barrier that helps prevent the spread of infection from the anterior to the posterior compartment.

Lateral pharyngeal infections can be caused by tonsillitis, otitis media, mastoiditis, or parotitis; most commonly they occur secondary to an odontogenic pathology. Involvement of the LPS can also occur via spread through lymphatic vessels and subsequent rupture of a node. Lymphatic drainage from the nose and paranasal sinuses, ear, or oral cavity can involve this area. Infection can also spread from retropharyngeal, sublingual, submandibular, or masticator space infections. Peritonsillar abscesses that rupture through the superior constrictor muscle can also cause entry and infection of the LPS directly.

Symptoms of LPS involvement vary according to whether the anterior or posterior compartment is involved. The four most common signs of involvement of the anterior compartment are:

1. Trismus
2. Induration or swelling at the angle of the jaw
3. Pharyngeal bulging with or without deviation of the uvula
4. Fever

Deviation of the uvula with bulging of the pharyngeal wall can also be seen with peritonsillar abscesses; however, trismus is usually absent. With LPS infections, trismus is seen secondary to involvement of the adjacent medial pterygoid muscle. It can be difficult to differentiate a pterygomandibular space abscess from an LPS infection, but this distinction may be of academic interest only, because treatment would be similar. Involvement of the posterior compartment may show posterior tonsillar deviation and retropharyngeal bulging. In this scenario, palsies of cranial nerves IX through XII may be seen, in addition to ipsilateral Horner's syndrome (ipsilateral blepharoptosis, pupillary miosis, and facial anhidrosis). A common sign of LPS involvement is the presence of swelling of the lateral neck just above the hyoid and just anterior to the sternocleidomastoid muscle. This is the point at which the LPS is closest to the skin and where dependent edema or exudate is constrained by binding of the fascial layers to the hyoid bone.

Significant upper airway edema may require the patient to remain in an upright position, because assuming the supine position may lead to airway obstruction. Also, depending on the severity of the obstruction, patients may present with breathing with the mouth open or in the "sniffing position," with extension of the neck, stridor, labored breathing, intercostal retractions, tracheal tug, sore throat, or globus. Changes in voice also provide a clue to the location of airway involvement. A muffled, or "hot potato," voice usually signifies a supraglottic process, whereas hoarseness is a sign of vocal cord involvement.

Bibliography

Brook I: Microbiology and management of peritonsillar, retropharyngeal and parapharyngeal abscesses, *J Oral Maxillofac Surg* 62:1545-1550, 2004.

Dzyak W, Zide MF: Diagnosis and treatment of lateral pharyngeal space infections, *J Oral Maxillofac Surg* 42:243-249, 1984.

Flynn T: What are the antibiotics of choice for odontogenic infections and how long should the treatment course last? *Oral Maxillofacial Surg Clin North Am* 23:519, 2011.

Flynn TR: Surgical management of orofacial infection, *Atlas Oral Maxillofac Surg Clin North Am* 8:77-99, 2000.

Flynn TR, Shanti RM, Levi MH, et al: Severe odontogenic infections. Part 1. Prospective report, *J Oral Maxillofac Surg* 64:1093-1103, 2006.

Hollinshead W: *Anatomy for surgeons.* Vol 1. The head and neck, Philadelphia, 1982, Lippincott-Raven.

Miller WD, Furst IM, Sandor GK, et al: A prospective blinded comparison of clinical examination and computed tomography in deep neck infections, *Laryngoscope* 109:1873-1879, 1999.

Munoz A: Acute neck infection: prospective comparison between CT and MRI in 47 patients, *J Comput Assist Tomogr* 25:733-741, 2001.

O'Grady NP, Barie PS, Bartlett JG, et al: Guidelines for evaluation of new fever in critically ill adult patients: 2008 update from the American College of Critical Care Medicine and the Infectious Diseases Society of America, *Crit Care Med* 36(4):1330-1349, 2008.

Potter JK: Tracheotomy versus endotracheal intubation for airway management in deep neck space infections, *J Oral Maxillofac Surg* 60:349-354, 2002.

Ray JM, Triplett RG: What is the role of biofilms in severe head and neck infections? *Oral Maxillofac Surg Clin North Am* 23:497, 2011.

Rega AJ: Microbiology and antibiotic sensitivities of deep neck space infections, *J Oral Maxillofac Surg* 62:25-26, 2004.

Soma VR: Contrast-associated nephropathy, *Heart Dis* 4:372-379, 2002.

Storoe W: The changing face of odontogenic infections, *J Oral Maxillofac Surg* 59:739-748, 2001.

Styer TE: Peritonsillar abscess: diagnosis and treatment, *Am Fam Physician* 65:95, 2002.

Osteomyelitis

Martin Salgueiro, Jaspal Girn, and Chris Jo

CC

A 49-year-old man returns to your office 3 months after extraction of his mandibular third molars complaining that, "I still have some swelling and drainage from my mouth." (Osteomyelitis is more common in the mandible than in the maxilla due to the relatively lower blood supply).

HPI

The patient presents with a history of persistent pain and swelling on the left side of his face, which has increased during the past month. He had four full bony impacted third molars removed 3 months ago without any acute complications. He returned 2 weeks after surgery for follow-up with a complaint of tenderness of the lower left extraction socket. The socket was noted to be filled with debris but without purulence and was irrigated clear. Instructions for follow-up were given, but the patient did not return for reevaluation. He now returns 3 months later due to the increasing pain, swelling, and some drainage from the left lower socket. He has not seen any other doctors and has not been on any antibiotics. He denies having fever or chills, difficulty swallowing (dysphagia), or difficulty talking (dysphonia).

PMHX/MEDICATIONS/ALLERGIES/SH/FH

Noncontributory. The patient has no risk factors for osteomyelitis.

Although osteomyelitis has a higher incidence in patients who are immunocompromised (diabetes, HIV/AIDS, chemotherapy), intravenous drug users, patients with compromised splenic function or splenectomy, patient undergoing radiation therapy, or patients who use tobacco, it can occur in patients with no risk factors.

The macrophages in the reticuloendothelial system of the spleen are involved in sequestration of encapsulated organisms (e.g., *Haemophilus influenzae, Streptococcus pneumoniae,* and *Salmonella* and *Klebsiella* species); therefore, an absent spleen or a compromised splenic function is a risk factor for osteomyelitis secondary to these organisms. Patients with sickle cell anemia are at risk because during a sickle cell crisis, the splenic reticuloendothelial system is overwhelmed and becomes "clogged" by sickled red blood cells, which can lead to splenic infraction or abscess requiring a splenectomy. Also, chronic splenomegaly in these patients can lead to splenic atrophy and eventual "autosplenectomy." A history of

radiation therapy or bisphosphonate use should also be noted, to rule out possible osteoradionecrosis (ORN) or bisphosphonate-related osteonecrosis of the jaws.

EXAMINATION

General. The patient is a well-developed and well-nourished man in no apparent distress.

Vital signs. His blood pressure is 132/81 mm Hg, heart rate 80 bpm, respirations 16 per minute, and temperature 37.1°C (afebrile).

Maxillofacial. There is mild left facial swelling, erythema, and tenderness at the inferior border of the mandible. No fistulous tract is present (*Actinomyces israelii* infections commonly cause cutaneous fistulas). The lymph nodes are palpable in the left submandibular area (secondary to chronic infection). The inferior alveolar nerve is intact bilaterally (altered sensation can be commonly seen in osteomyelitis of the mandible).

Intraoral. The maximal interincisal opening is 25 mm (decreased due to guarding secondary to pain). The left retromolar pad is tender to palpation, with moderate erythema and swelling. There is a small draining fistula distal to the left mandibular second molar in the attached gingiva. The oropharynx is clear, the uvula is midline, and the floor of the mouth is soft and nonelevated. The dentition is in good repair. The occlusion is stable and reproducible (occlusal change would be suggestive of a pathologic fracture).

IMAGING

Several imaging modalities are available for the evaluation of suspected osteomyelitis. A panoramic radiograph is the initial diagnostic study of choice when dealing with postextraction complications (e.g., retained tooth fragments, local wound infections, mandibular fractures, foreign bodies, bony sequestra, and pathology of adjacent teeth) or osteomyelitis. The destructive process of osteomyelitis must extend at least 1 cm and demonstrate 30% to 50% bone demineralization before it becomes radiographically apparent. The radiograph would show a loss of definition and lytic changes within the trabecular patterns of the involved bone. Eventually, radiopaque sequestra (fragments of bone that have become devitalized) may become visible, demonstrating a "mottled" radiolucent appearance.

Two-dimensional CT with contrast material is useful for visualizing soft tissue abnormalities, such as the presence of

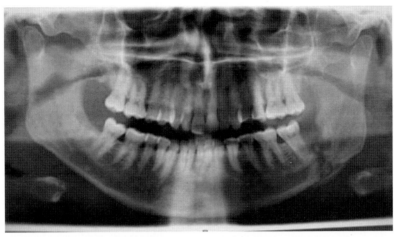

Figure 4-11   Panoramic radiograph showing mottled radiolucency at the extraction socket extending down to the inferior border. Extracortical reactive bone formation is seen at the inferior border. The proximal segment is not rotated or telescoped, suggesting that a pathologic fracture has not occurred.

an abscess, and for assessing bony integrity or cortical disruptions. MRI can be useful for the evaluation of osteomyelitis due to the superior imaging of soft tissue, defining the extent and location of osteomyelitis. However, MRI has limited ability to discriminate edema from outright infection and can result in nonspecific findings in posttraumatic and postsurgical patients. Nuclear medicine imaging modalities can detect osteomyelitis 10 to 14 days earlier than conventional radiographic imaging. Scintigraphy with technetium 99m scanning is very sensitive in detecting increased bone turnover, and its specificity in detecting osteomyelitis is improved with the use of gallium 67 or indium 111.

In the current patient, a panoramic radiograph (Figure 4-11) reveals a mottled radiolucent appearance in the area of the extracted left mandibular third molar that extends to the inferior border of the mandible. There is evidence of reactive extracortical bone formation at the inferior border of the mandible. The proximal segment is not rotated superiorly (a rotated proximal segment would indicate a pathologic fracture).

LABS

A CBC is necessary to evaluate the initial WBC count and to monitor the response to surgical and antibiotic therapy (the WBC count may be elevated in acute or subacute osteomyelitis). The current patient had a WBC count of 15,000 cells/mm^3 (elevated).

ASSESSMENT

Acute suppurative osteomyelitis of the left mandible.

Although a 3-month duration may indicate a chronic state, acute suppurative osteomyelitis is the corrected diagnosis based on the fact that this disease process has not yet been managed either medically or surgically. Suppuration indicates that the body has mounted an immune response to the infection.

Several classification systems have been proposed, but no one scheme has gained acceptance. In the simplest form, osteomyelitis can be classified as acute or chronic. It is further characterized as suppurative or nonsuppurative. Waldvogel and associates proposed the staging of osteomyelitis into three separate groups based on the etiology: osteomyelitis related to a hematogenous source, secondary to a contiguous focus of infection, or associated with vascular insufficiency. The Cierny-Mader staging system is the most commonly used classification system for long-bone osteomyelitis. It divides the disease into four stages of osseous involvement and then combines it with three physiologic host categories, resulting in 12 discrete clinical stages. In addition, chronic diffuse sclerosing osteomyelitis is a unique form of osteomyelitis that is described as a painful disease state that occurs only in the mandible and is more often seen in younger female patients.

TREATMENT

Osteomyelitis is treated with a combination of surgical and medical interventions. Nonsurgical management of true osteomyelitis is futile and only allows for exacerbation of the existing condition and delay of more extensive surgical interventions.

If feasible, empiric antibiotic therapy should not be initiated until cultures are taken (purulent exudate and/or bone cultures) to accurately identify the causative organism or organisms. A bone culture has higher bacterial counts than swabs or purulent drainage and is preferable for identification of the causative organism or organisms. Specimens should be sent to the laboratory as soon as possible, especially to prevent the loss of anaerobic species, which can happen in as little as 15 minutes. Osteomyelitis caused by a contiguous focus of infection is often polymicrobial; therefore, one or more empiric broad-spectrum antibiotics are initiated (more than 90% of cases of osteomyelitis of the jaws have a polymicrobial ethology). Once culture and sensitivity results are available, antibiotic regimens should be adjusted to target the causative organism or organisms. The course and route (intravenous or oral) of antibiotic therapy are debatable and are frequently determined by clinical judgment. It has been generally accepted that a 4-week course of intravenous antibiotics is necessary, especially when dealing with chronic or refractory osteomyelitis. However, earlier stages of osteomyelitis may require only a short course of intravenous antibiotics (if needed), followed by a 1- to 2-week course of oral antibiotics based on serial clinical examinations. Consultation with an infectious diseases specialist may be prudent to assist in effective antibiotic therapy.

Penicillin remains the empiric antibiotic of choice for osteomyelitis of tooth-bearing bone. However, many organisms responsible for osteomyelitis of the jaws are penicillin resistant, including *Prevotella, Porphyromonas, Staphylococcus,* and *Fusobacterium* spp. Therefore, it may be prudent to use a penicillin combined with a β-lactamase inhibitor (clavulanate) in combination with metronidazole (Flagyl) to improve anaerobic coverage. In patients who are allergic to β-lactam antibiotics, clindamycin is recommended due to its effectiveness against penicillinase-producing staphylococci, streptococci, and anaerobic bacteria. However, clindamycin is ineffective against *Eikenella corrodens* (a common organism in osteomyelitis and odontogenic infections), for which additional coverage is required. It is important to recognize that anaerobic organisms are difficult to culture, resulting in frequent false-negative anaerobic growth (therefore empiric anaerobic coverage may be prudent despite a negative anaerobic culture).

Surgical management of osteomyelitis should be planned in conjunction with medical treatment. In the early stages, surgical interventions should be limited to extraction of grossly loose teeth, debridement of fragments of bone, and incision and drainage of fluctuant areas. If the infection persists, further surgical procedures, such as sequestrectomy, saucerization, decortication, or resection, followed by reconstruction, should be considered.

Sequestra are devitalized pieces of bone, which act as a nidus of infection. Sequestra are eventually resorbed, removed, or spontaneously expelled through the mucosa or skin, but they may persist and propagate a host response. Due to the avascular nature of necrotic sequestra, they are poorly penetrated by antibiotics and should be removed with minimal trauma, intraorally and/or transcutaneously. Saucerization is the "unroofing" of bone to expose the medullary cavity. The buccal cortex of the mandible is removed until bleeding bone is encountered at all margins of the surgical defect, thus producing a saucerlike defect. The purpose of this is to decompress the bone to allow extrusion of pus, debris, and any bony sequestra. The defect can be packed with a medicated dressing, changed several times over subsequent days, and irrigated daily to ensure that no fragments of necrotic bone are left behind as the wound heals by secondary intention (or is simply left open for irrigation). The lingual aspect of the mandible rarely requires reduction, because it has a rich blood supply from the mylohyoid muscle. In the maxilla, saucerization is rarely needed, because the cortex is thin and formed sequestra can be easily removed. Decortication of the mandible refers to the removal of chronically infected cortical bone, which is usually extended 1 to 2 cm beyond the affected area. Corticocancellous bone grafting of osteomyelitis has traditionally not been advocated, but there is some recent evidence suggesting the feasibility of immediate bone grafting along with stabilization of the mandible.

Refractory cases or patients with a pathologic mandibular fracture (Figure 4-12) require resection of the diseased bone extending to a bleeding bone margin. Stabilization of the segments is accomplished with immediate placement of rigid internal fixation plates or, in rare cases, a Joe Hall Morris biphasic external fixator. After resolution of the infection, bony reconstruction can be completed with corticocancellous bone grafts or vascularized free flaps. Hyperbaric oxygen has been shown to be effective in treating osteomyelitis and should be considered in severe or refractory cases. Dental rehabilitation can be achieved after adequate bone and healing and reconstruction.

The current patient underwent a bone culture (antibiotic therapy was not initiated until cultures had been obtained) and local debridement via an intraoral approach. Intraoperatively, it was noted that the buccal and lingual cortices were intact.

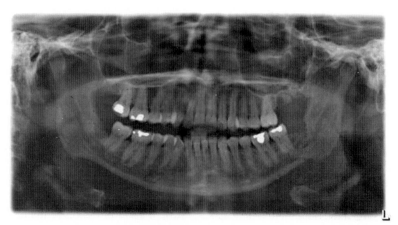

Figure 4-12   Panoramic radiograph of another patient with osteomyelitis of the left mandible after extraction of a third molar. Note that there is a pathologic fracture of the left mandible, with the proximal segment telescoped with the distal segment and rotated superiorly.

There were multiple loose fragments of devitalized bone (sequestra) and abundant granulation tissue tracking down to the inferior border of the mandible. After the wound had been debrided, a round burr was used to remove the surrounding affected bone until normal-appearing, bleeding bone was encountered. The patient was started on empiric intravenous antibiotics (ampicillin/sulbactam and metronidazole) and remained hospitalized until the initial culture and sensitivity results were available. Cultures demonstrated growth of *Streptococcus anginosis* that was pansensitive, with negative anaerobic cultures. The patient was discharged home on oral amoxicillin with clavulanic acid and metronidazole, in addition to chlorhexidine mouthwash. He was kept on a liquid diet until soft tissue healing occurred to prevent retention of food debris in the wound. He was subsequently switched to a soft diet for 8 weeks after surgery to prevent a postoperative pathologic fracture. Final cultures did not grow any additional organisms; therefore, the antibiotic regimen was not changed during the course of his treatment. He healed without any complications.

COMPLICATIONS

Osteomyelitis is a complication of various oral and maxillofacial surgical procedures, and its incidence is related to both host factors and the virulence of the infecting organisms. Treatment of osteomyelitis can itself be compounded by further complications. These include a persistent refractory infection of the bone, pathologic fractures (at presentation, intraoperatively, or postoperatively), the need for resection of chronically infected bone, disfigurement, neurosensory impairment, and systemic spread of the infection.

Antibiotic therapy is associated with side effects such as diarrhea and *Clostridium difficile* pseudomembranous colitis, in addition to the emergence of resistant microorganisms. Methicillin-resistant *Staphylococcus aureus* (MRSA) has become a very common community-acquired organism in many communities. MRSA osteomyelitis requires intravenous vancomycin until sensitivity profiles (antibiogram) are available. If the organism is sensitive to only vancomycin, a peripherally inserted central catheter (PICC) line can be used to allow delivery of intravenous antibiotics at home. Local antibiotic delivery systems have been used in an attempt to obtaining constant, higher local drug concentrations. The gentamycin-polymethylmethacrylate delivery system was introduced in the late 1970s. Despite some benefits, multiple shortcomings, including the need for additional surgery for removal, have limited its use. New research is focusing on delivery systems using reabsorbable carriers (polylactic acid, polyglycolic acid, and collagen sponges).

Uncontrolled diabetes mellitus presents a special challenge. Tight glycemic control (blood glucose 90 to 110 mg/dl) is paramount for recovery from any infection. Noncompliant patients may require extended hospitalization to achieve glycemic control and delivery of intravenous antibiotics. Some patients may require an insulin pump, and critically ill patients may require an insulin drip. Sliding scale insulin is generally not regarded as adequate treatment, because it is designed to treat hyperglycemia rather than to prevent it (therefore, it is always one step behind the hyperglycemia). Baseline insulin regimens need to be adjusted to prevent hyperglycemic episodes.

Pathologic fractures of the mandible (see Figure 4-12) occur with sufficient destruction of cortical bone, primarily due to osteolytic changes associated with osteomyelitis and/or the result of periosteal stripping during an aggressive debridement (at 2 to 3 weeks postdebridement, the mandible is at greatest risk of fracture due to the critical phase of remodeling/resorption). Maxillomandibular fixation (6 to 8 weeks) should be considered for patients at higher risk for postoperative pathologic fractures. A liquid or soft diet is prudent for those at moderate risk.

DISCUSSION

Osteomyelitis is an inflammatory condition involving the medullary cavity of bone. It begins as a bacterial infection and can cause significant bony destruction. The microorganisms cause host tissue injury from direct cellular attack and through enzymatic degradation. The host responds by recruiting neutrophils to the area to digest the pathogens via release of enzymes and phagocytosis. When purulence (composed of necrotic tissue, dead bacteria, and WBCs) accumulates, it causes an increase in the intramedullary pressure, causing collapse of the vessels, venous stasis, and congestion. Vessels in the haversian system and Volkmann's canals of the cortical bone may undergo thrombosis or experience stasis and congestion; as a result, the surrounding bone becomes ischemic, thereby permitting the extension of osteomyelitis. If purulence continues to accumulate, the periosteum is penetrated and mucosal or cutaneous fistulas develop.

The establishment of an infection in bone is related to the compromise in the bone's vascular supply. However, other factors (e.g., the virulence of the organism and the integrity of the host's defenses, diabetes), blood dyscrasias (e.g., sickle cell disease), immunosuppression (e.g., HIV infection, post-transplant patients), and collagen vascular disorders or bone dysplasias (e.g., osteopetrosis) are also important.

Initially, *S. aureus* and *Staphylococcus epidermidis* accounted for 80% to 90% of cases of osteomyelitis of the jaws. However, the frequency of *S. aureus* involvement in osteomyelitis has decreased due to the improved culture methods used to identify organisms, especially anaerobes. Anaerobes are frequently associated with aerobic organisms in osteomyelitis. Currently, osteomyelitis is recognized as a disease commonly caused by streptococci (β-hemolytic) and oral anaerobes such as *Peptostreptococcus, Fusobacterium,* and *Prevotella* spp.

Bibliography

Adekeye EO, Cornah J: Osteomyelitis of the jaws: a review of 141 cases, *Br J Oral Maxillofac Surg* 23:24-35, 1985.

Benson PD, Marshall MK, Engelstad ME, et al: The use of immediate bone grafting in reconstruction of clinically infected mandibular fractures: bone grafts in the presence of pus, *J Oral Maxillofac Surg* 64:122-126, 2006.

Cieny G, Mader JT, Pennick H: A clinical staging system of adult osteomyelitis, *Contemp Orthop* 10:17-37, 1985.

Cohen MA, Embil JM, Canosa T: Osteomyelitis of the maxilla caused by methicillin-resistant *Staphylococcus aureus*, *J Oral Maxillofac Surg* 61:387-390, 2003.

Flynn TR: Anatomy and surgery of deep space infections of the head and neck. In the American Association of Oral and Maxillofacial Surgeons: *Knowledge updates*, Rosemont, Ill, 1993, the Association.

Lew DP, Waldvogel FA: Osteomyelitis, *N Engl J Med* 336:999-1007, 1997.

Marx RE: Chronic osteomyelitis of the jaws, *Oral Maxillofac Clin North Am* 3:367-381, 1991.

Marx RE, Carlson EC, Smith BR, et al: Isolation of *Actinomyces* species and *Eikenella corrodens* from patients with chronic diffuse sclerosing osteomyelitis, *J Oral Maxillofac Surg* 52:26-33, 1994.

Mercuri LG: Acute osteomyelitis, *Oral Maxillofac Surg Clin North Am* 3:355, 1991.

Paluska S: Osteomyelitis, *Clin Fam Pract* 6:127-156, 2004.

Peterson LJ: Microbiology of head and neck infections, *Oral Maxillofac Surg Clin North Am* 3:247, 1991.

Vibhagool A, Calhoun J, Mader JP, et al: Therapy of bone and joint infections, *Hosp Formul* 28:63, 1993.

Waldvogel FA, Medoff G, Swartz MN: Osteomyelitis: a review of clinical features, therapeutic considerations and unusual aspects, *N Engl J Med* 282:316-322, 1970.

CHAPTER 5

Dentoalveolar Surgery

This section addresses:
- Third Molar Odontectomy
- Alveolar Osteitis (Dry Socket)
- Surgical Exposure of an Impacted Maxillary Canine
- Lingual Nerve Injury
- Displaced Root Fragments During Dentoalveolar Surgery

Dentoalveolar surgery is the surgical procedure that oral and maxillofacial surgeons perform most often. These procedures are associated with the dentate segment of the maxilla or mandible, termed the *alveolar ridge.* They include a variety of procedures, including simple tooth extractions, alveoplasty (recontouring of the alveolar bone), removal of tori, exposure of impacted teeth for orthodontic treatment, and extraction of impacted third molars. The origins and the current practice of oral and maxillofacial surgery are heavily based on dentoalveolar surgery. Such procedures account for more than 50% of the practice of oral and maxillofacial surgeons worldwide. Recently, placement of dental implants was added to the rehabilitative and reconstructive options for the maxillofacial region, replacing the more traditional preprosthetic procedures.

Since its establishment in 1918, the American Association of Oral and Maxillofacial Surgeons (AAOMS) has gone through extensive change, reflecting progressive changes in the specialty. Initially called the American Society of Exodontists, it was originally formed by a group of oral surgeons in Chicago after the National Dental Association meeting. As it has grown, the association has gone through several name changes, each reflecting the expansion of the specialty. Despite the wide scope of training of graduating oral and maxillofacial surgeons, as evidenced by the sections in this book, dentoalveolar surgery remains the foundation of our specialty.

In this chapter we present teaching cases representing some of the important aspects of this branch of oral and maxillofacial surgery. Three cases focus on complications of dentoalveolar surgery (dry socket, lingual nerve injury, and displacement of a tooth fragment during surgery), and two discuss the current issues in the treatment of impacted canines and third molars.

Third Molar Odontectomy

Shahrokh C. Bagheri and Sandeep V. Pathak

CC

A 17-year-old boy is referred to your clinic for consultation regarding his third molars.

HPI

The patient recently completed his orthodontic therapy. For the past few weeks, he had experienced increasing discomfort in the posterior mandible. He was subsequently referred by his orthodontist for evaluation. He denies any fever, swelling, or drainage from the area.

PMHX/PDHX/MEDICATIONS/ALLERGIES/SH/FH

Noncontributory. Thorough past medical and dental histories are important to determine any potential concerns with general health, fitness for anesthesia, and possible anesthetic or surgical morbidities. The patient does not report any symptoms suggestive of temporomandibular joint dysfunction (TMD) and does not take any medications. Certain medications may promote bleeding risk (e.g., aspirin, warfarin, and clopidogrel) or delay or impede healing (e.g., steroids or bisphosphonates). The patient smokes approximately one pack of cigarettes per day (risk factor for the development of dry sockets). Al-Belasy has reported that the incidence of dry sockets to be reduced with smoking cessation.

EXAMINATION

General. The patient is a well-developed and well-nourished man in no apparent distress (higher levels of anxiety may require a deeper level of sedation/anesthesia).

Maxillofacial. There is no soft tissue abnormality or lymphadenopathy (LAD). The patient has a good range of mandibular motion with an maximal interincisal opening (MIO) of 45 mm. Examination of the TMJ reveals no abnormalities (clicks or pain upon palpation). The muscles of mastication are nontender to palpation (important to detect preexisting symptoms of TMD).

Intraoral. Oral soft tissue is free of lesions, and there is no evidence of acute infection. The mandibular third molars are partially erupted, with approximately 20% of the crown visible in the oral cavity with insufficient room for functional eruption. The overlying operculum appears slightly inflamed, with evidence of food debris and periodontal pockets of greater than 6 mm on the distal of the left and right mandibular second molars. The right and left maxillary third molars are partially erupted. Oral hygiene is fair. An examination of the oropharynx is without tonsillar hypertrophy, and the patient has a Mallampati score of 1.

Indications for the removal of third molars include tooth malposition, periodontal conditions (e.g., probing lengths greater than 4 mm at distal of second molars or third molars), pericoronitis, symptoms of pain, evidence of infection or caries, orthodontic considerations, lack of space, associated pathology, and inability to maintain oral hygiene, especially when the third molars are incompletely erupted. Although some controversy exists as to the timing of or necessity for removal of asymptomatic third molars, there is evidence that younger patients (under 25 years old) have a decreased risk of complications and improved recovery after surgery. The decision to remove asymptomatic third molars should be driven by evidence-based decision making; the predominant guiding principle should be the patient's preference. The clinical findings should be the main driving factors in treatment decisions.

IMAGING

A panoramic radiograph is the minimum imaging modality necessary for the evaluation and treatment of impacted third molars. Computed tomography (CT) scans are not necessary for the routine evaluation, but they may be used in select cases of suspected maxillofacial pathology or for accurate determination of the inferior alveolar nerve anatomy. Partial odontectomy (coronectomy) may at times be an alternative treatment in patients requiring removal of a third molar that is in close proximity to the inferior alveolar nerve; however, this procedure does not eliminate the risk of inferior alveolar nerve injury and possible future infectious complications due to retention of root fragments.

In the current patient, the panoramic radiograph reveals a partial lack of space to accommodate the eruption of the mildly mesioangularly impacted mandibular molars with 75% root development (Figure 5-1). The roots are not fused and do not extend below the level of the neurovascular bundle. The outlines of mandibular canals are easily discerned on the radiograph. There is no diversion of the inferior alveolar canal, darkening of the third molar root, or interruption of the cortical white line (risk factors associated with inferior alveolar nerve injury) (Box 5-1). The maxillary third molars are vertically positioned with partial bony impaction. The

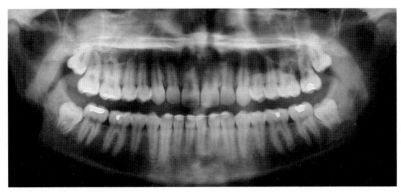

Figure 5-1 Panoramic radiograph demonstrating impacted maxillary and mandibular third molars (orthodontic retainer appliance is noted in the mandibular anterior incisors).

Box 5-1   **Rood's Radiographic Predictors of Potential Tooth Proximity to the Inferior Alveolar Canal**

- Darkening of the root
- Deflection of the root
- Narrowing of the root
- Dark and bifid root apex
- Interruption of the white line of the canal
- Diversion of the canal
- Narrowing of the canal

Modified from Rood JP, Shehab BA: The radiological prediction of inferior alveolar nerve injury during third molar surgery, *Br J Oral Maxillofac Surg* 28(1):20-25, 1990.

maxillary sinuses and the remainder of the radiograph are within normal limits.

LABS

No routine laboratory tests are indicated for the routine evaluation of impacted third molars unless dictated by underlying medical conditions.

ASSESSMENT

Partial bony impaction of the right and left maxillary and mandibular third molars with insufficient room for eruption; localized gingivitis and early periodontal pocketing noted around the left and right mandibular third molars.

TREATMENT

Two major professional organizations have made contradictory recommendations on the prophylactic removal of impacted third molars. The researchers for AAOMS Third Molar Clinical Trials published several scientific articles that linked third molars to future health problems in adults. In light of these findings, in 2005 the AAOMS suggested that removal of the third molars during young adulthood may be the most prudent option. In contrast, the National Health Service

(NHS) of Great Britain and an associated agency, the National Institute of Clinical Excellence (NICE), published a series of guidelines recommending that "the practice of prophylactic removal of pathology-free impacted third molars should be discontinued in the NHS." These guidelines, made public in 2000, did acknowledge the ongoing AAOMS Third Molar Clinical Trials. In 2012 Renton and colleagues published an article chronicling the United Kingdom's experience with retention of third molars. They concluded that "admissions for M3 [third molar] surgery activity under the NHS have decreased from the mid-1990s and into the 2000s, in association with professional and policy guidelines." They found that the average age for third molar surgery had risen, and the indications for the surgery were "increasingly associated with other pathologic features such as dental caries or pericoronitis, in line with NICE guidelines."

Although in some regions of the world, socioeconomic and available resources play a major role in the determination of guidelines for third molar extractions, current scientific evidence remains unchanged. The cumulative financial costs of treating the health complications of retained third molars in the older population should be considered. Although there is cost associated with the procedure to remove third molars, there is also the cost of monitoring retained third molars. Subsequent removal at an older age may also be associated with the cost of lost income in recuperation time, in addition to the greater risks of removal at an older age.

It is clear that the extraction of third molars poses some risks to the patient. However, the determination of extraction versus nonextraction of asymptomatic third molars must compare the cost and risks of surgical extraction with the lifetime health and cost benefits of preventing and eliminating any pathologic processes associated with retention of the third molars.

The effectiveness, safety, and relatively minimal cost of extraction of third molars using outpatient, office-based anesthesia, along with the currently available scientific evidence linking asymptomatic third molars to multiple health hazards, generally support the extraction of asymptomatic third molars in young adults; however, as mentioned, the patient's preference and an informed decision arrived at by the surgeon and patient are the most important deciding factors.

The current patient was seen in the clinic for extraction of his teeth under intravenous sedation. Monitors (pulse oximetry, capnography, blood pressure, and three-lead electrocardiography) were placed, and oxygen was delivered via a nasal mask at 4 L/min, followed by nitrous oxide. Midazolam and fentanyl were slowly titrated until a comfortable state of conscious sedation was achieved. A local anesthetic with epinephrine was injected, and adequate time was allowed for the local anesthetic block. A bite block was place for TMJ stabilization. An oral screen with loosely packed, moist gauze was placed to protect the airway from accidental aspiration. A full mucoperiosteal flap was elevated using a buccal envelope incision with a distal hockey-stick extension for the mandibular third molars. Special consideration was given to preventing trauma to the lingual tissue.

A buccal trough was made using a high-speed instrument (impaction drill and burr with irrigation), and the teeth were elevated and extracted. Careful attention must be given to avoiding violation of the lingual cortex (although at times, disrupting the lingual cortex is unavoidable). The neurovascular bundle was not visualized, and there was no excessive hemorrhage from the socket (visualization of the neurovascular bundle and excessive hemorrhage from the socket are associated with an increased risk of inferior alveolar nerve injury). The wound was irrigated with normal saline, and the flaps were closed with chromic suture, with careful attention paid to suturing only the superficial lingual mucosa and thus preventing lingual nerve injury.

The upper third molars were removed through an envelope mucoperiosteal flap. Care was taken to avoid the roots of the maxillary second molars (a possible complication). There was no evidence of an oral antral communication. The tooth follicles were removed, and the sites were irrigated. Gauze was placed between the teeth to promote hemostasis, and the patient was monitored in the recovery room until he was fully awake and alert.

COMPLICATIONS

As mentioned, third molar extraction is the surgical procedure that oral and maxillofacial surgeons perform most often. A well-planned surgical approach, with the goal of prevention, is the best way to minimize complications. Yet, despite our best efforts, complications are expected, and it is best to counsel patients preoperatively for potential risks. Clinicians need to be aware of the risk factors associated with an increased risk of complications for this commonly performed procedure.

Pogrel concluded, "The age of 25 years appears in many studies to be a critical time after which complications increase more rapidly." No studies indicate that complications decrease as age increases. In fact, the older a patient is, the more likely it is that the recovery from complications will be prolonged, less predictable, and less complete.

Sensory nerve injury is well documented. Injury to the inferior alveolar nerve can lead to a range of symptoms along its distribution (anesthesia, hypoesthesia, dysesthesia,

or paresthesia). A review of the literature demonstrates an incidence of nerve injury between 0.4% and 5%. In one large study with 367,170 patients, the incidence of nerve injury was 0.4% (22% of whom had symptoms lasting longer than 12 months). The risk of nerve injury is greater with increasing patient age, degree of root development, degree of impaction, and the radiographic relationship of the roots to the inferior alveolar canal. The incidence of injury to the inferior alveolar nerve is slightly higher than that for the lingual nerve, but the inferior alveolar nerve has a higher incidence of spontaneous recovery (due to its position in the bony canal, which allows a greater possibility that the nerve endings will reapproximate); however, older patients are more likely to have incomplete recovery. Injury to the long buccal nerve is also possible, but it is less of a concern, causing minimal to no subjective disability. Patients with severe inferior alveolar nerve or lingual nerve injury should be referred to a microneurosurgeon for prompt evaluation and potential surgical intervention (decompression, neurolysis, or neurorrhaphy). Complications from local anesthesia also have been reported, probably due to direct needle trauma to the inferior alveolar nerve. The reported incidence ranges from 1 in 400,000 to 1 in 750,000 patients.

Not unlike with any other procedure, infections are commonly associated with third molar removal, both preoperatively and postoperatively. This appears to be more common after removal of partial and full bony impactions. Infections can occur as early as several days after the procedure, or they may present late (within several weeks). They can be localized to the area of the third molar or occasionally can spread to adjacent fascial spaces to cause life-threatening conditions. Most infections are easily managed with local measures and the use of antibiotics. The incidence of postoperative infection is approximately 3%. Increasing evidence supports the use of antibiotic prophylaxis, which has been shown to decrease the risk of postoperative infection. However, the decision on whether to prescribe antibiotics is multifactorial.

Localized osteitis (dry socket) is a well-known complication of tooth extractions and is discussed in detail elsewhere (see Alveolar Osteitis [Dry Socket] later in this chapter). Other complications associated with third molar surgery include periodontal complications, maxillary sinus involvement (oral antral communications, displacement of a fragment into the sinus), displacement of a tooth into adjacent fascial spaces, breaking of instruments, aspiration or swallowing of foreign objects, TMJ pain, maxillary tuberosity fractures, root fracture, injury to adjacent teeth, hemorrhage/hematoma, wound dehiscence, mandible fracture, and soft tissue emphysema.

DISCUSSION

Indications for the removal of third molars are variable and influenced by many factors. Insufficient room for adequate eruption of the teeth can create difficulty with maintenance of oral hygiene in these areas, affecting the adjacent soft tissues and teeth. The increased difficulty and risks of third molar removal with increasing age, inadequate oral hygiene, and tooth position, in addition to periodontal health and orthodontic considerations, should be taken into account. Erupted or partially erupted third molars have been shown to have a negative impact on periodontal health. In a study by Dodson, attachment levels and probing depths improved after third molar removal. Pogrel reported that a periodontal condition may persist or may be created on the distal aspect of the second molar after third molar removal, especially in some older patients. Dodson has suggested that in this subgroup of patients, immediate reconstruction may be beneficial in the long term. However, the relationship between third molars and periodontal disease pathogenesis requires further study. There is no clear consensus on the ability of mandibular third molars to cause crowding of the anterior teeth. Although some investigators have shown a statistical association of third molars and late anterior crowding, this association is not strong. The majority of the literature does not support this hypothesis.

Offenbacher and colleagues published a study on periodontal disease and the risk of preterm delivery. The study involved 1,020 pregnant women who received antepartum and postpartum periodontal examinations. The findings clearly demonstrated that maternal periodontal disease increases the relative risk of preterm or spontaneous preterm birth. The mothers with third molar periodontal pathology had elevated serum markers of systemic inflammation (C-reactive protein, isoprostanes). Periodontal disease was also a predictor of more severe adverse pregnancy outcomes.

For extraction of third molars, there is a wide range of choices of anesthetic and surgical techniques related to the surgeon's training and experience. As the common dictum proclaims, "There is more than one way to do it." Many different surgical flaps and instruments have been developed over the years. A variation of the buccal hockey-stick incision appears to be the most commonly used and has the lowest incidence of permanent neurosensory injury. Similarly, the choice of anesthesia can vary from local anesthesia, to intravenous sedation using a variety of medications, to general anesthesia with endotracheal intubation. This choice is influenced by many factors, including the patient's preference, available resources, surgeon's training, and practice patterns in the region. Various regimens of perioperative care are also followed. Common practices include the use of a long-acting local anesthetic (e.g., 0.5% Marcaine), corticosteroids, and nonsteroidal antiinflammatory drugs (NSAIDs) to improve postoperative pain management.

The anatomy of the inferior alveolar nerve is variable, but the canal is usually located inferior and buccal to the impacted mandibular third molars. In the largest cadaveric study of lingual nerve anatomy, by Behnia and associates, 669 nerves from 430 fresh cadavers were examined. In 94 cases (14%), the nerve was above the lingual crest, and in one case the nerve was in the retromolar pad region. In the remaining 574 cases (86%), the mean horizontal and vertical distances of the nerve to the lingual plate and the lingual crest were 2.1 mm and 3 mm, respectively. In 149 cases (22%), the nerve was in direct contact with the lingual plate of the alveolar process. The unpredictable anatomy of the lingual nerve in relation to the mandibular third molar increases this nerve's susceptibility to injury.

Bibliography

Al-Belasy FA: The relationship of "Shisha" (water pipe) smoking to postextraction dry socket, *J Oral Maxillofac Surg* 62:10, 2004.

Alling CC: Dysesthesia of the lingual and inferior alveolar nerves following third molar surgery, *J Oral Maxillofac Surg* 44:454, 1986.

Alling C, Helfrick J, Alling R: *Impacted teeth*, Philadelphia, 1993, Saunders.

American Association of Oral and Maxillofacial Surgeons: Research study links wisdom teeth to health problems in young adults, September 20, 2005 (news release).

Bagheri SC, Khan HA: Extraction versus non-extraction management of third molars, *Oral Maxillofac Surg Clin North Am* 19(1):15-21, 2007.

Behnia H, Kheradvar A, Shahrokhi M: An anatomic study of the lingual nerve in the third molar region, *J Oral Maxillofac Surg* 58(6):649-651, discussion, 652-653; 2000.

Blaeser BF, August MA, Donoff RB, et al: Panoramic radiographic risk factors for inferior alveolar nerve injury after third molar extraction, *J Oral Maxillofac Surg* 61(4):417-421, 2003.

Blakey GH, Jacks MT, Offenbacher S, et al: Progression of periodontal disease in the second/third molar region in subjects with asymptomatic third molars, *J Oral Maxillofac Surg* 64(2):189-193, 2006.

Blakey GH, Marciani RD, Haug RH, et al: Periodontal pathology associated with asymptomatic third molars, *J Oral Maxillofac Surg* 60(11):1227-1233, 2002.

Cilasun U, et al: Coronectomy in patients with high risk of inferior alveolar nerve injury diagnosed by computed tomography, *J Oral Maxillofac Surg* 69:1557-1561, 2011.

Dodson TB: Management of mandibular third molar extraction sites to prevent periodontal defects, *J Oral Maxillofac Surg* 62(10):1213-1224, 2004.

Dodson TB: Management of asymptomatic wisdom teeth: an evidence-based approach. In Bagheri SB, Bell RB, Khan HA (eds): *Current therapy in oral and maxillofacial surgery*, pp 122-126, Philadelphia, 2011, Elsevier/Saunders.

Dodson TB: Surveillance as a management strategy for retained third molars: Is it desirable? *J Oral Maxillofac Surg* 70(9):S20-S24, 2012.

Elter JR, Cuomo CJ, Offenbacher S, et al: Third molars associated with periodontal pathology in the Third National Health and Nutrition Examination Survey, *J Oral Maxillofac Surg* 62(4):440-445, 2004.

Hall HD, Bildman BS, Hand CD: Prevention of dry socket with local application of tetracycline, *J Oral Surg* 29:35, 1971.

Herpy AK, Goupil MT: A monitoring and evaluation study of third molar surgery complications at a major medical center, *Military Medicine* 156:1, 1991.

Kiesselbach JE, Chamberlain JG: Clinical and anatomic observations on the relationship of the lingual nerve to the mandibular third molar, *J Oral Surg* 42:565, 1984.

Koumaras GM: What costs are associated with the management of third molars? *J Oral Maxillofac Surg* 70(9):S8-S10, 2012.

Long H, Zhou Y, Liao L, et al: Coronectomy vs total removal for third molar extraction: a systematic review, *J Dent Res* 91(7):659-665, 2012.

Nakamori K, Fujiwara K, et al: Clinical assessment of the relationship between the third molar and the inferior alveolar canal using panoramic images and computed tomography, *J Oral Maxillofac Surg* 66:2308-2313, 2008.

Nakayama K, Nonoyama M, Takaki Y, et al: Assessment of the relationship between impacted mandibular third molars and inferior alveolar nerve with dental 3-dimensional computed tomography, *J Oral Maxillofac Surg* 67:2587-2591, 2009.

National Institute for Clinical Excellence: Guidance on the extraction of wisdom teeth. Available at: www.nice.org.uk/pdf/wisdomteethguidance.pdf. Accessed February 5, 2013.

Offenbacher S, Boggess KA, Murtha AP, et al: Progressive periodontal disease and risk of very preterm delivery, *Obstet Gynecol* 107(1):29-36, 2006.

Offenbacher S, Beck JD, Moss KL, et al: What are the local and systemic implications of third molar retention? *J Oral Maxillofac Surg* 70(9):S58-S65, 2012.

Osborn TP, Frederickson G, Small IA, et al: A prospective study of complications related to mandibular third molar surgery, *J Oral Maxillofac Surg* 43:767-771, 1985.

Patel V, Gleeson CF, Kwok J, et al: Coronectomy practice. Paper 2. Complications and long term management, *Br J Oral Maxillofac Surg* 50(8):739-744, 2012.06.008.

Piecuch JF: What strategies are helpful in the operative management of third molars? *J Oral Maxillofac Surg* 70(9):S25-S32, 2012.

Pogrel MA: Complications of third molar surgery. In Kaban LB, Pogrel MA, Perrott DH (eds): *Complications of oral and maxillofacial surgery*, Philadelphia, 1997, Saunders.

Pogrel MA: What are the risks of operative intervention? *J Oral Maxillofac Surg* 70(9):S33-S36, 2012.

Pogrel MA: What is the effect of timing of removal on the incidence and severity of complications? *J Oral Maxillofac Surg* 70(9):S37-S40, 2012.

Renton T, et al: What has been the United Kingdom's experience with retention of third molars? *J Oral Maxillofac Surg* 70(9):S48-S57, 2012.

Rood JP, Shehab BA: The radiological predictors of inferior alveolar nerve injury during third molar surgery, *Br J Oral Maxillofac Surg* 28:20, 1990.

Sweet JB, Butler DP: Predisposing and operative factors: effect on the incidence of localized osteitis in mandibular third molar surgery, *J Oral Surg* 46:206, 1978.

White RP Jr, Madianos PN, Offenbacher S, et al: Microbial complexes detected in the second/third molar region in patients with asymptomatic third molars, *J Oral Maxillofac Surg* 60(11):1234-1240, 2002.

Alveolar Osteitis (Dry Socket)

Eric P. Holmgren and Shahrokh C. Bagheri

CC

A 19-year-old woman presents to your clinic 5 days after removal of four impacted third molars. She complains of increasing pain that is difficult to control with prescription pain medications.

HPI

The patient underwent removal of four difficult full bony impactions. Postoperatively, she was given a prescription for an opioid/acetaminophen combination medication for pain control. On the fifth postoperative day, she describes a worsening, dull, aching pain that radiates to her left ear. She complains of a bad odor (halitosis) and taste in her mouth emanating from her lower jaw. She reports that she adhered closely to the postoperative instructions and that this pain is different from her immediate postoperative pain.

PMHX/PDHX/MEDICATIONS/ALLERGIES/SH/FH

The patient uses birth control pills and smokes one pack of cigarettes per day (both risk factors for the development of alveolar osteitis) (Box 5-2).

EXAMINATION

General. The patient appears to be in mild distress secondary to pain. The accompanying parent is very concerned.

Vital signs. Her vital signs are within normal limits (dry sockets do not cause fever).

Box 5-2	Factors Implicated in the Development of Alveolar Osteitis

Increased Risk
- Smoking
- Birth control pills
- History of pericoronitis
- Increased age
- Traumatic extraction (inexperienced surgeon)
- Inadequate irrigation

Decreased Risk
- Prerinsing with chlorhexidine
- Maintenance of good oral hygiene perioperatively
- Thorough intraoperative lavage

Maxillofacial. There is bilateral edema of the lower face consistent with the patient's surgery. There are no cranial nerve deficits.

Intraoral. The extraction sockets of the maxillary third molars and the right mandibular third molar appear to be healing adequately with no evidence of exposed alveolar bone. The extraction socket of the left mandibular third molar shows evidence of exposed bone, food debris, and sensitivity upon irrigation. There is no purulence (alveolar osteitis is not an infection).

IMAGING

A panoramic radiograph is not routinely indicated for the evaluation of alveolar osteitis; it is used if there is suspicion of retained bony or tooth fragments in the sockets. Nonresorbable dry socket packs must contain a radiopaque material to ensure removal of any packing material upon subsequent visits, which can be confirmed with radiographs.

The preoperative panoramic radiograph should be evaluated for the proximity of the inferior alveolar nerve before application of eugenol-based medicaments because of the possible neurotoxic effects of this medication.

LABS

No laboratory tests are indicated for the routine management of alveolar osteitis.

ASSESSMENT

Alveolar osteitis (dry socket) of the extraction socket of the left mandibular third molar.

TREATMENT

The primary goal of treatment is relief of pain through this phase of delayed healing. Medicaments such as eugenol and lidocaine jelly have been advocated for packing the socket, although dry sockets resolve with symptomatic therapy alone. If the clinician chooses to use packs, they can be changed every day or every other day for approximately 3 to 6 days until the pain has resolved. It is imperative to avoid using eugenol-based packs if the alveolar nerve is suspected to be in close proximity, as mentioned, because of eugenol's neurotoxic properties. It is important to evaluate the preoperative panoramic radiograph and the operative note for evidence of close proximity to or exposure of the inferior alveolar nerve to the roots and/or sockets of the third molars. In such cases, alternatives such as in $\frac{1}{4}$-inch gauze strips saturated with lidocaine jelly may be used. Once the pain has subsided, the packing should be removed to avoid the development of a foreign body reaction.

Previously it was thought that curettage of the socket could induce bleeding and therefore healing. This has not been shown to promote healing. Aggressive curettage of the socket is unnecessary and contraindicated. There is no indication for the use of antibiotics for treatment of dry sockets.

In the current patient, treatment involved gentle irrigation with warm saline (without curettage), placement of iodoform/eugenol-based packing into the socket, and prescription anti-inflammatory medication. The patient had improvement of her pain within minutes, and she returned 48 hours later with a marked reduction of pain. The packing was removed, and the socket was gently irrigated. She was instructed to maintain good oral hygiene and rinse with warm saline until the socket no longer collected debris.

COMPLICATIONS

The vast majority of cases of alveolar osteitis heal without any intervention. Most medicaments placed in the socket (which usually contain eugenol) are palliative and may not necessarily expedite recovery. However, the clinician must identify chronic nonhealing extraction sockets, especially in patients at risk for the development of osteomyelitis (diabetes or chronic steroid use), osteoradionecrosis (history of radiation therapy to the surgical site), or bisphosphonate-induced osteonecrosis. Patients who do not respond to routine care of diagnosed alveolar osteitis must undergo further evaluation for other pathologic processes.

DISCUSSION

The onset of alveolar osteitis is variable but commonly occurs 3 to 7 days after extraction. The etiology, prevention, and treatment of alveolar osteitis are up for debate. The prevailing theory of the pathogenesis of alveolar osteitis is that the initial clot is destroyed by fibrinolytic activity, impairing the production of granulation tissue that in turn promotes the formation of the initial fibrillar bone and ultimately mature bone. Bacteria may play an important but not clearly defined role. The incidence of alveolar osteitis is between 1% and 3% of all extraction sockets. The condition is most common with mandibular molars; the next most commonly involved teeth are the mandibular premolars, followed by the maxillary premolars, molars, canines, and incisors.

It is well known that smoking, oral contraceptive pills, a history of existing pericoronitis, traumatic extractions (correlating with the surgeon's experience), older age, and inadequate irrigation at the time of surgery are strongly associated with the development of alveolar osteitis. Based on several studies, preoperative rinsing with chlorhexidine and thorough intraoperative lavage with physiologic saline reduce the incidence of alveolar osteitis by up to 50%. The findings of studies on the efficacy of topical/intra-alveolar antibiotics and their benefits are the subject of debate. Recent studies have not demonstrated any benefit. Similarly, the use of systemic perioperative antibiotics has not been shown to be of any benefit. At present, the literature does not support the use of perioperative antibiotics in reducing the incidence of alveolar osteitis.

Contrary to current thinking, factors such as the use of a vasoconstrictive drug, seasonal allergies, bacterial load in the socket, flap design, and negative pressure dislodgement of the clot (use of a straw or spitting) have not been shown to increase the incidence of dry socket. As mentioned, there is evidence that the use of oral contraceptives is a risk factor, but female gender alone is not.

Bibliography

Alexander RE: Dental extraction wound management: a case against medicating postextraction sockets, *J Oral Maxillofac Surg* 58(5):538-551, 2000.

Betts NJ, Makowski G, Shen YH, et al: Evaluation of topical viscous 2% lidocaine jelly as an adjunct during the management of alveolar osteitis, *J Oral Maxillofac Surg* 53(10):1140-1144, 1995.

Caso A, Hung LK, Beirne OR: Prevention of alveolar osteitis with chlorhexidine: a meta-analytic review, *Oral Surg Oral Med Oral Pathol Oral Radiol Endod* 99(2):155-159, 2005.

Garcia AG, Grana PM, Sampedro FG, et al: Does oral contraceptive use affect the incidence of complications after extraction of a mandibular third molar? *Br Dent J* 194(8):453-455, 2003.

Halabi D, Escobar J, Munoz C, et al: Logistic regression analysis of risk factors for the devel0pment of alveolar osteitis, *J Oral Maxillofac Surg* 70:1040-1044, 2012.

Hermesch CB, Hilton TJ, Biesbrock AR, et al: Perioperative use of 0.12% chlorhexidine gluconate for the prevention of alveolar osteitis: efficacy and risk factor analysis, *Oral Surg Oral Med Oral Pathol Oral Radiol Endod* 85(4):381-387, 1998.

Larsen PE: Alveolar osteitis after surgical removal of impacted mandibular third molars: identification of the patient at risk, *Oral Surg Oral Med Oral Pathol* 73(4):393-397, 1992.

Poeschl PW, Eckel D, Poeschl E: Postoperative prophylactic antibiotic treatment in third molar surgery—a necessity? *J Oral Maxillofac Surg* 61(1):3-8, 2004.

Rood JP, Shehab BA: The radiological prediction of inferior alveolar nerve injury during third molar surgery, *Br J Oral Maxillofac Surg* 28(1):20-25, 1990.

Sanchis JM, Sáez U, Peñarrocha M, et al: Tetracycline compound placement to prevent dry socket: a postoperative study of 200 impacted mandibular third molars, *J Oral Maxillofac Surg* 62(5):587-591, 2004.

Surgical Exposure of an Impacted Maxillary Canine

Bruce W. Anderson and Shahrokh C. Bagheri

CC

A 14-year-old boy is referred to your office by his orthodontist for exposure and bracketing of an impacted left maxillary canine (the canines normally erupt between 11 and 12 years of age). The maxillary canines are the second most commonly impacted teeth (the most common are the third molars).

HPI

The patient has a history of premature loss of the primary left maxillary canine secondary to trauma (premature loss of teeth with subsequent arch length reduction is one of the many causes of impaction). Orthodontic treatment has begun, and sufficient arch space has been accommodated for the guided eruption of the impacted canine. The patient has no history of any other impacted or congenitally missing teeth and presents with an otherwise full dentition.

PMHX/PDHX/MEDICATIONS/ALLERGIES/SH/FH

Noncontributory.

EXAMINATION

General. The patient is a well-developed and well-nourished boy in no apparent distress.

Maxillofacial. He has a symmetrical facial appearance with no obvious skeletal abnormalities.

Intraoral. Orthodontic bands, brackets, and arch wires are in place. A well-healed edentulous space is present in the area of the left maxillary cuspid with an adequate alveolar ridge. A small, painless, palpable bony buccal protuberance can be noted in the area of the left maxillary cuspid, consistent with the crown of the impacted canine (clinical evaluation to determine palatal or buccal impaction is important and often sufficient to determine the approach for access to the tooth). The gingival and palatal tissues both appear healthy, with no notable periodontal defects.

IMAGING

A panoramic radiograph is the initial screening study of choice for evaluating impacted teeth. It provides an excellent overview of the dentition, associated dentoalveolar structures, and location of impacted teeth. Periapical "shift shots" can help determine whether the tooth is buccal/labial or palatal/lingual (the SLOB rule [*same lingual, opposite buccal*] is frequently used to determine the position of the tooth on the subsequent x-ray film as the cone of the x-ray machine is moved anteriorly or posteriorly). Occlusal films, lateral cephalometric films, or CT scans can be used for precisely locating the position and orientation of impacted teeth.

In-office, small field cone-beam computed tomography (CBCT) provides perhaps the most convenient and valuable imaging method; it demonstrates not only the canine position, but also the details of angulation, orientation, and relationship to adjacent structures (see the figures in the section on cone-beam computed tomography [CBCT] in Chapter 1). This information can be beneficial for the surgeon's treatment plan and the choice of surgical approach, in addition to aiding the orthodontist in determining the path of eruption. CBCT may also detect root resorption of adjacent teeth that is not evident on panoramic radiographs. Haney reported significant changes in position diagnosis, root resorption detection, orthodontic vector determination, and surgical access planning by a group of orthodontists and oral surgeons who reviewed CBCT images compared with review of traditional radiographs of the same patients.

In the current patient, the panoramic radiograph shows a fully formed impacted left maxillary cuspid with a mesioangular orientation. Figure 5-2 demonstrates the position of the impacted canine before the initiation of orthodontic therapy. The crown of the canine appears to have a pericoronal radiolucent lesion consistent with a hyperplastic dental follicle (although a dentigerous cyst or other pathologic processes are also possible). No crestal bone loss is noted in the surrounding region. The full bony impacted third molars are also noted.

LABS

No laboratory studies are indicated for routine exposure and orthodontic bracket placement of impacted teeth unless dictated by the medical history.

ASSESSMENT

Full bony mesioangular labially impacted left maxillary canine.

TREATMENT

Current popular treatments of impacted canines can be divided into open and closed surgical techniques, differing slightly in

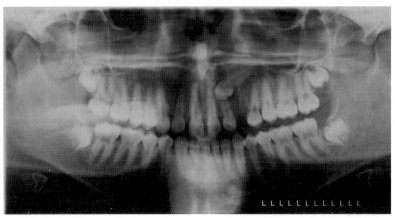

Figure 5-2 Panoramic radiograph demonstrating the horizontal impaction of the left maxillary canine before orthodontic therapy. The full bony impacted third molars are also noted.

regard to palatal versus labial impactions. Autotransplantation and extraction with implant replacement are less commonly used techniques and are described later with other historical techniques. Extraction of the primary canine may be considered if the patient is between 10 and 13 years old and sufficient arch space has been created, allowing observation for normal eruption of the permanent canine. Serial radiographs can be used to monitor eruption, and if no movement is observed over 12 months, alternative techniques should be performed.

Open techniques. These surgical techniques are indicated when the crown of the impacted canine is in an appropriate location near the alveolar process, allowing exposure and access for orthodontic bracket placement. For palatal impactions, the excision of overlying soft tissue may be performed with a surgical blade or electrocautery as a "window." Care should be taken to preserve sufficient soft tissue between the "window" and the cervical margin of surrounding erupted teeth to avoid potential tissue necrosis and periodontal complications. Bone removal may be performed with a rotary instrument, rongeurs, or hand instruments to expose the crown to the level of the cervical margin. Complete exposure of the crown may not be feasible in cases in which the crown is in close proximity to incisor roots. Any dental follicle remnants should be excised at this time, and gentle luxation of the tooth may be performed to rule out ankylosis. An orthodontic bracket with gold chain may be etched and bonded to the crown with the chain attached passively to existing orthodontic arch wires. The wound may be left open or packed with a periodontal dressing for a period of 4 to 5 days. It is generally accepted that a period of 6 to 8 weeks is observed for both palatal and labial impactions to allow for spontaneous eruption prior to the application of orthodontic forces. The apically repositioned flap is the open technique of choice for labially impacted canines. Electrocautery, or a "window" excision of overlying soft tissue, should be avoided with labial impactions, because it usually results in a lack of attached gingiva after eruption, with a possible need for a secondary graft procedure. A full thickness mucoperiosteal flap with vertical releasing incisions is raised to the level of the vestibular

sulcus, followed by bone removal, follicle removal, and crown exposure and luxation as previously described. The distal aspect of the flap is positioned apically and sutured with chromic gut at the level of the cervical margin, thus placing attached gingiva at the level of the cementoenamel junction. Again, the bracket with chain may be bonded at this time.

Closed techniques. These surgical techniques are indicated when the crown is not near the alveolar process or is in a position that inhibits the apical repositioning of a flap (Figures 5-3 and 5-4). In both palatal and labial impactions, a full thickness mucoperiosteal flap is raised, allowing subsequent crown exposure, gentle luxation, and bonding of the orthodontic bracket with a chain. At this point, the chain may be brought through the distal aspect of the flap (or through a stab incision in the body of the flap), and the full flap is repositioned and sutured. In closed techniques, orthodontic forces may be applied after 1 week to allow for soft tissue healing.

COMPLICATIONS

The most prevalent complication associated with surgical exposure of impacted canines is failure of the orthodontic bracket bond or fracture of the chain. This is of greater consequence in closed techniques, because it requires surgical reexposure of the crown before replacement of the bracket. Moisture in the surgical field during bracket bonding may be the likely cause of this complication. Reexposure also is required with the occurrence of gingival overgrowth in open techniques.

Periodontal defects may occur as a result of inappropriate flap design and/or bone loss adjacent to the surgical site. Damage to the erupting tooth and adjacent tooth roots, including root resorption, may occur secondary to difficulty controlling the path of eruption. Devitalization of the pulp of the impacted tooth or neighboring incisors requires cessation of orthodontic movement and evaluation for possible endodontic treatment.

Ankylosis of the impacted tooth should be considered if no movement is observed after sufficient application of orthodontic forces and adequate time. Intrusion of the anchoring

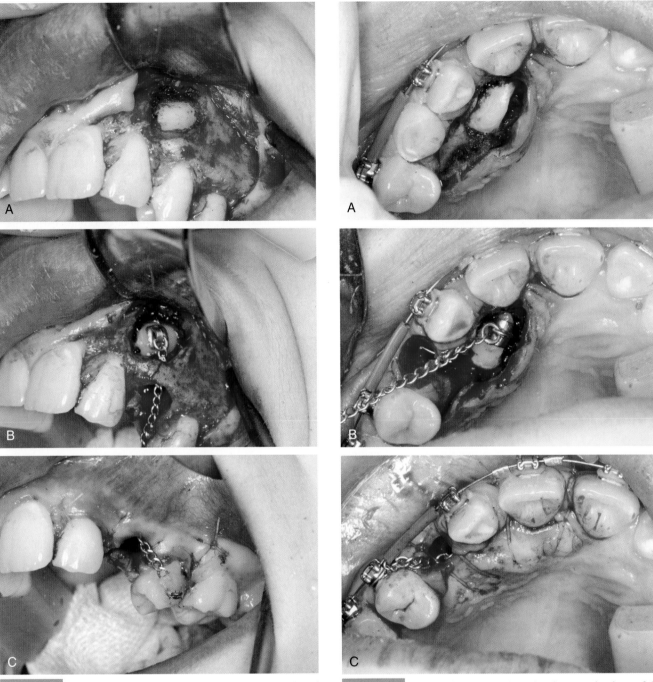

Figure 5-3   A labially impacted tooth #11 managed with a closed tunnel technique. *(From Bagheri SC, Bell B, Khan HA: Current therapy in oral and maxillofacial surgery, St Louis, 2012, Saunders.)*

Figure 5-4   A palatally impacted tooth #6 exposed using a full thickness palatal flap. *(From Bagheri SC, Bell B, Khan HA: Current therapy in oral and maxillofacial surgery, St Louis, 2012, Saunders.)*

dentition may be observed in this situation. Some suggest that the act of gently luxating the tooth at the time of exposure may cause ankylosis as a result of subsequent bleeding and inflammation.

Other complications include infection, flap necrosis secondary to poor design or contact with acid etch, lack of keratinized tissue secondary to poor flap design, and paresthesia of the palate (if the nasopalatine nerve is injured) or of the lower lip, chin, mandibular incisors, and gingiva in the case of impacted mandibular canines.

DISCUSSION

Excluding third molars, canines are the most commonly treated impactions by the oral and maxillofacial surgeon. The frequency of impacted canines has been reported as 2% to 5%, with palatal impactions occurring more frequently than labial impactions. The male to female ratio is commonly reported as 1:2, and mandibular impactions have a 0.4% reported frequency. Most impacted canines have an unknown etiology; however, numerous etiologies have been suggested, including mechanical obstruction by adjacent teeth, pathology, arch length discrepancy (more prevalent in labial impactions), premature loss of deciduous teeth, associated syndromes, questionable genetic predispositions, and endocrine abnormalities, such as hypothyroidism and hypopituitarism.

Historical treatments of impacted canines include the placement of crown forms or cervical wires. Adapted aluminum or plastic crown forms were commonly placed after exposure using a closed technique, with resulting erosion of overlying soft tissue secondary to a foreign body reaction. Once visible in the oral cavity, the crown form was removed and orthodontic brackets were placed. Wires secured around the cervical neck of the canine were also popularly used, but this was a more technically demanding procedure, sometimes requiring excessive manipulation of the tooth, and erosion of the canine at the cervical neck has been reported with this technique.

Additional surgical options include autotransplantation, segmental osteotomy, and extraction with subsequent implant placement. Autotransplantation may be indicated in circumstances of deep impactions and involves the creation of a bony socket for the extracted and transplanted canine. Survival rates have been reported at 70%, and as high as 94% when the periodontal membrane is intact at the time of transplantation. This technique, however, is not commonly used, because it is less predictable, and several cases of external root resorption have been reported. Segmental osteotomy is seldom performed and carries the risks of a more technical procedure. The incidence of extraction and replacement with osseointegrated implants has increased in recent years, but the use of implants in growing children is still controversial. Implants have been shown to migrate and may become submerged as growth continues vertically. The latter complication may be avoided by placement of the implant after vertical growth of the alveolus is complete. Despite these concerns, successful restoration using implants has been demonstrated in numerous studies and warrants further investigation.

The decision between an open or a closed technique is often left up to the practitioner and may be one of personal choice. As mentioned previously, certain physical location factors of the involved impacted tooth may dictate one technique over another. Some studies have reported a twofold higher rate of complications for closed techniques compared with open techniques. The primary complication with closed techniques is bond or wire failure, and the primary complication with open techniques is soft tissue overgrowth. More recent studies show no significant differences in surgical outcomes. Bond failure in open techniques is a minor complication, and some suggest delaying bracket placement until after the observational period, allowing greater control of moisture in the surgical field. No significant differences in subsequent periodontal complications have been reported between the two groups. The consensus appears to be that both techniques are acceptable and provide predictable results for the treatment of impacted canines.

Bibliography

Alberto PL: Management of the impacted canine and second molar, *Oral Maxillofac Surg Clin North Am* 19:59-68, 2007.

Bass T: Observation on the misplaced upper canine tooth, *Dent Pract Dent Rec* 18:25-33, 1967.

Caminiti MF, Sandor GK, Giambattistini C, et al: Outcomes of the surgical exposure, bonding and eruption of 82 impacted maxillary canines, *J Can Dent Assoc* 64(8):572-579, 1998.

Celikoglu M, Kamak H, Oktay H, et al: Investigation of transmigrated and impacted maxillary and mandibular canine teeth in an orthodontic patient population, *J Oral Maxillofac Surg* 68:1001-1006, 2010.

Chaushu S, et al: Patient's perception of recovery after exposure of impacted teeth: a comparison of closed- versus open-eruption techniques, *J Oral Maxillofac Surg* 63:323-329, 2005.

Felsenfeld AL, Aghaloo T: Surgical exposure of impacted teeth, *Oral Maxillofac Surg Clin North Am* 14:187-199, 2002.

Ferguson JW, Parvizi F: Eruption of palatal canines following surgical exposure: a review of outcomes in a series of consecutively treated cases, *Br J Orthod* 24(3):203-207, 1997.

Haney E, Gansky SA, Lee JS, et al: Comparative analysis of traditional radiographs and cone beam computed-tomography volumetric images in the diagnosis and treatment planning of maxillary impacted canines, *Am J Orthod Dentofacial Orthop* 137:590-597, 2010.

Jacobs SG: The impacted maxillary canine: further observations on aetiology, radiographic localization, prevention/interception of impaction, and when to suspect impaction, *Aust Dent J* 41(15):310-316, 1996.

Johnson W: Treatment of palatally impacted canine teeth, *Am J Orthod* 56(6):589-596, 1969.

Moss JP: Autogenous transplantation of maxillary canines, *Br J Oral Surg* 26:775, 1968.

Parkin NA, Deery C, Smith AM, et al: No difference in surgical outcomes between open and closed exposures of palatally displaced maxillary canines, *J Oral Maxillofac Surg* 70:2026-2034, 2012.

Pearson MH, Robinson SN, Reed R, et al: Management of palatally impacted canines: the findings of a collaborative study, *Eur J Orthod* 19(5):511-515, 1997.

Pogrel MA: Evaluation of over 400 autogenous tooth transplants, *J Oral Maxillofac Surg* 45:205-211, 1987.

Tiwanna PS, Kushner GM: Management of impacted teeth in children, *Oral Maxillofac Surg Clin North Am* 17:365-373, 2005.

Lingual Nerve Injury

Shahrokh C. Bagheri and Roger A. Meyer

CC

An 18-year-old female is referred to a microneurosurgeon for evaluation of numbness of her left tongue.

HPI

The patient had all four third molars surgically removed by an oral and maxillofacial surgeon 13 weeks before presentation. Upon follow-up at 7 days with the referring surgeon, the patient complained of persistent loss of feeling in her left tongue and altered taste sensation. No neurosensory testing was done at that time. Six weeks after surgery, the patient continued to report profound numbness of the left tongue and no improvement in taste perception. All surgical wounds were healed. Neurosensory testing (NST) of the tongue (pinprick and light touch) demonstrated total anesthesia (absence of perception of any stimulation of the mucosa) of the anterior two thirds of the left tongue, floor of the mouth, and lingual gingiva. Photographic documentation of the affected area of the tongue was obtained. An appointment was made for reevaluation of the patient in 4 weeks. At follow-up (10 weeks postsurgery), repeat NST revealed no change (persistent total anesthesia) from the previous examination. The patient was subsequently referred to a microneurosurgeon for evaluation of left lingual nerve (LN) injury.

The patient also complained of pain radiating into her left tongue when chewing food or brushing her left lower teeth (allodynia) and frequent accidental biting of her tongue. (*Allodynia* is defined as pain due to a stimulus that does not normally produce pain. *Dysesthesia* is an unpleasant abnormal sensation, either spontaneous or evoked, and *anesthesia dolorosa* is pain in an area or a region that is anesthetic.)

PMHX/PDHX/MEDICATIONS/ALLERGIES/SH/FH

Noncontributory.

EXAMINATION

General. The patient is a well-developed and well-nourished adolescent female in no apparent distress.

Maxillofacial. There is no cervical lymphadenopathy. Maximum interincisal opening is 51 mm without mandibular deviation, and all extraction/surgical sites are healed. There are no oral masses or ulcerations; no fasciculations, deviation, or atrophic changes of the tongue; and no evidence of recent tongue trauma (scars or lacerations). Inspection of the lingual and buccal aspects of the mandible reveals no abnormalities (texture, color, and consistency of mucosa are within normal limits). Palpation and percussion of the lingual surface of the posterior mandible adjacent to the third molar area produced a localized painful sensation that radiated to the left tongue (positive Tinel's sign: a provocative test of regenerating nerve sprouts in which light percussion over the nerve elicits a distal tingling sensation; it is often interpreted as a sign of small fiber recovery, but following LN injury with complete severance, this response likely represents proximal stump neuroma formation and phantom pain).

Clinical neurosensory. This examination is performed at three levels: A, B, and C (Box 5-3). Cranial nerves II through XII were intact except for the left LN distribution, mandibular division (V3 of the left trigeminal nerve [CN V]). The patient showed no response to any of the three levels of NST, which supports a diagnosis of anesthesia.

In patients with abnormal pain sensations (allodynia, anesthesia dolorosa, dysesthesia), a local anesthetic block of the involved nerve may be helpful in making treatment decisions. If the pain is abolished during the duration of the local anesthetic block, there is a reasonable possibility of pain relief from microneurosurgical repair of the injured nerve.

IMAGING

Panoramic radiograph (11 weeks postsurgery) reveals no evidence of retained root fragment or foreign bodies. The outline of the socket of the right mandibular third molar is well demarcated and is appropriate for the stage of healing.

Box 5-3	**Performance Levels for Clinical Neurosensory**

Level A (directional and two-point discrimination): Patient unable to feel the direction of the stimulus applied with a cotton swab and unable to feel a single- versus two-point stimuli applied to the affected side. Control side within normal limits (inability to discriminate two points farther than 6.5 mm apart is considered abnormal).

Level B (contact detection): Patient does not experience pain upon repetitive application of touch/pressure. Control side is within normal limits.

Level C (pain sensitivity): Patient shows no response to pinprick, noxious pressures, and heat on the left lingual nerve distribution. Control side is within normal limits.

Table 5-1	Nerve Injury Classification		
Seddon	**Sunderland**	**Histology**	**Outcomes**
Neurapraxia	First degree	No axonal damage, no demyelination, and no neuroma	Rapid recovery (days to weeks)
Axonotmesis	Second, third, and fourth degree	Some axonal damage, demyelination, possible neuroma	Loss of sensation; slow, incomplete recovery (weeks to months); microsurgery may help
Neurotmesis	Fifth degree	Severe axonal damage, nerve discontinuity, neuroma formation	Loss of sensation; spontaneous recovery unlikely; microsurgery may help

Table 5-2	Steps in Microsurgical Peripheral Nerve Repair
Procedural Steps*	**Description**
1. External decompression	Removal of bone, scar tissue, and foreign material (e.g., root canal filling material, missile fragments, internal fixation wires, screws or plates); exposure of nerve
2. Internal neurolysis	Incision of epineurium, inspection of internal nerve structure, removal of scar tissue, repair of individual fascicles
3. Preparation of nerve stumps	Excision of neuroma or scar tissue, exposure of viable nerve tissue in nerve stumps, mobilization of proximal and distal nerve limbs to allow approximation
4. Neurorrhaphy	Approximation and suturing of nerve stumps without tension
5. Reconstruction of nerve gap	Autogenous nerve graft; processed allogeneic nerve graft; alloplastic nerve guide
6. Nerve-sharing procedure	When proximal nerve is not available, anastomosis of proximal stump of nearby nerve (e.g., great auricular nerve) to viable distal stump of injured nerve, using a bridging autogenous nerve graft (e.g., sural nerve)
7. Irreparable nerve injury	Nerve capping; nerve redirection; neurectomy (only for pain of terminal malignancy)

*All steps are performed in consecutive order, as shown. The operation can be concluded at any step at which the surgeon decides the procedure has been completed.

Assessment of the LN is possible with an MRI study, but this is not generally necessary in making treatment decisions.

LABS

No routine or special laboratory tests are indicated for microneurosurgical evaluation unless dictated by the medical history.

ASSESSMENT

Left LN injury, exhibiting complete anesthesia to NST at 13 weeks after injury, is a neurotmesis, or Sunderland fifth-degree injury (i.e., nerve injury with anatomic disruption of all axonal and sheath elements and/or physiologic block of all impulse transmission, producing wallerian degeneration and probable neuroma formation) (Table 5-1).

Surgical intervention is indicated for microrepair of the left LN (i.e., excision of the proximal stump neuroma and, most likely, neurorrhaphy [repair of a severed nerve by suturing the two nerve ends together] or, less likely, reconstruction of a nerve gap with a graft).

TREATMENT

The two most important factors in successful decision making regarding treatment of peripheral trigeminal nerve injuries are prompt evaluation of suspected nerve injuries and correct patient selection (diagnosis). There is a time constraint on the interval after injury in which a peripheral nerve can be repaired with reasonable expectation of success. After injury, severed axons in the nerve undergo wallerian degeneration over a period of 1 to 2 months. If the distal endoneurial sheaths of the necrotic axons are not recannulated with new axonal sprouts from the proximal nerve stump within a critical interval (probably 9 to 12 months after injury), the endoneurial sheaths collapse and are replaced with scar tissue, making reinnervation unlikely or impossible. The selection of patients who might benefit from surgical intervention is based on a standardized neurosensory examination. Patients suffering from unacceptable partial or complete loss of sensation, with or without pain symptoms, are most likely to benefit from microsurgical repair of nerve injuries.

Surgical treatment of peripheral nerve injuries follows a stereotypical series of steps, performed in order. These include external decompression, internal neurolysis, preparation of nerve stumps (including excision of scar tissue and neuromas), neurorrhaphy, reconstruction of a nerve gap, and other steps, if the nerve is found not to be repairable) (Table 5-2). Specific intraoperative findings dictate the surgical treatment modality.

In the current patient, under general nasal endotracheal anesthesia, bupivacaine with epinephrine was injected into the soft tissue of the operative field (in addition to an inferior alveolar nerve block for vasoconstriction of the associated proximal vessels). Using ×3.5 loop magnification (or an operating microscope can be used) and fiberoptic lighting, incisions were made along the gingival margins of the premolar and molar teeth on both the buccal and lingual aspects of the left mandible and extended posterolaterally up the ascending ramus. The mucoperiosteum was elevated from the region of the bicuspids and posteriorly. There was a defect in the lingual cortex of the left mandible. The lingual periosteum was sharply incised with microscissors, and the left LN was identified and dissected free to reveal a total transection adjacent to the previously removed third molar with a stump (or amputation) neuroma on the proximal segment. The distal and proximal nerve stumps were freed of surrounding scar tissue, the proximal neuroma was excised, and the distal nerve stump was freshened to visualize viable fascicles (Figure 5-5, *A*). The proximal and distal nerve limbs were mobilized by dissecting them free of surrounding scar and connective tissue. This dissection enabled the nerve endings to be brought together without tension and sutured (neurorrhaphy) using 8-0 ophthalmic nylon (Figure 5-5, *B*). (Tension across the suture line of greater than 25g significantly compromises regeneration.) The anastomosis was encircled with a resorbable flexible collagen nerve cuff to prevent fibrous tissue ingrowth (Figure 5-5, *C*). The mucosal incision was closed with chromic sutures, and the patient was extubated.

Postoperatively, the patient was closely monitored for adequate wound healing, and physical therapy was prescribed to restore normal mandibular opening and range of motion. Four months after the operation, the patient began to experience spontaneous tingling sensations in her left tongue, and she could perceive the hot or cold temperature of ingested liquids. One month later, the anterior two thirds of the left tongue and lingual mandibular gingiva responded to painful stimuli (level C) and static light touch (level B). At that time, daily sensory reeducation exercises (SREs) were prescribed for the tongue and lingual gingiva, which the patient performed three times daily. At 1-year follow-up, the patient demonstrated both subjective and objective signs of left lingual nerve sensory function. She continued the SREs for several more months, after which two-point discrimination (level A) in the left tongue was equal to that in the normal right tongue. Subjectively, the left tongue seemed nearly normal to the patient, and she was dismissed from care.

COMPLICATIONS

Like other surgical procedures, microneurosurgical intervention is not without risks. Careful patient selection is of paramount importance. The indications for microneurosurgical intervention are not always consistent in the literature. However, common indications for surgical exploration and repair of the lingual nerve include the following:

- Spontaneous or stimulus-evoked hyperesthesia (a group of painful responses to stimuli that includes allodynia [a painful response to a stimulus that is ordinarily not painful, such as stroking with a cotton wisp],

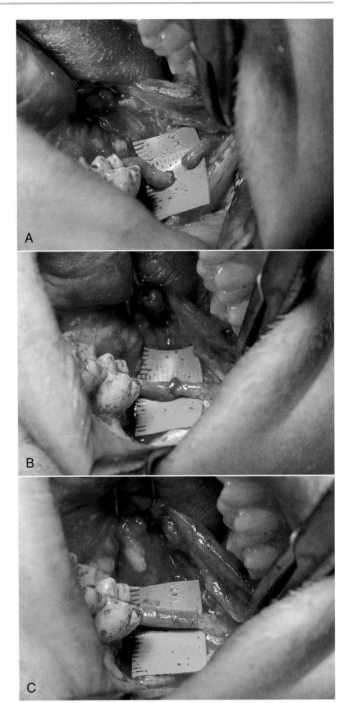

Figure 5-5   **A,** Proximal and distal nerve stumps before reanastomosis. **B,** Neurorrhaphy with 8-0 nylon sutures. **C,** Repair protected by a resorbable flexible collagen nerve cuff.

hyperpathia [delayed onset of pain in response to repetitive stimuli, such as tapping with a blunt object, with continuation of the pain for seconds or minutes after withdrawal of the stimulus], and hyperalgesia [an increased response to a stimulus that is normally painful]) that is abolished temporarily by a local anesthetic block of the suspected nerve

- Constant, deep pain in an anesthetic (anesthesia dolorosa) or a hypoesthetic area (e.g., the tongue) that is abolished by a local anesthetic block of the suspected nerve

- Intolerable or unacceptable (to the patient) anesthesia or hypoesthesia, with or without pain, that shows no signs of recovery (as determined by interval NST) and persists beyond 3 months after injury

Patients with acceptable anesthesia/hypoesthesia or with satisfactory neurosensory recovery without intolerable pain or dysfunction are generally not candidates for surgical nerve exploration. It is possible for such patients to experience a worse outcome, such as the development of anesthesia dolorosa in a previously anesthetic but nonpainful region. Fortunately, this appears to be a rare event. Likewise, most patients with nerve injury whose presurgical symptom is numbness rather than pain do not develop painful sensations after microsurgical nerve repair. More commonly, failure of peripheral trigeminal microneurosurgery is related to inability to restore the preinjury sensory function. In cases of total nerve severance (neurotmesis, or Sunderland fifth-degree injury), the time lapse from injury to repair, proper surgical technique (e.g., tension-free closure), and the patient's age and health status are among the most important factors influencing success. Best results are seen when repair is performed within 6 months of the date of injury. In cases of a witnessed nerve severance, immediate primary nerve repair is indicated unless the surgical site is contaminated (e.g., gunshot wound), the patient's current medical status is compromised, or the surgeon does not have the training or instrumentation to complete the repair at that time. In such instances, either a delayed repair is done, after the injury site shows early signs of healing without infection, or the patient is referred to a surgeon with microsurgical training for completion of the nerve repair. This delay of a few days or weeks seems not to result in a statistically significant reduction in the success rate of repair of peripheral nerve injuries.

DISCUSSION

The inferior alveolar nerve and the lingual nerve are the sensory nerves most commonly injured during surgical treatment by oral and maxillofacial surgeons. Injury to these nerves is not always avoidable, despite a good knowledge of the anatomy and meticulous surgical technique. The lingual nerve has a more variable and less predictable course. Studies based on anatomic cadaveric dissections show that the lingual nerve is positioned above the lingual alveolar crest at the retromolar area in 14% of cases (see the section on third molar odontectomy earlier in this chapter). In other instances, the lingual nerve travels through or inferior to the submandibular salivary gland and courses anteriorly adjacent to the submandibular salivary duct. Removal of a mandibular third molar tooth (M3) is the surgical procedure most commonly associated with injuries to the LN and the inferior alveolar nerve (IAN), with those to the LN occurring less frequently than those to the IAN. However, the lingual nerve, which is located entirely within soft tissue, is less likely to spontaneously recover from injury compared with the inferior alveolar nerve. This is hypothesized to be due to the position of the inferior alveolar nerve in the bony canal, which might serve as a conduit for nerve regeneration, although successful spontaneous regeneration of the IAN does not occur predictably.

The total encasement of the LN within soft tissue offers one important advantage in the surgical repair of this nerve. The LN has a rather tortuous course, especially distally from the adjacent third molar area into the floor of the mouth. By identifying and carefully dissecting the distal limb of a severed LN, the surgeon can straighten this tortuosity, thereby gaining up to 2 cm of length. This additional length often allows the proximal and distal nerve limbs to be brought together without tension. Therefore, the vast majority of LN injuries, except in cases of substantial avulsive or ablative loss of nerve tissue, can be repaired by neurorrhaphy, rather than requiring the additional surgery needed for reconstruction of a nerve gap with a nerve graft.

The reported incidence of temporary paresthesia of the lingual nerve from third molar surgery is between 2% and 6%; fewer than about 1% of these injuries result in a permanent deficit. Several factors may be associated with an increased risk of lingual nerve injury, including lingual bone–splitting technique, aggressive curettage of the follicular sac or granulation tissue, excessive lingual bone removal, lingual plate perforation by a drill or an instrument, and deeply placed lingual sutures. Placement of a lingual retractor increases the incidence of temporary lingual nerve paresthesia but most likely decreases the incidence of permanent nerve injury.

Upon injury to a nerve, the distal nerve segment undergoes wallerian degeneration. The severed distal axons rapidly become necrotic and are phagocytosed within 1 to 2 months, leaving the endoneurial superstructure initially intact. New axonal sprouts extend from the proximal nerve stump and attempt to recannulate the distal endoneurial tubules. If this does not occur within a variable period of time (estimated in humans to be between 9 and 15 months), the endoneurial tubules progressively degenerate and are replaced by scar tissue. Once scar tissue has fully replaced the connective tissue framework, the regenerating proximal axons can no longer recannulate the endoneurial tubules and reinnervate their target tissue. Therefore, the best results for microneurosurgical repair of nerve severance are achieved when surgery is performed as soon as the diagnosis is confirmed and the patient is willing to proceed with the procedure, given the risks and benefits. Within 6 months of the injury, repair has a reasonable chance of success (80% to 90%) (defined as response to pressure and light touch at normal thresholds, two-point discrimination at a threshold of less than 15 mm, and no hyperesthesia), whereas beyond 12 months, the likelihood of success is very low.

Bibliography

Bagheri SC, Meyer RA, Ali Khan H, et al: Microsurgical repair of the peripheral trigeminal nerve after mandibular sagittal split ramus osteotomy, *J Oral Maxillofac Surg* 68(11):2770, 2010.

Bagheri SC, Meyer RA, Ali Khan H, et al: Retrospective review of microsurgical repair of 222 lingual nerve injuries, *J Oral Maxillofac Surg* 68(4):715, 2010.

Bagheri SC, Meyer RA: Management of trigeminal nerve injuries. In Bagheri SC, Bell RB, Khan HA (eds): *Current therapy in oral and maxillofacial surgery*, pp 224-237, St Louis, 2011, Saunders.

Essick GK: Comprehensive clinical evaluation of perioral sensory function, *Oral Maxillofac Surg Clin North Am* 4(2):503, 1992.

Gregg JM: Surgical management of lingual nerve injuries, *Oral Maxillofac Surg Clin North Am* 4(2):417, 1992.

LaBanc JP: Classification of nerve injuries, *Oral Maxillofac Surg Clin North Am* 4(2):285, 1992.

Meyer RA: Applications of microneurosurgery to the repair of trigeminal nerve injuries, *Oral Maxillofac Surg Clin North Am* 4(2):405, 1992.

Meyer RA, Bagheri SC: Clinical evaluation of nerve injuries. In Miloro M (ed): *Trigeminal nerve injuries*, Heidelberg, 2013, Springer.

Meyer RA, Bagheri SC: Clinical evaluation of peripheral trigeminal nerve injuries, *Oral Maxillofac Surg Clin North Am* 19(1):15, 2011.

Meyer RA, Bagheri SC: Etiology and prevention of nerve injuries. In Miloro M (ed): *Trigeminal nerve injuries*, Heidelberg, 2013, Springer (in press).

Meyer RA, Bagheri SC: Nerve injuries from mandibular third molar removal, *Oral Maxillofac Surg Clin North Am* 19(1):63, 2011.

Meyer RA, Rath EM: Sensory rehabilitation after trigeminal injury or nerve repair, *Oral Maxillofac Surg Clin North Am* 13(2):365, 2001.

Miloro M, Kolokythas A: Inferior alveolar and lingual nerve imaging, *Oral Maxillofac Surg Clin North Am* 19(1):35, 2011.

Phillips C, Blakey G, Essick GK: Sensory retraining: a cognitive behavioral therapy for altered sensation, *Oral Maxillofac Surg Clin North Am* 19(1):109, 2011.

Robert RC, Bacchetti P, Pogrel MA: Frequency of trigeminal nerve injuries following third molar removal, *J Oral Maxillofac Surg* 63(6):732-735, 2005.

Ziccardi VB: Microsurgical techniques for repair of the inferior alveolar and lingual nerves, *Oral Maxillofac Surg Clin North Am* 19(1):79, 2011.

Zuniga JR, Meyer RA, Gregg JM, et al: The accuracy of clinical neurosensory testing for nerve injury diagnosis, *J Oral Maxillofac Surg* 56:2, 1998.

Displaced Root Fragments During Dentoalveolar Surgery

Danielle M. Cunningham and Shahrokh C. Bagheri

CC

A 41-year-old man is referred to your office for extraction of a nonrestorable left maxillary first molar.

HPI

Four years earlier the patient had undergone a root canal procedure because of extensive caries on the left maxillary first molar, without any complications (extractions of endodontically treated teeth have a greater probability of root fracture and displacement). He did not pursue restoration of the tooth due to financial reasons and has now been referred for extraction of the failed root canal. He presented to his general dentist with a complaint of pain and mild gingival swelling adjacent to the left maxillary first molar.

PMHX/PDHX/MEDICATIONS/ALLERGIES/SH/FH

Noncontributory. The patient does not use tobacco.

Medical comorbidities that compromise wound healing (e.g., chronic steroid therapy, smoking cigarettes, diabetes, radiation therapy, and malnutrition) may increase the likelihood of persistent oral antral communications, requiring repeat surgical closure. However, the regional anatomy of the area, such as the length of the roots, extent of sinus pneumatization, and amount and quality of surrounding bone, is also important.

EXAMINATION

Intraoral. The patient has localized gingival edema and erythema of the left maxillary first molar, with no vestibular fluctuance. There is a 2-mm draining fistula on the buccal gingiva. A large carious lesion is present on the mesialocclusal surface of the tooth. The left maxillary second and third molars (teeth #15 and #16) are missing, with significant resorption of the posterior maxillary ridge.

IMAGING

The periapical or panoramic radiograph is the minimal imaging modality necessary before the extraction of a tooth. The panoramic radiograph allows better evaluation of the surrounding structures (e.g., the maxillary sinus). Evaluation of the size and shape of the tooth, degree of sinus pneumatization, and amount of bone is important for assessment of possible risks for oral antral exposure or root fracture.

For the current patient, the panoramic radiograph reveals a long palatal root of the left maxillary first molar that appears to partially project into the sinus. There is a loss of continuity of the maxillary sinus in the area of the palatal root (suggestive of a periapical scar secondary to the previous root canal or a pathologic process involving the maxillary sinus).

LABS

No laboratory testing is indicated before routine dentoalveolar surgery unless dictated by the medical history.

ASSESSMENT

Nonrestorable carious left maxillary first molar requiring extraction.

Preoperative assessment of this patient should alert the surgeon to the increased likelihood of root fracture and/or oral antral communication upon surgical removal of the left maxillary first molar. Well-informed patients are more accepting of necessary secondary procedures (e.g., oral antral closure, root retrieval from the sinus, or nerve repair).

TREATMENT

After injection of a local anesthetic with epinephrine, extraction of the left maxillary first molar was attempted using an elevator and forceps. Removal of the tooth revealed fracture of the palatal root with the root fragment retained within the palatal socket. A root tip pick was used to retrieve the fragment. During elevation, the root tip suddenly disappeared from the surgical field. Evaluation of the socket revealed a dark hole, suggesting that the fragment has dislodged into the maxillary sinus.

Upon diagnosis of a displaced root into the maxillary sinus, several maneuvers may be attempted to retrieve the fragment. It is possible for a fragment to be displaced below the schneiderian membrane without actual dislodgment into the maxillary antrum. If the membrane appears intact, this diagnosis should be considered. In cases of dislodgment into the sinus, a perforation into the antrum may be visible. Asking the patient to exhale while pinching the nose may demonstrate air or bubbles exiting the socket, confirming the diagnosis of sinus perforation. Immediately upon diagnosis, a small suction tip can be placed at the apex of the extraction socket in an attempt to remove the fragment. The procedure can be repeated with the patient placed in an upright position. If this maneuver fails, the maxillary sinus can be irrigated with normal saline, followed by suctioning to allow root retrieval. If the root fragment cannot be visualized, the procedure should be aborted. The following two treatment approaches should be considered:

- Closure of the sinus communication, leaving the root fragment in place. The patient is subsequently monitored with panoramic radiographs to document the position of the root. In patients who are asymptomatic, with small fragments that are fixed in the antrum, it is possible to simply observe the root with serial radiographs.
- Closure of the sinus perforation, followed by immediate or delayed removal of the root fragment via a Caldwell-Luc, transalveolar, or endoscopic sinus surgery.

These treatment options are addressed in more detail in the Discussion section.

COMPLICATIONS

Displacement of a tooth or root fragment into the maxillary sinus in a known complication of maxillary dentoalveolar surgery. Although several preoperative findings (described earlier) can identify patients at risk, this complication can occur in any patient. Other possible complications of dentoalveolar surgery are listed in Box 5-4.

Pain and swelling are inevitable consequences of any surgical intervention. However, measures to minimize pain and swelling (preoperative steroids, short operative time, and careful surgical technique) may increase the patient's comfort and satisfaction.

DISCUSSION

The palatal root of the maxillary first molar is the most likely root to be pushed into the maxillary sinus. There is some controversy regarding the optimal management of root fragments displaced into the maxillary sinus. Many surgeons advocate removal of all root fragments from the sinus, regardless of any preexisting sinus or periapical pathology. It is hypothesized that a root tip may act as a foreign body in the sinus, leading to polyps or sinusitis. No randomized trials have evaluated this issue, and most authors argue that the decision needs to be made on a case-by-case basis. It is recommended that if the root tip is small (less than 3 mm) and the sinus and the tooth demonstrate no preexisting pathology, only minimal attempts should be made to retrieve the root. The majority of root fragments are fibrosed into the sinus membrane, without any long-term sequelae. Case reports of retrieved maxillary implants that had migrated or perforated the sinus mucosa have demonstrated no inflammatory changes in the mucosa (both clinically and radiographically). However, other case reports have found that migration of a cover screw has caused acute sinusitis.

| Box 5-4 | **Complications of Dentoalveolar Surgery** |

Intraoperative Complications
- Root fracture (increased incidence with age and root canal therapy)
- Injury to adjacent structures (lingual nerve, inferior alveolar nerve, mental nerve, greater palatine artery and vein, and injury to adjacent teeth and restorations)
- Maxillary tuberosity fracture (seen with maxillary second and third molar extractions, with an increasing incidence with age)
- Oral antral communication
- Displacement of the tooth fragments (or entire tooth) outside of the tooth socket. Root fragments can be displaced into the maxillary sinus, inferior alveolar canal, infratemporal fossa (uncommon complication of maxillary third molar extractions), sublingual space (perforation of the lingual cortex above the mylohyoid attachment), or the submandibular space (perforation below the mylohyoid attachment)
- Hemorrhage (bleeding in an otherwise noncoagulopathic patient is almost always easily controlled with local measures)
- Temporomandibular joint pain (secondary to acute temporomandibular joint muscle spasm, especially with preexisting internal derangement)
- Mandibular fracture (an uncommon but known complication of mandibular third molar extractions)
- Failure to achieve adequate local anesthesia

Postoperative Complications
- Alveolar osteitis (dry socket)
- Wound infection
- Periodontal complications (loss of gingival attachment levels or development of periodontal pockets)
- Poor wound healing, causing delayed recovery
- Alveolar bone abnormalities/irregularities (may require repeat minor alveoloplasty)
- Osteoradionecrosis
- Bisphosphonate-induced osteonecrosis of the jaws

A standard procedure used to retrieve foreign bodies from the maxillary sinus is the Caldwell-Luc procedure. A vestibular incision is used to access the canine fossa. A perforation is made in the anterior maxillary wall, allowing visualization of the sinus. This can be enlarged to gain access to the sinus as needed. Careful attention to the infraorbital nerve prevents postoperative hypoesthesia.

Access to the maxillary sinus can also be gained via a transalveolar approach, by extending the opening of the extraction socket. Removal of buccal bone beyond the apex of the socket allows exposure of the antral mucosa. If the membrane has not been violated, this tissue plane may be explored; otherwise, an opening can be made through the membrane to allow sinus exploration. The opening is closed primarily using a buccal flap. This technique provides superior exposure to the antral floor (exposing the most likely position of the dislodged tooth). However, if the patient is interested in replacing the edentulous area with an implant, this approach would compromise the alveolar ridge bone, which is important for implant restorations.

Prevention of root displacement is the best treatment. If a root tip is fractured and the clinician suspects the possibility of displacement into the sinus, blind attempts at elevation of the fragment should be avoided. The use of adequate lighting (headlight) and full exposure of the area usually allow successful retrieval of the root from the socket. A variety of methods, including the use of endodontic files to remove root tips, have been described.

It is generally recommended that exposure of the sinus via the oral cavity warrants antibiotic therapy and "sinus precautions," regardless of the decision to retain or retrieve a tooth fragment. The sinus flora includes the bacteria *Haemophilus influenzae*, *Streptococcus pneumoniae*, and *Moraxella catarrhalis*. Nasal decongestants, such as oxymetazoline (Afrin) or pseudoephedrine, are used to improve sinus drainage. Topical application of oxymetazoline (an α-agonist) causes arteriolar vasoconstriction, resulting in nasal mucosal shrinkage, which allows for improved drainage. Oxymetazoline should not be used for longer than 3 to 5 days secondary to the development of rhinitis medicamentosa, causing rebound nasal congestion. Decongestants containing pseudoephedrine (a sympathomimetic, α-adrenergic agonist) cause vasoconstriction by selectively acting on the peripheral α-receptors, without the central nervous system side effects. These medications are frequently available in combination with an antihistamine or antitussive agents.

In addition to root tip displacement into the maxillary sinus, case reports have found displacement of implants, either during placement or at a later time (Figure 5-6). The same techniques have been reported for retrieval as those used for root tips; however, waiting is not recommended. Generally either immediate or early retrieval is warranted, because the

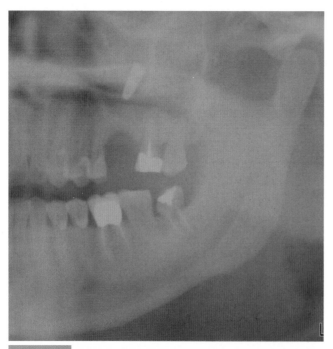

Panoramic radiograph showing displaced maxillary implant into the sinus 4 months after placement of the implant.

implant can act as a nidus of infection. There is a limitation on the size of the objects that can be removed using an endoscopic technique. A transnasal approach is limited both by the endoscope's inability to pick up an object greater than 20 mm and by the inability to remove such an object through the narrow and complicated pathway. An endoscope can be used in combination with a Caldwell-Luc access to minimize the amount of surgical trauma. It is possible to retrieve the implant via the initial osteotomy site; however, this could compromise future implant placement.

Although commonly discussed but rarely reported, displacement of the maxillary third molar into the infratemporal fossa is a potential complication. A number of case reports have discussed various treatment techniques. The infratemporal fossa is the space inferior and medial to the zygomatic arch, with possible superior extension superficial or deep to the temporalis muscle. A CBCT scan can demonstrate the position of the tooth (it also shows whether the tooth was displaced into the maxillary antrum or the infratemporal fossa); however, MRI or contrast-enhanced CT can better determine the location of the tooth in relation to the muscular (and soft tissue) anatomy. Upon displacement of the tooth, the surgical incision can be enlarged to attempt extraction of the tooth via the displacement tract. If the tooth can be palpated, a spinal needle can also be used to push the tooth inferiorly toward the oral cavity for retrieval. If this is not successful, the patient can be placed on antibiotics, and retrieval can be attempted in the operating room using endotracheal intubation. If possible, delaying the procedure for 6 weeks allows fibrosis and encapsulation of the tooth, which minimizes movement during removal. Other techniques include a coronal approach (including a Gilles approach) and intraoral access by removal of the coronoid process. Intraoperative navigation guided by CT can be used via an intraoral or a small temporal incision, or a combination of the two. This approach is technique sensitive and may be more costly.

Extraction of mandibular molars can be complicated by displacement of root tips through a perforated lingual cortex into the submandibular or sublingual space (depending on the attachment of the mylohyoid muscle). The lingual plate at the area of the mandibular third molars can be very thin and, in some instances, fenestrated. Upon identification of a tooth fragment that is likely to be dislodged from the socket, placement of a finger along the medial aspect of the lingual cortex can frequently prevent this complication.

If a tooth becomes dislodged into the submandibular/sublingual space, attempts at removal should be made through the extraction socket or the perforation. If this maneuver is unsuccessful, a lingual mucoperiosteal flap can be elevated to allow exploration of the immediate region. Care should be taken not to injure the lingual nerve. In the event of failure to identify the tooth, the procedure should be aborted and the patient placed on antibiotics. A waiting period of 4 to 6 weeks has been recommended to allow the development of fibrosis around the tooth to facilitate removal. A CT scan may be obtained to visualize the exact position of the tooth, allowing careful preoperative planning. For small root fragments (less than 5 mm) that are not associated with any pathology, the surgeon may elect to observe the tooth and remove the fragment only if it becomes symptomatic.

Bibliography

Barclay JK: Root in the maxillary sinus, *Oral Surg Oral Med Oral Pathol* 64:162-164, 1987.

Bodner L, Zion B, Puterman M: Removal of a maxillary third molar from the infratemporal fossa. a case report, *J Med Cases* 3(2):97-99, 2012.

Campbell A, Costello B: Retrieval of a displaced third molar using navigation and active image guidance, *J Oral Maxillofac Surg* 68:480-485, 2010.

Chrcanovic B, Custódio A: Surgical removal of dental implants into the maxillary sinus: a case report, *Serbian Dental Journal* 56:139-144, 2009.

Friedlich J, Rittenberg BN: Endoscopically assisted Caldwell-Luc procedure for removal of a foreign body from the maxillary sinus, *J Can Dent Assoc* 71:2000-2001, 2005.

Gulbrandsen SR, Jackson IT, Turlington EG: Recovery of a maxillary molar from the infratemporal space via a hemicoronal approach, *J Oral Maxillofac Surg* 45(3):279-282, 1987.

Iida S, Tanaka N, Kogo M, et al: Migration of dental implant into the maxillary sinus: a case report, *Int J Oral Maxillofac Surg* 29(5):358-359, 2000.

Lee FM: Management of the displaced root in the maxillary sinus, *Int J Oral Maxillofac Surg* 7:374-379, 1978.

Nakamura N, Mitsuyasu T, Ohishi M: Endoscopic removal of a dental implant displaced into the maxillary sinus: technical note, *Int J Oral Maxillofac Surg* 33:195-197, 2004.

Peterson LJ, Ellis E, Hupp JR, et al: *Contemporary oral and maxillofacial surgery*, pp 279-280, St Louis, 1993, Mosby.

Selvi F, Cakarer S, Keskin C, et al: Delayed removal of a maxillary molar accidentally displaced into the infratemporal fossa, *J Craniofac Surg* 22(4):1391-1393, 2011.

Speilman AI, Laufer D: Use of a Hedstrom file for removal of fractured root tips, *J Am Dent Assoc* 111(6):970, 1985.

Ueda M, Kaneda T: Maxillary sinusitis caused by a dental implant: report of two cases, *J Oral Maxillofac Surg* 50:285-287, 1992.

CHAPTER 6

Dental Implant Surgery

This chapter addresses:
- Posterior Mandibular Implant Supported Fixed Partial Denture
- Posterior Maxillary Implant Supported Fixed Prostheses
- Sinus Grafting for Implants
- Zygomatic Implants
- Contemporary Treatment Options for Edentulism
- Computer Assisted Implant Surgery
- Extraction Socket Preservation for Implant Placement
- Implants for the Esthetic Zone

The number of different dental professionals who place dental implants has increased dramatically during the past decade. This is likely to continue due to many changing healthcare and economic trends. Oral and maxillofacial surgeons remain the only specialists who can offer the full spectrum of dental implant surgery, encompassing complex implant reconstruction of the atrophic mandible and maxilla, restoration of the dentition after tumor resections, grafting for small and large defects, and esthetic implantology. Our specialty is also well positioned to provide safe and effective anesthesia, either in the office or in the operating room, for healthy patients and for those with complex medical comorbidities.

Although cone-beam computed tomography (CBCT) is not the standard of care for placement of dental implants, its use can have significant diagnostic and treatment planning implications. CBCT can improve the accuracy of implant placement and outline anatomic boundaries to reduce the risk of complications.

In this chapter we include eight cases that cover some of the contemporary issues related to dental implants. Two cases representing the routine placement of maxillary and mandibular implants are presented, followed by six cases that discuss sinus augmentation, zygoma implants, treatment of edentulism, guided implant surgery, extraction socket preservation, and implantology for the esthetic zone.

Posterior Mandibular Implant Supported Fixed Partial Denture

Sam E. Farish

CC

A 61-year-old man who is missing most of his upper and lower molars and premolars is referred by his prosthodontist for restoration using an implant-supported prosthesis in the posterior dentition to create first molar occlusion.

HPI

The patient lost the posterior teeth due to failed restorations, failed endodontic therapy, and advanced periodontal disease. The periodontal condition of the remaining dentition is considered stable.

PMHX/PDHX/MEDICATIONS/ALLERGIES/SH/FH

The patient is in excellent general and oral health except for the partial edentulism. He has been a one pack a day cigarette smoker for over 40 years. He is allergic to penicillin. He currently takes metoprolol (Lopressor), a selective β_1-receptor blocker. He specifically denies a history of diabetes mellitus.

There is support in the literature for implant treatment in patients with well-controlled type 2 diabetes. However, a qualified contraindication to such treatment must be considered to exist for patients with type 1 diabetes, because the variable success rates reported in this population are affected markedly by the quality of glycemic control. There are studies illustrating implant success in individuals with type 1 diabetes, but in most of these the numbers are small and the follow-up short. Early studies showed a markedly increased failure rate for implants in smokers; however, more recent techniques, in which the implants had oxidized rather than machined surfaces, do not show such glaring disparities. Good healthcare mandates smoking cessation in any patient, and the possibility of an increased risk of failure of osseointegration in smokers should be discussed with the patient and included in the consent as a shared liability.

Cardiovascular diseases, hypertension included, pose a considerable risk of stroke, heart failure, myocardial infarct, and renal failure; however, if a patient is able to undergo minor oral surgery, there is no increased risk of implant failure. The β-blocker this patient is on should be continued.

There are several other general risk factors affecting implant success that warrant discussion. There is little evidence regarding recommendations for implants in patients with other autoimmune disorders. Reasonable success rates have been obtained in patients who are osteoporotic with extended healing times. Implants in patients on bisphosphonate therapy have been studied on a very limited basis; although osteonecrosis of the jaw has a low incidence, its morbidity is extremely high. If implants are to be placed in these patients, it should be done with thorough informed consent and ongoing monitoring. Radiotherapy is a significant risk factor for implant failure, and the evidence for hyperbaric therapy in reducing this risk is inconclusive. There is limited evidence linking a history of periodontitis with an increase in peri-implant pathology, although the periodontal health of the remaining dentition affects the success of implant restoration. A higher implant failure rate is seen in poor-quality bone, in the maxilla, and in the posterior jaw. Bruxism and other paraoral habits are associated with increased implant failure rates due to increased load. Implant oral rehabilitation is a successful and predictable modality for most patients.

EXAMINATION

Examination of both the quality and quantity of bone is essential for successful implant placement.

Clinical examination of the posterior mandible indicates that the form of the ridge is rounded and wide (6 to 8 mm) in the buccal and lingual aspect. The anteroposterior ridge space is adequate for placement of several implants posterior to the most distal mandibular tooth on each side of the mandible. For this discussion we will concentrate on the posterior mandibular quadrant on the right. The distance from an implant to an adjacent natural tooth and between adjacent implants should be 1.5 mm and 2 mm, respectively. In the current patient, because first molar occlusion is planned, the distal implant will be placed about 12 mm or so from the front implant, and a three-unit bridge will be constructed. An interarch space greater than 5.5 mm already exists, and this is adequate for the restorative stack. No soft tissue or bony abnormalities are noted, and the patient opens 50 mm (restricted mouth opening can pose a problem for implant placement).

IMAGING

Although implant surgery can be planned on a panoramic radiograph with a surgical planning template coupled with bone mapping techniques, a far simpler and much more predictable methodology involves CBCT (Figure 6-1, *A*). The

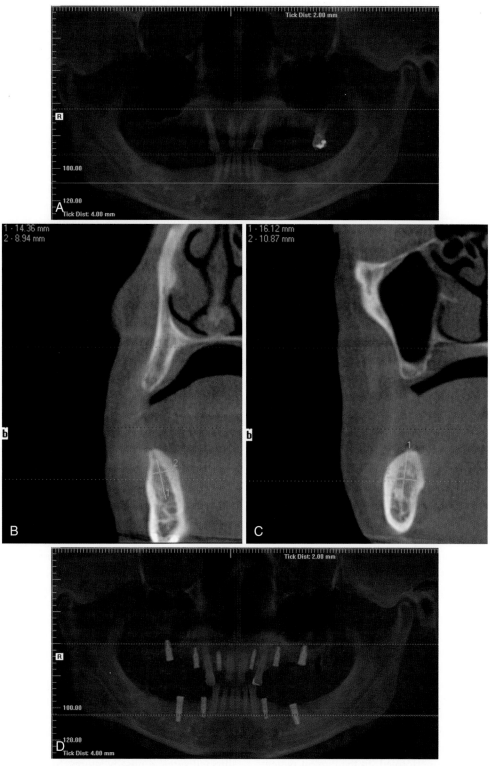

Figure 6-1   **A,** CBCT panoramic image showing proposed implant sites in the right mandible posterior. **B,** CBCT coronal cut showing anatomic features of the proposed anterior implant site, in addition to the proposed posterior implant site **(C),** and the measurements generated by the implant planning software. **D,** CBCT panoramic image showing implant placement completed as planned.

preoperative films show that the anterior implant site is 8.9 mm wide in a buccolingual dimension, 14.4 mm above the inferior alveolar neurovascular bundle, and 1.5 mm distal to the lower right mandibular cuspid tooth (Figure 6-1, *B*). At the proposed location of the more posterior implant, the

buccolingual distance is 10.9 mm and the inferior alveolar neurovascular bundle lies 16.1 mm below the ridge crest (Figure 6-1, *C*). The bone quality is type II (Box 6-1). A surgical guide can be generated from the data contained in the CBCT if the surgeon feels it is necessary, and instrumentation

---

| Box 6-1 | **Bone Classification Based on Radiographic and Clinical Parameters** |

Type I: Entire jaw composed of homogenous compact bone. Has the tactile sense of drilling into oak or maplewood.
Type II: A thick layer of compact bone surrounding a core of dense trabecular bone. Has the tactile sense of drilling into white pine or spruce.
Type III: A thin layer of cortical bone surrounding a core of dense trabecular bone of favorable strength. Has the tactile sense of drilling into balsa wood.
Type IV: A thin layer of cortical bone surrounding a core of low-density trabecular bone. Has the tactile sense of drilling into Styrofoam.

---

keyed to this guide can be applied for precision placement; otherwise, a surgical guide is prepared on the study models.

LABS

No laboratory testing is indicated for implant placement unless dictated by the medical history or anesthesia concerns.

ASSESSMENT

A healthy, 61-year-old man who desires mandibular posterior implants bilaterally for the restoration of the affected quadrants by fixed implant–supported partial dentures

The work-up reveals that a 4-mm by 13-mm implant can be placed in the most anterior site, and a 5-mm wide by 15-mm implant can be placed posteriorly on the right. A distance of 2 mm from the mandibular canal is recommended to avoid injury to the neurovascular bundle. The procedure would be appropriate under intravenous sedation with local anesthesia in the office setting.

TREATMENT

The planned treatment was discussed in detail with the patient and the restorative dentist. A surgical guide prepared by the restorative dentist was used, indicating the ideal position for the implants in the planned restorative schema. Underlying bone dictates where implants can be placed; if bone is not present where implants need to be placed, various grafting or distraction techniques (which are beyond the scope of the current discussion) can be performed. In the current patient, it was predetermined that no such additional surgery was indicated. Chlorhexidine mouth rinse was used before surgery. No preoperative prophylactic antibiotics were prescribed for this patient, because there is no literature support for this practice in low- and moderate-risk dental implant patients.

Under intravenous sedation and local anesthesia, implant surgery was performed according to the particular system protocol. The wound was sutured with nonresorbable sutures, and a gauze sponge was placed to obtain hemostasis. The

patient was recovered and discharged with detailed instructions for home care, analgesics, and a return appointment in 1 week for suture removal. Postoperative CBCT images (see Figure 6-1, *D*) revealed satisfactory placement of implants well above the mandibular canal, with adequate spacing for a three-unit fixed partial denture. A final restoration was placed 4 months later, and a satisfactory cosmetic and functional outcome resulted, with contours and emergence similar to those of the replaced natural dentition.

Although research indicates equally satisfactory results, during the first 16 weeks of healing after implant placement, for implants placed under three different loading regimens (loaded immediately, early [6 weeks], or using conventional/delayed timing [12 weeks]), the decision was made to follow the conventional/delayed plan in this patient.

COMPLICATIONS

The direct anchorage of dental implants to the host surrounding bone (osseointegration) is a good indication of clinical success, and although a high success rate is seen in implantology, endosseous implants do fail. Early implant failure is associated with a lack of primary stability (possibly aggravated by early loading protocols), surgical trauma, and infection. Infection noted early is much more problematic than infection later in the course of treatment because of the disturbance in primary bone healing associated with the former. Occlusal overburden and peri-implantitis are the most important factors associated with delayed or late implant failure. The primary limiting factor for lower premolar and molar implants is the height of bone above the mandibular canal. If it is determined that an implant has been placed in contact with the mandibular canal, causing postoperative hypoesthesia or anesthesia, the implant should be backed off of this structure as soon as possible or removed and replaced with a shorter implant (Figure 6-2). CBCT, unlike a panoramic film, can differentiate superimposition from direct contact with the nerve. In the presence of symptoms (e.g., paresthesia) and a CBCT scan showing no direct contact with the nerve, removal of the implant is unlikely to resolve the paresthesia, and interval neurosensory testing determines whether microneurosurgical exploration is indicated.

Perforation with the implant drill and direct injury to the mandibular nerve are possible (Figure 6-3). Hemorrhage, salivary gland involvement, painful impingement of implants on the lingual surface of the mandible, and associated misalignment are all complications associated with lingually directed surgical misadventures. Such problems can be minimized by careful attention to the anatomic features of the lower posterior jaw as depicted on the CBCT. Frequently a slight buccal inclination of posterior mandibular implants is necessary to avoid lingual perforation, and this fact is best determined and discussed preoperatively with the restorative dentist to minimize misunderstandings. Should infection occur in the early postoperative period, conservative management, including antibiotics, debridement, incision and drainage, and irrigation, is indicated, with implant removal as a last

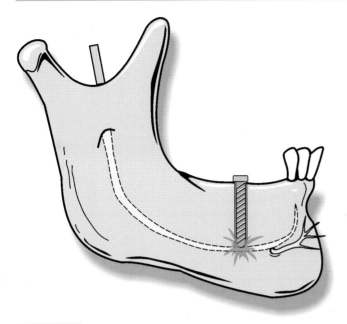

Figure 6-2 Injury to or contact with the inferior alveolar neurovascular bundle by an implant fixture.

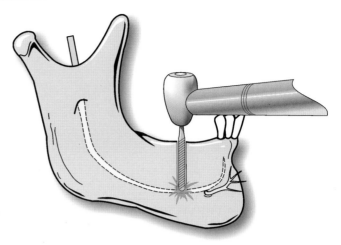

Figure 6-3 Direct injury to the inferior alveolar neurovascular bundle by the implant drill.

resort. Occasionally, inflammation and the development of a fistula over an implant site occur, and this frequently indicates that the cover screw has loosened. In this case the implant site should be exposed, the screw removed, the site debrided and irrigated, and a new, sterile cover screw placed and tightened.

Other complications with implant surgery include aspiration or swallowing of instruments or implant components. This can be prevented by paying close attention to positioning, using a well-placed gauze curtain, and attaching a 12- to 16-inch floss cord to such instruments as screwdrivers so retrieval is possible should the instrument be dropped.

DISCUSSION

Implant surgeons can choose from a wide range of implant designs, materials, and surfaces, although a detailed analysis of these variables is beyond the scope of this discussion. Currently, a textured-surface titanium alloy implant is indicated, because such surfaces have been shown to be better receptors for fibrin strands forming initial attachments of implants to bone in the microgap. A recently reported, long-term outcome study of titanium implants with a sand-blasted and acid-etched (SLA) surface in a large cohort of partially edentulous patients showed a 10-year implant survival rate of 98.8% and a restoration success rate of 97%. In addition, the prevalence of peri-implantitis in this large cohort of orally healthy patients was low (1.8% during the 10-year period).

Several techniques that can increase inadequate bone volume above the inferior alveolar canal and in the buccal and lingual dimensions have been documented, including onlay block or particulate grafting, guided tissue regeneration techniques, distraction osteogenesis, and nerve repositioning. When any technique is used other than what is considered standard implant surgery (as described in this discussion), there are tradeoffs, with additional potential complications associated with each of these techniques. Discussion of the particulars of these techniques is beyond the scope of the present text.

Bibliography

Ahmad N, Saad N: Effects of antibiotics on dental implants: a review, *J Clin Med Res* 4:1-6, 2012.

Barewal RM, Stanford C, Weesner TC: A randomized controlled clinical trial comparing the effects of three loading protocols on dental implant stability, *Int J Oral Maxillofac Implants* 27:945-956, 2012.

Buser D, Janner SF, Wittneben JG, et al: Ten-year survival and success rates of 511 titanium implants with a sand-blasted and acid-etched surface: a retrospective study in 303 partially edentulous patients, *Clin Implant Dent Relat Res* 14(6):839-851, 2012.

Lambert PM, Morris HF, Ochi S: The influence of 0.12% chlorhexidine digluconate rinses on the incidence of infectious complications and implant success, *J Oral Maxillofac Surg* 55(12 Suppl 5):25-30, 1997.

Liddelow G, Klineberg I: Patient-related risk factors for implant therapy: a critique of pertinent literature, *Aust Dent J* 56:417-426, 2011.

Marchand F, Raskin A, Dionnes-Hornes A, et al: Dental implants and diabetes: conditions for success, *Diabetes Metab* 38:14-19, 2012.

Misch CE: Density of bone: effect on treatment plans, surgical approach, healing and progressive bone loading, *Int J Oral Implantol* 6:23-31, 1990.

Renouard F, Rangert B: *Risk factors in implant dentistry: simplified clinical analysis for predictable treatment*, ed 2, Hanover Park, Ill, 2008, Quintessence.

Sakka S, Baroudi K, Nassani MZ: Factors associated with early and late failure of dental implants, *J Investig Clin Dent* 3(4):258-261, 2012.

Posterior Maxillary Implant Supported Fixed Prostheses

Sam E. Farish

CC

A 48-year-old man presents with the complaint that he is unable to eat with his removable partial dentures and desires fixed prostheses. He is missing both bicuspids and all molars on the maxillary left.

HPI

The patient states that he lost most of his posterior maxillary and mandibular dentition due to aggressive caries as a young man coupled with failed endodontic therapy on many of the aforementioned carious teeth. He has worn increasingly unsatisfactory removable partial dentures (RPD) for the past 10 years. The recent extraction of tooth #13 (removed 2 months prior) has made RPD function more difficult. The remainder of the upper and lower dentition is in good repair, and his periodontal status is excellent.

PMHX/PDHX/MEDICATIONS/ALLERGIES/SH/FH

The patient has a significant past medical history. He had an ST-elevated myocardial infarction (STEMI) 3 years earlier and had three-vessel coronary bypass 2 years ago for angina that interfered with his ability to work. He also has hypertension and hyperlipidemia. He denies any chest pain or exercise intolerance since his surgery and works as a structural engineer on outdoor jobs, where he is regularly engaged in physical exertion. For his hypertension he takes benazepril (Lotensin), an angiotensin-converting enzyme inhibitor (ACE inhibitor); for his hyperlipidemia he takes simvastatin (Zocor), a 3-hydroxy-3-methylglutaryl coenzyme (HMG-CoA) reductase inhibitor. Both of these medications can be given preoperatively in their usual dosages. In addition, he takes clopidogrel (Plavix), along with an 81-mg aspirin (low dose) for prophylaxis against thromboembolic events.

Clopidogrel reduces thrombosis by blocking adenosine diphosphate receptors on platelet cell membranes, thereby preventing platelet adhesion and aggregation. Aspirin irreversibly inhibits platelet-dependent cyclooxygenase (COX), which decreases platelet aggregation for the life of the platelet. Aspirin is a much more potent inhibitor of COX-1 than COX-2, so higher doses also inhibit endothelial cell synthesis of prostacyclin, a vasodilator that serves a protective role against ischemia (higher aspirin doses may be deleterious). It is suggested that clopidogrel be discontinued 5 days before elective surgery. Low-dose aspirin should have no clinically significant effect on bleeding and can be continued. The patient has no known drug allergies and no additional medical problems. He is a nonsmoker with excellent oral hygiene.

EXAMINATION

The quality and quantity of bone must be adequate for successful implant placement.

Clinical examination reveals that the posterior right maxilla has a rounded form and is free of soft tissue abnormalities. In the bicuspid region, the width of the ridge is about 7 mm, with a minimal facial undercut; in the molar region, 8 mm of width is noted. Because of the buccal undercut, perforation may occur at implant placement; however, if this happens, the defect can be augmented or repaired with a xenograft and collagen membrane. The mesiodistal dimension is a free end, so adequate room is present for three implants (two 4-mm-diameter anterior implants and one 5-mm-diameter posterior implant); however, the decision was made to place only two implants, spaced to allow for a three-unit bridge, as an economy measure. The interarch space is adequate, because the opposing dentition is absent (5 mm or more is needed for placement of the restorative stack). The patient opens 52 mm (limited opening can make implant placement difficult).

IMAGING

A cone-beam computed tomography (CBCT) panoramic image (Figure 6-4, *A*) reveals that there is adequate bone for placement of implants in both areas selected, without the necessity of a sinus graft. The bone quality is judged to be type II. Bone quality is determined by radiographic appearance and also by the tactile feeling on drilling (see Box 6-1). If CBCT is not available, an implant tracing template at 25% larger than normal size (due to a 25% magnification factor on a panoramic radiograph) can be used with a panoramic radiographic image for surgical planning. CBCT helps to accurately determine the position of the floor of the maxillary sinus and the condition of the sinus membrane, which aids in determining the necessity and feasibility of sinus grafting. Coronal CBCT images in the area planned for the placement of the more anterior implant in this case (2 mm posterior to tooth #11) demonstrates that the buccolingual dimension is 7.55 mm, and a vertical height of 18.8 mm is available (Figure 6-4, *B*). In the area proposed for the placement of the more posterior implant, 8.16 mm is noted as the buccolingual dimension, and 12.65 mm of bone is present from the crest

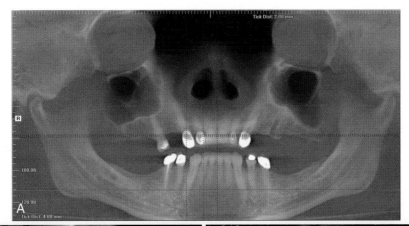

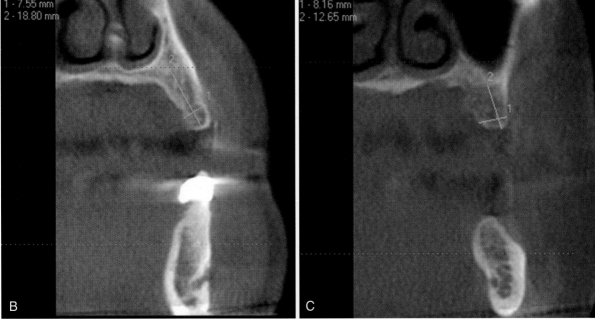

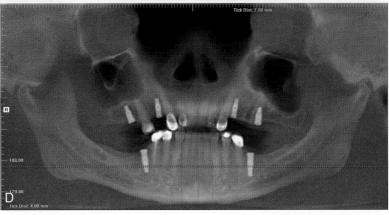

Figure 6-4 **A,** CBCT panoramic view showing proposed implant sites in right maxilla posterior. Quadrant CBCT coronal views showing the more anterior right maxillary implant site **(B)** and the more posterior right maxillary implant site **(C),** both with measurement data. **D,** Postoperative CBCT panoramic view showing implant placement in the right maxillary posterior, in addition to other fixtures placed at surgery (no sinus grafting was necessary).

of the ridge to the floor of the right maxillary sinus (Figure 6-4, *C*). It is relatively uncommon to have adequate bone below the maxillary sinus for placement of implants of satisfactory length, as is seen in this case. Various strategies can be used when adequate volume is absent. Bone graft

augmentation by open and closed technique using various graft materials (e.g., onlay grafting with particulate and/or block grafts of various natures), sinus membrane elevation followed by implant placement without grafting, and short implants are all methodologies used to overcome inadequate bone stock below the sinus floor in posterior maxillary constructs. Immediate, rather than delayed, implant placement in grafted sinuses is determined by the presence of at least 5 mm of bone, which allows for initial stability of immediately placed implants. In the case of two-stage sinus grafts, the primary graft placement is followed 4 months later by secondary implant surgery, with or without immediate loading as determined by initial stability at placement.

LABS

No routine laboratory studies are indicated for implant placement unless dictated by the medical history.

In the current patient, because hyperlipidemia is a risk factor for atherosclerosis and associated cardiovascular disease, in addition to an increased risk of stroke, it would be pertinent to evaluate the most recent total body cholesterol level, LDL, HDL, and triglyceride levels. The patient's total cholesterol was 167 mg/dl (a value below 200 mg/dl is associated with a relatively low risk of myocardial infarction unless other risks factors are present). The LDL was 70 mg/dl (normal range, 70 to 130 mg/dl, although lower values are better), the HDL was 64 mg/dl (normal range, 40 to 60 mg/dl, higher values are better), and triglycerides were 58 mg/dl (normal range, 10 to 150 mg/dl, lower values are better).

ASSESSMENT

A 48-year-old male with chronic hyperlipidemia and asymptomatic atherosclerotic heart disease who desires an implant-based, fixed partial denture in the right posterior maxilla.

The work-up reveals that a 4 × 15-mm implant can be placed anteriorly and a 5 × 11-mm implant can be placed posteriorly. No grafting procedure will be required as an adjunct to this surgery. There are no contraindications to the planned procedure in the office setting with intravenous sedation and local anesthesia.

TREATMENT

The planned surgery was discussed in detail with the restorative dentist, who showed the patient on a diagnostic wax-up what the final restoration will look like and has provided a surgical guide indicating the desired position and inclination for the implants. The patient had been off of clopidogrel for 6 days on presentation. He was given 2 gm of amoxicillin by mouth 1 hour before surgery, and chlorhexidine oral rinse was used immediately before surgery. Under intravenous sedation and local anesthesia, the implant surgery was performed in accordance with the manufacturer's protocol. After the osteotomies were performed, the sites were probed with a blunt instrument, and the sinus floors were found to be intact at both sites. The implants were placed, and wound closure was obtained with 4-0 polyglactin (Vicryl) sutures. The patient recovered and was discharged with instructions for home care, analgesics, and a return appointment in 1 week for suture removal. Postoperative CBCT

panoramic imaging revealed satisfactory implant placement (Figure 6-4, *D*).

Although there is research indicating good results with immediate placement of healing caps and even immediate loading, fewer problems can be expected from implants submerged and unloaded for 4 months in the mandible and 6 months in the maxilla and in grafts (two-stage placement).

COMPLICATIONS

Success rates for fixed partial dentures on implants in the posterior maxilla have been reported to be about 95% at 5 years and about 93% at 10 years, and the quality of bone appears to have little influence on the success rate. Patients should be informed of the risks associated with the surgical placement of implants in the posterior maxilla, including sinus penetration, buccal perforation, infection, and failure to integrate, even though survival data suggest an adequate success rate for this application of dental implants. The most common implants lost in the posterior maxilla are shorter fixtures; wide fixtures show the lowest failure rates. Other complications associated with implants used to treat partial posterior maxillary edentulism are fractures of the occlusal surface of restorations and loose anchorage components.

DISCUSSION

Implant surgeons can choose from a wide range of implant designs, materials and surfaces. Although a detailed analysis of the array of implant variables is beyond the scope of this discussion, a textured-surface, titanium alloy implant is currently indicated, because it is known to improve initial attachment of implants to bone in the microgap between the bone and the implant. Immediate loading, one-stage placement, and the traditional two-stage implant surgery all have their proponents. In the posterior maxilla, two-stage placement seems ideal, because no cosmetic considerations come into play. There are several techniques that can increase inadequate bone volume for implant placement below the maxillary sinus, decrease buccal undercuts, or treat buccal perforations. Onlay grafting of particulate or block bone or bone substitute, guided tissue regeneration, distraction, and sinus grafting are well documented. However, when any technique is used other than standard implant surgery, there are tradeoffs, with potential complications specific to the technique used.

Bibliography

Bahat O: Brånemark system implants in the posterior maxilla: clinical study of 660 implants followed for 5 to 12 years, *Int J Oral Maxillofac Implants* 15:646-653, 2000.

Benavides E, Rios HF, Ganz SD, et al: Use of cone beam computed tomography in implant dentistry: the International Congress of Oral Implantologists consensus report, *Implant Dent* 21:78-86, 2012.

Cheng-Ching E, Samaniego EA, Reddy Naravetla B, et al: Update on pharmacology of antiplatelets, anticoagulants, and thrombolytics, *Neurology* 79(13 Suppl 1):S68-S76, 2012.

Cho-Lee GY, Naval-Gias L, Castrejon-Castrejon S, et al: A 12-year retrospective analytic study of the implant survival rate in 177 consecutive maxillary sinus augmentation procedures, *Int J Oral Maxillofac Implants* 25:1019-1027, 2010.

Dent CD, Olsen JW, Farish SE, et al: The influence of preoperative antibiotics on success of endosseous implants up to and including stage II surgery: a study of 2,641 implants, *J Oral Maxillofac Surg* 55(Suppl 5):19-24, 1997.

Felice P, Soardi E, Pellegrino G, et al: Treatment of the atrophic edentulous maxilla: short implants versus bone augmentation for placing longer implants: five-month post-loading results of a pilot randomised controlled trial, *Eur J Oral Implantol* 4:191-202, 2011.

Kaufman E: Maxillary sinus elevation surgery: an overview, *J Esthet Restor Dent* 15:272-282, 2003.

Lambert PM, Morris HF, Ochi S: The influence of 0.12% chlorhexidine digluconate rinses on the incidence of infectious complications and implant success, *J Oral Maxillofac Surg* 55(12 Suppl 5):25-30, 1997.

Liddelow G, Klineberg I: Patient-related risk factors for implant therapy: a critique of pertinent literature, *Aust Dent J* 56:417-426, 2011.

Renouard F, Rangert B: *Risk factors in implant dentistry: simplified clinical analysis for predictable treatment*, ed 2, Hanover Park, Ill, 2008, Quintessence.

Sinus Grafting for Implants

Sam E. Farish

CC

A 47-year-old man was referred by a restorative dentist for evaluation of his posterior maxilla for implant placement. The patient requests restoration of his maxillary posterior teeth using a modality that will allow him to have a fixed restoration, because he has great difficulty with his existing removable partial dentures.

HPI

The patient lost most of his posterior teeth at a younger age due to decay and failed endodontics. Early loss of posterior maxillary teeth is associated with increased pneumatization of the maxillary sinus, and frequently inadequate bone for satisfactory implants does not exist below such a sinus. The patient has found himself at a point in life where he can seek optimal care, and his case has been followed by a periodontist, who believes that the patient's periodontal condition is stable. All remaining teeth are sound except for tooth #15, which shows extensive restoration. The referring dentist has informed the patient that he may require a "sinus lift" procedure. The patient wants to know the details of this surgery, and he wants treatment planned for implant-based restorations, because he is unable to wear his existing removable partial dentures comfortably.

PMHX/PDHX/MEDICATIONS/ALLERTGIES/SH/FH

The medical history is significant for paroxysmal supraventricular tachycardia (PSVT), for which he takes metoprolol (Lopressor), and for chronic maxillary sinusitis. He is a one-half pack per day smoker with a 10 pack-year history.

Cigarette smoking (nicotine) increases platelet adhesiveness, raises the risk of microvascular occlusion, and causes tissue ischemia. Tobacco smoking causes catecholamine release and associated vasoconstriction, resulting in decreased tissue perfusion. Smoking is additionally believed to suppress the immune responses by affecting the function of neutrophils. A perioperative smoking cessation program has been shown to reduce respiratory and wound-healing complications. Good health care mandates smoking cessation in any patient, and the possibility of an increased risk of failure of osseointegration in smokers should be discussed with the patient and included in the consent as a shared liability.

The risk of PSVT is increased with alcohol or caffeine use and with smoking. It can be associated with bothersome palpitations, anxiety, chest tightness, and shortness of breath. This patient takes metoprolol (Lopressor), a β-blocker, to prevent PSVT episodes, and he reports very infrequent episodes in the recent past. PSVT is typically a benign disease but can be associated with profound hypotension and require emergency management; therefore, it is an anesthesia consideration.

A history of acute or chronic sinusitis may be problematic for an implant surgery with an associated sinus graft procedure planned. Prolonged inflammation and/or infection creates an inappropriate environment for the procedure. Maxillary sinusitis results from a secondary bacterial infection of an obstructed sinus. The mucosal edema, increased mucous production, bacterial accumulation, and inflammatory debris associated with sinusitis create an unfavorable environment for surgery and subsequent healing. Infections of the maxillary sinus after sinus grafting surgery occur in a small percentage of cases and are usually managed conservatively, with preservation of uninfected graft and subsequent implant success. The two most common bacteria involved in acute maxillary sinusitis are *Haemophilus influenzae* and *Streptococcus pneumoniae*. *Staphylococcus aureus*, α-hemolytic streptococci, and *Bacteroides* and *Pseudomonas* spp. are most frequently found in chronic bacterial sinusitis. Any form of sinus infection should be treated with decongestants and antibiotics, and some infections require functional endoscopic sinus surgery (FESS) before performance of a sinus grafting procedure can be contemplated. A broad-spectrum antibiotic, such as amoxicillin with clavulanic acid (Augmentin), is often the initial antibiotic used in the management of infections caused by nasal or sinus flora.

EXAMINATION

The patient is a well-developed, well-nourished man in no acute distress. There are no signs or symptoms of sinus infection currently.

The patient is missing all of his lower posterior teeth (teeth #22 through #27 remain). In the maxilla he is missing teeth #1 through #5, #7, #10, #12 through #14, and #16. Tooth #15 is present but is considered nonrestorable and slated for removal. No lesions or bony irregularities are noted in the oral cavity, and the remaining teeth, except for tooth #15, are in satisfactory condition. In the maxilla the ridge form in the posterior is rounded without undercuts and is of adequate width clinically for implant placement. The maximal incisal opening is 48 mm (limited opening may prevent ideal implant placement and angulation, especially of posterior implants). There is adequate interarch space for the restorative stack because the patient is edentulous in the mandibular arch in the posterior, and full mouth, implant-based rehabilitation is planned.

IMAGING

A panoramic cone-beam computed tomography (CBCT) image showed that there was inadequate bone beneath the maxillary sinus bilaterally (especially on the right) in the posterior maxilla to allow for adequate implant placement (Figure 6-5, *A*). A coronal CBCT cut (Figure 6-5, *B*) determined that an implant of 5 mm in diameter could be placed in the most posterior right maxilla site; however, only 3.6 mm of bone is present below the sinus membrane. Consequently, a sinus graft must be completed to place an implant of adequate length to support a fixed partial denture on two implants in this area of relatively high occlusal load. On the left side at the site of the more posterior implant, 9.7 mm of bone in the buccolingual dimension is seen, and 10 mm of bone is noted below the sinus floor in the area of the most posterior implant placement site (Figure 6-5, *C*). An 8-mm implant could be placed in this site; however, because this implant will be the posterior stop in a high occlusal force area, it was determined that a longer implant with a sinus graft was indicated here. It should be noted that on both the right and the left, the more anterior implant site showed adequate bone for fixtures of 4 mm in diameter and 13 mm or greater in length and no need for a sinus graft (Figure 6-5, *D* and *E*). Implants will be placed at the time of grafting, because adequate bone for initial stability (greater than 4 mm) is present in all sites planned for fixtures.

LABS

No routine laboratory testing is indicated for a sinus graft and implant placement surgery unless dictated by the medical history. A call to the patient's cardiologist regarding the implications of the PSVT diagnosis would be appropriate.

ASSESSMENT

The patient presents with a resorbed edentulous posterior maxilla bilaterally with increased pneumatization of the maxillary sinus and insufficient bone available below the sinus for implant placement.

TREATMENT

Treatment with dental implants is initiated with a thorough physical examination, appropriate radiology (CBCT), and a coordinated treatment plan devised in cooperation with the restorative dentist. Numerous modalities for the management of the atrophic posterior maxilla in different clinical circumstances are available to oral and maxillofacial surgeons; these techniques include maxillary sinus augmentation, zygomatic implants, LeFort I downfracture osteotomy, distraction osteogenesis, onlay cortical or cancellous grafting associated with various containment protocols, and guided tissue regeneration with various membrane technologies. Maxillary sinus floor augmentation has become the most popular strategy among surgeons due to its predictability, low morbidity, and technical simplicity. Various methods can be used to augment the excessively pneumatized maxillary sinus to accommodate an implant of at least 10 mm in length. Sinus membrane elevation followed by implant placement without grafting has its advocates also. A lateral wall antrostomy, or window (open technique), is the most common technique used to expose the sinus floor. Alternatively, the Summer osteotome technique (closed technique) can be used for selected cases when less than 4 mm of sinus floor elevation is needed. The grafting material or materials are selected based on the surgeon's preference. If a decision is made to use autogenous bone, the harvest technique planned must be explained to the patient so that informed consent can be obtained (the tibial plateau bone harvesting technique is discussed later). The decision on simultaneous or staged augmentation and implant placement is made based on the quality and quantity of host bone at the surgical site.

There are four primary types of grafting material available for sinus augmentation:

- Autogenous bone
- Allogenic bone
- Alloplastic materials
- Xenogenic materials

These materials can be used alone or in combination (composite graft) for sinus augmentation. Autogenous bone (cancellous marrow or cortical shavings) is a popular and predictable material for sinus grafting. Donor sites for bone harvest include intraoral sites (maxillary tuberosity, zygomatic buttress, mandibular ramus, posterior body or symphysis) and extraoral sites (the tibial plateau and anterior iliac crest are the most commonly used). Donor site selection is based on the clinical situation and the amount and type of bone needed. Intraoral sites must be considered a limited source of cancellous marrow but are a good source of surface-derived autogenous cortical bone (cortical shavings). Extraoral sites can provide sufficient autogenous cancellous marrow for large, bilateral augmentations. Some surgeons prefer to construct a composite graft by mixing autogenous bone with allogenic, alloplastic, or xenogenic graft materials, especially when inadequate autogenous bone is available.

Another alternative modality for maxillary sinus floor augmentation is the use of recombinant human bone morphogenetic protein 2 (rhBMP-2), which has been shown to induce de novo bone formation. rhBMP-2 in combination with a collagen sponge (Infuse; Medtronic, Inc. Minneapolis, Minnesota) is placed on the sinus floor in a fashion similar to bone graft material; it acts as an osteoinductive factor that stimulates undifferentiated mesenchymal cells to transform into osteoprogenitor cells and produce bone. De novo bone formation for sinus augmentation and placement of functional implants has been shown to be predictable and

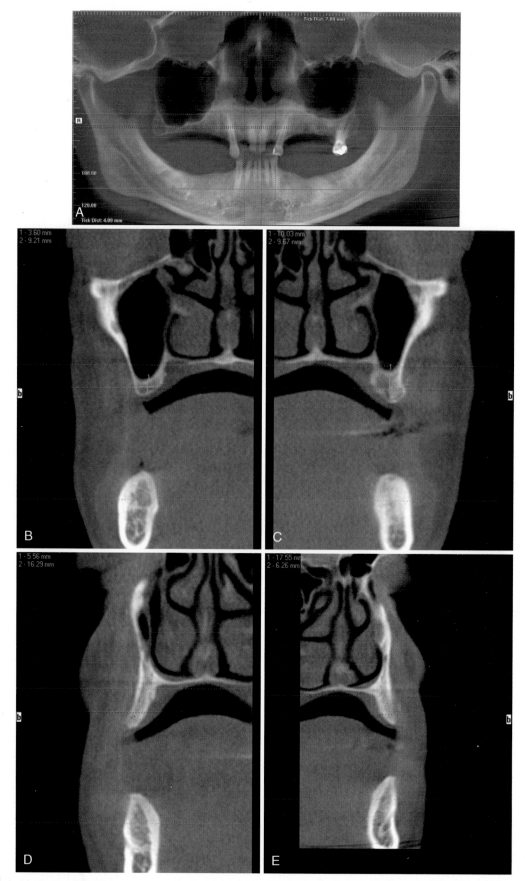

Figure 6-5   **A,** Panoramic CBCT showing proposed implant sites. Coronal CBCT cuts detailing area proposed for placement of the most posterior right maxillary implant **(B)** and the most posterior left maxillary implant **(C).** Coronal CBCT cuts detailing area proposed for placement of the more anterior right maxillary implant **(D)** and the more anterior left maxillary implant **(E).**

comparable to that seen with autogenous bone grafting; however, recent reports of increased adverse events with this modality have been published.

The technique of tibial bone harvest can be briefly discussed by pointing out that cancellous bone marrow of the tibial plateau can be approached by a medial or lateral route. Because the medial approach seems now to be the preferred method, this technique is discussed. The patient is placed in the supine position in the operating room or in the recumbent position in a dental chair if the procedure is performed in a clinic setting. A broad-spectrum antibiotic (generally a cephalosporin) is given as prophylaxis, and the surgical site is prepped and draped appropriately. The tibial tuberosity is located, and lines perpendicular and parallel to its long axis, intersecting at the center of the tuberosity, are scribed. A point 15 mm medial to the vertical line and 15 mm superior to the horizontal line is marked; this is the center of the incision. A 1- to 1.5-cm oblique incision is made over this point to the underlying bone (Figure 6-6). The periosteum is reflected, and a 1-cm circular osteotomy is prepared. The thin cortical window is removed, and cancellous bone is harvested with a curette. The upper boundary is 1 cm above the window to avoid the articular surface of the tibial plateau. Lateral and medial harvesting is done until the cortical bone is reached. Lower harvesting can proceed as far as the curette will reach. The wound is closed in layers, with attention paid to not tightly closing the periosteum. A pressure wrap is placed to

complete the procedure. About 15 cc of noncompressed bone can be obtained in such a harvest. The strength of the tibia is unaffected by the surgery.

In the current case, because the bone quantity needed was minimal, the decision was made to use a human bone allograft in a putty combination (RegenerOss; Biomet 3-I, LLC, Palm Beach Gardens, Florida). For this type of surgery, the maxillary sinus wall (just below the zygomatic buttress) is exposed with a crestal incision and vertical releases as needed. An antrostomy, or window to access the maxillary sinus, is created with a carbide or diamond burr (a piezosurgery unit may be used if preferred). The bony window can be completely removed or infractured, as preferred, and the sinus membrane is carefully elevated off of the antral floor and walls and positioned medially and superiorly. Occasionally septae can be encountered that make dissection of the membrane more difficult and increase the risk of membrane perforation. If sinus membrane perforations occur, they can be enfolded (if small) or repaired using a collagen membrane (if larger). After reflection of the sinus membrane, the implant osteotomies are completed, the graft is placed, and the implants are inserted. The antrostomy osteotomy is covered with a slow-resorbing collagen membrane, and closure is obtained with resorbable sutures.

For the current patient, the immediate postoperative CBCT is shown in Figure 6-7, *A*. Subsequently, when the implants were uncovered and the healing caps placed (about 4 months after surgery), the sinus grafts demonstrated good consolidation (Figure 6-7, *B*). A CBCT cut from the area of the most posterior fixture on the right (Figure 6-7, *C*) further demonstrated graft remodeling and consolidation.

COMPLICATIONS

Complications of sinus grafting can be divided into intraoperative and postoperative types. Significant intraoperative complications are unusual; however, considerable bleeding can occasionally be encountered. Sinus membrane perforation occurs in more than 20% of cases but is not considered a risk factor for implant survival generally. Infection is the most consistent and serious postoperative complication, although most series report an occurrence rate of less than 5%. Infections are managed by incision and drainage, along with antibiotic therapy; many respond to this conservative management and heal uneventfully. However, infection is the major cause of implant fixture loss in most series reported. If tibial harvesting is performed, the complication rate is similarly low, and most problems associated with this procedure resolve with conservative management.

DISCUSSION

Implant cases involving sinus grafting show a cumulative implant survival rate of more than 93% up to 5 years. Prosthesis survival rates are reported to be even higher. The patient's age, gender, health status, and smoking habits; the implant's size, shape, and surface; the residual ridge height;

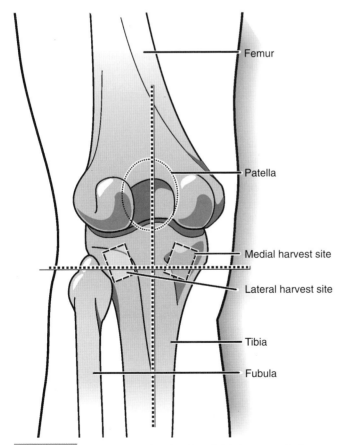

Figure 6-6 Surgical landmarks for tibial bone graft harvest techniques.

Femur

Patella

Medial harvest site

Lateral harvest site

Tibia

Fubula

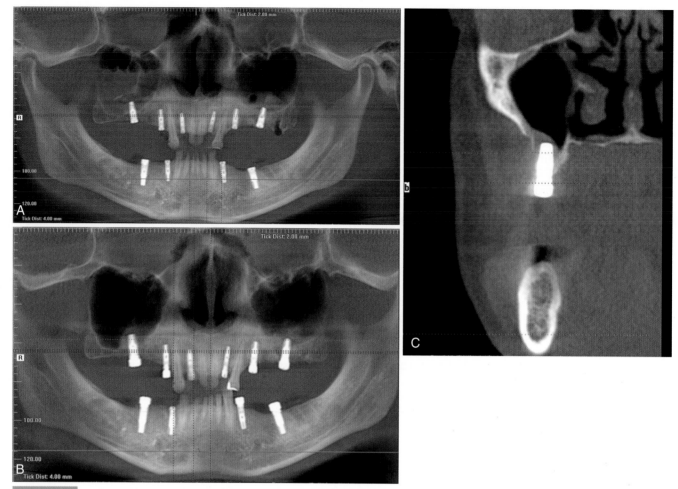

A, Panoramic CBCT immediately after grating and implant placement. **B,** Panoramic CBCT at implant exposure and placement of healing abutments (stage II). Note graft consolidation and return of aeration of maxillary sinuses. **C,** Coronal CBCT cut of most posterior implant site in the right maxilla, detailing graft consolidation.

the timing of implant placement with respect to grafting; the graft material; and the occurrence of surgical complications have been evaluated in analyses in an attempt to identify significant risk factors for implant failure in sinus grafting. Smoking more than 15 cigarettes per day and a residual ridge height of less than 4 mm are reported to be associated with significant reductions in implant survival rates. Smoking habits and residual ridge height should be carefully evaluated prior to sinus elevation procedures.

Bibliography

Balaji SM: Tobacco smoking and surgical healing of oral tissues: a review, *Indian J Dent Res* 19:344-348, 2008.

Herford AS, King BJ, Audia F, et al: Medial approach for tibial bone graft: anatomic study and clinical technique, *J Oral Maxillofac Surg* 61:358-3563, 2003.

Jensen OT (ed): *The sinus bone graft,* ed 2, Chicago, 2006, Quintessence.

Jensen T, Schou S, Svendsen PA, et al: Volumetric changes of the graft after maxillary sinus floor augmentation with Bio-Oss and autogenous bone in different ratios: a radiographic study in mini-pigs, *Clin Oral Implants Res* 23:902-910, 2012.

Liddelow G, Klineberg I: Patient-related risk factors for implant therapy: a critique of pertinent literature, *Aust Dent J* 56:417-426, 2011.

Lin IC, Gonzalez AM, Chang HJ, et al: A 5-year follow-up of 80 implants in 44 patients placed immediately after the lateral trap-door window procedure to accomplish maxillary sinus elevation without bone grafting, *Int J Oral Maxillofac Implants* 26:1079-1086, 2011.

Padmanabhan TV, Gupta RK: Comparison of crestal bone loss and implant stability among the implants placed with conventional procedure and using osteotome technique: a clinical study, *J Oral Implantol* 36:475-483, 2010.

Renouard F, Rangert B: *Risk factors in implant dentistry: simplified clinical analysis for predictable treatment,* ed 2, Hanover Park, Ill, 2008, Quintessence.

Rodriguez-Argueta OF, Figueiredo R, Valmaseda-Castellon E, et al: Postoperative complications in smoking patients treated with implants: a retrospective study, *J Oral Maxillofac Surg* 69:2152-2157, 2011.

Singh D, Teo SG, Poh KK: Regular narrow complex tachycardia, *Singapore Med J* 52:146-149, 2011.

Testori T, Weinstein RL, Taschieri S, et al: Risk factor analysis following maxillary sinus augmentation: a retrospective multicenter study, *Int J Oral Maxillofac Implants* 27:1170-1176, 2012.

Triplett RG, Nevins M, Marx RE, et al: Pivotal, randomized, parallel evaluation of recombinant human bone morphogenetic protein-2/absorbable collagen sponge and autogenous bone graft for maxillary sinus floor augmentation, *J Oral Maxillofac Surg* 67:1947-1960, 2009.

Urban IA, Nagursky H, Church C, et al: Incidence, diagnosis, and treatment of sinus graft infection after sinus floor elevation: a clinical study, *Int J Oral Maxillofac Implants* 27:449-457, 2012.

Vittayakittipong P, Nurit W, Kirirat P: Proximal tibial bone graft: the volume of cancellous bone and strength of decancellated tibias by the medial approach, *Int J Oral Maxillofac Surg* 41:531-536, 2012.

Wallace SS, Tarnow DP, Froum SJ, et al: Maxillary sinus elevation by lateral window approach: evolution of technology and technique, *J Evid Based Dent Pract* 12(3 Suppl):161-171, 2012.

Wong J, Lam DP, Abrishami A, et al: Short-term preoperative smoking cessation and postoperative complications: a systematic review and meta-analysis, *Can J Anaesth* 59:268-279, 2012.

Woo EJ: Adverse events reported after the use of recombinant human bone morphogenetic protein 2, *J Oral Maxillofac Surg* 70:765-767, 2012.

Zygomatic Implants

Eric Dierks and Jeremiah Johnson

CC

A 57-year-old female would like to discuss options for improving the retention and stability of her upper denture. She had been previously told that she "doesn't have enough bone for implants."

HPI

The patient required extraction of her entire maxillary dentition at age 20 due to caries and facial trauma and subsequent removal of her lower molars. Five years ago she had an unspecified ridge augmentation procedure, performed elsewhere. This was considered unsuccessful, because the patient observed that her maxillary denture continued to lose its retention. She believes that the resorptive process had continued and voiced concern that this will continue "up to her nose."

PMHX/PDHX/MEDICATIONS/ALLERGIES/SH/FH

The patient has a history of migraine headaches and osteoarthritis. Her surgical history is otherwise significant only for tonsillectomy. She denies medication allergies and does not smoke, use drugs, or drink alcohol. She has no history of paranasal sinus pathology and specifically denies polyps, chronic or recurrent rhinosinusitis, nasal breathing difficulties, and septal deviation, although these conditions do not necessarily preclude the application of a zygomatic implant. Preoperative ENT consultation was deemed unnecessary for this patient.

EXAMINATION

General. Alert and in no distress; noticeably anxious about the examination.

Vital signs. BP 152/80 mm Hg; pulse 88 bpm; respirations 14 per minute; weight 140 lb.

Maxillofacial. No abnormalities.

Intraoral. Oral examination reveals range of opening to be at least 40 mm. The maxilla is edentulous, with anterior greater than posterior alveolar ridge atrophy. The mandibular dentition is present from first premolar to the contralateral first premolar and is extensively restored. Gingival recession is present, as is significant attrition on the remaining teeth.

IMAGING

A recent panoramic radiograph demonstrates significant maxillary sinus pneumatization of the alveolar processes, extensively thinning the atrophic maxillary alveolar ridges bilaterally (Figure 6-8). The mandible demonstrates moderately advanced alveolar atrophy in the edentulous areas with periodontal bone loss around the remaining teeth. A radiopaque material is noted bilaterally in the maxilla and posterior mandible at the level of the alveolar

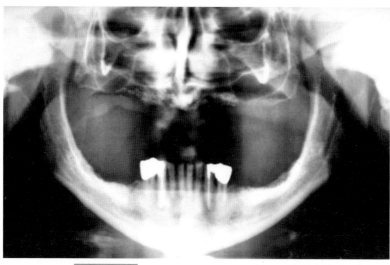

Figure 6-8 Preoperative orthopantogram (OPG).

ridge crests, consistent with previous hydroxyapatite augmentation.

A CBCT scan demonstrates the residual alveolar vertical dimension to be 2 mm in the posterior maxilla and 9 mm in the anterior maxilla at the nasomaxillary buttresses. The paranasal sinuses are otherwise radiographically normal. In the bilateral posterior mandible, the measurement from the inferior alveolar canal to the alveolar crest is 4 to 7 mm.

LABS

No routine laboratory testing is specifically necessary for the placement of zygomatic implants, other than those studies deemed prudent for a specific patient prior to the administration of IV sedation or general anesthesia.

ASSESSMENT

Advanced maxillary alveolar atrophy and sinus pneumatization, in addition to failing mandibular dentition with posterior alveolar atrophy.

TREATMENT

The goal of treatment for this patient is to restore a functional occlusion with adequate stability and retention of her prostheses, and to do so with a minimum number of operations and at a reasonable cost. Whether secondary to postextraction atrophy, traumatic loss, surgical resection, or congenital absence, the atrophic maxilla presents a clinical quandary for the reconstructive surgeon and prosthodontic team. Such interdisciplinary consultation and planning are mandatory, because surgical placement and restoration are technically more exacting for zygomatic implants than for conventional implants.

In many cases of maxillary atrophy, the maxillary dentition can be restored with optimal prosthodontic therapy with or without the use of endosseous implants. When implants are required, a variety of bone grafting and sinus augmentation techniques have been described to overcome the problem of limited maxillary bone stock, potentially enabling conventional implant placement. Even in patients with severe atrophy, zygomatic implants can provide an effective, predictable option that allows implant placement in a single surgical procedure, without preliminary sinus lift bone grafting. Immediate restoration and loading of zygomatic implants is an option. Contraindications are few (Box 6-2).

The operation is performed under general endotracheal anesthesia on an outpatient basis. The placement of zygomatic implants under IV sedation and local anesthesia has been described and is an option for healthy patients who can open the mouth widely and who lack a mandibular dentition. As was done in the current patient, an appropriate preoperative antibiotic is administered intravenously. After induction and nasal intubation, the mouth and face undergo a standard antiseptic prep. The oral surgical sites and the nasal floor are injected with 0.5% Marcaine containing 1:200,000

Box 6-2   Relative and Absolute Contraindications to Zygomatic Implants

Relative contraindications to zygomatic implants:
- Presence of mandibular anterior teeth (making proper alignment of the drill difficult)
- Active maxillary sinus pathology or sinusitis (chronic sinusitis is not a contraindication)

Absolute contraindications to zygomatic implants:
- Medical condition making the patient an unsuitable candidate for this surgery and general anesthesia or IV sedation
- Restricted mouth opening

---

epinephrine. The nose is packed with 0.05% oxymetazoline-soaked cottonoid sponges to vasoconstrict and shrink the mucosa.

The mouth is opened maximally to allow both visualization and access for the necessarily long instrumentation of the zygomatic implants. A crestal incision is created with an anterior midline and bilateral posterolateral releasing incisions to aid in tissue reflection. Subperiosteal exposure of the anterior maxillary sinus wall to the zygomatic buttress is completed. Three conventional implants are placed in the atrophic anterior maxilla. Two are placed beneath the piriform rim, and these include a limited elevation of the lateral nasal floor with bone grafting around the implant. The midline anterior implant is placed through the incisive foramen into the base of the nasal crest of the maxilla. Much of the hydroxyapatite material was removed. The zygomatic implants are placed according to the sinus slot technique described by Stella and Warner, which allows emergence of the fixture at the alveolar crest rather than on the palatal aspect of the alveolus, as in the original Brånemark technique (Figure 6-9, *A*).

The "slot" refers to the access slot through the maxillary sinus wall that is created to allow visualization of the trajectory of the implant. An emergence hole is drilled at the crest of the alveolus in the second premolar/first molar area. The slot then begins above the alveolus superior and lateral to this hole and extends along the crest of the zygomaticomaxillary buttress toward the body of the zygoma (Figure 6-9, *B*). The apex of the slot is flattened horizontally with a round bur, and a dimple is drilled into this flat area to allow drilling of the hole into the body of the zygoma for the implant. Attention is paid to adequate retraction and protection of the lips prior to drilling. It is impractical to protect the sinus membrane, and attempts to do so are unnecessary. A pistol grip orthopedic drill is used. The implant drill is then placed through the access hole and into the "slot," terminating in the dimple at the base of the zygomatic body. External digital pressure is used to identify the zygomatic notch; the implant drills are oriented to the zygomatic body, and retraction is optimized. The 2.9-mm-diameter drill bit is used first, and the surgeon drills obliquely until the tip of the drill bit is palpated as it exits the zygomatic body near the zygomatic arch. This is followed by a transitional drill. Last, the 3.5-mm drill bit

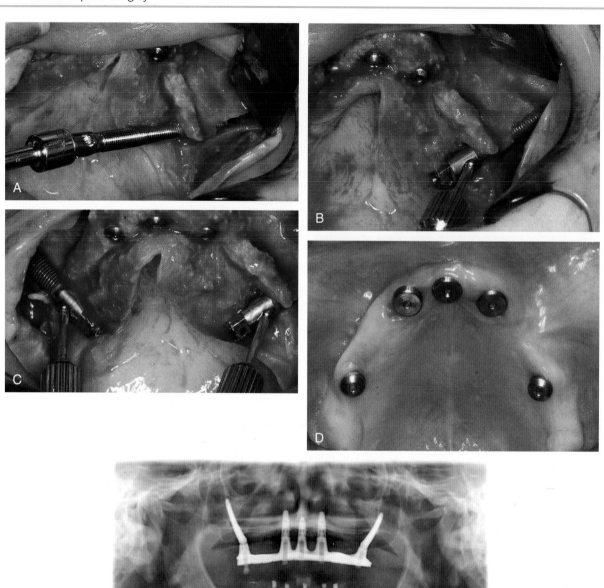

Figure 6-9   **A,** Insertion of the zygomatic implant showing the "slot" in the anterior maxillary sinus wall to aid visualization of the implant body. **B,** Removing the transfer abutment of the zygomatic implant. **C,** After placement of the anterior standard implants and bilateral zygomatic implants. **D,** After integration demonstrating the correct location of the zygomatic implant abutments on the palatal aspect of the alveolar crest at a location just anterior to the first molar position. **E,** Postoperative, postrestoration OPG showing stability at 2 years.

is passed. The depth gauge is used to determine the length of implant needed. Upon removal of the implant from its container, the screw retaining the transfer abutment should be preemptively loosened and retightened prior to placement of the implant. The zygoma implant is threaded into position without tapping. The long axis of the screw that retains the transfer abutment is aligned with the long axis of the anterior implants by placing the driver into its hex and assessing the long axis of the driver. The transfer abutment is removed, exposing the 45-degree orientation of the external hex implant platform, which now parallels the fixture surfaces of the anterior implants. In some patients, the sinus slot technique results in the exposure of implant threads outside the maxillary sinus wall rather than within the sinus. This is expected and does not affect stability. Closure is performed with 4-0 polyglactin sutures placed in horizontal mattress fashion (Figure 6-9, *C*).

Zygoma implants range in length from 30 to 55 mm. The shaft diameter tapers from 4 mm superiorly to 5 mm at the fixture level. Implant integration occurs within the thick bone in the body of the zygoma, which produces an integrated length in the range of 15 to 20 mm (Figure 6-9, *D*). The acquisition of an additional zone of integration at the level of the alveolus is welcome but unnecessary. The fixture is angulated at 45 degrees (Nobelbiocare, Zürich, Switzerland) or 55 degrees (Southern Implants, Irene, South Africa) and oriented roughly parallel to the occlusal plane. The long moment arm of the zygoma implant makes it inappropriate to use without cross-arch stabilization to other conventional implants or to anterior conventional implants plus a zygoma implant on the opposite side.

The mandibular teeth are then removed, and the vertical height of the anterior mandibular alveolus is reduced. Five conventional implants are placed between the mental foramina using standard technique. In the current case, the patient was extubated and recovered without incident. Postoperative medications include analgesics and chlorhexidine oral rinse. A postoperative antibiotic was prescribed for this patient in light of the anterior maxillary and nasal floor bone grafting. The use of nasal decongestants and antibiotics is optional.

A postoperative Panorex (OPG) is routinely obtained (Figure 6-9, *E*). Lateral and PA cephalograms are optional. Restoration of the zygoma implants can be initiated immediately after placement or after waiting for a period of integration. If restoration is delayed, an interim denture can be worn over the zygoma implants.

COMPLICATIONS

Complications of zygomatic implants can be divided into surgical failures and prosthetic failures. Infection is no more likely than with conventional root-form implants. Sinus pathology after implant placement is not expected, and although there may be radiographic mucosal thickening in up to 20% of cases, this does not affect the stability of the implant or necessitate intervention by an otolaryngologist. Ecchymosis is less common with the sinus slot technique than with the traditional Brånemark approach because of the limited soft tissue dissection. The surgeon should avoid placing the implant emergence point too lateral, because this may predispose to mucosal dehiscence over the threads. Prosthetic failures are more likely to be related to inadequate cross-arch stabilization, with resultant loosening of the fixture.

DISCUSSION

Bedrossian's classification of maxillary atrophy identifies three zones of potential atrophy. Zone 1 corresponds to the alveolus in the incisor region of the arch; zone 2 to the premolars; and zone 3 to the molars. Inadequate bone in zone 3 is a contraindication to conventional implants. Although a combination of sinus augmentation and bone grafting prior to implant placement is an option, the success of implants in this situation is not what can be expected under other circumstances. The 1994 Academy of Osseointegration Sinus Graft Consensus Conference reviewed the results of 2,997 implants placed among 1,007 grafted sinuses. After a minimum 3-year follow-up postrestoration, a 61% failure rate was found when implants were placed simultaneously with sinus lift bone grafts. The success of zygomatic implants has been well established. In a prospective 16-center evaluation with 3-year follow-up, Kahnberg and colleagues reported a 96.3% survival rate. Malevez and co-workers published a 100% survival rate with 103 zygoma implants in 55 patients, retrospectively, following 6 to 48 months of loading. Brånemark described his outcome results for 28 consecutive patients with severely resorbed edentulous maxillae involving 52 zygoma implants followed for 5 to 10 years with a survival rate of 94% with no significant complications.

In summary, the zygomatic implant is an underused resource that provides a cost-effective, single-stage solution to the problem of inadequate posterior maxillary bone. It merits careful consideration in the treatment planning for the patient with an atrophic maxilla who requires multiple implants.

Bibliography

Bedrossian E, Sullivan RM, Fortin Y, et al: Fixed-prosthetic implant restoration of the edentulous maxilla: a systematic pretreatment evaluation method, *J Oral Maxillofac Surg* 66:112-122, 2008.

Brånemark P-I, Gröndahl K, Öhrnell L-O, et al: Zygoma fixture in the management of advanced atrophy of the maxilla: technique and long-term results, *Scand J Plast Reconstr Surg Hand Surg* 38:70-85, 2004.

Davó R, Malevez C, López-Orellana C, et al: Sinus reactions to immediately loaded zygoma implants: a clinical and radiographic study, *Eur J Oral Implantol* 1:53-60, 2008.

Davó R, Malevez C, Rojas J: Immediate function in the atrophic maxilla using zygoma implants: a preliminary study, *J Prosthet Dent* 97(6 Suppl):44-51, 2007.

Garg A: Augmentation grafting of the maxillary sinus for placement of dental implants: anatomy, physiology, and procedures, *Implant Dent* 8:36-46, 1999.

Hirsch J-M, Öhrnell L-O, Henry PJ, et al: A clinical evaluation of the zygoma fixture: one year of follow-up at 16 clinics, *J Oral Maxillofac Surg* 62(Suppl 2):22-29, 2004.

Jensen O, Adams M, Cottam J, et al: The all-on-4 shelf: maxilla, *J Oral Maxillofac Surg* 68:2520-2527, 2010.

Kahnberg KE, Henry P, Hirsch J-M, et al: Clinical evaluation of the zygoma implant: 3-year follow-up at 16 clinics, *J Oral Maxillofac Surg* 65:2033-2038, 2007.

Malevez C, Abarca M, Durduf F, et al: The zygomatic implant: a 6-48 month follow-up study, *Clin Oral Implants Res* 15(1):15-18, 2004.

Malik N, Kumar V, Bora P: Lefort 1 distraction osteogenesis of the edentulous maxilla, *Int J Oral Maxillofac Surg* 40:430-433, 2011.

Petruson B: Sinuscopy in patients with titanium implants in the nose and sinuses, *Scand J Plast Reconstr Surg Hand Surg* 38(2):86-93, 2004.

Shulman LB, Jensen OT: Academy of Osseointegration: Sinus Graft Consensus Conference, *Int J Oral Maxillofac Implants* 13(Suppl):4, 1998.

Stella J, Warner M: Sinus slot technique for simplification and improved orientation of zygomaticus dental implants: a technical note, *Int J Oral Maxillofac Implants* 15:889, 2000.

Contemporary Treatment Options for Edentulism

Kumar J. Patel and Shahrokh C. Bagheri

CC

A 61-year-old female is referred from a prosthodontist for implant restoration with a complaint of "my dentures are loose."

HPI

The patient has been wearing the existing prostheses for more than 20 years without any follow-up.

The prosthodontist fabricated interim dentures at the correct vertical dimension. These prostheses help establish function, improve tissue health, and assist in diagnosing esthetic needs and lip support. For patients with facial antero-posterior desorption greater than 10 to 11 mm, the prosthodontist may elect to provide them with a flange to support the lips. This may limit the use of fixed maxillary prostheses. Interim prostheses are also used to assess interocclusal space. Restoring the vertical dimension of occlusion allows for resolution of angular cheilitis. These interim prostheses can be duplicated and used as a scanning guide to aid treatment planning using a cone-beam computed tomography (CBCT) scan. They can also be used as radiographic stents or as a surgical guide.

PMHX/PSHX/MEDICATIONS/ALLERGIES/SH/FH

Noncontributory.

EXAMINATION

General. Mild obesity.

Maxillofacial. The interincisal opening and lateral jaw movements were normal. A collapsed vertical dimension of occlusion and reduced lower facial height were noted (Figure 6-10). At correct occlusal vertical dimension (OVD), the patient demonstrated a class I skeletal jaw relationship. No asymmetry was noted.

INTRAORAL EXAMINATION

The occlusion was overclosed, and the existing prosthesis had a poor fit, with overextension and significant wear contributing to instability and poor function. The maxillary ridge showed significant resorption. The palatal mucosa was erythematous and had signs of denture stomatitis due to the poorly fitting prostheses.

The mandibular arch had moderate resorption due to prolonged edentulism.

IMAGING

The panoramic radiograph remains a good initial diagnostic tool. In many cases it will suffice, depending on the anticipated treatment plan. A CBCT or CT scan can be used in select cases for advanced planning and detailed analysis of the bony anatomy. A CBCT scan was obtained for the current

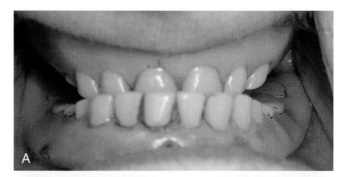

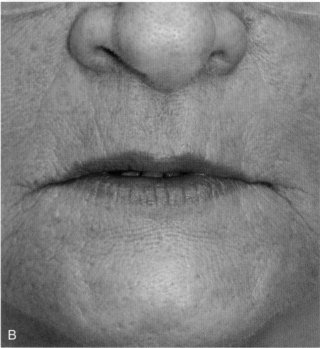

Figure 6-10 Preoperative photographs of the patient with "loose dentures." **A,** The old prosthesis has collapsed. **B,** Extraoral photograph shows collapsed vertical dimension.

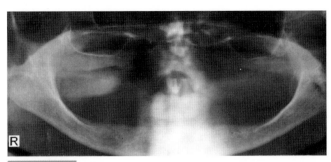

Figure 6-11   Preoperative panoramic radiograph. Moderate maxillary and mandibular resorption of the edentulous residual ridges can be seen.

patient. In this case there was adequate maxillary and mandibular bone height and width for most contemporary treatment options. No other noticeable pathology was observed in the edentulous ridges, and the temporomandibular joints were normal radiographically. The radiograph showed moderate maxillary and mandibular resorption of the edentulous residual ridges (Figure 6-11).

LABS

No routine laboratory studies are indicated unless dictated by the medical history in preparation for surgical intervention.

ASSESSMENT

Edentulous atrophic maxilla and mandible with poorly fitting dentures requiring prosthetic rehabilitation.

TREATMENT

Several options are available for patients with adequate bone height and width. Patients with inadequate bone require bone grafting (see chapters on bone grafting elsewhere in this text) prior to surgical placement of implants or consideration for zygoma implants (see Zygoma Implants in this chapter). CBCT imaging and additional preprosthetic planning can be helpful for determination of bony anatomy and delineation of vital structures. A team approach involving the oral and maxillofacial surgeon and the prosthodontist or restorative dentist is critical to achieving the treatment objectives. The following options were presented to the current patient by the referring prosthodontist.

1. Conventional upper and lower dentures. The use of implants for restoration of edentulism is the contemporary consensus. However, the option of conventional upper and lower dentures should be presented to the patient, along with its shortfalls, which include instability, discomfort, and inadequate function. The main advantage of this option is its lower cost and noninvasive nature.

2. Conventional maxillary denture with a mandibular overdenture retained by two implants (Figure 6-12).

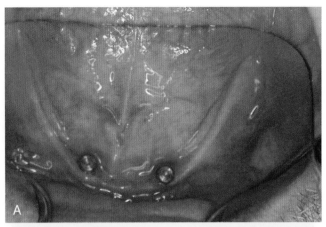

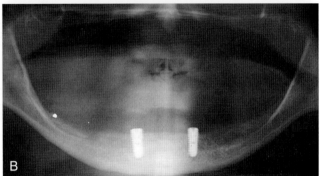

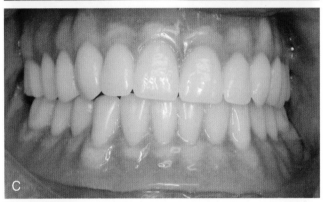

Figure 6-12   Conventional maxillary denture with mandibular overdenture retained by two implants. **A,** Two implants in place to retain the mandibular overdenture. **B,** Panoramic radiograph showing the two implants in the mandibular arch. **C,** Intraoral view of the conventional maxillary denture and mandibular overdenture (retained by two implants) in place.

This is the most cost-effective option with the use of implants.

3. Maxillary overdenture over four implants and mandibular overdenture using two, three, or four implants (Figure 6-13). (Two is the minimum number of implants for a mandibular overdenture [Figure 6-13, *B* and *D*].) Using three or four implants in the mandible (Figure 6-13, *H* and *I*) provides superior retention, although it can be more difficult for some patients to remove the prosthesis, and it is more costly.)

4. Maxillary overdenture ("snap in") retained and supported by four to six implants with limited palatal

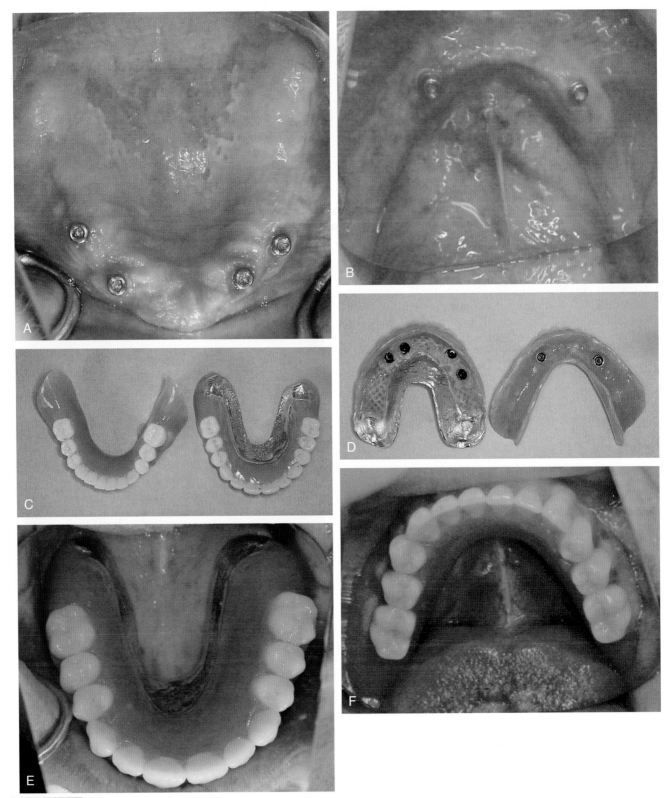

Figure 6-13 Maxillary overdentures retained with four implants and examples of mandibular overdentures retained by both two and three implants. **A,** Maxillary arch with four Locator abutments/attachments (patrix) on the implants. **B,** Mandibular arch with two Locator abutments/attachment (patrix) on the implants. **C,** The maxillary and mandibular prostheses. Note the partial metal coverage in the maxillary arch. **D,** Tissue surface (intaglio surface) of the maxillary and mandibular prostheses showing the attachment matrix (the matrix receives the patrix). **E,** Intraoral view of the maxillary prosthesis retained and supported by four implants. **F,** Intraoral view of a mandibular prosthesis retained by two implants.

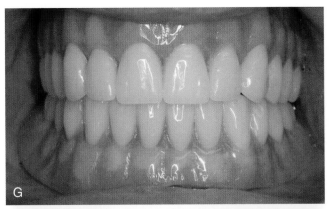

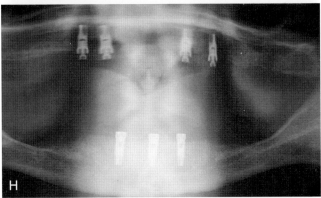

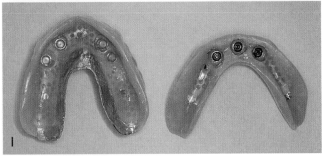

Figure 6-13, cont'd **G,** Intraoral view of the prostheses in place. **H,** Radiograph demonstrating the use of three implants to stabilize a lower denture and four to retain a maxillary overdenture. **I,** The maxillary and mandibular prostheses.

coverage and a mandibular fixed denture/prostheses (also known as a hybrid).

5. Maxillary and mandibular implant supported by a hybrid with four or six implants, with immediate placement and immediate or delayed loading (Figure 6-14).
6. Implant-supported crown and bridge (Figure 6-15).

A number of factors need to be considered in treatment planning for edentulism, including the patient's expectations and medical condition, the cost, and the expertise and comfort level of the restoring clinician.

TREATMENT

The patient chose option 4, using four maxillary and five mandibular implants. The following treatment was sequenced

between the prosthodontist and the oral and maxillofacial surgeon. This option presents an excellent balance of cost, practicality, bone preservation, and ease of posttreatment prosthetic maintenance, and it is minimally invasive compared with the other surgical options.

Phase 1: Prosthetic/Diagnostic Phase

The patient was prescribed an oral antifungal rinse (Nystatin), followed by an antifungal ointment applied to the intaglio (tissue surface of the prosthesis) on the newly made upper interim denture, for the resolution of denture stomatitis. The newly fabricated prostheses were allowed to function for 4 weeks to establish function and comfort at the new vertical dimension.

A CBCT was obtained to delineate the anatomy and enable treatment planning for four endosteal implants in the maxillary arch and five implants in the anterior mandible, with fabrication of a maxillary overdenture and a mandibular hybrid (Figure 6-16). "Hybrid" is a term frequently used to describe fixed yet removable prostheses. The prosthesis is typically screw retained and can be removed by the clinician. It also may be cement retained.

Phase 2: Surgical Phase

Four endosteal implants were placed in the maxilla, and five implants were placed in the mandible. The interim prostheses were relined with soft relining. The patient was prescribed 1 week of amoxicillin 500 mg with chlorhexidine mouthwash and appropriate analgesics. The patient was followed at 1, 2, 7, and 14 days postoperatively. Necessary denture adjustments and relining were performed as needed. At the 1 week postoperative visit, the patient had a mild wound dehiscence at one of the mandibular implant sites (most common complication). This was resolved, through local wound care, by 3 weeks, with no implant loss. The dentures were relined on two occasions during the healing period (performed as needed). At 12 weeks the implants were uncovered for fabrication of a definitive prosthesis.

Phase 3: Prosthetic Phase

Two weeks after the implants were uncovered, the lower interim denture was converted into a fixed interim hybrid prosthesis by the prosthodontist, and subsequently the definitive maxillary overdenture and lower fixed hybrid prostheses were fabricated. The maxillary overdenture was retained by use of Locator attachments (Figure 6-17).

For postoperative care, the patient was followed up every 6 months for soft tissue and prosthetic maintenance. This is a critical factor in the long-term success of implant-supported prostheses. The lack of adequate follow-up can result in greater failure rates.

COMPLICATIONS

Complications can be divided into prosthetic-related and surgery-related complications. Surgical complications of implant surgery are discussed elsewhere in this text.

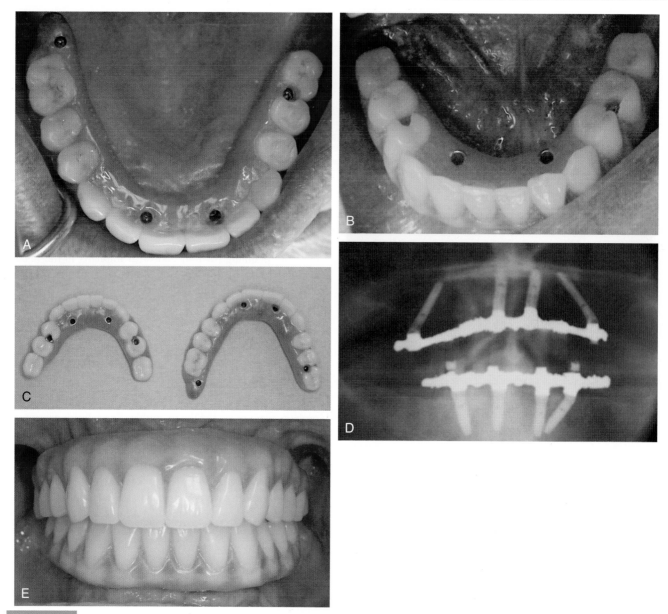

Figure 6-14 A maxillary and mandibular hybrid prosthesis supported by four implants. **A,** A maxillary prosthesis; note the access holes, which have been restored with composite. **B,** A mandibular hybrid prosthesis supported by four implants. The access holes have been restored with composite. **C,** Maxillary and mandibular hybrid prostheses. **D,** Postoperative panoramic radiograph (surgery performed by Dr. Wade Diab). Note the tilted posterior implants, which allow for better anteroposterior spread and avoid the need for sinus grafting. **E,** Intraoral view of the maxillary and mandibular hybrid prostheses in place.

The most common complications involve soreness and mild ulcerations associated with denture wear on the surgical sites. This can be minimized by the application of a soft liner, which is adjusted and changed periodically by the treating prosthodontist. A well-fitting set of dentures is paramount, because it minimizes the number of adjustments necessary and serves as a pressure bandage. Breakage of the prosthetic teeth and occasionally of the denture base is possible, especially if the base is made too thin to accommodate the soft liner. Simple planning and regular follow-up can help prevent this.

The temporary fixed prosthesis is weak and not adequate for any long-term use. In the opinion of the author (KJP),

a temporary fixed prosthesis should not be used for more than 6 months. They should not extend beyond the most posterior implant, to prevent breakage due to cantilever forces. Upon delivery of the definitive prosthesis, the temporary fixed prosthesis should be kept for emergency use.

Failure of an implant during the healing phase can be easily managed by replacing the implant. If implants fail years after treatment, the prosthesis should be evaluated. In the maxillary arch, when possible, this can be managed by replacing the implant or implants and fabricating or modifying the existing prosthesis. Loss of implants in the mandible may not require refabrication of a new prosthesis, depending on the position of the failed implant. A minimum of four implants is

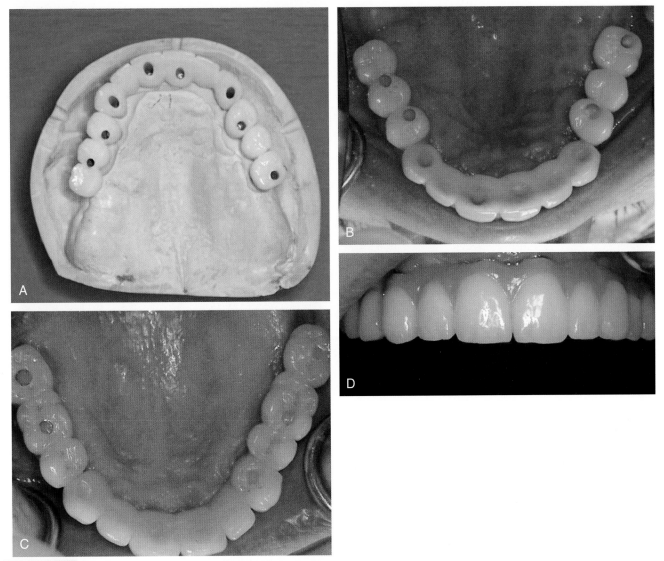

Figure 6-15 Implant-supported crown and bridge using eight implants in the maxilla. **A,** Screw-retained crowns and bridges on the model; there are three segments of teeth. Posterior segments are comprised of three units supported by two implants. The anterior six units are connected to facilitate esthetics. **B,** Intraoral view of the prostheses. **C,** Eight implants support three segments of fixed screw-retained bridges (fixed partial dentures). **D,** Frontal view with lips retracted. Note the use of pink porcelain.

necessary to support a mandibular fixed prosthesis. However, modification of the existing prostheses may be required. It is highly recommended that the prosthetic superstructure be well fitting, because a poor fit may cause screw loosening and undesirable forces on the implants. The patient should be encouraged to follow up regularly to maintain hygiene around the implants and to allow the clinician to assess stability and occlusal contacts.

DISCUSSION

Edentulism can be classified as a form of disability. About 26% of the U.S. population between the ages of 65 and 74 years are completely edentulous. Edentulous patients demonstrate a relatively lower intake of dietary fibers, and foods with folate and vitamin C. Lin and colleagues investigated the relationship between chewing ability and diet among elderly

edentulous patients; approximately 58% of the subjects reported dissatisfaction with their dentures, and 51% reported discomfort on chewing. A 6-year study on institutionalized elderly patients compared physical activity and mortality between groups of edentulous patients without dentures and those who were partially edentulous. The study suggested that there is a decline in physical ability and increase in mortality rates for patients with no replacement dentures.

Extractions of teeth are followed by reduction of the residual ridge (RRR). Bone loss is a continuing process, and the mandibular ridge may resorb at approximately four times the rate of the maxillary ridge. Although conventional dentures are prescribed to many patients as a form of replacement for teeth, there is increasing evidence suggesting that the first choice of treatment should include at least two implants in the mandibular arch to stabilize a mandibular prosthesis. The McGill Consensus Statement/Report (2002) recommended

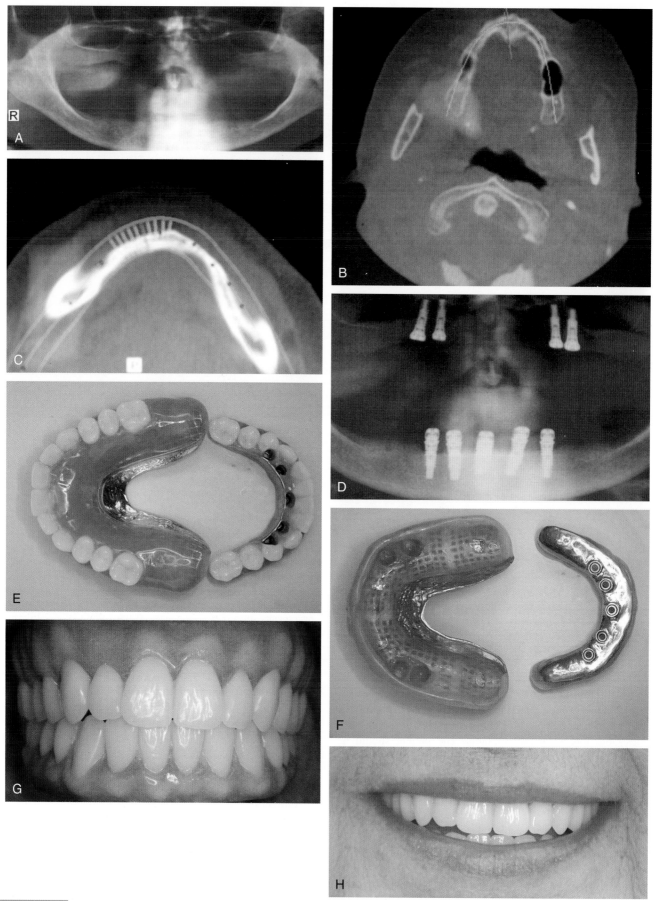

Figure 6-16 **A,** Preoperative panoramic radiograph showing moderate resorption. **B,** CBCT of the maxilla. **C,** CBCT used for treatment planning. **D,** Panoramic radiograph showing the implants in place. **E,** Occlusal view of the maxillary overdenture and mandibular hybrid. **F,** Maxillary overdenture and mandibular hybrid showing the tissue surface (intaglio surface). **G,** Intraoral view of the prostheses in place. **H,** Final smile of the patient at restored vertical.

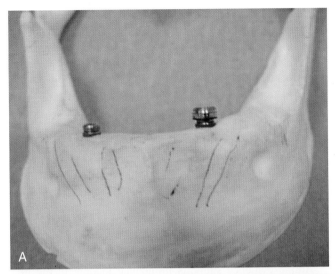

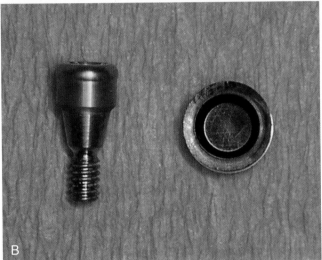

Figure 6-17 Implant and attachment components. The portion of the attachment that is screwed into the implant body is a prefabricated attachment (Locator; Zest Anchors, Escondido, California), also known as the "patrix." The housing (silver cap) that snaps onto this part is known as the "matrix." The matrix and patrix together form an attachment. **A,** Implant with a prefabricated Locator attachment/abutment/matrix and patrix. **B,** Locator attachment/abutment (matrix and patrix).

that an implant-retained mandibular overdenture should be the first-choice standard of care for patients who are edentulous. This statement was supported by the British Society for the Study of Prosthetic Dentistry in 2009. Das and colleagues reported similar findings in a 2012 survey of academic prosthodontists in the United States.

Dental implants provide stability and retention for the prostheses, and they help maintain bone volume. Endosseous implants are thought to maintain width and height, as long as the implant remains anchored in bone with healthy, biologic attachments. High levels of patient satisfaction have been reported for implant-retained and implant-supported prostheses. In a review, Felton reported a success rate of 92% to 100% for implant-retained mandibular overdentures, with a follow-up period ranging from 7 to 10 years.

The best choice of attachments between implant and denture base remains controversial. Use of more implants and a bar is associated with more retention. However, Burns and colleagues reported that patients preferred the independent implant attachment. Bars are also used when implant angulations are not favorable; however, they typically require more interocclusal room and should not be recommended without a full prosthetic evaluation. All attachments come with maintenance and require follow-up visits. Attachment retention forces from 5 to 7 N should be sufficient to stabilize overdentures. Most attachment systems suffer from wear during insertion and removal. In the authors' opinion, resilient independent attachments with nylon inserts are cost-effective and easy to maintain.

A few studies and some reports justify the use of four implants in the maxillary arch, with limited palatal coverage. Krennmair and colleagues reported a success rate greater than 97% on 179 implants followed for up to 5 years. Cavallaro and Tarnow reported 100% success on five patients, with 4 years' follow-up. Romeo and co-workers reported a 92.5% success rate for 40 implants with 7 years' follow-up. In the combined experience of the authors (KJP, SCB), a success rate of 95% has been seen over 4 years with more than 100 implants that used the prostheses design illustrated in the current case. In most reports, bars are used to connect implants or solitary attachments with or without metal reinforcement. Many authors have recommended full palatal coverage when four or fewer implants are used. Rodriguez and co-workers reported that the design using six implants with a bar has the highest success rates for maxillary implants. Eckard and Carr have advocated the use of six maxillary implants to ensure prosthetic success. In an in vitro evaluation, Damghani and colleagues (2012) concluded that using four Locator attachments produced significantly less force on the palate compared to using zero or two Locator attachments. There was a significant reduction in the force measured when the distance between the four Locator attachments increased from 8 to 16 mm. The use of eight Locators produced the least amount of force on the palate, but this was not significantly different compared with four Locators with a distance of 16 to 24 mm between implants. Based on a review of the work of Ekfeldt and co-workers, Kronstrom and co-workers, Lewis and colleagues, and Mericske-Stern, Drago and colleagues (2011) concluded that there appears to be consensus that a minimum of four implants yields a favorable long-term prognosis for prosthetic treatment options without palatal coverage. In the opinion of the authors, the use of partial palatal coverage with four well-distributed implants provides a retentive maxillary overdenture to improve function. Partial palatal coverage using a metal base provides for additional support and strength and reduced thickness.

The decision whether to use a fixed or removable prosthesis requires evaluation of numerous factors. Anteroposterior resorption of more than 10 mm in the maxilla may be an indication for the use of an implant-retained/removable prosthesis. The patient may require a flange for lip support; however, the procedure still can be accomplished if at least a minimum of lip support is available and the ridge lap is modified.

Mandibular fixed hybrid prostheses have shown very predictable success rates. Rodriguez and co-workers reported success rates of 98.1% for a mandibular fixed hybrid prosthesis followed up for 36 months. Gallucci and colleagues reported implant survival rates of 100% and prosthesis survival rates of 95.5% for mandibular hybrid prostheses on four to six implants with an average cantilever of 15.6 mm, followed up for 5 years. Aglietta and colleagues conducted a systemic review to assess the survival rates of implant-supported, cantilever fixed prostheses after an observation of 5 years. They reported success rates of 94.3% at 5 years and 88.9% at 10 years. Some of the complications seen were peri-implantitis (5.4%), veneer fracture (10.3%), screw loosening (8.2%), and abutment/screw fractures (2.1%). Although framework fracture was not reported, it is a known to be a complication.

The use of four to six implants for maxillary rehabilitation with a fixed prosthesis has been well reported. Capelli and co-workers reported success rates of 97.6% for immediately loaded maxillary implants followed up for 40 months. The study included 246 implants in 41 maxillae restored with a six implant–supported hybrid prosthesis. The same study reported 100% success rates for mandibular prostheses supported by four implants. Tealdo and colleagues followed 21 patients in whom 111 implants had been placed in the maxillary arch, followed by immediate loading of the full arch prostheses supported by four to six implants. They reported 92.8% implant survival at 12 months and a prosthesis survival rate of 100%.

Several studies support immediate implant loading of full arch maxillary and mandibular ridges. In 2012 Ghoul and co-workers reported that to load immediately, three important clinical criteria must be met: (1) micromotion must be reduced to 50 to 150 μm; (2) connecting several implants reduces this motion and provides cross-arch stabilization to counteract the bending effect of lateral forces; and (3) insertion torque values of implants should exceed at least 30 N cm^2 at the time of placement. Two different protocols are used:

1. Fabricating a temporary prosthesis, which is worn by the patient during the healing phase. In the authors' opinion, it is better to have a screw-retained prosthesis. Advantages include easy removal for maintenance. The prosthesis may be removed after 10 days for suture removal or for the addition of acrylic to adapt to tissues. This will not jeopardize implant stability during bone remodeling. As Borges and colleagues found, macro-movements are not recorded and micromovements are within the acceptable range with this approach. Ghoul and co-workers suggested that a cement-retained prosthesis should not be removed for 3 to 4 months to allow for healing. Residual cement removal can be difficult with these prostheses. Common complications include food trapping and breakage of teeth or the prosthesis. The patient should be advised to avoid hard food for 4 to 6 weeks. Ghoul and co-workers also suggested that the occlusion for these prostheses (which include a narrow occlusal platform for posterior teeth) should

have flat cusps that are distributed over a large area and occlusal contacts that are inside (lingual/palatal) of the implant. No cantilever extension should be present in these interim prostheses. This interim phase also allows for the management of any implant failure prior to fabrication of the definitive prosthesis.

2. Fabricating and delivering definitive prostheses the day of surgery. Despite the obvious advantages in time and the elimination of numerous steps, this approach does have disadvantages. Ghoul and co-workers reported in their review that early complications include bony interference that could prevent complete seating. Despite the use of CT-guided surgery, these types of prostheses have a failure rate of 9%. Ghoul and colleagues, in addition to many others, suggest insertion of an interim prosthesis before a definitive prosthesis is made.

Ample evidence supports immediate loading in the first protocol described. Malo and colleagues reported success rates of 97% in 32 patients treated with four implants in the maxillary arch, for a total of 128 implants. Capelli and co-workers reported success rates of 97% and 100% with use of four to six implants in the maxilla and mandible. Bergkvist and associates reported a success rate of 98.2% for 168 implants placed in the maxilla in 28 patients. Each patient received a hybrid prosthesis supported by six implants. Weinstein and colleagues and Agliardi and co-workers reported a success rate of 100% for four interforaminal implants with two axial and two tilted implants placed in the mandibular arch. Agliardi and colleagues further reported success rates of 98.36% for the maxilla and 99.73% for the mandible when both arches received four implants, two placed axially and two distal implants placed in tilted position. Evidence supporting immediate loading of maxillary overdentures is lacking, and this should not be done. Limited evidence supports immediate loading of a mandibular overdenture when a bar overdenture is used.

When adequate bone is present and the patient does not need lip support, consideration should be given to an implant-supported crown and bridge (see Figure 6-15). Screw-retained or cement-retained prostheses can be used. They are easy to maintain but costly to fabricate. This procedure may be performed using an interim fixed prosthesis to provide interim function or by using a delayed loading protocol. Atrophic maxilla and mandible, which lack adequate bone for the placement of standard implants, deserve separate discussion.

CONCLUSION

The first choice for treatment of a mandibular edentulous arch is an implant-retained overdenture. Implants improve the stability, and hence function, of the prosthesis. They also have been advocated to preserve bone. In general, maxillary overdentures should use four to six implants, and they should not be loaded immediately until more evidence is available. Delayed loading, along with partial palatal coverage with a metal base, has shown promising results and is a viable economic option for patients who gag. In addition, this option has the advantage of ease of fabrication and maintenance. Resilient independent attachments are preferred over bar and other nonresilient attachments; they are simple to maintain and change. Keeping the prosthesis simple should be considered for long-term success.

Bibliography

Agliardi E, Clerico M, Ciancio P, et al: Immediate loading of full-arch fixed prostheses supported by axial and tilted implants for the treatment of edentulous atrophic mandibles, *Quintessence Int* 41:285-293, 2010.

Agliardi E, Panigatti S, Clerico M, et al: Immediate rehabilitation of the edentulous jaws with full fixed prostheses supported by four implants: interim results of a single cohort prospective study, *Clin Oral Implants Res* 21:459-465, 2010.

Aglietta M, Siciliano VI, Zwanhlen M, et al: A systemic review of the survival and complication rates of implant supported fixed dental prosthesis with cantilever extension after an observation period of at least 5 years, *Clin Oral Implants Res* 20(5):441-451, 2009.

Attard NJ, Zarb GA: Long-treatment outcomes in edentulous patients with implant overdentures: the Toronto Study, *Int J Prosthodont* 17:425-433, 2004.

Atwood DA: Reduction of residual ridge: a major oral disease entity, *J Prosthet Dent* 26:266-279, 1971.

Bergkvist G, Nilner K, Sahlholm S, et al: Immediate loading of implants in the edentulous maxilla: use of an interim fixed prosthesis followed by a permanent fixed prosthesis—a 32 month prospective radiological and clinical study, *Clin Implant Dent Relat Res* 11:1-10, 2009.

Borges A, Dias Pereira L, Thome G, et al: Prostheses removal for suture removal after immediate load: success of implants, *Clin Implant Dent Relat Res* 12:244-248, 2010.

Burns DR, Unger J, Coffey JP, et al: Randomized, prospective, clinical evaluation of prosthodontic modalities for mandibular implant overdenture treatment, *J Prosthet Dent* 106(1):12-21, 2011.

Burns DR, Unger JW, Elswick RK Jr, et al: Prospective clinical evaluation of mandibular implant overdentures. II. Patient satisfaction and preferences, *J Prosthet Dent* 73:364-369, 1995.

Capelli M, Zuffetti F, Del Fabbro M, et al: Immediate rehabilitation of completely edentulous jaw with fixed prostheses supported by either upright or tilted implants: a multicenter clinical study, *Int J Oral Maxillofac Implants* (4):639-644, 2007.

Cavallaro JS Jr, Tarnow D: Unsplinted implants retaining maxillary overdentures with partial palatal coverage: reports of 5 consecutive cases, *Int J Oral Maxillofac Implants* 22:808-814, 2007.

Centers for Disease Control and Prevention (CDC): *National health interview survey*, Hyattsville, Md, 1997, Government Printing Office.

Das K, Jahangiri L, Katz R: The first-choice standard of care for an edentulous mandible, *J Am Dent Assoc* 143(8):881-889, 2012.

Degidi M, Piatelli A: Comparative analysis study of 702 dental implants subjected to immediate functional loading and immediate non functional loading to traditional healing periods with a follow-up of 24 months, *Int J Oral Maxillofac Implants* 20:99-107, 2004.

D'haese J, Van De Velde T, Komiyama A, et al: Accuracy and complications using computer-designed stereolithographic surgical guides for oral rehabilitation by means of dental implants: a review of the literature, *Clin Implant Dent Relat Res* 14(3):321-335, 2010.

Dietrich T, Jimenez M, Krall Kayes EV, et al: Age-dependent associations between chronic periodontitis/edentulism and risk of coronary heart disease, *Circulation* 117(13):1668-1674, 2008.

Drago C, Carpentieri J: Treatment of maxillary jaws with dental implants: guidelines for treatment, *J Prosthod* 20:336-346, 2012.

Drago C, Howell K: Concepts for designing and fabricating metal implant frameworks for hybrid implant prostheses, *J Prosthodont* 21:413-424, 2012.

Ekfeldt A, Christiansson U, Eriksson T, et al: A retrospective analysis of factors associated with multiple implant failures in maxillae, *Clin Oral Implants Res* 12:462-467, 2001.

Feine JS, Carlsson GE, Awad MA, et al: The McGill consensus statement on overdentures, *Int J Prosthodont* 15(4):413-414, 2002.

Felton D: Edentulism and comorbid factors, *J Prosthodont* 18:88-96, 2009.

Gallucci GO, Doughtie CB, Hwang JW, et al: Five year results of fixed implant–supported rehabilitations with distal cantilevers for the edentulous mandible, *Clin Oral Implants Res* 20(6):601-607, 2009.

Jemt T: Single implants in the anterior maxilla after 15 years of follow up: comparison with central implants in the edentulous maxilla, *Int J Prosthodont* 21:400-408, 2008.

Joshipura KJ, Rim EB, Douglas CW, et al: Poor oral health and coronary heart disease, *J Dent Res* 75(9):1631-1636, 1996.

Krennmair G, Kraninhofner M, Piehslinger E: Implant-supported maxillary overdentures retained with milled bars: maxillary anterior versus maxillary posterior concept—a retrospective study, *Int J Oral Maxillofac Implants* 23:343-353, 2008.

Kronstrom M, Widbom C, Soderfeldt B: Patient evaluation after treatment with maxillary implant-supported overdentures, *Clin Implant Dent Relat Res* 8(1):39-43, 2006.

Lewis S, Sharma A, Nishimura R: Treatment of edentulous maxillae with osseointegrated implants, *J Prosthet Dent* 68:503-508, 1992.

Lin YC, Chen JH, Lee HE, et al: Self-reported oral health and denture satisfaction in partially and completely edentulous patients, *Int J Prosthodont* 24:9-15, 2011.

Malo P, Rangert B, Nobre M: All-on-4 immediate-function concept with Brånemark system implants for completely edentulous maxillae: a 1-year retrospective clinical study, *Clin Implant Dent Relat Res* 7:S88-S94, 2005.

Mericske-Stern R: Treatment outcomes with implant-supported overdentures: clinical consideration, *J Prosthet Dent* 79:66-73, 1998.

Naert I, Gizani S, Van Steenbergh D: Rigidly splinted implants in the resorbed maxilla to retain a hinging overdenture: a series of clinical reports for up to 4 years, *J Prosthet Dent* 79:156-164, 1998.

Patterson A, Komiyama A, Hultin M, et al: Accuracy of virtually planned and template guided implant surgery on edentate patients, *Clin Implant Dent Relat Res* 14(4):527-537, 2010.

Rodriguez AM, Orenstein IH, Morris HF, et al: Survival of various implant-supported prosthesis designs following 36 months of clinical function: five-year results of fixed implant-supported rehabilitations with distal cantilevers for the edentulous mandible, *Ann Periodontol* 5(10):101-108, 2000.

Romeo E, Lops D, Margutti E, et al: Long-term survival and success of oral implants in the treatment of full and partial arches: a 7 year prospective study with the ITI dental implant system, *Int J Oral Maxillofac Implants* 19:247-259, 2004.

Shimazaki Y, Soh I, Saito T, et al: Influence of dentition status on physical disability, mental impairment and mortality in institutionalized elderly people, *J Dent Res* 80:340-345, 2001.

Tallgren A: The continuing reduction of the residual alveolar ridges in complete denture wearer: a mixed longitudinal study covering 25 years, *J Prosthet Dent* 89:427-435, 2003.

Tealdo T, Bevilacqua M, Pera F, et al: Immediate function with fixed implant supported dentures: 12 month pilot study, *J Prosthet Dent* 99(5):351-360, 2008.

Thomason JM, Feine J, Exley C, et al: Mandibular two implant–supported overdentures as the first choice standard of care for edentulous patients: the York consensus statement, *Br Dent J* 207(4):185-186, 2009.

Weinstein R, Agliardi E, Fabbro M, et al: Immediate rehabilitation of extremely atrophic mandible with fixed full-prosthesis supported by four implants, *Clin Implant Dent Relat Res* 14(3):434-441, 2010.

Wham EL, Ghoul J, Chiliad J: Prosthetic requirements for immediate implant loading: a review, *J Prosthodont* (21):141-154, 2012.

World Health Organization: WHO international classification of functioning, disability and health. Available at: www.who.int/classification/icf/en/. Accessed June 20, 2012.

Zarb G, Schmidt A: Edentulous predicament. Part 1. A prospective study of the effectiveness of implant supported fixed prostheses, *J Am Dent Assoc* 127:59-72, 1996.

Computer-Assisted Implant Surgery

A. Michael Sodeifi and Shahrokh C. Bagheri

CC

A 62-year-old female is referred to an oral and maxillofacial surgeon for consultation regarding extraction of nonrestorable tooth #28 and replacement of teeth #28, #29, and #30 with dental implants (Figure 6-18).

HPI

The patient previously had a bridge extending from tooth #28 to tooth #31 to replace missing teeth. The recent failure of tooth #28 has led to the loss of her bridge. She finds it difficult to function, because she is missing most of her posterior teeth on the right side. Chewing and eating have become very difficult for her.

PMHX/PDHX/MEDICATONS/ALLERGIES/SH/FH

The patient takes 125 mcg of levothyroxine for hypothyroidism, with routine care provided by her primary care physician. She does not have any history of bruxism (lateral forces of bruxism can lead to failure of the implants).

Each patient's medical history needs to be individually considered in preparation for implant surgery. Among the most common medical variables confronted today, which may affect treatment and outcomes, include smoking, uncontrolled diabetes, use of bisphosphonates, cardiac (including valvular) disease, anticoagulation, immune-compromised patients, a history of radiation therapy to the head and neck region, or a history of severe mental disorder.

The literature is conflicting regarding the implications of smoking and placement of dental implants. However, it is well established that smoking is a major risk factor for periodontal disease. Smoking has also been associated with an increased risk for peri-implantitis. The number of cigarettes smoked per day and the patient's overall hygiene need to be taken into consideration. It is the authors' opinion that dental implants should be generally avoided in heavy smokers. Responsible consumption of alcohol is not a contraindication.

Difficult or poorly controlled diabetes is a contraindication to implant surgery. Patients with well-controlled diabetes should be considered for dental implants. Diabetes leads to serum hyperosmolarity, metabolic disorders, and vascular damage. This leads to a compromise in both the ability of the tissue to heal and the body's ability to fight infection.

EXAMINATION

The maximum incisal opening is 53 mm (important for posterior implant placement, especially when using guided surgery). The intraoral exam reveals that the right mandibular ridge is rounded and reasonably wide (more than 7 mm) in the buccal to lingual dimension. There is enough interarch vertical room to accommodate the future crown height. Thick and adequate attached gingiva is present on the ridge. There is no clinical evidence of bruxism or unusual attrition on the dentition. No other soft or hard tissue abnormalities are seen.

IMAGING

A panoramic radiograph reveals missing teeth in the lower right quadrant (see Figure 6-18). The patient is also missing the left maxillary second molar, further limiting her posterior function. The mandibular canal cannot be adequately visualized.

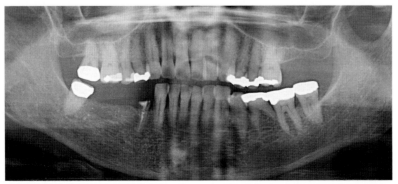

Figure 6-18 Preoperative panoramic radiograph showing nonrestorable tooth #28 and missing teeth #29, and #30.

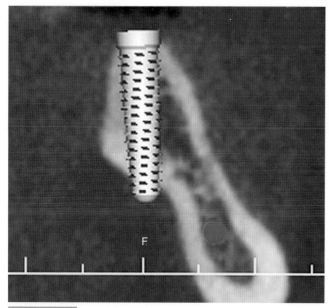

Figure 6-19 CBCT showing the implant perforating the lingual cortex.

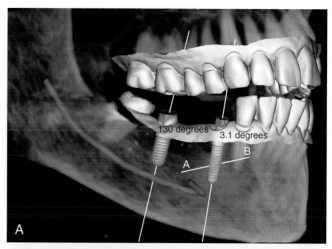

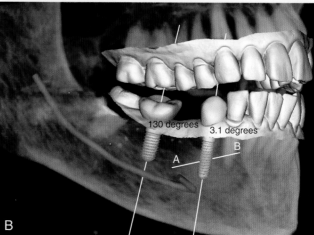

Figure 6-20 **A,** Anatomic landmarks, such as the mandibular canal, can be precisely mapped using CBCT. **B,** Prosthetically driven dental implant placement can be planned on the software when the limitations of the bone volume are recognized prior to surgery.

An important limitation of the panoramic radiograph is spatial distortions, which can vary from one type of equipment to another. This increases the risk of accidental injury to nearby vital structures. In addition, this imaging modality does not demonstrate anatomic landmarks, such as the mylohyoid ridge on the lingual aspect of the mandible. If left unrecognized, this anatomic variation may result in perforation of the lingual plate, which can lead to injury to the lingual nerve or vascular structures of the floor of the mouth (Figure 6-19).

Computed tomography (CT) or cone-bean computed tomography (CBCT) scans can help resolve many of the limitations of the two-dimensional imaging. The DICOM images provided by the CBCT can be exported to several versions of sophisticated, interactive software for implant treatment planning. Anatomic landmarks, such as the mandibular canal, can be precisely mapped (Figure 6-20, *A*). Details of soft tissue and surface dental anatomy can be obtained with an optic scan (obtained either directly with an intraoral scanner, as was used in this case, or from an optic scan of a stone model) and merged onto the CT images on the software (see Figure 6-20, *A*); this augments accuracy and the details of structures that are not effectively picked up by plain x-ray films due to distortions from existing dental restorations. Prosthetically driven dental implant placement is planned on the software, with recognition of the limitations of the bone volume prior to surgery (Figure 6-20, *B*). From this point, a precise surgical guide is generated for computer-guided implant placement (Figure 6-21).

LABS

No routine laboratory testing is required for placement of dental implants unless indicated by the medical history.

ASSESSMENT

Failed and nonrestorable tooth #28. Edentulous areas number #29 and #30. The patient desires implant restoration of the area.

TREATMENT

The risks, benefits, and alternative treatment plans were fully discussed with the patient. She choose treatment with dental implants. A CBCT scan was obtained on a well-calibrated machine (if the scanner is not calibrated correctly, incorrect dimensions on the software and inaccuracy in guided surgery can result, creating the risk of complications). Based on the CBCT scan and the location of the mental foramen, it was determined that extraction and immediate placement of the dental implant was a reasonable option for tooth #28. A presurgical work-up determined that a 4 mm × 13 mm implant for site #28 (Figure 6-22) and a 5 mm × 10 mm implant for site #30 (Figure 6-23) were appropriate. The apex of implant

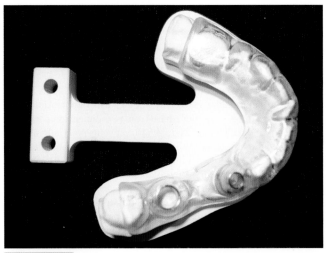

Figure 6-21 A precise surgical guide generated for computer-guided implant placement.

#30 was kept 2 mm away from the inferior alveolar nerve (IAN) to generate a safe zone (this is the minimum recommended distance to avoid injury to the inferior alveolar neurovascular bundle). It is important to recognize that many osteotomy drills have a tapered tip of approximately 0.5 mm beyond their established marked measurement lines; this can lead to osteotomy site preparations beyond the anticipated depth.

For the current patient, the dental implants were placed on the software. The abutments and crowns were digitally added to verify appropriate restorability based on the position of the implants. The restorative dentist approved the virtual prosthetic design and positioning on the implants (see Figures 6-22 and 6-23).

Subsequently, reference model intraoral scans were obtained to pick up soft tissue anatomy and the dental details that are missed with the CBCT. These are saved in an STL file format (this can also be done by taking a traditional impression of the patient and then scanning the stone models with an optic scanner).

The virtual surgical plan (in vivo) is uploaded, along with the STL files, from the intraoral scan (Itero) via the Internet to the company or laboratory that fabricated the surgical guide (see Figure 6-21).

Under intravenous anesthesia, tooth #28 was extracted with the use of periotomes to maintain the buccal plate. Because the implant site had demonstrated adequate attached gingiva at the tooth #30 site, a flapless surgery technique was performed using the surgical guide. The prescription protocol provided by the planning software was followed using the Navigator surgical kit. The implants were placed, and final stability was achieved at about 40 N/cm² of torque. A cover screw was placed on implant #28 to allow allograft bone placement in the areas void of bone. The cover screws on both implants were removed and replaced with healing abutments. Intraoperative periapical x-ray films where taken to ensure

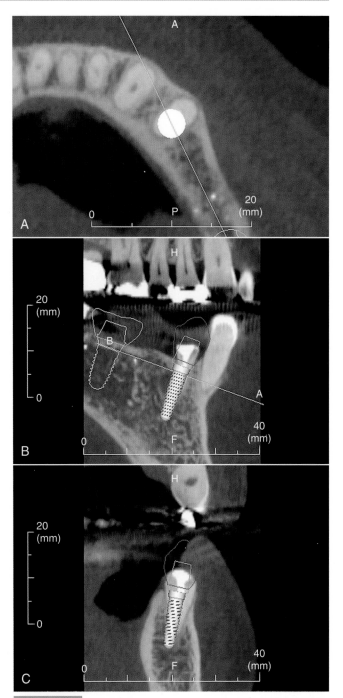

Figure 6-22 Presurgical work-up determined a 4 × 13 mm implant for site #28.

that the abutments were fully seated. The tissue around tooth #28 was closed and sealed around the healing abutment of #28 with 4-0 chromic suture. The patient did not want to wear an interim partial denture, because she could not tolerate it in her mouth. She was discharged with a prescription for amoxicillin and appropriate analgesics. A postoperative panoramic radiograph revealed satisfactory placement of the dental implants. The final restoration was delivered at 3 months. At the 6-month postoperative visit, the panoramic

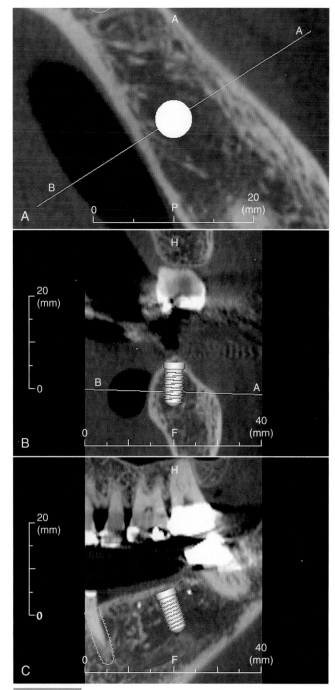

Presurgical work-up determined a 5 × 10 mm implant for site #30.

and periapical radiographs revealed stable, adequate bone (Figure 6-24, *A* and *B*) and excellent clinical esthetic and functional results (Figure 6-24, *C*).

COMPLICATONS

Complications of dental implant surgery are discussed elsewhere in this text. It is paramount to educate patients about the risks and benefits of these procedures. The risks include but are not limited to failed integration, infection at the

---

| Box 6-3 | **Benefits of Guided Surgery** |

1. It allows for minimally invasive surgery, which can result in less pain, decreased morbidity, and less soft tissue and osseous trauma.
2. It facilitates placement of implants in areas of high bone density and volume. This may allay an early impression that bone grafting is needed, based on two-dimensional radiographs and the clinical exam. It also prevents poor judgments, made on the basis of traditional two-dimensional imaging, in the placement of dental implants in areas of inadequate bone.
3. It allows the surgeon to more confidently place the implants in areas such as over the nerve, in narrow spaces between the mandibular incisors, and in the anterior maxilla, where the oblique angle of the bone can lead to unexpected perforation of labial bone in esthetically critical regions.
4. It is prosthetic driven, depending on the software, which allows optimal implant placement while considering the position of the bone.
5. It allows for predictable results with esthetics, function, and cost.
6. The three-dimensional work-up allows for better communication with patients and the referring dentist and better case acceptance.

---

implant site, nerve injury (despite the use of CBCT technology), damage to the roots of adjacent teeth, and complications related to the maxillary sinus.

The success of dental implants depends on patient selection, the surgeon's skill, the quality and quantity of bone, and host factors (e.g., oral hygiene, smoking, patient health, compliance); however, complications may occur even with correct surgical technique and meticulous surgical and medical preparation of the patient. The overall success rate for dental implants is considered to be greater than 90%. The failure rate further decreases when implants are placed and restored by experienced providers or specialists and other factors are optimized (e.g., bone volume).

Some inherent factors can lead to complications with guided surgery. An understanding of the possible pitfalls can minimize the additive effect of these factors that can lead to an undesirable outcome. These pitfalls include errors arising from the CT scanner due to lack of calibration, incorrect mapping of vital structures or treatment planning on the software by the surgeon, an unstable surgical guide during surgery, technical errors by the lab, surgeon error during surgery, inadequate interocclusal space for implant placement, and heat generation due to difficulty delivering irrigation through the guide. Despite these factors, this technology, when used with careful planning, has proven to have substantial benefits in the treatment of simple to complex cases, leading both to improved outcomes and a reduction in risks (Boxes 6-3 and 6-4; Figure 6-25).

DISCUSSION

CT and CBCT provide DICOM images that can be imported into several versions of sophisticated, interactive software.

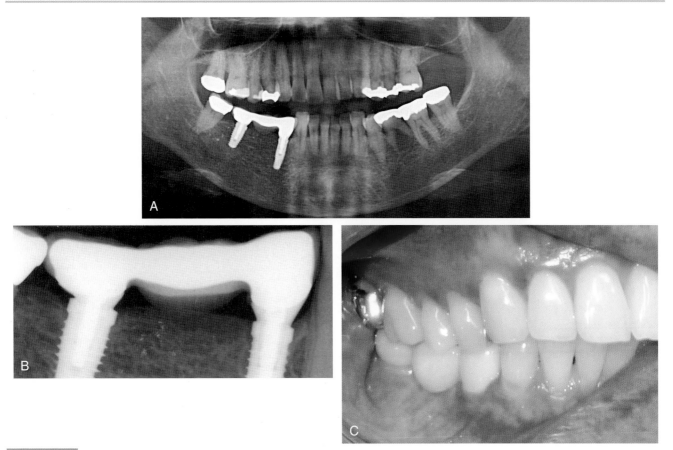

Figure 6-24   A 6-month postoperative panoramic radiograph (**A**) and periapical radiograph (**B**) show stable, adequate bone. **C,** A 6-month postoperative clinical photograph shows excellent esthetic and functional results.

Box 6-4   Benefits of Combining Guided Surgery with Use of the Intraoral Scanner

1. In many cases only digital impressions are taken for planning of guided surgery; this avoids the use of traditional impressions, which are less favorable to the patient.
2. There is no need to take a CBCT scan of the stone models, because the software can merge the intraoral scanner and CBCT images.
3. There is no need to send the patient through the CBCT scanner or x-ray machine again with a splint in the mouth.
4. In many cases, all the data needed for treatment planning and guided surgery can be collected in only one visit that involves a CBCT and intraoral scan impression.
5. The digital scanner can provide more accurate reference models than can traditional impressions.

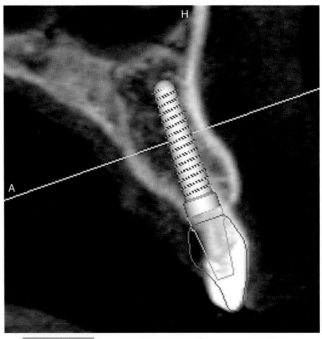

Figure 6-25   Correct placement of implant using CBCT.

Virtual planning of implant treatment and surgery can be performed on the software. Interactive three-dimensional visualization allows many different cross sections (e.g., axial, coronal, and sagittal views) to be considered simultaneously when placing the dental implants in ideal bone. Compared with traditional medical CT scanning, CBCT uses less than 2% of the radiation dose.

Bibliography

Block M, Chandler C: Computed tomography–guided surgery: complications associated with scanning, processing, surgery, and prosthetics, *J Oral Maxillofac Surg* 67(Suppl 3):13-22, 2009.

Heitz-Mayfield LJ: Peri-implant disease: diagnosis and risk indicators, *J Clin Periodontol* 35:292-304, 2008.

Lindquist LW, Ekelund JA, Carlsson GE, et al: A prospective 15-year follow-up study of mandibular fixed prostheses supported by osseointegrated implants: clinical results and marginal bone loss, *Clin Oral Implants Res* 7:329-336, 1996.

Ludlow JB: Regarding "Influence of CBCT exposure conditions on radiation dose," *Oral Surg Oral Med Oral Pathol Oral Radiol Endod* 106(5):627-628; author reply, 628-629; 2008.

McCoy G: Recognizing and managing parafunction in the reconstruction and maintenance of the oral implant patient, *Implant Dent* 11(1):19-27, 2002.

Pankaj S, Cranin N: *Atlas of oral implantology*, St Louis, 2010, Mosby.

Stefan R, Giovannoli J: *Peri-implantitis*, Paris, 2012, Quintessence.

Strietzel FP, Reichart PA, Kale A, et al: Smoking interferes with prognosis of dental implant treatment: a systematic review and meta-analysis, *J Clin Periodontol* 34:523-544, 2007.

Viegas VN, Dutra V, Pagnoncelli RM, et al: Transference of virtual planning and planning over biomedical prototypes for dental implant placement using guided surgery, *Clin Oral Implants Res* 21(3):290-295, 2010.

Extraction Socket Preservation for Implant Placement

A. Michael Sodeifi and Shahrokh C. Bagheri

CC

A 37-year-old female is referred by her general dentist for consultation to have tooth #19 extracted. She is interested in a dental implant.

HPI

Tooth #19 had had previous endodontic therapy. Recently the patient started to have pain while chewing. Endodontic evaluation found a poor prognosis due to root fracture. She denies any swelling or other symptoms.

PMH/PDH/MEDICATIONS/ALLERGIES/SH/FS

The medical history is not contributory. The patient has had routine dental care by her general dentist.

EXAMINATION

Examination of the TMJ is within normal limits (good range of motion is important in placement of posterior dental implants). There are no extraoral or intraoral soft tissue lesions, swelling, or masses. Tooth #19 is missing the crown and has a temporary restoration (Figure 6-26).

IMAGING

On the panoramic radiograph, a periapical radiolucency can be seen associated with mesial and distal roots of the endodontically treated tooth #19. The radiolucency appears to be a few millimeters away from the inferior alveolar nerve (Figure 6-27).

ASSESSMENT

Failed root canal therapy and nonrestorable tooth #19 with a periapical abscess

The patient is interested in a dental implant. The clinical and radiographic findings are fully explained to the patient. The risks, benefits, and alternative treatment considerations are discussed. Alternative options include extracting the tooth

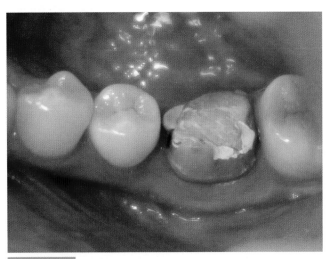

Figure 6-26 Preoperative photo showing the missing crown and defective temporary restoration on tooth #19.

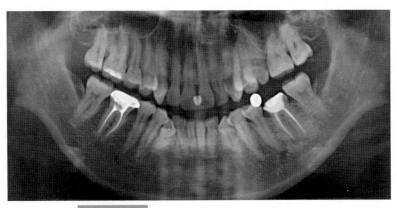

Figure 6-27 Preoperative panoramic radiograph.

without replacement or receiving a bridge or a partial denture. The plan for extraction, site preservation (with human allograft), and delayed implant placement is presented and accepted by the patient.

TREATMENT

Under intravenous sedation anesthesia, a sulcular incision is made and a buccal mucoperiosteal flap is elevated (Figure 6-28, *A*) to visualize and protect the buccal cortical plate. Vignoletti and colleagues report better outcomes when the flap is elevated for socket preservation than with a flapless technique.

A 1702 burr is used under loop magnification, and the tooth structure is removed from the buccal aspects of the roots under copious saline irrigation (to prevent overheating of the bone, which can lead to further bone loss). In essence, instead of a buccal trough alveolectomy, a buccal odontotomy is performed to keep the buccal cortical bone fully intact. The crown and the roots are sectioned from buccal to lingual (Figure 6-28, *B*).

Next, a periotome (Figure 6-28, *C*) is used on the mesial and distal of each root to loosen the segment (Figure 6-28, *D*). The roots are completely removed (Figure 6-28, *E*), and the granulation tissue in the apex is fully cleaned with a curette. Throughout the process care was taken not to damage the cortical buccal plate. The extraction site is irrigated with chlorhexidine. A round burr is used to decorticate the inside of the socket to induce bleeding. This leads to better early vascularization and release of osteoprogenitor cells.

A demineralized freeze-dried bone allograft (DFDBA) cortical allograft was prepared in advance by adding a small amount of amoxicillin powder and hydrating it with mixture of saline and the patient's blood, which was drawn from the IV site (this can also be harvested from a clean extraction site). This was done before the extraction to allow enough time for the allograft to hydrate (Figure 6-28, *F*).

The bone is grafted in the extraction socket (Figure 6-28, *G*). A 5-mm subperiosteal pocket was made on the buccal and lingual to allow the membrane to be tucked underneath the flaps. Studies have demonstrated a statistically significant difference in favor of use of membrane (Lekovic and colleagues). In the current case, a nonresorbable, high-density polytetrafluoroethylene (d-PTFE) membrane is chosen and used to cover the graft. d-PTFE membrane does not need primary closer over it; this minimizes displacement of the keratinized tissue, which is beneficial for keeping better-attached gingiva around the future implant. d-PTFE has extensive cardiovascular applications in heart valves and vascular grafts. It does not induce secondary inflammation. The flaps are sutured closed (Figure 6-28, *H*).

After recovery the patient was discharged to her husband. She was provided detailed instructions and prescribed amoxicillin (500 mg) three times per day for one week. The d-PTFE membrane will be removed in 3 weeks, and the site should be ready for placement of the dental implant in 4 months.

COMPLICATIONS

The main complication of socket grafting is infection (which also causes loss of graft). Fortunately, infections are rare (appearing in fewer than 5% of cases); however, when they occur, removal of the graft material typically is required. Optimizing the patient's oral hygiene and appropriate use of postoperative antibiotics may help decrease the incidence of infection. Most often, teeth removed during the extraction are very compromised and endodontically treated. Therefore, it is common for the roots to break into small segments. Remnants of roots accidentally left in place can lead to delayed infection or can compromise the future implant.

Periotomes can be driven into adjacent vital structure, such as the inferior alveolar nerve or sinus cavity, or can damage the adjacent teeth. It is essential that the periotomes be navigated with the utmost care and control. Copious irrigation is mandatory during the odontotomy to minimize heat generation. Excessive heat can damage the buccal plate and lead to unfavorable bone resorption.

Tension-free closure of the flap and appropriate use of membrane can reduce the incidence of flap retraction or dehiscence and subsequent loss of grafted bone granules. Wound healing can be compromised secondary to pressure applied by a removable partial denture. All attempts should be made to minimize pressure on the grafted site from a removable prostheses. Patients need to be taught to modify their diet to avoid function on the surgical site for 4 weeks and to undertake appropriate hygiene measures.

DISCUSSION

Preservation of hard and soft tissue at the time of extraction is essential in achieving better esthetic and long-term results for dental implants. After removal of a tooth, three-dimensional resorption of the alveolar ridge is expected. Most of the resorption takes place in the first 3 months; however, changes are seen up to 1 year after surgery, resulting in approximately 50% reduction in the buccolingual dimensions of the alveolar ridge, according to Schropp and colleagues.

The potential benefits of the different materials and techniques used for socket preservation are still debatable, and very few well-designed studies address these issues. No scientific guidelines have been established with regard to biomaterials or surgical techniques to date. It is the authors' opinion that the technique used at the time of extraction to keep the buccal bone intact is the most important step taken, when possible. Araujo and Lindhe also report that resorption of the buccal bone plate is a main cause of the bone loss. The approach used to remove the tooth and preserve the site substantially affects the quality of the bone and soft tissue at the time of implant placement. The rationale behind extraction site preservation with bone grafting is to provide a stable environment for osteoconduction to take its natural course. Allograft used in this case is just a scaffold, which still requires the natural turnover of bone as the adjacent osteocytes migrate from the native tissue to lay new vital bone

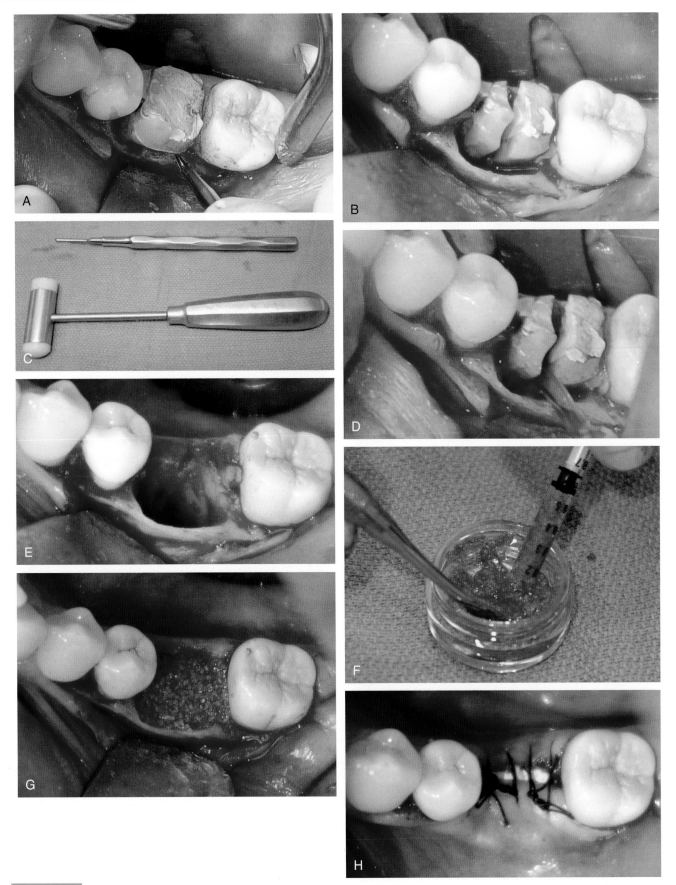

Figure 6-28 **A,** Sulcular incision and an elevated buccal mucoperiosteal flap. **B,** Crown and the roots are sectioned from buccal to lingual. **C,** Periotome and mallet. **D,** Periotome used on the mesial and distal of each root to loosen the segment. **E,** Roots are completely removed. **F,** Demineralized freeze-dried bone allograft (DFDBA) cortical allograft is prepared in advance. **G,** Bone is grafted in the extraction socket. **H,** Flaps are sutured closed.

within the graft and ultimately replace it. This cannot effectively take place without having healthy and vital neighboring bone. The ultimate goal is preservation of the soft tissue volume and architecture at the site by having a stable bony foundation to support it.

A systematic review by Vignoletti and colleagues reports that the changes in the horizontal dimension have benefited the most by the socket preservation techniques evaluated. They found the bone loss in the horizontal dimension to be the most important consequence during the first 3 to 6 months of healing after tooth extraction; this loss ranged from −0.16 to −4.50 mm. The results of their meta–regression analysis of nine studies concluded that some degree of bone modeling and remodeling occurs after tooth extraction; however, different ridge preservation procedures resulted in significantly less vertical and horizontal alveolar bone contraction. This review could not make a recommendation for the type of biomaterial or surgical procedure used, but the use of barrier membranes and flap (rather than flapless) surgical procedures demonstrated better results. In conclusion, these researchers found a difference (D) of −1.47 mm in height and −1.83 mm in width, with more significant bone loss seen in the control group without bone grafting.

There is no one graft material that can be recommended over others for every case. An understanding of the physical and biologic properties of the graft material and individualization of treatment planning are necessary in choosing the most appropriate material in each case.

Graft Material Classification

Autograft

Autograft refers to viable cortical or cancellous bone grafting when the source of the graft is the patient. This is the "gold standard," and it has osteoconductive, osteoinductive, and osteogenesis benefits. However, a second surgical site usually is required to obtain the bone, and this can lead to increases in morbidity, recovery time for the patient, and cost. At times it is possible to simply harvest bone from adjacent bony tissue without a significant increase in morbidity.

Allograft

Allograft refers to bone graft from cadavers in the same species. These are available from licensed tissue banks. The cadavers are screened for malignancy, HBV, HCV, HIV and lifestyle factors, which may place the donor at a higher risk category for transmittable diseases. The bone is obtained in an aseptic setting in the operating room. Patients should be advised of the remote possibility of disease transmission despite the lack of any documented cases. The patient's religious preference also needs to be considered. The graft material is available in the demineralized freeze-dried form, mineralized freeze-fried form, or a mixture of the two forms. It can also be selected in cortical or cancellous forms. These

differ in the time it takes for the grafted bone to remodel and be replaced by the patient's own vital bone. In general, demineralized bone is remodeled faster, and mineralized cortical bone takes longest to turn over. Therefore, the surgeon's understanding of these properties is important in choosing the right graft for a particular case.

Alloplast

Alloplast refers to synthetic biomaterials that function as scaffolding for osteoconduction and volume expanders. Examples of alloplast include hydroxylapatite, calcium phosphate, calcium sulfate, and bioactive glass.

Xenograft

Xenograft represents naturally derived hydroxylapatite from a cattle source. Even though there are no reported cases of transmittable disease from a bovine source, some have expressed concern about the possible risk of transmission of bovine spongiform encephalopathy. However, this risk is thought to be extremely low. Just as does the allograft, the xenograft provides scaffolding for osteoconduction.

Bibliography

Araujo M, Linder E, Wennstrom J, et al: The influence of Bio-Oss collagen on healing of an extraction socket: an experimental study in the dog, *Int J Periodontics Restorative Dent* 28:123-135, 2008.

Araujo MG, Lindhe J: Dimensional ridge alterations following tooth extraction: an experimental study in the dog, *J Clin Periodontol* 32:212-218, 2005.

Araujo MG, Lindhe J: Ridge alterations following tooth extraction with and without flap elevation: an experimental study in the dog, *Clin Oral Implants Res* 20:545-549, 2009.

Araujo MG, Lindhe J: Socket grafting with the use of autologous bone: an experimental study in the dog, *Clin Oral Implants Res* 22:9-13, 2011.

Bartee B: *Implant site development and extraction site grafting. Osteogenics clinical education*, Osteogenics Biomedical, Inc. 2011.

Bartee BK, Carr JA: Evaluation of a high-density polytetrafluoroethylene (nPTFE) membrane as a barrier material to facilitate guided bone regeneration in the rat mandible, *J Oral Implantol* 21:88-95, 1995.

Bartee BK: The use of high density polytetrafluoroethylene to treat osseous defects: clinical reports, *Implant Dent* 4:21-26, 1995.

Lekovic V, Camargo PM, Klokkevold PR, et al: Preservation of alveolar bone in extraction sockets using bioabsorbable membranes, *J Periodontol* 69:1044-1049, 1998.

Lekovic V, Kenney EB, Weinlaender M, et al: A bone regenerative approach to alveolar ridge maintenance following tooth extraction: report of 10 cases, *J Periodontol* 68:563-570, 1997.

Schropp L, Wenzel A, Kostopoulos L, et al: Bone healing and soft tissue contour changes following single-tooth extraction: a clinical and radiographic 12-month prospective study, *Int J Periodontics Restorative Dent* 23:313-323, 2003.

Sclar A: *Soft tissue and esthetic considerations in implant therapy*, Hanover Park, Ill., 2003, Quintessence.

Implants in the Esthetic Zone

Edward R. Schlissel

CC

A 42-year-old woman presents to the dental office complaining of a fractured maxillary incisor. She states that she suffered the injury in an automobile accident 2 days earlier and that she is not in pain.

Fracture of an anterior tooth in an otherwise intact dentition is a traumatic event for any person. In addition to acute pain and the possibility of infection, there are always concerns about cosmetic replacement and problems in the future. Immediate replacement with a provisional restoration and the fabrication of a final restoration that has an excellent long-term prognosis should be the goals of the dentist.

HPI

The maxillary left central incisor was fractured during an automobile accident. The patient was a passenger in the vehicle. She was drinking from a travel mug when the impact occurred. The tooth had endodontic treatment 3 years before the accident and was restored with a ceramic crown. No endodontic post had been placed.

PMHX/PDHX/MEDICATIONS/ALLERGIES/SH/FH

The patient has an unremarkable medical history. She has no known allergies and takes no medications that would have an impact on her dental treatment. She has had regular dental care and has several restorations in the area of the injury, including full crowns and porcelain veneers.

It is imperative to obtain a complete medical history when evaluating alternative treatment options for the replacement of a tooth. Systemic medications, including bisphosphonates and antineoplastic agents, and medical conditions such as uncontrolled diabetes are known to have deleterious effects on wound healing and bone metabolism and may be contraindications to implant placement.

EXAMINATION

The left maxillary central incisor was fractured at the level of the alveolar crest of bone and was out of the mouth (Figure 6-29). The patient had no pain and had not taken any analgesic medications. She was upset about her injury and the prospects for replacement of the fractured tooth. There was no radiographic evidence of injury to adjacent teeth or bone. Intraoral and extraoral examination revealed no other injuries in either

arch. There was no injury to the lips or other soft tissue. The anterior teeth were normal in appearance and showed neither discomfort on percussion nor abnormal mobility. Periodontal pocket depths were 3 mm or less, and there was no bleeding on probing. Oral health care was excellent. When making a full smile, the patient displayed the cervical lines of the maxillary incisors.

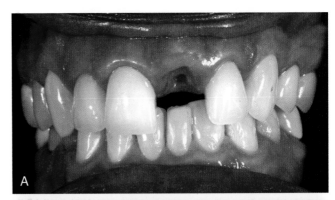

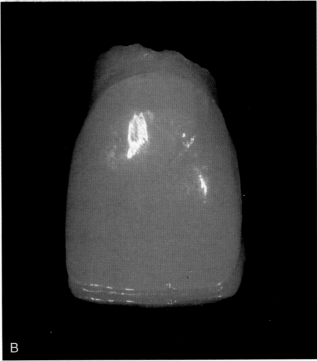

Figure 6-29 **A,** Intraoral, retracted view of the fractured incisor. **B,** Fractured incisor, out of the mouth.

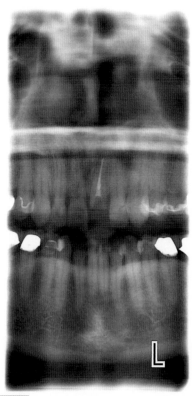

Figure 6-30   Periapical radiograph of fractured incisor.

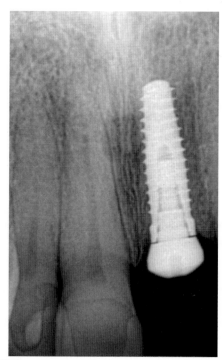

Figure 6-31   Radiograph of implant and healing abutment at time of placement.

When a patient suffers trauma to an anterior tooth, there is often injury to adjacent tissues or in the opposite arch. A complete examination is necessary to determine whether there is damage to the teeth, bone, or soft tissue. Follow-up evaluations should be conducted to detect undisclosed damage to other teeth or bone. Fractures that are not displaced may not be evident on clinical or radiographic examination. The patient should be advised that additional problems might become evident in the future and that more treatment may be needed.

IMAGING

Panoramic and periapical (intraoral) radiographs (Figure 6-30) were made and evaluated. There was no evidence of injury to the adjacent teeth or bone.

Consideration should be given to the use of cone-beam computed tomography (CBCT) to assess for damage to bony structures in the area of an injury. If there is evidence of soft tissue damage, the field of interest should be adequate to include all areas of concern. If this patient had suffered injury to the maxillary incisor as a result of impact to the mandible, it would have been appropriate to use additional imaging to evaluate the mandible, including the body, ramus, and condyle on both sides of the mouth.

LABS

No laboratory tests were indicated in the treatment of the current patient. If the patient had been on injectable or long-term oral bisphosphonate therapy, a serum C-terminal telopeptide (CTx) test may have been appropriate. If the patient had been diabetic, the appropriate test to measure blood glucose levels would be in order.

TREATMENT

Irreversible hydrocolloid (alginate) impressions were made of the upper and lower arches, and a shade was selected for a provisional prosthetic replacement. The patient was referred to an oral and maxillofacial surgeon for removal of the remainder of the fractured tooth and evaluation of the buccal plate of the alveolar bone, with a request that an endosseous dental implant be placed at the time of extraction. The surgical appointment was the next day. At that visit the surgeon used minimally invasive techniques to remove the root fragment. It was determined that the alveolar bone was intact and that there was sufficient bone volume for immediate placement of the implant. A tapered titanium implant (4 mm in diameter, 13 mm long) was placed in the osteotomy site. Insertion torque was 50 Ncm, and no bone graft was necessary. A healing abutment was selected and placed. It had an emergence profile of 5 mm and was 2 mm high. The superior surface of the healing abutment was just below the level of the crest of the ridge. Before placement of the healing abutment an index of the implant position was made with polyvinyl siloxane material and an open-tray impression transfer assembly. A periapical radiograph was made to verify the seating of the healing abutment (Figure 6-31). The provisional restoration made for the patient was an Essix-type retainer. There was no load on the implant at the time of surgery. The

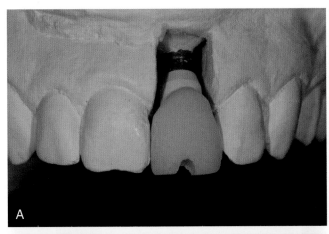

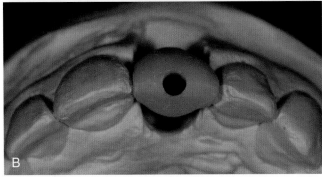

Figure 6-32 Facial view (**A**) and incisal view (**B**) of provisional restoration on the model.

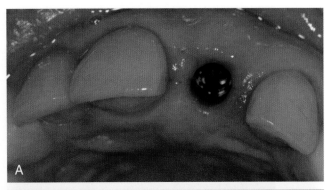

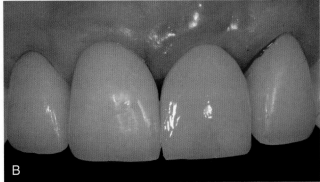

Figure 6-33 **A,** Implant platform exposed. **B,** Provisional restoration at placement.

surgical index was placed on a modified study model, and a screw-retained provisional restoration was made but was not placed on the implant at the time of surgery (Figure 6-32).

The patient was monitored for 4 months after surgery. No additional injuries were detected, and the implant was deemed ready for restoration. A small amount of gingival tissue was removed with a tissue punch, and the healing abutment was removed (Figure 6-33, *A*). The provisional restoration, which had been made during the healing phase, was tried in and adjusted. The contours of the provisional were modified until the emergence profile gave the correct tissue support and the interproximal contact areas had correct pressure and were located less than 5 mm from the levels of bone on the adjacent teeth (Figure 6-33, *B*). The height of the papilla on the mesial side of the provisional restoration was noted to be inadequate at the time of placement. The access cavity of the provisional restoration was closed, and a bruxism splint was delivered.

The patient returned periodically over the next 3 months. It was noted that the papilla on the mesial aspect filled the space below the contact area. A custom impression coping was fabricated (Figure 6-34, *A* and *B*) and an impression made of the maxillary arch. The color was selected for the final restoration. Using CAD/CAM technology, the laboratory made a custom zirconia abutment (Figure 6-34, *C*). The margins of the crown preparation were located 0.5 mm below the free gingival margin. A prosthetic crown was made of lithium silicate in the color specified. The abutment and crown

were tried in the mouth; seating and adaptation were verified with a radiograph (Figure 6-34, *D*). Occlusal and interproximal contacts were evaluated and adjusted. Impressions were made for a bruxism splint, which was delivered the next day. Follow-up examinations were conducted, and photographs were taken 4 months after placement of the crown and abutment (Figure 6-35). The patient was satisfied with the outcome.

COMPLICATIONS

There are many complications that can be associated with implants in the esthetic zone. They include implant location and angulation, soft tissue defects, and the consequences of not removing excess cement. Improper placement of the implant or poorly designed abutments or crowns may lead to results that are not esthetically acceptable. Proper surgical and restorative techniques and good communication between the surgeon and restorative dentist are essential to a good outcome.

DISCUSSION

Several alternatives were possible for the treatment of this patient's problem. These included options for the type of restoration and the timing of the steps in the implant reconstruction. Instead of an implant-supported individual crown, the missing tooth could have been replaced with a fixed partial denture (FPD) or an individual restoration after crown lengthening surgery. However, crown lengthening surgery would have resulted in an unfavorable crown-to-tooth ratio,

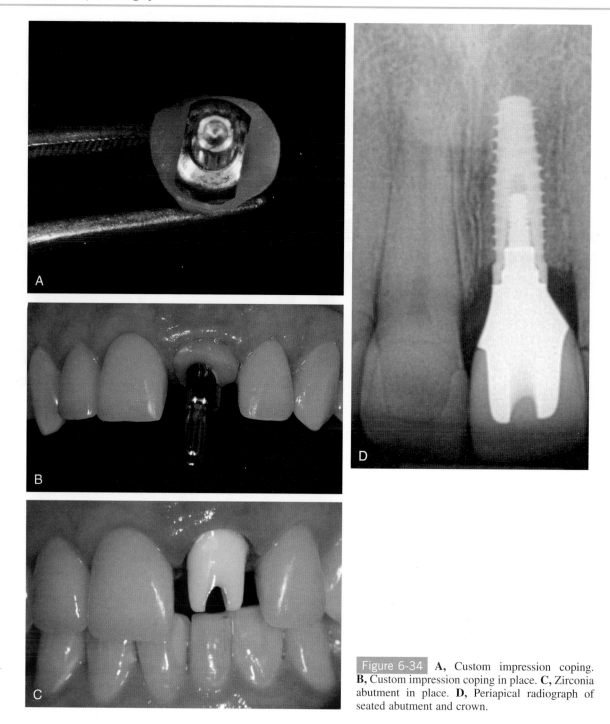

Figure 6-34 **A,** Custom impression coping. **B,** Custom impression coping in place. **C,** Zirconia abutment in place. **D,** Periapical radiograph of seated abutment and crown.

unacceptable esthetics, and a poor prognosis. Considering the age of the patient and the predicted lifetime of an FPD, it was thought that an implant restoration offered the better choice. If the alveolar plate had been fractured or deficient, implant placement would have been delayed. If there had been a gap between the implant and the surrounding bone, graft material would have been placed. Because circumstances were favorable, the implant was placed immediately after extraction of the root. This procedure is associated with retention of the buccal plate of bone, which leads to good esthetic results.

The patient had a Class I occlusion, with approximately 50% overbite and no overjet. This precluded placement of a provisional restoration at the time of surgery, because it would have been impossible to avoid contacts in centric occlusion or protrusive movement, which are mandatory conditions for immediate provisionalization of individual teeth. The provisional restoration is essential for developing tissue contours. It is more efficient to make the provisional restoration during the healing period than at a patient appointment.

Using a custom impression post allows capture of the properly developed soft tissue profile, which is essential for the

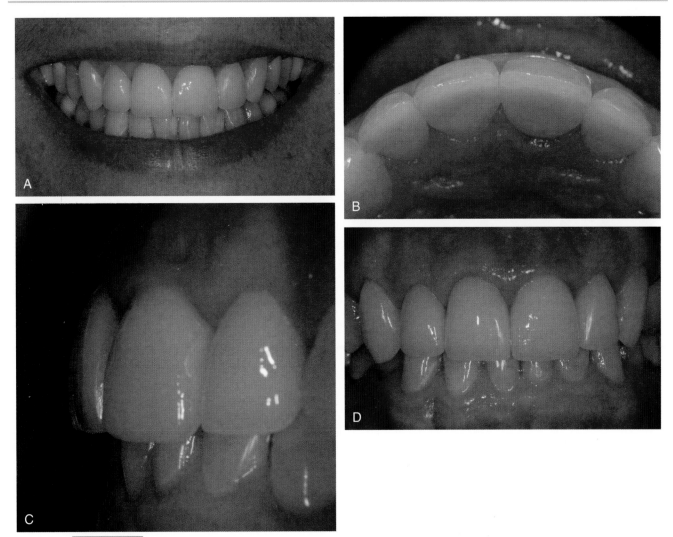

Figure 6-35 Final restoration. **A,** View of the high smile. **B,** Incisal view. **C,** Lateral view. **D,** Retracted view.

fabrication of the custom abutment. The zirconia abutment does not darken the appearance of the gingiva below the crown margins. The margins of the crown were located just below the free gingival margin to facilitate removal of cement. The interproximal contacts were located in accordance with well-established guidelines, and the tissue responded as expected. The restorative material was selected for its translucency and strength.

For clinicians, following well-established clinical procedures leads to predictable results. Also, a thorough understanding of the biologic and technical aspects of implant dentistry can lead to patient satisfaction and long-term success.

Bibliography

Al-Sabbagh M: Implants in the esthetic zone, *Dent Clin North Am* 50(3):391-407, 2006.

Potashnick SR: Soft tissue modeling for the esthetic single-tooth implant restoration, *J Esthet Dent* 10(3):121-131, 1998.

Saadoun AAP, LeGall M, Touati B: Selection and ideal tridimensional implant position for soft tissue aesthetics, *Pract Periodontics Aesth Dent* 11(9):103-172, 1999.

Tarnow DP, Magner AW, Fletcher P: The effect of the distance from the contact point to the crest of bone on the presence or absence of the interproximal dental papilla, *J Periodontol* 63:995-996, 1992.

CHAPTER 7

Head and Neck Pathology

This chapter addresses:
- Pleomorphic Adenoma
- Mucocele and Fibroma
- Acute Herpetic Gingivostomatitis
- Aphthous Ulcers
- Sialolithiasis
- Acute Suppurative Parotitis
- Differential Diagnosis of a Neck Mass
- Oral Leukoplakia
- Osteoradionecrosis

Pathologic disease of the head and neck encompasses a wide spectrum of disorders with associated maxillofacial or systemic involvement. The increasing number of disorders and surgical treatments further challenge our profession, often demanding additional training and continuing education courses.

Several categories of disorders can be identified, which can frequently assist in formulation of a differential diagnosis:

1. Infectious (e.g., bacterial, viral, fungal infections)
2. Traumatic etiology (e.g., irritation fibroma)
3. Neoplastic: epithelial, connective tissue, glandular, lymphatic, osseous, muscle, and vascular tumors, which can be characterized as benign or malignant. Metastatic disease to the head and neck, by definition, is malignant.
4. Immunologically mediated disorders (e.g., rheumatoid arthritis)
5. Side effects of other medical or surgical therapy (e.g., osteoradionecrosis)
6. Cysts of the head and neck (inflammatory and noninflammatory cysts)
7. Pathologic processes related to the regional anatomy (e.g., sialolithiasis)
8. Congenital malformations (cleft lip and palate)
9. Degenerative disorders (osteoarthritis)
10. Iatrogenic (e.g., intraoperative damage to a cranial nerve)
11. Idiopathic (e.g., aphthous ulcers)
12. Vasculitis (e.g., temporal arteritis)

Several of these categories are addressed elsewhere in this book. This chapter illustrates eight teaching cases, representing disorders of infectious, traumatic, neoplastic, anatomic, and idiopathic etiology, that are common in the oral and maxillofacial region. A teaching case discussing the differential diagnosis of a neck mass also is provided. The case that discusses osteoradionecrosis outlines the current controversies and management issues arising from this complex complication of head and neck irradiation. Drug-induced osteonecrosis of the jaws (DIONJ) was discussed in Chapter 2.

Pleomorphic Adenoma

Ketan Patel and Deepak Kademani

CC

A 53-year-old woman (pleomorphic adenoma is most common in the fourth to sixth decades of life, with a slight female predilection), who is a schoolteacher, is referred for evaluation of a mass inferior to her right ear.

HPI

Over the past 8 months, the patient had noticed a progressively enlarging mass anterior and inferior to her right ear. (Pleomorphic adenoma is the most commonly occurring benign tumor of the major salivary glands. It typically grows slowly, at a rate of less than 5 mm per year). The patient explained that the mass has slowly enlarged, prompting her to bring it to her dentist's attention. There is no associated pain, paresthesias, or motor deficits (motor and sensory nerve deficits are not commonly seen with benign salivary neoplasms). She denies any constitutional symptoms, including fever, chills, night sweats, appetite changes, and weight loss (systemic symptoms associated with inflammatory or malignant processes).

PMHX/PSHX/MEDICATIONS/ALLERGIES/SH/FH

The patient sees her dentist yearly for routine maintenance. She drinks alcohol on social occasions and has never smoked. (Tobacco use and alcohol consumption are not known to be risk factors for the development of pleomorphic adenomas. A potential risk factor is exposure to certain chemicals and dyes, but this association is very weak.)

There is no previous history of head and neck cancer or facial cosmetic surgery (it is important to be aware of previous surgeries in the area of the pathology). The patient has completed all her childhood immunizations, including the mumps vaccine as part of the MMR vaccine (therefore mumps are less likely to be the cause of the parotid swelling).

EXAMINATION

General. The patient is a well-developed and well-nourished, 53-year-old woman in no apparent distress.

Vital signs. Blood pressure is 135/90 mm Hg, heart rate 80 bpm, respirations 16 per minute, and temperature 36.9°C.

Maxillofacial. Examination of the eyes and ears is unremarkable. The tympanic membranes are clear bilaterally. Cranial nerves II to XII are intact, with no weakness of the muscles of mastication (V). There is no sensory deficit in the V1-V3 distributions. Facial mimetic muscles are intact and symmetrical (involvement of the facial or trigeminal nerve would be suggestive of a malignant process).

There is a visible swelling in the right subauricular area that distorts the facial contour (Figure 7-1). Palpation reveals a well-circumscribed, freely moveable, firm, rubbery, 1- to 1.5-cm, nontender mass above the angle of the mandible. (Benign processes are typically slow growing and push, rather than infiltrate, local structures, such as the overlying skin; adjacent structures, such as blood vessels and nerves, are usually not involved). There is no warmth, erythema, ulceration, or induration of the overlying soft tissue (signs of an inflammatory or a malignant process).

Intraoral. The parotid papillae appear noninflamed bilaterally, with expression of clear saliva from Stensen's duct (purulent drainage from the duct would be indicative of suppurative parotitis). No mucosal ulcerations are present, and there is no intraoral extension of the mass (consistent with a benign process).

Neck. No palpable submandibular or cervical lymphadenopathy (palpable lymph nodes would be indicative of a malignant neoplastic process).

IMAGING

Several imaging modalities may be used for the evaluation of a parotid mass, including ultrasound, computed tomography (CT), magnetic resonance imaging (MRI), and sialography. The most commonly used initial studies of choice are CT and MRI.

Histologic confirmation is ideally performed preoperatively by means of fine-needle aspiration (FNA). This is best performed by an experienced cytopathologist and can provide diagnostic information guiding definitive treatment. FNA can have a high false-negative rate; therefore, ultrasonographic or CT guidance can be used to recheck when results are inconclusive. Should the FNA results continue to be inconclusive, the clinician should proceed with definitive surgical resection of the tumor with facial nerve preservation, if possible. It is not necessary to perform an open biopsy of the parotid gland, because 80% of parotid masses are benign; therefore, a parotidectomy is appropriate as a diagnostic and treatment modality. Patients should be prepared preoperatively for the possibility of facial nerve deficit. If the integrity of the nerve is maintained during the procedure, facial nerve function returns.

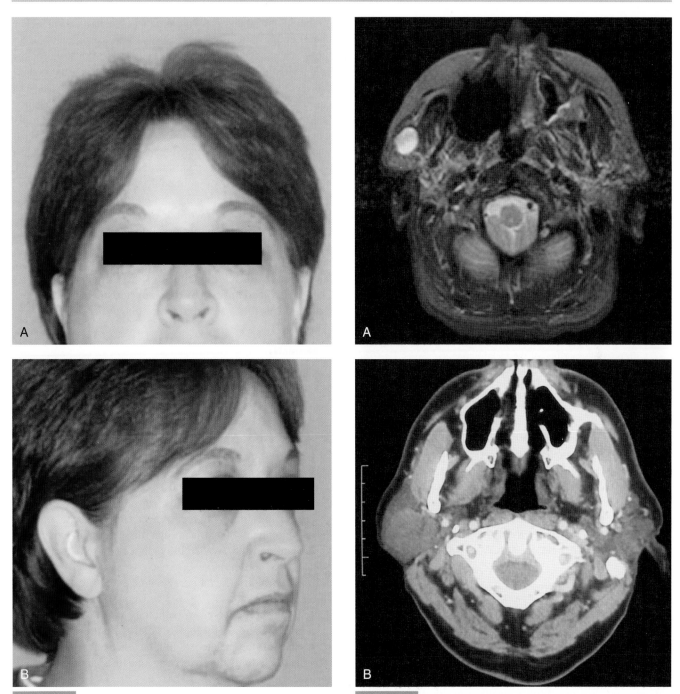

Figure 7-1 Frontal (**A**) and side (**B**) views showing the swelling over the right ear.

Figure 7-2 MRI (**A**) and CT (**B**) scans showing a pleomorphic adenoma of the right parotid in the T2 window.

Sialography can be used to identify sialoliths and ductal obstruction and to differentiate parenchymal from nodal disease. A CT scan can also help differentiate nodal from parenchymal disease and is particularly useful in assessing larger lesions with atypical ultrasonic features. However, it is not as reliable as sialography for identification of ductal pathology. MRI offers excellent visualization of the glandular pathology and tumors. It is often the imaging modality of choice. Neither CT nor MRI can reliably outline the surgical anatomy of the mass relative to cranial nerve VII.

A panoramic radiograph can be used as a surveillance imaging tool to exclude the presence of intraductal or glandular calcifications; however, it is not particularly useful in the evaluation of parotid gland lesions.

For the current patient, a panoramic radiograph confirmed no observable pathology. An MRI scan demonstrated a well-circumscribed mass within the substance of the parotid gland, measuring 1.5 cm in diameter, with no homogeneous enhancement (Figure 7-2). There was no evidence of enlarged intraparotid lymph nodes.

<table>
<tr><td>Box 7-1</td><td>**Differential Diagnosis of a Slow-Growing Parotid Mass**</td></tr>
</table>

- **Pleomorphic adenoma** (most likely diagnosis, given the presentation). This is the most common tumor of the major salivary glands, with 75% occurring in the tail of the parotid.
- **Warthin's tumor (papillary cystadenoma lymphadenosum).** This is also a benign, slow-growing tumor, typically seen in the elderly male population older than 50 years. About 10% of these tumors can present bilaterally at the time of diagnosis.
- **Monomorphic adenoma.** This is a benign tumor affecting the major or minor salivary glands, accounting for 6% of all benign salivary tumors. There are two histologic variants: canalicular adenoma, which predominantly affects the minor salivary glands of the lips, and basal cell adenoma, which is most often seen in the parotid gland.
- **Malignant salivary gland neoplasms.** These include mucoepidermoid carcinoma, adenoid cystic carcinoma, acinic cell carcinoma, polymorphous low-grade adenocarcinoma, and squamous cell carcinoma. All these tumors may present as a mass within the parotid gland. These tumors frequently involve the facial nerve and require more extensive treatment, with possible sacrifice of the facial nerve.

LABS

No routine laboratory tests are indicated in the work-up of a parotid mass. A complete blood cell count (CBC) may be obtained to evaluate for an elevation of the white blood cell (WBC) count secondary to an infectious process. The minimum preoperative laboratory examination should include the hematocrit and hemoglobin levels. Further laboratory tests would be dictated by the medical and surgical histories.

For the current patient, the CBC was within normal limits.

DIFFERENTIAL DIAGNOSIS

In the current case, the slow, circumscribed growth, lack of fixation, and absence of cranial nerve involvement or adenopathy associated with the lesion suggest a benign process. In addition, the absence of any erythema, pain, or warmth, together with a normal WBC count, implies a noninfectious/inflammatory process. With a swelling in this region, a differential for proliferative processes includes pleomorphic adenoma, subcutaneous lipoma, Warthin's tumor, monomorphic adenoma, and malignant salivary gland neoplasms (Box 7-1).

ASSESSMENT

FNA demonstrates a combination of ductal cells, chondromyxoid matrix, and dispersed plasmacytoid and lymphocyte-like myoepithelial cells (classic histology for pleomorphic adenoma), confirming the diagnosis of pleomorphic adenoma.

A pleomorphic adenoma is characterized by a variety of morphologic and histologic patterns. It is considered a true "mixed" tumor, referring to the biphasic proliferation of both ductal epithelial and myoepithelial (mesenchymal) cells. The ductal epithelial cells give rise to glandlike epithelial structures, whereas the myoepithelial cells are responsible for the characteristic pleomorphic extracellular matrix (myxochondroid connective tissue). Within a single tumor there may be cellular, glandular, myxoid, cartilaginous, and even ossified features. This morphologic diversity may be evident only when the lesion is excised and examined in its entirety. Histologically, pleomorphic adenomas may resemble polymorphous, low-grade adenocarcinoma, adenoid cystic carcinoma, basal cell adenoma, or epithelial-myoepithelial carcinoma. The connective tissue lining, or "pseudocapsule," is an important feature limiting growth but may be incomplete or infiltrated by tumor cells (tumor pseudopodia).

FNA may show various combinations of three elements: ductal cells, chondromyxoid matrix, and myoepithelial cells. An aspirate with more than one of these components, especially when accompanied by the characteristic clinical presentation, makes this a straightforward diagnosis.

TREATMENT

Enucleation of a pleomorphic adenoma of the parotid gland is associated with recurrence rates of up to 40%. The treatment of choice is a superficial parotidectomy, which has resulted in low morbidity, with recurrence rates of less than 2% to 3%. An attempt should be made to remove the tumor en bloc while maintaining the integrity of the capsule, with a 5-mm cuff of normal tissue. When the capsule is encountered on the deep aspect, it must be carefully dissected from the facial nerve. Maintaining the capsule is thought to be the key factor in minimizing recurrence. This observation led to the development of extracapsular dissection, in which the tumor and capsule are carefully dissected from the parotid gland. This conservative approach is associated with low rates of morbidity (facial nerve damage and Frey syndrome) and recurrence rates of 2% to 3%. Upon excision, the specimen should be delivered to pathology intact, to allow macroscopic evaluation of the integrity of the capsule. Pleomorphic adenomas of the palate should be excised with a 5-mm margin, including the overlying mucosa and underlying periosteum.

For the current patient, a superficial parotidectomy with cranial nerve VII preservation was performed through a facelift incision. The tumor was excised with a 5- to 10-mm margin of uninvolved surrounding tissue, with the exception of the deep margin, where the capsule was carefully dissected off of the facial nerve.

The procedure is usually initiated by making a modified Blair incision with a no. 15 scalpel blade. The dissection is taken down to the subdermal plane, and the flap is elevated in the preauricular region. The neck extension is dissected through the platysma, and the great auricular nerve is identified and preserved if possible. The anterior border of the sternocleidomastoid muscle is identified, and the proximal third is dissected. The muscle belly is retracted laterally, and the posterior belly of the digastric muscle identified deep to the sternocleidomastoid muscle. The preauricular portion of the dissection is deepened in the pretragal plane to the extent of the bony-cartilaginous junction of the external auditory meatus. The upper and lower portions of the dissections are then joined, and the root of the facial nerve is identified, approximately 4 mm above the posterior belly of the digastric muscle. A nerve stimulator is used for verification. The roots of the facial nerve are then identified, from the frontal, zygomatic, buccal, marginal mandibular, and cervical aspects. The parenchyma of the parotid is then elevated in a superficial plane over the preserved nerve roots. The parotid gland is mobilized anteriorly to include the pleomorphic adenoma. The external carotid artery is usually identified at the deep aspect and left intact. The specimen is removed en bloc and submitted for pathologic examination. The branches of the facial nerve are usually tested after the surgery.

The wound is thoroughly irrigated, and Jackson-Pratt (JP) drains are placed in a dependent fashion. The skin is closed in a layered fashion consisting of deep 3-0 and 4-0 Vicryl sutures, with particular attention to closure of the superficial musculoaponeurotic system to prevent Frey syndrome. The skin can be closed with nonresorbable 5-0 Prolene sutures, which are usually removed about 1 week after surgery.

COMPLICATIONS

Early complications can include facial nerve paralysis, hemorrhage, hematoma, infection, skin flap necrosis, trismus, salivary fistula, sialocele, and seroma formation. Long-term complications include Frey syndrome, hypoesthesia of the greater auricular nerve, tumor recurrence, and cosmetic deformity from the soft tissue defect (Box 7-2).

DISCUSSION

Salivary gland tumors are rare, with an annual overall incidence of 2.5 to 3 per 100,000 population. The majority of parotid (80%) and submandibular gland (60%) tumors are benign. Fifty percent of tumors originating from the minor salivary glands, but only 10% of tumors of the sublingual gland, are benign. Pleomorphic adenoma compromises about 40% to 70% of all salivary gland tumors. It is the most frequent salivary gland tumor in both children and adults and the most common tumor of both major and minor salivary glands. Approximately 75% of pleomorphic adenomas occur in the parotid gland. Ten percent are found in the submandibular gland, and another 10% are found in the palate. Pleomorphic adenomas make up 60% to 70% of all parotid neoplasms, 40% to 60% of submandibular gland tumors, and 40% to 70% of minor salivary gland tumors.

A pleomorphic adenoma classically presents as a painless, firm swelling. It may be lobulated, irregularly dome shaped, or smooth. The consistency is typically rubbery or semisolid, and there may be isolated areas that are softer. If untreated, it enlarges slowly over months or years. The connective tissue capsule generally limits growth, but tumors can become very large if neglected.

Box 7-2   Complications of Parotidectomy for Pleomorphic Adenoma

- **Facial nerve injury.** Cranial nerve VII can be preserved in most parotidectomies in the setting of benign disease. However, despite correct surgical technique, paresis of this nerve can occur. Careful handling, with minimal skeletonization of the branches, can help reduce anoxia and ischemia intraoperatively. If major trauma to the nerve is avoided, deficits are usually transient (seen in 14% to 40% of cases) and can be expected to resolve.

- **Recurrence.** In a review of 52 studies (804 cases of pleomorphic adenoma), Hickman and co-workers reported a 5-year recurrence-free rate of 96.6% and a 10-year recurrence-free rate of 93.7%. There is a higher risk of multifocal recurrence (20% to 40% of cases), of which 25% are malignant, when the surrounding tissues are seeded by inappropriate handling of the tumor, such as with open biopsy of major glands or attempts at enucleation. Such recurrences usually occur within the first 10 years after the original surgery. Some recent immunohistochemical studies (Bankamp and Bierhoff, 1999) have claimed that recurrent tumors are characterized by differentiation of the epithelial components, which is related to greater proliferation.

- **Malignancy and metastasis.** The overall rate of malignant transformation for a pleomorphic adenoma has been estimated at about 6%. There are three distinct histologic types of mixed tumor with the potential for metastasis:
  (1) A benign-appearing lesion may become a benign metastasizing pleomorphic adenoma. These lesions tend to recur locally, often multiple times, before metastasizing. This is a rare occurrence.
  (2) There is a 2% to 3% risk of malignant transformation to carcinoma ex-pleomorphic adenoma. This usually occurs in larger and longstanding benign pleomorphic adenomas (usually about twice the size and present for about twice as long). The average age for presentation of carcinoma ex-pleomorphic adenoma is 60 years, and usually the original pleomorphic adenoma has been present for more than 15 years.
  (3) Very rarely, malignant change in both ductal and myoepithelial elements gives rise to a true mixed malignant pleomorphic adenoma or carcinosarcoma.

- **Frey syndrome (auriculotemporal nerve syndrome or gustatory sweating).** This is a relatively common long-term complication of parotidectomy. It is characterized by localized sweating and dermal flushing during salivary stimulation. This is thought to be caused by aberrant connections between severed secretomotor parasympathetic fibers as they anastomose with severed postganglionic sympathetic fibers that supply the sweat glands of the face in the auriculotemporal region. Frey syndrome has been reported in as many as 30% to 60% of patients undergoing parotidectomy. However, only 10% of patients have symptoms requiring treatment. Treatment options include surgical disruption of the aberrant neural connections or use of botulinum toxin.

From Bankamp DG, Bierhoff E: Proliferative activity in recurrent and nonrecurrent pleomorphic adenoma of the salivary glands, *Laryngorhinootologie* 78(2):77-80, 1999.

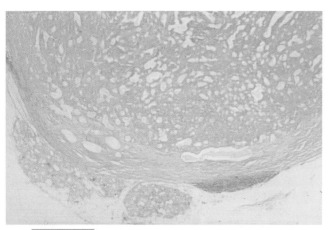

Figure 7-3 Histopathology of pleomorphic adenoma.

In the parotid gland, pleomorphic adenoma most commonly presents in the inferior aspect of the superficial lobe. Deep lobe invasion may manifest as a mass of the soft palate or lateral pharyngeal space. CT or MRI scans can help localize tumor or differentiate lymph nodes from tumor.

The most common intraoral sites are the palate and upper lip. When arising from minor glands of the palate, pleomorphic adenomas are most commonly located lateral to the midline at the junction of the hard and soft palate. Minor gland tumors may cause localized pressure resorption of the palate but do not tend to invade the underlying bone.

Histopathologically, permanent hematoxylin- and eosin–stained sections demonstrate typical histology, including glandlike epithelial cells forming nests, chords, and ductlike structures within a heterogeneous stromal background of myxoid, chondroid, and mucoid material, along with a distinct fibrous connective tissue lining (Figure 7-3).

Bibliography

Allison GR, Rappoport I: Prevention of Frey's syndrome with superficial musculoaponeurotic system interposition, *Am J Surg* 166:407-410, 1993.

Bankamp DG, Bierhoff E: Proliferative activity in recurrent and nonrecurrent pleomorphic adenoma of the salivary glands, *Laryngorhinootologie* 78(2):77-80, 1999

Garcia-Perla A, Munoz-Ramos M, Infante-Cossio P, et al: Pleomorphic adenoma of the parotid in childhood, *J Craniomaxillofac Surg* 30:242-245, 2002.

Hickman RE, Cawson RA, Duffy SW: The prognosis of specific types of salivary gland tumors, *Cancer* 54(8):1620-1624, 1984.

Howlett DC, Kesse KW, Hughes DV, et al: The role of imaging in the evaluation of parotid disease, *Clin Radiol* 57:692-701, 2002.

Jorge J, Pires FR, Alves FA, et al: Juvenile intraoral pleomorphic adenoma: report of five cases and review of the literature, *Int J Oral Maxillofac Surg* 31:273-275, 2002.

Kwon MY, Gu M: True malignant mixed tumor (carcinosarcoma) of parotid gland with unusual mesenchymal component: a case report and review of the literature, *Arch Pathol Lab Med* 125:812-815, 2001.

Nadershah M, Salama A: Removal of parotid, submandibular, and sublingual glands, *Oral Maxillofacial Surg Clin North Am* 24(2):295-305, 2012.

Salama AR, Ord RA: Clinical implications of neck in salivary gland disease, *Oral Maxillofacial Surg Clin North Am* 20(3):445-458, 2008.

Schreibstein JM, Tronic B, Tarlov E, et al: Benign metastasizing pleomorphic adenoma, *Otolaryngol Head Neck Surg* 112(4):612-615, 1995.

Shashinder S, Tang IP, Velayutham P, et al: A review of parotid tumors and their management: a ten-year-experience, *Med J Malaysia* 64(1):31-33, 2009.

Speight PM, Barrett AW: Salivary gland tumours, *Oral Dis* 8:229-240, 2002.

Stanley MW: Selected problems in fine needle aspiration of head and neck masses, *Mod Pathol* 15(3):342-350, 2002.

Valentini V, Fabiani F, Perugini M, et al: Surgical techniques in the treatment of pleomorphic adenoma of the parotid gland: our experience and review of literature, *J Craniofac Surg* 12(6):565-568, 2001.

Mucocele and Fibroma*

Ketan Patel, Deepak Kademani, and Shahrokh C. Bagheri

CC

A 20-year-old patient presents to the office complaining of a painless mass in her lower lip. (Mucoceles are more common in young adults but can be seen in all age groups, including infants. There is no gender predilection.) Irritation fibromas can also be present on the commissure or lower lip but are more commonly found on the cheek with repeated trauma. Both fibromas and mucoceles are a result of repeated trauma to the intraoral mucosal lining.

HPI

The patient was recently evaluated by her general dentist and was subsequently referred for evaluation and treatment of a persistent mass in her lower lip. The lesion was noticed 1 month earlier and has gradually increased to its current size (some patients give a history of recurrent swelling that periodically ruptures). The mass developed after trauma to the lower lip during function and has proved to be a site of continued trauma due to its persistence. Although trauma (e.g., lip biting) has been associated with mucoceles, a positive history of trauma is frequently lacking.

PMHX/PDHX/MEDICATIONS/ALLERGIES/SH/FH

Noncontributory. There is no association between preexisting medical conditions and the incidence of mucoceles or irritation fibromas.

EXAMINATION

Maxillofacial. There is asymmetrical prominence of the patient's lower lip (most common site). There are no other areas of swelling or lymphadenopathy.

Intraoral. Examination reveals no pathology of the hard or soft palate, tongue, floor of the mouth, or buccal mucosa. A soft, 1-cm, painless mass is appreciated just inferior and medial to the right labial commissure (Figure 7-4). The mass is fluctuant, soft, and nontender with a bluish mucosal discoloration. There is some evidence of trauma to the mass from the adjacent dentition. The tissue overlying the mass has become fibrotic as a result of repetitive trauma.

IMAGING

No imaging studies are indicated unless there is suspicion of other pathologic processes.

LABS

No routines labs are indicated unless dictated by underlying medical conditions.

DIFFERENTIAL DIAGNOSIS

Despite the classic characteristic clinical findings, salivary gland tumor needs to be considered on the differential diagnosis. Salivary gland tumors of the minor glands can occur on the lips but are more commonly seen in the upper lip rather than the lower lip.

The differential diagnosis also includes an irritation fibroma. This lesion is commonly pink and nonfluctuant and does not have history of intermittent swelling and rupturing (as opposed to a mucocele). An irritation fibroma usually presents as a pedunculated, round, nonulcerated lesion that is frequently found along the linea alba in patients with chronic cheek biting. The lesion is slightly pale but has the same consistency as the surrounding mucosa, with no erythema.

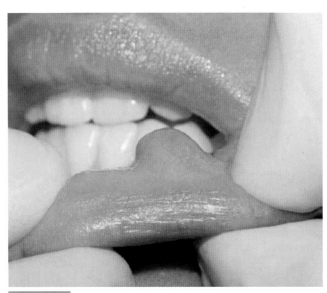

Figure 7-4 A 1-cm, painless mass seen just inferior and medial to the left labial commissure.

*The authors and publisher wish to acknowledge Dr. Aric Murphy and Dr. David M. Weber for their contribution on these topics in the previous edition.

193

BIOPSY

Although the clinical examination can be highly suspicious of a mucocele, histopathologic analysis is the only confirmatory test. An excisional biopsy (removal of the entire lesion) is both diagnostic and the definitive treatment.

ASSESSMENT

An excisional biopsy was performed under local anesthesia confirming the diagnosis of a mucocele.

Histopathologic examination of a mucocele demonstrates spillage of mucin surrounded by dense granulation tissue, which may be seen in association with minor salivary glands. An inflammatory response (neutrophils) may be observed.

TREATMENT

The current patient was seen in the clinic for excisional biopsy under local anesthesia. Care was taken to evert the lower lip with finger pressure against the skin. This provides increased exposure of the mass on the mucosal surface. A straight-line incision is made perpendicular to the vermillion border over the length of the mass on the mucosal surface. This is followed with careful blunt and sharp dissection around the mucocele and the offending gland. The surgical specimen was labeled and sent to pathology, and a diagnosis of a mucocele was confirmed.

An alternative surgical approach to treatment of a mucocele includes excision or marsupialization with a carbon dioxide laser. Cryotherapy has also been used for the treatment of mucoceles. Direct application of liquid nitrogen is made with a cotton-tip applicator. A major advantage of this technique is compliance in pediatric patients.

COMPLICATIONS

The most common complication associated with treatment of a mucocele is recurrence. This can be minimized by the removal of any adjacent minor salivary glands. For patients who experience problematic recurrence, a carbon dioxide laser can be used to ablate the surgical field, which is left to heal by secondary epithelialization. Excision or dissection of larger mucoceles of the lower lip can pose a risk to the labial branch of the mental nerve, resulting in postoperative neurosensory dysfunction.

DISCUSSION

Mucoceles, also called *mucus retention cysts* or *mucus extravasation phenomenon,* by definition are cavities filled with mucus produced by trauma to minor salivary glands. With functional trauma to the soft tissue and underlying glands, mucus leaks into the adjacent tissues, creating a mucocele. It is the most common lesion affecting the oral mucosa. It can grow to a few millimeters in size and rarely is larger than 1.5 cm. The lower lip is the most common site of a mucocele due to its susceptibility to trauma. Seldom are these lesions seen in the upper lip, even though it has an equivalent number of minor salivary glands. In a recent study of the distribution of mucoceles in 263 patients, 78% occurred in the lower lip and 3% occurred in the upper lip. These findings are consistent with previous studies. Mucoceles do not have an epithelial lining (in contrast to salivary duct cysts). The extravasation of mucus produces a wall of inflamed fibrous tissue.

The oral fibroma (irritational or traumatic) is one of the most common exophytic, soft tissue lesions seen in the oral cavity, with an incidence of 12 lesions per 1,000 population. It is considered a reactive hyperplasia of fibrous connective tissue in response to local irritation or trauma. These lesions have limited growth potential, and the lesion may even decrease in size after prolonged removal of irritation or trauma.

Clinically, the fibroma can occur anywhere in the oral cavity, but it is most common in the buccal mucosa along the occlusal plane. Other common sites are the labial mucosa, tongue, and gingiva. Fibromas often appear pink due the absence of vascularity. Most commonly, they appear as a well-circumscribed nodule that is often pedunculated or sessile. Rarely do the lesions exceed 2 cm in the greatest dimension. In some cases, the lesion can appear white due to hyperkeratosis from continual irritation. Occasionally, the fibroma can appear mildly erythematous and even ulcerated, if recently traumatized. Fibromas most commonly occur between ages 30 and 50 years, favoring females to males in a 2 : 1 ratio in cases submitted for biopsy. Treatment is conservative surgical excision, and the prognosis is excellent, with rare recurrence. It is important to submit the lesion for histopathologic diagnosis, because some benign, and even malignant, tumors can mimic the clinical appearance of the fibroma.

Histologically, the lesion appears as a nodular mass of fibrous connective tissue covered by stratified squamous epithelium; this is consistent with the diagnosis of a traumatic (irritation) fibroma of the buccal mucosa

Occasionally, chronic inflammatory infiltrates can be seen in the connective tissue portion of the lesion.

Bibliography

Bahadure RN, Fulzele P, Thosar N, et al: Conventional surgical treatment of oral mucocele: a series of 23 cases, *Eur J Paediatr Dent* 13(2):143-146, 2012.

Baurmash H: Mucoceles and ranulas, *J Oral Maxillofac Surg* 61:369-378, 2003.

Bouquot JE, Gundlach KK: Oral exophytic lesions in 23,616 white Americans over 35 years of age, *Oral Surg Oral Med Oral Pathol* 62(3):284-291, 1986.

Harrison JD: Salivary mucoceles, *Oral Surg Oral Med Oral Pathol* 39:268-278, 1975.

Ishimaru M: A simple cryosurgical method for treatment of oral mucous cysts, *Int J Oral Maxillofac Surg* 22:353-355, 1993.

Jinbu Y: Mucocele of the glands of Blandin-Nuhn: clinical and histopathologic analysis of 26 cases, *Oral Surg Oral Med Oral Pathol Oral Radiol Endod* 95:467-470, 2003.

Kopp WK, St-Hilaire H: Mucosal preservation in the treatment of mucocele with CO_2 laser, *J Oral Maxillofac Surg* 62:1559-1561, 2004.

Mandel L, Baurmash H: Irritation fibroma: report of a case, *NY State Dent J* 36(6):344-347, 1970.

Martins-Filho PR, Santos Tde S, da Silva HF, et al: A clinicopathologic review of 138 cases of mucoceles in a pediatric population, *Quintessence* 42(8):679-685, 2011.

Marx RE, Stern D: *Oral and maxillofacial pathology: a rational for diagnosis and treatment*, p 395, Carol Stream, Ill, 2003, Quintessence.

Neville BW, Damm DD, Allen CM: *Oral and maxillofacial pathology*, ed 2, pp 438-439, Philadelphia, 2002, Saunders.

Regezi JA, Courtney RM, Kerr DA: Fibrous lesions of the skin and mucous membranes which contain stellate and multinucleated cells, *Oral Surg Oral Med Oral Pathol* 39(4):605-614, 1975.

Regezi JA, Sciubba JJ: Connective tissue lesions. In Regezi JA, Sciubba JJ (eds): *Oral pathology*, p 191, Philadelphia, 1995, Saunders.

Sela J, Ulmansky M: Mucous retention cyst of salivary glands, *J Oral Surg* 27(8):619-623, 1969.

Acute Herpetic Gingivostomatitis*

Ketan Patel and Deepak Kademani

CC

A 4-year-old boy presents to the pedodontist because he has had a sore mouth and decreased oral intake for the past 2 days.

Acute herpetic gingivostomatitis is an infection that typically affects children. The most common age of onset is 6 months to 5 years. A second peak occurs in the early 20s. The majority (90%) of primary infections are asymptomatic. By adulthood about 60% to 95% of the population is affected by a herpes virus.

HPI

The patient's mother reports that he has been in distress with mouth pain and has not been eating well for the past few days (pain is the most common presenting symptom). The parents noticed multiple vesicles and ulcers in his mouth 2 days earlier. He has had a low-grade temperature over the past 2 days, which they have treated with acetaminophen (in the pediatric population, decreased oral intake is often the first sign of a developing infectious/pathologic process).

It is important to distinguish primary and recurrent infection. Primary infection tends to be more severe and can occur anywhere in the oral cavity. Symptoms typically last 1 week and can be associated with malaise, lymphadenopathy, and fever. Recurrent disease occurs sporadically and tends to be limited to the keratinized mucosa.

PMHX/PSHX/MEDICATIONS/ALLERGIES/SH/FH

The patient has never been to the dentist. He does not have any known drug allergies and is not on any medications. The mother admits to having recurrent herpes labialis several weeks ago.

Herpes simplex virus (HSV) is transmitted via direct contact with infected secretions from the saliva and other bodily fluids. The main risk factor is a known exposure to the virus. When HSV-1 comes into contact with the host, the virus migrates to the sensory nerve endings and frequently to the trigeminal ganglia. The virus then enters a latent phase for 7 to 10 days before replication. Recurrent disease with HSV-1 characteristically involves the distribution of the trigeminal nerve.

*The authors and publisher wish to acknowledge Dr. Matthew J. Karban for his contribution on this topic in the previous edition.

EXAMINATION

General. The patient is an uncooperative, anxious boy in otherwise good health.

Vital signs. His blood pressure is 105/70 mm Hg, heart rate 100 bpm, respirations 18 per minute, and temperature 38.9°C (febrile).

Maxillofacial. He has palpable cervical lymph nodes (this is commonly seen with acute herpetic gingivostomatitis). The face is symmetrical, with no other obvious signs of infection or edema.

Intraoral. Multiple vesicles and ulcerations extend over the buccal and labial alveolar mucosa and dorsal tongue (Figures 7-5) (primary acute herpetic gingivostomatitis can affect both the keratinized and nonkeratinized mucosa, but recurrent infection preferentially involves the keratinized tissue). Ulcerations measure from 1 to 3 mm in diameter and

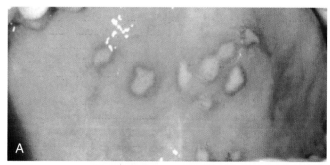

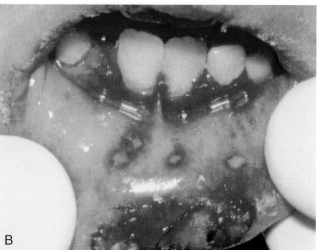

Figure 7-5 Herpetic lesions on the ventral tongue **(A)** and lower lip **(B)**.

are covered by a pseudomembrane and an erythematous border. The gingiva is erythematous and painful, and there is copious saliva production with drooling. The ulcers present as foul-smelling ulcers when they rupture due to the friable pseudomembrane.

Extremities. Right thumb displays similar erythematous vesicles and ulcerations (consistent with herpetic whitlow).

IMAGING

No imaging modalities are necessary for the diagnosis and management of acute herpetic gingivostomatitis.

LABS

The diagnosis of acute herpetic gingivostomatitis is mainly a clinical diagnosis, but several laboratory tests are available for detecting an active herpes viral infection. Some of these tests include viral cultures, direct immunofluorescence, and a Tzanck smear. The Tzanck smear involves unroofing the vesicles and scraping of the tissue bed for cytologic examination. Identification of multinucleated epithelial giant cells with eosinophilic viral inclusions is the hallmark feature.

ASSESSMENT

Acute (primary) herpetic gingivostomatitis.

TREATMENT

Acute herpetic gingivostomatitis is a self-limiting condition usually resolving within 3 weeks from the onset of symptoms. Treatment predominantly involves observation and palliative care. This may involve topical anesthetics and over-the-counter pain relief, such as acetaminophen or ibuprofen. Fluids and electrolyte status should be monitored as needed to avoid dehydration.

Pharmacologic treatment is often minimal due to the self-limiting course of the herpes virus. In more severe cases, pharmacotherapy can be of use if administered appropriately. Conventional antiviral therapy (e.g., acyclovir, valacyclovir, and penciclovir) has proved effective and can shorten the healing times by several days.

Primary acute herpetic gingivostomatitis can be managed on an outpatient basis with aggressive oral hydration, analgesia, and topical and systemic antiviral therapy. The main criteria for hospital admission include severe dehydration and pain.

Adult patients are typically managed on an outpatient basis. Severe disease refractory to treatment may indicate an underlying cause of immunosuppression that may require further evaluation for recurrent, persistent, or refractory disease.

COMPLICATIONS

The main complications include potential nutritional deficiencies and inadequate fluid intake leading to dehydration, ocular involvement, herpetic whitlow, and central nervous system involvement.

Ocular herpes is relatively rare, affecting 50,000 patients in the United States per year. Stromal keratitis occurs in 25% of patients affected with ocular symptoms, involves inflammation of the deep layers of the cornea, and can lead to globe rupture and blindness. Herpetic whitlow is an intense, painful infection of the hand, involving one or more fingers, that typically affects the terminal phalanx. HSV-1 is the cause in approximately 60% of cases of herpetic whitlow, and HSV-2 is the cause in the remaining 40%. In children, HSV-1 is the most likely causative agent. Infection involving the fingers usually is due to autoinoculation from primary oropharyngeal lesions as a result of finger-sucking or thumb-sucking behavior in patients with herpes labialis or herpetic gingivostomatitis. In the general adult population, herpetic whitlow is most often due to autoinoculation from genital herpes; therefore, it is most frequently secondary to infection with HSV-2. Before the use of gloves, herpetic whitlow was common among dentists, transmitted by the infected oropharyngeal secretions of patients. Transmission easily can be prevented by the use of gloves and by scrupulous observation of universal fluid precautions.

Although a prodrome of fever and malaise may be observed, most often the initial symptoms are pain and burning or tingling of the infected digit. This usually is followed by erythema, edema, and the development of 1- to 3-mm grouped vesicles on an erythematous base over the next 7 to 10 days. These vesicles may ulcerate or rupture and usually contain clear fluid, although the fluid may appear cloudy or bloody. Lymphangitis and epitrochlear and axillary lymphadenopathy are not uncommon. After 10 to 14 days, symptoms usually improve significantly, and lesions crust over and heal.

After the initial infection, the virus enters cutaneous nerve endings and migrates to the peripheral ganglia and Schwann cells, where it lies dormant. They are protected from antibody detection due to the blood-brain barrier and therefore lie dormant in the cell bodies of the gasserian ganglion. The primary infection usually is the most symptomatic. Recurrences observed in 20% to 50% of cases are usually milder and shorter in duration.

More than 2,100 cases of herpetic encephalitis are seen in the United States per year, making it a rare but extremely serious brain disease. HSV-1 is almost always the culprit, except in newborns. In about 70% of infant herpes encephalitis, the disease occurs when a latent HSV-2 virus is activated. Untreated, herpes encephalitis is fatal in more than 70% of cases. Fortunately, rapid diagnostic tests and treatment with acyclovir have significantly improved both survival rates (up to about 80%) and complication rates.

DISCUSSION

Acute gingivostomatitis is an oral presentation of HSV-1. The virus typically presents in children between the ages of 6 months and 5 years, with a peak incidence at 2 to 3 years of age. Infection is rare before 6 months of age due to the presence of maternal anti-HSV antibodies. Manifestations rarely present into adulthood.

The initial clinical presentation includes fever, nausea, and cervical lymphadenopathy, although it is thought that 90% of all primary infections are subclinical. Patients may proceed to display multiple small, yellow- or white-filled vesicles, which develop into 1- to 3-mm ulcers after a few days and ultimately heal with some scarring. These vesicles and ulcers can present on attached and unattached gingiva and the tongue. Affected gingiva is erythematous, enlarged, and painful, often leading to constitutional symptoms such as dehydration from lack of adequate oral intake. In adults, acute herpetic gingivostomatitis can also present as pharyngotonsillitis. Diagnosis is primarily based on clinical presentations, along with the absence of any previous clinical symptoms and confirmatory laboratory studies.

Bibliography

Ajar AH, Chauvin PJ: Acute herpetic gingivostomatitis in adults: a review of 13 cases, including diagnosis and management, *J Can Dental Assoc* 68(4):247-251, 2002.

Blevins JY: Primary herpetic gingivostomatitis in young children, *Dermatol Nurs* 29(3):199-202, 2003.

Fatahzadeh M: Primary oral herpes: diagnosis and management, *J N J Dent Assoc* 83(2):12-13, 2012.

McDonald RE, Avery DR, Weddell JA, et al: Gingivitis and periodontal disease. In Dean JA, Avery DR, McDonald RE (eds): *Dentistry for the child and adolescent*, ed 9, pp 366-402, St Louis, 2011, Mosby.

Aphthous Ulcers*

Ketan Patel, Ma'Ann C. Sabino, and Deepak Kademani

CC

A 25-year-old woman is referred for evaluation of painful ulcerations inside her mouth (aphthous ulcerations affect 20% of the population, with a slight female predilection).

HPI

The patient reports that for the past 5 years, she has had episodes of ulcers that occur spontaneously and typically last for 3 weeks, with intervals of up to 1 to 3 months between episodes. She does not have any history of trauma or known infectious diseases. The ulcers occasionally occur at multiple sites simultaneously. The hallmark feature is that they are slow healing with visible scarring, extremely painful, and can take as long as 3 weeks to heal.

PMHX/PDHX/MEDS/ALLERGIES/SH/FH

There is no known history of immunosuppression, HIV, malnutrition, cancer, or previous infections of the head and neck region (potential risk factors).

A careful history may identify contributing etiologic factors. In some individuals, the ulcers are a secondary or hypersensitivity response to an antigenic stimulus, especially foods, whereas in other cases the ulcers represent a primary autoimmune disorder. Patients with aphthae have a decreased ratio of T-helper (CD4$^+$) cells to T-suppressor/cytotoxic (CD8$^+$) cells in their circulation, and the ulcer bed itself has a high level of CD8$^+$ cytotoxic T cells. Although this is a likely contributor to the cellular destruction caused by these ulcers, initiating causes are variable due to multiple contributing factors: familial predisposition, allergy, nutritional imbalances, infectious agents, hormones, trauma, stress, and blood dyscrasias. Individuals with comorbid extraoral diseases, such as Behçet disease (ulcerations of the genitalia and ocular and oral mucous membranes), Crohn's disease, celiac disease, ulcerative colitis, psoriasis, and ankylosing spondititis are at increased risk of developing aphthous ulcerations. Cyclic neutropenia is responsible for a subgroup of patients with aphthous stomatitis, with the ulcers occurring at points of minor trauma during times when the number of circulating neutrophils is low. Stress may be indirectly responsible for the sores, which were once called "stress ulcers," through its modulation of the immune system. Paradoxically, tobacco smoking, with its own immune modulation, is often protective, probably because of the increased keratinization resulting from local irritation of the oral mucous membranes.

EXAMINATION

General. The patient is a well-developed and well-nourished woman in no apparent distress.

Vital signs. Vital signs are stable, and the patient is afebrile (fever is usually not seen with aphthous ulcers).

Maxillofacial. There is no facial swelling or cervical lymphadenopathy.

Intraoral. There are multiple ulcerations at various stages of healing in the oral mucosa measuring 6 to 12 mm. Two ulcers at the right buccal mucosa appear to coalesce. There is also a 7-mm ulcer of the left lateral tongue. The lesions demonstrate a central zone of ulceration covered by a fibrinopurulent membrane that is surrounded by a varying degree of erythema along the margins. There does not appear to be any source of trauma in association with the ulcers (sharp dental restorations or fractured dental cusps). Figures 7-6 and 7-7 show examples of minor and major aphthous ulcers on the mucosa of the commissure and the palate.

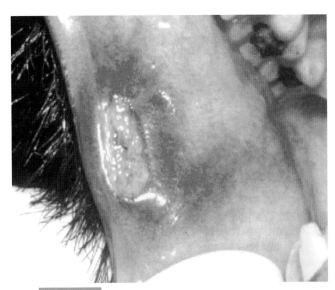

Figure 7-6   Major ulcer of the commissure of the lip.

*The authors and publisher wish to acknowledge Dr. Anthony A. Indovina, Jr., for his contribution on this topic in the previous edition.

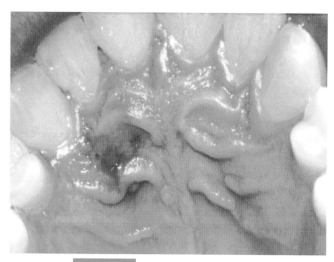

Figure 7-7 Minor ulcer in the palate.

IMAGING

No imaging studies are indicated for the evaluation of aphthous ulcers.

LABS

Routine laboratory tests are not indicated unless dictated by other underlying medical conditions.

ASSESSMENT

Multiple minor and major aphthous ulcers in an otherwise healthy 25-year-old woman.

The diagnosis of aphthous ulcers is usually a clinical diagnosis. In cases of chronic nonhealing ulcers, a biopsy may be indicated to exclude viral and/or neoplastic etiologies. Therefore, all lesions should be followed for observation for adequate healing. Diagnosis is established by clinical history without the need for routine histopathology. Should a biopsy be performed, it would likely show surface mucosal ulceration with an intense inflammatory infiltrate. The ulcer bed would likely have an increased concentration of CD8+ cytotoxic T cells.

TREATMENT

There is no definitive cure for aphthous ulcerations. Treatment is directed toward symptomatic relief and is based on the type of ulcer and response to topical versus systemic therapy. Aphthous ulcers are categorized into three types based on clinical course, size, and shape and are designated as minor, major, and herpetiform (Box 7-3).

Topical corticosteroid therapy. Topical therapy should be discontinued within 2 weeks if no improvement is observed. Clinicians should be cautious with prolonged use of topical steroids, because pseudomembranous candidiasis may develop.

| Box 7-3 | **Categorization of Aphthous Ulcers** |

- **Minor aphthous ulcer (Mikulicz aphthae).** Less than 10 mm in size, requiring no treatment and resolving within 7 to 10 days without scarring. Should the ulcer remain after 2 weeks, topical corticosteroid therapy is indicated. Palliative therapy in the form of a topical local anesthetic, such as 2% viscous lidocaine, diphenhydramine elixir (12.5 mg/ml), or topical benzocaine, may be indicated in cases of severe pain associated with minor aphthous ulcers.
- **Major ulcers (periadenitis, mucosa necrotica recurrens, Sutton disease).** Major aphthous ulcers, by definition, are greater than 10 mm in diameter with deeper penetration than minor ulcers and therefore heal with scarring. Resolution of major aphthous ulcers may take longer than several weeks. Treatment of more severe forms of major aphthous ulcers includes the use of topical or systemic corticosteroid therapy. A protocol has been established by Kerr and Ship in the management of aphthous ulcers, especially with reference to those seen in HIV-infected patients.
- **Herpetiform ulcers.** Herpetiform ulcers occur as many (10 to 100) small ulcerations coalescing within a large area of nonkeratinized mucosa that can extend to keratinized mucosa. In name and clinical characteristics, these ulcers resemble ulcerations resulting from primary herpes simplex infection. Herpetiform ulcers are distinct from herpetic ulcers in that they lack viral particles and are not preceded by the formation of vesicles. Healing occurs within 7 to 10 days.

- Fluocinonide 0.05% ointment or gel over ulcer four times daily
- Clobetasol propionate 0.05% ointment over ulcer three times daily
- Dexamethasone elixir 0.5 mg/5 ml swish for 3 minutes and expectorate three times daily

First-line systemic therapy. If topical corticosteroid therapy fails to resolve the pathology, intralesional or systemic corticosteroid therapy is indicated. Intralesional injection of 20 to 40 mg triamcinolone has been shown to be efficacious in reducing pain and resolving recurrent and major aphthous ulcers in HIV-positive patients. Additionally, short-course, high-dose ("short-burst") prednisone (40 to 80 mg) therapy for 3 to 7 days without taper has been described with excellent clinical results. Clinicians should be cautioned about the use of systemic corticosteroid therapy during active infections, such as tuberculosis, which is prevalent in the HIV-positive population.

Second-line systemic therapy. Thalidomide has been shown to be a potent immunomodulator that is efficacious in the treatment of severe forms of recurrent aphthous ulcers. Treatment with thalidomide 200 mg daily for 1 month resulted in a significantly greater number of individuals with complete or partial resolution of ulcers and decreased pain compared with control subjects. However, its use is limited by adverse effects, including constipation, drowsiness, peripheral neuropathy, and excessive fatigue.

COMPLICATIONS

The most common complication of aphthous ulceration is pain leading to difficulty eating. Scar formation can be seen with major aphthous ulcers.

DISCUSSION

Recurrent aphthous ulcerations remain one of the most common oral mucosal disorders. Despite their prevalence, their etiology is largely unknown. The differentiation of aphthous ulcers into minor, major, and herpetiform categories does not have an etiologic basis. Mucosal ulcerations may also be manifested in chronic diseases related to immunosuppression, malnutrition, infection, and neoplasm. A distinction between major and minor aphthous ulcers can also be made histopathologically based on the depth of involvement of inflammation. Major aphthous ulcers tend to be deeply infiltrative, thereby leading to the scarring that is often seen after these lesions heal.

Chronic irritation of nonkeratinized oral mucosa by dental appliances (ill-fitting dentures or orthodontic wires), fractured dental cusps, or dental treatment may cause ulcerations to occur; this needs to be differentiated from aphthous ulcerations. Removal of the source of irritation usually allows for resolution of the ulcer.

Deficiencies of iron, vitamin B_{12}, and folate have been implicated in the pathogenesis of chronic aphthous ulcers. According to a study by Scully and colleagues, 18% to 28% of cases of recurrent aphthous ulcers occurred in patients with these deficiencies compared with 8% in healthy cohorts. In some cases, replacement of the deficiencies results in clinical improvement.

Varicella zoster virus and cytomegalovirus antibody titers have been isolated in patients with recurrent aphthous ulcers, but studies are conflicting. The association between the presence of varicella zoster virus or cytomegalovirus and the development of aphthous ulcers has not been demonstrated. The gram-negative organism *Helicobacter pylori* was previously implicated in the formation of recurrent aphthous ulcers in children and adolescents, but it is no longer considered an important etiologic factor. HIV infection has been shown to increase the propensity for developing recurrent aphthous ulcers, especially the major aphthous variant. The relationship between HIV infection and ulcer formation may be related to the decrease in circulating CD4 T lymphocytes (fewer than 100 cells/mm^3) and resultant immunosuppression related to this disease.

Although multiple regimens have been advocated for the treatment of these lesions, a recent Cochrane review suggests that there is no difference in the outcome between patients treated with any regimen, whether antiinflammatory, immunomodulatory, or another form of treatment.

Bibliography

Brocklehurst P, Tickle M, Glenny AM, et al: Systemic interventions for recurrent aphthous stomatitis (mouth ulcers), *Cochrane Database Syst Rev* 12:9, 2012.

Friedman M, Brenski A, Taylor L: Treatment of aphthous ulcers in AIDS patients, *Laryngoscope* 104(5):566, 1994.

Fritscher AM, Cherubini K, Chies J, et al: The association between *Helicobacter pylori* and recurrent aphthous stomatitis in children and adolescents, *J Oral Pathol Med* 33(3):129, 2004.

Jacobson JM, Greenspan JS, Spritzler J, et al: Thalidomide for treatment of oral aphthous ulcers in patients with human immunodeficiency virus infection: National Institute of Allergy and Infectious Diseases AIDS Clinial Trial Group, *N Engl J Med* 336(21):1487, 1997.

Kerr AR, Ship JA: Management strategies for HIV-associated aphthous stomatitis, *Am J Clin Dermatol* 4(10):669, 2003.

Natah SS, Kontinen YT, Enattah NS, et al: Recurrent aphthous ulcers today: a review of the growing knowledge, *Int J Oral Maxillofac Surg* 33:221, 2004.

Scully C, Grosky M, Lozada-Nur F: The diagnosis and management of recurrent aphthous stomatitis: a consensus approach, *J Am Dent Assoc* 134(2):200, 2003.

Sialolithiasis*

Ketan Patel, Deepak Kademani, and Shahrokh C. Bagheri

CC

A 48-year-old woman reports to your office complaining of pain and swelling of the right submandibular region (sialoliths, or salivary stones, within the salivary gland ductal system, tend to occur more commonly in the elderly population, with a slight female predominance).

HPI

The patient reports having episodes of mild discomfort of the right submandibular area over the past 7 months (it is not uncommon for symptoms to wax and wane, especially during mealtime, coinciding with gland function). Her pain and swelling increased significantly 2 days earlier, which has prompted her to seek care.

Decreased salivary flow is the most significant risk factor for the development of sialolithiasis (salivary gland stones within a gland or duct) and sialadenitis (inflammation of the salivary gland). Dehydration, poorly controlled diabetes mellitus, certain medications, and radiation therapy are among several factors that can lead to xerostomia (dry mouth) secondary to decreased salivary flow.

PMHX/PSHX/MEDICATIONS/ALLERGIES/SH/FH

Major depression diagnosed 5 years earlier (some of the medications used to treat depression have anticholinergic side effects that include decreased production of saliva).

Type 1 diabetes mellitus was diagnosed 7 years ago. The patient's most recent HbA_{1c} was 9%, and her blood glucose levels range between 200 and 300 mg/dl (both indicative of poorly controlled diabetes, which is associated with an increased risk of sialolithiasis secondary to osmotic diuresis causing dehydration. The decreased immune function seen with diabetes is also a risk factor for the development of sialadenitis).

She has no known history of autoimmune disorders, such as Sjögren syndrome, or a history of radiation therapy (both are risk factors for xerostomia).

Medications include amitriptyline (tricyclic antidepressant with anticholinergic side effects, including xerostomia) and regular and NPH insulin as adjusted by her endocrinologist. The patient admits to drinking alcohol socially (chronic excessive alcohol consumption may predispose to the development of sialoliths secondary to frequent episodes of dehydration. Alcohol suppresses the antidiuretic hormone [ADH], causing polyuria).

EXAMINATION

General. The patient is a well-developed and well-nourished alert woman in mild discomfort (secondary to pain).

Vital signs. Her blood pressure is 143/89 mm Hg (elevated secondary to anxiety), heart rate 110 bpm (tachycardia secondary to anxiety), respirations 15 per minute, and temperature 37.1°C (sialadenitis can present with fever secondary to inflammation of the gland).

Neck. There is mild to moderate tender right submandibular swelling (Figure 7-8). The area is firm and warm to the touch on the overlying skin (dolor, tumor, calor, and rubor secondary to localized inflammation). Several palpable cervical lymph nodes are detected on the ipsilateral neck. (Enlarged lymph nodes are not uncommon secondary to localized inflammation of the submandibular gland. Lymphadenopathy due to a neoplastic process is also possible, but these are usually nontender due to the noninflammatory etiology.)

Intraoral. Bimanual palpation reveals a 2- to 3-cm palpable tender mass of the right posterior floor of the mouth consistent with the location of the submandibular gland. Decreased salivary flow is observed relative to the

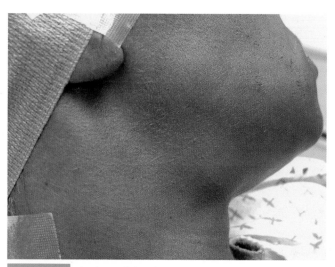

Figure 7-8 A view of the right neck demonstrating swelling of the right submandibular region.

*The authors and publisher wish to acknowledge Dr. Derek H. Lamb for his contribution on this topic in the previous edition.

contralateral gland at the opening of Wharton's duct (strong evidence of dysfunction or obstruction of the right submandibular gland). Any intraoral sources of infection, such as decayed teeth, should be ruled out as a source of submandibular swelling.

IMAGING

The majority of sialoliths are radiopaque and are visible on plain radiographs (panoramic or occlusal radiograph) or CT scans. Some calculi may be radiolucent (not visible radiographically) secondary to the lack of mineralization or smaller size. If there is a high index of suspicion for a sialolith despite negative imaging, a sialogram may be considered. This was frequently used in the past, but it has been largely replaced by CT and ultrasound imaging. Sialography is contraindicated in the setting of acute infection due to a chance of rupturing the duct, and also it can cause significant pain. Ultrasonography and magnetic resonance sialography are other imaging modalities that have been more recently applied for identification of sialoliths.

In the absence of documented caliculi, kinks and strictures should be considered as possible causes of salivary obstruction. Sialography and sialoendoscopy can be useful in diagnosing such anatomic impediments to salivary flow.

For the current patient, a panoramic radiograph revealed a 1-cm radiopaque lesion of the right submandibular area consistent with a sialolith (Figure 7-9, *A*). (It is not uncommon, however, for the sialolith to be undetectable on a panoramic radiograph due to overlap with the body of the mandible or due to the radiolucent nature of a sialolith). A CT scan with intravenous contrast was also obtained to outline the anatomy of the submandibular gland in preparation for surgical excision. The CT scan also revealed a 10-mm stone within the body of the submandibular gland (Figure 7-9, *B*).

LABS

No laboratory studies are indicated in the evaluation and treatment of sialolithiasis unless dictated by the medical history. In the management of sialadenitis, a WBC count may be beneficial for monitoring the progression of an infectious process. In cases of suspected sepsis, adjunctive laboratory studies, such as blood cultures and complete metabolic panels, can be obtained to guide medical and supportive therapy.

ASSESSMENT

Sialolithiasis within the right Wharton's duct with associated localized chronic sialadenitis (inflammation of the submandibular gland).

TREATMENT

There is a considerable body of literature with regard to the treatment of sialolithiasis. Methods have included transductal

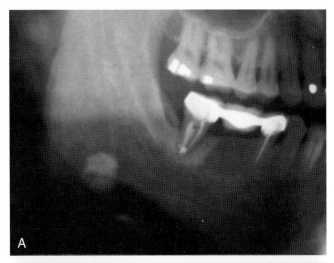

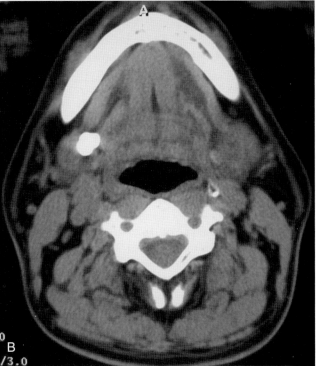

Figure 7-9 **A,** Panoramic radiograph demonstrating a well-demarcated radiopaque lesion in the area of the right mandibular angle. **B,** Contrast-enhanced CT scan demonstrating an 10-mm radiopaque lesion within the body of the submandibular gland consistent with a sialolith.

surgical removal, ductal dilation, lithotripsy, laser ablation, endoscopic retrieval, sialadenectomy (submandibular gland excision), or a combination of these approaches. The size and location of the stone, history of prior treatments, existing medical conditions, availability of resources, and surgeon's preference are among the factors to be considered for optimal treatment planning. Transductal surgical removal is probably the most common technique; up to 70% of sialoliths can be removed by this method. Surgical access to the proximal portion of the duct and the risk for injury to the lingual nerve are among factors limiting the use of this technique.

In select cases, small stones along the anterior portion of Wharton's duct can be managed conservatively with antiinflammatory agents and antibiotics. Moist heat; sialogogues (cholinergic agonists); and certain foods, such as hard, tart candies or sour lemon drops, can be used adjunctively to ameliorate symptoms. Palpable sialoliths can often be "massaged" out, relieving symptoms and alleviating the need for further treatment (although recurrence is not uncommon). Anticholinergics (which decrease salivary gland production) should be avoided when possible. If these measures are unsuccessful, ductal dilation followed by manual expression of the stone may be used to facilitate stone removal. Larger stones in the proximal third of the duct or within the glandular parenchyma that foresee problematic transoral surgical access may be best served by removal of the submandibular gland and ligation of Wharton's duct.

The choice of treatment is based on individual clinical and radiographic findings and surgical judgment. The most important factor in the treatment of sialolithiasis is the presence or absence of clinical symptoms. In the absence of symptoms, treatment may not be necessary. In the presence of signs and symptoms (pain, swelling, purulent drainage) of ductal or glandular obstruction, treatment is typically medical with hydration, systemic antibiotics, and sialogogues to stimulate salivary flow for cleansing of the ductal system.

In this case, given the diagnosis of chronic sialadenitis and the presence of a large sialolith, it was elected to excise the submandibular gland transcutaneously (intraoral removal of the submandibular gland has been reported, but the transcutaneous approach is the most commonly used procedure), along with removal of the existing sialolith. With the patient under general endotracheal anesthesia, an incision was made 1.5 to 2 cm below the inferior border of the mandible (to avoid the marginal mandibular branch of the facial nerve) and dissection was carried through the platysma muscle. The investing layer of deep cervical fascia was incised at the inferior-most extent of the dissection. The facial artery and vein were ligated, and the gland was removed, along with the capsule (which is an extension of the fascia that surrounds the gland). The submandibular duct was identified, and the duct was ligated. The lingual nerve was identified as it courses from lateral to medial (passing inferior to Wharton's duct) by using a vein retractor to reflect the mylohyoid muscle superiorly and anteriorly. The crossing of these two structures takes place in the area of the first and second molars, lateral to the hypoglossal nerve. The surgical specimen (submandibular gland) was sent to pathology for histologic examination (Figure 7-10). A drain was placed to prevent hematoma formation (the decision to place a drain is not uniform among surgeons and depends on intraoperative bleeding due to inflammation of the surrounding tissue and patient-related factors). This was removed the next day. The pathology report confirmed the presence of submandibular calculi within the gland parenchyma that showed extensive fibrosis and destruction of glandular architecture.

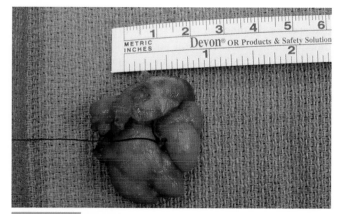

Figure 7-10 Gross specimen of the excised submandibular gland, demonstrating the enlarged and firm gland structure consistent with sialadenitis.

COMPLICATIONS

Depending on the severity of the presenting symptoms and the chronology of the disease process, sialolithiasis may be treated with a variety of methods. A common complication in all modalities that spare the submandibular gland is recurrent, new-onset, or nonresolving sialadenitis. The initial pathologic insult may irreversibly damage the gland (fibrosis of glandular architecture), rendering it incapable of function and thereby prone to sialadenitis. Therefore, in cases of multiple recurrences with nonsurgical therapy or in patients with significant comorbid medical conditions, such as diabetes, that increase the risk of infection, consideration should be given to excision of the gland. In select cases, excision of the gland may be the treatment of choice at the initial presentation. In either scenario, most surgeons elect not to remove the gland during acute episodes of infection, because the existing inflammation can complicate surgical dissection and increase the chances of nerve injury, postoperative infection, and fistula formation. If there is clinical or radiographic evidence of purulence around the gland, an incision and drainage may be performed initially to gain control of the acute process.

A significant complication associated with surgical excision of major salivary glands is nerve injury. Removal of the submandibular gland may be associated with damage to the lingual and hypoglossal nerves or the marginal mandibular branch of the facial nerve. Facial nerve injury is also a complication of parotidectomy (although sialolithiasis of this gland is far less common).

The submandibular glands produce up to 70% of the saliva, so decreased salivary output may be one consequence of sialadenectomy. Patients sometimes complain of subjective xerostomia after submandibular gland excision. This is rarely of any clinical consequence, especially in cases in which the contralateral gland is functioning well.

Postoperative pain and swelling should be managed as with other maxillofacial procedures using a combination of opioids, over-the-counter analgesics (e.g., nonsteroidal antiinflammatory drugs), and steroids as deemed necessary by the treating surgeon. The use of postoperative antibiotics should be based on the status of host factors, preexisting infections, clinical findings, and the experience of the surgeon. Postoperative infection should be managed with antibiotics using culture and sensitivity studies when available and incision and drainage as needed.

DISCUSSION

Sialolithiasis is the most common nonneoplastic disease of the salivary glands and the most common cause of salivary gland obstruction. Patients frequently complain of recurrent pain and swelling of the gland, particularly around mealtimes. Salivary gland calculi are estimated to occur in 1% to 2% of the population. However, the prevalence of symptomatic sialolithiasis is 0.45%. Sialoliths are most common within the body of the submandibular gland or Wharton's duct (80% to 90%). From 5% to 10% of sialoliths occur in the parotid gland/duct, and the remaining 0% to 5% are located within the sublingual or minor salivary glands.

The higher incidence of submandibular sialoliths is likely secondary to the thicker, mucoid secretions of the gland and the long, convoluted, and superiorly directed path of the duct along the anterior floor of the mouth. Wharton's duct has two noteworthy bends (areas more likely to develop sialolithiasis): the genu (knee area), which is located at the posterior border of the mylohyoid muscle, and around the punctum, where the duct makes an acute turn before emptying into the oral cavity. The diameter of the duct ranges from 2 to 4 mm and is narrowest at the punctum.

The etiology of sialolithiasis is not clear. A popular theory is that mineralization occurs around a nidus of organic matter and may be the initial etiologic factor. Bacteria, foreign bodies, ductal epithelial cells, and collections of mucus are thought to be probable sources of this organic matrix. Their retention in the gland and ductal system is likely due to morphoanatomic abnormalities, such as ductal stenosis (obstruction), strictures (constriction), or diverticula (outpouching). Irregular salivary composition is thought to contribute to mineralization around these structures. High concentrations of substances such as calcium combined with low levels of crystallization inhibitors in the saliva are thought to play a role in the continued growth of the calculi, which ultimately may result in obstruction.

In conclusion, a brief mention should be made for the recent advances that have been made with sialoendoscopy and lithotripsy. The procedure is usually initiated by dilating the duct first with lacrimal probes and dilators. Balloon dilatation can also be completed with salivary duct balloon dilators or Fogarty catheters. A sialoendoscope is usually introduced into the duct with continuous irrigation with lactated Ringer's solution under pressure to dilate the duct. Once the sialolith has been visualized within the duct, several methods can be used to dislodge the obstruction. Sialolithectomy is usually performed on sialoliths that are smaller than 7 mm in diameter. When the sialoliths are larger, lithotripsy is indicated, using an intracorporeal or an extracorporeal technique. Lasers (erbium or holmium YAG) are used to generate energy directly over the sialolith, leading to fragmentation in the intracorporeal technique. The smaller fragments can be delivered by a grasping forceps or wire stone removal baskets. Extracorporeal lithotripsy involves applying extraoral acoustic pulses in the direction of the sialolith through an aqueous gel into the soft tissues. The potential energy of the shock wave is transformed to kinetic energy, causing cavitation and fissuring in the stone. Multiple such pulses lead to the fragmentation of the sialolith, and these fragments are removed if they are large or washed out in the saliva.

Postoperative complications with sialoendoscopy and sialoendoscopy-assisted sialolithectomy include failure to remove the calculi, postoperative infection, changes in peripheral nerve function, intraductal adhesion formation, and sialocele or ranula formation. Although gland-sparing treatments have generally been thought to be involved with recurrent infections and the development of new calculi, a review of approximately 1,154 patients treated with sialoendoscopy showed the overall success rate and the long-term symptom-free rate were greater than 90%.

Bibliography

Berini-Aytes L, Gay-Escoda C: Morbidity associated with removal of submandibular gland, *J Craniomaxillofac Surg* 20:216-219, 1992.

Escudier MP, McGurk M: Symptomatic sialoadenitis and sialolithiasis in the English population: an estimate of the cost of hospital treatment, *Br Dent J* 186:463-469, 1999.

Fritsch MH: Sialendoscopy and lithotripsy: literature review, *Otolaryngol Clin North Am* 42(6):915-926, 2009

Grases F, Santiago C, Simonet BM, et al: Sialolithiasis: mechanism of calculi formation and etiologic factors, *Clin Chim Acta* 334(1-2):131-136, 2003.

Jacob RF, Weber RS, King GE: Whole salivary flow rates following submandibular gland resection, *Head Neck* 18:242, 1996.

Marchal F, Dulguerov P: Sialolithiasis management: the state of the art, *Arch Otolaryngol Head Neck Surg* 129:951, 2003.

Marchal F, Kurt AM, Dulguerov P, et al: Histopathology of submandibular glands removed for sialolithiasis, *Ann Otol Rhinol Laryngol* 110:494-499, 2001.

McGurk M, Escudier MP, Brown JE, et al: Modern management of salivary calculi, *Br J Surg* 92(1):107-112, 2005.

Nahlieli O, Shacham R, Shlesinger M, et al: Diagnosis and treatment of strictures and kinks in salivary gland ducts, *J Oral Maxillofac Surg* 59(5):484-490, discussion 490-492; 2001.

Turner M: Sialoendoscopy and salivary gland sparing surgery, *Oral Maxillofac Surgery Clinic North Am* 21(3):323-329, 2009.

Zenk J, Koch M, Klintworth N, et al: Sialendoscopy in the diagnosis and treatment of sialolithiasis: a study on more than 1000 patients, *Otolaryngol Head Neck Surg* 147(5):858-863, 2012.

Acute Suppurative Parotitis*

Ketan Patel, Deepak Kademani, and Shahrokh C. Bagheri

CC

A 25-year-old man presents to the emergency department complaining of right facial swelling. You are consulted for management of a presumed odontogenic infection.

HPI

The patient reports awakening with painful right facial swelling 48 hours earlier. He has noticed a foul taste in his mouth (secondary to oral mucosal dehydration and purulent drainage from Stensen's duct) and has had no appetite. He admits to limited oral intake over the past 24 hours. Over the past 12 hours, he has begun to feel weak and lightheaded and has developed chills. He has not been to a dentist in more than 10 years and acknowledges having several "bad teeth."

PMHX/PDHX/MEDICATIONS/ALLERGIES/SH/FH

The patient is a known alcoholic (risk factor for acute suppurative parotitis) who is presently living in a homeless shelter. He is unaware of any major medical problems or allergies and is not currently taking any medications. There has also been an association between diabetes and parotitis caused by viral infections (mumps), especially in children. Medications that decrease saliva secretion, such as antihistamines and tranquillizers, can also lead to parotitis. Some other nidus of infection, such as chronic tonsillitis or dental abscess, should be ruled out, because these could extend into the periparotid region, mimicking parotitis.

EXAMINATION

General. The patient is a thin man (dehydration and malnutrition) who appears older than his stated age; he is trembling (chills) and appears to be in pain.

Vital signs. His blood pressure is 128/85 mm Hg, heart rate 110 bpm (mild tachycardia secondary to elevated temperature), respirations 16 per minute, and temperature 39.5°C (febrile).

Maxillofacial. He has obvious facial asymmetry, with swelling of the soft tissues over the right preauricular area and angle of the mandible (Figure 7-11). The tissue is indurated, erythematous, and exquisitely tender to palpation (signs of inflammation). He has palpable, mobile, tender lymph nodes in the right precervical chain. His maximum interincisal opening is 25 mm (trismus).

Intraoral. He is partially edentulous, and most of his remaining teeth are grossly carious, including the right mandibular second and third molars. The oral mucous membranes are dry (consistent with dehydration). There is no visible or palpable fluctuance, suppuration, or swelling around any teeth or in the buccal vestibules or floor of the mouth. The uvula is midline, with no fullness of the lateral pharyngeal spaces. Palpation of involved tissues extraorally produces purulence from Stensen's duct on the right. The contralateral duct produces clear saliva, as do both submandibular ducts.

Skin. There is decreased skin turgor with tenting (sign of dehydration, a predisposing factor for acute suppurative parotitis).

IMAGING

A panoramic radiograph is the initial screening study of choice to rule out possible odontogenic sources of infection.

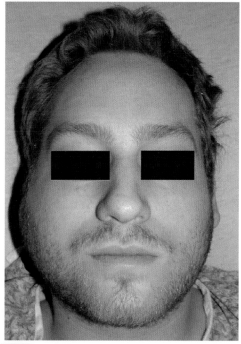

Figure 7-11 Frontal view showing facial asymmetry, with swelling of the soft tissues over the right preauricular area and angle of the mandible.

*The authors and publisher wish to acknowledge Dr. David G. Molen for his contribution on this topic in the previous edition.

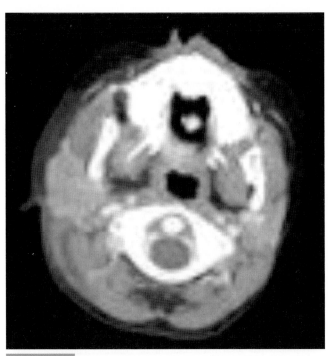

Figure 7-12 Contrast-enhanced CT showing diffuse enlargement of the right parotid parenchyma with stranding.

CT with intravenous contrast is indicated when the source and extent of infection are unclear. Contrast-enhanced CT assists in determining the proper management strategies.

In this patient, the panoramic radiograph reveals multiple grossly carious teeth, consistent with the clinical examination. There are no frank periapical lesions, and no other pathology is noted. Contrast-enhanced CT (which can be rapidly performed and delineates the suspected infectious process when performed with intravenous contrast) shows diffuse enlargement of the right parotid parenchyma with stranding. There are no discrete lesions or loculations in the gland and no involvement of the adjoining potential fascial spaces (Figure 7-12). A sialogram is contraindicated in this setting. (It would pose an increased risk of ductal or glandular rupture and typically is extremely painful in the patient with acute parotitis.)

LABS

A CBC with differential is indicated to evaluate the presenting WBC count. A basic metabolic panel is indicated to rule out metabolic and electrolyte derangements associated with chronic alcohol abuse, dehydration, and malnutrition. Liver function tests may be indicated in chronic alcohol abusers. Blood cultures may be indicated in patients presenting with signs of sepsis. Gram stain and culture and sensitivity of the purulent exudates (if present) ensure that proper antibiotic coverage is maintained.

In the current patient, the WBC count was elevated: $17 \times 10^9/L$. Serum electrolytes were: Na^+ 153 mEq/L (hypernatremia), K^+ 3.6 mEq/L, Cl^- 112 mEq/L, HCO_3^- 20 mEq/L, blood urea nitrogen 28 mg/dl, creatine 1.4 mg/dl, and Mg^{2+} 1.3 mg/dl.

Liver function tests. Aspartate amino transferase 180 U/L, alanine aminotransferase 90 U/L, gamma-glutamyl transpeptidase 90 U/L, and alkaline phosphatase 98 U/L.

Serum amylase and C-reactive protein (CRP) tests can also be performed and usually show marked elevation. A CRP value obtained weekly postoperatively can be used as a marker for resolution of infection.

Microbiology.
- **Gram stain.** Gram-positive cocci in clusters and gram-negative bacilli.
- **KOH.** Few hyphae noted (normal finding).
- **Cultures of purulence from Stensen's duct.** *Staphylococcus aureus* identified after 48 hours.

The patient's electrolyte values are consistent with dehydration (elevated Na^+, blood urea, and creatine), which is common in alcoholics (alcohol suppresses ADH, causing water loss from the kidneys). Low magnesium and elevated liver enzymes, with the aspartate amino transferase/alanine aminotransferase ratio 2:1 or greater, are also common with chronic alcohol abuse.

ASSESSMENT

Acute suppurative parotitis with associated dehydration in an alcoholic patient.

TREATMENT

The management of patients with acute suppurative parotitis is primarily medical, consisting of rehydration with intravenous fluids, initiation of empiric antibiotic therapy, nutritional support, and stimulation of salivary flow (sialogogues). Surgical intervention may be necessary when demonstrated areas of loculation are present within the gland. More than 80% of cases are caused by *S. aureus;* therefore, empiric first-line antibiotic treatment includes the β-lactamase–resistant penicillins, first-generation cephalosporins, or clindamycin. A review by Brook found strict anaerobes to be the causative agent in 43% of cases of acute suppurative parotitis; cultures and sensitivities should be followed closely and antibiotic therapy adjusted accordingly, for a total course of 10 to 14 days. Most patients should respond to aggressive medical management within 3 to 5 days. Extraoral incision and drainage of the capsule of the parotid may be indicated for failure to respond to medical therapy. Follow-up after resolution with sialography and/or repeat CT scan to determine possible underlying treatable explanations for the episode (stones, duct strictures, or tumor) may be indicated.

COMPLICATIONS

There are rare reports of patients with acute suppurative parotitis developing cervical necrotizing fasciitis. Possible infectious complications also include facial nerve dysfunction, septicemia, mastoiditis/osteomyelitis, and spread into adjacent fascial spaces, with possible airway compromise. The reported mortality rate of acute suppurative parotitis

| Box 7-4 | **Categorization of Parotitis to Guide Management** |

- **Acute (bacterial) suppurative parotitis (ASP).** This is caused by colonization of the gland by oral bacteria that have migrated in a retrograde fashion through Stensen's duct. Patients almost invariably have a comorbid state, causing decreased salivary flow and/or immunosuppression. Common contributors to this relatively uncommon condition are diabetes, alcoholism, autoimmune disorders (e.g., Sjögren's disease), medications (e.g., tricyclic antidepressants, anticholinergics, or diuretics), dehydration, malnutrition, neoplasm, or ductal obstruction. It is most common in debilitated elderly patients (nursing home or hospitalized patients) but has been described in all populations. The hallmark of ASP is frank suppuration, along with the cardinal signs of inflammation: tumor (swelling), rubor (redness), calor (heat), dolor (pain), and *functio laesa* (loss of function). Sialography can be beneficial at follow-up in diagnosing ductal disorders or obstructions. However, it should be avoided in the acute stage, because the increased pressure can be exquisitely painful and may rupture an already dilated duct.
- **Nonsuppurative parotitis (NSP) (parotid sialadenitis).** The list of other causes of parotid inflammation and swelling that will not cause frank suppuration is lengthy and includes viruses, granulomatous inflammation, and autoimmune disorders. Although frank suppuration is not present, the gland can still be milked for discharge, which can be sent for viral or microbial studies. The most common viral cause of parotitis is paramyxovirus (mumps), although others must be considered (Epstein-Barr virus, coxsackievirus, herpes simplex, cytomegalovirus). HIV can cause bilateral parotid enlargement secondary to intraglandular lymphadenopathy. The most common cause of granulomatous parotid inflammation is *Mycobacterium tuberculosis*. Other mycobacterium, *Actinomycosis* species, and cat-scratch disease *(Bartonella henselae)* may need to be considered. Autoimmune states head the list of "other" causes and usually lead to bilateral parotid swelling. Common culprits are Sjögren's

disease, systemic lupus erythematosus, diabetes, cystic fibrosis, and collagen vascular disease. Nonsuppurative infectious states should be treated accordingly; noninfectious inflammation is usually addressed by treating the underlying disease state and avoiding low-flow salivary states and antisialagogue medications whenever possible.
- **Chronic recurrent parotitis (CRP).** This entity has been described as a nonspecific parotid sialadenitis with episodes of swelling and remission or persistent swelling with recurrent infection, either unilaterally or bilaterally. The overlap with the two previously discussed disease states is the cause of much confusion, and often the diagnosis of CRP is delayed until further investigations and resolution of the presenting complaint, especially with recurrent episodes. A state of CRP can also be initiated by many of the same diseases that contribute to ASP and NSP. Diagnosis is made upon discovery of characteristic changes in the ductal and parenchymal architecture of the gland. These changes can be noted on sialography, CT, MRI, scintigraphy, or combinations thereof. Early findings include ectasia and dilatation of peripheral ducts, progressing to "sausaging" of the primary duct and continuing to destruction of parenchyma, with extravasation of contrast material in late stages. Treatment is usually supportive when patients are symptomatic and includes antibiotics when appropriate, sialogogues, short-term oral steroids (dexamethasone), and dilatation of Stensen's duct with lacrimal probes to encourage drainage. Lavage with normal saline or penicillin solutions has been advocated to facilitate resolution of symptoms due to stasis of salivary flow or the presence of sialoliths. The treatment of last resort for troublesome recurrent or refractory cases is parotidectomy, either superficial or total, and should not be entertained until conservative treatment options have been exhausted. Both operations have risks of facial nerve dysfunction, with a slightly greater risk with total parotidectomy.

approaches 25%. Acute suppurative parotitis is also seen as a complication of chronic recurrent parotitis, which may ultimately necessitate superficial or total parotidectomy (see Discussion). In the setting of acute suppurative parotitis, the criterion for parotidectomy is recurrence after two episodes of medical management; elective parotidectomy should be performed only after a period of 4 to 6 weeks of quiescence to allow for identification and preservation of the facial nerve in a noninflamed surgical field.

DISCUSSION

The term "parotitis" is a generic designation for parotid swelling with an inflammatory component. The aim of diagnosis should be to categorize the patient with parotitis into one of three possible subcategories to guide management (Box 7-4):

- Acute (bacterial) suppurative parotitis
- Nonsuppurative parotitis (parotid sialadenitis)
- Chronic recurrent parotitis

Organisms involved in acute suppurative sialadenitis of the parotid gland include aerobic, facultative, and anaerobic bacteria. In a study conducted by Brooks and colleagues, the main aerobic bacterial species isolated was *S. aureus,* and the main anaerobic organisms were *Peptostreptococcus* spp. When culturing for anaerobic organisms, specimens from Stensen's duct should be avoided due to oropharyngeal contamination. Needle aspiration of the purulent gland can yield a better specimen that is free of contamination.

Bibliography

Antoniades D, Harrison J, Epivatianos A, et al: Treatment of chronic sialadenitis by intraductal penicillin or saline, *J Oral Maxillofac Surg* 62(4):431-434, 2004.

Baurmash H: Chronic recurrent parotitis: a closer look at its origin, diagnosis, and management, *J Oral Maxillofac Surg* 8(62):1010-1018, 2004.

Brook I: Acute bacterial suppurative parotitis: microbiology and management, *J Craniofac Surg* 14(1):37-40, 2003.

Brook I: Non-odontogenic abscesses in the head and neck region, *Periodontology 2000* 49:106-125, 2009.

Brook I: The bacteriology of salivary gland infections, *Oral Maxillofacial Surg Clin North Am* 3(21):267-274, 2009.

Fattahi T, Lyu P, Van Sickels J: Management of acute suppurative parotitis, *J Oral Maxillofac Surg* 60(4):446-448, 2002.

Marioni G, Bottin R, Tregnaghi A, et al: Craniocervical necrotizing fasciitis secondary to parotid gland abscess, *Acta Otolaryngol* 123(6):737-740, 2003.

Motamed M, Laugharne D, Bradley PJ: Management of chronic parotitis: a review, *J Laryngol Otol* 117(7):521-526, 2003.

Nahlieli O, Bar T, Shacham R, et al: Management of chronic recurrent parotitis: current therapy, *J Oral Maxillofac Surg* 62(9):1150-1155, 2004.

O'Brien CJ, Murrant NJ: Surgical management of chronic parotitis, *Head Neck* 15(5):445-449, 1993.

Pou AM, Johnson JT, Weissman J: Management decisions in parotitis, *Compr Ther* 21(2):85-92, 1995.

Differential Diagnosis of a Neck Mass

Kevin L. Rieck and Shahrokh C. Bagheri

CC

A 63-year-old man is referred for evaluation of a mass in his neck.

HPI

The patient reports a several-month history of a midline submandibular neck swelling that he associated with an abscessed tooth. A mandibular tooth was subsequently removed by his dentist, but the patient indicates no improvement. He reports that the area is slightly tender (swellings of neoplastic origin are unlikely to be painful or tender). He further indicates the swelling under his jaw had been present for many months (chronic process) but became bothersome over the past several weeks. There are no associated symptoms of hoarseness or dysphagia (as would be seen with impingement of a mass on the vocal cords or posterior oropharynx). There is no history of recent weight loss (cachexia could be a sign of a malignant process). He does not have any complaints of airway obstruction or difficulty breathing (an expanding mass could progressively impinge on the airway).

PMHX/PDHX/ MEDICATIONS/ALLERGIES/SH/FH

The patient has no significant past medical or surgical history. There is no family history of similar presentations. He does not have any risk factors for neoplastic causes of his neck mass (smoking, alcohol). His abscessed tooth could cause submandibular swelling, but this would be unlikely due to persistence of symptoms after removal of the infectious source.

Patients should be questioned regarding a history of malignancies that may present with a metastatic lesion in the neck.

EXAMINATION

General. The patient is a well-developed and well-nourished male in no apparent distress.

Vital signs. Vital signs are stable, and he is afebrile (fever and the associated elevation in baseline heart rate can be secondary to an infectious etiology). Tumors can also cause fever either secondary to associated inflammation/infection or due to the release of inflammatory mediators, such as tumor necrosis factor.

Maxillofacial. There is a soft, doughy midline swelling of the submandibular area measuring 6 cm in diameter. The mass is freely movable subcutaneously with no clear attachment to the overlying skin. No fluctuance or frank fluid component is appreciated within the mass upon bimanual examination. It is not warm to palpation (seen with inflammation). The overlying skin appears normal (Figure 7-13). No palpable cervical adenopathy is noted (palpable adenopathy may be a harbinger of metastasis or inflammation).

Intraoral. Partial edentulism is noted, with no gross areas of decay in the remaining dentition. There are no soft tissue lesions in the oral cavity. Salivary flow appears normal and without evidence of obstruction or erythema at the orifices of the submandibular and parotid ducts (an important finding that makes sialadenitis unlikely). The muscles of mastication

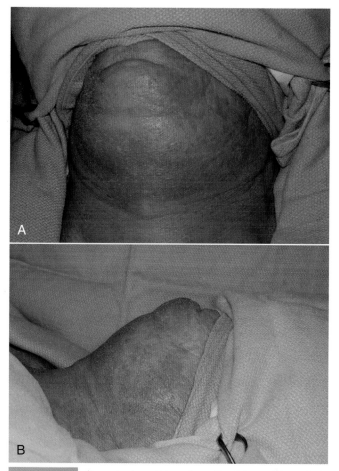

A

B

Figure 7-13 Frontal view (**A**) and profile (**B**) swelling of the submandibular area measuring 6 cm in diameter. The overlying skin appears normal.

and temporomandibular joints are unremarkable. Bimanual intraoral examination also reveals a palpable mass in the midline floor of the mouth that appears to be contiguous with the anterior neck mass. The mass does not elevate with tongue protrusion or swallowing (elevation of the mass would be consistent with a thyroglossal duct cyst).

IMAGING

Panoramic, lateral cephalometric or lateral neck films are rarely used in evaluating a neck mass. The panoramic radiograph should be used as a screening tool for evaluation of the dentition if there is suspicion of an odontogenic source of infection.

For the current patient the panoramic radiograph demonstrated no source of odontogenic or osseous pathology. The contrast-enhanced CT scan showed a 5-cm, cystic-appearing mass in the anterior midline neck between the mandible and the hyoid bone (Figure 7-14). Several spherical densities were noted within the lesion. There was no evidence of adenopathy. The mass appeared discrete and not attached to the overlying skin.

LABS

No specific laboratory tests are indicated in the absence of pertinent medical history.

DIFFERENTIAL DIAGNOSIS

The differential diagnosis of a neck mass can be quite extensive and can include any or all of the intricate structures in the neck. There are several considerations in distinguishing

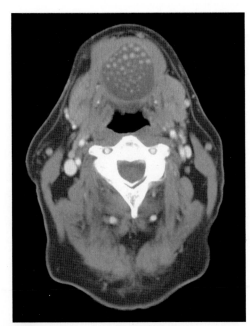

Figure 7-14 Contrast-enhanced CT scan showing a 5-cm, cystic-appearing mass in the anterior midline neck between the mandible and the hyoid bone.

between inflammatory and/or infectious causes, anatomic variants, congenital lesions, and benign or malignant processes. One of the most important aspects in assessing a neck mass is a thorough patient history. The age of the patient is an important initial consideration. An adult patient over the age of 40 has an 80% chance that a nonthyroid neck mass will be neoplastic; of these, 80% of cases are metastatic squamous cell carcinoma from the aerodigestive tract. Figure 7-15 presents a flow chart for the diagnosis of a neck mass that incorporates age and location as distinguishing factors.

In general, for differential diagnosis of a neck mass, it is useful to consider four broad categories: anatomic, inflammatory and/or infectious, congenital, and neoplastic (Box 7-5).

The clinician must maintain a high index of suspicion for metastatic disease processes. These commonly include squamous cell cancers of the head and neck, in addition to lung, thyroid, and salivary gland malignancies. Melanoma may also present in this area. Primary neck tumors presenting as a neck mass typically result from salivary gland lesions, lymphoma, or thyroid masses. Benign masses result from several of the tissues in the neck. These can include lipomas, neural tumors, vascular lesions, sebaceous cysts, and fibromas.

ASSESSMENT

A well-circumscribed soft tissue mass of the anterior midline neck.

Fine-needle aspiration (FNA) was performed and revealed scant cellular material. Diagnosis would require surgical exploration with an excisional biopsy.

TREATMENT

The current patient underwent a cervical exploration under general anesthesia in the hospital. Prior to any incision, the lesion was aspirated and returned several milliliters of a viscous, yellowish fluid. A transverse incision was made in the anterior neck well below the mass. Subcutaneous skin flaps were raised, and the platysma muscle was identified. Blunt dissection was performed around the mass. The mylohyoid muscle was identified and divided in the midline. No communication with the oral cavity was encountered. The mass was removed and submitted for permanent histopathologic examination (Figure 7-16). A drain was placed in the neck defect, and the wound was closed in standard layered fashion.

The pathologic diagnosis revealed the lesion to be a dermoid cyst. These cysts can have tremendous histologic variability. There is a connective tissue wall that may have a thin lining of epithelial cells. This can exhibit keratinization, and the lumen may be filled with keratin and a sebaceous fluid. Glandular components from apocrine or sebaceous tissue may also be present.

COMPLICATIONS

Several complications can occur in performing neck surgery. Hematomas; seromas; wound infections; injury to branches

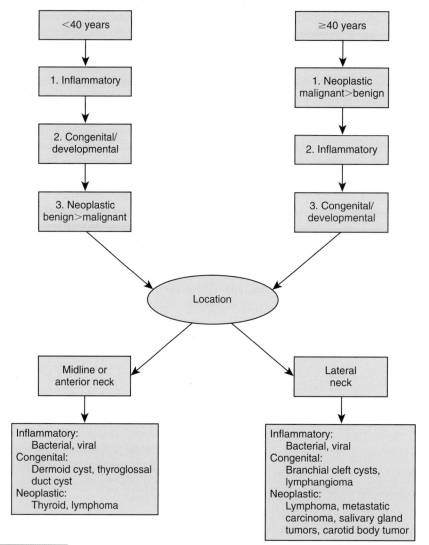

Figure 7-15   Evaluation of a neck mass using age and location as distinguishing factors.

of the facial, trigeminal, or hypoglossal nerves; and atypical scar formation are all possible sequelae. Surgeons must have a thorough understanding of anatomy to effectively recognize and manage lesions and complications in this complex area.

DISCUSSION

The diagnostic challenge in assessing a neck mass can be overwhelming. It is important to have a consistent system in both history taking and examination aspects in the approach to this complex anatomic region. Onset, duration, size fluctuations, or progression and any associated symptoms must be elucidated from the patient when possible. Similarly, the association of squamous cell carcinoma with alcohol and tobacco abuse has been well documented, and the patient's present and past use of these products should be noted. Any recent exposure to infectious diseases, trauma, animals (cats), dental work, or surgical intervention should be determined.

The adult patient presenting with a neck mass should have a thorough history taken to assist the diagnosis. Supplemental

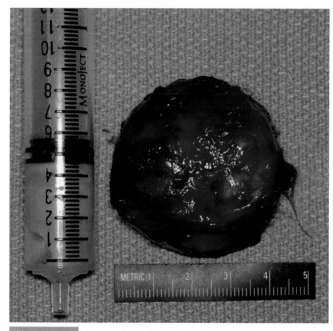

Figure 7-16   Surgical specimen, later diagnosed as a dermoid cyst.

| Box 7-5 | **Four Major Categories for Differential Diagnosis of a Neck Mass** |

- **Anatomic.** Several anatomic structures are palpable in certain patients. These include the transverse process of C1, the hyoid bone, the thyroid and cricoid cartilages, and prominent or atherosclerotic carotid bulbs.
- **Inflammatory and/or infectious.** This category encompasses several causes for a neck mass, which is generally a reactive process. Cervical adenitis can arise from bacterial, viral, parasitic, and fungal sources. *Staphylococcus aureus,* cutaneous skin infections, Epstein-Barr virus, and herpes simplex viruses are frequent culprits. Other inflammatory causes include infectious and/or obstructive lesions of the salivary glands. Sialadenitis and associated sialolithiasis of the major salivary glands can cause significant swelling in the neck.
- **Congenital lesions or masses.** These are frequently recognized at an early age but may also present later in life with the onset of new symptoms. Several common disorders are encountered: thyroglossal duct cyst, branchial cleft cyst or fistula, cystic hygroma, dermoid cyst, lymphangioma, and ranula. Other rare conditions, such as thymic mass, laryngoceles, and teratomas, also can occur.
  - **Thyroglossal duct cysts** are midline or anterior neck masses. These frequently appear post upper respiratory tract infection. The mass itself moves with swallowing or tongue protrusion. The cyst, thyroglossal tract, and midportion of the hyoid bone are removed in the Sistrunk procedure to treat this condition.
  - **Dermoid cysts** are midline masses that lie deep to the cervical fascia and tend to be slow growing. They are above the hyoid bone and do not move with protrusion of the tongue.
  - **Branchial cleft cysts** are remnants of the branchial arch apparatus present during embryogenesis.
  - **First branchial cleft cysts** (two types are possible):
    - (a) **Type I cysts** tend to occur in the preauricular or postauricular region and connect the skin to the external auditory canal.
    - (b) **Type II cysts** are near the mandibular angle and closely associated with the parotid gland.
  - **Second branchial cleft cysts** are the most common of the branchial cleft cysts. The cyst or opening to the cyst is usually found at the anterior edge of the sternocleidomastoid muscle.
  - **Third branchial cleft cysts** are very rare. These are also found along the anterior border of the sternocleidomastoid muscle but ultimately empty into the piriform sinus.
  - **Fourth branchial cleft cysts** can occur and have an extensive course through the neck, looping around the hypoglossal nerve and aortic arch.
- **Neoplastic.** Neoplastic lesions in the neck are common and have certain characteristics that set them apart from other conditions. Masses fixed to the underlying structures and matted nodes are ominous findings for malignancy.

evaluation with ultrasound, CT, MRI, or positron emission tomography (PET) scans, in addition to FNA of the mass, can be extremely useful in further defining the lesion. Suspected inflammatory or infectious conditions should respond to broad-spectrum antibiotics. Suspected neoplastic masses should be evaluated with contrast-enhanced CT scans and FNA of the mass.

The current patient tolerated the surgical procedure well and had an uneventful postoperative course. Histopathologic evaluation confirmed the diagnosis of a dermoid cyst. This is thought to result from entrapment of midline epithelial tissue during the closure of the mandibular and hyoid branchial arches. In this location, they are rarely present at birth and typically present in young adulthood. As in this case, these cysts typically feel doughlike, but this can vary with the actual contents of the cyst. They can be either above or below the mylohyoid.

Bibliography

Armstrong WB, Giglio MF: Is this lump in the neck anything to worry about? *Postgrad Med* 104(3):63-78, 1998.

Cummings CW, Fredrickson JM, Harker LA, et al: *Otolaryngology: head and neck surgery,* ed 2, vol 2, pp 1543-1565, St Louis, 1993, Mosby.

Gujar S, Gandhi D, Mukherji SK, et al: Pediatric head and neck masses, *Top Magn Reson Imaging* 15(2):95-101, 2004.

Lee J, Fernandes R: Neck masses: evaluation and diagnostic approach, *Oral Maxillofacial Clin North Am* 20:321-337, 2008.

Prakash PK, Hanna FW: Differential diagnosis of neck lumps, *Practitioner* 246(1633):252-254, 259, 2002.

Prisco MK: Evaluating neck masses, *Nurse Pract* 25(4):50-51, 2002.

Rosa PA, Hirsch DL, Dierks EJ: Congenital neck masses, *Oral Maxillofacial Clin North Am* 20:339-352, 2008.

Schwetschenau E, Kelley DJ: The adult neck mass, *Am Fam Physician* 66(5):831-838, 2002.

Shafer WG, Hine MK, Levy BM, editors: *Textbook of oral pathology,* ed 4, pp 75-79, Philadelphia, 1983, Saunders.

Thawley SE, Panje WR, editors: *Comprehensive management of head and neck tumors,* vol 2, pp 1230-1240, Philadelphia, 1987, Saunders.

Oral Leukoplakia*

Ketan Patel, Deepak Kademani, and Shahrokh C. Bagheri

CC

A 53-year-old man is referred to your office by his general dentist for evaluation of an intraoral lesion that was found during a routine dental examination. (The prevalence of oral leukoplakia increases with age and has a strong male predilection.)

HPI

The patient presents with a painless, asymptomatic white lesion (leukoplakia) of the right buccal mucosa (lip vermilion, buccal mucosa, and gingiva are the most common sites) (Figure 7-17). He was not aware of the lesion until his general dentist detected it during a routine oral exam. The lesion has been present for an unknown duration. He denies any history of trauma, cheek biting (morsicatio buccarum), or parafunctional habits (chewing tobacco, snuff, sunflower seeds, or other foreign objects that may cause frictional keratosis). He denies any history of fevers, weight loss, dysphagia, or other constitutional symptoms.

PMHX/PSHX/MEDICATIONS/ALLERGIES/SH/FH

The patient's history is significant for a 44-pack-per-year history of smoking (higher incidence in patients using tobacco on a routine basis).

EXAMINATION

General. The patient is a white man who appears his stated age. He is well nourished with no signs of cachexia (seen with advanced malignant disease or malnutrition).

Maxillofacial. There is a 1.3×0.8 cm, well-circumscribed, slightly elevated white plaque of the right midbuccal mucosa just inferior to the occlusal plane (presents as linea alba on the buccal mucosa). The lesion is soft, nonindurated, nonulcerated, and nonadherent to underlying tissues (firm, indurated, ulcerated, and/or fixed lesions can be a sign of invasive carcinoma). The lesion does not rub off with gauze (white lesions that can be scraped off have a separate differential diagnosis) and does not form a bulla with firm pressure (negative Nikolsky sign). No Wickham striae are present (seen in

lichen planus). The lesion does not diminish or disappear when stretched (seen in leukoedema). No other lesions or masses are noted. He is partially edentulous with poor oral hygiene and no grossly carious teeth.

Neck. No cervical or submandibular lymphadenopathy is noted.

IMAGING

Imaging for soft tissue lesions is based on the clinical presentation and differential diagnosis. This lesion is a superficial mucosal lesion that does not appear to invade underlying structures; therefore, no imaging studies are required.

LABS

No routine laboratory studies are indicated for a planned biopsy or workup of a white lesion in an otherwise healthy patient.

DIFFERENTIAL DIAGNOSIS

The working differential diagnosis of a white lesion of the buccal mucosa that cannot be scraped off should include hyperkeratosis with or without dysplasia (histologic diagnosis), lichen planus, morsicatio buccarum (chronic cheek biting), frictional keratosis, nicotine stomatitis, leukoedema, and white sponge nevus. The diagnosis of leukoplakia is one of exclusion; the lesion presents as a white plaque that cannot

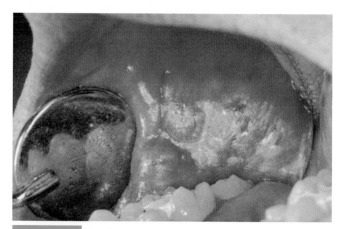

Figure 7-17 Leukoplakia of the right buccal mucosa. (*From Rose LF, Mealey BL, Genco RJ, et al: Periodontics: medicine, surgery and implants, St Louis, 2004, Mosby.*)

*The authors and publisher wish to acknowledge Dr. Derek H. Lamb for his contribution on this topic in the previous edition.

be removed and requires biopsy for histologic confirmation. Because leukoplakia is considered a premalignant lesion with a risk of malignant transformation, squamous cell carcinoma is included in the differential diagnosis.

BIOPSY

Definitive diagnosis requires an incisional or excisional biopsy, depending on the size and character of the lesion. Typically, lesions less than 1 cm can be easily excised and closed primarily, whereas an incisional biopsy is indicated for larger lesions or when a malignancy is suspected.

In this patient, an excisional biopsy was performed under local anesthesia (direct infiltration into the lesion should be avoided to prevent distortion of the specimen). The specimen showed full-thickness (from basal layer to surface mucosa) epithelial dysplasia with cellular atypia, loss of rete peg formation with mucosal atrophy, and superficial parakeratosis. The integrity of the basement membrane was maintained, indicating carcinoma in situ (if the dysplastic cells invaded through the basement membrane into the underlying submucosa, invasive squamous cell carcinoma would be the correct diagnosis).

ASSESSMENT

Oral leukoplakia with biopsy-proved diagnosis of carcinoma in situ (T is N_0 M_0, stage 0 squamous cell carcinoma) of the right buccal mucosa.

TREATMENT

Traditionally, the first line of treatment of white oral lesions has been identification and elimination of possible etiologic factors. This is followed by a 2-week period of observation. Persistent lesions with no identifiable cause are biopsied to establish a diagnosis. The resulting diagnosis should dictate the subsequent management. Toluidine blue may be used to identify potential biopsy sites that are more likely to exhibit dysplastic changes. Exfoliative cytology can be used for the evaluation of mucosal lesions (this has the advantage of being less invasive and of not requiring local anesthesia). However, a biopsy is required for a definitive diagnosis.

Current treatment is aimed at prevention of malignant transformation and resolution of the lesion. Biopsy-proved hyperkeratosis (gives the lesion its white, textured appearance) without dysplasia can be closely observed for changes, whereas hyperkeratosis with mild to moderate dysplasia can be treated with carbon dioxide laser ablation. Severe dysplasia or carcinoma in situ requires wide local excision. Laser excision, ablation, or a combination of the two can also be performed, depending on the location of the leukoplakia.

Chemopreventive measures (β-carotene, vitamin A, or retinoids) have been shown to reverse leukoplakias; however, there are limitations (therapy must be maintained indefinitely, patient compliance is low). Although there are a variety of clinical trials underway for several potential agents, such as rapamycin, celecoxib, and pioglitazone, no randomized controlled trials have proven the efficacy of these drugs.

Lasers are widely used for the treatment of premalignant and malignant lesions. The CO_2 lasers are by far the highest power, continuous wave lasers currently available. They are useful in oral surgical procedures, because the energy is maximally absorbed by water in the oral tissues. The advantages of lasers include minimal damage to adjacent tissues, delayed acute inflammatory reaction, and reduced myofibroblastic activity, leading to reduced wound contraction and scarring. The laser-treated wound bed can be left exposed to granulate without the need of a skin graft. Several studies have shown good results with laser ablation of leukoplakias, with a 90% efficacy and a low rate of recurrence.

The current patient underwent an excisional biopsy of the lesion under local anesthesia. An elliptical incision was made around the entire lesion and into the submucosa (the junction of the basement membrane and submucosa is important in the evaluation for possible invasive carcinoma). Normal-appearing tissue surrounding the area is also included in the biopsy specimen to ensure clear margins. Electrocautery is used to provide hemostasis of the surgical bed. The wound is closed primarily. The surgical specimen is oriented with sutures of different length placed at the anterior and superior margins.

The histopathologic report confirmed carcinoma in situ, which requires a wide local excision of the entire lesion for histologic documentation.

COMPLICATIONS

The main concern with oral leukoplakia is the risk of malignant transformation. Leukoplakia is a premalignant lesion, implying that it is "a morphologically altered tissue in which cancer is more likely to occur than in its normal counterpart." The rate of malignant transformation of oral leukoplakia (homogeneous type) is between 3% and 6%. Erythroplakia, which is much less common than leukoplakia, has a much higher transformation rate (20% to 90%) and always requires surgical excision. Consequently, it is very important for these patients to be followed closely for any mucosal changes so that prompt treatment can be provided to reduce the morbidity and mortality from malignant transformation.

DISCUSSION

The World Health Organization defines leukoplakia as "a white patch or plaque that cannot be characterized clinically or pathologically as any other disease." It is, therefore, a diagnosis of exclusion. Leukoplakia is a condition that is frequently encountered in the oral cavity and is most commonly found on the lip vermillion, buccal mucosa, and gingiva. However, lesions of the floor of the mouth, tongue, and lower lip are most likely to exhibit dysplasia and are associated with a higher rate of malignant transformation. The prevalence in the general population is estimated to vary from less than 1% to greater than 5%. The presence of leukoplakia has been associated with tobacco smoking (although the rate of malignant transformation with smokeless tobacco has not definitively been shown to be higher), sanguinaria, ultraviolet radiation, and microorganisms, such as *Treponema pallidum* (mucous patch of stage 2 syphilis), *Candida albicans,* and human papilloma virus.

Lesions may present as a white patch (leukoplakia), a white patch with red dots (speckled leukoplakia), or a mixed red and white lesion (erythroleukoplakia). Lesions with areas of mixed erythema frequently contain advanced dysplasia or invasive squamous cell carcinoma (biopsy of mixed lesions should include the red component). Leukoplakic lesions are classified histopathologically according to the degree of dysplasia or histology of the cellular and other epithelial elements. Mild dysplasia is cellular atypia that is limited to the basilar and parabasilar epithelial layers. Moderate dysplasia involves the basal layer up to the midportion of the spinous layer. Severe dysplasia is atypia that extends more than halfway through the epithelium but does not involve the full thickness. Carcinoma in situ is defined as dysplasia of the entire epithelial layer without invasion of the basement membrane into the underlying tissue.

Most leukoplakias do not transform into carcinomas, and recent studies have attempted to identify molecular markers for malignant transformation. Potential areas that have been explored are DNA ploidy status; loss of heterozygosity, using microsatellite markers, p53 mutations, and aberrant expression; inappropriate expression of other oncogenes (e.g., cyclin D1); and differentiation markers, such as keratins and cell surface carbohydrates, including blood group antigens.

Another aggressive form of this disease is proliferative verrucous leukoplakia. Interestingly, proliferative verrucous leukoplakia is not associated with tobacco use, and it has a strong female predilection. It has a high recurrence rate and a tendency to slowly spread to involve multiple oral sites. Proliferative verrucous leukoplakia has a high rate of malignant transformation (to verrucous or squamous cell carcinoma).

Figure 7-18 shows a case of severe leukoplakia under denture-bearing tissue in another patient. There was evidence of moderate dysplasia on biopsy of the midpalatal area.

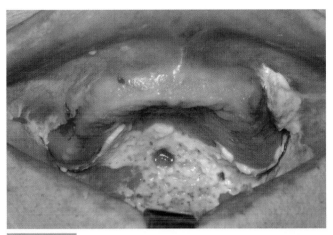

Figure 7-18 Extensive leukoplakia of the palate in a different patient, who showed evidence of moderate dysplasia upon biopsy.

Bibliography

Chandu A, Smith AC: The use of CO_2 laser in the treatment of oral white patches: outcomes and factors affecting recurrence, *Int J Oral Maxillofac Surg* 34(4):396-400, 2009.

Jerjes W, Hamdoon Z, Hopper C, et al: CO_2 lasers in the management of potentially malignant and malignant oral disorders, *Head Neck Oncol* 4:17, 2012.

Jerjes W, Upile T, Hamdoon Z, et al: CO_2 lasers for oral dysplasias: clinicopathological features or recurrence and malignant transformation, *Lasers Med Sci* 27(1):169-179, 2012.

Rhodus NL: Oral cancer: leukoplakia and squamous cell carcinoma, *Dent Clin North Am* 49:143-165, 2005.

Saito T, Suguira C, Hirai A, et al: Development of squamous cell carcinoma from preexisting oral leucoplakia with respect to treatment modality, *Int J Oral Maxillofac Surg* 30:49-53, 2001.

Silverman S Jr: Leukoplakia, dysplasia, and malignant transformation [editorial], *Oral Surg Oral Med Oral Pathol* 82:117-125, 1996.

Slaughter DP, Southwick HW, Smejkal W: Field cancerization in oral stratified squamous epithelium: clinical implications of multicentric origin, *Cancer* 6(5):963-968, 1953.

Van der Hem PS, Nauta JM, van der Wal JE, et al: The results of CO_2 laser surgery in patients with oral leukoplakia: a 25 year follow up, *Oral Oncol* 41(1):31-37, 2005.

Vigliante CE, Quinn PD, Alwai F: Proliferative verrucous leukoplakia: a case report with characteristic long term progression, *J Oral Maxillofac Surg* 61:626-631, 2003.

Osteoradionecrosis

Shahrokh C. Bagheri and Abtin Shahriari

CC

A 67-year-old man is referred to your office for evaluation of exposed bone of the left posterior mandible subsequent to full-mouth extraction. (Osteoradionecrosis [ORN] is more commonly seen in the elderly and in the posterior mandible.)

HPI

The patient has a history of squamous cell carcinoma of the left tonsillar fossa, which had been treated with a total dose of 7,300 centiGrays (cGy) of external radiation 1 year earlier (cGy is the unit for radiation that has replaced the equivalent unit of rad). Full-mouth extraction was performed 9 months after completion of radiation therapy. During the past 3 months, the patient has developed a nonhealing, painful wound of the left mandible. He has been on several different antibiotics and oral chlorhexidine, with no apparent resolution. His current pain level has been difficult to manage with opioid analgesics. In addition, he reports that he has lost more than 10 pounds in the past 2 months (due to decreased oral intake). One month ago, he heard a cracking noise on his left mandible, with associated pain (suggestive of a pathologic fracture). More recently, the skin overlying his mandible has developed an orocutaneous fistula.

The risk for development of ORN after radiation therapy has been declining in recent years. The incidence has been reported to range from 4.7% to 37.1%. A more recent review by Nabil and Samman placed the risk at 2.7%. This reduction may be attributed to modification of risk factors. The most important risk factor for the development of osteoradionecrosis is the radiation dose. High-dose radiotherapy (above 7,200 cGy) is likely to reach the clinical threshold for the development of ORN, compared to a moderate dose (5,000 cGy to 6,400 cGy). Patients are generally at a progressively increasing risk with doses above 5,000 cGy.

The risk of developing ORN is also related to other factors, including location of the primary tumor, size of the tumor, proximity of the tumor to bone, condition of the dentition, and type of treatment (external beam radiotherapy, brachytherapy, surgery, or chemotherapy). Other medical comorbidities that influence wound healing (e.g., nutritional status, oral hygiene, prior mandibulectomy or osteotomy) and extrinsic factors (e.g., tobacco or alcohol abuse) are likely to play a role. However, the radiation dose and the time elapsed since radiation therapy are the most significant risk factors. The size of the tumor is also important, because there is a higher incidence with T3 and T4 tumors.

The incidence of osteoradionecrosis increases with increased proximity of the primary tumor to the mandible. The highest incident is seen with tumors of the posterior lateral tongue, floor of the mouth, alveolar ridge, and retromolar trigone area. Maxillary osteoradionecrosis is more common with sinonasal and nasopharyngeal carcinoma.

There are three basic types of radiotherapy protocols. External beam radiotherapy is the most common (this includes intensity-modulated radiation therapy [IMRT]), followed by interstitial (or implant-seeded) radiotherapy. The third type is neutron beam radiotherapy, which is the most damaging both to normal tissue and to tumor cells. The latter is rarely used due to its complications. Radiation entails high linear energy transferred to tissue with the intent to kill cancer cells. External beam radiotherapy is usually achieved with cobalt-60 radiation-emitting beta-particles that collide with water molecules, splitting them into free radicals, such as superoxide O·, and hydroxyl OH·, which react with DNA, RNA, enzyme systems, and cell membranes. Most cells survive but incur internal damage to the cell structures, resulting in impairment of cell division. Consequently, the tissue becomes progressively less cellular, less vascular, and hypoxic. The frequency of radiation therapy, such as accelerated fractionation (shortening of the intervals between radiation therapy sessions) or hyperfractionation (increasing the total dose but decreasing the dose per fraction), affects the risk for osteoradionecrosis remains unclear.

IMRT uses dose-volume relationships and computer imaging to substantially localize the delivered radiation and reduce the dose received by the mandible, with the goal of reducing the risk of ORN. The advantages of IMRT include (1) delivery of high doses to the target volume; (2) relative sparing of normal structures in the head and neck because of the sharp dose gradient, and (3) accurate delivery of radiation. The main disadvantages are the greater preparation required, compared to conventional plans, with regard to physician contouring and physics design, and the need for the treating physician to have a thorough understanding of target selection and delineation. The use of IMRT is expected to translate into a further reduction of the risk of ORN.

More recently, chemotherapy has been combined with radiation therapy. Chemotherapy may be introduced prior to radiation therapy (induction), at the same time (concomitant), or after radiation therapy (adjuvant). Conflicting reports have emerged on whether chemotherapy increases or has no effect on the incidence of osteoradionecrosis.

PMHX/PDHX/MEDICATIONS/ALLERGIES/SH/FH

The patient has a 40-year history of tobacco and alcohol use (risk factors for oral squamous cell carcinoma). He has no history of oral or intravenous bisphosphonate use or adjuvant chemotherapy.

Osteonecrosis of the jaws secondary to bisphosphonate use can have a clinical presentation similar to that of osteoradionecrosis, despite its different pathophysiology (see Chapter 2, sections on bisphosphonate related osteonecrosis of the jaws). Metastatic disease to the mandible (from the prostate or kidney) is rare but can present as a nonhealing wound. Primary malignant tumors of bone, osteomyelitis, and fibro-osseous lesions can present as exposed bone, but most of these conditions are distinguished from osteoradionecrosis by an accurate history and physical examination.

EXAMINATION

General. The patient is a cachectic, thin man in mild distress (generalized muscle wasting is an indication of poor nutritional status but is also related to the wasting associated with advanced malignant processes).

Vital signs. Vital signs are stable, and he is afebrile (lack of fever is not uncommon with osteoradionecrosis).

Maxillofacial. There is minimal left facial edema, with hyperemic skin (secondary to the effects of radiation) overlying the mandible posteriorly. The left mandible is painful to palpation. The maximal jaw opening is less than 25 mm (due to radiation fibrosis and pain). There is no cervical or submandibular lymphadenopathy (positive nodes may be seen with acute infections or recurrence of the primary tumor). There is a draining orocutaneous fistula of the left neck, with surrounding erythema.

Intraoral. Oral hygiene is poor. The extraction sockets of the posterior left mandible have not healed, and there is approximately 1.5 cm of exposed bone. The oral mucous membranes are dry (radiation-induced xerostomia secondary

to the effects of radiation on salivary glands). The mandible shows intersegmental mobility across the area of exposed bone (indicative of mandible fracture).

Pulmonary. The patient has a barrel-shaped chest, with distant breath sounds and mild, bilateral, scattered rhonchi (physical findings consistent with emphysema secondary to prolonged tobacco use).

Although this patient is edentulous, radiation caries is commonly seen on teeth remaining in the path of radiation and is probably related to pulpal necrosis combined with the effects of xerostomia from radiation.

IMAGING

The panoramic radiograph is the initial imaging study of choice for evaluation of the mandible, and it may be the only study necessary for suspected osteoradionecrosis. A CT scan of the mandible may also be used to more accurately delineate the areas of bony involvement. A low marrow signal on T1 MRI or a high-intensity signal on T2 MRI may be indicative of osteoradionecrosis. Although technetium methylene diphosphonate and gallium scans have been used for osteoradionecrosis, they have not been found to be superior to a CT scan.

For the current patient, the panoramic radiograph demonstrates an undefined, poorly demarcated, sclerotic radiolucent lesion with a fracture at the left angle (Figure 7-19).

LABS

Laboratory tests for the preoperative work-up of osteoradionecrosis should include a CBC to assess for leukocytosis secondary to any acute infection and baseline hematocrit and hemoglobin levels. Other tests are ordered based on the medical history and extent of anticipated surgery. Albumin and prealbumin levels may be obtained if there is a suspicion of malnutrition (as seen with chronic alcohol use). Nutritional status should be supplemented as needed.

The current patient had a WBC count of 11,000 cells/mm^3. The prealbumin level was 8 mg/dl, which is consistent with malnutrition (normal range, 16 to 30 mg/dl). The basic metabolic panel was within normal limits.

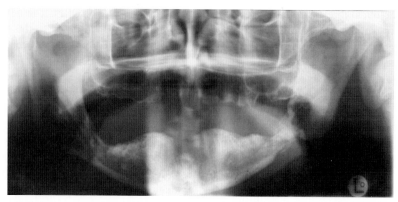

Figure 7-19   Panoramic radiograph demonstrates an undefined, poorly demarcated sclerotic radiolucent lesion with a fracture at the left angle.

ASSESSMENT

Stage III osteoradionecrosis of the left posterior mandible, with a pathologic fracture and an orocutaneous fistula compounded by generalized malnutrition.

TREATMENT

There is some controversy regarding the optimal treatment of osteoradionecrosis. The description of the pathophysiology of osteoradionecrosis by Marx in 1983 (hypoxia, hypocellular, hypovascular) is generally well accepted. As radiation energy passes through normal tissue, it immediately kills a small number of cells, which incur internal damage to their DNA, RNA, enzyme systems, and cell membranes. These cells may not be replaced when they die (due to impaired cell division). Consequently, the tissue become less cellular (hypocellular), less vascular (hypovascular), and less oxygenated (hypoxic). Marx has further popularized the use of hyperbaric oxygen therapy for treatment of early and advanced osteoradionecrosis using a hyperbaric oxygen protocol (described later). Hyperbaric oxygen therapy is administered in a pressurized chamber most commonly at 2.4 atmospheres (ATA), which is equal to the pressure under 45 feet of water. The patient breathes 100% oxygen for a predetermined amount of time (90 minutes at 2.4 ATA is considered one dive). The increase in partial pressure (PaO_2) of the inspired air increases the amount of oxygen dissolved in blood and subsequently increases the oxygen delivered to tissue. The increased oxygen gradient at the cellular level stimulates angiogenesis, and therefore vascularity. Hyperbaric oxygen may also have a oxygen-dependent bactericidal function affecting the function of leukocytes (oxygen tension less than 30 mm Hg significantly impairs the ability of the leukocytes to kill the phagocytosed organism). Absolute contraindications to hyperbaric oxygen include untreated pneumothorax, optic neuritis, fulminant viral infections, and congenital spherocytosis. Complications of hyperbaric oxygen include seizures, decompression sickness, and ear barotrauma.

With the advent of microvascular surgery and the recent advances in this field, many surgeons have recommended resection of the necrotic mandibular (or maxillary) segment and immediate reconstruction using microvascular free flaps without the use of hyperbaric oxygen. Until further studies regarding the outcome, morbidity, cost, and effectiveness of these two dramatically different treatment philosophies are available, the optimal treatment of osteoradionecrosis remains partially unclear. The two methodologies are briefly described next.

Hyperbaric oxygen protocol. This protocol, developed by Marx, is based on categorizing osteoradionecrosis into three stages. Patients presenting with exposed bone are designated as having stage I osteoradionecrosis. These patients would receive 30 dives of hyperbaric oxygen. If the bone softens and granulation tissue develops, the patient is designated as a stage I responder and is treated by minimal local debridement followed by 10 more dives. However, if the patient does not respond, he is designated as having stage II, which is treated by surgical debridement followed by 10 additional dives. If there is persistence of dehiscence and exposed bone, he is designated as having stage III osteoradionecrosis. This requires a continuity resection, jaw stabilization, and soft tissue flap as needed. Patients presenting with a pathologic fracture, orocutaneous fistula, or osteolysis of the inferior border of the mandible are also designated as having stage III osteoradionecrosis.

Microvascular techniques. A vast body of literature supports the treatment of early and late osteoradionecrosis using free vascular tissue transfer into the irradiated field; success rates are greater than 95%. Microvascular surgery (free flaps) allows the surgeon to bring in hard and soft tissues with an independent blood supply anastomosed outside of the radiated field. Commonly used donor sites include the free fibular osteocutaneous flap (see the section on fibular free flaps for mandibular reconstruction in Chapter 11), radial forearm fasciculocutaneous flap (see the section on radial forearm free flaps in Chapter 11), the deep circumflex iliac artery osteomyocutaneous flap using the iliac crest, and the anterolateral thigh (soft tissue transfer). The arterial and venous blood supply of the transferred tissue (flap) is anastomosed into the available vessels in the head and neck (most commonly, the carotid or associated branches and the jugular venous system).

An advantage of microvascular flaps in osteoradionecrosis is the ability to bring in a new blood supply independent of the compromised host bed. This eliminates the need for multiple, costly hyperbaric oxygen treatments.

The current patient was taken to the operating room for resection of the fracture segment and associated necrotic tissue and fistula (Figure 7-20, *A*). A free fibular flap was harvested (Figure 7-20, *B*) and inserted into the defect, followed by anastomosis of the vessels to the facial artery and internal jugular vein. The postoperative panoramic radiograph and clinical photograph demonstrate the position of the fibular graft and soft tissue closure 4 weeks postsurgery (Figure 7-20, *C* and *D*).

Pentoclo, a combination of an anti-TNF-α agent (pentoxifylline), vitamin E, and clodronate (biphosphonate), has resulted in some success in the treatment of ORN. The success of this treatment is based on fibroatrophic therapy; the induction of fibroblastic activity resulting in atrophy and breakdown of tissue.

COMPLICATIONS

Radiotherapy can be highly effective in the treatment of head and neck cancer. However, direct and scattered radiation on adjacent normal tissue is associated with significant side effects that further affect the already compromised quality of life of a cancer patient. Radiation-induced damage should be anticipated and prevented whenever possible. Early management can ameliorate the long-term effects. Radiation-induced damage is the result of the deleterious effects of radiation, not only on the oral mucosa, but also on the adjacent salivary glands, bone, dentition, and masticatory musculature.

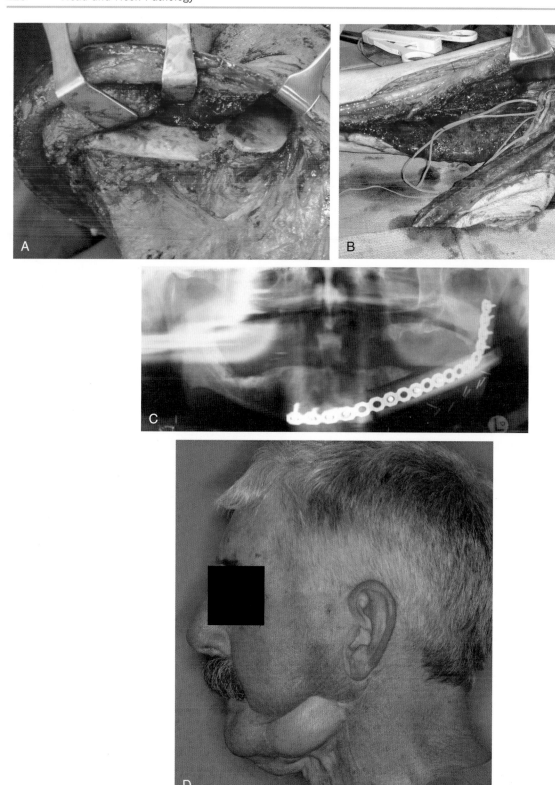

Figure 7-20   **A,** Intraoperative view demonstrating the pathologic fracture of the angle of the mandible with adjacent necrotic bone. **B,** Harvest of a free fibula osteomyocutaneous flap. **C,** Postoperative panoramic radiograph showing inset of the free fibula for mandibular reconstruction. **D,** Profile view of the patient showing the inset of the soft tissue flap and closure of the orocutaneous fistula. *(Courtesy R. Bryan Bell, DDS, MS.)*

Radiation mucositis is an acute complication representing the inflammatory response to acute radiation injury. This is a self-limiting condition that may develop in the last 3 weeks of radiotherapy and may persist for about 1 month thereafter. During this period, topical viscous 2% lidocaine gel and a systemic analgesic may be needed for pain control, along with the use of chlorhexidine gluconate antiseptic rinses. Radiation caries is seen as hard, black erosions of the tooth structure, mostly at the gingival margin, cusp tips, and incisal surfaces, presenting only in the direct path of radiation. Even the best oral hygiene, dental care, and fluoride treatment cannot totally prevent this condition.

The chronic complications of radiotherapy include mucosal fibrosis and atrophy, salivary gland dysfunction, soft tissue necrosis, osteoradionecrosis, dysgeusia (distortion or decrease in the sense of taste), ageusia (loss of taste function), muscular fibrosis (causing trismus), xerostomia, and fungal and bacterial infections. Radiation-induced xerostomia is caused by the direct damaging effects of radiation on both major and minor salivary gland structures in the path of radiation. Dysphagia (difficulty swallowing) is one of the most troubling and least treatable chronic complications of radiation. Radiation also can have significant effects on jaw growth and the development of teeth in the younger population.

Complications directly related to osteoradionecrosis include chronic pain, drug dependency, trismus, nutritional deficiencies, pathologic fractures, orocutaneous fistulas, disfigurement due to loss of soft tissue and bone, loss of time from work and family, and the psychological stigma of having a nonhealing wound.

DISCUSSION

Osteoradionecrosis is defined as a radiation-induced necrosis of bone and associated soft tissue. This is a well-known complication of radiation therapy that predominantly involves the mandible, although it can be seen in the maxilla. This condition has frustrated maxillofacial surgeons and radiation oncologists since the 1950s and the popularization of radiation therapy for head and neck cancer. Osteoradionecrosis, initially described by Regaude in the 1920s, was thought to have an infectious etiology (it was described as a triad of radiation, trauma, and infection by Meyer), but subsequent studies have shown infection to be a secondary process related to the hypovascular, hypoxic, and hypocellular nature of radiated tissue and the subsequent inability to resist infection.

Osteoradionecrosis can be categorized into three different types based on etiology and chronology:

1. Early trauma-induced osteoradionecrosis, which develops either soon after irradiation or months afterward (attributed to the combined effects of radiation injury with surgical trauma and the physiologic demands of wound healing)
2. Spontaneous osteoradionecrosis (unassociated with any surgical or traumatic event, occurring secondary to high-dose irradiation)

3. Late trauma–induced osteoradionecrosis, usually associated with surgical procedures performed more than 2 years after radiotherapy

Prevention of osteoradionecrosis is currently the best modality of treatment. Upon diagnosis of head and neck cancer, radiation therapy is usually initiated as soon as possible. General dental evaluations should be conducted promptly to treat and control for caries and to initiate fluoride tray treatments. It is generally recommended that grossly carious and periodontally diseased mandibular teeth that would be in the direct path of radiation of 5,000 cGy or greater be removed at least 14 to 21 days before initiation of radiation therapy. Restorable maxillary teeth that do not have severe periodontal disease do not require preradiation extraction. A retrospective study by Curi and Dibb reviewed 104 patients who were treated for osteoradionecrosis of the jaws. All patients had a history of osteoradionecrosis of at least 3 months' duration, with a minimum follow-up of 1 year. In this group, osteoradionecrosis was seen predominantly in the mandible compared with the maxilla (20:1). This is attributed to the greater blood supply and thinner bone of the maxilla. If a severe toothache or a dental abscess occurs during radiation therapy, treatment should not be interrupted. The decayed tooth should be restored with noninvasive methods, such as pulpotomies, pulpectomies, endodontic treatment, and analgesics. In cases of an acute odontogenic abscess, the recommended treatment is incision and drainage, in addition to endodontic therapy and antibiotics. There generally is a 4-month period after radiation, the "golden window," that allows for definitive care, including extractions. The effects of radiation damage to the tissue are time dependent and take several months to affect wound healing.

There has been some controversy over the prophylactic use of hyperbaric oxygen therapy before extraction of teeth in a previously irradiated field. Hyperbaric oxygen therapy dates back to 1930s, when the U.S. Navy studied the use of oxygen to treat divers who had decompression sickness and arterial gas embolism. In clinical practice it has been used both for treatment and prophylactically for management and prevention of compromised wound healing. The benefit of prophylactic hyperbaric oxygen therapy before the extraction of teeth in previously irradiated tissue has been questioned, given the lower incidence of osteoradionecrosis reported in recent years. Despite the growing body of scientific evidence supporting hyperbaric oxygen therapy in wound healing, its precise application remains a controversial issue. This controversy has resulted in continuing skepticism among some practitioners. Further scientific studies are necessary to address the optimal application of hyperbaric oxygen therapy in the prevention and treatment of osteoradionecrosis.

Bibliography

Ang E, Black C, Irish J, et al: Reconstructive options in the treatment of osteoradionecrosis of the craniomaxillofacial skeleton, *Br J Plast Surg* 56:92, 2003.

Annane D, Depondt J, Aubert P, et al: Hyperbaric oxygen therapy for radionecrosis of the jaw: a randomized, placebo-controlled, double-blind trial from the ORN96 Study Group, *J Clin Oncol* 22(24):4893-4900, 2004.

Buchbinder D, St Hilaire H: The use of free tissue transfer in advanced osteoradionecrosis of the mandible, *J Oral Maxillofac Surg* 64:961, 2006.

Cordeiro PG, Disa JJ, Hidalgo DA, et al: Reconstruction of the mandible with osseous free flaps: a 10 year experience with 150 consecutive patients, *Plast Reconstr Surg* 104:1314, 1999.

Curi MM, Dib LL: Osteoradionecrosis of the jaws: a retrospective study of the background factors and treatment in 104 cases, *J Oral Maxillofac Surg* 55:540, 1997.

Delanian S, Chatel C, Porcher R: Complete restoration of refractory mandibular osteoradionecrosis by prolonged treatment with a Pentoxifylline-Tocopherol-Clodronate Combination (PENTO-CLO): a phase II trial, *Int J Radiat Oncol Biol Phys* 80:832-839, 2011.

Delanian S, Lefaix JL: The radiation-induced fibroatrophic process: therapeutic perspective via the antioxidant pathway, *Radiother Oncol* 73:119-131, 2004.

Feldmeier JJ: Hyperbaric oxygen for delayed radiation injuries, *Undersea Hyperb Med* 31:133-135, 2004.

Hermans R: Imaging of the mandible, *Neuroimaging Clin N Am* 13:597-604, 2003.

Hidalgo DA: A review of 716 consecutive free flaps for oncologic surgical defects: refinement in donor site selection and technique, *Plast Reconstr Surg* 102:722, 1998.

MacCombe WS: Necrosis in treatment of intraoral cancer by radiation therapy, *Am J Roentgenol Radium Ther Nucl Med* 87:431-440, 1962.

Marx RE: A new concept in the treatment of osteoradionecrosis, *J Oral Maxillofac Surg* 41:351, 1983.

Meyer I: Infectious disease of the jaws, *J Oral Surg* 28:17, 1970.

Nabil S, Samman N: Risk factor for osteoradionecrosis after head and neck radiation: a systemic review, *Oral Surg Oral Med Oral Pathol Oral Radiol Endod* 113:54-69, 2012.

O'Dell K, Sinha U: Osteoradionecrosis, *Oral Maxillofac Surg Clin North Am* 23:255-464, 2011.

Peleg M, Lopez EA: The treatment of osteoradionecrosis of the mandible: the case of hyperbaric oxygen and bone graft reconstruction, *J Oral Maxillofac Surg* 64:956, 2006.

Puri DR, Chou W, Lee N: Intensity-modulated radiation therapy in head and neck cancers: dosimetric advantages and update of clinical results, *Am J Clin Oncol* 28:415, 2005.

Reuther T, Schuster T, Mende U, et al: Osteoradionecrosis of the jaws as a side effect of radiotherapy of head and neck tumour patients: a report of a thirty year retrospective review, *Int J Oral Maxillofac Surg* 32:289-295, 2003.

Schwartz HC, Kagan AR: Osteoradionecrosis of the mandible: scientific basis for clinical staging, *Am J Clin Oncol* 25:168-169, 2002.

Sciubba PJ, Goldenberg D: Oral complications of radiotherapy, *Lancet Oncol* 7:17, 2006.

Studer G, Studer SP, Zwahlen RA, et al: Osteoradionecrosis of the mandible: minimized risk profile following intensity-modulated radiation therapy (IMRT), *Strahlenther Onkol* 182:283, 2006.

Sulaiman F, Huryn MJ, Zlotolow MI: Dental extractions in the irradiated head and neck patient: a retrospective analysis of Memorial Sloan-Kettering Cancer Center protocols, criteria, and end results, *J Oral Maxillofac Surg* 61:10, 2003.

Wahl MJ: Osteoradionecrosis prevention myths, *Int J Radiat Oncol Biol Phys* 64:661, 2006.

Withers HR, Peters LJ, Taylor JM, et al: Late normal tissue sequelae from radiation therapy for carcinoma of the tonsil: patterns of fractionation study of radiobiology, *Int J Radiat Oncol Biol Phys* 33:563-568, 1995.

CHAPTER 8

Craniomaxillofacial Trauma Surgery

Editors: Shahrokh C. Bagheri and Martin B. Steed

This chapter addresses:
- Dentoalveolar Trauma
- Subcondylar Mandibular Fracture
- Combined Mandibular Parasymphysis and Angle Fractures
- Zygomaticomaxillary Complex Fracture
- Zygomatic Arch Fracture
- Nasal Fracture
- Frontal Sinus Fracture
- Naso-Orbital-Ethmoid Fracture
- Le Fort I Fracture
- Le Fort II and III Fractures
- Orbital Trauma: Fracture of the Orbital Floor
- Panfacial Fracture

Oral and maxillofacial surgeons are the only specialists who have the training to provide complete craniomaxillofacial trauma care that includes medical and dental management and the capability to address reconstruction of all elements of the face. However, only with continued training, participation in trauma care, and observation of one's own "personal residency" beyond formal training can surgeons maintain current skills for management of facial trauma. As specialists, we should endorse and support this essential component of oral and maxillofacial surgery (OMFS), because it has had a crucial impact on the advancement of the profession and has contributed to our gaining our rightful seat among other surgical disciplines.

The modern management of maxillofacial trauma has evolved with the advent of new biomaterials, improved diagnostic imaging, and refined instrumentation with associated techniques. The approach to maxillofacial trauma is in part related to the surgeon's training and the available facilities; however, the basis of evaluation of the trauma patient who has sustained maxillofacial injuries remains unchanged. The importance of adherence to advanced trauma life support (ATLS) protocols and a comprehensive physical examination cannot be overemphasized. The use of bone grafts and the placement of dental implants put our specialty in the unique position of being able to offer complete rehabilitation beyond the immediate surgical repair of the fractured segments. An

understanding of occlusion and the related musculoskeletal apparatus is essential for correct management of facial fractures, many of which involve the dentate segments. The goal of maxillofacial trauma surgery is restoration of the preinjury level of function and optimal cosmetic outcome.

In this chapter we present a series of cases representing the spectrum of maxillofacial injuries as they are encountered in the most classic way. Although most of the cases presented (except for the panfacial trauma case) represent isolated injury patterns, it is important to recognize that injuries can present in any combination.

It is not our intent to provide an exclusive approach to the evaluation and management of these injuries, but rather to emphasize common patterns of presentation, treatment options, and complications and to discuss other pertinent factors. In clinical practice three interdependent factors are related to a successful outcome; the patient, the injury, and the surgeon. These are different every time.

The Facial Injury Severity Scale (FISS) is a tool recently devised for designation of the severity of facial injuries (Box 8-1). The result is a numeric value that is the sum of all facial fractures and fracture patterns. The FISS is a predictor of the severity of facial injury as measured by the operating room charges required for treatment and the length of hospital stay.

The Glasgow Coma Score is a universally used system for evaluation of neurologic status (Box 8-2).

Box 8-1 Facial Injury Severity Scale (FISS)	
Facial Area	**Points**
Mandible	
Dentoalveolar fracture	1
Each fracture of body/ramus symphysis	2
Each fracture of condyle/coronoid	1
Midface*	
Dentoalveolar fracture	1
Le Fort I[†] fracture	2
Le Fort II fracture	4
Le Fort III fracture	6
Naso-orbital-ethmoid (NOE) fracture	3
Zygomaticomaxillary complex fracture	1
Nasal fracture	1
Orbital floor/rim fracture	1
Upper Face	
Orbital roof/rim fracture	1
Displaced frontal sinus/bone fracture	5
Nondisplaced frontal sinus/bone fracture	1
Facial Laceration > 10 cm long	1
The FISS is the sum of the points assigned.	

From Bagheri SC, Dierks EJ, Kademani D, et al: Application of a facial injury severity scale in craniomaxillofacial trauma, *J Oral Maxillofac Surg* 64:404-414, 2006.
*Each midfacial fracture is assigned 1 point unless it is part of a complex.
[†]Unilateral Le Fort fractures are assigned half the value shown.

Box 8-2   Glasgow Coma Scale (GCS) Score

Eye Opening (E)
4 = Spontaneous
3 = To voice
2 = To pain
1 = None

Verbal Response (V)
5 = Normal conversation
4 = Disoriented conversation
3 = Words but not coherent
2 = No words, only sounds
1 = None

Motor Response (M)
6 = Normal
5 = Localizes to pain
4 = Withdraws to pain
3 = Decorticate posture
2 = Decerebrate
1 = None

GSC Score = E + V + M

Dentoalveolar Trauma

Patrick J. Louis, Anthony B. P. Morlandt, and Somsak Sittitavornwong

CC

A 22-year-old male presents to the oral and maxillofacial surgery office complaining of anterior facial pain, swelling, oral bleeding, and mobile teeth.

HPI

The patient reports that he was riding his mountain bike when an abrupt bump resulted in him striking his lower face against the handlebars. He dismounted the bicycle without other injuries and drove himself to an outside emergency department. He denies loss of consciousness, nausea, vomiting, visual disturbances, or headache (indicative of head trauma with intracranial injury). He further denies stridor, dyspnea, or increased work of breathing (suggestive of foreign body aspiration resulting from dislodged teeth, dental restorations, or orthodontic appliances). He notes several dental fractures, profound mobility of the lower teeth, and gingival bleeding. He undergoes primary and secondary surveys, according to the ATLS protocol, that are found to be negative. A computed tomography (CT) scan is obtained, and the patient is given instructions to report by private car to your office for evaluation.

PMHX/PDHX/MEDICATIONS/ALLERGIES/SH/FH

The patient denies any significant cardiac, pulmonary, renal, hepatic, or neurologic diseases.

EXAMINATION

General. The patient is a well-developed, well-nourished adult male in mild distress secondary to pain and oral bleeding. He is neurologically intact.

Maxillofacial. There are no lacerations, contusions, or abrasions of the scalp, midface, or chin. The pupils are equal at 4 mm, round, and reactive to light and accommodation. The nasal dorsum is midline and stable. There is no rhinorrhea (a concern for violation of the cribriform plate with cerebrospinal fluid [CSF] leakage) and no septal hematoma on speculum examination. The ears are symmetric and without injury to the pinnae. Examination of the external auditory meatus reveals no otorrhea (also a concern for CSF leakage) or disruption of the tympanic membrane. There is no mastoid ecchymosis noted (Battle's sign, significant for occult skull base fracture). The orbits, midface, and mandible are without step deformity or crepitus on palpation. Cranial nerves II through XII are intact.

Intraoral. There is a 1-cm abrasion of the upper lip skin without significant laceration. Intraorally, there is profound ecchymosis of the upper lip mucosa with a laceration extending into the sublabial vestibule (Figure 8-1). Teeth #7 and #8 are mobile as a single unit with displacement of the buccal cortical plate on manipulation. Tooth #9 is grossly mobile and subluxed several millimeters. It also demonstrates an oblique coronal fracture with pinpoint pulp exposure (Ellis class III). In addition, tooth #9 is sensitive to mechanical stimulation with a cotton-tipped applicator and tender to percussion. There is occlusal prematurity with interference of the maxillary anterior teeth on attempted intercuspation.

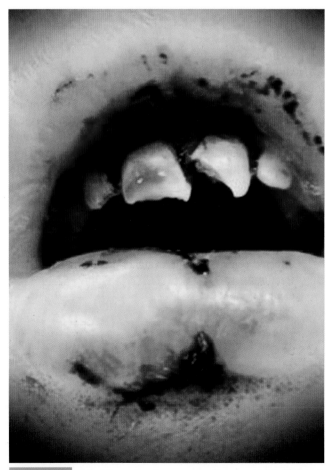

Figure 8-1 Maxillary alveolar segment fracture involving teeth #7, #8, and #9, with coronal fractures involving teeth #8 and #9.

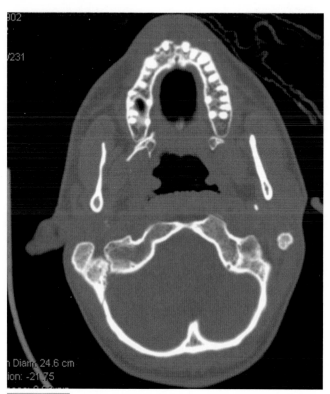

Figure 8-2 Axial CT scan showing displacement of teeth #7, #8, and #9 due to alveolar segment fracture.

IMAGING

A maxillofacial CT scan demonstrates an alveolar segment fracture involving teeth #7 and #8, with subluxation of tooth #9 and fracture of the alveolar plate (Figure 8-2). There are otherwise no injuries to the maxillofacial skeleton, cervical spine, brain, or cranium. The minimum radiographic study necessary for diagnosis of dentoalveolar fractures is a periapical radiograph, although the diagnosis can often be made with a physical examination alone. Based on availability, other radiographic studies may include:

- Computed tomography
- Cone-beam CT (CBCT)
- Periapical radiograph with horizontally and laterally directed central beam to evaluate traumatized roots for fractures
- Occlusal view
- Panoramic radiograph

LABS

No routine laboratory tests are indicated for the work-up and diagnosis of dentoalveolar injuries in the healthy individual. If coagulopathy is suspected based on the medical history and physical exam, a coagulation profile, including the prothrombin time/partial thromboplastin time (PT/PTT), international normalized ratio (INR), and platelet count, may be obtained.

ASSESSMENT

Anterior maxillary alveolar segment fractures involving teeth #7 through #9, with lateral luxation and an Ellis class III fracture of tooth #9, and an intraoral laceration of the upper lip.

TREATMENT

Initial stabilization includes reduction of the teeth and splinting (Figure 8-3). With the current patient, bonded flexible wire splinting was not available, so the teeth were splinted with an arch bar. The occlusion was checked, and the teeth were not in occlusion during maximum intercuspation. The patient's tetanus status was up to date. He was given a prescription for amoxicillin and chlorhexidine and discharged home. The teeth were splinted for 8 weeks because of the alveolar segment fracture. Root canal therapy was initiated on day 10 with calcium hydroxide therapy.

COMPLICATIONS

In the past, only about 25% to 40% of replanted, avulsed teeth show periodontal ligament (PDL) healing. This has been attributed to poor handling of the tooth. Three different types of posttraumatic external root resorption have been distinguished in the literature: surface resorption (repair-related root resorption), inflammatory resorption (infection-related root resorption) and replacement resorption (ankylosis-related root resorption). Surface resorption has no significant clinical consequences and can be observed. However, the other types of resorption can ultimately result in tooth loss. In the avulsed tooth, if the PDL that is still attached to the tooth does not dry out, the cells can remain viable for an extended period, depending on the storage medium. Once the tooth has been reimplanted and stabilized, the viable PDL cells reattach to the PDL within the socket. When the injury to the cementum of the root is localized, there is minimal destructive inflammation, allowing for new cementum to be laid down after the inflammation resolves. When there is poor handling of the avulsed tooth (e.g., drying or storage in nonphysiologic solutions), damage and necrosis of the PDL occur. Subsequently, there is a large area of inflammation to remove the damaged PDL and cementum. This must be replaced by new tissue. The slower moving cementoblasts compete with the osteoblasts in the replacement process, resulting in some areas of the root surface being replaced by bone. Over time, through osseous remodeling, this can result in osseous or replacement resorption. Internal root resorption can occur through persistent inflammation or metaplastic replacement of normal pulp tissue. This can result in late tooth fractures. Root surface treatments and root canal therapy are directed toward prevention of this complication. Ideal management of dentoalveolar trauma may have to be delayed due to life-threatening injuries that must be managed first (Figure 8-4). This may result in resorptive complications.

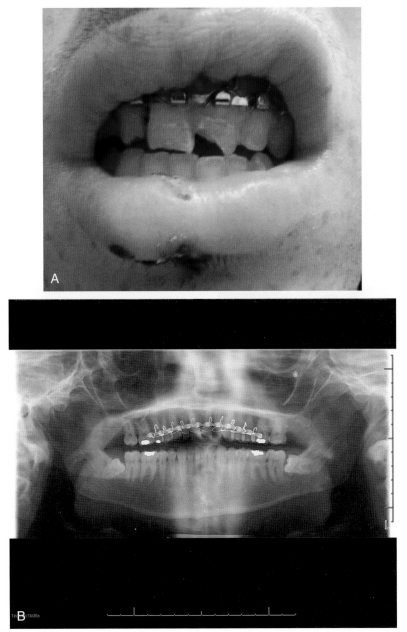

Figure 8-3   **A** and **B,** Maxillary alveolar segment fracture involving teeth #7, #8, and #9, reduced with Erich arch bar and circumdental ligature wiring.

DISCUSSON

Appropriate diagnosis is critical in identifying and treating dentoalveolar injuries, which are known to affect one fourth of all children and one third of all adults. Depending on the mechanism of injury, a number of maxillofacial injuries may present with concomitant intracranial or cervical spine injuries, despite normal neurologic findings on physical examination. After a thorough physical examination that follows the ATLS protocol, attention is directed to the head and neck. Contaminated facial wounds should be irrigated with normal saline if available, although tap water has been shown to be as effective as saline. Patients with grossly contaminated

wounds or facial injuries caused by dog or human bites should be considered for tetanus immunization based on their vaccination history. If an adult has an ambiguous immunization history or has received fewer than three prior doses of tetanus toxoid, he or she should receive tetanus immune globulin (TIG) and the tetanus-diphtheria (Td) or tetanus-diphtheria-acellular pertussis (Tdap) vaccine. Prior tetanus disease is inadequate at providing immunity, because a small amount of the highly potent toxin is sufficient to cause clinical neuromuscular weakness and airway compromise. Antibiotic coverage must be based on the mechanism and extent of injury. It is indicated in contaminated wounds with significant soft

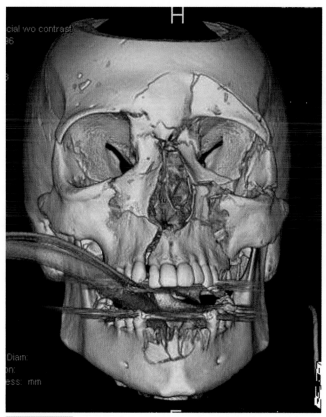

Figure 8-4 Mandibular alveolar segment fractures associated with panfacial fractures from a high-speed motor vehicle injury. Management of the dentoalveolar trauma can be deferred to allow management of the more life-threatening injuries.

tissue injury, luxated teeth, avulsed teeth, pulp exposures, root fractures and alveolar fractures. Amoxicillin is usually chosen unless the patient is allergic to penicillin; in such cases, clindamycin can be substituted. Chlorhexidine oral rinse is an excellent choice for most oral injuries to help prevent infection.

The cause of dentoalveolar trauma varies among different demographics, but it generally results from falls, playground accidents, domestic violence, bicycle accidents, motor vehicle accidents, assaults, altercations, and sports injuries. Gassner and colleagues reported an incidence of 48.25% in all facial injuries, 57.8% in play and household accidents, 50.1% in sports accidents, 38.6% in accidents at work, 35.8% in acts of violence, 34.2% in traffic accidents, and 31% in unspecified accidents. Falling is the primary cause of dentoalveolar trauma in early childhood. Andreasen reported a bimodal trend in the peak incidence of dentoalveolar trauma in children aged 2 to 4 and 8 to 10 years.

Dentoalveolar injuries have been classified by the International Association of Dental Traumatology, which regularly reviews and updates its guidelines and publishes them online at *www.dentaltraumaguide.org*. Broadly, the discrete categories of dentoalveolar injury include:

- Injuries to the periodontium
- Injuries to the dental crown and root
- Injuries to the supporting alveolar bone

| Box 8-3 | **Splinting Schedule** |

- Subluxation—Flexible splint for up to 2 weeks for patient comfort only
- Extrusive luxation—Flexible splint for 2 weeks
- Lateral luxation—Flexible splint for 4 weeks
- Intrusive luxation
  - *Incomplete root formation:* Eruption without intervention; if no movement within a few weeks, orthodontic therapy (if intruded > 7 mm, reposition surgically or with orthodontics)
  - *Complete root formation:* If < 3 mm of intrusion, eruption without intervention. If there is no movement within 2-4 weeks, reposition surgically or with orthodontics (before ankylosis develops); stabilize with orthodontics, or stabilize surgically repositioned tooth with flexible splint × 4-8 weeks.
- Alveolar segment—Rigid stabilization × 8-12 weeks
- Avulsed teeth—Flexible splint × 7-10 days
- Root fracture—Flexible splint × 4 weeks (if fracture is near cervix, stabilize × 4 months)

From Diangelis AJ, et al: International Association of Dental Traumatology guidelines for the management of traumatic dental injuries. Part 1. Fractures and luxations of permanent teeth, *Dent Traumatol* 28(1):2-12, 2012.

Injuries to the periodontium resulting from forces directed through the tooth and to the surrounding bone and periodontal attachment are the most common types of dental trauma in the primary dentition.

Periodontal Injuries

Periodontal injuries may be classified according to the following system.

Concussion. No visible trauma to tooth or alveolar structures but pain on percussion. Treatment is conservative, with a no-chew diet only and surveillance of pulpal vitality.

Subluxation. Increased mobility of the tooth without dislocation. Treatment is conservative, although a flexible splint may be applied for the patient's comfort for up to 2 weeks (Box 8-3).

Extrusion. Coronal dislocation of the tooth due to separation of the periodontal ligament without alveolar bone disruption. Treatment involves repositioning the tooth into the socket, stabilizing the tooth for 2 weeks with a nonrigid, flexible splint, and performing root canal therapy in teeth with closed apices. If the marginal alveolar bone demonstrates radiographic signs of breakdown at follow-up, prolonged splinting is recommended, for up to 6 weeks after the injury.

Lateral luxation. Tooth displacement with fracture of the alveolar process. Treatment includes flexible splinting for 4 weeks; root canal therapy is indicated for cases of pulpal necrosis to prevent root resorption.

Intrusion. Apical dislocation of the tooth, with crushing injury of supporting alveolar bone. Treatment depends on the status of the root apex. Incomplete root formation is treated conservatively, allowing several weeks for passive eruption. If no spontaneous movement is appreciated, orthodontic repositioning may be attempted after several weeks of conservative treatment. Teeth with complete apical development undergo immediate orthodontic repositioning if intruded more than 3 mm and conservative observation if intruded less than 3 mm, with application of orthodontic forces after 2 to 4 weeks. Teeth with 7 mm or greater of intrusive displacement should undergo immediate surgical repositioning regardless of the root apex development. Repositioned teeth must then undergo stabilization using a flexible splint for 4 to 8 weeks. Teeth with complete root formation that are intruded will likely develop pulpal necrosis and must undergo root canal therapy 2 to 3 weeks after injury. Formal obturation may be preceded by calcium hydroxide canal treatment if the tooth is actively being repositioned.

Avulsion/extrarticulation. The complete loss of tooth from alveolar supporting bone. The most commonly avulsed tooth is the maxillary central incisor, and the condition most often affects children 7 to 10 years of age. In most cases, replantation of avulsed permanent teeth should be attempted. Contraindications to replantation include an immunosuppressed patient after transplant surgery and patients with cardiac valve replacement. When possible, teeth should be positioned back into the socket immediately and stabilized. If this is not possible, the prognosis of the avulsed tooth depends on how it was handled. The prognosis is improved if there is no dry time, the tooth is stored in physiologic solution, and replantation is performed within 1 hour. Organ transport solution allows the PDL cells to survive for 1 week, Hank's Balanced Salt Solution (HBSS) allows cells to survive for 24 hours, but milk allows only 6 hours of survival. Water is a poor storage medium for teeth. Because it is hypotonic, it results in rapid lysis of the PDL cells. For teeth with a closed apex and no dry time, stored in HBSS for less than 24 hours, or in milk or saliva for less than 6 hours, the tooth should be placed in doxycycline (0.05 mg/ml) for 5 minutes and then replanted. In animal studies, Cvek and colleagues and Yanpiset and Trope demonstrated that the use of doxycycline in this fashion significantly enhanced revascularization. Tetracycline has antiresorptive and antimicrobial properties. Tetracycline has a direct inhibitory effect on collagenase activity and osteoclasts. Its antimicrobial effects help to eliminate bacteria that have contaminated the alveolus, PDL, and pulpal tissues. The tooth is stabilized with flexible wire and composite for 7 to 10 days. At the 7- to 10-day follow-up visit, root canal therapy is started. The pulp is extirpated, and calcium hydroxide therapy is started. Calcium hydroxide is an effective antimicrobial agent that decreases resorption and promotes healing. The more alkaline environment in the dentin slows the resorptive cells and promotes hard tissue formation. Therapy continues usually until a viable PDL is radiographically demonstrated (6 to 24 months). The root canal can then be obturated with the final filling material, such as gutta percha. For teeth with an open apex and dry time less than 1 hour, the goal is to encourage revascularization, continued root formation, and apex closure. For these teeth, soaking in doxycycline (0.05 mg/ml) for 5 minutes is recommended. The tooth is stabilized with a flexible wire and composite and monitored for signs of pulpal

necrosis. Apexification therapy should be performed with calcium hydroxide treatment if pulpal necrosis develops. Teeth that have been out of the mouth for longer than 1 hour and have not been kept in a storage medium will have a necrotic PDL and a poorer prognosis, with a greater risk of root resorption. To improve the prognosis, the PDL is debrided by placing the tooth in a sodium hypochlorite solution for 30 minutes. Extraoral root canal therapy is completed with gutta percha. The tooth is then placed sequentially in citric acid solution for 3 minutes, 1% stannous fluoride solution for 5 minutes, and 0.005% doxycycline solution for 5 minutes. The tooth is then replanted and splinted for 7 to 10 days. A study using Emdogain (Straumann; Basel, Switzerland) has shown some beneficial effects for teeth with extended dry times. Emdogain is an enamel matrix protein that has been shown to make the root more resistant to resorption and also to stimulate new PDL formation from the socket. The prognosis for teeth with an open apex and longer than 1 hour dry time is poor. No attempt should be made at revascularization. Instead, calcium hydroxide therapy for apexification can be initiated. An alternative treatment is to perform root canal therapy prior to replantation of the tooth; this allows for better sealing of the open apex. Treatment of the root surface is the same as for the closed apex. The tooth will likely undergo resorption, but it can allow for maintenance of alveolar width and height until the patient is old enough for implant placement.

Prominent maxillary central incisors that protrude beyond the confines of the upper lip are associated with a higher incidence of dental trauma in these children. Children are more challenging to examine and treat, and the parents' cooperation is required. Injuries in the primary dentition, especially intrusion, can result in crown deformation or enamel hypoplasia of the underlying permanent teeth. For these reasons, primary teeth, if avulsed, should not be replanted for fear of injury to the underlying permanent teeth. Luxated and intruded teeth should likewise be removed.

Bonded composite with flexible wire is the treatment of choice for injuries to the periodontium and root fractures. This technique permits flexible stabilization that allows some movement of the tooth in relation to the alveolus. This in turn allows for healing of the PDL and reduces the risk of ankylosis or resorption. The recommended fixation time for an injury to the periodontium is 7 to 10 days. Arch bars are more rigid and provide better stabilization for alveolar segment fractures; they also may be less technically challenging to place. The disadvantages of the arch bar technique are that it car produce an eruptive or extrusive force because of the placement of the wire beneath the height of contour of the tooth; also, the rigid nature of this technique can facilitate ankylosis and resorption.

Dental Crown and Root Injuries

Injuries to the dental crown and root are classified as follows:
- Ellis classification of fractures
  - I—within the enamel
  - IV—root fracture

- Other dental fractures
  - Crown fractures that extend onto the root without pulp exposure
  - Crown fractures that extend onto the root with pulp exposure

Crown fractures are common, and many times treatment is delayed to allow management of more severe injuries. Treatment is based on the extent of the crown-root involvement and/or pulpal involvement. Crown fractures that extend longitudinally onto the root below the level of the bone require extraction. Crown lengthening or orthodontic extrusion can be used to salvage some teeth. Treatment of root fractures depends mainly on the location of the fracture. Horizontal root fractures in the apical one third have the best prognosis. If the tooth is stable, it may not require treatment. Teeth that are mobile must be splinted for 12 weeks or extracted. Fractures in the cervical one third are usually extracted. Crown lengthening or orthodontic extrusion may also be performed.

The two types of treatment for pulpal injuries are direct pulp cap and root canal therapy. Direct pulp cap therapy is indicated for small, pinpoint exposures treated within 24 hours for mature teeth with a closed apex, and also for small and large pulp exposures in teeth with an open apex, to encourage apexification. Calcium hydroxide is used to seal small exposures. For teeth with an open apex and a large exposure, or exposure for longer than 24 hours, or deciduous teeth, a pulpotomy is performed first and then the calcium hydroxide therapy. Root canal therapy, with pulp extirpation, instrumentation of one or more canals, and sealing of the root, is recommended for pulpal injuries in mature teeth for large exposures or exposures exceeding 24 hours.

Injuries to the Alveolar Bone

Injuries to the supporting alveolar bone are classified as follows:

- *Comminution of the alveolar socket:* Crushing and comminution can be isolated or associated intrusive and lateral luxation.
- *Fracture of the alveolar socket wall:* Fracture of the alveolar socket isolated to the facial or lingual wall.
- *Fracture of the alveolar process:* May be isolated or associated with the socket wall.
- *Fracture of the mandible or maxilla:* Fracture involving the base of the mandible or maxilla combined with the alveolar process.

Alveolar fractures associated with intrusion or luxation are managed by immediate closed reduction of the fracture to realign the segments, reduce the teeth, and set the teeth into the best occlusion. Splinting with a rigid splint using acid-etched resin or orthodontic brackets and wire on either side of the fractured alveolus for 4 to 6 weeks is an option. In isolated alveolar segment fractures with no associated luxation injury, closed reduction is performed, followed by fixation with a single arch bar and 24- or 26-gauge wire for 4 weeks. Rigid fixation with titanium mini-plates and screws is generally reserved for alveolar fractures associated with fractures involving the basal bone and requiring open repair.

Bibliography

Andersson LJ, Friskopp J, Blomlof L: Fiber-glass splinting of traumatized teeth, *ASDC J Dent Child* 50(1):21-24, 1983.

Andreasen JO: Effect of extra-alveolar period and storage media upon periodontal and pulpal healing after replantation of mature permanent incisors in monkeys, *Int J Oral Surg* 10(1):43-53, 1981.

Andreasen JO: *Traumatic dental injuries: a manual*, ed 3, Chichester, West Sussex, UK, 2011, Wiley-Blackwell.

Andreasen JO, Borum MK, Jacobsen HL, et al: Replantation of 400 avulsed permanent incisors. 4. Factors related to periodontal ligament healing, *Endod Dent Traumatol* 11(2):76-89, 1995.

Andreasen JO, Andreasen FM, Andersson L, et al: *Textbook and color atlas of traumatic injuries to the teeth*, ed 4, Oxford, UK, 2007, Blackwell Munksgaard.

Andreasen JO, et al: The dental trauma guide, 2012. Available from: www.dentaltraumaguide.org. Accessed December 2012.

Blomlof L: Milk and saliva as possible storage media for traumatically exarticulated teeth prior to replantation, *Swed Dent J Suppl* 8:1-26, 1981.

Bystrom AR, Claesson R, Sundqvist G: The antibacterial effect of camphorated paramonochlorophenol, camphorated phenol and calcium hydroxide in the treatment of infected root canals, *Endod Dent Traumatol* 1(5):170-175, 1985.

Centers for Disease Control and Prevention; Atkinson W, Wolfe S, Hamborsky J (eds): *Epidemiology and prevention of vaccine-preventable diseases*, ed 12, Washington DC, 2012, Public Health Foundation.

Chen JW: Cervical spine injuries, *Oral Maxillofac Surg Clin North Am* 20(3):381-391, 2008.

Cohenca N, Simon JH, Roges R, et al: Clinical indications for digital imaging in dento-alveolar trauma. Part 1. Traumatic injuries, *Dent Traumatol* 23(2):95-104, 2007.

Cvek M, Cleaton-Jones P, Austin J, et al: Pulp revascularization in reimplanted immature monkey incisors: predictability and the effect of antibiotic systemic prophylaxis, *Endod Dent Traumatol* 6(4):157-169, 1990.

Cvek M, Cleaton-Jones P, Austin J, et al: Effect of topical application of doxycycline on pulp revascularization and periodontal healing in reimplanted monkey incisors, *Endod Dent Traumatol* 6(4):170-176, 1990.

Diangelis AJ, Andreasen JO, Ebeleseder KA, et al: International Association of Dental Traumatology guidelines for the management of traumatic dental injuries. Part 1. Fractures and luxations of permanent teeth, *Dent Traumatol* 28(1):2-12, 2012.

Elias H, Baur DA: Management of trauma to supporting dental structures, *Dent Clin North Am* 53(4):675-689, vi, 2009.

Filippi A, Pohl Y, von Arx T: Treatment of replacement resorption with Emdogain: preliminary results after 10 months, *Dent Traumatol* 17(3):134-138, 2001.

Fuss Z, Tsesis I, Lin S: Root resorption: diagnosis, classification and treatment choices based on stimulation factors, *Dent Traumatol* 19(4):175-182, 2003.

Gassner R, Bösch R, Tuli T, et al: Prevalence of dental trauma in 6,000 patients with facial injuries: implications for prevention, *Oral Surg Oral Med Oral Pathol Oral Radiol Endod* 87(1):27-33, 1999.

Gazelius B, Olgart L, Edwall L: Non-invasive recordings of blood flow in human dental pulp, *Endod Dent Traumatol* 2:219-221, 1986.

Gonda F, Nagase M, Chen RB, et al: Replantation: an analysis of 29 teeth, *Oral Surg Oral Med Oral Pathol* 70(5):650-655, 1990.

Hiltz J, Trope M: Vitality of human lip fibroblasts in milk, Hanks balanced salt solution, and Viaspan storage media, *Endod Dent Traumatol* 7(2):69-72, 1991.

Iqbal MK, Bamaas N: Effect of enamel matrix derivative (EMDOGAIN) upon periodontal healing after replantation of permanent incisors in beagle dogs, *Dent Traumatol* 17(1): 36-45, 2001.

Jamal BT, Diecidue R, Qutob A, et al: The pattern of combined maxillofacial and cervical spine fractures, *J Oral Maxillofac Surg* 67(3):559-562, 2009.

Karayilmaz H, Kirzioğlu Z: Comparison of the reliability of laser Doppler flowmetry, pulse oximetry and electric pulp tester in assessing the pulp vitality of human teeth, *J Oral Rehabil* 38(5):340-347, 2011. doi: 10.1111/j.1365-2842.2010.02160.x. (Epub September 26, 2010.)

Kehoe JC: Splinting and replantation after traumatic avulsion, *J Am Dent Assoc* 112(2):224-230, 1986.

Kloss F, Laimer K, Hohlrieder M, et al: Traumatic intracranial haemorrhage in conscious patients with facial fractures: a review of 1,959 cases, *J Craniomaxillofac Surg* 36(7):372-377, 2008.

Malmgren B, Andreasen JO, Flores MT, et al: International Association of Dental Traumatology guidelines for the management of traumatic dental injuries. Part 3. Injuries in the primary dentition, *Dent Traumatol* 28(3):174-182, 2012.

Mithani SK, St.-Hilaire H, Brooke BS, et al: Predictable patterns of intracranial and cervical spine injury in craniomaxillofacial trauma: analysis of 4,786 patients, *Plast Reconstr Surg* 123(4):1293-1301, 2009.

Needleman HL: The art and science of managing traumatic injuries to primary teeth, *Dent Traumatol* 27(4):295-299, 2011.

Reynolds JS, Reynolds MT, Powers MP: Diagnosis and management of dentoalveolar injuries. In Fonseca RJ, Walker RV, Barber HD (eds): *Oral and maxillofacial trauma*, ed 4, pp 248-292, St Louis, 2013, Saunders.

Sjögren U, Figdor D, Spangberg L, et al: The antimicrobial effect of calcium hydroxide as a short-term intracanal dressing, *Int Endod J* 24(3):119-125, 1991.

Soder PO, Otteskog P, Andreasen JO, et al: Effect of drying on viability of periodontal membrane, *Scand J Dent Res* 85(3):164-168, 1977.

Tronstad L, Andreasen JO, Hasselgren G, et al: pH changes in dental tissues after root canal filling with calcium hydroxide, *J Endod* 7(1):17-21, 1981.

Trope M: Root resorption of dental and traumatic origin: classification based on etiology, *Pract Periodontics Aesthet Dent* 10(4):515-522, 1998.

Trope M: Avulsion and replantation, *Refuat Hapeh Vehashinayim* 19(2):6-15, 76, 2002.

Trope M, Friedman S: Periodontal healing of replanted dog teeth stored in Viaspan, milk and Hanks balanced salt solution, *Endod Dent Traumatol* 8(5):183-188, 1992.

Valente JH, Forti RJ, Freundlich LF, et al: Wound irrigation in children: saline solution or tap water? *Ann Emerg Med* 41(5):609-616, 2003.

Wilder-Smith PEEB: A new method for the non-invasive measurement of pupal blood flow, *Int Endod J* 21:307-312, 1988.

Wolfe RM: Update on adult immunizations, *J Am Board Fam Med* 25(4):496-510, 2012.

Yanpiset K, Trope M: Pulp revascularization of replanted immature dog teeth after different treatment methods, *Endod Dent Traumatol* 16(5):211-217, 2000.

Subcondylar Mandibular Fracture

Timothy M. Osborn and Brett A. Ueeck

CC

A 21-year-old man comes to the local emergency department, stating, "I fell and cut my chin." You are asked to evaluate this patient.

Falls show a greater proportion of subcondylar fractures compared with other fracture patterns; the role of the dentition and the influence of open versus closed mouth position are likely of minor importance. The force from direct blunt trauma at the chin (symphysis) in a fall is transmitted to the condylar region and, given the reduced cross-sectional area, a fracture is most likely to occur at this site.

HPI

The patient reports that during routine daily exercise, he jumped over a fence, tripped, and landed on his chin and right hand. He was seen at a local emergency department for the deep laceration on his chin. He also complains of inability to open wide and pain in front of his right ear. The patient did not lose consciousness, and no bleeding from the ear canal, auditory dysfunction, dizziness, tinnitus, nausea/vomiting, or visual changes are present. There is no dyspnea, stridor, or inability to manage secretions. The patient states that he is unable to get the teeth to interdigitate, he has reduced ability to open the mouth, and he feels intense pain when attempting excursive movements. There are no neurosensory changes in the lip, chin, tongue, or midface.

A thorough review of systems is essential when evaluating these patients, as is ensuring appropriate advanced trauma life support (ATLS) evaluation. Traumatic force to the mandible is transmitted to the skull base. A review of symptoms related to intracranial injury and closed head injury, as mentioned previously, allows the surgeon to determine additional studies, evaluations, or referrals. The surgeon must also be diligent about investigating signs of cervical injury; the association between mandibular fractures and cervical spine injuries is well established (although these two types of injuries infrequently occur together), and any neck pain warrants further evaluation. In addition, the surgeon must evaluate for signs of concomitant mandibular fractures, because more than half of fractures are associated with contralateral parasymphysis or body/angle fracture. A significant impact to the chin, as occurred in the current patient, raises concern for bilateral subcondylar fracture with the potential for airway compromise; therefore, a review of symptoms related to airway obstruction must be performed.

PMHX/PDHX/MEDICATIONS/ALLERGIES/SH/FH

Noncontributory.

EXAMINATION

General. The patient is a well-developed and well-nourished man in no apparent distress.

Maxillofacial. There is a 3-cm hemostatic laceration at the submental region with no foreign body or signs of obvious fracture. Upon opening, the mandible deviates to the right (due to the unopposed contralateral lateral pterygoid muscle and impaired rotation and translation on the affected side). The maximal interincisal opening is limited to 20 mm, with associated pain. There is edema of the right preauricular region, no deformity of the ear, no blood at the external auditory canal (EAC), no hemotympanum, and normal auditory acuity (hemotympanum and blood at the EAC may indicate perforation of the anterior tympanic plate). There is no otorrhea or Battle's sign (which may indicate basilar skull fracture and CSF leakage). Palpation of the right preauricular region also elicits pain (pain in the preauricular area with a history of trauma to the symphysis is highly suggestive of a subcondylar fracture).

Intraoral. Left lateral excursive movement is limited to 2 mm (excursive movement of the mandible to the left requires the function of the right lateral pterygoid against an intact condylar neck). There are no associated intraoral lacerations and no dental trauma (fractures of the teeth are not uncommon with forceful closure of the mandible at the time of trauma). Occlusal examination shows premature contacts on the right side, with a posterior left open bite (secondary to collapse of the vertical height of the mandible on the right). The airway is patent with no obstruction or reduction in airflow.

Extremities. There is pain to passive range of motion (ROM) of the right wrist. A palpable radial pulse and normal capillary refill in the nail beds are present (vascular compromise from a distal radial fracture or a carpal bone fracture, or in a compartment system, is a surgical emergency).

IMAGING

Depending on the facility, initial imaging for evaluation of the mandible may include a computed tomography (CT) scan, cone-beam CT scan, panoramic radiograph, or plain view mandibular series that includes lateral and posteroanterior cephalometric films, a reverse Towne's view, and oblique views of the mandible. Many rural hospitals still use a plain view series of the mandible. Most hospitals use a CT scan, which has become the gold standard imaging modality. A CT scan allows the entire face to be evaluated in one study. The mandible can also be evaluated in several different anatomic planes. The axial and coronal planes are the two most commonly used views. The coronal plane can be very helpful for condylar process fractures and for determining dislocation and orientation; the axial planes are useful for intracapsular fractures and the remainder of the mandible. Direct coronal imaging requires hyperextension of the neck and should not be obtained in patients with a suspicion of cervical spine injury. Three-dimensional reconstructions are extremely valuable and allow preoperative planning in a more sophisticated manner for complex cases such as gunshot wounds or severely comminuted fractures. A panoramic film is the single best plain film for evaluating the entire mandible at once. In combination with a reverse Towne's view, the sensitivity for detecting a condylar process fracture increases. However, all modalities have limitations, and surgeons should use imaging studies based on individual cases and available resources.

For the current patient, a CT scan was obtained as the initial study. It demonstrated a right subcondylar fracture on coronal and axial views (Figure 8-5). A plain wrist film was also obtained, which revealed a right-sided fracture of the distal radius (Colles fracture).

LABS

No routine laboratory testing is indicated unless dictated by the medical history.

ASSESSMENT

Right subcondylar fracture of the mandible and associated chin laceration; Colles fracture of the right wrist; FISS score of 1.

TREATMENT

The treatment of fractures of the mandibular condyle is one of the most widely debated topics in the maxillofacial literature. Several variables should be considered when determining treatment and predicting the prognosis, including the level of fracture, degree and direction of displacement, age and medical status of the patient, concomitant injuries, and status of the dentition. Assael has developed a comprehensive list of considerations affecting treatment selection and outcome, all of which should be included in the evaluation of the patient prior to the institution of therapy. Although comprehensive discussion of these considerations is beyond the scope of this chapter, the variables can be divided into patient, surgeon, and third-party categories. Age, gender, medical status, compliance, associated injuries, and fracture type are a few of the patient-specific variables. The surgeon's ability and resources, in addition to resources to cover the expense of treatment, are also pertinent to successful treatment.

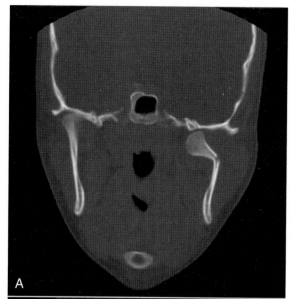

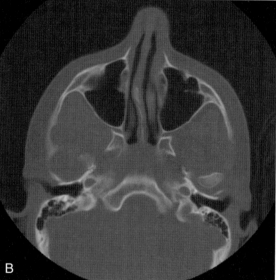

Figure 8-5   **A,** Coronal view of the ramus and condyle showing anteromedially displaced subcondylar fracture on the right side. **B,** Axial view at the level of the glenoid fossae. Notice the absence of the condyle from the fossa on the right.

The primary goal in the treatment of any fracture is adequate stabilization that allows for fracture healing and primary osseous union. In the treatment of mandibular condyle fractures, the goals of treatment are:

- Pain-free mouth opening with return to an acceptable interincisal opening
- Pain-free functional movement
- Restoration of occlusion
- Facial and jaw symmetry and establishment of facial height
- Minimal visible scarring

Preinjury alignment of the mandibular condyle within the glenoid fossa is not essential for adequate rehabilitation after mandibular condyle fractures. The pull of the lateral pterygoid muscle characteristically displaces the condyle anteriorly and medially; therefore, closed reduction (more correctly termed "closed treatment") typically does not reduce the condyle into its original position.

The treatment options are categorized into surgical and nonsurgical modalities. Surgical treatment includes open reduction with or without internal fixation; however, most agree that if an open approach is taken, fixation should be applied. Endoscopic reduction and fixation of condylar fractures has gained popularity during the past decade. The use of this technique requires familiarity with the endoscope and the ability to convert the procedure to an open method if endoscopic reduction fails to successfully complete the procedure. The options for nonsurgical treatment include closed reduction (closed treatment) with maxillomandibular fixation (CR-MMF) and dietary modification with ROM exercises. In the treatment of facial fractures, patients older than 10 years are treated in a manner similar to that for adults; however, it is rarely advocated that children and teenagers undergo open reduction of condylar fractures. A soft diet with mobilization is the treatment of choice in patients 15 years old or younger. If the occlusion is unstable and not reproducible, a short period of intermaxillary fixation (2 weeks) can be advocated.

For the current patient, the occlusion was reestablished easily with minimal manipulation, and after extensive discussion of procedures, alternatives, risks, and benefits, the patient was placed in maxillomandibular fixation (MMF) for 4 weeks, After the 4 weeks, an aggressive post-treatment physiotherapy program was instituted, with active and passive range of motion exercises. Return to full function occurred within 4 weeks of release from MMF. There were no postoperative complications and, the patient returned to full function with stable and repeatable occlusion.

COMPLICATIONS

The complications of treating fractures of the mandibular condyle are well described in the literature and are often used as the basis of comparison for surgical and nonsurgical treatment. One of the most severe late complications can be temporomandibular joint (TMJ) ankylosis (fusion between the mandibular condyle and the glenoid fossa). Patients with TMJ ankylosis often have a history of facial trauma. Prevention of ankylosis was discussed by Zide and Kent in 1983. They advocated appropriate physiotherapy early in the phase of nonsurgical treatment. Other types of late mandibular dysfunction have been cited as complications of closed reduction, including chronic pain, malocclusion, internal derangement, asymmetry, limited mobility, and gross radiographic abnormalities (however, radiographic abnormalities in the absence of pain or functional impairment have no clinical significance). Long-term complications of open reduction and internal fixation (ORIF) are scar perception, facial nerve palsy/paralysis, loss or failure of fixation, Frey's syndrome, avascular necrosis, TMJ dysfunction, and facial asymmetry. The early complications are few and can include early failure of fixation, malocclusion, pain, and infection.

DISCUSSION

As is common with most traumatic injuries, fractures of the mandibular condyle occur in men (78%) between the ages of 20 and 39 (60%). The majority of the fractures are unilateral (84%); fewer are bilateral (16%); 14% of fractures are intracapsular, 24% are in the condylar neck, and 62% are subcondylar fractures. Adults have a relatively narrow condylar neck and thick articular surface, whereas the pediatric patient has a relatively broad condylar neck and thin articular surface in an active osteogenic phase (pediatric fractures are discussed later in the chapter).

Many studies have compared various outcomes of surgical and nonsurgical therapy, with most of the debate centering on ORIF and CR-MMF (closed treatment). The outcomes studied included perception of pain, occlusal function, asymmetry, maximal interincisal opening/ROM, muscle activity, malocclusion, midline deviation, radiographic changes, and nerve dysfunction. Brandt and Haug in 2003 conducted a review of the literature (Table 8-1) regarding open versus closed treatment and suggested indications for closed and open reduction. If a patient has an acceptable ROM, good occlusion, and minimal pain, observation or CR-MMF is preferred, regardless of the level of the fracture. They also suggested that condylar displacement and ramus height instability are the only orthopedic indications for ORIF of condylar fractures. Based on their review, they concluded that under similar indications and conditions, ORIF is the preferred approach. In 2009, Ellis developed a method for determining which patients would not benefit from ORIF using preoperative imaging and intraoperative clinical evaluation. This method demonstrated that patients with fractures that did not easily drop back into a malocclusion with digital pressure would not require either open reduction and can be treated with elastics to attain an acceptable occlusion.

Haug and Assael described the indications and contraindications for open treatment of condylar fractures in 2001. Their absolute indications for ORIF are patient preference (when no absolute or relative contraindications coexist); cases in which manipulation and closed reduction cannot reestablish pretraumatic occlusion and/or excursion; cases in which rigid internal fixation is used to address other fractures, affecting the occlusion; the rare instance of intracranial impaction of the proximal condylar segment; and cases in which stability of the occlusion is limited. Among the absolute contraindications are condylar head fractures (including single fragment, comminuted, and medial pole) and patients in whom medical illness or systemic injury adds undo risk to an extended general anesthesia. Condylar neck fractures were among the relative contraindications.

With nonsurgical techniques, there is no consensus on the use or duration of immobilization. Literature is available supporting anywhere from 0 to 6 weeks of closed treatment. A period of MMF is typically instituted for one of three reasons:

Table 8-1	Open Versus Closed Treatment of Mandibular Subcondylar Fractures: Review of the Literature		
Author	**Total Number of Patients**	**Follow-Up**	**Results**
Hidding et al.	20 ORIF/54 CR-MMF	5 yr	Deviation: 64% CR-MMF; 10% ORIF
			Anatomic reconstruction: 93% ORIF; 7% CR-MMF
			No differences in headaches, mastication, or MIIO
Konstantinovic and Dimitrijevic	26 ORIF/54 CR-MMF	2.5 yr	ORIF: 100% were 81% to 100% of ideal
			CR-MMF: 77.7% were 81% to 100% of ideal
			No difference in deviation or MIIO
Oezman et al.	20 ORIF/10 CR-MMF	2 yr	ORIF: MRI revealed 10% disc displacement
			CR-MMF: MRI revealed 30% disc displacement; also, MRI revealed 80% of CR-MMF with maligned or deformed condyles
Worsae and Thorn	61 CR-MMF/40 ORIF	2 yr	CR-MMF: 39% complication rate (asymmetry, malocclusion, reduced MIIO, headaches, pain)
			ORIF: 4% complication rate (malocclusion, impaired mastication, pain)
Haug and Assael	10 CR-MMF/10 ORIF	6 yr	ORIF/CR-MMF: No statistically significant differences in ROM, occlusion, contour, or motor or sensory function
			ORIF: Associated with perceptible scars
			CR-MMF: Associated with chronic pain
Throckmorton et al.	14 CR-MMF/62 ORIF	3 yr	ORIF/CR-MMF: No perceivable differences in mandibular motion or muscle activity
Palmieri et al.	74 CR-MMF/62 ORIF	3 yr	ORIF: Greater mobility
Ellis et al.	65 CR-MMF	6 wk	Position of condylar process is not static
Ellis et al.	61 ORIF	6 mo	Anatomic reduction possible, but changes in condylar process position may result from loss of fixation
Ellis et al.	77 ORIF/65 CR-MMF	3 yr	CR-MMF: Significantly greater percentage of malocclusion
Ellis and Throckmorton	81 CR-MMF/65 ORIF	3 yr	CR-MMF: Shorter posterior facial and ramus heights on injured side
Ellis et al.	93 ORIF/85 CR-MMF	3 yr	ORIF: 17.2% facial nerve weakness at 6 weeks with 0% at 6 mo and 7.5% scarring judged as hypertrophic
Ellis and Throckmorton	91 CR-MMF/64 ORIF	3 yr	ORIF/CR-MMF: No difference noted in maximum bite forces

From Brandt MT, Haug RH: Open versus closed reduction of adult mandibular condyle fractures: a review of the literature regarding the evolution of current thoughts on management, J Oral Maxillofac Surg 61:1324-1332, 2003.
CR-MMF, Closed reduction with maxillomandibular fixation; *MIIO,* maximal interincisal opening; *ORIF,* open reduction and internal fixation; *ROM,* range of motion.

1. Patient comfort
2. To promote osseous union and restore premorbid occlusion
3. To help reduce the fractured segment

One method for treating fractures with no occlusal disturbances, acceptable ROM, and minimal pain is to place the patient in early full function, along with functional physiotherapy. If the patient demonstrates occlusal discrepancy, Erich arch bars can be placed for MMF or guiding elastics. For pediatric patients in a mixed dentition stage who demonstrate an occlusal discrepancy, there may be a need for circummandibular wires and/or circumzygomatic or piriform wires to obtain adequate stabilization.

Regardless of the type of treatment, patients should undergo postoperative physical therapy. Functional therapy is needed to improve ROM, asymmetric movements, scarring within the joint, or other TMJ dysfunctions. If there is limitation in mouth opening, tongue blades or other sequentially enlarging devices to gradually improve the range of mandibular opening can be used. For patients with asymmetric mouth opening, it is recommended that they function on the contralateral side.

Patients can be encouraged to observe their opening and closing in the mirror and to use their hand to help correct any asymmetric movement. The overall goal is to achieve early full function and restoration to symmetric, pain-free mandibular motion.

When the decision is made to use ORIF, many advocate a retromandibular approach. This approach affords excellent exposure to the ramus-condyle unit for reduction and fixation. The approach was first described by Hinds and Girotti in 1967 and later adapted for use in the treatment of mandibular condylar fractures. An incision of 3 cm is made parallel to the posterior border of the mandible starting 1 cm below the earlobe. Dissection proceeds through skin, subcutaneous tissue, and platysma down to the parotid capsule. The tail of the parotid is released and elevated with blunt dissection, if necessary, to avoid violation of the parotid capsule. The posterior mandible and pterygomasseteric sling are identified. The periosteum at the posterior border of the mandible is incised and dissected in a subperiosteal plane. Both sides of the fracture are exposed to facilitate reduction and fixation. A similar approach can be used with endoscopy. This approach

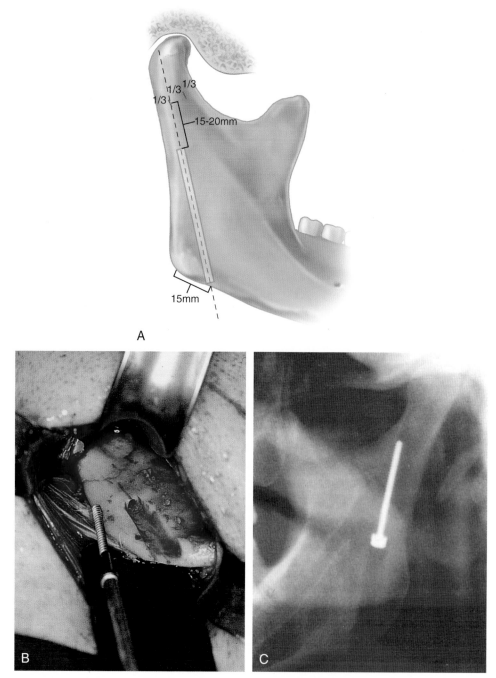

allows excellent exposure to the ramus-condyle unit, minimal visible scarring, and a low incidence of facial nerve damage. Other surgical approaches to the mandibular condyle include a preauricular (or endaural) incision, intraoral incision, or Risdon-type incision, depending on the fracture pattern and location.

Multiple modalities have been used to rigidly fix mandibular condylar fractures. Studies have evaluated the biomechanical behavior of dynamic compression plates, locking plates, mini–dynamic compression plates, adaptation plates, and single and double miniplates. Both mini–dynamic compression plates and double miniplates have been shown to

be stable for fixation. It has also been shown that resorbable plates are effective and provide reliable stability in ORIF of condylar fractures. Many surgeons recommend that fixation be applied with the use of one or two 2-mm plates with two or three bicortical screws on both sides of the fracture. Lag screw fixation can be used in appropriate situations (Figure 8-6).

As is true for most conditions, the treatment of pediatric patients requires special consideration. Up to 40% of mandibular fractures in pediatric patients involve the condyle. Anatomically, pediatric patients have a relatively broad condylar neck and a thin articular surface; this accounts for the fact that 41% of the fractures are intracapsular. Clinical suspicion and accurate diagnosis are crucial in the early stages, because missed or delayed diagnosis may not be apparent until further growth leads to morphologic or occlusal disturbance. Because pediatric patients are often in the mixed dentition stage, occlusal changes may not be as readily detected. Imaging of children is of particular concern; panoramic imaging is useful, but coronal CT has been found to be highly diagnostic in the pediatric population. Historically, nonsurgical treatment of condylar fractures has involved MMF followed by physiotherapy; given the greater osteogenic potential and faster healing rates in children than in adults, the duration of MMF has been decreasing over time and often is not even used. We recommend that a soft diet, aggressive physiotherapy, and growth monitoring be used and that closed treatment be reserved for open bite or malocclusion. Although many are proponents of open reduction even in a pediatric population, there is little role for this treatment modality, and no functional benefit has been shown. Growth disturbance has been associated with pediatric condylar fractures, and growth surveillance should be provided for all patients with these injuries.

Airway

Acute airway obstruction after bilateral mandibular fractures is typically associated with symphyseal injuries, in which lack of bony continuity causes collapse of the genioglossus and intrinsic tongue musculature and obstruction into the oropharynx. Medical personnel involved in primary and secondary surveys often are concerned about airway obstruction in patients with bilateral condylar fractures. Although the airway should be rapidly and continuously evaluated in any patient with maxillofacial injuries, condylar injuries have never been shown to be a cause of airway obstruction.

The treatment of fractures of the mandibular condyle requires consideration of many factors. Many techniques are available to surgeons and patients. Always, the best course is to use the simplest approach with the lowest risk of morbidity to accomplish the goals of treatment.

Bibliography

Assael LA: Open versus closed reduction of adult mandibular condyle fractures: an alternative interpretation of the evidence, *J Oral Maxillofac Surg* 61:1333-1339, 2003.

Beekler DM, Walker RV: Condylar fractures, *J Oral Surg* 27:563, 1969.

Behnia H, Motamedi MHK, Tehranchi A: Use of activator appliances in pediatric patients treated with costochondral grafts for temporomandibular joint ankylosis: an analysis of 13 cases, *J Oral Maxillofac Surg* 55:1408, 1997.

Brandt MT, Haug RH: Open versus closed reduction of adult mandibular condyle fractures: a review of the literature regarding the evolution of current thoughts on management, *J Oral Maxillofac Surg* 61:1324-1332, 2003.

Chacon GE, Dawson KH, Myall RW, et al: A comparative study of two imaging techniques for the diagnosis of condylar fractures in children, *J Oral Maxillofac Surg* 61:668, 2003.

Chatzistavrou EK, Basdra EK: Conservative treatment of isolated condylar fractures in growing patients, *World J Orthod* 8:241, 2007.

Choi BH, Yi CK, Yoo JH, et al: Clinical evaluation of three types of plate osteosynthesis for fixation of condylar neck fractures, *J Oral Maxillofac Surg* 59:734-737, 2001.

Chossegros C, Cheynet F, Blanc JL, et al: Short retromandibular approach of subcondylar fractures: clinical and radiologic long-term evaluation, *Oral Surg Oral Med Oral Pathol Oral Radiol Endod* 82:248-252, 1996.

Chrcanovic BR: Open versus closed reduction: mandibular condyle fractures in children, *Oral Maxillofac Surg* 16:245, 2012.

Ellis E, McFadden D, Simon P, et al: Surgical complications with open treatment of mandibular condylar process fractures, *J Oral Maxillofac Surg* 58:950, 2000.

Ellis EE: Method to determine when open treatment of condylar process fractures is not necessary, *J Oral Maxillofac Surg* 67:1685, 2009.

Ellis EE, Dean J: Rigid fixation of mandibular condyle fractures, *Oral Surg Oral Med Oral Pathol Oral Radiol Endod* 76:6-15, 1993.

Ellis EE, Throckmorton GS: Treatment of mandibular condylar process fractures: biologic considerations, *J Oral Maxillofac Surg* 63:115-134, 2005.

El-Sheikh MM, Medra AM, Warda MH: Bird face deformity secondary to bilateral temporomandibular joint ankylosis, *J Craniomaxillofac Surg* 24:96, 1996.

Eppley BL: Use of resorbable plates and screws in pediatric facial fractures, *J Oral Maxillofac Surg* 63(3):385-391, 2005.

Haug RH, Assael LA: Outcomes of open versus closed treatment of mandibular subcondylar fractures, *J Oral Maxillofac Surg* 59:370-375, 2001.

Haug RH, Gilman PP, Goltz M: A biomechanical evaluation of mandibular condyle fracture plating techniques, *J Oral Maxillofac Surg* 60:73-80, 2002.

Hinds EC, Girotti WJ: Vertical subcondylar osteotomy: a reappraisal, *Oral Surg Oral Med Oral Pathol Oral Radiol Endod* 80:394-397, 1967.

Ikemura K: Treatment of condylar fractures associated with other mandibular fractures, *J Oral Maxillofac Surg* 43:810, 1985.

Ivy RH, Curtis L: *Fractures of the jaws*, p 78, Philadelphia, 1931, Lea & Febiger.

Manisali M, Amin M, Aghabeigi B, et al: Retromandibular approach to the mandibular condyle: a clinical and cadaveric study, *Int J Oral Maxillofac Surg* 32:253-256, 2003.

Posnick JF, Wells M, Pron GE: Pediatric facial fractures: evolving patterns of treatment, *J Oral Maxillofac Surg* 51:836, 1993.

Schüle H: Injuries of the temporomandibular joint. In Krüger E, Schilli W (eds): *Oral and maxillofacial traumatology*, vol 2, pp 45-70, Chicago, 1986, Quintessence.

Silovennoinen U, Iizuka T, Lindqvist C, et al: Different patterns of condylar fractures: an analysis of 382 patients in a 3-year period, *J Oral Maxillofac Surg* 50:1032,1992.

Suzuki T, Kawamura H, Kasahara T, et al: Resorbable poly-L-lactide plates and screws for the treatment of mandibular condyle process fractures: a clinical and radiologic follow-up study, *J Oral Maxillofac Surg* 62:919-924, 2004.

Thoren H, Hallikainen D, Iizuka T, et al: Condylar process fractures in children: a follow-up study of fractures with total dislocation of the condyle from the glenoid fossa, *J Oral Maxillofac Surg* 59:768-773, 2001.

Villareal PM, Monje F, Junquera LM, et al: Mandibular condyle fractures: determinants of outcome, *J Oral Maxillofac Surg* 62:155-163, 2004.

Zide MF, Kent JN: Indications for open reduction of mandibular condyle fractures, *J Oral Maxillofac Surg* 41(2):89-98, 1983.

Combined Mandibular Parasymphysis and Angle Fractures

Michael Wilkinson, Brett A. Ueeck, and Shahrokh C. Bagheri

CC

You are asked by the trauma physician at your local emergency department (ED) to evaluate a 23-year-old male patient for facial fractures (mandibular fractures are more common in males in the third decade of life). His chief complaint is, "My jaw hurts, and my teeth do not come together like before."

HPI

The patient was riding his motocross bike earlier today when he crashed and landed on his face. He was not wearing a helmet; however, he denies any loss of consciousness. He was able to get up from the scene and ride his bike to the ED. He explains that his lower face and jaw are painful, his teeth do not occlude correctly, and his left lip is anesthetic.

Assault, motor vehicle accidents, and sporting injuries are the most common etiologies of mandibular fractures. Malocclusion is the single most important historic information suggestive of a mandibular or dentoalveolar fracture. Paresthesia of the distribution of the third division of the trigeminal nerve (V3) is common and can be due to neuropraxia, axonotmesis, or neurotmesis of the mental or inferior alveolar nerve at the fracture site.

PMHX/PDHX/MEDICATIONS/ALLERGIES/SH/FH

The patient smokes one pack of cigarettes a day and drinks alcohol on the weekends. He denies all other habits (both alcohol and tobacco use have been associated with an increased risk of infectious complications with mandibular fractures).

EXAMINATION

Primary Survey

Airway and cervical spine control. Speaking without difficulty (in cases of multiply fragmented mandibular fractures, the upper airway can become acutely compromised due to posterior collapse of the tongue with loss of a stable genioglossus insertion at the genial tubercle). The cervical spine examination is within normal limits (WNL) (Haug and colleagues report an association between cervical spine injuries and mandibular fractures. The stability of the cervical spine is crucial throughout the care of the patient).

Breathing and oxygenation. Unlabored. Oxygen saturation of 97% on room air.

Circulation. No active bleeding.

General. Semisupine on ED bed with O_2.

Vital signs. Blood pressure 116/78 mm Hg, heart rate 70 bpm, respirations 12 per minute, T 37°C.

Secondary Survey

Neurologic. Alert and oriented × 3. Glasgow Coma Scale score (GCS) 15.

Maxillofacial. The facial structures are grossly symmetric. Examination of the eyes (pupils, visual acuity, visual fields, and extraocular movements) is WNL. External ears are without deformity. Tympanic membranes (TMs) are clear (external auditory canal lacerations, tympanic plate rupture, and fracture of the posterior wall of the joint should be ruled out). The remainder of the facial bones are stable except for the mandible, which demonstrates mobility in the parasymphysis region on the right and in the left angle region. Facial edema is present bilaterally, with tenderness to palpation at the fracture sites. This movement causes pain. Cranial nerves II through XII are intact, with the exception of anesthesia of V3 on the left side. The neck is nontender and demonstrates full range of active movement with no neck pain (it is important to rule out cervical spine injury).

Intraoral. The dentition is in moderate repair. The patient has obvious steps in the occlusal plane between teeth #25 and #26 and distal to tooth #18. There are multiple lacerations involving the gingiva in the associated areas. He has an obvious malocclusion. There is hematoma formation in the anterior floor of the mouth.

IMAGING

Most practitioners consider computed tomography (CT) scans to be the gold standard imaging modality for evaluation of mandibular fractures. A CT scan allows the entire face to be evaluated in one study. Facial bones, including the mandible, can be evaluated in several different anatomic planes. The axial and coronal planes are the two most commonly used views. The coronal plane can be very helpful for condylar process fractures, whereas the axial views are useful for the corpus. Patients with suspicion of cervical spine injury should not have the neck hyperextended for direct coronal imaging. Instead. digitally reconstructed coronal images can be used.

Despite the popularity of CT imaging, in many facilities the initial imaging studies may consist of a panoramic radiograph or a plain view series of the mandible (posterior-anterior, reverse Towne's, bilateral lateral oblique radiographs).

Many hospitals still use a plain view series of the mandible; therefore, familiarity with plain radiographs is important.

A panoramic radiograph is the imaging modality of choice for patients presenting at the surgeon's office. This radiograph is inexpensive and is the single best plain film for evaluation of the entire mandible. However, nondisplaced or minimally displaced fractures of the condyle or the symphyseal area may be difficult to detect on a panoramic radiograph. The combination of a reverse Towne's view and an anterior-posterior radiograph of the mandible results in a sensitivity and specificity similar to that of a CT scan. The decision to order different imaging modalities should be based on available resources, physical exam findings, and the cost and knowledge of limitations related to particular studies. When available, in-office cone-beam CT scans are excellent for evaluating mandibular fractures.

For the current patient, a panoramic radiograph demonstrates fractures at the left angle and in the right parasymphysis area (Figure 8-7, *A*). A anterior-posterior view of the mandible shows severe displacement at the left angle (which explains the anesthesia of the left V3) and fracture at the right parasymphysis (Figure 8-7, *B*); note that the degree of lateral displacement is not evident on the panoramic radiograph.

LABS

Routine laboratory testing is not mandatory prior to surgical correction of mandibular fractures unless dictated by underlying medical conditions. In cases of infected mandibular fractures, a white blood cell count should be obtained.

ASSESSMENT

Open mandibular fractures at the right parasymphysis (nondisplaced), and left angle (severely displaced). Facial Injury Severity Scale (FISS) score of 4. Also, an associated injury to the left inferior alveolar nerve most consistent with neurotmesis or a Sunderland's class 5 injury.

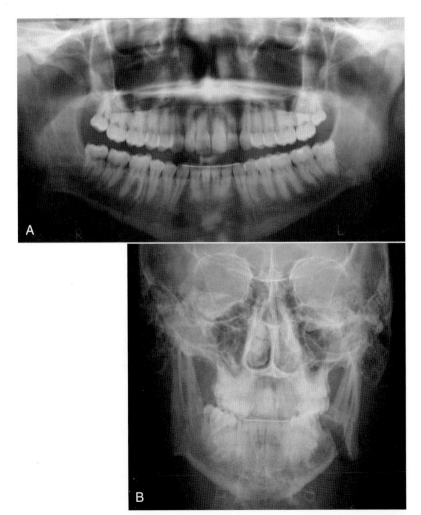

Figure 8-7   **A,** Panoramic radiograph demonstrating a fracture at the left angle and right parasymphysis area. **B,** Anterior-posterior (AP) radiograph of the skull showing severe lateral displacement of the mandibular angle on the left. The fracture at the right parasymphysis is also evident.

TREATMENT

The treatment of mandibular fractures has a long and complicated history, dating back to 1600 B.C. The mandible is unique in that it is singled out as the bone in the face requiring special attention for various aspects of treatment (occlusion, esthetics, function) to achieve a good result. The important points in treating mandibular fractures are immobilizing fractures, appropriate use of antibiotics, and restoration of form and function.

Mandibular fractures at the angle and parasymphysis involving the teeth-bearing segments are considered open fractures. Treatment should be rendered in a timely fashion, as soon as the patient is stable and operating room facilities are available. Preoperative antibiotics have been shown to decrease the incidence of postoperative infectious complications and should be initiated regardless of the time interval before definitive surgery can be completed. The use of postoperative antibiotics remains largely practitioner dependent, and no good evidence exists guiding its necessity and potential benefits or the duration of treatment.

More important in the prevention of infection is the proper application of fixation. Movement at the fracture site increases not only the chance of infection but also the development of fibrous union, malunion, or nonunion. Rigid fixation is the key to a good outcome. However, semirigid fixation techniques, when correctly applied, can also provide a successful outcome. In addition, lag screws are a strong form of fixation and provide very good rigidity; however, the technique is not applicable to all fractures. Locking (rather than nonlocking) fixation plates provide continued rigidity if the contact area at the screw or plate–to–bone interface is reduced due to bony remodeling. In addition, locking plates do not require precise adaptation to the bony anatomy, because the screw is "locked" into special threads in the plate. Closed reduction of mandibular fractures continues to be an acceptable form of treatment and in certain patients is the best option. Closed reduction does not offer the benefit of early function, and the patient must tolerate a prolonged period of intermaxillary fixation.

If the mandible has more than one fracture, consideration should be given to the sequence of fixation. It is generally advocated to fixate the fracture segments involving dentate segments, to ensure correct occlusal relationship, prior to fixation of nondentate segments. In the current patient, the parasymphysis facture was repaired first to correctly establish arch form and occlusion.

The patient was treated with open reduction and rigid internal fixation (ORIF) under general anesthesia in an ambulatory care facility (Figure 8-8). Arch bars were applied, and subsequently the occlusion and arch form were reestablished. Fixation at the parasymphysis fracture was completed by placing a plate at the superior border (zone of tension) and a plate at the inferior border (zone of compression). The fracture at the angle was reduced and fixated using rigid fixation plates at the superior and inferior borders. No postoperative maxillomandibular fixation (MMF) was used. The patient was allowed to function and maintain a soft-chew diet. The use of antibiotics consisted of perioperative intravenous penicillin. The patient was sent home with a prescription for Peridex and oral analgesics. The postoperative course was otherwise uncomplicated.

This type of fracture can also be treated using a single lag screw placed according to the Niederdellman method (Figure 8-9).

COMPLICATIONS

Mandibular angle fractures are generally more prone to the development of complications compared with the body, symphyseal, or parasymphyseal areas. Multiple complications may arise, but the most common are loose hardware, necessitating removal; infection; malocclusion; delayed union; and fibrous union. Damage to the inferior alveolar and lingual

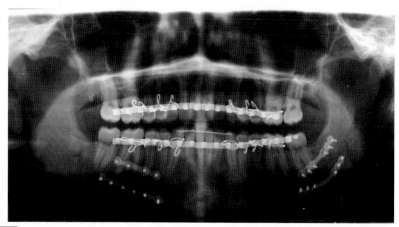

Figure 8-8 Postoperative panoramic radiograph demonstrating rigid fixation of the fracture segments.

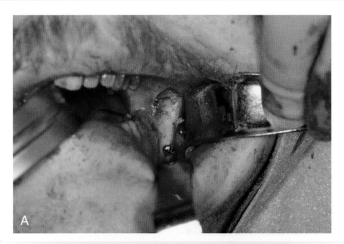

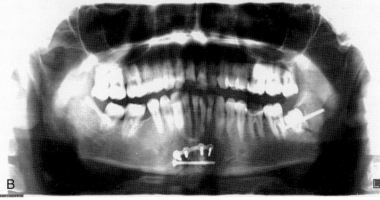

Figure 8-9   Different patient with angle and parasymphysis fractures. **A,** Intraoperative view of angle fracture treated with a single lag screw. **B,** Postoperative panoramic radiograph showing fixation at the angle using a lag screw and fixation of the parasymphysis using a lag screw and a superior border plate.

nerves can be a complication of the initial injury or a consequence of treatment. Infection rates for angle fractures reportedly range from 2% to more than 19%.

DISCUSSION

There is a variety of options for the treatment of mandibular fractures, and these options primarily differ in the method of fixation (number, size, and location of fixation plates and screws). Traditionally, mandibular fractures have been successfully treated with closed reduction using intermaxillary fixation. This method results in relatively few complications. However, it is associated with a delay in functional rehabilitation compared with the more modern ORIF techniques.

Open reduction and internal fixation failed to attain widespread use prior to the 1960s mainly due to early reports of metal corrosion of steel plates and screws, metal fatigue, and screw loosening. The advent of biocompatible materials (e.g., Vitallium and titanium), along with orthopedic biomechanical studies describing the benefits of compression osteosynthesis, increased interest in open treatment of mandibular fractures. Today many practitioners prefer open to closed reduction of parasymphysis/angle fractures of the mandible. The treatment

of subcondylar fractures has caused a series of controversies that are addressed in a separate chapter.

Considerable variation is seen when methods of fixation are compared. For example, dynamic compression plating (Schmoker and Spiessl), monocortical noncompression miniplate (Michelet), superior border mandibular angle plate (Champy) (Figure 8-10), lag screw (Niederdellmann and colleagues), and rigid locking reconstruction plate techniques have all been described in the literature. Consensus on the optimal treatment of mandibular parasymphysis/angle fractures remains elusive; each method has its pros and cons, and few prospective, randomized trials have been done for direct comparison.

Angle fractures produce the highest frequency of complications among mandibular fractures. Infection, malunion, nonunion, and damage to adjacent structures (nerve, tooth) all plague reduction of this anatomic site. Thus many practitioners advocate absolute rigidity of the bony segments for rapid, uncomplicated healing. Early on, the *Arbeits-gemeinschaft für Osteosynthesefragen*/Association for the Study of Internal Fixation (AO/ASIF) established principles recommending superior and inferior border dynamic compression plates. On the other end of the spectrum, Champy recommended a single

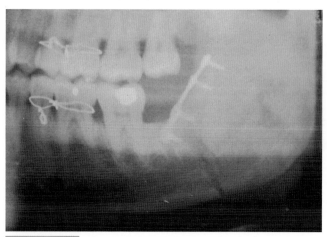

Figure 8-10 Postoperative panoramic radiograph of a patient with a left angle mandibular fracture. The left angle is treated using the Champy technique, with semirigid fixation with a four-hole plate.

noncompression miniplate at the superior border for angle fractures, based on his studies demonstrating the tendency of the superior border to separate from unfavorable muscle pull (tension zone) and the inferior mandibular border to compress (compression zone), with an interposed neutral zone or "line of zero force." Contrary to the principles of interfragment rigidity for optimal healing, some studies describe decreased complications with less rigid techniques, such as the Champy technique.

Niederdellmann in the 1970s described the use of lag screws for the treatment of mandibular angle fractures, with placement of the screw through the impacted third molar, if present, and subsequent removal of the tooth and screw after healing. Due to technique sensitivity and difficulty, the Niederdellmann lag screw technique remains less popular.

Several studies have found an increased risk of angle fractures associated with the presence of impacted third molars. Management of teeth in the line of fracture had previously sparked some controversy. Extraction is undoubtedly indicated when the tooth in the line of fracture is deeply carious, harbors periodontal or pericoronal infection, prevents bony reduction of the fracture, demonstrates severe root exposure, or is fractured. However, in the absence of these conditions, extraction of the tooth has not been shown to have a statistically significant benefit. Ellis reported a relatively increased, but statistically not significant, risk of postoperative complications (namely, infection) with teeth left in the line of fracture, resulting in the need for infection management and/or removal of hardware. Other studies recommend that tooth buds in the line of fracture be preserved unless infection occurs, requiring subsequent removal.

Overall, mandibular angle fractures are common and relatively easily treated with a variety of conventional techniques. The surgeon should keep in mind the potential complications and adhere strictly to sound principles of treatment, regardless of the technique selected.

Bibliography

Alpert B: Complications in the treatment of facial trauma, *Oral Maxillofac Clin North Am* 11(2):255, 1999.

Barber DH, Smith BM, Deshmuck DD, et al: Mandibular fractures. In Fonseca RJ, Barber HD, Walker RV, et al (eds): *Oral and maxillofacial trauma*, ed 4, pp 293-330, St Louis, 2013, Elsevier.

Champy M, Lodde JP, Schmitt R, et al: Mandibular osteosynthesis by miniature screwed plates via a buccal approach, *J Maxillofac Surg* 614-621, 1978.

Ellis E: Treatment methods for fractures of the mandibular angle, *J Craniomaxillofacial Trauma* 2:28, 1996.

Ellis E: Lag screw fixation of mandibular fractures, *J Craniomaxillofac Trauma* 3:16, 1997.

Ellis E: Outcomes of patients with teeth in the line of mandibular angle fractures treated with stable internal fixation, *J Oral Maxillofac Surg* 60:863, 2002.

Ellis E, Walker L: Treatment of mandibular angle fractures using two noncompression miniplates, *J Oral Maxillofac Surg* 52:1032, 1994.

Gear A, Apasova E, Schmitz JP, et al: Treatment modalities for mandibular angle fractures, *J Oral Maxillofac Surg* 63:655, 2005.

Halmos D, Ellis E, Dodson TB: Mandibular third molars and angle fractures, *J Oral Maxillofac Surg* 62:1076, 2004.

Haug RH, Wible RT, Likavec MJ, et al: Cervical spine fractures and maxillofacial trauma, *J Oral Maxillofac Surg* 49:725, 1991.

Lamphier J, Ziccardi V, Ruvo A, et al: Complications of mandibular fractures in an urban teaching center, *J Oral Maxillofac Surg* 61:745, 2003.

Leonard MS: History of the treatment of maxillofacial trauma, *Oral Maxillofac Clin North Am* 2(1):1, 1990.

Michelet FX, Dessus B, Benoit JP, et al: Mandibular osteosynthesis without blocking by screwed miniature stellite plates, *Rev Stomatol Chir Maxillofac* 74:239-245, 1973.

Murthy A, Lehman J: Symptomatic plate removal in maxillofacial trauma: a review of 76 cases, *Ann Plast Surg* 55:603, 2005.

Niederdellmann H, Akuamoa-Boateng E, Uhlig G: Lag-screw osteosynthesis: a new procedure for treating fractures f the mandibular angle, *J Oral Surg* 39:938, 1981.

Niederdellmann H, Schilli W, Düker J, et al: Osteosynthesis of mandibular fractures using lag screws, *Int J Oral Surg* 5(3):117-121, 1976.

Potter J, Ellis E: Treatment of mandibular angle fractures with a malleable noncompression miniplate, *J Oral Maxillofac Surg* 57:288, 1999.

Prein J (ed): *Manual of internal fixation in the cranio-facial skeleton*, Heidelberg, 1998, Springer Verlag.

Schmoker R, Spiessl B: Excentric-dynamic compression plate. Experimental study as contribution to a functionally stable osteosynthesis in mandibular fractures, *SSO Schweiz Monatsschr Zahnheilkd* 83(12):1496-1509, 1973. German.

Schmoker R, Spiessl B, Tschopp HM, et al: Functionally stable osteosynthesis of the mandible by means of an excentric dynamic compression plate. Results of a follow-up of 25 cases, *SSO Schweiz Monatsschr Zahnheilkd* 86(2):167-185, 1976. German.

Tate GS, Ellis E, Throckmorton G: Bite forces in patients treated for mandibular angle fractures: implications for fixation recommendations, *J Oral Maxillofac Surg* 52:734, 1994.

Zygomaticomaxillary Complex Fracture

Shahrokh C. Bagheri and Chris Jo

CC

A 28-year-old (peak incidence is in the second or third decade) man (male to female ratio is 4:1) is admitted to the local emergency department 4 hours after he was hit on the left side of the face with a fist (left zygoma is most commonly affected). He complains of left-sided facial pain, blurry vision, and inability to open his mouth fully (trismus is present in about one third of patients).

HPI

The patient claims that he was minding his own business when he was suddenly "jumped" and punched in the face by an unknown individual. He does not report losing consciousness. He was subsequently brought to the emergency department by the emergency medical services (EMS) personnel.

PMHX/PDHX/MEDICATIONS/ALLERGIES/SH/FH

The patient has a positive history of alcohol abuse (more common in the trauma population) and an 8 pack-year history of tobacco use.

EXAMINATION

The patient's advanced trauma life support (ATLS) primary survey is negative, and his Glasgow Coma Scale (GCS) score is 15.

General. The patient is alert and oriented × 3. He is a well-developed and well-nourished man in mild distress.

Vital signs. His blood pressure is 130/84 mm Hg, heart rate 120 bpm (tachycardia), respirations 16 per minute, and temperature 37.6°C.

Maxillofacial. There is tenderness over the left zygoma and subconjunctival ecchymoses and edema around the left eye (present in 50% to 70% of cases). There is a palpable step along the zygomaticofrontal (ZF) suture and infraorbital rim, with flattening over the zygomatic arch, in addition to visible depression over the malar eminence and hypoesthesia of the left maxillary branch (V2) of the trigeminal nerve (50% to 90% of cases).

Eyes. The pupils are equal, round, and reactive to light and accommodation (PERRLA) (cranial nerves II and III), with no ptosis (cranial nerve III). There is no proptosis (tense proptosis may be indicative of a retrobulbar hematoma, a surgical emergency). Careful examination of the pupils reveals a downward displacement of the left pupil suggestive of loss of osseous support along the orbital floor and/or an increase in orbital volume. The lateral palpebral fissure appears grossly displaced inferolaterally (producing an anti-mongoloid slant). Examination of the extraocular muscles demonstrates a decrease in range of motion in the extremes of upward and downward gaze (mostly due to edema). Visual fields are intact by confrontation (cranial nerve II). Examination of the left eye confirms binocular diplopia (10% to 40% of cases). Visual acuity is 20/25 bilaterally (cranial nerve II); there is no hyphema (blood in the anterior chamber of the eye); and the fundoscopic examination is within normal limits.

Intraoral. There is ecchymosis of the maxillary buccal sulcus on the left.

IMAGING

The CT scan (bony windows) is the gold standard for evaluation of zygomatic fractures, using axial and coronal sections. Reconstructed parasagittal views through the orbit can be valuable for assessing the orbital floor in the anteroposterior dimension. Direct coronal imaging may not be feasible, given the status of the cervical spine in the acute setting.

In the current patient, axial sections (Figure 8-11, *A*) reveal a significantly displaced left zygoma with fractures at the anterior maxillary wall and zygomaticotemporal (ZT) and zygomaticosphenoid (ZS) sutures. Coronal CT (Figure 8-11, *B*) reveals fractures at the right ZF suture and zygomaticomaxillary (ZM) buttress and disruption of the left orbital floor with displacement of orbital contents into the maxillary sinus. A three-dimensional computer reconstruction, although not necessary, can also be helpful in treatment planning (Figure 8-11, *C*).

Three-dimensional reconstructed CT or cone-beam computed tomography (CBCT) scans can also be most valuable in the diagnosis and visualization of ZMC fractures. Figure 8-12 demonstrates a more severe comminuted and displaced orbito-ZMC fracture.

LABS

No routine laboratory testing is necessary for the management of isolated zygomaticomaxillary complex (ZMC) fractures unless dictated by the medical history. A blood alcohol level and urine drug screen should be obtained in cases of suspected alcohol or drug intoxication.

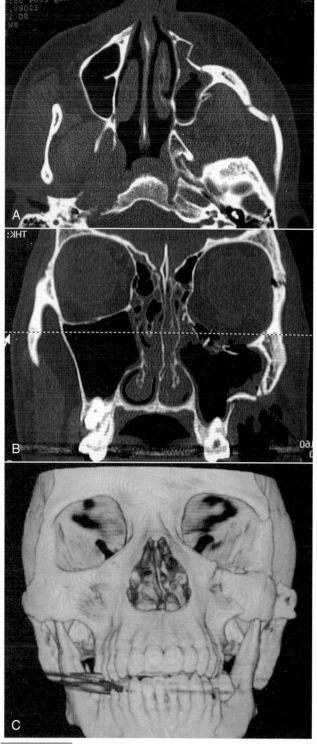

Figure 8-11 **A,** Axial bony window CT scan demonstrating a depressed left ZMC fracture. **B,** Reformatted coronal CT scan demonstrating a left ZMC fracture with mild herniation of orbital contents through the displaced orbital floor fracture. **C,** Three-dimensional reconstruction CT scan demonstrating the degree of displacement of the left ZMC.

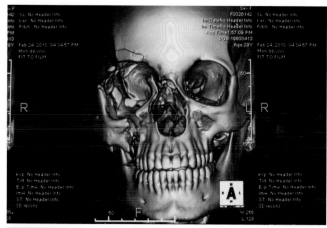

Figure 8-12 Severely fragmented and displaced right ZMC fracture.

The current patient had a blood alcohol level of 150 mg/dl (alcohol is commonly implicated in the trauma population) and a negative urine drug screen.

ASSESSMENT

Isolated fracture of the left ZMC; FISS score of 1.

TREATMENT

The goal of treatment is reduction of the fracture to its anatomic position to achieve optimal functional and aesthetic rehabilitation. The ZS is not commonly fixated, but adequate reduction at this suture is a good indicator of the overall three-dimensional position of the zygoma. The degree of displacement and comminution, the age of the patient, and preexisting skin creases or lacerations, in addition to the status of the globe, should be taken into account for surgical treatment planning. As with any surgery, the best treatment is that which achieves the best outcome with the least intervention. Extensive dissection and plating at multiple sutures may provide a very stable zygoma, yet the anatomic demands on the zygoma may be equally met with more conservative approaches in select cases. In a study by Zachariades and colleagues, 1,270 patients with ZMC fractures were reviewed; the researchers concluded that the best results are achieved with semirigid fixation with miniplates at one or more sites.

The current patient was taken to the operating room for open reduction with internal fixation (ORIF). Fixation was used at the ZF suture via an upper blepharoplasty (supratarsal fold) incision and at the maxillary buttress via the maxillary buccal vestibular approach. The zygomatic arch was reduced via the same incision using a Goldman elevator. Subsequently, the orbital floor and rim were explored and reconstructed via the transconjunctival approach using a titanium mesh and plate. A bilateral forced duction test was performed at beginning and the completion of the procedure.

CT-guided intraoperative navigation has gained some role in the treatment of complex midfacial fractures. This allows

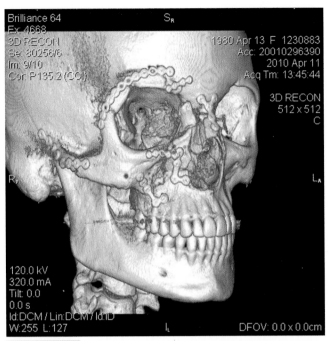

Brilliance 64
Ex: 4668
3D RECON
Se: 30256/6
Im: 9/10
Cor P135.2 (COI)

1980 Apr 13 F 1230883
Acc: 20010296390
2010 Apr 11
Acq Tm: 13:45:44

3D RECON
512 x 512
C

120.0 kV
320.0 mA
Tilt: 0.0
0.0 s
Id:DCM / Lin:DCM / Id:ID
W:255 L:127

DFOV: 0.0 x 0.0cm

Figure 8-13 Right ZMC fracture reduction using CT-guided intraoperative navigation.

three-dimensional intraoperative visualization of the anatomy, for more accurate reconstruction, especially when multiple comminuted fragments complicate the stable landmarks for reduction. The patient in Figure 8-12 was treated using CT-guided intraoperative navigation and subsequent anatomic reduction (Figure 8-13).

COMPLICATIONS

Complications of ORIF of ZMC fractures can be divided into functional and aesthetic categories, which can be related to the surgical approach. The most feared, but fortunately rare, complication is blindness secondary to retrobulbar hemorrhage (0.3%). Retrobulbar hematoma may present as tense proptosis, eye pain, elevated intraocular pressures, and visual disturbances (decreased red-green color perception, followed by decreased visual acuity) that may require surgical decompression via a lateral canthotomy and inferior cantholysis. The initial trauma also may irreversibly affect the vision. Orbital complications, such as ectropion and enophthalmos, can be a significant concern to the patient and the surgeon. The incidence of ectropion after a subciliary incision varies considerably in the literature. However, most series have reported a greater incidence of ectropion with this incision compared with the transconjunctival approaches. A great majority of cases of ectropion are transient and resolve with nonsurgical interventions.

Enophthalmos can be a difficult aesthetic problem to correct and predict. Our ability to predict the incidence of enophthalmos (based on clinical and radiographic parameters) is a key measure in determining the need for orbital floor exploration. This is weighed against the aesthetic and functional risks to the eye and periorbital tissue from orbital floor exploration and reconstruction. It is unclear what amount of orbital floor disruption would predictably cause enophthalmos. However, it is generally accepted that disruption of more than 50% of the floor, along with loss of support at the equator of the globe, causes future enophthalmos if left untreated. Therefore, careful consideration must be given to orbital floor exploration in treatment planning.

Dysfunction of the infraorbital nerve is common and intuitively related to the severity of the initial trauma, the status of the nerve, and the complexity of dissection and stretching of the soft tissue. Persistent diplopia is uncommon, because most cases of binocular diplopia resolve after the resolution of edema; however, persistent diplopia beyond 7 days requires further investigation to rule out inferior rectus entrapment.

It is important to distinguish between monocular diplopia (double vision with the unaffected eye closed) and binocular diplopia (double vision with both eyes open). Monocular diplopia may be caused by trauma to the globe, such as lens dislocation or retinal detachments. This requires emergent ophthalmologic consultation. Binocular diplopia (which is far more common) is generally caused by extraocular muscle dysfunction secondary to edema or entrapment or globe malposition.

Aesthetic complications, such as hypertrophic scars and inadequate bony reduction, can be addressed surgically at the appropriate time.

DISCUSSION

An understanding of the anatomy of the zygoma is essential in the treatment of ZMC fractures. By definition, the four articulating sutures (ZF, ZT, ZM, and ZS) are disrupted in this fracture. Therefore, the commonly applied term "tripod fracture" is a misnomer and does not correctly describe this fracture.

Much controversy exists regarding the optimal treatment of ZMC fractures. Not unlike any other condition, treatment needs to be individually tailored to both the patient and the surgeon's experience. In the preoperative evaluation of the patient with a ZMC fracture, the ophthalmologic examination is of paramount importance. An ophthalmology consultation should be obtained on select cases as dictated by the physical examination findings.

Another area of controversy is the amount of fixation necessary for adequate reduction (ranging from none to four-point fixation). The ZF and ZM sutures are the most commonly fixated areas. All ZMC fractures involve the orbital floor (composed of the orbital segment of the maxilla, zygomatic bone, and orbital process of the palatine bone). However, as mentioned, not all ZMC fractures warrant orbital floor exploration and reconstruction. Entrapment of the extraocular muscles warrants orbital floor exploration. On evaluation of the eye, however, the examiner should be careful to distinguish impaired extraocular movement secondary to generalized edema, which is very common and frequently impairs all directions of gaze, from inferior rectus entrapment, which is rare and usually demonstrates strict impairment of upward gaze.

Bibliography

Adekeye DO: Fractures of the zygomatic complex in Nigerian patients, *J Oral Surg* 38:596, 1980.

Bell RB, Bustani SA: Orbital fractures. In Bagheri SC, Bell RB, Khan HA (eds): *Current therapy in oral and maxillofacial surgery*, pp 304-323, Philadelphia, 2011, Elsevier/Mosby.

Bui TG, Bell RB, Dierks EJ: Technological advances in the treatment of facial trauma, *Atlas Oral Maxillofac Surg Clin North Am* 20(1):81-94, 2012.

Colletti G, Valassina D, Rabbiosi D, et al: Traumatic and iatrogenic retrobulbar hemorrhage: an 8-patient series, *J Oral Maxillofac Surg* 70(8):e464-468, 2012.

Ellis E, El-Attar A, Moos KF: An analysis of 2,067 cases of zygomatico-orbital fractures, *J Oral Maxillofac Surg* 43:428, 1985.

Fisher-Brandeis E, Dielert E: Treatment of isolated lateral midface fractures, *J Maxillofac Surg* 12:103, 1984.

Foo GC: Fractures of the zygomatic malar complex: a retrospective analysis of 76 cases, *Singapore Dent J* 9:1, 1984.

Haggarty CJ, Demian N, Marchena JM: Zygomatic complex fractures. In Bagheri SC, Bell RB, Khan HA (eds): *Current therapy in oral and maxillofacial surgery*, pp 324-333, St Louis, 2011, Mosby.

Kim JH, Lee JH, Hong SM, et al: The effectiveness of 1-point fixation for zygomaticomaxillary complex fractures, *Arch Otolaryngol Head Neck Surg* 138(9):828-832, 2012.

Larsen OD, Thompsen M: Zygomatic fractures. II. A follow-up study of 137 patients, *Scand J Plast Reconstr Surg* 12:59, 1978.

Lundin K, Ridell A, Sandberg N: One thousand maxillofacial and related fractures at the ENT clinic in Gothenburg: a two year prospective study, *Acta Otolaryngol* 75:359, 1973.

Nysingh JG: Zygomaticomaxillary fractures with a report of 200 consecutive cases, *Arch Chir Neerl* 12:157, 1960.

Ord RA: Postoperative retrobulbar hemorrhage and blindness complicating trauma surgery, *Br J Oral Surg* 19:202, 1981.

Rake PA, Rake SA, Swift JQ, et al: A single reformatted oblique sagittal view as an adjunct to coronal computed tomography for the evaluation of orbital floor fractures, *J Oral Maxillofac Surg* 62(4):456-459, 2004.

Wisenbaugh JM: Diagnostic evaluation of zygomatic complex fractures, *J Oral Surg* 28:204, 1970.

Zachariades N, Mezitis M, Anagnostopoulos D: Changing trends in the treatment of zygomaticomaxillary complex fractures: a 12-year evaluation of methods used, *J Oral Maxillofac Surg* 56:1152-1156; discussion, 1156-1157; 1998.

Zygomatic Arch Fracture

Justine Moe, Jaspal Girn, and Martin B. Steed

CC

A 33-year-old man presents to the emergency department complaining of left facial swelling, pain, and difficulty opening his mouth.

The epidemiology of isolated midfacial fracture varies greatly, depending on the geographic region, population density, socioeconomic status, and type of facility in which the research was conducted. Generally, an increased incidence is seen in the third decade of life and over the age of 50. Primary mechanisms of injury are interpersonal violence and motor vehicle collisions in the younger population and falls in the older population. A preponderance of left-sided injuries is seen when the etiology involves a personal altercation, because most assailants are right-handed and use this hand to strike the opponent on the left side.

HPI

The patient reports that he was assaulted on the way home several hours earlier by an unknown individual and was hit once on the left side of the face with a hard object (isolated zygomatic arch fractures are most frequently due to assault). He denies any loss of consciousness, nausea, or vomiting and has experienced no changes in his vision (it is important to question the patient about any signs of transient or progressive neurologic impairment for suspicion of possible intracranial injury). He explains that he has difficulty opening his mouth, and any attempt to stretch open his mouth causes severe pain.

PMHX/PDHX/MEDICATIONS/ALLERGIES/SH/FH

The patient denies any significant past medical history and takes no medications. He admits to drinking several glasses of beer that night. (A history of alcohol abuse is frequently elicited in the trauma population. The clinician should also maintain an index of suspicion for other drugs of abuse).

EXAMINATION

Evaluation of the patient as dictated by the advanced trauma life support (ATLS) protocol revealed no findings except for the maxillofacial injuries outlined later (despite obvious isolated maxillofacial injuries, the evaluation of the patient should be comprehensive).

General. The patient is a well-developed and well-nourished man in no apparent distress.

Vital signs. Vital signs are stable, and he is afebrile (abnormal vital signs in an otherwise healthy patient may be due to anxiety or autonomic stimulation secondary to substance abuse).

Neurologic. The patient is alert and oriented × 4 (to person, place, time, and event) and has a GCS score of 15.

Maxillofacial. There are no scalp lacerations or contusions. Examination of the eyes reveals no abnormalities (visual acuity, visual fields, extraocular movements, and pupillary size, shape, and response to light and accommodation). There are no palpable step deformities of the orbital rims, nasal bones, maxilla, or mandible. There is no evidence of posterior or anterior epistaxis (bleeding from the nose [epistaxis] and subconjunctival hemorrhage can be seen with zygomatic arch fractures). There is mild left facial edema and tenderness anterior to the tragal cartilage of the ear (a palpable step deformity may or may not be present at initial presentation, but an indentation and loss of normal convex curvature would be evident in the left malar area after the acute edema subsides). The temporomandibular joints (TMJs) are not painful to palpation or with function. Findings are normal on otoscopic visualization of the external auditory canals and tympanic membranes. The cranial nerves, including the sensory branches of the trigeminal nerve (V1, V2, and V3), are intact bilaterally (gross sensory deficits can be evaluated by asking the patient to identify soft and sharp sensations at different regions of the face).

Intraoral. Maximal interincisal opening is measured at 15 mm (trismus associated with zygomatic arch fractures is seen in 45% of cases). The maxilla and mandible are stable, and the occlusion is reproducible. There is tenderness on palpation of the posterior aspect of the left maxillary vestibule. Mandibular lateral excursive movements demonstrate limitation of the right side (less than 5 mm) and normal lateral excursion toward the left (11 mm) (limitation of movement of the left mandibular condyle secondary to a fractured zygomatic arch impairs excursive movement of the mandible to the contralateral side).

IMAGING

Many radiologic studies are available for evaluation of the zygomatic arch; the gold standard is the non-contrast-enhanced maxillofacial CT scan. Axial images are ideal for assessment of fractures of the zygomatic arch. Reformatted or direct coronal views can also allow visualization of the segments. Three-dimensional reconstructed views are not essential but

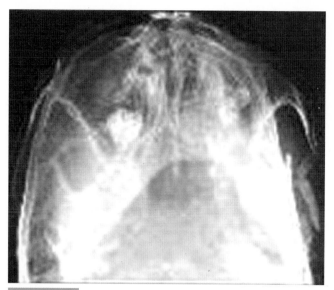

Figure 8-14 Plain radiograph submentovertex view showing a left zygomatic arch fracture.

permit visualization of the displaced fractures in all planes. If facial CT is not available, standard plain-film facial series should be obtained, including the submentovertex view (SMV) (Figure 8-14) which, when correctly obtained, allows for excellent visualization of the zygomatic arch. The SMV is directed from the submandibular region toward the vertex (top) of the skull. The film is placed behind the patient's head in the supine position, and the cone is directed from underneath the genial region so that the beam bisects the mandibular angles, capturing the entire skull. This film should not be obtained in the trauma patient with suspicion of cervical spine injury, because it requires hyperextension of the neck.

In the current patient, a facial CT scan (Figure 8-15, *A*) revealed an isolated, medially displaced fracture of the left zygomatic arch that is clearly demonstrated on the three-dimensional reconstructed view (Figure 8-15, *B*) (this is the most common pattern of zygomatic arch injury and includes fractures at three points).

LABS

No routine laboratory tests are indicated for the evaluation and treatment of isolated zygomatic arch injuries unless dictated by other systemic injuries or medical conditions. A blood alcohol level and a urine drug screen should be considered in cases of suspected substance abuse.

ASSESSMENT

Isolated medially displaced fracture of the left zygomatic arch; FISS score of 1.

TREATMENT

Various intraoral and transcutaneous approaches have been advocated for reduction of zygomatic arch fractures.

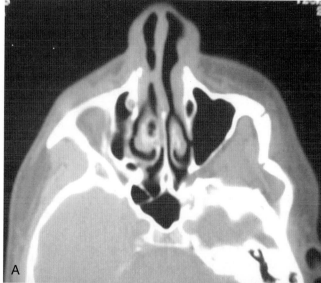

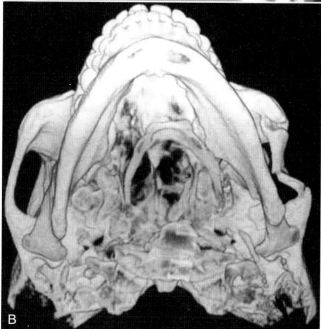

Figure 8-15 **A,** Axial CT scan bony window cut of a depressed left zygomatic arch fracture. **B,** Reconstructed facial CT scan bony window cut showing a depressed left zygomatic arch fracture.

Transcutaneous approaches include the Gillies (temporal) approach, described first in 1927, which has been a popular technique for reduction of the zygomatic arch (described later). Alternatively, incisions in the area of the zygomatico-frontal (ZF) suture (lateral brow or supratarsal fold incisions) can be used to gain access for placement of an instrument medial to the arch. Several methods for reduction of the arch through a percutaneous approach have been described, including:

- Using a J-shaped bone hook elevator through a preauricular stab incision
- Towel clip reduction using two stab incisions superior and inferior to the fractured arch

- Passing a wire or heavy suture medial to the arch to allow lateral force for reduction

Open reduction with internal fixation (ORIF) can be done via a hemicoronal approach, but this should be reserved for severely displaced or comminuted fractures that are not amendable to more conservative approaches. In endoscopically assisted reduction, preauricular, lateral orbital, or temporal scalp incisions are made; an optical cavity is created between the superficial and deep temporalis fascial layers; the periosteum of the arch is incised; and fracture reduction, with or without fixation (in or ex vivo), is completed.

Transoral approaches include the Keen, or buccal sulcus, approach, in which a small incision is made in the mucobuccal fold beneath the zygomatic buttress of the maxilla. A periosteal elevator is inserted into the incision, and subperiosteal dissection is completed superiorly and posteriorly along the lateral maxilla until contact is made with the infratemporal surface of the maxilla, zygoma, and zygomatic arch in a supraperiosteal manner. Subsequently, a heavier instrument can be inserted medial to the zygomatic arch and, using lateral and anterior controlled force, the fracture is reduced. Another intraoral technique is the lateral coronoid or Quinn approach. In this approach, a 3- to 4-cm incision is made intraorally along the anterior border of the ramus. The incision is deepened superiorly, following the lateral aspect of the temporalis muscle, with blunt dissection. A flat-bladed, heavy instrument is inserted to elevate the arch. Care must be taken to ensure that the instrument is lateral to the coronoid process.

If reduction of the arch is questioned, intraoperative plain x-ray films (SMV), CT, cone-beam CT (CBCT), portable or C-arm fluoroscopy, and ultrasonography have all been used to assess the adequacy of reduction. Regardless of the method used, protection is required to prevent displacement of the reduced zygomatic arch for 3 to 5 days postoperatively. Commonly used materials include metal eye patches or aluminum finger splints, which are secured in place with tape.

The current patient was taken to the operating room for closed reduction of the right zygomatic arch fracture using the Gillies (temporal) approach. A temporal incision (2 cm in length) was made behind the hairline. The incision was made through the skin and subcutaneous tissue, angled from the anterosuperior to posteroinferior direction, down to the glistening white deep temporal fascia. The temporal fascia was incised horizontally to expose the temporalis muscle. Next, the broad end of a no. 9 periosteal elevator was inserted between the temporalis muscle and the temporalis fascia and swept back and forth until the medial aspect of the zygomatic arch was felt. At this point, the periosteal elevator was removed and a Rowe zygomatic elevator was inserted and pulled laterally and superiorly for reduction of the zygomatic arch (other commonly used instruments include the urethral sound, Kelly hemostat and Dingman elevator). Reduction was confirmed by palpation with the nonoperating hand. The Rowe elevator was then swept back and forth to ensure reduction of the arch. The incision was closed in layers.

Attempts to reduce isolated arch fractures more than 10 days after the initial injury may be difficult secondary to progressive healing. Severely comminuted and displaced zygomatic arch fractures and displaced fractures that present late may require ORIF through either a hemicoronal approach or an extended preauricular incision. Postoperative reduction may be confirmed by SMV or CBCT. Restoration of normal mandibular opening and midface projection and width should also be assessed postoperatively.

COMPLICATIONS

Early complications of zygomatic arch injuries include damage to the temporal branch of the facial nerve, because it runs tangentially in a superior-anterior direction at the level of the zygomatic arch. Intraoperative bleeding may be encountered if the superficial temporal artery is injured.

Long-term complications can be categorized as functional or cosmetic. Cosmetic deformities due to asymmetry of the malar region may result if a depressed zygomatic arch fracture is not diagnosed or if it is inadequately elevated. A rare functional complication is ankylosis between the coronoid process and the zygomatic arch, causing limitation of mouth opening.

DISCUSSION

The zygomatic arch is formed by the temporal process of the zygoma and the zygomatic process of the temporal bone, which are joined at the zygomaticotemporal (ZT) suture. The glenoid fossa and articular eminence are located at the posterior aspect of the zygomatic process of the temporal bone. The point of least resistance to fracture is not at the ZT suture, but approximately 1.5 cm more posterior in the zygomatic process of the temporal bone.

Isolated zygomatic arch fractures constitute 10% to 20% of all zygomatic fractures. The most common symptoms associated with zygomatic arch fractures are indentation or flattening over the zygomatic arch and limitation of mouth opening. This limitation is most likely due to spasm of the temporalis muscle from impinging displaced fragments and not from the direct impingement of the translating coronoid process by zygomatic arch fragments. Most often, fractures of the zygomatic arch are incomplete, or greenstick fractures, and may require no surgical intervention if minimally displaced. Depending on the severity of the fracture, medical comorbidities, associated injuries, and the experience of the surgeon, arch fractures can be treated either under general anesthesia in the hospital or using intravenous sedation techniques in the office setting.

Bibliography

Carter T, Bagheri S, Dierks EJ: Towel clip reduction of the depressed zygomatic arch fracture, *J Oral Maxillofac Surg* 63:1244, 2005.

Chen CT, Lai JP, Chen YR, et al: Application of endoscope in zygomatic fracture repair, *Br J Plast Surg* 53(2):100-105, 2000.

Czerwinski M, Lee C: The rationale and technique of endoscopic approach to the zygomatic arch in facial trauma, *Facial Plast Surg Clin North Am* 14(1):37-43, 2006.

Dingman RO, Natvig P: *Surgery of facial fractures*, pp 211-245, Philadelphia, 1964, Saunders.

Ellis E, El-Attar A, Moos KF: An analysis of 2,067 cases of zygomatico-orbital fractures, *J Oral Maxillofac Surg* 43:417, 1985.

Gillies HD, Kilner TP, Stone D, et al: Fractures of the malar-zygoma compound, with a description of a new x-ray position, *Br J Surg* 14:651, 1927.

Griffin JE Jr, Max DP, Frey BS: The use of the C-arm in reduction of isolated zygomatic arch fractures: a technical overview, *J Craniomaxillofac Trauma* 3(1):27-31, 1997.

Hwang K, Kim DHL: Analysis of zygomatic fractures, *J Craniofac Surg* 22(4):1416-1421, 2011.

Keen WW: *Surgery: its principles and practice*, Philadelphia, 1909, Saunders.

McLoughlin P, Gilhooly M, Wood G: The management of zygomatic complex fractures: results of a survey, *Br J Oral Maxillofac Surg* 32:284, 1994.

Ogden GR: The Gillies method for fractured zygomas: an analysis of 105 cases, *J Oral Maxillofac Surg* 49:23, 1991.

Quinn JH: Lateral coronoid approach for intra-oral reduction of fractures of the zygomatic arch, *J Oral Surg* 35:321, 1977.

Yamamoto K, Murakami K, Sugiura T, et al: Clinical analysis of isolated zygomatic arch fractures, *J Oral Maxillofac Surg* 65(3):457-461, 2007.

Zingg M, Laedrach K, Chen J, et al: Classification and treatment of zygomatic fractures: a review of 1025 cases, *J Oral Maxillofac Surg* 50:778, 1992.

Nasal Fracture

Eric P. Holmgren and Samuel L. Bobek

CC

A 22-year-old man presents to the emergency department complaining, "I think I broke my nose, and I can't breathe out of it."

Nasal bone fracture is the most common facial fracture, due to the relatively little force required to fracture this bone and its prominent position in the face. The most common cause of nasal fractures is blunt trauma to the face from interpersonal violence and sporting injuries.

HPI

The patient was involved in an altercation at a bar several hours before presentation. He received a single blow from a right fist to the left side of his nose. He does not report falling to the ground or losing consciousness. Immediately post injury, he experienced approximately 30 minutes of brisk epistaxis (highly suggestive of nasal bone or septal fractures and lacerations of the nasal mucosa), which progressively slowed down. His pain is localized to his nasal complex. He complains of difficulty breathing through both nostrils but otherwise denies any diplopia, visual changes, or paresthesias. He states that his nose now appears crooked and was perfectly straight before this injury (preinjury appearance can be determined by a detailed history or ideally by evaluation of preinjury photographs). He also denies neck or back pain, headache, nausea, vomiting, dizziness, or malocclusion. (The review of systems should include questions about symptoms suggestive of possible intracranial, ocular, or perinasal injury.)

PMHX/PDHX/MEDICATIONS/ALLERGIES/SH/FH

The patient has an unremarkable medical history. A thorough nasal history is important when evaluating nasal or nasal-septal fractures. There is no previous history of facial fractures, nasal surgeries, or preexisting nasal deformities (preexisting nasal form and function are paramount for surgical treatment planning). He denies a prior history of chronic nasal obstruction (this would be suggestive of prior septal deviation). He denies any history of cocaine use (cocaine compromises nasal mucosal blood flow and predisposes to septal perforation).

EXAMINATION

The patient's advanced trauma life support (ATLS) primary survey is negative, and his Glasgow Coma Scale (GCS) score is 15.

General. The patient is a well-developed and well-nourished man in mild distress from pain and nasal obstruction.

Eyes. The pupils are equal, round, and reactive to light and accommodation (PERRLA), and the extraocular muscles are intact. Visual acuity is 20/20 in both eyes (OS [ocular sinister, or left eye], OD [ocular dexter, or right eye]). Visual fields are intact by confrontation, without monocular or binocular diplopia. There is no evidence of hyphema (blood in the anterior chamber of the eye), no chemosis (subconjunctival edema), or subconjunctival hemorrhage. The patient exhibits bilateral infraorbital edema that is more severe on the left. There is no epiphora (large "crocodile" tears suggestive of lacrimal apparatus injury). The intercanthal distance is normal, measuring 31 mm (range, 30 to 33 mm) (increased intercanthal distance is suggestive of a naso-orbito-ethmoid [NOE] fracture).

Maxillofacial. There is minimal edema of the nose with an obvious deviation of the dorsum to the right (Figure 8-16)

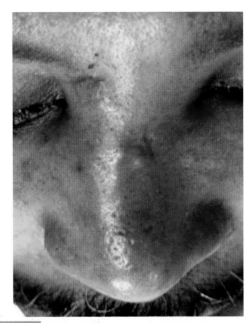

Figure 8-16 Preoperative photograph (bird's eye view) showing displacement of the nasal complex to the right.

(with moderate to severe edema, treatment may be best delayed to allow for resolution of the edema). The bony nasal dorsum is tender to palpation, with bony crepitus over the radix and upper dorsum. The alar base appears normal and coincident with the remainder of the face. Nasal tip projection is adequate, with no signs of lateral or columellar collapse (this suggests there is no septal fracture). The upper, middle, and lower thirds of the nose do not collapse with digital pressure (Brown-Gruss provocation). There is no evidence of cerebrospinal fluid rhinorrhea (cerebrospinal fluid leakage is indicative of fracture of the cribriform plate).

Intranasal. Using a fine suction, several blood clots were evacuated from the nares. Nasal speculum examination using a headlight and prior application of a topical vasoconstrictor (oxymetazoline [Afrin] spray or 4% cocaine) reveals a 2-cm left nostril mucosal laceration over the cartilaginous septum with obvious lateral displacement. There is no septal hematoma (blood collection between the perichondrium and quadrangular cartilage, which can disrupt the blood supply to the cartilage, resulting in septal necrosis, septal abscess formation, and a subsequent saddle nose deformity). The turbinates are intact, and the inferior meatus is identified. (Endoscopic intranasal examination provides the most information when evaluating the nasal septum.)

IMAGING

Although imaging studies may not be necessary to diagnose nasal fractures, studies are recommended to evaluate the degree of displacement and comminution (especially of the nasal septum) and to rule out other facial fractures. The CT scan is the gold standard imaging modality for the evaluation of nasal bones and associated structures. Clinical examination of acute nasal fractures in the setting of edema is often difficult, and accurate diagnosis using CT imaging becomes important. Routine plain films are rarely used in the diagnosis and characterization of nasal fractures unless CT imaging is unavailable. Plain films have a low specificity (false-positive rates as high as 66%) and are limited in their ability to distinguish old from new fractures (only 15% of nasal bone fractures heal by ossification). Additionally, plain films cannot detect cartilaginous injuries, which occur more often in the pediatric population.

In the current patient, a facial CT scan demonstrated bilateral nasal bone fracture with deviation to the right and bowing of the septum (Figure 8-17) (bowing of the septum can be a result of fracture displacement and typically reduces as the fracture is reduced). Preinjury photographs can be extremely helpful for delineating injury displacement and can serve as a guide in surgical correction.

LABS

No routine laboratory tests are necessary for the diagnosis and management of nasal fractures unless dictated by the medical history. In patients with suspicion of drug or alcohol abuse, a toxicology screen (including cocaine metabolites) and a blood

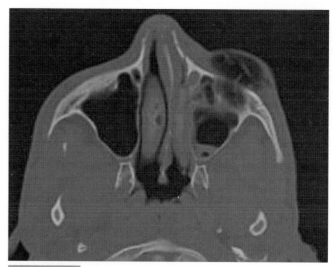

Figure 8-17 Axial CT scan demonstrating fracture of the nasal bones and septal deviation to the left.

alcohol level should be obtained. In patients with unusual bleeding that cannot be controlled with nasal packs, coagulation studies (partial thromboplastin time [PTT], prothrombin time [PT], international normalized ratio [INR], and platelet count) should be obtained to evaluate for underlying blood dyscrasias (von Willebrand disease is the most common previously undiagnosed bleeding disorder).

ASSESSMENT

Bilateral nasal bone and nasal septal fracture; FISS score of 1.

TREATMENT

Treatment for nasal bone fractures begins with a detailed nasal history and control of hemorrhage. Information regarding previous nasal trauma, surgery, deviation, and obstruction should be obtained. The mechanism, injuring agent, direction of blows, timing of injury, and postinjury epistaxis should be determined. A preinjury photograph can be very helpful. A detailed history allows the surgeon to better evaluate the extent of the nasal deformity, including septal deviation. Preexisting nasal deformities can complicate the reduction of the bony nasal pyramid, which may potentially drift back toward the preinjury state (the key to fracture stabilization is septal alignment). This is especially true in cases of a preinjury deviated nasal septum (see Discussion later in this section). The anticipated difficulty of reduction is an important factor in the choice of anesthesia (local versus general).

Control of epistaxis can be achieved with one of the many choices of nasal packings, with or without the aid of vasoconstrictors or electrocautery. The placement of anterior and posterior nasal packing should be precise, and the surgeon must be aware of potential complications, such as infection, dehydration, and altered ventilation from obstructive and physiologic derangements in pulmonary mechanics. Ribbon gauze or Merocel sponges can be used to pack off anterior bleeding. Posterior bleeding usually requires an anteroposterior pack, which frequently includes a balloon as a means of tamponade. Nasal packs are usually left in place for a maximum of 24 to 48 hours. The patient is admitted to the hospital for observation, and antibiotics are initiated. If the epistaxis is persistent, FloSeal (Baxter) or other local hemostatic agents can be considered. Adequate control of blood pressure and the patient's pain can assist in the management of epistaxis. Silver nitrate or electrocautery is usually not helpful in traumatic bleeding if the hemorrhage is not from a punctuate source.

A thorough external and internal nasal examination precludes the need for any adjunctive radiographic studies. Undetected and untreated septal injuries have been found to cause postreduction nasal deformities, and a thorough endonasal examination with a rigid endoscope or a speculum examination is recommended. This should be done after adequate anesthesia and decongestion of the nasal mucosa has been achieved with 2% lidocaine with oxymetazoline or 4% cocaine.

Treatment options include open or closed reduction. The timing of repair can be immediate or delayed. Immediate repair should be done if there is no significant edema that would compromise the assessment of surgical intervention. With significant edema, surgery should be postponed to allow the edema to resolve (typically 3 to 5 days). In cases of delayed repair, it is generally recommended that nasal bone fractures be treated within 10 days of injury for optimal results (earlier in the pediatric population).

The surgeon should have an algorithm to follow in the case of a difficult or unstable closed reduction. An uncomplicated displaced nasal bone fracture with no preexisting nasal or septal deformity is most amenable to closed reduction. This can be attempted with any number of instruments (e.g., Boies elevator, Walsham's forceps, Asch forceps). If the nasal pyramid snaps into position and is stable, an external nasal splint is applied (either an Aquaplast thermal splint or a Denver metal splint). If there is continued memory or drift of the nasal pyramid, further intervention is indicated until a stable reduction has been achieved. First, a septoplasty procedure should be considered, especially in patients with a prior history of nasal obstruction. Nasal osteotomies are performed if there is continued drift. The upper lateral cartilages can be released from the nasal septum if there continues to be drift of the nasal structures. (The upper lateral cartilages splint bones toward the initial preexisting deformity; therefore, release of the upper lateral cartilages from the septum allows the nasal bones to remain midline.) This can be followed by fracturing of the bony septum (the anterior extension of the perpendicular plate of the ethmoid and vomer) opposite the deviation by pushing the bony pyramid toward the contralateral lateral canthus. The final attempt at correcting any residual deformity can be accomplished with a cartilage camouflage graft in the depressed area. An external nasal splint, worn for 1 to 2 weeks, and the use of endonasal packing (bacitracin-impregnated, $\frac{1}{2}$-inch NuGauze [Johnson & Johnson; New

Brunswick, New Jersey]) for 2 to 3 days assist in further stabilizing the fractures.

In the current patient, the nasal bones were treated with closed reduction using a Boies elevator. The nasal bony pyramid was reduced into correct anatomic position with a distinct "snapping" sound and remained in stable position. The nasal-septal fracture was treated with closed reduction back to a stable midline position. There was no immediate memory or drift noted after reduction (preinjury nasal and nasal septal deformities predispose the nasal complex to drift). An external nasal splint was applied for 1 week (Figures 8-18 and 8-19).

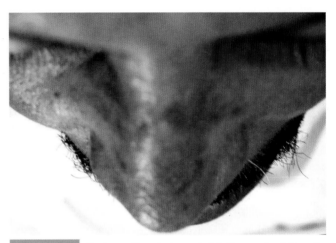

Figure 8-18 Postoperative photograph (bird's eye view) 6 weeks after closed reduction.

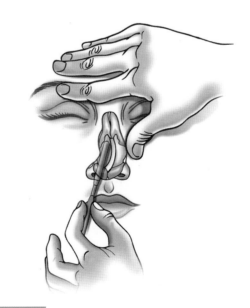

Figure 8-19 Closed reduction of nasal fracture. An elevator is placed inside the nostril to support the septum as the nasal bones are reduced toward the midline. *(Courtesy of Dr. Benham Bohlouli.)*

COMPLICATIONS

The most common and problematic postinjury or postoperative complication is a postreduction nasal deformity. Most authors believe that an undiagnosed or untreated nasal-septal fracture or deviation plays a significant role in causing this complication. The incidence of posttraumatic nasal deformity has been reported at 14% to 50%. The algorithm presented here is aimed at reducing the incidence of postreduction deformities with special attention to the nasal septum. Nasal obstruction due to collapse of the nasal valve and formation of synechiae can cause significant breathing and chronic sinus problems.

The presence of a septal hematoma is an urgent complication in the setting of nasal trauma. The mucosa overlying the nasal septum is highly vascular. Kiesselbach's plexus (Little's area) is a vascular area in the anterior septum where terminal branches of the internal and external carotid arteries meet. The anterior ethmoidal, septal branches of the superior labial, sphenopalatine, and greater palatine arteries compose this plexus. Injury to this area can cause a septal hematoma in the subperichondrial plane, disrupting the vascular supply to the septum. A septal hematoma requires immediate evacuation, with dependent drainage and intranasal packing to prevent reaccumulation. Undetected or untreated septal hematomas can lead to abscess formation, septal necrosis, and resultant fibrosis and deformity (saddle-nose deformity).

Other complications include unremitting epistaxis, synechiae formation, scar contracture, nasal airway obstruction, cerebrospinal fluid rhinorrhea, and toxic shock syndrome (the latter is very rare).

DISCUSSION

The nasal bone is reported to be the most common facial fracture. The nose can be divided into three vaults. The upper vault is comprised of the paired nasal bones, frontal processes of the maxilla, and the perpendicular plate of the ethmoid bone. This structure is also referred to as the *bony pyramid.* The middle vault includes the upper lateral cartilages and the midportion of the nasal septum (quadrangular cartilage). The lower vault includes the nasal tip, lower lateral (alar) cartilages, and the inferior portion of the nasal septum. These vaults can be tested individually for stability by applying digital pressure, which will cause the vault to collapse if it is unstable; this is called the *Brown-Gruss provocation.*

It is important to remember that the nasal septum is attached to both the bony nasal pyramid and the upper and lower lateral cartilages. Any septal deformity has the potential to transmit forces to the bony and cartilaginous portions of the nose and cause a postreduction deformity. The nasal septum is composed of the perpendicular plate of the ethmoid bone, vomer, nasal crests of the maxilla, palatine bones, and the quadrangular cartilage. Treatment of nasal fractures in the pediatric patient should follow the same protocol as for adults, because normal growth resumes after septal repair and surgery.

The indications for primary open reduction of nasal fractures include the following:

- Inability of the septum to remain in the reduced position
- Considerable displacement of cartilaginous structures
- Bilateral fractures with dislocation of the nasal dorsum and septal pathology
- Fractures of the cartilaginous pyramid, with or without dislocation of the upper lateral cartilages
- Anticipation of cartilage or bone grafting

Nasal fractures should be diagnosed and treated with careful consideration of function and esthetics. The simplicity of closed reduction techniques should not replace more invasive surgical interventions. Untreated septal injuries can significantly complicate airway flow and the aesthetic outcome.

Bibliography

Chegar B, Tatum S: Nasal fractures. In Flint PW, Haughey BH, Lund VJ (eds): *Cummings otolaryngology: head and neck surgery,* ed 4, pp 962-979, Philadelphia, 2005, Elsevier.

Deeb G, Dierks E: Use of CT in diagnosing nasal fractures. Paper presented at the 82nd Annual Meeting of the American Association of Oral and Maxillofacial Surgeons, San Francisco, October, 2000.

de Vries N, van der Baan S: Toxic shock syndrome after nasal surgery: is prevention possible? A case report and review of the literature, *Rhinology* 27(2):125-128, 1989.

Frodel JL: Avoiding and correcting complications in perinasal trauma, *Facial Plast Surg* 28(3):323-332, 2012.

Indreasano AT, Beckley ML: Nasal fractures. In Fonseca RJ (ed): *Oral and maxillofacial trauma,* ed 3, pp 737-750, Philadelphia, 2004, Saunders.

Logan M, O'Driscoll K, Masterson J: The utility of nasal bone radiographs in nasal trauma, *Clin Radiol* 49(3):192-194, 1994.

Mondin V, Rinaldo A, Ferlito A: Management of nasal bone fractures, *Am J Otolaryngol* 26(3):181-185, 2005.

Oluwasanmi AF, Pinto AL: Management of nasal trauma: widespread misuse of radiographs, *Clin Perform Qual Health Care* 8(2):83-85, 2000.

Reddy LV, Haithem EM: Nasal fractures. In Fonseca RJ (ed): *Oral and maxillofacial surgery,* ed 2, pp 270-282, St Louis, 2009, Saunders.

Rhee SC, Kim YK, Cha JH, et al: Septal fracture in simple nasal bone fracture, *Plast Reconstr Surg* 113(1):45-52, 2004.

Ridder GJ, Boedeker CC, Fradis M, et al: Technique and timing for closed reduction of isolated nasal fractures: a retrospective study, *Ear Nose Throat J* 81(1):49-54, 2002.

Rohrich RJ, Adams WP Jr: Nasal fracture management: minimizing secondary nasal deformities, *Plast Reconstr Surg* 106(2):266-273, 2000.

Weber R, Keerl R, Hochapfel F, et al: Packing in endonasal surgery, *Am J Otolaryngol* (5):306-320, 2001.

Frontal Sinus Fracture

Justine Moe, Martin B. Steed, and Shahrokh C. Bagheri

CC

You are called by the trauma team to evaluate a 25-year-old man status post high-speed motor vehicle collision and to manage his facial trauma.

HPI

The patient was the unrestrained driver in a high-speed, head-on collision with another vehicle. No air bag was deployed, and there was subsequent significant steering wheel and windshield damage. The patient was found unconscious and was not arousable. He was intubated at the scene due to a Glasgow Coma Scale (GCS) score of 7 (high index of suspicion for a severe intracranial injury) and was brought to your Level I trauma center by air medical transport for evaluation and treatment.

PMHX/PDHX/MEDICATIONS/ALLERGIES/SH/FH

All histories are unknown (when possible, the history should be obtained from available family members).

EXAMINATION

Primary Survey

The primary survey is accomplished via the advanced trauma life support (ATLS) protocol. The patient is sedated and intubated with spontaneous respirations. A transport cervical collar is in place (correctly sized and positioned), and his pupils are equal and reactive. His Glasgow Coma Scale (GCS) score is 10T on arrival. He is otherwise hemodynamically stable.

Secondary Survey

Vital signs. Blood pressure is 115/64 mm Hg, heart rate is 115 bpm (tachycardia), respirations are 12 per minute, and temperature is 37.6°C.

Maxillofacial. There is a 10-cm stellate laceration through the frontalis muscle in the left forehead and supraorbital region. Bony crepitus and step deformities are noted on palpation of the supraorbital rims, nasal bones, and frontal bone (indicative of comminuted fractures). There is a flow of clear, blood-tinged fluid from the left naris (possible cerebrospinal fluid rhinorrhea). The maxilla is stable. The dental occlusion is difficult to assess secondary to oral endotracheal intubation.

Eyes. OU (bilateral) pupils are equal, round, and reactive to light (5 to 2 mm; direct and consensual light reflexes intact OU). There is bilateral subconjunctival hemorrhage and no evidence of hyphema (blood in the anterior chamber of the eye, which may be difficult to detect in the supine patient). Fundoscopic exam shows mild papilledema OD (optic disc edema secondary to increased intracranial pressure). The bilateral intraocular pressures measured with a portable tonometer are normal at 16 mm Hg.

IMAGING

The imaging modality of choice for evaluation of frontal sinus injuries is a noncontrast axial computed tomography (CT) scan with 1 mm or less slice thickness. However, CT is not a reliable predictor of nasofrontal duct injury.

In the current patient, head and facial helical CT scans were obtained after the primary and secondary surveys. The head CT scan revealed a 3 × 1-cm left subarachnoid hemorrhage with no midline shift and two 1 × 1-cm areas of hyperdensity in the left frontal lobe (frontal sinus fractures are commonly associated with intracranial injury). Axial views of the facial CT scan revealed a displaced, comminuted frontal bone fracture involving both the anterior and posterior tables of the bilateral frontal sinuses (Figure 8-20, *A*). There were also fractures of the nasal bones, bilateral supraorbital rims, and left infraorbital rim. Three-dimensional reconstruction allows assessment of the overall fracture patterns and orientation of fracture segments (Figure 8-20, *B*). A plain radiographic trauma series also was obtained, including cervical spine, anteroposterior chest, and anteroposterior pelvis views, which are all negative (the incidence of facial fractures accompanied by spinal injuries is a significant concern for the craniomaxillofacial surgeon).

LABS

Standard laboratory tests for the evaluation of multisystem trauma patients include a complete blood cell count (CBC), complete metabolic panel, arterial blood gas analysis, urine analysis, and coagulation studies (prothrombin time [PT], partial thromboplastin time [PTT], and international normalized ratio [INR]). A urine drug screen and blood alcohol level are indicated in patients with decreased mental status.

For the current patient, laboratory values were within normal limits except for a slightly low hemoglobin and hematocrit (secondary to blood loss from the scalp laceration and

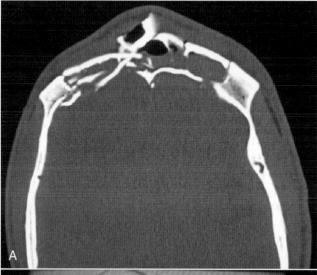

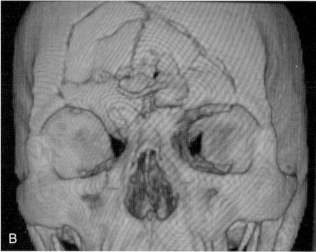

Figure 8-20   **A,** Preoperative axial CT scan demonstrating comminuted displaced anterior and posterior sinus wall fractures. **B,** Three-dimensional reconstruction of preoperative CT scan demonstrating a comminuted frontal bone fracture with a step deformity at the supraorbital rims bilaterally. There is also evidence of fractures at the inferior orbital rims bilaterally.

fluid resuscitation). One milliliter of the blood-tinged transudate from the patient's left naris was collected and sent for laboratory analysis. The sample tested positive for β_2 transferrin (diagnostic of cerebrospinal fluid).

ASSESSMENT

Subarachnoid hemorrhage with left frontal lobe intracerebral contusion; bilateral comminuted frontal sinus fracture with significant displacement of the anterior and posterior tables; bilateral nasal bone, left infraorbital rim, and bilateral supraorbital rim fractures; left frontal stellate skin laceration, evidence of cerebrospinal fluid rhinorrhea, possible nasofrontal duct injury or obstruction, possible elevated ICP; FISS score of 10 (displaced frontal sinus fracture [5], bilateral supraorbital rim fractures [2], left infraorbital rim fracture [1], nasal bone fracture [1], and forehead laceration over 10 cm [1]).

TREATMENT

Three components of frontal sinus fractures must be considered when determining the proper treatment: the anterior sinus wall, posterior sinus wall, and nasofrontal outflow tract (NFOT). In general, fractures of the anterior or posterior table are considered significantly displaced when bony segments are found at a distance of greater than one table thickness. Indications for surgical management are given in the following sections. However, these indications are not absolute, and each case needs treatment planning on an individual basis.

Displaced anterior sinus wall fractures without NFOT involvement. The goal of treatment is to prevent cosmetic deformity. After reduction, internal fixation is completed with titanium or resorbable microplates. Surgical access may be accomplished through a coronal or local approach (existing lacerations, open sky incision). Endoscopic repair through a transnasal or transcutaneous approach (brow or coronal incisions) may be used for minimally displaced anterior table fractures. Bone grafting should be considered for avulsed fragments or extensive comminution. Isolated, nondisplaced anterior table fractures do not require surgical reduction and may be managed conservatively.

NFOT injury without significantly displaced posterior table fracture. The outflow tract is not often injured with minimally displaced anterior table fractures; it more commonly presents with significantly displaced frontal sinus fractures or concomitant naso-orbito-ethmoid (NOE) and Le Fort fractures. An untreated, obstructed NFOT injury prevents evacuation of mucin from the frontal sinus and may lead to mucocele or mucopyocele formation, osteomyelitis, sinusitis, meningitis, or brain abscess. Treatment goals are complete debridement of sinus mucosa from the sinus and upper outflow tract, using a curette or high-speed burr, and obliteration of the frontal sinus and nasofrontal duct with various materials, including bone, temporalis muscle, fat, fascia, Gelfoam (Pfizer; New York, New York), and hydroxyapatite cement. The anterior table segments are replaced and stabilized with rigid fixation. For an isolated, mild NFOT injury, some authors advocate observation, NFOT reconstruction, or stenting; however, reocclusion has been reported in up to 30% of patients. Endoscopic frontal sinusotomy or a modified endoscopic Lothrop procedure may also be considered for a mild NFOT injury or persistent obstruction after conservative management. Less commonly used surgical techniques include trephination, a frontoethmoidectomy (Lynch or Knapp procedure), and a frontal sinus collapse (Reidel) procedure.

Displaced posterior table fractures. These fractures can present with intracranial injury or dural tear and CSF leakage. Goals of treatment are acute management of intracranial injury (often with a craniotomy), dural repair, and cranialization (removal of the posterior table, allowing the brain parenchyma to occupy the frontal sinus). NFOT obliteration prior to cranialization is achieved with a variety of materials, including temporal fascia, temporal muscle, bone, and tissue sealants. A pedicled pericranial flap placed after cranialization facilitates separation of the brain from the nasal environment.

Open reduction and internal fixation of the anterior table segments and reconstruction of the craniotomy defect with rigid fixation plates or mesh is completed. Management of isolated and minimally displaced fractures of the inner table without an obvious dural tear is more controversial, and conservative management or sinus obliteration may be considered.

The ability of the surgeon to evaluate the patency and function of the NFOT is critical. For fractures treated nonsurgically and those in which the nasofrontal ducts are not obliterated, interval CT imaging must be performed to assess duct function over time. Intraoperatively, patency may be assessed by injecting dye into the duct and observing its emergence in the nasal cavity. However, the accuracy of this test is questionable.

In the current patient, the presence of a displaced posterior table fracture, dural tears, and cerebrospinal fluid leak warranted cranialization through a bicoronal flap, in coordination with the neurosurgical team. A craniotomy was performed, the subarachnoid hematoma was evacuated, and an external ventriculostomy drain (EVD) was placed. The supraorbital rims and nasal bone were reconstructed and rigidly fixated with titanium plates (Figure 8-21, *A*). The posterior table was removed, and the dural tears were repaired by primary closure (a fascial graft and fibrin glue may be used if primary closure is not possible). The sinus mucosa was removed from the sinus and upper outflow tract using a pear-shaped burr. The remaining NFOT mucosa was inverted into the nose, and the outflow tracts were occluded with a small amount of free temporalis fascia. An anteriorly based pericranial flap (based on deep branches of the supratrochlear and supraorbital vessels) was placed into the frontal sinus (Figure 8-21, *B*). The anterior table was reduced and stabilized with titanium microplates (Figure 8-21, *C*).

The patient did well postoperatively. A postoperative CT scan demonstrated excellent restoration of frontal region contour and projection (Figure 8-22). The neurologic examination results improved, the EVD was removed 5 days postoperatively, and the patient was discharged home 11 days after surgery.

COMPLICATIONS

The reported overall complication rates for frontal sinus fracture repair range from 4% to 18%. Early complications often present within the first 6 weeks after surgical intervention. They include CSF leakage, wound infection, meningitis, brain abscess, iatrogenic brain injury (cerebral contusion), NFOT obstruction, supraorbital nerve paresthesia, diplopia, headache, and chronic forehead pain.

Meningitis is the most worrisome early postoperative complication and has an incidence as high as 6%. Prompt diagnosis and treatment are essential to minimize morbidity and mortality. Alteration in mental status, fever, and/or neck rigidity should prompt the clinician to obtain a head CT scan, which is followed by lumbar puncture. Diagnosis may be delayed in trauma patients with impaired neurologic status. If meningitis is suspected, the patient should be stabilized

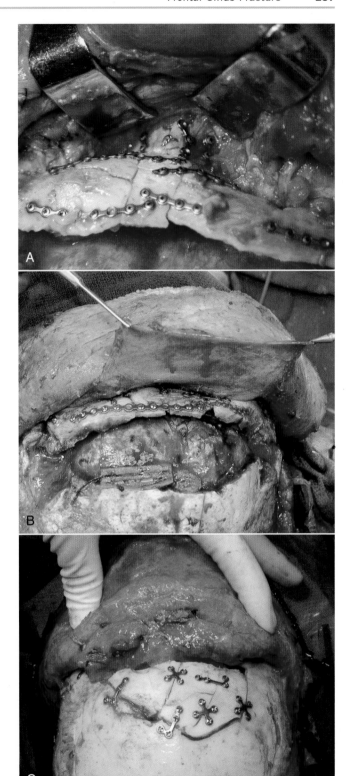

Figure 8-21 **A,** Intraoperative photograph demonstrating cranialization (posterior table has been removed, and supraorbital bar has been reconstructed. **B,** Anterior-based pericranial flap: anteriorly pedicled pericranial flap (based on the supratrochlear and supraorbital vessels) before insetting. **C,** Intraoperative photograph demonstrating inset anterior-based pericranial flap and restoration of superior frontal region contour.

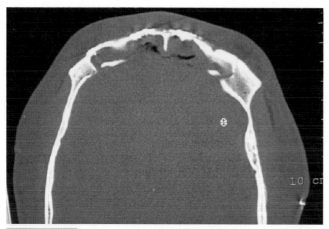

Figure 8-22 Postoperative axial CT scan demonstrating removal of the posterior sinus wall and cranialization of the frontal lobe into the previous sinus space, with good reduction of the anterior sinus wall and restoration of proper contour.

medically and should receive empirically administered, broad-spectrum antibiotics with high CSF penetrance (e.g., nafcillin). The choice of antibiotic should be guided by Gram stain and culture results, when available.

Late frontal sinus fracture complications occur after 6 weeks and may present over 10 years after the surgical repair. They include cosmetic defects (which are common and result from inadequate reduction or stabilization of the anterior table), mucocele or mucopyocele formation, pneumocephalus, osteomyelitis, and intracerebral abscess. Mucocele formation can result from retained sinus mucosa or compromised sinus ventilation (even partial obstruction of the duct from traumatic disruption can result in stasis of secretions). Mucopyoceles develop upon bacterial contamination and can cause the infection to spread to the orbit and brain. Treatment goals are complete surgical removal of the mucocele or mucopyocele and reconstruction to isolate the splanchnocranium (the part of the skull derived from the branchial [or pharyngeal] arches that comprises the bones of the face) from the orbit and nasal cavity. Endoscopic marsupialization of mucoceles has been reported, with limited success rates.

DISCUSSION

Frontal sinus fractures comprise 5% to 12% of all facial fractures and are most commonly found in adults. These injuries usually result from blunt trauma to the anterior skull at the glabella. The most common mechanism is automobile accidents, and the next most common is assault. The force necessary to fracture the anterior wall of the frontal sinus (800 to 1600 N) is two to three times greater than that required to fracture the zygoma, mandible, or maxilla. Significant intracranial injury occurs more often with frontal sinus injuries than with injury to the maxilla or mandible secondary to the proximity to the brain and the force necessary to fracture the frontal bone.

Primary pneumatization of the frontal sinus occurs around the sixteenth week of gestation. The frontal sinus develops as a smooth mucosal pocket from single or multiple extensions of the frontal recess or ethmoid infundibulum in the middle meatus. Secondary pneumatization into the frontal bone begins between the ages of 6 months to 2 years. The frontal sinus is radiographically detectable by age 7 and reaches complete development in adolescence. The sinus may be a single or paired structure, with one or several vertical septa. The adult sinus is rarely symmetric and varies in size, averaging 24.3 mm in height, 29 mm in width, and 20.5 mm in depth. A frontal sinus may be absent in 4% of the population and may be rudimentary or completely lack pneumatization on one side in approximately 12%.

The nasofrontal outflow tract is often erroneously referred to as the nasofrontal duct. This is a misnomer, because the NFOT is a passive space with walls formed by surrounding structures and thus is not a true duct. The 1995 International Conference on Sinus Disease established the current preferred nomenclature and a clear description of the functional units of the outflow tract, which, from superior to inferior, include the frontal sinus infundibulum (found posteromedially in the sinus), frontal sinus osteum, and frontal recess (in the middle meatus). Drainage of the frontal sinus in the nasal cavity is highly variable. In most cases, it drains superior and medial to the ethmoid infundibulum; in some cases, it drains directly into the ethmoid infundibulum; and in a few cases, it drains into the suprabulbar recess (superior and medial to the ethmoid bulla).

The chief blood supply to the frontal sinus is by the anterior ethmoidal branch and, less commonly, the supraorbital branch of the ophthalmic artery. The supraorbital and supratrochlear arteries may also penetrate the frontal sinus. Venous drainage occurs by the diploic veins of Breschet, which coalesce anteriorly to drain into the facial and superior ophthalmic veins. Posteriorly, the diploic veins communicate directly with the dural sinuses and marrow cavity of the frontal bone via the foramen of Breschet (intracranial infection may occur by this route).

Detection of a CSF leak is critical in determining the management of a frontal sinus fracture. Measurement of electrolyte levels has been proposed in the past, because CSF has a higher glucose level and lower levels of protein, sodium, and potassium than do nasal secretions (compared to serum, CSF has a lower glucose level and a higher chloride level). However, these levels are variable and are not reliable for identifying cerebrospinal fluid. The "halo" test is performed by placing a drop of the fluid onto a clean bed sheet or filter paper. A positive test result is the formation of a clear halo around the central stain.

The best test for identifying CSF in serum or secretions is the β_2 transferrin test using immunofixation electrophoresis. However, β_2 transferrin is also present in aqueous humor and perilymph fluid, and false-positive test results may occur in patients with inborn errors of glycoprotein metabolism, chronic liver disease, or genetic variants of transferrin. Still, the reported sensitivity for this test is 94% to 100% and specificity is 98% to 100%; therefore, the β_2 transferrin test is currently the gold standard for detection of CSF in otorrhea or rhinorrhea.

Bibliography

Bagheri SC, Dierks EJ, Kademani D, et al: Application of a Facial Injury Severity Scale (FISS) in cranio-maxillofacial trauma, *J Oral Maxillofac Surg* 64:408-414, 2006.

Bell RB, Dierks EJ, Brar P, et al: A protocol for the management of frontal sinus fractures emphasizing sinus preservation, *J Oral Maxillofac Surg* 65(5):825-839, 2007.

Bell RB, Dierks EJ, Homer L, et al: Management of cerebrospinal fluid leak associated with craniomaxillofacial trauma, *J Oral Maxillofac Surg* 62(6):676-684, 2004.

Gerbino G, Roccia F, Benech A, et al: Analysis of 158 frontal sinus fractures: current surgical management and complications, *J Craniomaxillofac Surg* 28:133, 2000.

Gonty AA, Marciani RD, Adornato DC: Management of frontal sinus fractures: a review of 33 cases, *J Oral Maxillofac Surg* 57(4):372-379, 1999.

Gossman DG, Archer SM, Arosarena O: Management of frontal sinus fractures: a review of 96 cases, *Laryngoscope* 116(8):1357-1362, 2006.

Helmy ES, Koh ML, Bays RA: Management of frontal sinus fractures, *Oral Surg Oral Med Oral Pathol* 69:137-148, 1990.

Holt GR: Ethmoid and frontal sinus fractures, *Ear Nose Throat J* 62:33-42, 1983.

Koudstaal MJ, van der Wal KG, Bijvoet HW, et al: Post-trauma mucocele formation in the frontal sinus; a rationale of follow-up, *Int J Oral Maxillofac Surg* 33(8):751-754, 2004.

Lang J: *Clinical anatomy of the nose, nasal cavity and paranasal sinuses*, New York, 1989, Thieme.

Lee D, Brody R, Har-El G: Frontal sinus outflow anatomy, *Am J Rhinol* 11:283, 1997.

Manolidis S: Frontal sinus injuries: associated injuries and surgical management of 93 patients, *J Oral Maxillofac Surg* 62:882-891, 2004.

Marshall AH, Jones NS, Robertson JA: CSF rhinorrhea: the place of endoscopic sinus surgery, *Br J Neurosurg* 15(1):8-12, 2001.

McLaughlin RB Jr, Rehl RM, Lanza DC: Clinically relevant frontal sinus anatomy and physiology, *Otolaryngol Clin North Am* 34(1):1-22, 2001.

Metzinger SE, Metzinger RC: Complications of frontal sinus fractures, *Craniomaxillofac Trauma Reconstr* 2(1):27-34, 2009.

Nahum AM: The biomechanics of maxillofacial trauma, *Clin Plast Surg* 2:59-64, 1975.

Rice DH: Management of frontal sinus fractures, *Curr Opin Otolaryngol Head Neck Surg* 12:46-48, 2004.

Roelandse FW, van der Zwart N, Didden JH, et al: Detection of CSF leakage by isoelectric focusing on polyacrylamide gel, direct immunofixation of transferrins, and silver staining, *Clin Chem* 44(2):351-353, 1998.

Schultz RC: Frontal sinus and supraorbital fractures from vehicle accidents, *Clin Plast Surg* 2:93-106, 1975.

Smith TL, Han JK, Loehrl TA, et al: Endoscopic management of the frontal recess in frontal sinus fractures: a shift in the paradigm? *Laryngoscope* 112(5):784-790, 2002.

Stammberger HR, Kennedy DW: Paranasal sinuses: anatomic terminology and nomenclature: the Anatomic Terminology Group, *Ann Otol Rhinol Laryngol Suppl* 167:7-16, 1995.

Strong EB, Pahlavan N, Saito D: Frontal sinus fractures: a 28-year retrospective review, *Otolaryngol Head Neck Surg* 135(5):774-779, 2006.

Van Alyea OE: Frontal sinus drainage, *Ann Otol Rhinol Laryngol* 55:267-277, 1946.

Wallis A, Donald PJ: Frontal sinus fractures: a review of 72 cases, *Laryngoscope* 98(6 Part 1):593-598, 1988.

Naso-Orbital-Ethmoid Fracture

Martin B. Steed and Shahrokh C. Bagheri

CC

A 21-year-old man arrives via EMS responders to the emergency department status post high-speed motor vehicle collision.

HPI

The EMS personnel report that the patient was an unrestrained driver traveling at 60 mph through a red light at an intersection when he hit an oncoming vehicle. The driver's side airbag did not deploy, resulting in the direct collision of the upper midface with the steering wheel, causing a positive "steering wheel deformity." (The incidence of naso-orbital-ethmoid [NOE] fractures has decreased since the advent of airbags. However, the impact of the midface with the steering wheel continues to be a common cause of NOE fractures). The patient had a transient loss of consciousness but remained coherent, alert, and oriented during transport to the emergency department He complains of a severe headache, poor vision, and pain in the midface (a history of severe headache, loss of consciousness, or declining mental status should raise suspicion of intracranial injury/hemorrhage). The trauma team has requested a consultation for management of the patient's midfacial soft tissue lacerations and evaluation for facial fractures.

PMHX/PDHX/MEDICATIONS/ALLERGIES/SH/FH

The patient has a prior history of substance abuse (cocaine), according to the patient and telephone contact with a family member.

A history of cocaine abuse is important to the reconstructive maxillofacial surgeon, because it may imply previous nasal septal perforation or compromised local vasculature of the nasal structures due to repeated episodes of vasoconstriction from nasal cocaine abuse. In addition, a chronic or recent history of cocaine abuse has cardiovascular implications, putting the patient at increased risk for coronary vasospasm and cardiac arrhythmias. Illicit drugs are commonly implicated in motor vehicle accidents.

EXAMINATION

The initial evaluation of a trauma patient should follow the advanced trauma and life support (ATLS) protocol.

Primary Survey

The patient's primary survey is intact, and he has a Glasgow Coma Scale (GCS) score of 15. The patient is alert and oriented to person, place, time, and event and has been able to easily maintain his airway (severe posterior nasal hemorrhage can compromise the airway and be a significant source of blood loss).

Secondary Survey

General. The patient is a well-developed and well-nourished man in moderate distress, requesting pain medications and supporting a partially soaked 4 × 4 dressing held over the bridge of his nose and right eye.

Vital signs. His blood pressure is 150/84 mm Hg (hypertensive), heart rate 125 bpm (tachycardia), respirations 16 per minute, and temperature 37.6°C.

Maxillofacial. There is significant bilateral midfacial and periorbital edema with a 10-cm horseshoe (U)-shaped laceration to the frontal region down to bone. A second 8-cm horizontal laceration extends across the nasal bridge (nasion) and through both the right and left upper eyelids with no orbital fat herniation (open globe injury should be suspected with exposure of orbital fat) (Figure 8-23). There are several small

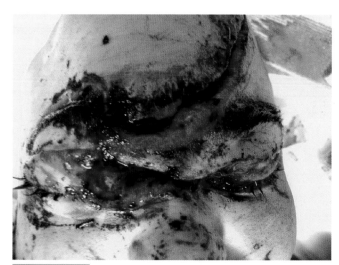

Figure 8-23 Preoperative photograph showing frontal and orbital/nasal bridge lacerations, increased intercanthal distance, severe depression of the nasal bridge unit, bilateral midfacial edema, and periorbital ecchymosis.

arterial bleeders within each laceration. Facial abrasions extend over the left malar (zygoma) region. The patient exhibits a positive result on the bowstring test on the left (movement of bone fragment at insertion of medial canthal tendon upon lateral pull on the upper eyelid). The intercanthal distance is 42 mm (the distance between the left and right medial canthus may be increased in NOE fractures), and the interpupillary distance is 62 mm (normal intercanthal distance is race dependent and ranges from 28.6 to 33 mm for women and 28.9 to 34.5 mm for men).

Nose. There is crepitus and tenderness of the nasal complex upon palpation (nasal bones are displaced and unstable), and movement with digital pressure over bilateral medial canthi (NOE complex instability requiring reduction and stabilization). There is a widened nasal bridge, upturned nasal tip, and depressed radix. Nasal speculum examination reveals bright red blood in the bilateral nares (epistaxis) and deviation of the nasal septum to the right with no evidence of a septal hematoma (this would require urgent decompression). Clear fluid was obtained from the right naris (rhinorrhea) and has been sent for laboratory evaluation for cerebrospinal fluid (the β_2 transferrin test and occasionally glucose and chloride levels are used to confirm CSF rhinorrhea).

Maxilla. Bilateral hypoesthesia of the infraorbital nerve distributions (cranial nerve V2) is present. The maxilla is nonmobile, and the patient's occlusion is intact. The patient has a full complement of teeth, with no grossly carious lesions and no mobile dentoalveolar segments.

Eyes. There is severe bilateral chemosis and subconjunctival hemorrhage. The patient is unable to open either eye, and examination requires careful lid elevation (a Desmarres retractor or disinfected paperclip retractor allows for gentle lid elevation). There is blunting of the bilateral medial palpebral fissures. There is no obvious epiphora (excessive tearing from the eye), but no attempts are made at primary probing of any of the canaliculi (the lacrimal drainage system is commonly injured with a NOE fracture).

Right eye (OD) examination reveals a reactive pupil with hyphema (blood in the anterior chamber of the eye). The OD pupil appears round, and visual acuity is limited to light perception. Left eye (OS) visual acuity is 20/200 with a round and reactive pupil and no hyphema (visual acuity should be tested with the patient's corrective lenses whenever present). Extraocular movements are intact bilaterally, and there is no enophthalmos (medial orbital wall fractures can cause enophthalmos in the setting of NOE fractures).

The physical examination of suspected NOE fractures should be detailed and directed toward assessing the degree of telecanthus and early identification of concurrent ocular and neurologic injuries. Soft tissue intercanthal distances greater than 35 mm are suggestive of a displaced NOE fracture, and distances greater than 40 mm are diagnostic. Crepitus or movement upon palpation of the medial orbital rim indicates instability and the presence of a fracture; clinical bowstring examinations can demonstrate whether the canthal-bearing bone fragment is displaced and mobile. Other tests include the Furness test (the degree of displacement is assessed by grasping the skin over the medial canthus with tissue forceps) and the bimanual exam (with an intranasally placed instrument applying lateral pressure to the NOE complex, the medial canthal tendon is digitally palpated for movement).

IMAGING

The imaging modality of choice in the diagnosis and evaluation of midface fractures is a noncontrast maxillofacial CT scan of the face. Due to overlapping bony architecture, plain films fail to demonstrate the degree and location of bony disruption. Thin cuts (1 to 1.5 mm) are usually required to determine the extent of the NOE injury. Of surgical importance is the determination of the position and status of the frontal process of the maxilla, because this region bears the insertion of the medial canthal tendon.

In the current patient, a facial helical CT scan without contrast was obtained. Axial bony windows showed bilateral fractures at the NOE region with avulsion of several bony segments and bilateral medial orbital wall fractures (Figure 8-24, *A*). The orbital floors appear intact bilaterally. There is evidence of a 1-cm punctate subarachnoid hemorrhage in the left temporal lobe, with no midline deviation. A three-dimensional reconstruction view permits visualization of the lines of fracture (Figure 8-24, *B* and *C*).

LABS

In the current patient, a complete trauma panel was obtained. The results were remarkable for an elevated WBC count of 15,100 cells/µl (may be secondary to demargination of leukocytes in the setting of acute trauma), and a urine toxicology screen that was positive for cocaine metabolites.

The β_2 transferrin test performed on the nasal fluid was negative (low likelihood of dural tear, which could cause CSF rhinorrhea).

ASSESSMENT

- *Type I NOE fracture of the right side (right medial canthal tendon attached to one large segment of bone)*
- *Type III NOE fracture of the left side (significant comminution and complete avulsion of left medial canthal tendon)*
- *11-cm U-shaped frontal region laceration through frontalis muscle to frontal bone, with no evidence of frontal sinus fracture*
- *10-cm linear horizontal laceration through both upper eyelids and probable left nasolacrimal duct injury*
- *OD grade I traumatic hyphema (less than one fourth of the height of the anterior chamber of the right eye is filled with blood)*
- *Punctate left temporal lobe subarachnoid hemorrhage*
- *Facial Injury Severity Scale (FISS) score of 5 (NOE = 3, facial laceration over 10 cm = 1 + 1)*

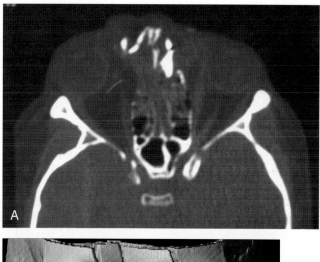

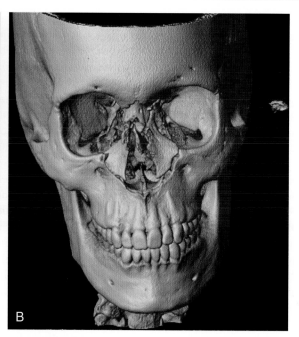

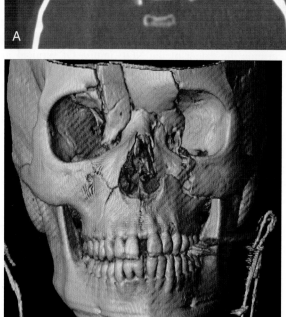

Figure 8-24 **A,** Preoperative axial bony CT window showing fracture of the nasal bones with severe displacement of the bilateral nasal bones and comminution of the frontal process of the maxilla. This view also shows the fracture of the lamina papyracea and bilateral medial orbital walls. **B,** Three-dimensional reconstruction CT of a different patient showing a NOE fracture with intact frontal bone. **C,** Three-dimensional reconstruction of a different patient showing a combined NOE fracture with frontal bone fracture.

TREATMENT

The goals of surgical correction of NOE fractures are to restore the patient to the preinjury levels of function and cosmesis. This becomes extremely challenging in the treatment of complex and comminuted NOE fractures with concomitant injuries.

Adequate exposure is essential for the precise reduction and fixation required for correction of NOE fractures. Most commonly, the combination of a coronal flap and lower eyelid incisions (or simply a coronal flap alone) is adequate. Placement of incisions in areas over the radix or lateral aspect of the nasal bridge should be avoided due to unfavorable scarring. Most often, the fractured segments can be fixated to a curved titanium plate that extends vertically from the nasofrontal junction along the frontal process of the maxilla onto the medial portion of the inferior orbital rim. The canthal tendon is rarely avulsed from bone and is usually attached to

a sizable bony fragment that can be reduced to a correctly adapted plate. When the medial canthal tendon is avulsed, a canthopexy must be performed, primarily through transnasal wiring or by securing a permanent suture to a transnasal wire that is directed superiorly and posteriorly, as described by Herford and colleagues.

The current patient was evaluated by the neurosurgical team and the ophthalmology service after the primary and secondary surveys and diagnostic imaging. The patient required no surgical intervention for the small subarachnoid hemorrhage and no intracranial pressure monitoring in light of consistently normal serial neurologic examinations. The ophthalmologic team concurred with the diagnosis of a grade I traumatic hyphema, which required no surgical intervention, and the high likelihood of a nasolacrimal apparatus injury, which would be formally evaluated under general anesthesia at the time of NOE repair. The patient was found to have no evidence of a ruptured globe or traumatic optic neuropathy.

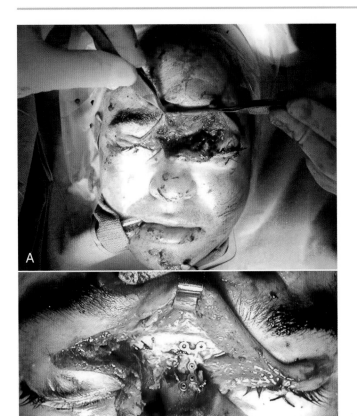

Figure 8-25 **A,** Intraoperative photograph showing access through facial lacerations. **B,** Intraoperative photograph after ORIF of the NOE complex.

He was taken to the operating room and orally intubated. A coronal flap was not used because of the excellent exposure through the existing lacerations (Figure 8-25, *A*). It must be stressed that this is usually not the case. Access is paramount in the proper reduction and fixation of NOE fractures, and a large number of comminuted NOE fractures benefit from immediate bone grafting. Each of these requirements is met through the use of a coronal incision, which provides large amounts of access and allows the concurrent harvest of cranial bone grafts for immediate grafting of the nasal dorsum or medial orbital walls.

Careful intraoperative examination revealed a 1 × 1-cm fiberglass foreign body within the right upper eyelid. A Jones type I test (fluorescein dye into eye) or Jones type II test (dye into the puncta/canaliculi) can be performed intraoperatively to assess the lacrimal function. The nasolacrimal apparatus may be injured in 20% of patients with NOE fractures. It is especially susceptible when telecanthus is present secondary to a loss of the protective influence provided by the anterior limb of the medial canthal ligament. Open reduction and anatomic fixation of the fracture segments usually result in reestablishment of the lacrimal drainage. Intraoperative repair may be completed through the use of a stent (e.g., a Crawford

tube), which acts to bridge the two severed ends of the canaliculi, and careful closure of the pericanalicular tissues. Delayed assessment may be done with fluorescein dye, instrument probing, or dacrocystography. Refractory or uncorrected epiphora often necessitates correction through a dacrocystorhinostomy at a later date. In this procedure, the tear drainage pathways are reconnected to the inside of the nose. A small incision is usually placed approximately midway between the corner of the eye and the bridge of the nose. The lacrimal sac is located, incised, and then connected to the nasal mucosa, creating a new tear drainage pathway. A stent is then placed in the newly created tear drainage pathway for a few months to prevent scarring of the tear drainage ducts, which might otherwise result in failure of the surgery. The tubes can usually be removed in the office with little if any discomfort or need for anesthesia.

In the current patient, the lacerations were meticulously washed out with pulse irrigation. The NOE fractures were confirmed to be a type I on the right side, with the medial canthus attached to a large segment of bone, and a type III on the left side, with complete avulsion of the medial canthal ligament attachment. A 2.0 X-shaped plate was applied to secure the nasal bones to the frontal bone (Figure 8-25, *B*). The medial orbital rims were also reconstructed using rigid minifixation plates. Twenty-six–gauge wires were used to directly secure the left and right medial canthal tendons to stable bone posterior and slightly superior to the insertion of the preinjured tendon. This is done to overcome the forces of migration, relapse, and telecanthus. Intranasal splints (i.e., Doyle splints) were placed and sutured in place anteriorly through the membranous septum. The lacerations were closed in layers, with special attention to the upper eyelid regions, where the levator muscle and its insertion were evaluated and maintained. An external nasal splint (e.g., Denver or Aquaplast splint) was placed for protection and to minimize edema. Postoperatively, the patient underwent serial neurologic checks. A second CT head scan, obtained on postoperative day 1, showed no change in the punctuate subarachnoid hemorrhage. The external and intranasal splints were removed, and the patient was discharged on the third postoperative day.

COMPLICATIONS

Intraoperative

Intraoperative complications are often best prevented by a thorough preoperative evaluation and examination. Concomitant ocular injuries must be identified and evaluated before general anesthetic induction and surgical manipulation of the globe and adnexal structures. Neurosurgical consultation must be obtained in case of neurologic changes and/or radiographic evidence of intracranial injury. In the case of severe epistaxis from midfacial injuries, the use of bilateral posterior nasal packs can be lifesaving.

Early

Nasolacrimal injury may present as epiphora secondary to inadequate tear drainage. Most cases of epiphora resolve within a few weeks after NOE reduction and/or lacrimal duct repair. However, persistent epiphora may require secondary correction with a dacrocystorhinostomy procedure.

Late

The majority of complications resulting from NOE fractures are cosmetic in nature and are the result of untreated or inadequately treated NOE fractures. Perhaps the most common is a residual "saddle defect," or shortened and retruded nose. This is secondary to the loss of dorsal nasal support in the upper bony and lower cartilaginous dorsum. The importance of immediate primary dorsal bone grafting has been emphasized in the literature. It is important when placing the graft as a strut to position it inferiorly underneath the lower lateral cartilage to provide support for the inferior portion of the nose and prevent palpation of the graft after healing is complete. The graft is secured superiorly with screws or plate fixation. Attention should be given to fixation of the graft superiorly to avoid overprojection at the nasofrontal region or at the nasal tip. Primary graft failure (infection) and long-term graft resorption can also occur.

Telecanthus is best managed at the time of initial surgery through correct reduction of the bone fragments that carry the medial canthal tendon insertions or, in the case of type III fractures, meticulous reduction of the insertions themselves with overcorrection. Septal deviation may require immediate correction or a septoplasty at a later date. Enophthalmos most often results from an increase in the orbital volume due to untreated medial orbital wall or orbital floor fractures. These injures should be addressed concurrently or secondarily with NOE reconstruction.

DISCUSSION

Fractures of the NOE region are among the most complex maxillofacial injuries in both diagnosis and treatment. The superior limits of this region are defined medially by the cribriform plate and laterally by the roof of the ethmoid sinuses. The anterior cranial fossa and contents lie above. The lateral limits comprise the medial orbital walls and are made up primarily of the lacrimal bone and the orbital plate of the ethmoid. The anterior limits consist of the frontal bone and, more laterally, the frontal process of the maxilla. Posteriorly lie the sphenoid bone and its sinus. The inferior limit is the lower border of the ethmoid sinuses. An NOE fracture involves the central midface—the nasal bones, frontal process of the maxilla, and ethmoid bones. In 1973 Epker coined the term "naso-orbito-ethmoid" to describe this midfacial injury. Prior to 1960, most textbooks offered little guidance in the treatment of these injuries, and early investigations focused on closed treatment using external nasal dressings after nasal manipulation. Open reduction with internal fixation (ORIF) has proved

to be an important advance in the management of these fractures and, combined with proper reduction of the medial canthal tendon and primary nasal dorsum bone grafting, has improved the cosmetic result even in severe injuries.

A detailed classification scheme by Markowitz and colleagues defined the injury pattern with respect to the medial canthal tendon and the fragment of bone upon which it inserts. Three distinct patterns have been identified. A type I injury is the simplest form of NOE fracture and involves only one portion of the medial orbital rim with its attached medial canthal tendon. Type II fractures have a comminuted central fragment with the fracture lines remaining external to the medial canthal tendon insertion. Type III fractures have comminution involving the central fragment of bone where the medial canthal tendon inserts. Variants of type I, II, and III fractures may occur in bilateral fractures.

In a 1985 study by Holt and Holt, 67% of 727 patients with facial fractures sustained some degree of ocular injury, although most series report the incidence to be in the range of 20% to 25%. A high degree of suspicion is warranted with significant NOE fractures, and a full fundoscopic examination should be performed. Slit-lamp examinations, when possible, allow evaluation of adnexal structures. The nasolacrimal apparatus may also be injured in about 20% of patients with NOE fractures.

NOE fractures are an uncommon but aesthetically challenging maxillofacial injury. The importance of precise reduction and primary bone grafting in the setting of inadequate dorsal nasal support and comminution cannot be overemphasized.

Bibliography

Ellis E III: Sequencing treatment for naso-orbito-ethmoid fractures, *J Oral Maxillofac Surg* 51:543-558, 1993.

Epker BN: Open surgical management of naso-orbital-ethmoid facial fractures, *Trans Int Conf Oral Surg* 4:323-329, 1973.

Fedok FG: Comprehensive management of nasoethmoid-orbital injuries, *J Craniomaxillofac Trauma* 1:36-48, 1995.

Gruss JS: Naso-ethmoid-orbital fractures: classification and role of primary bone grafting, *Plast Reconstr Surg* 75:303-317, 1985.

Herford AS, Ying T, Brown B: Outcomes of severely comminuted (type III) nasoorbitoethmoid fractures, *J Oral Maxillofac Surg* 63:1266-1277, 2005.

Holt GR, Holt JE: Nasoethmoid complex injuries, *Otolaryngol Clin North Am* 18:87-98, 1985.

Leipziger LS, Manson PN: Nasoethmoid orbital fractures: current concepts and management principles, *Clin Plast Surg* 19:167-193, 1992.

Markowitz BI, Manson PN, Sargent L, et al: Management of the medial canthal tendon in nasoethmoid orbital fractures: the importance of the central fragment in classification and treatment, *Plast Reconstr Surg* 87:843-853, 1991.

Sargent LA, Rogers GF: Nasoethmoid orbital fractures: diagnosis and management, *J Craniofac Trauma* 5:19-27, 1999.

Le Fort I Fracture

Martin B. Steed and Shahrokh C. Bagheri

CC

A 26-year-old man presents to the emergency department with the chief complaint of, "They hit my face with a brick and got my wallet. My face hurts … I was bleeding from my nose, but it has stopped."

HPI

You are called by the emergency department team to evaluate the patient. He reports being struck in the face at the level of his upper lip and teeth just below the nose by an unknown man who was walking the opposite way on the sidewalk (the vast majority of Le Fort I injuries are from blunt, as opposed to penetrating, trauma). He explains that he was hit one time in the face with a brick and subsequently fell to his knees, without any loss of consciousness (lower likelihood for intracranial injury in the absence of loss of consciousness).

PMHX/PDHX/MEDICATIONS/ALLERGIES/SH/FH

The patient smokes one pack of cigarettes daily and drinks alcohol regularly. (Both of these factors contribute to an increased relative risk of postoperative infections. A history of alcohol abuse is more frequently encountered in the trauma population). The remainder of his medical history is noncontributory.

EXAMINATION

The initial evaluation of a trauma patient should follow the advanced trauma life support (ATLS) protocol.

Primary Survey

The patient's primary survey is intact. (Control of the airway and hemorrhage are both part of the primary survey. Compromised airway and life-threatening hemorrhage are unlikely with isolated Le Fort I injuries; however, they can be seen with more complex facial fractures; that is, those with a higher Facial Injury Severity Scale [FISS] score).

Secondary Survey

General. The patient is a well-developed and well-nourished man in no apparent distress who is holding a blood-soaked cloth under his nose.

Vitals. His blood pressure is 115/64 mm Hg, heart rate 115 bpm, respirations 12 per minute, and temperature 37.6°C

(mild tachycardia can be due to a compensatory response to volume loss from prolonged oropharyngeal bleeding and/or from the sympathetic response associated with pain and anxiety).

Eyes. Pupillary response, visual acuity, visual fields, and extraocular movements are all within normal limits (a complete eye examination is mandatory in all midface fractures). There is no evidence of subconjunctival hemorrhage or hyphema (blood in the anterior chamber of the eye).

Maxillofacial. The patient has moderate bilateral midface edema with left facial abrasions extending over the lip region. There is mild hypoesthesia of the bilateral infraorbital nerve distributions (cranial nerve V2). The maxilla is mobile, with no simultaneous movement of the nasal bones upon palpation (as would be seen in Le Fort II and III injuries). Examination of the teeth reveals premature posterior occlusal contacts and a 5-mm anterior open bite (Figure 8-26). There is no evidence of mobile dentoalveolar segments. The remaining facial skeleton, including the nasal bones, is intact and stable upon palpation. Nasal speculum examination reveals a deviated nasal septum to the right, with no evidence of a septal hematoma (a septal hematoma needs to be drained to prevent subsequent necrosis of the quadrangular cartilage and possible saddle-nose deformity).

IMAGING

The imaging modality of choice for the diagnosis and evaluation of suspected maxillary Le Fort I fractures is a noncontrast maxillofacial CT scan with thin cuts (axial views with coronal reconstructions). Direct coronal imaging or coronal reconstructions are helpful (patients with suspected cervical

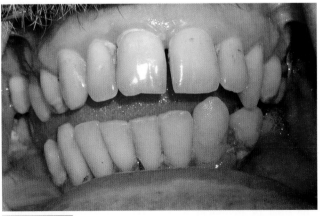

Figure 8-26 Posttraumatic anterior open bite and malocclusion.

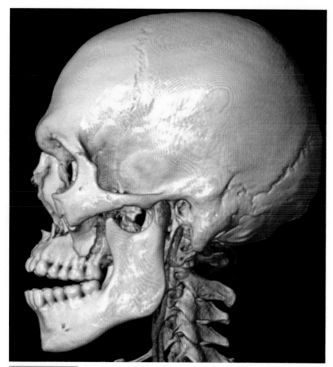

Figure 8-27 Preoperative three-dimensional lateral view of a different patient showing maxillary impaction anteriorly with resultant anterior open bite.

spine injuries should not hyperextend the neck for direct coronal imaging). Three-dimensional reconstructed CT can be useful to demonstrate the fracture anatomy (Figure 8-27).

For the current patient, a facial helical CT scan without contrast was obtained after the primary and secondary surveys were completed. Axial bony window cuts showed bilateral pterygoid plate, anterior and lateral maxillary wall, and posterior nasal septal fractures, with opacification of the maxillary antrum (Figure 8-28, *A*). A moderate amount of soft tissue edema and subcutaneous emphysema was noted. Coronal reconstruction views showed bilateral fractures through the lateral walls of the maxillary sinuses (Figure 8-28, *B*). A three-dimensional reconstruction view allowed clear visualization of the lines of fracture at the Le Fort I level (Figure 8-28, *C*).

LABS

For the current patient, a complete trauma panel was obtained. The results were remarkable for an elevated WBC count of 16,900 cells/μl (increased WBCs or leukocytosis in the acute setting is most likely secondary to physiologic stress due to catecholamine-induced demargination of WBCs).

ASSESSMENT

Isolated Le Fort I maxillary fracture; FISS score of 2.

TREATMENT

The goal of treatment of Le Fort I injuries is to reduce the displaced maxillary bone with its dentition to allow

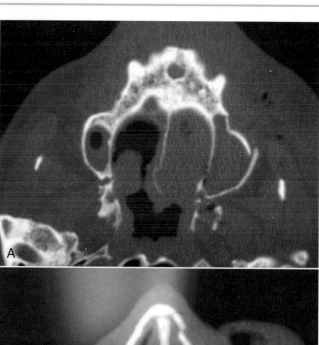

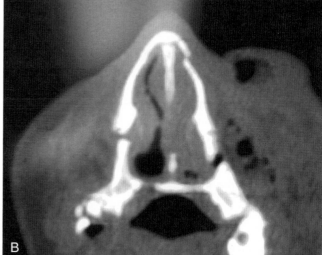

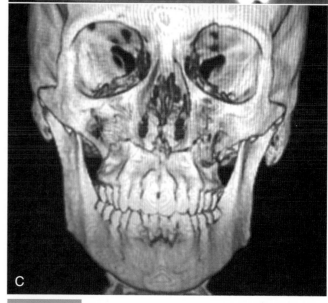

Figure 8-28 **A,** Preoperative axial bony CT window showing fractures of the pterygoid plates, anterior maxillary walls, and subcutaneous emphysema and opacification of the maxillary sinuses. **B,** Preoperative coronal bony CT window through the anterior maxilla and nasal vault showing fracture at the Le Fort I level. **C,** Preoperative anterior three-dimensional reconstruction showing a horizontal fracture of the maxilla at the Le Fort I level.

for uneventful healing, reestablishment of the patient's pre-existing occlusal function, and aesthetics. Treatment of a particular fracture needs to be individualized and includes several options, mainly either open reduction with internal fixation (ORIF) or closed reduction with maxillomandibular fixation (CR-MMF). The use of surgical splints should be considered, especially with segmental maxillary fractures. The degree of comminution at the anterior and lateral maxillary walls needs to be assessed for possible reconstructive measures.

Currently, most surgeons consider ORIF the gold standard. As a general principle, early reduction and fixation is preferable. After a 7- to 10-day period, some difficulty may be encountered in mobilizing the maxilla to achieve appropriate reduction, especially if the fracture is associated with significant impaction. Consideration should also be given to reosteotomy of the maxilla at the Le Fort I level (as in an orthognathic Le Fort osteotomy) if the fracture is incomplete or significant time has elapsed since the original insult. Attempting to mobilize the incompletely fractured maxilla can result in unfavorable fractures, often distant from the site of injury. After MMF has been established, it is critical to establish passive reduction of the maxilla (maxillomandibular complex) with the condyles seated in a correct position; otherwise, an anterior open bite will reemerge after rigid fixation has been applied and the intermaxillary fixation is released. If adequate bone contact is available, a plating system applied bilaterally at the piriform rims and zygomatic buttress areas is usually sufficient for stabilization. However, if more comminution is present and less bone contact is available, immediate bone grafting or secondary bone grafting reconstructive procedures should be considered.

The presence of palatal fractures complicates the treatment of Le Fort I fractures and deserves special attention. If there is a palatal fracture but no concurrent mandibular fractures, the mandibular arch is used to guide the width of the maxilla with arch bars and MMF. With concurrent mandibular fractures, two options exist: (1) the mandible can be reconstructed first anatomically, followed by the maxilla, or (2) alginate impressions can be obtained and model surgery carried out with the use of an intraoperative maxillary splint to reestablish the occlusion.

In the current patient, maxillomandibular arch bars were placed. An intraoral circumvestibular maxillary incision was made to gain access to the fractured segments. After appropriate mobilization of the maxilla, the patient was placed in MMF. The maxillomandibular complex was guided passively, using the arc of rotation of the condyle, into proper anatomic reduction while the patient was paralyzed to ensure that the condyles were appropriately positioned (failure to seat the condyles may result in postoperative anterior open bite). The deviated septum was reduced onto the nasal crest of the maxilla and sutured to a hole drilled through the anterior nasal spine. Subsequently, the maxilla was stabilized with fixation at the piriform rim and zygomaticomaxillary (ZM) buttress regions bilaterally (four plates). MMF was then released, and the occlusion was found to be intact and reproducible.

COMPLICATIONS

Complications of Le Fort I injuries are related to the severity of the initial injury and to host-related factors but can be categorized into intraoperative, early, and late complications.

Intraoperative

- Bleeding can occur as a result of damage to any number of the vessels in the vicinity, especially when significant disimpaction or an osteotomy is required for reduction of the segment. Potential sources of bleeding include the anterior and posterior superior alveolar, nasopalatine, and descending palatine arteries and, uncommonly, the internal maxillary artery. Packing, cauterization, and ligation are usually sufficient in controlling most situations. When hemorrhage cannot be controlled, external carotid artery ligation can be performed. Arterial angiography with embolization should also be considered.

- Maxillary hypoperfusion is uncommon but can occur, especially when the maxilla is fractured in multiple pieces and/or when surgical splints are used. Early reduction and stabilization with rigid internal fixation may help improve the outcome. In addition, consideration should be given to positioning the maxilla back into the preoperative position (in trauma situations). Postoperative use of hyperbaric oxygen has been suggested, but its benefits remain unclear. If prefabricated occlusal splints are used, they should be checked to prevent impingement on the soft tissues (and possibly the blood supply) of the palate.

- Malpositioning of the maxilla can occur when the bony interferences are not appropriately evaluated and the maxillomandibular complex is not seated passively with the condyles in the correct position; this results in a postoperative anterior open bite. Palatal fractures that are not reduced also result in improper maxillary segment positioning.

Early

- Control of nasal bleeding can be obtained in the immediate postoperative period by using a variety of techniques for nasal packing. A speculum and a good light source are essential for detecting an anterior versus a posterior origin. If adequate control is not achieved, exploration in the operating room or interventional radiology for angiographic evaluation may be necessary.

- Malocclusion can result from improper intraoperative maxillary positioning, early hardware failure, or undiagnosed mandibular or maxillary segmental fractures. Careful examination and appropriate imaging modalities help discern the etiology of malocclusion for surgical repositioning and refixation.

- Infraorbital nerve paresthesia can be the result of nerve injury at the initial trauma, especially when fracture patterns extend through the infraorbital foramen, or from intraoperative traction or manipulation for adequate reduction. Nasal septal deviation can result from improper repositioning of the nasal septum onto nasal crest of the maxilla, undiagnosed nasal septal injuries, or preoperative septal deformities. This can result in increased airway resistance, nasolacrimal obstruction, and aesthetic complaints by the patient.

- Loss of vision can result from an unfavorable fracture pattern of the maxilla or from the initial trauma, compounded by surgical manipulation of the segment during repositioning. The orbital process of the palatine bone makes up a portion of the bony orbit and has been hypothesized as a possible cause (this is very rare for Le Fort I fractures but more common with Le Fort III injuries).

- Early postoperative infection can result from foreign bodies, necrotic teeth, or bony segments but is also related to host factors (malnutrition, immunocompromised state, chronic alcohol use). Management should be directed at appropriate antibiotic selection, incision and drainage, and removal of any possible source.

Late

- Malocclusion, if not addressed early, typically presents with an anterior open bite, posterior premature contacts, and an overall Class III skeletal appearance. Once union has developed, small discrepancies can be treated with orthodontics; larger ones need to be addressed through orthognathic surgery.

- Late postoperative bleeding (especially with an intermittent pattern) should be taken seriously. Pseudoaneurysm formation should be high on the differential diagnosis list and can be evaluated by angiography.

- Epiphora (excessive tearing) can result from damage or obstruction of the nasolacrimal duct (the nasolacrimal duct drains beneath the inferior turbinate 11 to 17 mm above the nasal floor and 11 to 14 mm posterior to the piriform aperture). Epiphora can be managed by a dacryocystorhinostomy procedure.

- Nonunion or fibrous union causes the maxilla to demonstrate mobility, which can often be subtle. Management should be directed at refixating the maxilla with rigid internal fixation, skeletal fixation, extraskeletal fixation, and/or MMF.

DISCUSSION

Maxillary fractures most frequently occur as a result of blunt trauma from assault, sporting injuries, and motor vehicle accidents. They are frequently seen in conjunction with other facial and systemic injuries. The Le Fort classification is frequently used to describe midface fracture patterns. In 1901 Rene Le Fort published the results of his experiments based on 35 cadavers whose heads were subjected to different forms of force. Based on these findings, he concluded that the midface commonly fractures in three predictable patterns. A Le Fort level I fracture involves the anterior and lateral walls of the maxillary sinus, lateral nasal walls, the pterygoid plates, and the nasal septum (see Figure 8-30). It should be noted that isolated Le Fort fractures are relatively uncommon and that fractures occur in a variety of combinations of Le Fort I, II,

or III types, with unilateral (hemi–Le Fort) and bilateral fractures. The "pure" Le Fort I fracture is typically bilateral and is composed of the maxilla with associated alveolar bone and part of the palatine bone posteriorly. Unilateral fractures are seen with an additional fracture between the midpalatal suture.

The blood supply to the maxilla is from the descending palatine artery, which contributes to the greater and lesser palatine arteries and the terminal branch of the nasopalatine artery, and from the anterior, middle, and posterior superior alveolar arteries. Extensive research has been done with regard to the blood supply of the fractured maxilla, mostly in association with orthognathic maxillary procedures. In experiments done by Bell and later by Bays and by Dodson and colleagues, it has been shown that the maxilla (along with its associated dentition and periodontium) maintains an adequate blood supply even after complete downfracture and ligation of the descending palatine artery. The maxilla remains pedicled to the palate, receiving contributions from the ascending pharyngeal artery (a branch of the external carotid artery) and the ascending palatine artery (a branch of the facial artery), which in turn anastomose with the greater and lesser palatine arteries.

Patients suspected of having maxillary fractures should be evaluated according to the ATLS protocol. Because other bodily injuries may be present, the initial evaluation and stabilization of the patient are best performed by a trauma team experienced in the management of the multisystem trauma. Proper diagnosis should begin with a careful history and physical examination. The mechanism of injury should be considered. Symptoms associated with a Le Fort I fracture may include facial pain, infraorbital hypoesthesia, malocclusion, or epistaxis. Clinical signs suggestive of a Le Fort I fracture include facial edema, ecchymosis, abrasions, lacerations, active epistaxis, palpable crepitus, mobile maxilla, and step deformities. Intraoral examination could identify fractured teeth, vestibular ecchymosis, mucosal lacerations, palatal edema and/or ecchymosis (especially with fractures associated with midpalatal suture), and malocclusion (typically, an anterior open bite with posterior occlusal premature contacts secondary to the vector of impact and the pull of lateral and medial pterygoid muscles).

Bibliography

Bagheri SC, Dierks EJ, Kademani D, et al: Comparison of the severity of bilateral Le Fort injuries in isolated midface trauma, *J Oral Maxillofac Surg* 63:1123-1129, 2005.

Bagheri SC, Dierks EJ, Kademani D, et al: Application of a Facial Injury Severity Scale in craniomaxillofacial trauma, *J Oral Maxillofac Surg* 64:404-414, 2006.

Bays RA: Complications of orthognathic surgery. In Kaban LB, Pogrel MA, Perrott DH, et al (eds): *Complications in oral and maxillofacial surgery*, pp 193-221, Philadelphia, 1997, Saunders.

Bays RA, Reinkingh MR, Maron G: Descending palatine artery ligation in Le Fort osteotomies, *J Oral Maxillofac Surg* 51(Suppl):142, 1993.

Bell WH: Revascularization and bone healing after anterior maxillary osteotomy, *J Oral Surg* 27:249, 1969.

Bell WH, Fonseca RJ, Kennedy JW, et al: Bone healing and revascularization after total maxillary osteotomy, *J Oral Surg* 33:253, 1975.

Bell WH, Levy BM: Revascularization and bone healing after posterior maxillary osteotomy, *J Oral Surg* 29:313, 1971.

Cunningham LL Jr, Haug RH: Management of maxillary fractures. In Miloro M, Ghali GE, Larsen PE, et al (eds): *Peterson's principles of oral and maxillofacial surgery*, ed 2, pp 435-443, Hamilton, Ontario, 2004, BC Decker.

Dodson TB, Bays RA, Biederman GA: In-vivo measurement of gingival blood flow following Le Fort I osteotomy, *J Dent Res* 71:603, 1992.

Dodson TB, Bays RA, Neuenshwander MC: Maxillary perfusion during Le Fort I osteotomy after ligation of the descending palatine artery, *J Oral Maxillofac Surg* 55:51-55, 1997.

Dodson TB, Neuenschwander MC, Bays RA: Intraoperative measurement of maxillary gingival blood flow during Le Fort I osteotomy, *J Oral Maxillofacial Surg* 51(Suppl 3):138, 1993.

Dodson TB, Neuenschwander MC, Bays RA: Intraoperative assessment of maxillary perfusion during Le Fort I osteotomy, *J Oral Maxillofac Surg* 54:827, 1994.

Ellis E III: Passive repositioning of maxillary fractures, *J Oral Maxillofac Surg* 62:1477-1485, 2004.

Gruss JS, Mackinson SE: Complex maxillary fractures: role of buttress reconstruction and immediate bone grafts, *Plast Reconstr Surg* 78:9, 1986.

Gruss JS, Philips JH: Complex facial trauma: the evolving role of rigid fixation and immediate bone graft reconstruction, *Clin Plast Surg* 16:93-104, 1989.

Haug RH, Adams JM, Jordan RB: Comparison of the morbidity with maxillary fractures treated by maxillomandibular and rigid internal fixation, *Oral Surg* 80:629, 1995.

Iida S, Kogo M, Sugiura T, et al: Retrospective analysis of 1502 patients with facial fractures, *Int J Oral Maxillofac Surg* 30:286-290, 2001.

Morris CD, Tiwana PS: Diagnosis and treatment of midface fractures. In Fonseca RJ (ed): *Oral and maxillofacial trauma,* ed 4, pp 416-450, St Louis, 2013, Saunders.

Perciaccante VJ, Bays RA: Maxillary orthognathic surgery. In Miloro M, Ghali GE, Larsen PE, et al (eds): *Peterson's principles of oral and maxillofacial surgery*, ed 2, pp 1179-1204, Hamilton, Ontario, 2004, BC Decker.

Plaiser BR, Punjabi AP, Super DM, et al: The relationship between facial fractures and death from neurologic injury, *J Oral Maxillofac Surg* 58:708-712, 2000.

Top H, Aygit C, Sarikay A, et al: Evaluation of maxillary sinus after treatment of midfacial fractures, *J Oral Maxillofac Surg* 62:1229-1236, 2004.

Vaughan ED, Obeid G, Banks P: The irreducible middle third fracture: a problem in management, *Br J Oral Surg* 21:124, 1983.

You ZH, Bell WH, Finn RA: Location of the nasolacrimal canal in relation to the high Le Fort I osteotomy, *J Oral Maxillofac Surg* 50:1075-1080, 1992.

Le Fort II and III Fractures*

Justine Moe and Martin B. Steed

CC

A 41-year-old man is transported to the emergency department by EMS personnel status post motor vehicle accident (the most common etiology of Le Fort II and III injuries). You are called to the trauma bay to evaluate his facial injuries.

HPI

The patient was an unrestrained driver (higher risk for more severe facial injuries) involved in a high-speed, head-on collision with another vehicle. There was no rollover or ejection (lower risk of cervical, thoracic, and lumbar spine injury), but significant damage was done to the front side of the car, with 6-inch intrusion and a steering wheel deformity (evidence of significant energy transfer to the head and neck). Upon arrival of EMS personnel, the patient was hunched over the steering wheel; he had a Glasgow Coma Scale (GCS) score of 13.

Fifteen minutes later, at the emergency department (rapid transport time has reduced prehospital morbidity), the repeat GCS score was 11 (moderate head injury); vital signs were consistent with mild volume loss (tachycardia and hypotension); and there was active bleeding from both nares. The patient could not recall events surrounding the accident and admitted to loss of consciousness for an unknown period after striking the steering wheel with his face (indicative of intracranial injury, which can occur with up to 50% of midfacial fractures). Deteriorating mental status and uncontrolled nasopharyngeal hemorrhage necessitated a definitive airway, so the patient was orally intubated in the emergency department (approximately 40% of patients with Le Fort III injuries require advanced airway interventions). A cervical collar was placed for in-line cervical spine stabilization (the reported incidence of cervical spine fracture in patients with maxillofacial injuries is approximately 2%).

PMHX/PDHX/MEDICATIONS/ALLERGIES/SH/FH

The patient's histories are unknown (when possible, information may be obtained from family members).

EXAMINATION

Advanced Trauma Life Support (ATLS) Primary Survey

Airway and cervical spine control. The patient is orally intubated with a transport cervical collar in place. (Intubation is difficult with unstable midfacial fractures due to altered anatomy, soft tissue edema, expanding hematoma, and hemorrhage from the nasopharynx. An emergency surgical airway, including cricothyroidotomy, may be necessary should intubation fail).

Breathing and oxygenation. An oral endotracheal tube is in place, with mechanical ventilation on FiO_2 of 100%. The patient has bilateral chest rise, clear breath sounds bilaterally, and an oxygen saturation of 99%. Respirations are spontaneous and regular at 12 breaths per minute.

Circulation and hemorrhage control. Blood pressure is 107/90 mm Hg and heart rate is 115 bpm. Peripheral pulses are regular and thready. Extremities are pale and mildly diaphoretic, with delayed capillary refill. (Class II hypovolemic shock occurs with 15% to 30% blood volume loss and is characterized by normal mean arterial blood pressure, increased diastolic blood pressure, decreased pulse pressure, tachycardia, decreased urine output [20 to 30 ml/hour], peripheral vasoconstriction, and anxiety). Slow, active hemorrhage is observed in the nasopharynx with blood pooling in the oral cavity (uncontrolled nasal bleeding can be a source of significant blood loss and commonly arises from Woodruff's plexus posteriorly or Kiesselbach's plexus anteriorly). For posterior nasal packing, a Foley catheter (a nasal balloon catheter or cuffed endotracheal tube may also be used) is inserted into the nares and passed beyond the nasopharynx; the balloons are inflated, and the catheter/tube is advanced until the balloons occlude the posterior nasal aperture. Anteriorly, Merocel packing (Medtronic, Minneapolis, Minnesota) is coated with bacitracin, inserted along the floor of the nasal cavity, and expanded with a saline solution (many other forms of nasal packing are available, including ribbon gauze, sponges [Rhino Rocket; Shippert Medical Technologies Corp., Centennial, Colorado], biodegradable foam [Nasopore; Polyganics], and balloon catheters [Rapid Rhino, The Netherlands; ArthroCare, Austin, Texas]). The anteroposterior nasal packs effectively control the acute hemorrhage. The patient responds well to a 2-L bolus of lactated Ringer's solution. The control of hemorrhage and adequacy of fluid resuscitation are frequently reassessed.

Disability and dysfunction. On the AVPU scale (*A,* awake; *V,* responds to voice; *P,* responds to pain; *U,*

*The authors and publisher wish to acknowledge Dr. Chris Jo and Dr. Shahrokh C. Bagheri for their contributions on these topics in the previous editions.

unresponsive), the patient is responsive to pain. His GCS score is E2 + M5 + V1T = 8T. The right pupil is 4 mm and reactive, and the left pupil is 8 mm and nonreactive (a fixed, dilated pupil may be a sign of increased intracranial pressure or globe injury). There are no lateralizing signs.

Exposure and environmental control. The patient's clothing is removed, and a warm blanket or other warming devices are used to prevent hypothermia.

ATLS Secondary Survey

History. The AMPLE history (allergy, medications, past medical history, last meal, events leading to presentation) is taken from available sources.

General. The patient is a well-developed and well-nourished man who is intubated and sedated. He has a GCS score of 8T. A transport cervical collar is in place.

Neurologic. Sequential neurologic examination is more challenging in an intubated patient than in a conscious patient. Sedation should be discontinued for an accurate assessment of mental status. The use of propofol as the sedative drug allows for rapid emergence and facilitates hourly neurologic evaluations. AVPU and GCS scores, pupil size and responsiveness, and motor strength and responsiveness are assessed (weakness, hyporeflexia or hyperreflexia, and posturing can be indicative of intracranial or spinal derangement).

In the intubated patient, a high index of suspicion for intracranial hemorrhage and edema should be maintained. Any acute deterioration in neurologic status warrants a STAT head CT scan. An intracranial pressure–monitoring device is indicated in cases involving an initial low-yield neurologic examination (unconscious and unresponsive), deep sedation, paralysis, or severe head injury with evidence of elevated intracranial pressure.

Eyes. There is significant bilateral periorbital ecchymosis (raccoon eyes are indicative of anterior basilar skull fracture) and periorbital edema, with OS (left) greater than OD (right). There is chemosis (conjunctival edema) and subconjunctival hemorrhage OU (bilaterally). OD pupil is round, reactive, and sluggish (4 to 2 mm). OS pupil is large, irregular (the apex of a tear-shaped pupil points toward the site of rupture), and nonreactive. The globe is flaccid (ruptured globe) with a grade II hyphema (blood in the anterior chamber of the eye). Visual acuity cannot be assessed.

Maxillofacial. Examination shows significant facial edema and ecchymosis. Step deformities are palpated at the right lateral orbital rim, the left infraorbital rim, and at the naso-frontal junction. The intercanthal distance is 32 mm, with a negative bowstring test (the normal intercanthal distance is 30 to 34 mm and varies by race and gender [increased for those of African and Asian descent and for males]). There is no vertical or horizontal dystopia (disturbance in globe position). There is mild left enophthalmos (loss of anteroposterior projection of the globe) (however, enophthalmos and dystopia are difficult to assess in the presence of significant edema). Bimanual palpation yields gross mobility of the maxilla with associated mobility and crepitus at the nasofrontal junction, left lateral orbital rim, and right infraorbital rim (indicative of

maxillary/midfacial disjunction at the Le Fort II and III levels).

On otoscopic exam, tympanic membranes are clear and intact, and there is no evidence of CSF otorrhea. There is no Battle's sign (ecchymosis in the mastoid region, indicative of posterior basilar skull fracture). An 8-cm laceration of the lower face involving the full thickness of the lip and multiple other abrasions are present. Hypoesthesia along the infraorbital nerve distribution is present bilaterally (commonly seen after fractures of the anterior maxillary wall, inferior orbital rim, and orbital floor).

Intranasal. There is bright red blood in the bilateral nasal cavities. The nasal septum is deviated to the right, with no evidence of a septal hematoma. There is no evidence of CSF rhinorrhea.

Intraoral. Occlusion is difficult to assess secondary to orotracheal intubation. Ecchymosis is present along the posterior soft palate bilaterally (Guerin's sign, indicative of ptery-goid plate disjunction or fracture). The mandible is stable, without any signs of fracture (e.g., ecchymosis, step deformity, bony crepitus, mobility, or deviation). The dentition is in good repair.

IMAGING

For the trauma patient, the protocol for plain film radiographs includes cervical spine, anteroposterior chest, and anteroposterior pelvis radiographs. Other studies are completed if indicated, including a cervical spine series (suspected cervical spine injury), thoracic and lumbar spine series (motor vehicle accident with ejection or rollover or in symptomatic patients), and extremity radiographs (suspected fracture or dislocation).

To evaluate midfacial fractures, noncontrast, axial cut computed tomography (CT) with cuts of 1 mm or less is the gold standard imaging modality. Direct coronal CT should be avoided in patients with suspected cervical spine injury, because it requires hyperextended head positioning.

In the current patient, a maxillofacial CT scan reveals fracture lines extending from the nasofrontal suture through the medial wall of the orbit. On the right side, the fracture extends through the superior orbital fissure, lateral orbital wall along the zygomaticofrontal (ZF) suture, and along the zygomaticosphenoid (ZS) suture. There is a fracture of the right zygomatic arch near the zygomaticotemporal (ZT) suture. On the left side, a pyramidal fracture extends from the nasofrontal suture along the orbital floor, inferior orbital rim, and anterior and lateral maxillary walls. Sagittal and coronal views demonstrate a minimally displaced, left orbital floor defect. There is separation of the pterygomaxillary junction bilaterally (pterygoid plates). (This is a classic description of a pure right Le Fort III and a pure left Le Fort II fracture pattern.)

The anterior maxilla is grossly comminuted bilaterally (Le Fort fractures most commonly present in combination with other facial fractures). There are air-fluid levels in the bilateral maxillary sinuses (consistent with blood in the sinuses). A moderate amount of soft tissue edema and emphysema are also noted. A three-dimensional reconstruction provides the most graphic representation of the fractures, degree of displacement, and orientation of fragments.

Due to the patient's decrease in mental status (risk of intracranial injury), an initial head CT scan was obtained. It demonstrated bilateral frontal lobe contusions, with no evidence of skull fracture, epidural or subdural hematoma, or increased intracranial pressure. A repeat head CT scan after 24 hours showed no evolution of the intracranial injury (an initially negative head CT scan may also require a repeat scan at 12 to 24 hours, because closed head injuries may produce CT findings only after 24 hours).

LABS

Standard laboratory tests for the evaluation of multisystem trauma patients included CBC, complete metabolic panel, arterial blood gas, urine analysis, and coagulation studies (prothrombin time [PT], partial thromboplastin time [PTT], and international normalized ratio [INR]). A urine drug screen and blood alcohol level are indicated in patients with decreased mental status.

The current patient demonstrates decreased hemoglobin (11.2 g/dl) and hematocrit (32.6%) (true and relative anemia secondary to hypovolemia and hemodilution from fluid resuscitation). Arterial blood gas analysis shows a mild base deficit of −3.5 (base deficit is a reliable indicator of adequacy of resuscitation and mortality in trauma patients and is a better marker of blood loss than are the hemoglobin and hematocrit). There is also a mild elevation in blood urea nitrogen (BUN) and creatinine (Cr), with a BUN:Cr ratio of 15 (prerenal azotemia secondary to hypovolemia) and a positive blood alcohol level (common in the trauma patient). The remainder of the patient's laboratory values are within normal limits.

ASSESSMENT

Comminuted midfacial fractures consistent with a right Le Fort III and left Le Fort II pattern, with a concomitant left orbital floor fracture and displaced nasal septal fracture, complicated by significant nasopharyngeal hemorrhage, bilateral frontal lobe contusions, ruptured left globe, and laceration of the lower face and lip. Facial Injury Severity Scale (FISS) score is 6.

TREATMENT

A variety of treatment modalities have been advocated for the treatment of Le Fort II and III fractures. Techniques are generally categorized as open or closed reduction or a combination of the two. Commonly, Le Fort fractures are sustained at more than one level, and all combinations of Le Fort I, II, and III fractures are possible. Moreover, Le Fort fractures are usually comminuted and occur in conjunction with other facial fractures, including naso-orbito-ethmoid (NOE), orbital floor/rim, and zygomaticomaxillary complex (ZMC) fractures. As such,

these fractures should be considered by their individual components when developing a treatment plan. Medical comorbidities, associated systemic trauma, airway status, hemorrhage, and available resources further dictate the course of treatment in each case.

Intraoperative and perioperative airway management should allow for safe anesthetic administration, optimal surgical care, and decreased morbidity. Nasoendotracheal intubation facilitates intraoperative maxillomandibular fixation (MMF) and is considered if extubation is expected upon completion of the procedure. Care must be taken in placing nasoendotracheal tubes in patients with midfacial fractures that may have basilar skull components, because there have been isolated reports of intracranial placement of the endotracheal tube. However, there is insufficient evidence to exclude this technique in the hands of skilled personnel. Nasotracheal intubation may interfere with nasal septal correction.

Oral intubation is considered if the endotracheal tube may pass through an edentulous space, to allow for MMF, or for submental intubation, in which the endotracheal tube is passed through the anterior floor of the mouth and through a submental transcutaneous incision. Early tracheostomy is considered for severe midfacial fractures in which intubation is difficult and if prolonged postoperative intubation is expected (Figure 8-29).

Multiple surgical approaches are possible to access Le Fort II and III fractures. For Le Fort III fractures, the coronal incision provides complete access to the nasofrontal region, lateral orbital rim, and zygomatic arch for reduction and fixation. A coronal incision provides optimal visualization, which is essential for comminuted Le Fort III fractures. Releasing incisions in the coronal flap may be made to avoid intracranial monitoring devices, such as a Camino bolt or an external

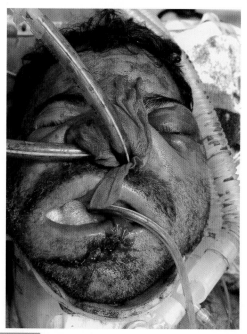

Figure 8-29 Patient with a Le Fort III fracture with multiple nasal and oral packing used to control posterior nasal and pharyngeal hemorrhage. The airway has been secured with a tracheostomy.

ventriculostomy drain. Lateral brow and upper blepharoplasty (supratarsal fold) incisions allow access to the lateral orbital rim but not to the zygomatic arch.

For Le Fort II fractures, the inferior orbital rim and floor may be accessed by various transcutaneous (lower lid, subtarsal, subciliary) or transconjunctival (with or without lateral canthotomy) incisions. A transmucosal incision in the maxillary vestibule provides access to the zygomaticomaxillary (ZM) buttress and inferior orbital rim for alignment and fixation. Existing lacerations may also be extended and used for access.

It should be noted that it is not always necessary to visualize all components of Le Fort II and III fractures. Isolated Le Fort II fractures may sometimes be reduced with disimpaction forceps and MMF for 4 weeks, although they usually require open reduction and internal fixation. Reduction should be achieved at the nasofrontal region, inferior orbital rim, and ZM buttress in Le Fort II fractures and at the nasofrontal region, lateral orbital rim (ZF suture area), and zygomatic arch (ZT suture area) in Le Fort III fractures. A key and often challenging step in the surgical correction of Le Fort fractures is disimpaction of the maxillofacial unit to allow passive positioning of the segment. This can be achieved by different techniques, such as using a Rowe disimpaction forceps or a wire passed through the anterior nasal spine.

If disimpaction cannot be achieved with these techniques, a Le Fort I osteotomy can be made unilaterally or bilaterally to mobilize and reduce the maxilla and dentate segment. Osteotomy should considered only for noncomminuted maxillary fractures in which rigid fixation with adequate bone buttressing is possible.

Internal rigid fixation with miniplate systems is the current standard of care for Le Fort fractures. Comminuted Le Fort patterns often require fixation of the fragmented segments in a "stable to unstable" fashion. In particular, Le Fort III fractures usually present as a component of panfacial fractures rather than as isolated fractures. Several sequencing methods have been advocated for panfacial fracture management, including "bottom up" and "outside in."

The location, amount, and size of rigid fixation also vary among surgeons and depend on the severity of displacement. Severe comminution or avulsed bony segments at the anterior and lateral maxillary walls may complicate reduction at the ZM buttress and, infrequently, immediate or secondary bone grafting may be indicated. In addition, Le Fort fractures complicated by a palatal fracture may benefit from the use of surgical splints to achieve an optimal postoperative occlusion.

It is not always necessary to fixate all reduced components of Le Fort II and III fractures for proper alignment of the segments. For example, adequate fixation at the bilateral ZM and/or orbital rim areas may alleviate the need for fixation at the nasofrontal suture, thereby avoiding a coronal or other unsightly incision. If the nasofrontal segment is unstable despite fixation at these areas, exposure of the nasofrontal area may then be necessary using a variety of approaches (coronal, upper blepharoplasty, Lynch, or open sky incisions).

A stable mandible and intact dentition greatly facilitate the treatment of midfacial fractures involving the dentate segment, particularly in the absence of direct visualization of fracture segments. After the maxillary segment has been mobilized, the patient is placed in MMF and the intact mandibular arc of rotation is used to determine the correct reduction of facial and cranial units. In the presence of a fractured mandible, treatment of midfacial fractures is dictated by anatomic reduction at stable segments.

COMPLICATIONS

Complications of Le Fort II and III injuries are related to the severity of the initial injury and host-related factors; they can be categorized as intraoperative, early, and late complications.

Intraoperative

- Bleeding can occur as a result of damage to any number of the vessels, particularly when significant disimpaction or an osteotomy is required for reduction of the midfacial segment. Potential sources of arterial bleeding include the anterior and posterior superior alveolar, sphenopalatine, descending palatine, and internal maxillary arteries. Injury to the pterygoid venous plexus presents as a steady flow of dark blood. In most cases, packing, cauterization, and ligation are sufficient for achieving hemostasis. If hemorrhage cannot be controlled locally, external carotid artery ligation or transcatheter arterial embolization should be strongly considered.
- Maxillary hypoperfusion is uncommon but may occur in comminuted maxillary fractures or with impingement of the palatal mucosa by surgical splints. Early reduction and stabilization with rigid internal fixation may help improve the outcome. Postoperative use of hyperbaric oxygen has been suggested, but its benefits remain unclear. Prefabricated occlusal splints should be checked to avoid impingement on the soft tissues of the palate.
- Improper reduction and malpositioning of the maxilla can occur when the bony interferences are not appropriately evaluated and the maxillomandibular complex is not seated passively with the condyles in correct position. This results in a postoperative anterior open bite. Infrequently, osteotomies are required to completely disimpact and reduce the midface.

Early

- Postoperative nasal bleeding can usually be controlled locally with nasal packs. A nasal speculum and a good light source are essential to determine the anterior or posterior origin. If adequate control is not achieved by local means, reexploration in the operating room or angiographic evaluation with interventional radiology may be necessary.
- Malocclusion can result from poor intraoperative maxillary reduction, early hardware failure, or undiagnosed mandibular or maxillary segmental fractures. Thorough examination and appropriate imaging modalities help

discern the etiology of the malocclusion. Surgical repositioning and refixation should be considered.

- Nasal septal deviation can result from improper repositioning of the nasal septum onto the septal crest of the maxilla, undiagnosed nasal septal injuries, or preoperative septal deformities. By definition, the nasal septum is fractured in Le Fort II injuries; thus special care must be taken to identify and reduce deviations.

- Loss of vision is rarely reported as a direct or an indirect optic nerve injury. Insult may result from bony compression, laceration, hematoma, or edema of the optic nerve and sheath after the initial trauma or after surgical manipulation of bony segments. Ideal management is controversial and may include conservative treatment with steroids or surgical decompression. Other orbital injuries include iatrogenic corneal or penetrating injuries.

- Local wound infection can result from retained foreign bodies, necrotic teeth, or avulsed bony segments and may be related to host factors. Management should be directed at appropriate antibiotic selection, incision and drainage and, when possible, removal of the source.

Late

- Malunion causes malocclusion, facial asymmetry, enophthalmos, and ocular dystopia. Malocclusion, if not addressed early, typically presents with midfacial retrusion, decreased midfacial height, anterior open bite, and mandibular overclosure. Secondary repair is difficult; small discrepancies may be treated with orthodontics, whereas larger deformities require orthognathic surgery.

- Nonunion or fibrous union causes the maxilla to demonstrate mobility, which may be subtle. Management should be directed at reduction and refixation with rigid internal fixation, with or without MMF.

- Late postoperative bleeding (especially with an intermittent pattern) is often serious and may suggest pseudoaneurysm formation. Future rupture of a false aneurysm presents as massive hemorrhage. A high index of suspicion should be maintained, and angiography should be considered for evaluation.

- Epiphora (excessive tearing) can result from ectropion or from nasolacrimal duct injury (the duct drains beneath the inferior turbinate, 11 to 17 mm above the nasal floor and 11 to 14 mm posterior to the piriform aperture). Ectropion is managed by a lid-tightening procedure; lacrimal injury requires lacrimal stents or a dacryocystorhinostomy procedure.

- Unrecognized CSF leakage is most commonly caused by fractures through the cribriform or fovea ethmoidalis. Meningitis, cerebral abscess, and epidural empyema have been reported up to several years after injury.

- Other complications include cosmetic deformity, unsightly scars, hair loss (secondary to coronal incision), facial nerve palsy (injury to temporal branch of facial nerve secondary to coronal incision), and trigeminal nerve injury (hypoesthesia, dysesthesia, or anesthesia of V1 secondary to

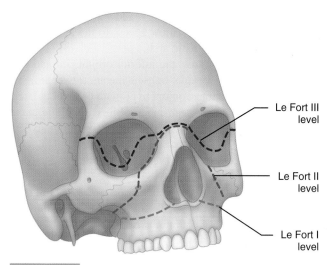

| Figure 8-30 | Fracture levels for Le Fort I, II, and III fractures.

coronal incisions or V2 secondary to Le Fort II injury and treatment).

DISCUSSION

The Le Fort classification system was originally described by Rene Le Fort in a 1901 human cadaver study. It continues to be used today to identify classic fracture patterns along three weak lines in the facial bony structure (Figure 8-30). The Le Fort II fracture results from blunt trauma at the level of the infraorbital rim and nasofrontal junction. It is a pyramidal fracture in which the central midface and maxilla are mobilized independently from the facial skeleton and cranial base. The Le Fort III fracture results from blunt trauma at the level of the nasofrontal junction and upper lateral orbital rims. It is termed *craniofacial disjunction,* because it causes disarticulation of the facial skeleton from the cranial base.

Knowledge of these fracture lines has been paramount in developing reconstructive strategies in trauma, craniofacial, and orthognathic surgery. In clinical practice, however, Le Fort II and III fractures rarely follow ideal fracture patterns and are often unilateral, comminuted, and found in combination with other Le Fort fractures and other facial fractures.

Initial management of patients with suspected maxillofacial fractures should follow ATLS protocol. Airway management in patients sustaining Le Fort II or III injuries is paramount, because altered mental status, changes in anatomy, airway edema, and active hemorrhage can compromise a patient's airway patency. The incidence of uncontrolled hemorrhage is greater in Le Fort II and III fractures than in all facial injuries (incidences of 5.5% versus 1.2% are reported by Bynoe and colleagues), and establishment of an emergent airway is often necessary. Clinicians treating midfacial trauma should be prepared to establish a surgical airway both acutely and in more controlled settings.

Ideally, surgical management of midfacial fractures should be completed as soon as the patient's status allows. Goals of treatment include reestablishing premorbid occlusion and facial width, projection, and height. Early reconstruction allows for better restoration of the preinjury appearance, as determined by the relationship of bone and soft tissue. Delayed reconstruction at 7 to 14 days after injury results in a second insult to the contused soft tissue and may increase subcutaneous fibrosis, rigidity, and hyperpigmentation. The introduction of rigid miniplate fixation has obviated the need for external fixation and interfragment wiring and has allowed for greater flexibility in the sequence of repair. In general, the management of Le Fort fractures follows the principles of wide exposure and direct viewing of fracture segments, the use of vertical and horizontal buttresses of the face for alignment and fixation, and immediate bone grafting to reconstruct comminuted or avulsed bony structures.

Bibliography

Bagheri SC, Dierks EJ, Kademani D, et al: Comparison of the severity of bilateral Le Fort injuries in isolated midface trauma, *J Oral Maxillofac Surg* 63:1123-1129, 2005.

Bagheri SC, Dierks EJ, Kademani D, et al: Application of a Facial Injury Severity Scale (FISS) in cranio-maxillofacial trauma, *J Oral Maxillofac Surg* 64:408-414, 2006.

Bähr W, Stoll P: Nasal intubation in the presence of frontobasal fractures: a retrospective study, *J Oral Maxillofac Surg* 50:445-447, 1992.

Bell RB, Dierks EJ, Homer L, et al: Management of cerebrospinal fluid leak associated with craniomaxillofacial trauma, *J Oral Maxillofac Surg* 62(6):676-684, 2004.

Bynoe RP, Kerwin AJ, Parker HH III, et al: Maxillofacial injuries and life-threatening hemorrhage: treatment with transcatheter arterial embolization, *J Trauma* 55(1):74-79, 2003.

Girotto JA, Gamble WB, Robertson B, et al: Blindness after reduction of facial fractures, *Plast Reconstr Surg* 102(6):1821-1834, 1998.

Haug RH, Savage JD, Likavek MJ, et al: A review of 100 closed head injuries associated with facial fractures, *J Oral Maxillofac Surg* 50:218, 1992.

Haug RH, Wible RT, Likavek MJ, et al: Cervical spine fractures and maxillofacial trauma, *J Oral Maxillofac Surg* 49:725, 1991.

Horellou MF, Mathe D, Feisse P: A hazard of naso-tracheal intubation, *Anaesthesia* 33:73-74, 1978.

Imola MJ, Ducic Y, Adelson RT: The secondary correction of post-traumatic craniofacial deformities, *Otolaryngol Head Neck Surg* 139(5):654-660, 2008.

Kelly KJ, Manson PN, Vander Kolk CA, et al: Sequencing Le Fort fracture treatment: organization of treatment for a panfacial fracture, *J Craniofac Surg* 1(4):168-178, 1990.

Khanna S, Dagum AB: A critical review of the literature and an evidence-based approach for life-threatening hemorrhage in maxillofacial surgery, *Ann Plast Surg* 69(4):474-478, 2012.

Kreiner B, Stevens MR, Bankston S, et al: Management of panfacial fractures, *Oral and Maxillofacial Surgery Knowledge Update* 3:63-81, 2001.

Le Fort R: Experimental study of fractures of the upper jaw. I, II, and II, *Rev Chir De Paris* 23:208-227, 360-379, 479-507, 1901; translated by Tessier P: *Plast Reconstr Surg* 50:497-506, 600-607, 1972.

Manson PN, Clark N, Robertson B, et al: Comprehensive management of pan-facial fractures, *J Craniomaxillofac Trauma* 1(1):43-56, 1995.

Manson PN, Hoopes JE, Su CT: Structural pillars of the facial skeleton: an approach to the management of Le Fort fractures, *Plast Reconstr Surg* 66:53-61, 1980.

Marlow TJ, Goltra DD, Schabel SI: Intracranial placement of a nasotracheal tube after facial fracture: a rare complication, *J Emerg Med* 15:187-191, 1997.

Ng M, Saadat D, Sinha UK: Managing the emergency airway in Le Fort fractures, *J Craniomaxillofac Trauma* 4:38, 1998.

Roccia F, Cassarino E, Boccaletti R, et al: Cervical spine fractures associated with maxillofacial trauma: an 11-year review, *J Craniofac Surg* 18(6):1259-1263, 2007.

Orbital Trauma: Fracture of the Orbital Floor

Martin B. Steed, Robert S. Attia, and Shahrokh C. Bagheri

CC

A 36-year-old man is seen in the emergency department status post assault. He explains that he was "jumped, robbed, beaten, and punched in the left eye." You are asked to evaluate the patient for maxillofacial injuries.

HPI

The patient was returning from work when he was assaulted. He received a right-handed blow with a fist to the left upper face (common pattern of injury). He reports no loss of consciousness but has difficulty seeing out of his left eye, and his cheek is numb (hypoesthesia of the V2 cutaneous distribution is suggestive of an orbital floor, zygomaticomaxillary complex [ZMC], or isolated anterior maxillary wall fracture).

PMHX/PDHX/MEDICATIONS/ALLERGIES/SH/FH

Noncontributory. The patient has no previous history of maxillofacial trauma.

Patients with a previous history of orbital floor reconstruction are at a higher risk of globe rupture with subsequent trauma to the globe, because the reconstructed orbital floor is less likely to fracture. The energy delivered to the eye is absorbed by the globe (as opposed to being dispersed by fracture of the floor), causing more devastating injuries (blindness).

EXAMINATION

The initial evaluation of a trauma patient should follow the advanced trauma life support (ATLS) protocol.

Primary Survey

The patient's primary survey is intact; he has a Glasgow Coma Scale (GCS) score of 15.

Secondary Survey

General. The patient is a well-developed and well-nourished man in no acute distress.

Vital signs. Blood pressure is 135/84 mm Hg, heart rate 108 bpm (tachycardia), respirations 16 per minute, and temperature 37.6°C.

Maxillofacial. There is moderate left midface edema with left V2 hypoesthesia. There is no loss of malar projection (seen with displaced ZMC fractures). The intercanthal distance is maintained at 32 mm with a negative bowstring test result (a positive bowstring test result is seen with naso-orbito-ethmoid [NOE] fractures).

Eyes. Examination of the left eye (OS) reveals subconjunctival hemorrhage (ruptured blood vessel that leaks into the space between the conjunctiva and sclera), chemosis (inflammation and edema of the conjunctiva), and mild periorbital edema (Figure 8-31).

Vision, pupil, and pressure are the "vital signs" of the eye. After a thorough medical history and adnexal exam, it is important to check these measurements before dilating the eye (vital signs may change with dilation). The vision assessment that is most important is the "best corrected vision."

The current patient's visual acuity was OD 20/20 and OS 20/40, determined using a 14-inch near card. The pupils were equal, round, and reactive to light (5 mm to 3 mm) with accommodation (PERRLA). Assessment of direct and consensual visual reflexes revealed no abnormalities. (The "swinging flashlight test" is based on the consensual light reflex and is the best method for diagnosing a relative afferent pupillary defect [RAPD], also called a *Marcus-Gunn pupil.* Illumination of one eye that results in failure to constrict in the pupils of both eyes suggests an RAPD of the illuminated eye or a defect of the afferent visual pathway of the illuminated eye.)

A tonometer pen revealed a globe tension pressure of 12 mm Hg. (Tonometry measures the intraocular pressure, which, when high, may raise suspicion for a retrobulbar hemorrhage. An extremely low value is suggestive of globe rupture. Normal intraocular pressure [IOP] ranges from 11 to

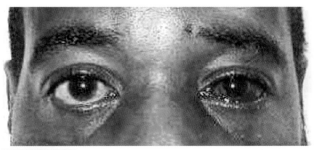

Figure 8-31 Preoperative view showing left subconjunctival hemorrhage and an incidental finding, arcus senilis (a cloudy, opaque arc or circle around the edge of the eye, often seen in the eyes of the elderly).

20 mm Hg. Gentle digital palpation of the closed upper lid is a crude assessment of IOP; although slight increases in IOP cannot be detected, a rock-hard eye should raise concern about a marked increase in IOP.)

An additional useful test is the red color saturation test, which is the most sensitive and best measure of optic nerve function. The two eyes are evaluated separately. A red object is held in front of the patient, who is asked whether the object seems to have the same color (hue) and brightness (intensity) in each eye. If the optic nerve has been damaged (e.g., by optic neuritis or increased IOP), the red object appears duller and more brown or grayish to the affected eye compared with the contralateral eye.

In the current patient, evaluation of the extraocular muscles of the left eye revealed restriction of upward gaze (suggestive of inferior rectus entrapment). There was no evidence of monocular diplopia within 30 degrees of primary gaze (monocular diplopia should be investigated for retinal detachment or lens dislocation). The patient reported binocular diplopia within 20 degrees of primary gaze. (This is commonly seen secondary to edema, neuromuscular paralysis, or extraocular muscle entrapment. To determine what muscle groups and nerves are involved, the clinician should determine what gaze directions improve and worsen the doubling.)

After administration of a topical mydriatic agent and fluorescein dye to the eye, a slit-lamp examination was performed with a cobalt blue light in an anterior-to-posterior sequence. This revealed no abnormalities of the bilateral adnexa (eyelids and lacrimal system) and no corneal abrasions, opacities, or foreign bodies. There was no evidence of blood within the anterior chamber (hyphema) and no evidence of injury to the iris (traumatic iridialysis) or lens (dislocation or subluxation). (Traumatic iridodialysis occurs when the iris is torn from its root. A red reflex can be seen through the tear. Surgical repair is indicated only if decreased visual acuity or diplopia persists. The use of mydriatic agents to dilate the pupil of the eye is relatively contraindicated in patients who have sustained head injuries due to the need for multiple-interval neurologic examinations.)

Fundoscopic examination of the posterior segment (vitreous, retina, and optic nerve) revealed no vitreous or retinal hemorrhage. There were no apparent tears or foreign bodies. A forced duction test was performed after administration of a topical anesthetic and revealed true incarceration of infraorbital contents. (For this test one or two fine forceps are used to carefully move the eye in the directions of gaze while feeling for mechanical restriction. Further measurements of globe position include those based on the surrounding bone [e.g., Hertel exophthalmeter using the zygomaticofrontal region or the Naugel exophthalmeter using the frontal bone]. If these bony landmarks are displaced or significant soft tissue edema is present, reliable readings are difficult to obtain.)

The remainder of the current patient's maxillofacial examination revealed hypoesthesia of the left V2 distribution. No palpable bony step deformities of the left orbital rim were noted.

IMAGING

Computed tomography is the gold standard for assessing the status of the bony orbit. For the current patient, a facial helical CT scan (1-mm cuts) without contrast was obtained after the primary and secondary surveys were completed. Coronal views (best view of the internal orbit) showed a fracture of the left orbital floor with complete opacification of the maxillary sinus (Figure 8-32, *A*). Sagittal views showed the location of the fracture in an anterior-posterior dimension (Figure 8-32, *B*). (Three-dimensional reconstruction views add little information for the preoperative planning of orbital floor fractures, except for teaching purposes.)

LABS

For the management of isolated orbital floor injuries, no routine laboratory testing is indicated unless dictated by the medical history. When evaluated as part of the treatment of a

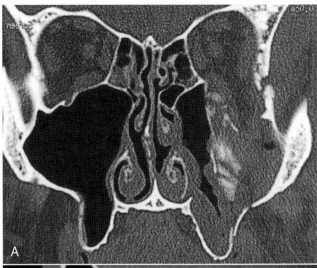

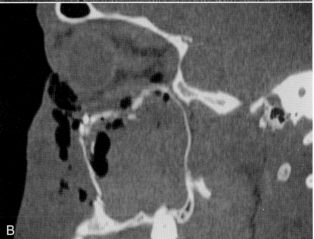

Figure 8-32 **A,** Preoperative CT scan (coronal cut/bony window) showing a left orbital floor fracture. **B,** Preoperative CT scan (sagittal cut) showing a left orbital floor fracture with evidence of an intact orbital rim.

multisystem trauma patient, routine laboratory tests include a CBC, complete metabolic panel, liver function tests, and coagulation studies.

ASSESSMENT

Isolated fracture of the left orbital floor with entrapment of the inferior rectus muscle; Facial Injury Severity Scale (FISS) score of 1.

TREATMENT

A much disputed topic is which orbital floor fractures require treatment. Surgical intervention may be required in two clinical situations: globe malposition and diplopia. A number of factors can be helpful in determining whether a pure blowout fracture requires internal orbital surgery; these factors can be broken down into absolute indications, relative indications, and contraindications to immediate repair.

Absolute Indications

- Globe malposition with acute enophthalmos and/or hypoglobus
- Immediate correction of diplopia in the setting of muscle (inferior rectus) incarceration and a positive forced duction test result, or unresolved diplopia with a positive forced duction test result
- Immediate correction in the symptomatic pediatric patient with an orbital floor "trapdoor" fracture that has elicited the oculocardiac reflex (the oculocardiac reflex can be seen with true entrapment)

Relative Indications

- Prevention of a cosmetic deformity. Disruption of greater than 50% of the orbital floor is likely to cause cosmetically apparent enophthalmos, especially with fractures in the critical area at the junction of the floor and medial wall.
- Correction of unresolved diplopia (7 to 11 days) in the setting of soft tissue prolapse

Contraindications to Immediate Repair

- Any condition that puts the globe in jeopardy, such as ocular injuries (e.g., hyphema, retinal tears, lens displacement). For example, a lacerated globe or hyphema may put the globe at increased risk because of the retraction necessary to perform orbital surgery.
- The status of the noninjured eye as a possible contraindication. Diplopia (binocular) would not be possible in a patient with one blind eye; therefore, the only reason to perform surgery, other than restriction of globe motion secondary to incarceration of soft tissues, would be to prevent globe malposition.

The current patient had binocular diplopia within 20 degrees of primary gaze, a positive forced duction test result with concurrent evidence of greater than 50% orbital floor disruption, and a high likelihood of cosmetically significant postinjury enophthalmos.

The patient was taken to the operating room 4 days after the assault, to allow for partial resolution of soft tissue edema. A preseptal (between the septum and the overlying orbicularis oculi muscle) transconjunctival incision was made, without the need for a lateral canthotomy (Figure 8-33, *A*). Once the bony defect had been isolated (Figure 8-33, *B*), a titanium mesh was fitted and then properly contoured and fixated (Figure 8-33, *C* and *D*). A forced duction test, which was confirmed with the contralateral side, showed full mobility of the eye in all directions. The incision was closed with 5-0 fast-absorbing gut suture, and a frost suture was placed. A postoperative CT scan (Figure 8-34) revealed proper positioning and contour of the reconstruction plate.

The patient did well postoperatively. with no apparent enophthalmos or diplopia on follow-up at 6 weeks.

COMPLICATIONS

Orbital floor fractures may be seen in isolation or in association with other facial injuries. Complications can be related to the impact or the initial injury, concomitant injuries, the surgical repair, or a combination of these elements and can be categorized as early or late complications.

Early

- **Corneal abrasion.** Clinical suspicion should be raised by a patient's complaint of ocular pain, photophobia, and a foreign body sensation. Corneal abrasions are diagnosed on clinical examination with fluorescent dye viewed under cobalt blue light. Treatment includes patching the eye (24 hours) and administration of a topical cycloplegic (e.g., homatropine 5%) for ciliary body spasm.
- **Hyphema.** This is defined as the presence of blood in the anterior chamber caused by damage to blood vessels in the ciliary body or rupture of blood vessels in the iris. Hyphema is graded according to the extent to which it vertically fills the anterior chamber. Grade I is designated as less than one third; grade II is between one third and one half; grade III is one half to near total; and grade IV is total (eight ball) filling of the anterior chamber. Treatment is directed toward controlling bleeding, and preventing rebleeding. This is especially important in patients with sickle cell anemia or sickle cell trait, because sickling (obstruction of blood flow in the microvasculature caused by the distorted red blood cells) leads to increased intraocular pressures and optic nerve damage.
- **Superior orbital fissure syndrome.** Compression of the contents of the superior orbital fissure accounts for the manifestations of this syndrome. Clinical findings include loss of forehead sensation, loss of corneal reflex, ophthalmoplegia, upper lid ptosis, edema (secondary to venous obstruction), and proptosis. This syndrome must be differentiated from orbital apex syndrome, which also involves the optic nerve, causing loss of vision.
- **Lens dislocation.** Subluxation of the lens may occur due to disruption of the lens zonule fibers. The lens margin is often visible, but visual acuity may be compromised, and

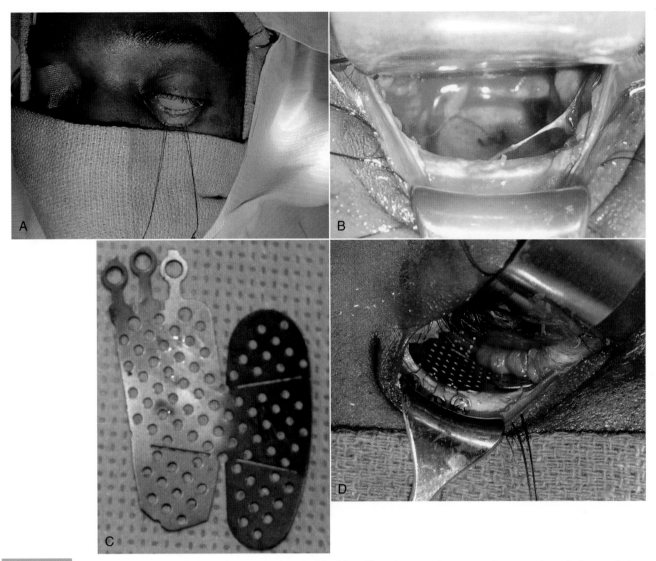

Figure 8-33   **A,** Intraoperative photograph of a transconjunctival incision. Note the retraction suture placement through the tarsal plate to minimize lower lid injury and the scleral shield to prevent inadvertent corneal abrasion. **B,** Orbital floor defect seen through the transconjunctival incision. **C,** Titanium mesh plate for reconstruction. **D,** Mesh implant in place, restoring the orbital floor contour.

monocular diplopia can be present. Zonular disruption can cause dislocation of the lens either posteriorly or anteriorly. Patients who are symptomatic with posterior dislocation can be treated with an aphetic contact lens or with intraocular lens implantation. An anteriorly dislocated lens is an ophthalmic emergency because of possible blockage of the aqueous flow, resulting in acute glaucoma. Attempts at repositioning the lens can be made by a skilled ophthalmologist; this involves maximally dilating the pupils, placing the patient in a supine position, and indenting the cornea with a gonioprism.

- **Retrobulbar hemorrhage.** Retrobulbar hemorrhage is an ocular emergency, and prompt diagnosis and treatment are essential to prevent loss of vision. This emergent clinical entity can occur after a traumatic injury to the orbit or postoperatively after orbital or eyelid surgery. The orbit is a relatively closed compartment, and orbital pressure can

rise rapidly with hemorrhage. If left untreated, orbital compartment syndrome may develop, causing ischemia of the optic nerve. Patients with increased orbital pressure present with pain, decreased vision, diplopia, ophthalmoplegia (restricted extraocular movements), proptosis, ecchymosis around the eye, chemosis, resistance to retropulsion, and an afferent pupillary defect. An emergent lateral canthotomy with inferior cantholysis is indicated, allowing the orbital contents to expand anteriorly.

- **Traumatic optic neuropathy.** Traumatic optic neuropathy presents as a sudden loss of vision secondary to either blunt or penetrating trauma to the orbit that cannot be explained by other ocular pathological changes. The damage to the nerve is either direct (hemorrhage or compression), shearing (acceleration of the nerve at the optic canal where it is tethered to the dural sheath), or through transmission of a shock wave through the orbit along the course of the optic

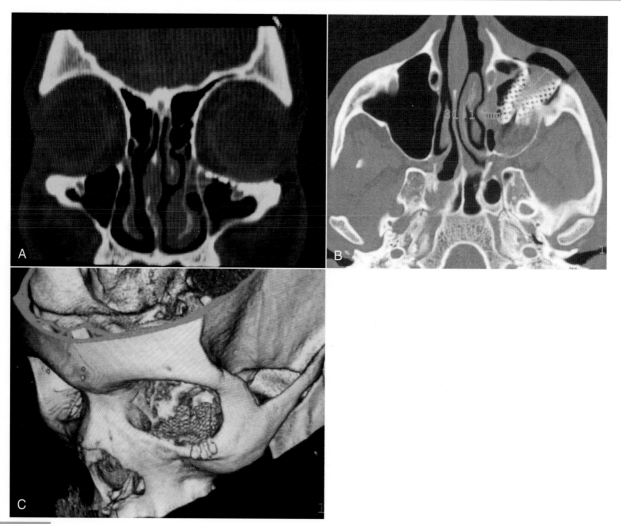

Figure 8-34 **A,** Postoperative CT scan (coronal view) demonstrating proper alignment and contour. **B,** Postoperative CT scan showing the length of the plate from the infraorbital rim. **C,** Postoperative CT scan (three-dimensional reconstruction) showing the contour of the titanium mesh.

nerve. Many treatment modalities have been advocated, including high-dose intravenous steroids, optic canal decompression, and optic nerve sheath fenestration. The largest study looking at traumatic optic neuropathy, the International Optic Nerve Trauma Study, was conducted by Levin and colleagues in 1999. They concluded that the use of corticosteroids in patients with traumatic optic neuropathy did not change the outcome (loss of visual acuity), compared with the control group that did not receive any steroid therapy.

• **Ruptured globe.** Globe rupture occurs when the integrity of the outer membranes is disrupted by blunt or penetrating trauma. A peaked, teardrop-shaped, or otherwise irregular pupil may indicate a ruptured globe. A full-thickness laceration to the cornea or sclera constitutes a globe perforation, requiring repair in the operating room. Prolapse of the iris through a full-thickness corneal laceration may be seen as a dark discoloration at the site of injury. Scleral buckling

is indicative of rupture with extrusion of ocular contents. Intraocular pressure will likely be low, but direct measurement is contraindicated to avoid pressure on the globe. Globe rupture is a major ophthalmologic emergency that requires surgical intervention.

• **Blindness.** This is a known but uncommon complication of facial trauma, with a reported incidence of only 2% to 5%. In a review of the University of Maryland shock trauma experience of facial trauma over 11 years, the researchers discovered that 2,987 of the 29,474 admitted patients (10.1%) sustained facial fractures and that 1,338 of these fractures (44.8%) involved one or both of the orbits. Operative repair of the facial fractures was performed in 1,240 of these patients. Three patients (0.24%) experienced postoperative complications that resulted in blindness. In 13 of 27 other patients (48%), blindness was attributed to intraorbital hemorrhage. Another 5 patients experienced visual loss with unspecified mechanisms related to increased intraorbital pressure. Within the restricted confines of the optic canal, even small changes in pressure may cause ischemic optic neuropathy.

Late

Late complications of orbital floor fractures and repair can be the result of injuries sustained at the time of the traumatic event or complications associated with the repair itself.

- **Lacrimal system injury.** Epiphora (excessive tearing due to impaired drainage) can occur. Eyelid lacerations, particularly those extending medially, should be thoroughly evaluated for lacrimal drainage system injury, canthal tendon disruption, or injury to the tarsal plate and levator aponeurosis. Fractures through the lacrimal apparatus (NOE) can also cause epiphora.
- **Unresolved diplopia.** Diplopia that has a neuromuscular origin (e.g., cranial nerve III palsy) should be observed for spontaneous recovery over 6 months. Elective strabismus surgery can be considered if the diplopia is unresolved. Acute entrapment of the extraocular muscles, causing diplopia, needs to be addressed soon after the injury.
- **Enophthalmos.** Enophthalmos results from an increase in orbital volume and persists if the orbital volume is not restored adequately. This occurs in large unrepaired fractures, particularly when multiple walls are involved. Defects at the junction of the floor and medial wall of the orbit are most prone to causing enophthalmos. Studies have shown that an increase in orbital volume of anywhere from 0.5 to 1 cc creates approximately 1 mm of enophthalmos.
- **Ectropion.** Ectropion is the outward eversion of the lid margin away from the globe. This can result in corneal irritation and exposure and abnormalities of lacrimal outflow. Prevention of ectropion begins with minimizing vertical tension when closing lid lacerations and/or periorbital skin incisions. Use of the transconjunctival incision, with resuspension of the suborbicularis oculi fat, and meticulous repair of lid lacerations reduce the incidence of this complication. Cicatricial ectropion results from scarring of the anterior lamella; involutional ectropion results from horizontal lid laxity, usually due to age-related weakness of the canthal ligaments and pretarsal orbicularis.
- **Entropion.** Entropion is malposition of the lid, resulting in inversion of the lid margin. Cicatricial entropion occurs as a result of scarring of the palpebral conjunctiva, with consequent inward rotation of the eyelid margin.
- **Unesthetic scar.** Cutaneous placement of periorbital incisions (e.g., an infraorbital incision) carries the risk of an unesthetic scar.

DISCUSSION

The management of orbital floor fractures remains controversial. The indications for and timing of surgical intervention have proved difficult to study and evaluate. Isolated orbital wall fractures account for 4% to 16% of all facial fractures. If fractures that extend outside the orbit (ZMC, NOE) are included, the proportion is 30% to 50% of all facial fractures.

The optimal management of orbital fractures necessitates an intimate knowledge of the complex anatomy of the region. The orbit is a quadrilateral pyramid, with an average volume of 30 cm^3 and a height and width at the rim averaging 40 mm and 35 mm, respectively. The average length of the medial wall is 40 to 45 mm (rim to optic canal). Seven bones make up the orbits: the sphenoid, maxillary, lacrimal, ethmoid, frontal, zygomatic, and palatine bones. The orbital process of the frontal bone and the lesser wing of the sphenoid make up its roof. The floor is made up of the orbital plates of the maxilla, zygoma, and palatine bone. The zygoma and the greater and lesser wings of the sphenoid form the lateral wall. The medial wall is formed by the frontal process of the maxilla and the lacrimal, sphenoid, and ethmoid (lamina papyracea) bones.

The distances to known orbital landmarks are crucial for preventing postoperative complications and aiding intraoperative dissection. These measurements are averages and may be altered by posttraumatic changes in the orbital rim. The average distance from the orbital rim to the orbital apex is 40 to 45 mm. The subperiosteal dissection along the orbital walls can safely be extended up to 25 mm posteriorly along the inferior and lateral rims.

Three theories have been advocated with regard to the physiologic mechanism of orbital floor fractures.

- The hydraulic theory, advocated by Smith and Regan in 1957, proposed that a generalized increased orbital content pressure resulted in direct compression of the orbital floor, thereby fracturing the thin orbital bone.
- The globe-to-wall contact theory, proposed by Raymond Pfeiffer in 1943, stated that a force is delivered to the globe, pushing it backward into the orbit, causing it to strike and fracture the bony walls. This theory is based on common sense and radiologic reasoning, but it is not evidence based. Erling and colleagues found that the size of the orbital wall defect exactly fit the size of the globe in many cases of blowout fractures analyzed with CT scans. They stated that it is the "displacement of the globe" that directly causes many orbital wall fractures.
- In 1974 Fujino proposed that a direct compression force or buckling force, transmitted via the orbital rim, was the causative factor in orbital floor fractures. This theory of a bone conduction mechanism of injury was first proposed by Le Fort and Lagrange at the turn of the twentieth century. In a series of dried human cadaver experiments during the mid-1970s, Fujino convincingly demonstrated the occurrence of orbital floor fractures with direct blows to the orbital rim without fracture of the orbital rim itself. Recent studies, such as that by Waterhouse and associates, have revealed that orbital fractures may occur by way of

the "buckling" or "hydraulic" mechanism, with a combination of the two mechanisms being the most likely etiology, depending on the direction of the striking force.

A recent study by Fan and colleagues demonstrated a high correlation between the increment of orbital volume and the degree of enophthalmos. An increase of 1 cm^3 of the orbital volume elicited 0.89 mm of enophthalmos. The authors concluded that the measurement of orbital volume in patients with orbital blowout fractures could be used to predict the degree of late enophthalmos and that this may be accomplished through the use of computer-assisted volumetric measurements.

The approaches to the orbit include the transconjunctival (often with a lateral canthotomy and inferior cantholysis), subciliary, lower lid crease, and transcaruncular approaches. The transconjunctival approach has been shown to result in fewer cases of postoperative ectropion and may be used in conjunction with the transcaruncular approach to gain further access to the medial orbit. Attention to the medial orbital wall is paramount in completely treating orbital fractures and preventing enophthalmos.

The literature provides support for notable clinical differences in orbital floor fracture patterns between pediatric patients and adults. Jordan and associates coined the term "white-eyed blowout fracture" for patients 16 years or younger with minimal soft tissue injury, severe diplopia, extraocular muscle limitation, and extremely small extrusion of tissue around the orbit seen on CT imaging. Diplopia, extraocular muscle limitation, and trapdoor fractures are more frequent in children than in adult patients and can be accompanied by nausea and vomiting.

The choices for reconstruction materials for repair of orbital bony contour are numerous and remain controversial. Many autogenous (split calvarial bone, iliac crest, septal cartilage or rib), alloplastic (titanium mesh, porous polyethylene [MEDPOR], PGA/PLLA, Gelfilm), and allogeneic (lyophilized cartilage or dura, banked bone) materials have been used and advocated. The use of autogenous materials is thought to decrease the risk of infection and/or extrusion; alloplastic materials offer superior ease in intraoperative handling and contouring.

When the entire orbit has been disrupted and there are no posterior landmarks to guide the reconstruction, accurate positioning of bone grafts or titanium mesh becomes exceedingly difficult. Especially in late repairs, there is a significant challenge to establishing proper orbital contour, volume, and medial bulge projection. The risk of encroachment on the orbital apex and optic nerve also exists. Presurgical virtual planning, patient-specific implants, and the use of intraoperative navigation (Box 8-4) can aid reconstruction in such cases, improving the predictability of a complex orbital reconstruction.

A multidisciplinary approach to complex orbital trauma is highly recommended, and consultation with ophthalmology and/or oculoplastic services should be considered. Many

---

Box 8-4 **Four Phases of Navigation-Assisted Computer-Aided Reconstruction**

1. **Data acquisition phase.** Visualization, orientation, and diagnosis of the orbital deformity. Clinical and radiographic diagnoses are made, and a high-quality CT scan of the orbits with 1-mm slices is obtained (Figure 8-35, *A*).
2. **Manipulation (simulation) phase.** Mirroring, segmentation, and virtual orbital implant insertion (Figure 8-35, *B*). CT data are imported into a proprietary software program for virtual planning before surgery.

3. **Surgical phase.** Surgery involves CAD/CAM-derived stereolithographic models and/or custom orbital implant insertion using intraoperative navigation (Figure 8-35, *C* and *D*).
4. **Assessment phase.** Evaluation of the accuracy of the treatment plan transfer using intraoperative or postoperative CT imaging (Figure 8-35, *E* and *F*).

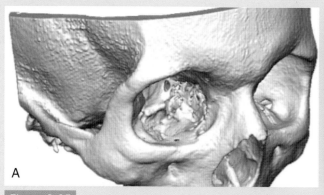
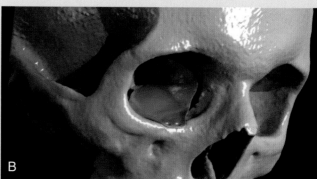

Figure 8-35 **A,** Data acquisition phase. Preoperative CT scan of the medial floor. **B,** Manipulation (simulation) phase. CT scan of specific implant inset.

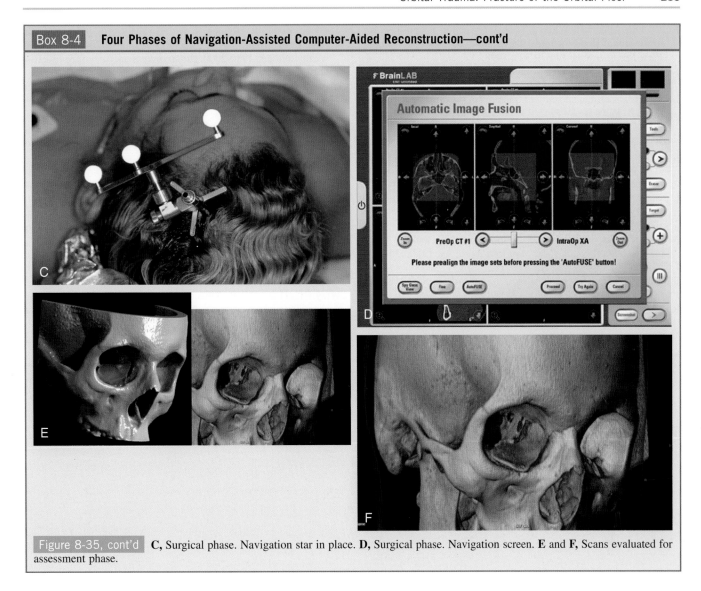

Box 8-4   **Four Phases of Navigation-Assisted Computer-Aided Reconstruction—cont'd**

Figure 8-35, cont'd   **C,** Surgical phase. Navigation star in place. **D,** Surgical phase. Navigation screen. **E** and **F,** Scans evaluated for assessment phase.

posterior segment injuries may be subtle and need to be identified before exploration and reconstruction of the bony orbital architecture.

Bibliography

Appling WD, Patrinely JR, Salzer TA: Transconjunctival approach vs subciliary skin-muscle flap approach for orbital fracture repair, *Arch Otolaryngol Head Neck Surg* 119:1000-1007, 1993.

Burnstine MA: Clinical recommendations for repair of orbital facial fractures, *Curr Opin Ophthalmol* 14:236-240, 2003.

Dulley B, Fells P: Long-term follow-up of orbital blowout fracture with or without surgery, *Mod Probl Ophthalmol*, 14:467-470, 1975.

Erling BF, Iliff N, Robertson B, et al: Footprints of the globe: a practical look at the mechanism of orbital blowout fractures, with a revisit to the work of Raymond Pfeiffer, *Plast Reconstr Surg* 103:1313-1316, 1999.

Fan X, Li J, Zhu J, et al: Computer-assisted orbital volume measurement in the surgical correction of late enophthalmos caused by blowout fractures, *Ophthal Plast Reconstr Surg* 9:207-211, 2003.

Feliciano DV, Mattox KL, Morre EE: *Trauma*, ed 6, New York, 2007, McGraw-Hill.

Friedrich RE, Heiland M, Bartel-Friedrich S: Potentials of ultrasound in the diagnosis of midfacial fractures, *Clin Oral Invest* 7:226-229, 2003.

Fujino T: Experimental "blow-out" fracture of the orbit, *Plast Reconstr Surg* 54:81-82, 1974.

Girotto JA, Gamble W, Robertson B, et al: Blindness after reduction of facial fractures. *Plast Reconstr Surg* 102(6):1821-1834, 1998.

Goldenberg-Cohen N, Miller NR, Repka MX: Traumatic optic neuropathy in children and adolescents, *J AAPOS* 8:20-27, 2004.

Hammer B: *Orbital fractures: diagnosis, operative treatment, secondary corrections*, Seattle, 1995, Hogrefe & Huber.

He D, Li Z, Shi W, et al: Orbitozygomatic fractures with enophthalmos: analysis of 64 cases treated late, *J Oral Maxillofac Surg* 70(3):562-576, 2012.

Holt JE, Holt GR, Blodgett JM: Ocular injuries sustained during blunt facial trauma, *Ophthalmology* 90:14-18, 1983.

Holtmann B, Wray RC, Little AG: A randomized comparison of four incisions for orbital fractures, *Plast Reconstr Surg* 67:731-737, 1981.

Jordan DR, Allen LH, White J, et al: Intervention within days for some orbital floor fractures: the white-eyed blowout, *Ophthal Plast Reconstr Surg* 14:379-390, 1998.

Lang GK: *Ophthalmology: a pocket textbook atlas*, ed 2, New York, 2000, Thieme.

Le Fort R: Experimental study of fractures of the upper jaw. Parts I, II and II. *Rev Chir De Paris* 23:208-227, 360-379, 479-507, 1901 [translated by Tessier P: *Plast Reconstr Surg* 50:600-607, 497-506, 1972].

Levin LA, Beck RW, Joseph MP, et al: The treatment of traumatic optic neuropathy: the International Optic Nerve Trauma Study, *Ophthalmology* 106:1268-1277, 1999.

Lorenz P, Longaker M, Kawamoto H: Primary and secondary orbit surgery: the transconjunctival approach, *Plast Reconstr Surg* 103:1124-1128, 1999.

Markiewicz MR, Bell RB: The use of 3D imaging tools in facial plastic surgery, *Facial Plast Surg Clin North Am* 19(4):655-682, 2011.

Pfeiffer RL: Traumatic enophthalmos, *Arch Ophthalmol* 30:718-726, 1943.

Rhee JS, Kilde J, Yoganadan N, et al: Orbital blowout fractures: experimental evidence for the pure hydraulic theory, *Arch Facial Plast Surg* 4:98-101, 2002.

Shere JL, Boole JR, Holtel MR, et al: An analysis of 3,599 midfacial and 1,141 orbital blowout fractures among 4,426 United States Army soldiers, 1980-2000, *Otolaryngol Head Neck Surg* 130:164-170, 2004.

Shorr N, Baylis HI, Goldberg RA, et al: Transcaruncular approach to the medial orbit and orbital apex, *Ophthalmology* 107:1459-1463, 2000.

Smith B, Regan WF Jr: Blow-out fracture of the orbit: mechanism and correction of internal orbital fracture, *Am J Ophthalmol* 44(6):733-739, 1957.

Soparkar CN, Patrinely JR: The eye examination in facial trauma for the plastic surgeon, *Plast Reconstr Surg* 120(7 Suppl 2):49s-56s, 2007.

Waterhouse N, Lyne J, Urdang M, et al: An investigation into the mechanism of orbital blowout fractures, *Br J Plast Surg* 52(8):607-612, 1999.

Westfall CT, Shore JW, Nunery WR, et al: Operative complications of the transconjunctival inferior fornix approach, *Ophthalmology* 98(10):1525-1528, 1991.

Wray RC, Holtmann B, Ribaudo JM, et al: A comparison of conjunctival and subciliary incisions for orbital fractures, *Br J Plast Surg* 30:142-145, 1977.

Panfacial Fracture

Chris Jo, Martin B. Steed, and Shahrokh C. Bagheri

CC

A 49-year-old man is transported to the emergency department by EMS personnel status post pedestrian-versus-automobile accident. You are called by the trauma team for the evaluation and management of his facial injuries.

HPI

The patient arrives at the emergency department intubated. The driver of the automobile and another eyewitness report that the patient was walking alongside a busy intersection and suddenly jumped into the path of a vehicle traveling at approximately 35 mph. The front end of the car struck his thighs, and then his face hit the hood and windshield, causing significant damage to the automobile. He was launched several feet into the air and landed in a prone position on the pavement. He had a Glasgow Coma Scale (GCS) score of 3 at the scene and was orally intubated by EMS personnel for airway protection (airway intubation is warranted for a GCS score of 8 or lower, which is indicative of a severe head injury). When you arrive in the emergency department, the patient is being actively resuscitated by the trauma team according to the advanced trauma life support (ATLS) protocol, and the orthopedic team is evaluating multiple extremity fractures.

PMHX/PDHX/MEDICATIONS/ALLERGIES/SH/FH

The patient's histories are unknown (information may be obtained from family members, when present).

EXAMINATION

The initial evaluation of a trauma patient should be dictated by the ATLS protocol.

Primary Survey

Airway and cervical spine control. The patient has been orally intubated, and a transport cervical collar is in place. (In a review of 563 patients with maxillofacial injuries, Haug and associates found that concomitant cervical spine fractures occurred in 2% of patients. Of those with cervical spine fractures, 91% had mandibular fractures. Bagheri and colleagues found a 1.5% incidence of cervical spine fractures in a series of 67 patients with isolated midfacial fractures.)

Breathing and oxygenation. Oral endotracheal tube is in good position (confirmed by portable chest radiograph) on mechanical ventilation. The right hemithorax shows no chest rise or breath sounds and is hypertympanic to percussion (indicative of a pneumothorax, also confirmed by portable chest radiograph). A chest tube is placed to re-expand the right lung. Oxygen saturation is 90% on 100% inspired oxygen (suggestive of a ventilation-perfusion mismatch).

Circulation and hemorrhage control. Blood pressure is 90/70 mm Hg, heart rate 125 bpm (moderate hypotension and tachycardia consistent with class III shock). (Class III hypovolemic shock is indicative of a 30% to 40% loss of blood volume, which is characterized by a heart rate over 120 bpm; decreases in systolic blood pressure, mean arterial blood pressure, pulse pressure, and urine output [5 to 15 ml/hour]; and altered mental status). A small amount of bleeding is observed from the nasopharynx and is easily controlled with bilateral nasal packs. The magnitude of bleeding does not clinically correlate with the estimated blood loss and volume depletion (raising suspicion for other sources of bleeding). The abdomen is soft and nondistended, and the focused abdominal sonography for trauma (FAST) is negative (FAST examination is used in the hypotensive blunt trauma patient and evaluates the perihepatic, pericardiac, perisplenic, and pelvic windows for the presence of free intraperitoneal fluid or cardiac tamponade); this rules out intraabdominal hemorrhage (hypovolemic) and cardiac tamponade (obstructive) as the source of shock. Bilateral femoral deformities (each femur fracture can be a source of 1.5 to 2 L of blood loss) and other open extremity fractures can be a source of significant blood loss and hypovolemic shock. Fractures should be reduced and stabilized to reduce the amount of hemorrhage in the initial resuscitation phases. Fluid resuscitation should begin with crystalloid intravenous fluid boluses to maintain organ perfusion. Transfusion of packed red blood cells should be considered in class III hemorrhagic shock.

Disability and dysfunction. On the AVPU scale (awake; responds to voice; responds to pain; unresponsive), the patient is unresponsive (off sedation) and has a GCS score of E1 + M1 + V1T = 3T. Pupils are equal, 7 mm with a sluggish reaction to light (large pupils with a sluggish reaction to light reflex may indicate a closed head injury and elevated intracranial pressures). Sedation should be discontinued for an accurate assessment of mental status as needed. Initial head CT scan reveals moderate contusions in the frontal and occipital lobes (coup, countercoup injury, indicative of a rapid acceleration-deceleration mechanism). A Camino bolt is placed to monitor the intracranial pressure, which reveals a mildly elevated opening pressure at 22 mm Hg (normal intracranial pressure is 15 mm Hg or below).

Exposure and environmental control. The patient's clothing has been removed, and a warm blanket and other warming devices are used to prevent hypothermia.

Secondary Survey

The AMPLE history (allergy, medications, past medical history, last meal, events leading to presentation) is taken from available sources.

General. The patient is a well-developed male who is intubated and sedated and has a cervical collar in place.

Neurologic. GCS score is 3T (off sedation). Pupils are 7 mm, equal, and sluggish (this parameter was covered during the primary survey but should be repetitively monitored for changes). The intracranial pressure–monitoring device (e.g., intraparenchymal Camino bolt or external ventriculostomy drain) gives a precise, moment-by-moment assessment of intracranial pressures. A sustained intracranial pressure of over 25 mm Hg warrants intervention to reduce the pressure (intravenous mannitol, hyperosmolar therapy with 3% NaCl, elevation of head of bed, hyperventilation to reduce the $Paco_2$ to the low range of normal). Therapy is aimed at not only reducing intracranial pressure (below 20 mm Hg) but also at maintaining cerebral perfusion pressures (Cerebral perfusion pressure = Mean arterial pressure − Intracranial pressure), which should be maintained greater than 70 mm Hg (35% reduction in mortality) to prevent secondary brain injury. Invasive hemodynamic monitoring is indicated when hyperosmolar therapy is initiated to maintain an acceptable blood pressure and cerebral perfusion pressure (mortality increases 20% for each 10 mm Hg loss of cerebral perfusion pressure).

Maxillofacial. There is significant upper and lower facial edema. A 2-cm full-thickness laceration extends over the bridge of the nose (indicating blunt trauma to the upper midface), and there is a 5-cm full-thickness stellate laceration over the lower lip and chin.

Eyes. There is significant periorbital edema. Visual acuity cannot be assessed. The patient has bilateral periorbital ecchymosis (raccoon eyes, indicative of anterior basilar skull fracture) and bilateral subconjunctival hemorrhage and chemosis. Intercanthal distance is 36 mm without blunting of the medial canthus. (An increased intercanthal distance is indicative of a naso-orbital-ethmoid [NOE] fracture or avulsion of the medial canthal tendon. Normal intercanthal distance is 30 to 34 mm and varies among races and genders). The bowstring test (a clinical test for evaluation of the medial canthal attachment) is negative. Bilateral step deformities are present at the lateral and inferior orbital rims (step deformity and bony crepitus indicate the presence of fractures).

Nose. The nasal bridge demonstrates crepitus with gross mobility. The endonasal examination reveals an edematous nasal mucosa with mild bleeding. The anterior nasal septum is midline with no septal hematoma (septal hematoma requires immediate incision and drainage to prevent necrosis of the septal cartilage and potential perforation and saddle-nose deformity). No cerebrospinal fluid rhinorrhea or otorrhea is noted. The maxilla is grossly mobile with bony crepitus at the anterior maxillary walls and the zygomaticomaxillary (ZM) buttresses. No step deformity or crepitus is appreciable at the zygomatic arches bilaterally (this does not exclude the possibility of fractures).

Intraoral. There is bilateral maxillary vestibular ecchymosis (indicative of fractures of the ZM buttresses). There are multiple missing maxillary teeth and a step deformity with an associated gingival laceration between the left mandibular lateral and central incisors (teeth #23 and #24), with gross mobility of the mandibular segments. The patient has an anterior open bite with no distinct mandibular posterior stop and bilateral posterior prematurities (indicative of bilateral condylar fractures and/or Le Fort level fracture), with the oral endotracheal tube exiting between the edentulous spaces. Ecchymosis at the posterior soft palate bilaterally (Guerin's sign, indicative of pterygoid plate disjunction/fracture).

IMAGING

A plain film radiograph series in the acute setting includes cross-table cervical spine, portable anteroposterior chest radiography and an anteroposterior pelvis radiograph. Other studies are added as needed, including cervical spine series (in suspected cervical spine injury), thoracic and lumbar spine series, and extremity radiographs (depending on the mechanism of injury).

Axial cut bony window CT scans (with coronal reconstructions) are the gold standard radiographic examination for midfacial fractures. Direct coronal views are useful but should be avoided in patients with suspected cervical spine injury (the patient's head needs to be hyperextended for a direct coronal CT scan). Three-dimensional reconstructions are helpful adjuncts, because they provide the most graphic representation of the fractures, degree of displacement, and orientation of fragments. A panoramic radiograph is always helpful; however, in the unstable patient with cervical-thoracic-lumbar (CTL) spine precautions, this is not likely to be possible.

In the current patient, head and facial helical CT scans without contrast were obtained after the primary and secondary surveys were completed. The head CT scan revealed moderate frontal lobe and occipital lobe contusions without evidence of intracerebral hemorrhage or midline shift (these scans should be repeated in 12 to 24 hours to monitor for any changes). The fine cut axial face CT scan revealed bilateral nasal bone fractures, fractures of the lateral orbital rims and walls, and bilateral zygomatic arch fractures (Figure 8-36, *A* and *B*). Fractures at the pterygoid plates and along the anterior and posterior maxillary sinus and lateral nasal walls also were seen (Figure 8-36, *C*). Coronal reconstruction views anteriorly demonstrated fractures at the nasofrontal junction, a Le Fort I fracture, and a midpalatal split (Figure 8-36, *D*). Coronal views of the midface demonstrated severe

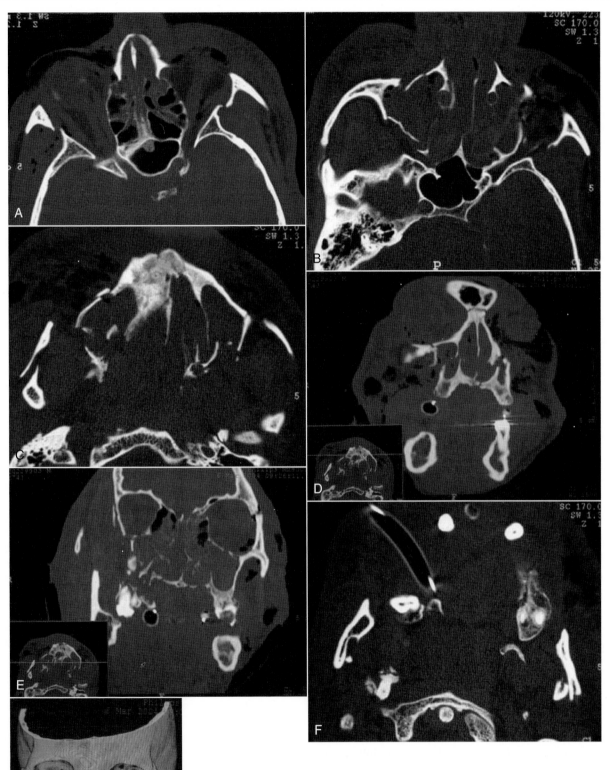

Figure 8-36   **A,** Axial cut bony window CT scan showing displaced bilateral lateral orbital wall fractures. **B,** Axial cut bony window CT scan showing the inferior component of the bilateral NOE type I fracture (inferior orbital rim fractures) and bilateral ZMC fractures. **C,** Axial cut bony window CT scan showing a right subcondylar fracture, a palatal split of the maxilla, pterygoid plate fractures/disjunction, and maxillary sinus wall comminution. **D,** Coronal reconstruction CT scan showing Le Fort I fracture with a palatal split and bilateral NOE type I fracture. **E,** Coronal reconstruction CT scan showing bilateral lateral orbital rim fractures, a comminuted Le Fort I fracture, nasal septal comminution, and nondisplaced orbital floor fractures. **F,** Axial cut bony window CT scan showing a left subcondylar fracture. **G,** Three-dimensional CT reconstruction demonstrating the spatial relationship of the fractures. The symphysis and anterior frontal sinus fractures are seen clearly in this view.

comminution of the midface, including at the NOE, orbital floors, and zygomaticofrontal (ZF) junction (Figure 8-36, *E*). Scans of the mandible demonstrated bilateral condylar neck fractures (Figure 8-36, *F;* also see *C*) and a midline mandibular symphysis fracture. Figure 8-36, *G,* shows the three-dimensional reconstructed view, which also demonstrated fracture of the anterior table of the frontal sinus, confirmed on the axial views.

The CT scan of the cervical spine was negative. The anteroposterior chest radiograph showed evolving bilateral pulmonary contusions and a chest tube in good position without any residual pneumothorax.

LABS

Standard laboratory tests for the evaluation of multisystem trauma patients include a CBC, complete metabolic panel, arterial blood gas values, urine analysis, and coagulation studies (prothrombin time [PT], partial thromboplastin time [PTT], and international normalized ratio [INR]). A urine drug screen and blood alcohol level are indicated in patients with decreased mental status.

The current patient demonstrated decreased hemoglobin (9.2 g/dl) and hematocrit (26.6%) (suggestive of blood loss; however, acutely, hemoglobin/hematocrit may not be an accurate measure due to a delay in volume redistribution). Arterial blood gas analysis showed a moderate base deficit of −5.5 mEq (base deficit is one of the parameters monitored for adequacy of resuscitation in hypovolemic shock and is a better indicator of acute blood loss than hemoglobin/hematocrit). The complete metabolic panel demonstrated a mild elevation in blood urea nitrogen (30 mg/dl) and creatinine (1.9 mg/dl) (indicative of prerenal azotemia secondary to blood loss) and a negative blood alcohol level and urine drug screen (alcohol and drug intoxication must be considered and ruled out as the source for altered mental status). The remainder of the patient's laboratory test results were within normal limits.

ASSESSMENT

Panfacial fracture involving the frontal bone, midface, and mandible—FISS of 17; complicated by class III hemorrhagic shock, closed head injury, multiple extremity fractures, and right pneumothorax with bilateral pulmonary contusions.

The maxillofacial injures are classified as follows (the FISS designation is given in parentheses):

Upper face	Fracture of the anterior wall of the frontal sinus and frontal bar (5)
Midface	Bilateral zygomaticomaxillary complex (ZMC) fractures (2 × 1)
	• Bilateral NOE fractures (type I) (3)
	• Le Fort I fracture (2), with a midpalatal split (1)
Mandible	Bilateral subcondylar (2 × 1) and symphysis (2) fractures

TREATMENT

Treatment begins with initiation of the ATLS protocol and stabilization of the patient. Maxillofacial injuries compromising the airway should be promptly evaluated. Tracheotomy should be readily considered for panfacial fractures. Submental intubation is also a viable alternative. A cricothyrotomy is usually reserved for an acute airway emergency. The control of hemorrhage from the maxillofacial region is part of the ATLS protocol. Nasal packing and pressure dressings should be applied as needed. Severe or life-threatening posterior nasal bleeding can be managed emergently with posterior balloon nasal packing or with Foley catheters placed bilaterally through the nares into the oropharynx and then inflated and pulled tight to the soft palate (Figure 8-37). If local packing measures are unsuccessful, interventional management is needed.

Treatment of panfacial fractures can be challenging and should begin, after completion of the ATLS protocol, with a thorough maxillofacial and radiographic examination. Often the patient requires significant resuscitation prior to facial surgery. Once the maxillofacial diagnosis has been made, a treatment plan must be developed to expose the necessary fractures for alignment and fixation. Selective exposure of necessary fractures is used for stabilization with rigid fixation (before the advent of rigid fixation, it was common for all fracture sites to be exposed). The surgeon must develop a preoperative plan to expose, examine, align, fixate, and reconstruct the facial skeleton in an orderly fashion. This may include immediate bony reconstruction with bone grafting techniques. If necessary, the entire facial skeleton can be visualized by combining multiple approaches.

Once the fracture sites have been exposed, the principle of using the buttresses of the facial skeleton to help align the fractures from "stable to unstable" segments is followed. Different concepts and strategies regarding the order of stabilization have been advocated in the past; these include progression from top to bottom, bottom to top, inside to out, and outside to in. With the advent of miniplates and rigid internal fixation, a broader range of reconstructive possibilities allows new definitions of optimal sequencing in facial reconstruction. Goals for linking fragmented bones came into existence. Starting with stable bone, fractured and displaced segments are fixated to adjacent stable, nondisplaced bone in a piecemeal fashion.

In the current patient, the following treatment sequence was used.
1. **Management of the airway.** Due to the severity of this patient's head injury and anticipation of prolonged mechanical ventilation, an open tracheotomy was initially performed.
2. **Exposure of fractures.** Maxillary and mandibular arch bars were applied but not tightened (leaving the arch bars slightly loose on the least dentate segment of the fracture allows for adjustment at a later time, when the proper occlusion and horizontal facial width have been established). Subsequently, all fractures necessary for alignment and fixation were exposed in a systematic fashion.

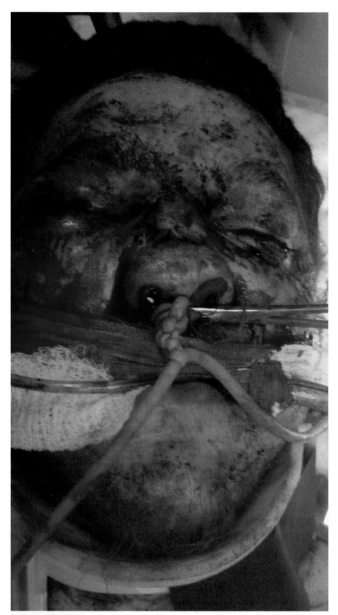

Figure 8-37 Clinical photograph demonstrating emergent bilateral placement of Foley catheters through the nose. The catheters were insufflated once they had been passed over the soft palate, then pulled back and tied together.

a. Transoral exposure of the maxillary and mandibular fractures was accomplished with a maxillary circumvestibular incision (from first molar to first molar) and a genioplasty-type incision (the midpalatal fracture can also be accessed via a parasagittal palatal incision if it needs to be rigidly fixated). The midface was degloved to expose the body of the zygomas, bilateral ZM buttress, the pyriform rim (nasomaxillary buttress), the inferior portion of the NOE fracture, and the inferior orbital rims (inferior orbital rims can be plated from this access) while skeletonizing and protecting the infraorbital neurovascular bundles. The mandibular symphysis fracture was exposed by degloving the anterior

mandible to the inferior border anterior to the mental foramina. Both mental nerves (and associated three branches) were identified and protected (some surgeons prefer an extraoral approach via a submental incision, which decreases mental nerve injury and gives better visualization of the lingual cortex reduction to prevent splaying). If a fracture exists in the posterior mandible (body, angle, or ramus), submandibular (Risdon), retromandibular (Hinds), or intraoral incisions can be used.

b. A coronal incision (also referred to as the *bicoronal incision* in the literature) was made to access the frontal bone and sinuses, superior and lateral orbital rims (supraorbital bar), the NOE complex, and the zygomatic arches. This incision also provides access for a cranial bone graft harvest, if needed (the parietal area offers the thickest bicortical width, reducing the risk of entry into the cranium). The incision was extended into bilateral preauricular incisions (some surgeons prefer an endoaural approach) for access to the mandibular condyle and better access to the zygomatic arch and body.

c. The inferior orbital rims and inferior component of the NOE fractures were exposed via a transconjunctival approach. Various periorbital incisions can be used for access to the inferior orbital rims, orbital floor and medial orbital walls, inferior components of the NOE, and lateral orbital rims. The lower eyelid incisions can be transcutaneous or transconjunctival. The transcutaneous approaches include the subciliary, subtarsal, and inferior orbital rim (unfavorable scarring) incisions. The subciliary incision can be a skin-only flap, skin-muscle flap, or stepped flap. The stepped flap is recommended when using this approach, because it has a lower incidence of postoperative lower eyelid malposition (ectropion, entropion, and scleral show). The transconjunctival incision can be done with or without a lateral canthotomy and inferior cantholysis, depending on the amount of access needed. This incision can be extended medially, via a transcaruncular incision, for greater exposure of the medial orbital wall. The transconjunctival incision is preferred by most surgeons, because it has the lowest incidence of transient and permanent postoperative lower eyelid malposition. If a coronal incision is not used, the lateral orbital rim can be exposed via an upper blepharoplasty incision or a lateral brow incision. Paranasal Lynch incisions can be used to access NOE fractures; however, this technique is associated with poor cosmesis.

3. **Alignment and fixation of fractures.** After all necessary fractures had been exposed, attention was turned to the dentoalveolar segments and occlusion. Fracture of the dentate segment (parasymphysis/symphysis) of the mandible, along with a maxillary palatal split, can make it difficult to restore proper lower facial width and occlusion. In the current patient, the surgeons chose to rely on proper reduction of the symphysis fracture (guided by direct visualization of the lingual cortex reduction and correct

position of the condylar heads in the glenoid fossa) to define the lower facial third width and occlusion. Proper horizontal width of the maxilla was obtained by placing the dentoalveolar segments into intermaxillary fixation with a properly reduced mandible. Typically, fractures through dentate segments are addressed first. However, when dealing with a symphysis (parasymphysis) and bilateral (or unilateral) subcondylar fractures, it may be wise to reduce and rigidly fixate the subcondylar fractures prior to addressing the symphysis fracture. This allows the surgeon to visualize and keep the condylar heads in the glenoid fossa as the symphysis fracture is reduced and fixated (assisted by gentle digital pressure at the mandibular angles). When subcondylar fractures are addressed after fixation of the symphysis, there may be undetected splaying of the lingual cortex at the symphysis, causing subsequent condylar displacement and fixation lateral to the fossa. With the occlusion set and the mandibular symphysis and condylar neck fractures reduced and fixated, the mandible's arc of rotation is used to guide the proper reduction of the midfacial fractures (the vertical dimension of the maxilla cannot be established by the mandible).

a. Following the "stable to unstable" principle, the most cephalad fractures were addressed next, using the anterior cranial vault as the stable point of fixation. The frontal bar and anterior table of the frontal sinus should be reconstructed first, starting at the lateral orbital rims (frontozygomatic suture area) and working medially toward the radix (the frontal sinus should also be addressed according to the type of injury and should be addressed after reconstructing the frontal bar [see the section Frontal Sinus Fracture in this chapter]). Then, the zygomatic arches are fixated bilaterally (accurate reduction of the zygomatic arches is important for restoring proper anteroposterior projection of the midface). The superior portion of the NOE fracture (near the nasofrontal junction) is then reduced and fixated to the stable frontal bar, and the inferior portion is addressed later via the periorbital and/or maxillary vestibular access (some surgeons prefer to use a long C-shaped plate to vertically span the entire NOE fracture and simultaneously fixate it to the inferior orbital rims and frontal bar). Otherwise, comminuted NOE fractures are typically addressed last, after reduction and stabilization of the surrounding bony structures.

b. The orbital rim fractures were reduced and fixated via the transconjunctival incisions. The orbital floor can be explored and reconstructed (cranial bone graft or alloplastic orbital floor plate/mesh) if indicated. In the current patient, the inferior component of the NOE fracture was coincident with the inferior orbital rim fracture, which was part of the ZMC fractures.

c. Once the upper and midface had been reduced and stabilized, the fractured maxilla at the Le Fort I level was reduced and fixated to the now-reduced and stable midface, using the buttresses (ZM and nasomaxillary) as a guide for reduction and with the patient in

maxillomandibular fixation (MMF). Miniplates were placed at the ZM buttresses and pyriform rims bilaterally. Further stabilization may be required for palatal split situations, such as this case. Palatal vault fixation, intermaxillary fixation, or a palatal strap splint can be used to prevent horizontal collapse of the maxilla.

4. **Primary bone grafting.** Primary bony reconstruction with immediate cranial bone grafts can be performed at this point. Areas that are highly comminuted or missing bony segments require one-piece bone grafts to replace the defects in bone volume and to support the overlying soft tissue. The need may arise to reconstruct the nasal dorsum, orbital rims, orbital floors, maxillary sinus walls, ZM buttress area (usually comminuted in high-impact injuries), and any other area of avulsed or severely comminuted bone.

5. **Soft tissue repair and resuspension.** Soft tissue injuries should be addressed last. Layered closure of incisions and lacerations and resuspension of stripped periosteum and suspensory ligaments of the face are important to provide a natural soft tissue drape.

COMPLICATIONS

Major complications secondary to the surgical correction of panfacial fractures can be difficult to assess and depend on the severity of the initial traumatic insult. Damage secondary to the initial trauma itself is usually the most devastating (e.g., death, loss of vision, intracranial injury, cranial nerve deficits, cervical spine injury). For the maxillofacial trauma surgeon, the most troubling complication is a poor cosmetic and/or functional outcome. Wide exposure for proper alignment of facial substructures, rigid fixation, and immediate bone grafting reconstructive techniques have significantly reduced the incidence of postoperative facial deformities. However, despite accurate reduction of facial fractures, the soft tissue envelope can exert undesirable forces in the form of scar formation and wound contracture. This can lead to a progressive migration of the bony infrastructure of the face and to late postoperative deformities. It is important for patients to realize that a full functional and cosmetic outcome may require multiple operations and revisions.

Other complications of panfacial repair include cerebrospinal fluid leaks, nonunion, malunion, cosmetic deformity (telecanthus, orbital dystopia, loss of malar projection, increased midfacial or lower facial width, nasal deformity), malocclusion, infection (local wound abscess, meningitis, cerebral abscess, epidural empyema), facial nerve palsy, anosmia, and trigeminal nerve injury (hypoesthesia, dysesthesia, anesthesia).

DISCUSSION

The term "panfacial fracture" is frequently used incorrectly. By definition, panfacial fractures involve the upper, middle, and lower thirds of the face. Traditionally, the facial skeleton is divided into thirds or upper and lower halves. More recently,

Manson and others have described four anatomic areas of the face: the frontal area (including the frontal bar), the upper midfacial area (including the ZMC and NOE), the lower midfacial area and occlusion (including the maxilla at the Le Fort I level and the maxillary and mandibular dentoalveolar segments), and the basal mandibular area (including the condyle, ramus, body, and symphysis). Nonetheless, when there is a fracture in each of these four anatomic areas, it is considered a true panfacial fracture. Comminution is a common feature of all midfacial fractures, especially at the anterior maxillary sinus wall and in the ZM buttress area.

It is of paramount importance to maintain the three dimensions of the facial skeleton: the height (from vertex to menton), the width (bizygomatic width), and the anteroposterior projection. Reconstruction of the anatomy using alignment and fixation of the facial vertical and horizontal buttresses is crucial. The horizontal buttresses, as described by Manson and associates, include the frontal bar, infraorbital rim, zygomatic arch, maxillary alveolar bone, and mandibular buttresses. The vertical buttresses include the orbital, frontonasomaxillary, frontozygomaticomaxillary, pterygomaxillary, and mandibular buttresses.

In the past, it has been advocated to wait until edema resolves before fixation of facial fractures. However, surgeons have found that waiting can make surgical efforts more difficult. Now, immediate repair, once the patient has been stabilized, is recommended. Panfacial fractures frequently occur concomitantly with closed head injuries, mandating neurosurgical evaluation and possible treatment prior to any maxillofacial intervention. A team approach, in conjunction with neurosurgeons, is important in cases requiring cranialization of the frontal sinus. It is important to reconstruct the frontal bar and superior aspect of the NOE fracture before placement of an anteriorly based pericranial flap, to allow access to this region.

The goal of modern panfacial fracture repair and reconstruction is achievement of the preinjury level of both function and cosmesis. The treatment of these complex fractures mandates a knowledge of facial bony anatomy and facial cosmetic surgery.

Bibliography

Bagheri SC, Dierks EJ, Kademani D, et al: Comparison of the severity of bilateral Le Fort injuries in isolated midface trauma, *J Oral Maxillofac Surg* 63:1123-1129, 2005.

Bagheri SC, Dierks EJ, Kademani D, et al: Application of a Facial Injury Severity Scale in craniomaxillofacial trauma, *J Oral Maxillofac Surg* 64:404-414, 2006.

Bähr W, Stoll P: Nasal intubation in the presence of frontobasal fractures: a retrospective study, *J Oral Maxillofac Surg* 50:445-447, 1992.

Bell RB, Dierks EJ, Homer L, et al: Management of cerebrospinal fluid leak associated with craniomaxillofacial trauma, *J Oral Maxillofac Surg* 62(6):676-684, 2004.

Bouma GJ, Muizelaar JP: Relationship between cardiac output and cerebral blood flow in patients with intact and with impaired autoregulation, *J Neurosurg* 73:368-374, 1990.

Bouma GJ, Muizelaar JP, Bandoh K, et al: Blood pressure and intracranial pressure-volume dynamics in severe head injury: relationship with cerebral blood flow, *J Neurosurg* 77:15-19, 1992.

Buehler JA, Tannyhill RJ: Complications in the treatment of midfacial fractures, *Oral Maxillofacial Surg Clin North Am* 15:195-212, 2003.

Changaris DG, McGraw CP, Richardson JD, et al: Correlation of cerebral perfusion pressure and Glasgow Coma Scale to outcome, *J Trauma* 27:1007-1013, 1987.

Haug RH, Wible RT, Likavek MJ, et al: Cervical spine fractures and maxillofacial trauma, *J Oral Maxillofac Surg* 49:725, 1991.

Horellou MF, Mathe D, Feisse P: A hazard of nasotracheal intubation, *Anaesthesia* 33:73-74, 1978.

Kreiner B, Stevens MR, Bankston S, et al: Management of panfacial fractures, *Oral and Maxillofacial Surgery Knowledge Update* 3:63-81, 2001.

Le Fort R: Experimental study of fractures of the upper jaw. I, II, and II, *Rev Chir De Paris* 23:208-227, 360-379, 479-507, 1901; translated by Tessier P: *Plast Reconstr Surg* 50:497-506, 600-607, 1972.

Manson PN, Clark N, Robertson B, et al: Comprehensive management of panfacial fractures, *J Craniomaxillofac Trauma* 1(1):43-56, 1995.

Manson PN, Hoopes JE, Su CT: Structural pillars of the facial skeleton: an approach to the management of Le Fort fractures, *Plast Reconstr Surg* 66:53-61, 1980.

Marion DW, Darby J, Yonas H: Acute regional cerebral blood flow changes caused by severe head injuries, *J Neurosurg* 74:407-414, 1991.

Marlow TJ, Goltra DD, Schabel SI: Intracranial placement of a nasotracheal tube after facial fracture: a rare complication, *J Emerg Med* 15:187-191, 1997.

Marmarou A, Anderson RL, Ward JD, et al: Impact of intracranial pressure instability and hypotension on outcome in patients with severe head trauma, *J Neurosurg* 75:S59-S66, 1991.

Ng M, Saadat D, Sinha UK: Managing the emergency airway in Le Fort fractures, *J Craniomaxillofac Trauma* 4:38, 1998.

Rosner MJ, Daughton S: Cerebral perfusion pressure management in head injury, *J Trauma* 30:933-941, 1990.

CHAPTER **9**

Orthognathic Surgery

This chapter addresses:
- Mandibular Orthognathic Surgery
- Maxillary Orthognathic Surgery
- Maxillomandibular Surgery for Apertognathia
- Distraction Osteogenesis: Mandibular Advancement in Conjunction with Traditional Orthognathic Surgery
- Inferior Alveolar Nerve Injury
- Computer-Assisted Surgical Simulation: Virtual Surgical Planning for Orthognathic Surgery

The practice of orthognathic surgery was popularized in the 1980s, especially after the blood supply of the maxilla became more clearly understood. The procedures have undergone several modifications in surgical technique, administration of anesthesia, and postoperative care. Over the past decade, two factors have influenced the practice of this surgical specialty. First, decreasing insurance reimbursement and limited coverage (at least in the United States) have created economic barriers for patients and surgeons. Second, the introduction of virtual surgical planning and surgery have revolutionized the accuracy and speed of treatment.

Correction of dentofacial deformities using combined orthodontic and surgical treatment can provide dramatic changes in both the cosmetic and functional aspects of the face. Patient commitment to an extended period of treatment and a close working relationship with the orthodontist are essential to a successful outcome.

An important component of the management of patients planning for orthognathic surgery is the correct diagnosis of both dental and skeletal abnormalities. Dental compensation can frequently mask an underlying skeletal deformity. Assessment of the maxilla and mandible should consider the three dimensions: anterior-posterior, vertical, and transverse. Evaluation at each dimension should account for cosmetic factors (e.g., amount of tooth/gingival show or size of the chin), growth abnormalities (hypoplasia or hyperplasia), and asymmetries.

Treatment is tailored to each patient based on the procedure that would achieve the best result while minimizing morbidity. Patient education about the procedure, postoperative healing, and potential complications of orthognathic surgery is by far the most important factor in patient satisfaction.

This section presents four teaching cases that address maxillary, mandibular, and bimaxillary surgery and severe mandibular horizontal hypoplasia treated with distraction osteogenesis surgery. In this new edition we have added two new cases — computer-assisted surgery and the neurologic complications of and microneurosurgery for orthognathic surgery.

Mandibular Orthognathic Surgery

Brett A. Ueeck, Shahrokh C. Bagheri, and Timothy M. Osborn

CC

A 23-year-old female is referred by her orthodontist for evaluation of a skeletal malocclusion and for recommendations regarding surgical correction. She states, "My lower jaw is too small for my face."

HPI

The patient reports having had braces twice when she was younger, but she notices this did nothing to change the appearance of her chin. She was referred to a different orthodontist, because her general dentist was concerned about the periodontal health of her lower incisors. Previous orthodontia had proclined the lower anterior teeth outside the alveolus, resulting in several millimeters of clinical attachment loss. The patient has completed presurgical orthodontic treatment to reverse the previous orthodontic camouflage and is now ready for surgical correction. She explains that she has difficulty eating foods with the front teeth and has become very self-aware of her retrusive chin and everted lower lip (both functional and cosmetic complaint). She does not have any symptoms of temporomandibular joint (TMJ) dysfunction (TMD) (although a relationship between malocclusion and TMD has been suggested, the scientific evidence is not clear).

PMHX/PSHX/MEDICATIONS/ALLERGIES/SH/FH

Noncontributory.

EXAMINATION

The examination of a patient for orthognathic surgery can be divided into four components: TMJ, skeletal, dental, and soft tissue components. Skeletal discrepancies (hypoplasia or hyperplasia) should be assessed in three dimensions: transverse (horizontal), anteroposterior, and vertical.

The maxillofacial examination of the current patient proceeded as follows.

1. **TMJ component**
   - There is full range of motion without significant deviation or joint noise.
2. **Skeletal component**
   - There is no facial asymmetry.
     a. *Transverse dimension*
        - Maxillary dental midline is coincident with the facial midline.
        - Mandibular dental midline is coincident with the maxillary dental midline.
        - Chin point is coincident with the maxillary and mandibular midlines.
        - Maxillary occlusal plane is canted down 1 mm on the right.
        - Mandibular angles are level.
        - Maxillary and mandibular arch widths are well coordinated (evaluated by handheld models or by having the patient posture the mandible forward into a Class I relationship).
     b. *Anteroposterior dimension*
        - Nasolabial angle is 110 degrees (normal is 100 degrees ± 10 degrees).
        - There is a convex facial profile.
        - Chin is microgenic.
        - Labiomental angle is deep (consistent with mandibular hypoplasia).
     c. *Vertical dimension*
        - Upper and middle facial thirds are equal. Lower facial third is deficient, most noticeably in its lower two thirds.
3. **Dental component (occlusion and dentition)**
   - Class II relationship is present at first molars and canines.
   - Overjet is 10 mm (Figure 9-1).
   - Overbite is 100%.
   - There is no crossbite.
   - The arch form is level with no crowding.
4. **Soft tissue component**
   - Upper lip has adequate thickness and length.
   - Lower lip is everted. (Depending on the amount of overbite and the mandibular plane angle, with a Class II malocclusion there can be a normal lower lip position, eversion, or labial incompetence combined with mentalis strain.)

IMAGING

The panoramic and lateral cephalogram are the minimum preoperative radiographs necessary for mandibular orthognathic surgery. The panoramic radiograph allows evaluation of the dentition, the mandibular bony anatomy, and the position of any impacted third molars. Some surgeons recommend surgical removal of the mandibular third molars at least 9 months prior to a sagittal split osteotomy (alternatively, third

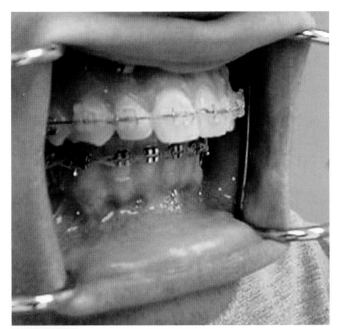

Preoperative occlusion demonstrating an overjet of 10 mm.

molars can be removed during the procedure). The PA cephalogram is useful in cases of asymmetry.

Other imaging for orthognathic surgery includes CT scans with conventional and three-dimensional views and videography. These imaging modalities can be useful in complex cases of skeletal asymmetry and cases requiring multiple surgical moves in the maxilla and mandible. There is also software that allows for manipulation of imaging in attempts to predict surgical changes and outcome. (The discussion of these tools is addressed in the section on computer-assisted surgical simulation later in this chapter.)

The lateral cephalogram is the standard film for evaluation of the anteroposterior position of the soft and hard tissue. Measurements of cephalometric norms are used for evaluation of the mandible (and maxilla) in the vertical and anteroposterior dimensions. Most current cephalometric analysis involves comparing the position of the mandible in reference to the cranial base (SNB) and the maxilla (ANB). A variety of other measurements are used to assess the vertical or horizontal abnormalities of the maxillomandibular complex (including teeth). Lateral cephalometric analysis does not assess mediolateral facial parameters. There are different techniques available to analyze a lateral cephalogram, and it is best to be consistent.

For the current patient, the preorthodontic cephalometric measurements and films are shown in Table 9-1 and Figure 9-2.

LABS

No preoperative laboratory tests are indicated for an otherwise healthy patient unless dictated by the medical history.

Before and after orthodontic treatment, maxillary and mandibular dental casts are obtained for treatment planning and construction of an occlusal splint.

Table 9-1	Assessment of Relationship of Maxilla and Mandible to Cranial Base and to Each Other	
Cephalometric Measurements for Patient in Figures 9-2 and 9-3	**Normal Parameters for Caucasians**	**Patient Notes**
SNB: 71 degrees	80 degrees (±3 degrees)	Suggestive of mandibular hypoplasia
ANB: 10 degrees	2 degrees (±2 degrees)	Maxillomandibular discrepancy due to mandibular hypoplasia
SNA: 81 degrees	82 degrees (±3 degrees)	
Vertical Facial Measurements		
Nasion to anterior nasal spine (N-ANS): 57 mm	Female: 53 mm Male: 58 mm	
ANS-Me: 60 mm	Female: 65 mm Male: 65 mm	
Mandibular plane angle: 19 degrees	27 degrees (±4 degrees)	
Relationship of the Teeth to the Skeletal Base		
Upper 1 to SN: 104 degrees	102 to 104 degrees	
Lower 1 to mandibular plane (MP): 109 degrees	90 to 95 degrees	Dental or orthodontic compensation for mandibular hypoplasia

ANB, A point, Nasion, B point; *SN,* Sella-Nasion; *SNB,* Sella, Nasion, B point.

ASSESSMENT

Mandibular hypoplasia resulting in a Class II skeletal and dental malocclusion.

TREATMENT

Treatment of mandibular hypoplasia or hyperplasia is dependent on any coexisting maxillary dentofacial abnormalities. If the position of the maxilla is deemed to be appropriate (clinical and radiographic analysis), mandibular surgery alone can be considered, because the final position of the mandible will be dictated by the occlusion and the position of the maxilla. If the maxilla is abnormally positioned, then maxillomandibular surgery is indicated. Setting the mandible anteriorly or posteriorly in the ideal occlusion may produce an unaesthetic chin position. Therefore the need for adjunctive surgical procedures (advancement/reduction genioplasty/submental liposuction/submentalplasty) should be considered, especially in mandibular setbacks.

The basic method of the sagittal split osteotomy has remained unchanged since it was first described in 1955; however, individual surgeons have developed different

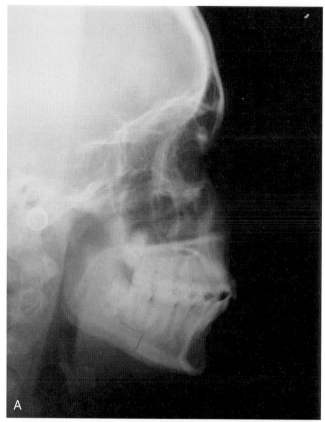

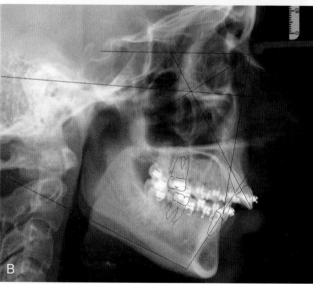

Figure 9-2   **A,** Preorthodontic lateral cephalogram demonstrating significant dental compensation (orthodontic camouflage). **B,** Preoperative cephalogram after completion of presurgical orthodontics (orthodontic compensation has been removed).

instrumentations and cutting sequences to complete the surgery. Similarly, practitioners differ in their preference for fixation (i.e., bicortical position screws, lag screws, or one or more rigid fixation plates).

Patients with mandibular asymmetry require special consideration related to correction of the deformity. Surgical implications include the uneven overlap of the osteotomized

distal and proximal segments. Similarly, the end position of the chin and the mandibular angles have to be anticipated for optimal results. Bony recontouring, genioplasty, or augmentation at the angles or chin may be required.

The overlying soft tissue response to mandibular osteotomies can be predicted. In general, the soft tissue (chin/lip) response for mandibular advancement or setback is about 90% of the skeletal move (e.g., advancing the mandible 10 mm advances the chin and lip about 9 mm). The status of facial growth also needs to be determined in younger patients. The gold standard for evaluation of facial growth is superimposition of interval (6 months apart) standard lateral cephalograms.

The current patient underwent a bilateral sagittal split osteotomy (Figure 9-3, *A*), resulting in a 10-mm advancement. The proximal and distal segments were fixated using three bicortical position screws at the superior border (Figure 9-3, *B*) on each side. Figure 9-4 shows the occlusion 9 months after the completion of surgery and 1 month after removal of the orthodontic appliances. Figure 9-5 shows the postoperative lateral cephalogram.

COMPLICATIONS

Complications of mandibular orthognathic surgery can be categorized into intraoperative, early, and late. The complications related to the sagittal split osteotomy are emphasized next.

Intraoperative. The most common intraoperative complication is an undesirable split or fracture of the segments, reported in 3% to 20% of cases. A common cause of proximal segment fractures is failure to complete the osteotomy at the inferior border, resulting in a free segment. Some proximal segment fractures can lead to fracture propagation up to the condylar head. Confirmation of the continuity of the condyle with the proximal segment detects this fracture. Undesirable fractures can be treated with rigid fixation or a period of 6 weeks of intermaxillary fixation.

Damage to the inferior alveolar nerve is a known complication of the sagittal split osteotomy. When possible, intraoperative transection of the nerve is best treated by immediate epineural repair. Retention of the neurovascular bundle in the proximal segment as the mandible is split is a common cause of injury to the nerve. If the nerve is observed to be in the proximal segment as the mandible is split, it should be gently dissected and positioned along the canal in the distal segment.

Uncontrollable intraoperative hemorrhage is uncommon for mandibular orthognathic surgery in an otherwise healthy patient. However, it can be seen in patients with vascular anomalies or undiagnosed coagulopathies. Damage to the facial artery or retromandibular vein is uncommon but can be caused by inadvertent laceration of the periosteal envelope.

Early. Early complications include malocclusion, wound infection, hardware failure, periodontal defects (more common with interdental osteotomies), and injury to teeth. Early postoperative neurosensory deficit (inferior alveolar nerve) is not considered a complication, because the majority of cases

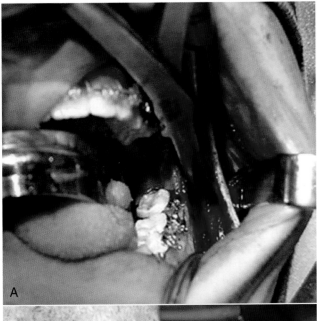

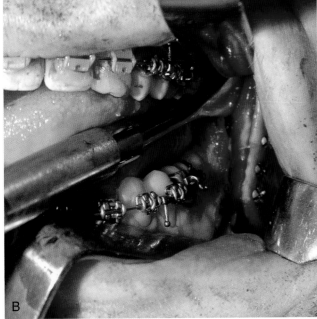

Figure 9-3 **A,** Intraoperative view immediately after completion of the left sagittal split osteotomy. **B,** Intraoperative view demonstrating placement of three bicortical position screws placed above the inferior alveolar canal.

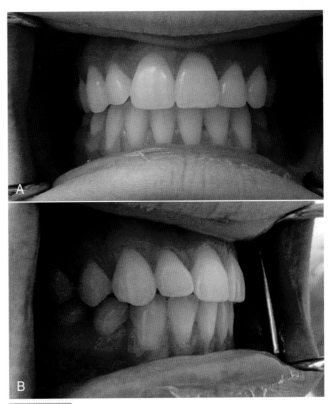

Figure 9-4 **A** and **B,** Postoperative occlusion after completion of the postoperative orthodontics.

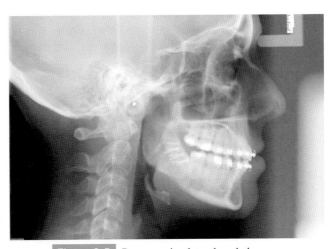

Figure 9-5 Postoperative lateral cephalogram.

(more than 85%) demonstrate some degree of paresthesia. Progressive improvement can be observed up to 9 to 12 months postoperatively.

The presence of immediate postoperative malocclusion can be indicative of hardware failure or intersegmental shifting. If this is not detected clinically or radiographically, it is most likely due to proximal (condylar) segment malpositioning during fixation (e.g., if the condyle is not seated in the fossa as it is fixated to the distal segment, upon release of intermaxillary fixation, the condyles reposition, resulting in an anterior open bite).

Infection is a rare complication (less than 3%) in otherwise healthy patients. Hardware removal commonly allows rapid resolution of a draining fistula or ongoing acute infection. Antibiotics may be used to hasten the recovery. Bone fragments that form a sequestrum (frequently a segment of the inferior border) should also be considered in the differential diagnosis of a nonhealing wound.

Late. Permanent neurosensory abnormalities (beyond 12 months) are seen in fewer than 10% of bilateral sagittal split osteotomies. Intraoperative nerve transection, placement of a screw through the nerve, and neurovascular encroachment by bony segments are possible etiologies of permanent nerve injury. Given the high incidence of prolonged postoperative hypoesthesia, the diagnosis of a permanent nerve injury is often very difficult. Due to the spontaneous recovery of the majority of cases, surgeons are generally inclined to observe postoperative hypoesthesia/anesthesia for extended periods. This may lead to permanent neurosensory deficits in a small number of patients who may benefit from early postoperative nerve exploration.

Relapse refers to late postoperative occlusal changes toward the preoperative occlusion. The etiology of relapse is not entirely clear; however, it is hypothesized to be related to postoperative changes in the mandibular bony architecture (e.g., condylar resorption) or to failure of the neuromuscular system to adjust to the new mandibular position, resulting in an unfavorable muscle pull. Relapse is seen in approximately 20% of mandibular advancements and is usually limited to about 15% of the total surgical advancement. It has been shown that larger surgical moves (greater than 7 mm) have a greater possibility of relapse, which supports the neuromuscular adaptation/pull etiology for relapse. Distraction osteogenesis should be considered in patients requiring moves greater than 10 mm.

DISCUSSION

The first description of mandibular osteotomy dates to Hullihen in 1849 (mandibular subapical osteotomy). Subsequently, several techniques and modifications were described, including the Blair ramus osteotomy, Limberg oblique ramus osteotomy, C-osteotomy, inverted L-osteotomy, and vertical ramus osteotomy. The vertical ramus osteotomy is still used by many surgeons via an intraoral approach (intraoral vertical ramus osteotomy). Mandibular orthognathic surgery was revolutionized by the development of the bilateral sagittal split osteotomy by Obegwesser in 1955 in Germany. The procedure has since undergone several modifications by Obegwesser, Dalpont, Hunsuk, and others. Today, the bilateral sagittal split osteotomy remains the most commonly used osteotomy for advancement or setback of the mandible. The Dalpont modification was one of the earlier changes that introduced the vertical cut through the cortex. Hunsuk suggested a shorter medial osteotomy posteriorly, resulting in a shorter split and allowing reduced soft tissue trauma and improved posterior mandibular contour, especially with larger setbacks.

Successful orthognathic surgery requires good communication between the surgeon and orthodontist, in addition to patient commitment to a long treatment period. The main goals of preoperative orthodontic treatment include leveling and aligning the arches, positioning the teeth over the basal bone, and achieving proper inclination of the teeth (dental decompensation), especially the incisors. Placement of molar bands and adequate orthodontic hardware is important for intraoperative maxillomandibular fixation.

Augmentation or reduction genioplasty is frequently used in conjunction with mandibular orthognathic surgery.

Similarly, some patients may elect to defer orthognathic surgery and undergo only chin surgery. A patient with mandibular hypoplasia may elect to "camouflage" the abnormality by an advancement genioplasty alone. Although this does not completely address the skeletal issue or alter the dental relationship, it can improve the aesthetic outcome.

The preoperative work-up is a combination of clinical and radiographic planning. The decision for the surgical movements should be predominantly determined from the patient, not the radiographs, in accordance with the adage, "Treat the patient, not the radiograph." Once the clinical and cephalometric plans are in place, preoperative dental casts should be made and mounted on an articulator with facebow transfer and occlusal registration. The casts should be trimmed anatomically so that measurements and moves on the casts can be accurately transferred to the operating room. Once the model surgery has been performed, based on the cephalometric predictions and clinical examination, the acrylic splint can be made. Measurements should be recorded and verified on the films and surgical casts.

Several adjuncts are used clinically during the operative period to enhance both the surgical field and the patient's recovery. The use of hypotensive anesthesia at the time of the osteotomy helps to minimize blood loss and increase visibility in the surgical field, allowing for more precise and timely surgery. In general, an increase of up to 500 ml of blood loss can be expected in patients not undergoing hypotensive anesthesia. Although the exact amount of blood loss and increase in visibility are still debated, several studies have shown this method to be effective. A reverse Trendelenburg (head up) position also aids reduction of venous congestion in the head and neck.

The use of antibiotics and steroids has been debated. A single preoperative prophylactic dose of antibiotic is probably useful in reducing the infection risk without undo adverse sequelae. Studies have shown an infection rate of less than 5% with a single preoperative antibiotic dose. Some surgeons suggest continuing antibiotics for 5 to 7 days postoperatively, but this practice is not supported by clinical studies. Continuing antibiotics beyond the preoperative dose is probably unwarranted in an otherwise healthy patient. Corticosteroids have been shown to decrease the total amount and duration of postsurgical edema. They are also beneficial antinausea medications.

Despite the decreases in reimbursement and insurance coverage, orthognathic surgery continues to be a viable tool for the treatment of a variety of clinical diagnoses, and it has a significant impact on both function and cosmesis. The skills required to perform these operations successfully are challenging and require continuing refinement and education.

Bibliography

Baqain ZH, Hyde N, Patrikidou A, et al: Antibiotic prophylaxis for orthognathic surgery: a prospective, randomised clinical trial, *Br J Oral Maxillofac Surg* 42(6):506-510, 2004.

Bays RA: Complications of orthognathic surgery. In Kaban LB, Perrot DH, Pogrel MA (eds): *Complications of oral and maxillofacial surgery*, Philadelphia, 1997, Saunders.

Dalpont G: Retromolar osteotomy for the correction of prognathism, *J Oral Surg Anesth Hosp Dent Serv* 19:42, 1961.

Frey DR, Hatch JP, Van Sickels JE, et al: Effects of surgical mandibular advancement and rotation on signs and symptoms of temporomandibular disorder: a 2-year follow-up study, *Am J Orthod Dentofacial Orthop* 133:490, 2008.

Gerressen M, Stockbrink G, Riediger D, et al: Skeletal stability following BSSO with and without condylar positioning device, *J Oral Maxillofac Surg* 65:1297, 2007.

Hullihen SP: Case of elongation of the under jaw and distortion of the face and neck, caused by a burn, successfully treated, *Am J Dent Sci* 9:157, 1849.

Hunsuk EE: Modified intraoral sagittal splitting technique for correction of mandibular prognathism, *J Oral Surg* 26:250, 1968.

Lee J: Bilateral sagittal split osteotomy for surgical management of mandibular deficiency. In Bagheri SC, Bell RB, Khan HA (eds): *Current therapy in oral and maxillofacial surgery*, St Louis, 2011, Saunders.

Obwegeser H: The indications for surgical correction of mandibular deformity by the sagittal split technique, *Br J Oral Surg* 1:157, 1962.

Praveen K, Narayanan V, Muthusekhar MR, et al: Hypotensive anaesthesia and blood loss in orthognathic surgery: a clinical study, *Br J Oral Maxillofac Surg* 39(2):138-140, 2001.

Shepherd J: Hypotensive anaesthesia and blood loss in orthognathic surgery, *Evid Based Dent* 5(1):16, 2004.

Zijderveld SA, Smeele LE, Kostense PJ, et al: Preoperative antibiotic prophylaxis in orthognathic surgery: a randomized, double-blind, and placebo-controlled clinical study, *J Oral Maxillofac Surg* 57(12):1403-1406; discussion, 1406-1407; 1999.

Maxillary Orthognathic Surgery

Brett A. Ueeck, Timothy M. Osborn, and Chris Jo

CC

A 19-year-old woman is referred by her orthodontist for combined surgical-orthodontic management of her Class III skeletal malocclusion and maxillary hypoplasia. She complains that, "My face looks sunken in and looks too short."

In treatment planning for patients presenting for orthognathic surgery, it is essential to differentiate the degree of cosmetic versus functional dissatisfaction. For elective surgical procedures, a successful outcome requires this distinction to be well integrated into the surgical plan. Although this patient's functional impairments are obvious, she focuses mostly on her appearance.

HPI

The patient admits to some difficulty and discomfort when chewing certain foods, but her main concern is her appearance. She presents to your office after finishing 3 years of orthodontic therapy. She was being monitored for cessation of mandibular growth and possible development of mandibular hyperplasia in conjunction with maxillary hypoplasia. Serial lateral cephalograms at 1-year intervals showed that her mandibular growth was complete (interval superimposition of standard lateral cephalograms is a reliable way to monitor facial growth). Her occlusion has been aligned and leveled for a single-piece Le Fort I osteotomy (if the curve of Spee cannot be leveled in the mandibular arch preoperatively, then postoperative tripod occlusion and postoperative leveling are planned). There is no history or symptoms of temporomandibular joint disorders. (A preexisting TMD should be recognized and addressed before orthognathic surgery, because the latter may exacerbate a preexisting TMD. Although some surgeons recommend simultaneous orthognathic and TMJ surgery in select cases of preexisting anterior disk displacement, this issue is highly controversial.)

PMHX/PSHX/MEDICATIONS/ALLERGIES/SH/FH

Noncontributory.

Elective orthognathic surgery should be carefully considered in patients classified ASA III or higher.

EXAMINATION

The examination of a patient for orthognathic surgery can be divided into four components: TMJ, skeletal, dental, and soft tissue. Skeletal discrepancies (hypoplasia or hyperplasia) should be assessed in three dimensions: transverse (horizontal), anteroposterior, and vertical. As for all surgical patients, the airway, cardiopulmonary, neurologic, and other organ systems should be assessed in anticipation of the use of general anesthesia.

The maxillofacial examination of the current patient proceeded as follows.

1. **TMJ component**
   - The muscles of mastication and the TMJ capsule are nontender, with no evidence of clicking or crepitus (seen with disk perforation). The maximal interincisal opening is 45 mm, with good excursive movements and no deviation upon opening or closing (normal TMJ examination).

2. **Skeletal component**
   - There is no vertical orbital dystopia. The intercanthal distance is 31 mm (normal). The nose is straight and coincident with the midline. Malar eminences are within normal limits.
   a. *Transverse dimension*
      - Maxillary dental midline is 1 mm right of the facial midline.
      - Mandibular dental midline is 1 mm left of the maxillary dental midline and coincident with the facial midline.
      - Chin point is coincident with the facial midline.
      - Maxillary occlusal plane is canted down 1 mm on the left at the canine.
      - Mandibular occlusal plane and angles are level.
      - Maxillary arch width is adequate (evaluated by handheld models).
   b. *Anteroposterior dimension*
      - Overjet is −6 mm.
      - Nasolabial angle is 45 degrees (normal is 100 degrees ± 10 degrees).
      - Labiomental fold is within normal limits.
      - Chin is relatively prognathic.
      - Profile is brachycephalic (Figure 9-6, *A*).
   c. *Vertical dimension*
      - Lower facial third is deficient (normal nasion-ANS-to–ANS-menton ratio is 7:8).
      - Maxillary incisor length is 10 mm.
      - Upper incisor show is 0 mm at rest (ideally, there is 2 to 4 mm of tooth show at rest) and 6 mm in full smile (in an esthetically pleasing smile line,

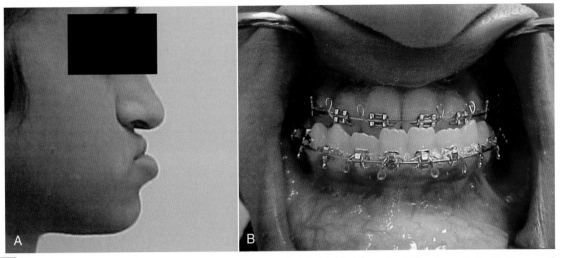

Figure 9-6   **A,** Preoperative profile view showing shortened lower facial third height and midface hypoplasia. **B,** Preoperative intraoral view showing Class III skeletal malocclusion.

the gingival papilla or 1 mm of gingival margin is visible at full smile).

3. **Dental component (occlusion and dentition)**
   * There is deep bite (Figure 9-6, *B*).
   * Overjet is −6 mm (normal is +3.5 mm ± 2.5 mm).
   * Class III relationship is present at the first molars and canines bilaterally.
   * Arch width is adequate on handheld models (transverse maxillary deficiencies may require a segmental Le Fort I osteotomy or surgically assisted rapid palatal expansion).
   * Curve of Spee has been appropriately leveled, and additional postoperative leveling will be required (1 to 1.5 mm of arch space is required for each 1 mm of curve of Spee leveled).
   * Maxillary and mandibular arch forms are ideal.
   * Dental compensations have been adequately decompensated without the need for bicuspid extractions (retracting proclined incisors requires 0.8 mm of arch space for each 1 degree retracted; proclining incisors 1.25 degrees gains 1 mm of arch space).
   * Dentition is in good repair, with no missing teeth (except for third molars).

4. **Soft tissue component**
   * Upper lip has adequate thickness and length.
   * Nasolabial angle is 40 degrees (normal is 100 degrees ± 10 degrees).
   * Nasal tip shows a downward rotation.

IMAGING

The panoramic radiograph and a lateral cephalometric radiograph are the minimum imaging modalities necessary for orthognathic surgery. Preoperative profile, frontal (upon smiling and rest), and occlusal photographs should be obtained. For patients with more complicated conditions, such as facial asymmetry or a cleft, and for those with other

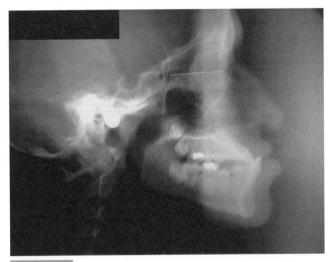

Figure 9-7   Preoperative lateral cephalogram showing maxillary hypoplasia and severe compensation of the maxillary incisors.

syndromes, a PA cephalogram, CT scan, or stereophotogrammetry may be obtained.

For the current patient, the panoramic radiograph shows normal bony architecture of the condylar head and no other pathology. The right and left maxillary and mandibular third molars (teeth #1, #16, #17, and #32) are full bony impacted with minimal root formation.

An initial lateral cephalogram was obtained with the patient in centric relation and lips in a relaxed/reposed position (Figure 9-7). Cephalometric analysis reveals anteroposterior maxillary hypoplasia. This preorthodontic lateral cephalogram illustrates the degree of skeletal discrepancies, in addition to the degree of dental compensations (proclined maxillary incisors); these are important considerations when calculating the adequacy of the existing arch space and determining the need for extractions (decompensating or retroclining flared incisors requires 0.8 mm of arch space for each

Table 9-2	Cephalometric Analysis	
Patient in Figures 9-6 to 9-8	**Normal Parameters for Caucasians**	**Patient Notes**
Cranial base angle: Normal	Sella-nasion (SN)-basion angle: 129 degrees ± 4 degrees Sella-nasion (SN) to Frankfurt horizontal (FH) angle: 7 degrees ± 4 degrees	
SNA: 79 degrees	82 degrees ± 3 degrees	Patient's value is suggestive of a maxillary anteroposterior deficiency relative to the cranial base.
SNB: 88 degrees	80 degrees ± 3 degrees	Patient's value is suggestive of an excessive anteroposterior position of the mandible relative to the cranial base.
Harvold difference*: Excessive	Females: 27 mm Males: 29 mm	Patient's value is suggestive of maxillary hypoplasia or mandibular hyperplasia.
Mandibular plane (MP): Flat	SN-MP: 32 degrees ± 10 degrees FH-MP: 22 degrees ± 6 degrees	
Long axis of upper incisor to SN angle: 134 degrees	104 degrees ± 4 degrees	Patient's value indicates severely compensated maxillary incisors
Long axis of lower incisor to MP angle: 100 degrees	90 degrees ± 5 degrees	
Upper lip to E-plane: −5 mm	−3 mm ± 2 mm	
Lower lip to E-plane: +3 mm	−2 mm	Patient's value shows retrusive soft tissue chin and concave profile.

SNA, Sella-nasion, A point; *SNB*, sella-nasion, B point.
*The Harvold difference is the distance from condylion to pogonion minus the distance from condylion to A point.

1 degree of retraction). It is important to note that measurements differ between Caucasians, Asians, and African Americans (normal values for Caucasian are listed in Table 9-2).

LABS

No preoperative labs are required for healthy patients classified ASA I. A pregnancy test (urine pregnancy test or serum β-hCG) is warranted for females of childbearing age if there is any question about the possibility of pregnancy.

ASSESSMENT

Maxillary retrognathia secondary to hypoplasia, resulting in a Class III skeletal facial deformity.

TREATMENT

Treatment of maxillary hypoplasia involves a combined orthodontic and surgical approach for stable results. A coordinated approach involving the orthodontist and the oral and maxillofacial surgeon requires a close working relationship to meet the needs of the patient. The goals of presurgical orthodontic therapy are to:
- Align and level the occlusion
- Coordinate the maxillary and mandibular arches (progress is monitored with handheld models)
- Eliminate dental compensations in preparation for surgical correction of the skeletal deformities

- Diverge the roots of adjacent teeth for planned segmental osteotomies (only the roots should be diverged; the crowns retain interproximal contact)

During the treatment planning phase, the need for dental extractions is determined. The surgeon should be aware of the rationale for arch space management during the presurgical orthodontic phase. It is important to avoid any unstable orthodontic movement (e.g., closing anterior open bites by extruding maxillary or mandibular anterior teeth or widening the posterior maxillary horizontal dimension by tipping the molars) that would later result in relapse. Postsurgical orthodontics is aimed at creating a final, stable occlusion and closing any posterior open bites that resulted from the surgical correction. Frequently, the orthodontist is not able to level the mandibular curve of Spee presurgically and sets up a tripod occlusion. The curve is leveled and spaces are closed postoperatively. Most orthodontists use a retainer for maintenance of the final occlusal relationship and alignment.

Orthognathic surgical treatment options and plans for maxillary hypoplasia are case specific but may include a Le Fort I osteotomy and advancement (single piece versus multiple piece) or bimaxillary surgery. During maxillary advancement, the surgeon can also control the vertical position of the maxilla and incisors, because the mandibular arc of rotation and model setup determine the final position of both the maxilla and mandible (mounted model surgery is paramount to determine the anteroposterior position of the maxillomandibular unit when it is set at the desired vertical position).

A Le Fort I osteotomy alone can be considered in the following situations:

- The mandible is in good position (dental midline and chin midline coincident with the facial midline).
- There is no mandibular occlusal cant.
- The mandible is aligned with the face (symmetrical).
- The mandibular arc of rotation positions the maxilla into a good anteroposterior position while maintaining an appropriate chin projection.

A segmental Le Fort I osteotomy is indicated when a transverse deficiency or a dual occlusal plane exists. Bimaxillary (maxillomandibular) surgery (Le Fort I and sagittal split or vertical ramus osteotomies) may be warranted when deformities exist in both the maxilla and mandible, and the mandibular position and arc of rotation cannot be used to position the maxilla (see Maxillomandibular Surgery for Apertognathia later in this chapter). Surgically assisted rapid palatal expansion should be considered when there is a maxillary transverse discrepancy or arch length discrepancy with no other vertical or anteroposterior discrepancies.

Once the surgical treatment plan has been developed, the surgeon can proceed with model surgery to fabricate one or more surgical splints on mounted models. If the open bite is to be closed with maxillary surgery alone, the maxillary cast is set to the ideal occlusion with the opposing mounted mandibular cast (occlusion set with a small posterior open bite maximizes the amount of incisor overlap and reduces relapse). Small posterior open bites can be easily closed orthodontically, especially in young patients (surgically created posterior open bites allow maximal overlap of the anterior teeth, reducing the risk of relapse). A thin interocclusal acrylic wafer (splint) is made to stabilize the occlusion intraoperatively during rigid fixation of the maxilla. If a segmental osteotomy is performed, the splint is made with a palatal strap and wired to the maxillary dentition during the healing phase to prevent horizontal collapse and relapse of the open bite. The maxilla is generally fixated with two-point fixation at the piriform buttress bilaterally using 1.5-mm maxillary orthognathic plates.

For a maxillary osteotomy, the surgeon should discuss with the anesthesiologist the need for hypotensive anesthesia to reduce intraoperative bleeding. When feasible, hypotension induced with β-blockers, rather than "deep anesthesia" produced by anesthetic gases, is preferred, because the former is more effective and easily titrated. After nasotracheal intubation, a local anesthetic with epinephrine is infiltrated into the maxillary buccal vestibule and internal nares (injection of a vasoconstrictor in the palate should be avoided). Incision design is a critical portion of the surgery, and the vascular perfusion of the hard and soft tissues is the most important factor in healing. The most common incision used during Le Fort I osteotomy is a horizontal incision through the mucosa well above the level of the keratinized gingiva (1 cm past the buccal sulcus), from first molar to first molar, made with a scalpel or electrocautery (the parotid papilla should be identified and protected before the incision). The incision is then carried down through the periosteum to bone. Keeping the periosteal incision perpendicular to the bone prevents extrusion of the buccal fat pad. Subperiosteal dissection is performed on the superior aspect of the incision, preserving the cuff of mucogingival tissue. Dissection is carried to the piriform rim, up to the infraorbital foramen, with exposure of the zygomaticomaxillary buttress. Dissection is then carried posteriorly with subperiosteal tunneling to the pterygomaxillary fissure. Attention is then turned to elevation of the nasal mucosa from the medial portion of the lateral wall and floor. After the maxilla has been exposed, vertical reference points can be established (both internal and external references have been used).

A curved retractor is placed at the pterygomaxillary junction, and a Freer or other retractor is placed under the nasal mucosa for protection during the osteotomy. The osteotomy is made using a reciprocating saw, with care taken to remain 5 to 6 mm above the root apices. A nasal septal osteotome is used to free the septal cartilage and vomer from the nasal floor. A spatula osteotome can be used to complete the lateral nasal osteotomies. A pterygoid osteotome is placed and angled slightly inferiorly to avoid inadvertent laceration of the internal maxillary artery, which is approximately 25 mm superior to the pterygomaxillary junction. The pterygomaxillary junction is then separated with the osteotome. Gentle pressure can be applied to the anterior maxilla as the nasal mucosa is elevated. With continuing downfracture, the descending palatine neurovascular bundle comes into view, and care should be taken to prevent injury to the vessels (some surgeons elect to ligate and section the descending palatine neurovascular bundle). Any areas of incomplete osteotomy can be identified and mobilized to completely free the mobilized segment. The maxilla should be completely mobilized so that it can be repositioned and stabilized as planned. If a multiple-piece Le Fort is planned, the interdental osteotomy is made before downfracture of the maxilla, and parasagittal (thinner bone and thicker soft tissue, compared with the midline) osteotomies are made after the downfracture. Also, inferior turbinate reduction should be considered when performing maxillary impactions.

Next, the surgical splint is inserted and secured to the dental arch. The maxillomandibular complex is then passively seated, and any bony interferences are selectively removed until the desired vertical height has been achieved (complete paralysis should be verified with train-of-four twitches by the anesthesiologist). If there are any large defects in the walls of the maxilla, bone grafts can be used. Rigid fixation with plates at the buttress and piriform region is the most commonly used method of stabilizing the maxilla. Once the maxilla has been rigidly fixed, the maxillomandibular fixation can be removed so that the occlusion can be checked. The mandible should seat passively into the splint, verifying proper stabilization as planned. Some surgeons place deep sutures in the muscular layer to reapproximate the facial and labial musculature prior to mucosal closure. The mucosal layer is closed with a running suture in a V-Y pattern to help maintain lip length. Upon completion of the procedure, the occlusion is verified, and light elastics are used as needed to guide the occlusion.

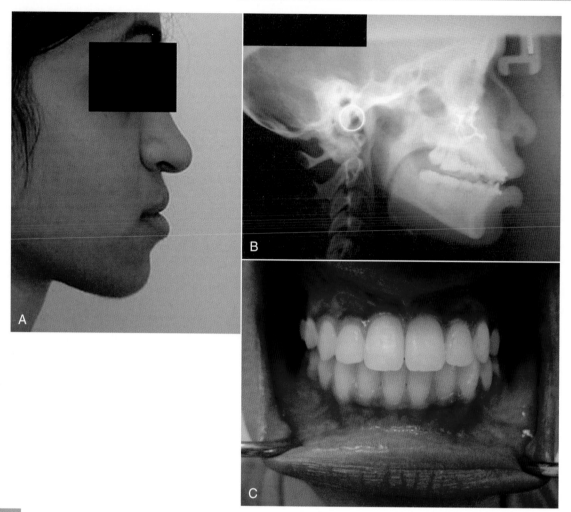

Figure 9-8 **A,** Postoperative profile showing correction of the midface hypoplasia and elongation of the short lower facial third. **B,** Postoperative lateral cephalogram showing correction of the maxillary hypoplasia and aesthetically pleasing facial profile. **C,** Postoperative intraoral view revealing the final occlusion.

The final results for the current patient are shown in Figure 9-8.

COMPLICATIONS

An important aspect of orthognathic surgery is management of complications. A well-informed patient and attention to detail cannot be overemphasized. The most important complications of maxillary orthognathic surgery are (Box 9-1):
- Hemorrhage
- Vascular compromise and maxillary necrosis
- Relapse and malpositioning
- Neurosensory deficits (greater and lesser palatine, nasopalatine, infraorbital nerves)
- Damage to the dentition (maxillary roots) and periodontal defects
- Postoperative nasal deformity

Other complications include infection, hardware failure, malunion, fibrous union, and pulpal necrosis (devitalization of the teeth; this is generally prevented if the osteotomy is at least 5 to 6 mm superior to the root apices).

DISCUSSION

The success of maxillary orthognathic surgery is based on the recognition of the blood supply to the maxilla, which was first investigated by Bell. The main blood supply is based on branches of the external carotid system, including the ascending palatine, ascending pharyngeal, palatine, nasopalatine, posterior superior, and infraorbital arteries. With a maxillary osteotomy, it has been shown that the buccal gingival and mucoperiosteal pedicle and the palatal soft tissue pedicle allow preservation of the blood supply and proper wound healing. Proper incision design and minimal dissection of the palatal soft tissues ensure an adequate blood supply.

Traditional methods of stabilizing the maxilla with wires and prolonged periods of maxillomandibular fixation have been replaced with rigid internal fixation using titanium plates and screws. Resorbable fixation materials have been studied successfully for orthognathic surgery, but they are not routinely applied by most surgeons. Direct bony contact, especially at the zygomaticomaxillary buttresses, is needed to improve immediate and long-term stability. When there are

| Box 9-1 | **Most Important Complications of Maxillary Orthognathic Surgery** |

- **Hemorrhage.** Intraoperative or postoperative hemorrhage can be life threatening (although rare). Hypotensive anesthesia (mean arterial pressure maintained at around 60 mm Hg) is used by most surgeons to reduce the amount of intraoperative bleeding and to improve visualization of the surgical field. Vascular injury to the pterygoid plexus of veins (most common) can result in a significant amount of blood loss (usually easy to control by packing the wound). An arterial injury (most often the descending palatine artery) is more difficult to control and can result in significant blood loss within a short period (the internal maxillary artery and its terminal branches are most susceptible during the osteotomy and downfracture of the maxilla). Typically, arterial bleeding can be controlled by controlling the blood pressure, proper visualization, pressure/packing, and electrocautery or hemoclips. Uncontrollable arterial hemorrhage warrants emergent angiography and embolization (a carotid cutdown and ligation of the external carotid artery can be performed but is less efficacious due to collateral arterial supply). Turvey and associates have shown that the internal maxillary artery is located 25 mm superior to the most inferior junction of the maxilla and pterygoid plate, leaving a 1-mm margin of safety if a 15-mm wide, curved osteotome is used. Late bleeding (usually preceded by sentinel bleeding) can arise from undetected injury to the descending palatine artery (most common source of postoperative bleeding), pseudoaneurysm formation, or ischemic necrosis of the descending palatine artery due to excessive stretching (especially if the descending palatine artery was not ligated and sectioned during the procedure) and warrants immediate angiography. When required, selective arterial embolization should be cautiously performed to avoid compromising the blood supply to the maxilla. Self-donated blood banking was previously advocated by some groups, but this practice is no longer used (severe bleeding that requires transfusion of packed red blood cells is very rare when appropriate transfusion thresholds are followed). The patient should be informed that intermittent small amounts of dark blood may drain from the nose, which may mimic epistaxis, because the blood collection is emptied from the maxillary sinuses.
- **Vascular compromise and maxillary necrosis.** Avascular necrosis of the maxilla is the most feared complication after maxillary orthognathic surgery (higher risk for segmental osteotomies and large advancements). The vascular supply to the maxilla arises from branches of the external carotid artery (ascending palatine artery from the facial artery; also, the ascending pharyngeal, greater and lesser palatines, descending palatine, and nasopalatine artery, all from the internal maxillary artery). Some surgeons elect to ligate and section the descending palatine neurovascular bundle, which has been shown to not significantly affect labial gingival perfusion. Vascular insult results from not only the incisions and osteotomies/downfracture, but also from repositioning of the maxilla. If signs of serious hypoperfusion (pale gingival or palatal mucosa with no capillary refill are early signs and mucosal sloughing is a late sign) are noted intraoperatively, the procedure should be aborted and the maxilla positioned and rigidly fixed into its original position. If poor perfusion is observed postoperatively, removal of splints (if wired to the maxilla for postoperative stability) and removal of rigid fixation to allow the maxilla back into its presurgical position may be required. Maxillary splints

with a palatal strap should be constructed with caution; if they impinge on the palatal mucosa, vascular compromise can result. Hyperbaric oxygen should be considered postoperatively for maxillary hypoperfusion. Smoking has also been implicated in an increased risk of avascular necrosis.
- **Relapse and malpositioning.** Long-term stability is one of the main goals of orthognathic surgery. Closing anterior open bites with posterior impaction of the maxilla is more stable than a mandibular osteotomy with surgical counterclockwise rotation of the mandible. However, more recent studies suggest that counterclockwise surgical rotation of the mandible is very stable, especially with the advent of rigid fixation. If anterior open bite occurs in the immediate postoperative period, it is likely due to incomplete seating of the condyles intraoperatively. This can be minimized by inducing complete paralysis during fixation and upward manual pressure at the angles of the mandible when positioning the maxillomandibular unit (the maxilla can pivot around a posterior bony prematurity, which will pull the condyle out of the glenoid fossa during positioning of the maxillomandibular complex). Bays introduced the rigid adjustable pin (RAP) system, which allows for postoperative three-dimensional adjustability. If relapse of the open bite occurs several weeks to months after surgery or release of maxillomandibular fixation, the most common cause is collapse of the horizontal dimension of the posterior maxilla (bony horizontal relapse for segmental Le Fort osteotomies or dental relapse of molars inappropriately tipped laterally). The RAP system can also be used when there is inadequate bone for miniplate fixation. Aggressive mobilization of the maxilla and passive repositioning with rigid internal fixation are also important for improved long-term stability. Widening and downward moves are the most unstable moves in maxillary surgery.
- **Neurosensory deficits (greater and lesser palatine, nasopalatine, infraorbital nerves).** Although the infraorbital nerve is not severed, traction and compression injuries to this nerve result in a reported 6% incidence of infraorbital nerve neurosensory deficits at 1 year after surgery. Nasopalatine and superior alveolar nerves (posterior, middle, and anterior) are severed during surgery (some surgeons also ligate and section the descending palatine neurovascular bundle). Sensory recovery of the palate is much slower and less complete and is likely due to collateral reinnervation. Neurosensory disturbances of the palate are generally well tolerated.
- **Damage to the dentition (maxillary roots) and periodontal defects.** This is especially a concern in segmental Le Fort I osteotomies (although there are no studies to suggest a higher incidence of periodontal defects in segmental osteotomies). The majority of these complications can be prevented by careful presurgical orthodontic preparation (diverging the roots at the interdental osteotomy sites) and careful surgical technique.
- **Postoperative nasal deformity.** Buckling of the cartilaginous nasal septum (quadrangular cartilage) can cause a nasal deformity (deviation of the nasal tip and buckling of the upper lateral cartilages). The nasal septum and the nasal spine of the maxilla and palatine bones should be appropriately trimmed (especially during maxillary impaction), and the caudal portion of the quadrangular cartilage should be trimmed during maxillary advancement. The nasal septum should be secured to the anterior nasal spine with a heavy resorbable suture to prevent displacement during the recovery phase.

bony gaps, bone grafts may be warranted (especially with large advancements or widening or downgrafting procedures). Egbert and colleagues studied patients undergoing maxillary advancement. These researchers looked at horizontal and vertical relapse and demonstrated improved stability with rigid fixation compared with wire fixation and maxillomandibular fixation.

The soft tissue changes associated with maxillary surgery are predominantly observed in the nasal and labial structures. The nasal changes depend on the type of movement: anterior repositioning results in widening of the nasal base and an increase in the supratip break; superior repositioning leads to elevation of the nasal tip and widening of the nasal base; inferior repositioning results in loss of tip support; and posterior movement results in loss of tip support (because of posterior movement of the anterior nasal spine [ANS]) with minimal change at the alar base. The labial changes include upper lip widening and lengthening of the philtral columns. With V-Y closure, shortening of the upper lip and loss of vermillion are minimized.

A hierarchy of stability in orthognathic surgery has been classically described by Profitt and associates, from most to least stable (modifications to the original description are given in parentheses):

- Maxilla up (non–open bite cases are more stable than open bite cases)
- Mandible forward (low mandibular plane angle is better)
- Maxilla forward
- Maxilla up/mandible forward
- Maxilla forward/mandible back
- Mandible back
- Maxilla down
- Maxilla wider

Bibliography

Bays RA: Maxillary osteotomies utilizing the rigid adjustable pin (RAP) system: a review of 31 clinical cases, *Int J Adult Orthod Orthognath Surg* 1:275, 1986.

Bays RA: Descending palatine artery ligation in LeFort osteotomies, *J Oral Maxillofac Surg* 8:142, 1993.

Bays RA, Bouloux GF: Complications of orthognathic surgery, *Oral Maxillofac Surg Clin North Am* 15:229-242, 2003.

Bell WH: Revascularization and bone healing after anterior maxillary osteotomy: a study using adult rhesus monkeys, *J Oral Surg* 27(4):110-115, 1969.

Bell WH, Proffit WR: Esthetic effects of maxillary osteotomy. In Bell WH, Proffit WR, White RP (eds): *Surgical correction of dentofacial deformities*, pp 368-370, Philadelphia, 1980, Saunders.

Betts NJ: Techniques to control nasal features, *Atlas Oral Maxillofac Surg Clin North Am* 8(2):53-69, 2000.

Betts NJ, Dowd KF: Soft tissue changes associated with orthognathic surgery, *Atlas Oral Maxillofac Surg Clin North Am* 8(2):1-11, 2000.

Betts NJ, Fonseca RJ, Vig P, et al: Changes in nasal and labial soft tissues after surgical repositioning of the maxilla, *Int J Adult Orthod Orthognath Surg* 8:7, 1993.

Brons S, van Beusichem ME, Maal TJJ, et al: Development and reproducibility of a 3D stereophotogrammetric reference frame for facial soft tissue growth of babies and young children with and without orofacial clefts, *Int J Oral Maxillofac Surg* 42:2-8, 2013.

Dodson TB, Bays RA, Neuenschwander MC: Maxillary perfusion during Le Fort I osteotomy after ligation of the descending palatine artery, *J Oral Maxillofac Surg* 55:51-55, 1997.

Egbert M, Hepworth B, Myall R, et al: Stability of Le Fort I osteotomy with maxillary advancement: a comparison of combined wire fixation and rigid fixation, *J Oral Maxillofac Surg* 53:243, 1995.

Guymon M, Crosby DR, Wolford LM: The alar base cinch suture to control nasal width in maxillary osteotomies, *Int J Adult Orthod Orthognath Surg* 3:89, 1988.

Ingersoll SK, Peterson LJ, Weinstein S: Influence of horizontal incision on upper lip morphology, *J Dent Res* 61:218, 1982.

Kau CH, Richmond S, Savio C, et al: Measuring adult facial morphology in three dimensions, *Angle Orthod* 76:773-778, 2006.

Lanigan DT: Vascular complications associated with orthognathic surgery, *Oral Maxillofac Surg Clin North Am* 9(2):231-250, 1997.

Milles M, Betts NJ: Techniques to preserve or modify lip form during orthognathic surgery, *Atlas Oral Maxillofac Surg Clin North Am* 8(2):71-79, 2000.

O'Ryan F, Schendel S: Nasal anatomy and maxillary surgery. I. Esthetic and anatomic principles, *Int J Adult Orthod Orthognath Surg* 4:75, 1989.

O'Ryan F, Schendel S: Nasal anatomy and maxillary surgery. II. Unfavorable nasolabial esthetics following LeFort I osteotomy, *Int J Adult Orthod Orthognath Surg* 4:157, 1989.

Proffit WR, Turvey TA, Phillips C: Orthognathic surgery: a hierarchy of stability, *Int J Adult Orthod Orthognath Surg* 11:191, 1996.

Quejada JG, Kawamura H, Finn RA, et al: Wound healing associated with segmental total maxillary osteotomy, *J Oral Maxillofac Surg* 44:366, 1986.

Radney LJ, Jacobs JD: Soft tissue changes associated with surgical total maxillary intrusion, *Am J Orthod* 80:191, 1981.

Tiner BD, Van Sickels IE, Schmitz JP: Life-threatening delayed hemorrhage after LeFort I osteotomy requiring surgical intervention: report of two cases, *J Oral Maxillofac Surg* 49:571, 1997.

Turvey TA, Fonseca RJ: The anatomy of the internal maxillary artery in the pterygopalatine fossa: its relationship to maxillary surgery, *J Oral Surg* 38:92-95, 1980.

Van Sickels JE: Treatment of skeletal open bite deformities, *OMFS Knowledge Update* 2:45-56, 1998.

Wolford ME: Management of transverse maxillary deficiency, *OMFS Knowledge Update* 1:15-20, 1995.

Zweig BE: Esthetic analysis of the cervicofacial region, *Atlas Oral Maxillofac Surg Clin North Am* 8(2):1-11, 2000.

Maxillomandibular Surgery for Apertognathia

Kevin L. Rieck, Chris Jo, and Shahrokh C. Bagheri

CC

A 17-year-old girl is referred by her orthodontist for combined surgical-orthodontic management of her anterior open bite (apertognathia) and mandibular hypoplasia. She complains that, "I have difficulty eating and would like to have my open bite fixed."

Patients presenting for orthognathic surgical correction of jaw deformities and/or malocclusions most frequently have functional problems. Correction of these issues also can have ramifications for the patient's facial appearance. It is essential to differentiate the degree of functional versus cosmetic dissatisfaction. Successful outcomes require this distinction to be well integrated into the surgical plan.

HPI

The patient reports difficulty chewing certain foods due to the anterior open bite and is also concerned about her facial profile and her retrusive chin. She completed extensive orthodontic therapy as a teenager to close her anterior open bite. This progressively relapsed over time (orthodontic closure of an anterior open bite has a high relapse rate). One week before her surgical consultation, she had orthodontic appliances placed by her orthodontist. She admits to a history of a thumb-sucking habit from childhood into her early teen years (thumb- or finger-sucking habits can cause apertognathia). There is no history of tongue thrusting. (Although this is a difficult parameter to rule out, an unrecognized tongue-thrusting habit can cause future relapse of surgical and orthodontic treatment. Macroglossia should be recognized and treated as needed by tongue reduction procedures.) She is congenitally missing the right maxillary third molar, but the remaining third molars are full bony impactions. (Most surgeons prefer that impacted mandibular third molars be extracted at least 6 months before mandibular sagittal split osteotomy procedures to avoid complications related to fixation. Maxillary molars do not need to be removed in advance.) The patient has no history or symptoms of temporomandibular joint disease (TMD). (Preexisting TMD should be recognized and addressed before orthognathic surgery, which may exacerbate preexisting TMD. Some prominent surgeons recommend simultaneous orthognathic and TMJ surgery in select cases of preexisting anterior disk displacement; however, this issue is highly controversial.)

PMHX/PSHX/MEDICATIONS/ALLERGIES/SH/FH

Noncontributory.

Elective orthognathic surgery should be avoided in patients classified ASA III or higher.

EXAMINATION

The examination of a patient for orthognathic surgery can be divided to four components: TMJ, skeletal, dental, and soft tissue. Skeletal discrepancies (hypoplasia or hyperplasia) should be assessed in three dimensions: transverse (horizontal), anteroposterior, and vertical. As for all surgical patients, the airway, cardiopulmonary, neurologic, and other organ systems should be fully assessed in anticipation of the use of general anesthesia.

The maxillofacial examination of the current patient proceeded as follows.

1. **TMJ component**
   - The muscles of mastication and the TMJ capsule are nontender, with no evidence of clicking or crepitus (seen with disk perforation). The maximal interincisal opening is 45 mm, with good excursive movements and no deviation upon opening or closing (normal TMJ examination).

2. **Skeletal component**
   - There is no vertical orbital dystopia. The intercanthal distance is 31 mm (normal). The nose is straight and coincident with the midline. Malar eminences are within normal limits.
   a. *Transverse dimension*
      - Maxillary dental midline is coincident with the facial midline.
      - Mandibular dental midline is 1 mm right of the maxillary dental midline.
      - Chin point is 2 mm right of the maxillary midline.
      - Maxillary occlusal plane is canted down 1 mm on the right at the canine.
      - Mandibular angles are level.
      - Maxillary arch width is adequate.
   b. *Anteroposterior dimension*
      - Overjet is 6 mm.
      - Nasolabial angle is 110 degrees (normal is 100 degrees ± 10 degrees).
      - Labiomental fold is deep.
      - Chin is retrognathic.
      - Profile is brachycephalic.

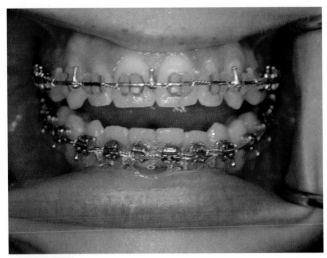

Figure 9-9 Preoperative intraoral view revealing anterior open bite. *(Courtesy Dr. Vincent J. Perciaccante.)*

c. *Vertical dimension*
  - Maxillary incisor length is 10 mm.
  - Upper incisor show is 3 mm at rest (ideally, there is 2 to 4 mm of tooth show at rest) and 8 mm in full smile (in an esthetically pleasing smile line, the gingival papilla or up to 1 mm of gingival margin is visible at full smile).
  - Anterior open bite is 7 mm.
3. **Dental component (occlusion and dentition)**
  - Open bite is 7 mm at incisors and 3 mm at canines, with single divergent occlusal planes (Figure 9-9).
  - Overjet is 6 mm (normal is 3.5 mm ± 2.5 mm).
  - Class II relationship is present at first molars and canines bilaterally.
  - Arch width is adequate on handheld models.
  - Curve of Spee has been leveled.
  - Dentition is in good repair, with no missing teeth (except for third molars).
  - Mandibular arch form is good. There is no mandibular occlusal cant.
4. **Soft tissue component**
  - Upper lip has adequate thickness and length.
  - Nasolabial angle is 85 degrees (normal is 100 degrees ± 10 degrees).
  - Nasal contour is within normal limits (dorsum, alar base, tip).

IMAGING

Panoramic radiograph and lateral cephalometric radiographs are the minimum imaging modalities necessary for orthognathic surgery. Preoperative profile, frontal (repose and smiling), and occlusal photographs should be obtained.

The current patient's panoramic radiograph showed normal bony architecture of the condylar head and no other pathology. The right maxillary third molar was missing, and the left maxillary and left and right mandibular third molars were full bony impacted with minimal root formation (Figure 9-10, *A*).

A lateral cephalogram was obtained with the patient in centric relation and the lips in a relaxed/repose position (Figure 9-10, *B*). Cephalometric analysis revealed anteroposterior maxillary hypoplasia (Table 9-3). It is important to note that measurements differ for Caucasians, Asians, and African Americans (normal values for Caucasians are listed in Table 9-3).

LABS

Baseline hemoglobin and hematocrit are the minimum preoperative laboratory values necessary for orthognathic surgery in the otherwise healthy patient, if required by anesthesia or hospital admissions. No blood work is required in a young, healthy patient classified ASA I or ASA II who has an otherwise negative medical history. Although blood loss requiring transfusion therapy is uncommon for orthognathic surgery, baseline hemoglobin and hematocrit values are helpful in cases of excessive blood loss to determine the need for transfusion or to guide fluid resuscitation. The current patient had normal values (hemoglobin of 13.1 mg/dl and hematocrit of 40.2%).

A pregnancy test (urine pregnancy test or serum β-hCG) is also warranted for females of childbearing age. Because the need for transfusion of blood products is rare, a type and screen is generally not indicated.

ASSESSMENT

Maxillary and mandibular hypoplasia, resulting in apertognathia and a Class II skeletal facial deformity.

TREATMENT

Treatment of a significant anterior open bite typically involves a combined orthodontic and surgical approach for stable results. A coordinated approach involving the orthodontist and the oral and maxillofacial surgeon requires a close working relationship to meet the needs of the patient. The goals of presurgical orthodontic therapy are to:
  - Align and level the occlusion
  - Coordinate the maxillary and mandibular arches (progress is monitored with handheld models)
  - Eliminate dental compensations in preparation for surgical correction of the skeletal deformities

It is important to avoid any unstable orthodontic movement (e.g., closing anterior open bites by extruding maxillary or mandibular anterior teeth or widening the posterior maxillary horizontal dimension by tipping the molars) that would later result in relapse. Postsurgical orthodontics is aimed at creating a final, stable occlusion and closing any posterior open bites that resulted from the surgical correction. Most orthodontists use a retainer for maintenance of the final occlusal relationship and alignment.

Orthognathic surgical treatment options and plans for closure of an anterior open bite include Le Fort I osteotomy with posterior impaction and anterior advancement

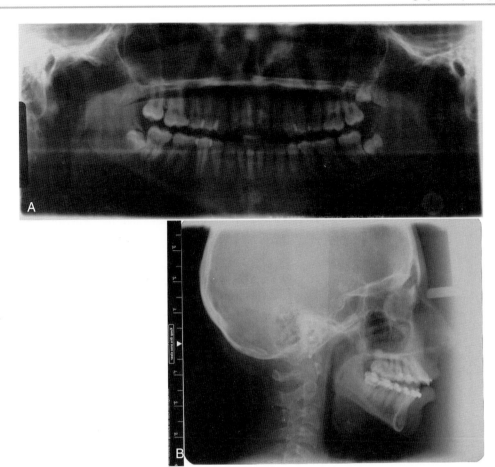

Figure 9-10   **A,** Preoperative panoramic radiograph demonstrating impacted left maxillary and mandibular third molars and an anterior open bite. **B,** Preoperative lateral cephalogram showing the apertognathia and degree of mandibular hypoplasia. *(Courtesy Dr. Vincent J. Perciaccante.)*

Table 9-3	Cephalometric Analysis		
Patient in Figures 9-9 to 9-12	**Normal Parameters for Caucasians**	**Patient Notes**
Cranial base angle: Normal	Sella-nasion (SN)-basion angle: 129 degrees ± 4 degrees	
	Sella-nasion (SN) to Frankfurt horizontal (FH) angle: 7 degrees ± 4 degrees	
SNA: 74 degrees	80 degrees ± 3 degrees	Patient's value is suggestive of a maxillary anteroposterior deficiency relative to the cranial base.
Harvold difference*: 18 mm	Females: 27 mm	Patient's value is suggestive of mandibular hypoplasia.
	Males: 29 mm	
SN-MP: 47 degrees	SN-MP: 32 degrees ± 10 degrees FH-MP:	Patient's mandibular plane (MP) is steep.
FH-MP: 33.5 degrees	22 degrees ± 6 degrees	
Long axis of upper incisor to SN angle: 102 degrees	104 degrees ± 4 degrees	
Long axis of lower incisor to MP angle: 95 degrees	90 degrees ± 5 degrees	
Upper lip to E-plane: −2 mm	−3 mm ± 2 mm	
Lower lip to E-plane: +2.5 mm	−2 mm	Patient's value shows retrusive soft tissue chin and concave profile.

SNA, Sella-nasion, A point.
*The Harvold difference is the distance from condylion to pogonion minus the distance from condylion to A point.

(clockwise rotation), allowing the mandibular arc of rotation to close the anterior open bite (determined by mounted model surgery). The surgeon can control the vertical position of the maxilla and incisors, because the mandibular arc of rotation and model setup determine the final position of both the maxilla and mandible (mounted model surgery is important to determine the anteroposterior position of the maxillomandibular unit when it is set at the desired vertical position). A Le Fort I osteotomy alone can be considered in the following situations:

- The mandible is in good position (dental midline and chin midline coincident with the facial midline)
- There is no mandibular occlusal cant
- The mandible is aligned with the face (symmetrical)
- The mandibular arc of rotation positions the maxilla into a good anteroposterior position while maintaining an appropriate chin projection

A segmental Le Fort I osteotomy is indicated when a transverse deficiency or a dual occlusal plane exists.

- Bimaxillary (maxillomandibular) surgery (Le Fort I and sagittal split or vertical ramus osteotomies) may be warranted when deformities exist in both the maxilla and mandible and the mandibular position and arc of rotation cannot be used to position the maxilla (see Discussion).
- Although controversial and historically considered an unstable move (especially before the advent of rigid fixation), mandibular osteotomies with surgical counterclockwise rotation of the dentate mandibular segment can be used in select clinical situations to close anterior open bites. Frequently, occlusal equilibration is required to remove any prematurities that can cause an unstable occlusion.

Once the surgical treatment plan has been developed, the surgeon can proceed with model surgery to fabricate one or more surgical splints on mounted models. Contemporary orthognathic surgical planning and splint fabrication can be done virtually. Preoperative records are obtained and correlated with either cone-beam computed tomography (CBCT) or medical-grade CT data for this analysis. The surgeon then plans the case virtually with a biomedical engineer. Appropriate splints are forwarded for the surgical procedure. (The details of this technique are discussed on p. 327.) If the open bite is to be closed with maxillary surgery alone, the maxillary cast is set to the ideal occlusion with the opposing mounted mandibular cast (occlusion set with a small posterior open bite maximizes the amount of incisor overlap and reduce relapse). Small posterior open bites can be easily closed orthodontically, especially in young patients (surgically created posterior open bites allow maximal overlap of the anterior teeth, reducing the risk of relapse). A thin interocclusal acrylic wafer (splint) is made to stabilize the occlusion intraoperatively during rigid fixation of the maxilla. If a segmental osteotomy is performed, the splint is made with a palatal strap and wired to the maxillary dentition during the healing phase to prevent horizontal collapse and relapse of the open bite. Various fixation techniques can be used, depending on the clinical situation and the surgeon's preference. The maxilla is generally fixated with four-point fixation (at the piriform rim and zygomaticomaxillary buttress bilaterally) using 1.5- or 2-mm plates. The mandible can be fixated using position screws (lag screws are contraindicated because of their tendency to torque the condylar head) and/or rigid fixation plates with monocortical screws.

In the current patient, a Le Fort I osteotomy and bilateral sagittal split osteotomies were used to correct the anterior open bite and to advance the hypoplastic mandible (Figure 9-11). The maxilla was advanced 2 mm at the incisors and 2.5 mm at the anterior nasal spine. The posterior maxilla was impacted 3 mm, and the anterior maxilla was impacted 0.5 mm. The mandible was allowed to autorotate and was surgically advanced. (It is important to realize the difference between net move [total change in position] and surgical move [surgical change in position after accounting for autorotation].) The patient underwent postoperative orthodontic treatment, and the orthodontic appliances were removed 6 months after surgery. Figure 9-12 shows the final occlusion.

COMPLICATIONS

Complications of maxillary and mandibular surgery are discussed in teaching cases elsewhere in this book. An important complication related to orthognathic surgery for closure of an anterior open bite is long-term stability of the final occlusion (relapse). Several measures can be taken to minimize this outcome:

- Sound orthodontic therapy
- Patient compliance with postoperative retainers
- Avoidance of unstable maxillary or mandibular surgical movements

Immediate postoperative malocclusion or anterior open bite usually results from failure of fixation; inadequate mandibular positioning (failure to seat the condyles during fixation); or inadequate maxillary impaction, causing the condyles to be malpositioned. It is generally recommended that any postsurgical malocclusion be corrected promptly, once the diagnosis has been confirmed, because maintaining the patient in intermaxillary fixation to treat the problem is simply delaying and complicating future treatment.

DISCUSSION

Depending on its etiology, an anterior open bite can be categorized as either predominantly of dental origin without a skeletal component (seen with thumb or finger sucking or abnormal tongue habits) or as a skeletal abnormality (most commonly, posterior maxillary hyperplasia) with or without a dental component. The skeletal deformity in skeletal open bite can be in the maxilla only (elongated posterior maxilla), mandible only (steep mandibular plane angle), or both the maxilla and mandible.

Closing a large anterior open with orthodontic therapy alone is frequently complicated by relapse. A combined orthodontic and surgical modality offers the most stable result.

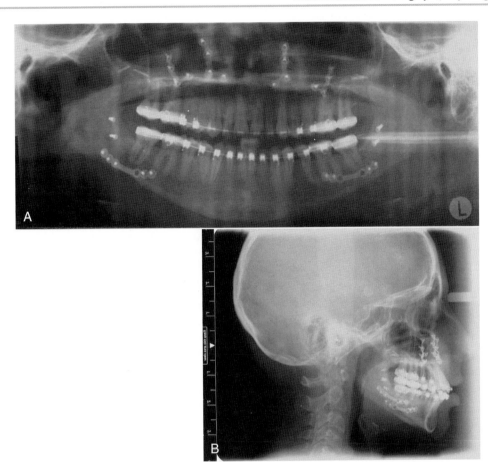

Figure 9-11 **A,** Postoperative panoramic radiograph showing the rigid fixation hardware. **B,** Postoperative lateral cephalogram showing correction of the apertognathia and an esthetically pleasing facial profile. *(Courtesy Dr. Vincent J. Perciaccante.)*

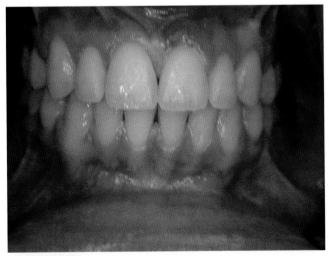

Figure 9-12 Postoperative intraoral view revealing the final occlusion. *(Courtesy Dr. Vincent J. Perciaccante.)*

Preoperative and postoperative orthodontic therapy is mandatory for most orthognathic surgical procedures (except for some cases involving sleep apnea surgery). During the preoperative orthodontic phase, the maxillary and mandibular arch forms are idealized. The occlusion is leveled by eliminating the curve of Spee. Dental compensations are reduced or eliminated by correcting proclined or retroclined incisors. Arch space is evaluated to predict whether it will allow these changes; leveling the curve of Spee, aligning the teeth to proper arch form, and retracting proclined incisors require more arch space. This can be accomplished by interproximal stripping or bicuspid extractions when crowding is an issue.

The Le Fort I osteotomy alone (without mandibular surgery) for correction of an anterior open bite is indicated when the mandible is in an ideal position (the mandibular midline is coincident with the facial midline, there is no mandibular occlusal cant, and the mandible's anteroposterior position is within normal limits) or it demonstrates only a mild anteroposterior hypoplasia (because posterior maxillary impaction allows autorotation of the mandible forward, increasing the anteroposterior projection). Closure of the open bite cannot be esthetically successful with maxillary surgery alone if the mandible is in an asymmetric position. Setting the maxilla to an asymmetric mandible produces poor esthetic results, especially if there is a maxillary anteroposterior discrepancy. When the mandible has a significant midline discrepancy or an occlusal cant, a double jaw procedure is necessary to correct the mandibular discrepancies. Also, the anteroposterior position of the mandible must allow autorotation of the maxilla to a possible and acceptable anteroposterior position, which can be verified only by mounted model surgery.

In cases of anterior open bite in which the maxilla is deficient in the anteroposterior dimension, advancing the maxilla and impacting it posteriorly closes the open bite, with improved long-term stability. Advancement and impaction of the maxilla represent the most stable long-term procedure of the hierarchy of possible orthognathic surgical movements. The posterior teeth may need to be positioned in slight infra-occlusion to allow for overcorrection of the overlap. When maxillary surgery alone is performed, the final maxillary position and occlusion are dictated by the position of the mandible and its arc of rotation. The desired tooth show at rest and during full smile dictates the anterior vertical position of the maxilla and the amount of impaction or disimpaction, using the mandible's arc of rotation. Closing an open bite with mandibular surgery alone is generally considered a less stable move and is not recommended by most surgeons, although it has been recently described for cases involving a smaller open bite. Rigid fixation must be used to secure the mandibular segments and thus minimize the risk of relapse.

Bibliography

Bays RA: Maxillary osteotomies utilizing the rigid adjustable pin (RAP) system: a review of 31 clinical cases, *Int J Adult Orthod Orthognath Surg* 1:275, 1986.

Bays RA, Bouloux GF: Complications of orthognathic surgery, *Oral Maxillofac Surg Clin North Am* 15:229-242, 2003.

Bell RB: Computer planning and intraoperative navigation in orthognathic surgery, *J Oral Maxillofac Surg* 69:592-605, 2011.

Betts NJ: Techniques to control nasal features, *Atlas Oral Maxillofac Surg Clin North Am* 8(2):53-69, 2000.

Betts NJ, Dowd KF: Soft tissue changes associated with orthognathic surgery, *Atlas Oral Maxillofac Surg Clin North Am* 8(2):1-11, 2000.

Dodson TB, Bays RA, Neuenschwander MC: Maxillary perfusion during Le Fort I osteotomy after ligation of the descending palatine artery, *J Oral Maxillofac Surg* 55:51-55, 1997.

Lanigan DT: Vascular complications associated with orthognathic surgery, *Oral Maxillofac Surg Clin North Am* 9(2):231-250, 1997.

McCormick SU, Drew SJ: Virtual model surgery for efficient planning and surgical performance, *J Oral Maxillofac Surg* 69:638-644, 2011.

Milles M, Betts NJ: Techniques to preserve or modify lip form during orthognathic surgery, *Atlas Oral Maxillofac Surg Clin North Am* 8(2):71-79, 2000.

O'Ryan F, Lassetter J: Optimizing facial esthetics in the orthognathic surgical patient, *J Oral Maxillofac Surg* 69:702-715, 2011.

Turvey TA, Fonseca RJ: The anatomy of the internal maxillary artery in the pterygopalatine fossa: its relationship to maxillary surgery, *J Oral Surg* 38:92-95, 1980.

Van Sickels JE: Treatment of skeletal open bite deformities, *OMFS Knowledge Update* 2:45-56, 1998.

Wolford ME: Management of transverse maxillary deficiency, *OMFS Knowledge Update* 1:15-20, 1995.

Zweig BE: Esthetic analysis of the cervicofacial region, *Atlas Oral Maxillofac Surg Clin North Am* 8(2):1-11, 2000.

Distraction Osteogenesis: Mandibular Advancement in Conjunction with Traditional Orthognathic Surgery

Lee M. Whitesides and Shahrokh C. Bagheri

CC

A 26-year-old woman is referred by her orthodontist for consultation regarding the correction of her maxillofacial skeletal deformity. She complains about the excessive amount of maxillary anterior gingiva visible upon smiling ("gummy smile"), and she is not pleased with the amount of overbite.

HPI

The patient has had her "gummy smile" (secondary to vertical maxillary excess) and excessive overbite (secondary to mandibular hypoplasia) since puberty. She explains that this has significantly influenced her appearance during adolescence and adulthood. In addition, she has difficulty biting into food with her front teeth. More recently, she has decided to pursue possible treatment options for her cosmetic and functional deformity. Her orthodontist has recommended a combined surgical/orthodontic correction of the dentofacial deformity.

It is not uncommon for patients with maxillofacial skeletal deformities to have both a cosmetic and a functional component related to the maxillofacial abnormality.

PMHX/PDHX/MEDICATIONS/ALLERGIES/SH/FH

Noncontributory.

EXAMINATION

The patient is a well-developed and well-nourished woman in no apparent distress. She appears to have realistic expectations regarding possible surgical interventions.

Maxillofacial. Evaluation of patients for dentofacial deformities should be done in three dimensions (transverse, vertical, and anteroposterior) for the maxilla and the mandible. The dentition is evaluated for occlusion, alignment, and the status of the periodontal tissue.

The maxillofacial examination of the current patient proceeded as follows.

1. **Transverse dimension**
   - Maxillary midline to facial midline: coincident.
   - Mandible midline to maxillary midline: mandible is to the left 1 mm.
   - Chin to maxillary midline: chin is to the left 2 mm.
   - Occlusal plane is level with no cant and no curve of Spee or Wilson.
   - Mandibular angles are level with no visible cant.
   - Arch width is adequate (as determined by examination of models).
2. **Anteroposterior dimension**
   - Overjet is −12 mm.
   - Nasolabial angle is 125 degrees (normal is about 100 degrees to 110 degrees).
   - Labiomental fold is deep (abnormal).
   - Chin is microgenic.
3. **Vertical dimension**
   - Upper central teeth show at rest is 8 mm (normal for females is 3 to 4 mm).
   - Upper central teeth show with speech is 7 to 9 mm (excessive).
   - Upper central teeth show with smiling is 5 mm of gingival show (gummy smile).
   - Open bite is Class II occlusion.

Examination of the temporomandibular joint (TMJ) reveals no abnormalities.

IMAGING

A lateral cephalogram, panoramic radiograph, and standard facial and dental photographs are the minimal imaging studies necessary in preparation for distraction osteogenesis in combination with orthognathic surgery. A three-dimensional, actual-size stereolithographic model can be reconstructed using high-resolution computed tomography (CT) scans. These models can be used in preparation for distraction osteogenesis to demonstrate the quantity and topography of the bone in the distraction site. They also assist the surgeon by delineating pertinent anatomic structures in the bone, such as the inferior alveolar nerve. This information is extremely helpful.

Cone-beam CT (CBCT) can be used to image the patient with a high degree of anatomic truth. This information may then be used to virtually plan the case by assisting in osteotomy design and placement and in distraction device placement and vector. Virtual three-dimensional planning of the surgery provides the surgeon with an accurate representation of the anticipated outcome and assists in uncovering any possible weaknesses in the surgical plan. Stereolithic templates made from CBCT permit the transfer of the three-dimensional planning to the patient during surgery.

The lateral cephalogram is used for analysis of cephalometric norms. By comparing a patient's values with normal values, the surgeon arrives at an appropriate diagnosis, and anticipated surgical movements in the anteroposterior and

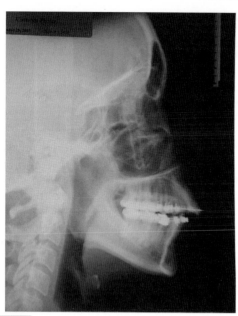

Figure 9-13 Preoperative lateral cephalogram demonstrating significant anteroposterior mandibular hypoplasia.

Table 9-4	Cephalometric Analysis	
Patient in Figures 9-13 and 9-14		**Normal Parameters for Caucasians**
Horizontal Skeletal Profile		
Nasion perpendicular to B point: −15 mm		−5.3 mm ± 6.7 mm
Nasion perpendicular to pogonion: −17 mm		−4.3 mm ± 8.5 mm
Vertical Skeletal Profile		
N-ANS: 60 mm		54.7 mm ± 3.2 mm
Posterior nasal spine (PNS) to nasion: 77 mm		53.9 mm ± 1.7 mm
Maxillary central incisor edge to nasal floor: 41 mm		30.5 mm ± 2.1 mm
Maxillary molar cusp tip to nasal floor: 40 mm		26.2 mm ± 2 mm
ANS to gnathion: 81 mm		68.6 mm ± 3.8 mm
Mandibular central incisor edge to MP: 50 mm		45 mm ± 2.1 mm
MP horizontal plane: 34 degrees		23 degrees ± 5.9 degrees

ANS, Anterior nasal spine; *MP,* mandibular plane; *N-ANS,* nasion-anterior nasal spine.

vertical dimensions can be predicted. This also allows evaluation of the facial soft tissue profile.

For the current patient, the preoperative lateral cephalogram is shown in Figure 9-13. Cephalometric analysis was performed using the COGS analysis (as described by Burnstone in 1978) prior to orthodontic therapy (Table 9-4). The two abnormal measurements from the horizontal skeletal profile are indicative of mandibular hypoplasia in the anteroposterior dimension. The first four values of the vertical skeletal profile indicate that the patient has an increased facial height (vertical maxillary excess). The anterior nasal spine (ANS) to gnathion, and the distance of the mandibular plane indicate that the patient has a "long face." The high mandibular plane angle (34 degrees) is typical of patients with vertical maxillary excess and long facial height.

The panoramic radiograph reveals no osseous or dental pathologic processes.

LABS

Baseline hemoglobin and hematocrit values are the minimum laboratory tests necessary in anticipation of orthognathic surgery. Although significant blood loss requiring transfusion is highly unlikely with the modern practice of maxillary and mandibular orthognathic surgery, hemoglobin and hematocrit values are important as baseline markers for all major surgical procedures. Other laboratory tests are indicated based on the medical history. A pregnancy test is highly recommended for all women of childbearing age.

The current patient had a hemoglobin of 13 mg/dl and a hematocrit of 39.5%. Her urine pregnancy test was negative.

ASSESSMENT

Maxillary hyperplasia, mandibular hypoplasia (anteroposterior), mild mandibular asymmetry, and microgenia.

TREATMENT

The goals of combined surgical/orthodontic treatment are to establish a functional and a cosmetic improvement in the dentofacial structures. Several surgical modalities are available for advancement of the mandible to correct the anteroposterior deficiency. Techniques of distraction osteogenesis are usually considered in cases in which a large mandibular advancement would be necessary to treat the mandibular hypoplasia.

The two most common methods of mandible advancement are the bilateral sagittal split osteotomy, as first described by Obwegeser, and mandibular osteotomy with application of bilateral distraction devices, as described by Guerrero and colleagues. The sagittal split osteotomy has been used by surgeons for more than 30 years and is described elsewhere in this text. Distraction osteogenesis surgery has been used for at least 10 years to treat deformities of the maxillofacial and craniofacial skeleton.

Distraction osteogenesis surgery can be divided into five phases:

Phase 1. *Surgery:* The sectioning of hard and soft tissue and application of a distraction device
Phase 2. *Latency:* The healing time between surgery and device activation
Phase 3. *Activation:* The process of gradually separating the tissue to increase length and mass

Phase 4. *Consolidation:* The primary healing of the distracted tissue and formation of the bony callus

Phase 5. *Remodeling:* The secondary healing of soft tissue and the change of immature bone into mature bone in the distraction gap

For the current patient, the left mandibular cuspid and the right mandibular first bicuspid (teeth #22 and #28) were extracted per the orthodontist to permit her to level and align the mandibular teeth before orthognathic/distraction osteogenesis surgery. The initial amount of overjet increased to 15 mm after the presurgical orthodontics, correcting the dental compensation. Additionally, surgical impaction of the maxilla increases the mandibular arc of rotation, further increasing the distance for mandibular advancement.

It was decided to address the skeletal deformity in two stages. First, correction of the maxillary hyperplasia, followed by distraction osteogenesis for mandibular advancement. In correction of the maxillary hyperplasia, a Le Fort I osteotomy is used to separate the maxilla from the cranial base to correct the vertical dimension. Bilateral distraction osteogenesis devices are placed in the posterior mandible, after mandibular sagittal split osteotomy, for forward distraction of the mandible.

While the patient was under general anesthesia, she underwent a standard Le Fort I osteotomy with reduction of the vertical height of the maxilla of approximately 5 mm. The maxilla was appropriately positioned on the cranial base and then rigidly fixed with plates and screws. Subsequently, mandibular sagittal split osteotomy was performed bilaterally, and a distraction device was applied across each osteotomy site. An advancement sliding genioplasty was also performed to correct for microgenia. The patient recovered uneventfully from the surgery and was discharged from the hospital 2 days later with oral analgesics and antibiotics. Figure 9-14, *A*, shows the postoperative lateral cephalogram.

After 6 days of latency, the distraction devices were activated at the rate of 1 mm per day until the patient's mandible had advanced into a Class I occlusion. During the activation process, the patient was permitted to activate the device herself unless she was seen in the clinic. She was monitored at least every 4 days at an office visit, where the surgeon activated the device to obtain a "feel" for how well the devices were working. The patient was maintained in Class II elastics bilaterally during the activation period and allowed to eat a soft diet. Figure 9-14, *B*, shows the distraction devices in position close to completion of the activation phase.

After 5 days of consecutive activation, the patient was permitted a day when the devices were not activated. Total time of the active phase of distraction was approximately 1 month.

At the end of distraction, the patient's mandible had advanced into a Class I occlusion. The total advancement measured 18 mm. Figure 9-14, *C*, demonstrates the postoperative lateral cephalogram after completion of the activation phase.

Six months after cessation of distraction, the patient underwent removal of bilateral distraction devices under intravenous sedation. Removal of the distraction devices was predicated on radiographic demonstration of adequate bone mass in the distraction gap and clinical confirmation of adequate healing.

COMPLICATIONS

Complications of mandibular advancement with traditional sagittal split osteotomies are discussed elsewhere in this text (see the section Mandibular Orthognathic Surgery earlier in this chapter).

Potential complications of mandibular advancement with distraction osteogenesis include those discussed for traditional mandibular osteotomies, in addition to failure of the device, infected hardware, and patient noncompliance. A complication unique to distraction osteogenesis surgery is placement of the device along the improper vector. When this occurs, the surgeon must either replace the device at a second surgery or use elastic traction to gradually influence the direction of the advancing segment. Such use of elastics is commonly called "molding the regenerate."

DISCUSSION

The use of distraction osteogenesis surgery dates to the late 1800s; however, Dr. Gavril Ilizarov is considered the "father" of modern distraction osteogenesis surgery. More recently, in the 1990s, McCarthy, Guerrero, Chin, Molina, and many others pioneered the use of distraction osteogenesis surgery to treat selected deformities of the maxillofacial and craniofacial skeletal. Since then, as the technology has improved and more surgeons have learned the technique, distraction osteogenesis surgery has gained popularity as a predictable method to treat selected deformities of the facial skeleton.

The process of distracting a healing wound to grow tissue takes advantage of the body's natural healing mechanisms. During the active distraction process, as the segments of bone are gradually separated, the body sends massive amounts of growth factors, bone morphogenic proteins, and precursor cells to the wound. These cells, which are the building blocks for new tissue, work to regenerate the missing hard and soft tissue in the gap created by the distraction.

As with any other surgical technique, certain principles must be respected in distraction osteogenesis surgery if the surgeon is to be successful. The basic surgical principles of maintaining excellent blood supply and conserving soft tissue in the area to be distracted are paramount for success. If either of these axioms is ignored, the body will not be capable of regenerating new tissue in the distraction gap, and/or the wound will undergo dehiscence.

Close attention to the wound as it heals is very important. Because the distraction device protrudes from the soft tissue mucosa, these wounds have an increased risk of infection.

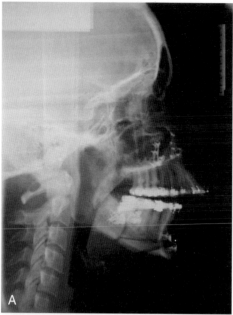

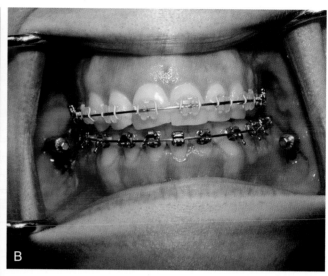

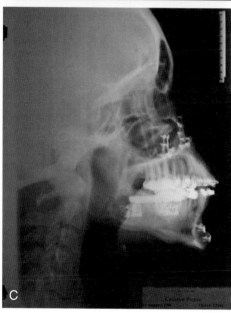

Figure 9-14 **A,** Immediate (2 days) postoperative lateral cephalogram after a mandibular osteotomy and placement of bilateral mandibular distraction device, Le Fort I osteotomy, and sliding genioplasty. The distraction device has not been activated. **B,** Intraoral view demonstrating the position of the bilateral distraction near completion of the active phase. **C,** Postoperative lateral cephalogram at 5 weeks after completion of anterior mandibular distraction osteogenesis and before completion of postsurgical orthodontics.

Last, the surgeon must be diligent in critically evaluating how the distraction process is proceeding. Frequent evaluations, both clinical and radiologic, must be done to examine the device, the vector of distraction, and the response of the soft tissue. This diligence permits anticipation of potential complications.

The advantages and disadvantages of each method should be considered in the presurgical planning phase. A bilateral sagittal split osteotomy with rigid fixation offers the patient an acute lengthening of the mandible into the desired position at the time of surgery. Drawbacks of this method in the current case included the likely need of a bone graft and/or maxillomandibular fixation in association with rigid fixation for large mandibular advancements. Additionally, the acute,

severe stretching of the inferior alveolar nerve has been reported to cause damage to the inferior alveolar nerve. Furthermore, large mandibular advancements are associated with a greater propensity for relapse.

Mandibular osteotomy, sagittal or vertical, with application of distraction devices can potentially produces less acute trauma, eliminates the need of a bone graft, and produces less damage to the inferior alveolar nerve. Additionally, mandibular advancement with distraction osteogenesis surgery allows the surgeon to fine-tune the advancement by gradually molding the regenerate with elastic forces as the patient's mandible is advanced. The long-term stability of the distracted mandible is considered to be reliable and predictable.

Many recent articles have addressed the modification of the distraction osteogenesis protocol by adding osteogenic substances, such as rh-BMP 2 and mesenchymal stem cells, to the distraction gap during the consolidation period. This has proven to accelerate the formation of bone in the distraction gap and thus permit earlier removal of the distraction device.

The addition of osteogenic substances to the distraction gap post activation is a logical progression in distraction histiogenesis. The distraction process is designed to stimulate the body's natural histiogenic mechanisms to generate both hard (bone) and soft (mucosa) tissue. Adding osteogenic substances in the distraction gap post activation allows new bone to form faster and in the appropriate location. This speeds the patient's recovery and lessens the opportunity for complications such as infection and malunion.

Bibliography

Burstone CJ, James RB, Legan H, et al: Cephalometrics for orthognathic surgery, *J Oral Surg* 36:269-277, 1978.

Cheung LK, Zheng LW: Effect of recombinant human bone morphogenic protein-2 on mandibular distraction at different rates in an experimental model, *J Craniofac Surg* 17(1):100-108, 2006.

Chin M, Toth BA: Distraction osteogenesis in the maxillofacial surgery using internal devices: review of five cases, *J Oral Maxillofac Surg* 54:453-485, 1996.

Choy JY, Hwang KG, Baek SH, et al: Original sagittal split osteotomy revisited for mandibular distraction, *J Craniomaxillofac Surg* 29:165-173, 2001.

Diner TA, Tomatt C, Soupre V, et al: Intraoral mandibular distraction: indications, technique, and long term results, *Ann Acad Med* 28:634-643, 1999.

Garey TM, Klotch DW, Sasse J, et al: Basement membrane of blood vessels during distraction osteogenesis, *Clin Orthop Relat Res* 301:132-138, 1994.

Guerrero CA, Bell WH, Gonzalez M, et al: Intraoral distraction osteogenesis. In Fonseca RJ (ed): *Oral and maxillofacial surgery*, pp 359-402, Philadelphia, 2000, Saunders.

Hwang YJ, Choi JY: Addition of mesenchymal stem cells to scaffold of platelet-rich plasma is beneficial for the reduction of the consolidation period in mandibular distraction osteogenesis, *J Oral Maxillofac Surg* 68:1112-1124, 2010.

Ilizarov GA: The tension-stress effect on the genesis and growth of tissues. I. The influence of stability and fixation and soft tissue preservation, *Clin Orthop Relat Res* 238:249, 1989.

Ilizarov GA: The tension-stress effect on the genesis and growth of tissues. II. The influence of rate and frequency of distraction, *Clin Orthop Relat Res* 239:263, 1989.

Ilizarov GA, Ledyaev VI: The replacement of long tubular bone defects by lengthening distraction osteotomy of defragments, *Clin Orthop Relat Res* 238:7, 1992.

Issa JPM, Nascimento C, Lamano T, et al: Effect of recombinant human bone morphogenic protein-2 on bone formation in the acute distraction osteogenesis of rate mandibles, *Clin Oral Implant Res* 20(11):1286-1292, 2009.

Kroczek A, Park J, Birkholz T, et al: Effects of osteoinduction on bone regeneration in distraction: results of a pilot study, *J Craniomaxillofac Surg* 38:334-344, 2010.

McCarthy JG: The role of distraction osteogenesis in the reconstruction of the mandible in unilateral craniofacial microsomia, *Clin Plast Surg* 21:625, 1994.

Molina F, Ortis-Monasterio F: Mandibular elongation and remodeling by distraction: a farewell to major osteotomies, *Plast Reconstr Surg* 96:825, 1995.

Quevedo LA, Ruiz JV, Quevedo CA: Using a clinical protocol for orthognathic surgery and assessing a three-dimensional virtual approach—current therapy, *J Oral Maxillofac Surg* 69:623-637, 2011.

Robiony M, Polini F, Costa F, et al: Osteogenesis distraction and platelet rich plasma for bone restoration of the severely atrophic mandible: preliminary results, *J Oral Maxillofac Surg* 60(6):630-635, 2002.

Robiony M, Zorzan E, Polini F, et al: Osteogenesis distraction and platelet-rich plasma: combined use in restoration of severe atrophic mandibles—long-term results, *Clin Oral Implant Res* 19:1202-1210, 2008.

Seeberger R, Davids R, Kater W, et al: Use of stereolithographic drilling and cutting guides in bilateral mandibulae distraction, *J Craniofac Surg* 22(6):2031-2035, 2011.

Whitesides LM, Meyer RA: Effect of distraction osteogenesis on the severely hypoplastic mandible and inferior alveolar nerve function, *J Oral Maxillofac Surg* 62(3):292-297, 2004.

Inferior Alveolar Nerve Injury

Roger A. Meyer and Shahrokh C. Bagheri

CC

A 24-year-old male is referred for evaluation and treatment of numbness and pain in his entire lower lip, chin, and gums.

HPI

The patient had a Le Fort I maxillary osteotomy (LF1), bilateral mandibular sagittal split ramus osteotomies (SSROs), and genioplasty for correction of maxillomandibular deformities 7 months ago. No injuries to the inferior alveolar nerves (IANs) or mental nerves (MNs) were noted in the operative report. After surgery, both sides of his lower lip, chin, and mandibular labial gingiva remained numb. Six weeks after surgery the numbness persisted, and clinical testing revealed that the entire lower lip, chin, and mandibular labial gingiva were anesthetic. In the past month, the patient began to notice that daily activities such as chewing food, brushing his lower teeth, washing his face, or shaving caused painful sensations in the numb areas. Kissing his girlfriend also caused these painful symptoms. There has been no improvement in the numbness, and the painful sensations seem to be getting more intense and longer in duration. He has noticed drooling of food and fluids, and he has accidentally bitten his lower lip several times while eating. He has been referred for further evaluation.

PMHX/PDHX/MEDICATIONS/ALLERGIES/SHX/FHX

The patient is in good general health. His only other previous surgery was removal of wisdom teeth at age 18 years. He takes no chronic medications and has no known allergies.

EXAMINATION

General. The patient is a well-developed, well-nourished young adult male with a normal facial profile. He is in no acute distress. His vital signs are normal, and his weight is 178 pounds.

Maxillofacial. There is no facial edema. There is no temporomandibular joint (TMJ) or masticatory muscle tenderness. The nasal passages are patent, and the nasal septum is in the midline. There is no evidence of recent trauma to the lower lip. Voluntary interincisal opening is 41 mm, and there is no mandibular deviation on opening. There are orthodontic appliances on both dental arches, and the dental occlusion is Class I with some minor rotational discrepancies. The surgical incisions in the maxillary and mandibular labiobuccal vestibules are well healed with minimal scarring. The level of oral hygiene is good except in the anterior mandible, where there is some accumulation of debris on the labiobuccal aspect of the incisor, canine, and premolar teeth and moderate inflammation of the associated gingiva (attributed to difficulty with hygiene due to pain). The tongue, palate, and pharynx are normal. There are no abnormal neck masses, and the carotid pulses are normal.

Cranial nerves. Cranial nerves II through XII are normal except for the mandibular divisions (V3) of the right and left trigeminal nerves. Within the V3s, the distributions of the right and left IANs and MNs are found to be abnormal. (These nerves are evaluated bilaterally using neurosensory testing [NST] at levels A, B, and C [see Lingual Nerve Injury in Chapter 5; also Box 5-3]). Both sides of the lower lip, chin, and mandibular labial gingiva are anesthetic to levels A (directional two-point discrimination), B (contact detection), and C (pain sensitivity). In addition, when any area of the lower lip, chin, or mandibular labial gingiva or mucosa is gently stroked with a cotton wisp, there is a definite pain response that disappears upon withdrawal of the stimulus (i.e., *allodynia,* a painful response to a stimulus that is ordinarily not painful). Repetitive tapping of these same areas produces a delayed-onset pain response that increases with intensity and persists for 20 to 30 seconds after discontinuation of the stimulus (i.e., *hyperpathia,* a painful response that is characterized by a delayed onset after initial application of the stimulus, that often builds in intensity with repeated application of the stimulus [so-called crescendo], and that persists for a variable period after discontinuation of the stimulus [so-called afterglow]).

IMAGING

A cone-beam computed tomography (CBCT) scan shows fixation screws and plates at the Le Fort I level, two plates with screws in the genioplasty area, plates and screws at the areas of the sagittal split osteotomies, bicortical positioning screws on each side of the mandible that were not superimposed on the inferior alveolar canals (IACs), and some loss of definition of osteotomy cuts (due to the healing process). The horizontal osteotomies for the genioplasty appear to traverse through both inferior alveolar canals (Figure 9-15).

318

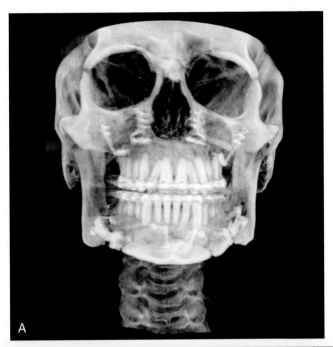

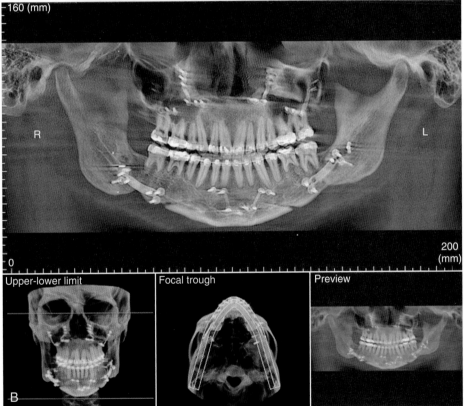

Figure 9-15   **A,** CBCT reconstruction showing internal fixation screws in the maxilla and mandible corresponding to the Le Fort I, bilateral sagittal split ramus osteotomy (BSSRO), and genioplasty surgery. Screws are located above the inferior alveolar canal in the right mandible. The genioplasty osteotomies appear to transect the inferior alveolar nerves bilaterally. **B,** CBCT panoramic reconstruction film demonstrates inappropriate horizontal osteotomy cuts that are too close to the mental foramina; these inadvertently crossed the inferior alveolar canals, causing bilateral inferior alveolar nerve injuries.

DIAGNOSTIC BLOCKS

Local anesthetic blocks (2% lidocaine with 1:100,000 epinephrine) of the right and left IANs were administered into both pterygomandibular spaces. In a few minutes the allodynia and hyperpathia were abolished, and this pain relief lasted for the duration of the blocks. This finding is suggestive of pain originating distal to the location of the blocks (either within the courses of the IANs or at the sites of injury to the MNs). With this result, there is a reasonable chance that microsurgical repair of these peripheral nerves will result in reduction, if not abolition, of the pain. This is in contrast to centralized pain that usually does not improve with a peripheral nerve block and is not favorably affected by peripheral nerve surgery.

LABS

There are no studies indicated for the routine evaluation of a peripheral nerve injury, and this patient has no medical history or physical findings that require specific blood or urine investigation.

ASSESSMENT

Right and left IAN/MN injuries, classified as a neurotmesis (Seddon classification) or fifth-degree injury (Sunderland classification) (see Table 5-1). This is complete anatomic (e.g., severance) and/or physiologic (conduction failure) disruption of all axonal and endoneurial elements of the nerves. In addition, the patient has developed bothersome painful symptoms (allodynia, hyperpathia).

In an injury in which there has been persistent anesthesia for longer than 3 months, the prognosis for meaningful spontaneous improvement or full recovery of sensory function is dismal. When painful symptoms develop, it is important to treat them early (i.e., within 6 to 9 months after injury) to minimize the chance of a chronic, intractable, benign pain syndrome developing. Such a condition is often seen in patients whose neuropathic pain is untreated or inadequately treated and allowed to persist beyond 12 months after nerve injury. The condition may become debilitating, interfering with the normal activities of daily living (e.g., eating, hygiene, sleeping, employment, normal social interactions), and intractable to medical or surgical intervention. The current patient is approaching that critical timeline; therefore, it is important that treatment for pain control be initiated forthwith.

TREATMENT

The initial goal of treatment in the current patient was pain control. He was started on clonazepam 0.5 mg every 8 hours, which brought him relief of allodynia and hyperpathia. There was some mild sedation effect, but this was well-tolerated in view of the adequacy of pain relief. Although the medication dose could be adjusted, it was not necessary in this patient, because the sedation resolved after 2 weeks. Other

medications available for control of neuropathic pain include gabapentin and pregabalin, among others. Narcotics are not efficacious for relief of acute neuropathic pain, which in some patients may require long-term management.

Surgical intervention is indicated for these IAN/MN injuries because they have failed to resolve or improve to an acceptable level for this patient within a reasonable period, and the symptoms (loss of sensation and pain) interfere with the patient's quality of life. Further expectant observation in the vain hope that meaningful spontaneous improvement will occur sometime in the distant future decreases the likelihood of a successful outcome of nerve repair and increases the patient's risk of developing an intractable pain syndrome.

The most difficult determination in the surgical approach to an IAN injury from SSRO is locating the site of the injury. During an SSRO, the IAN is exposed to surgical manipulation (and, therefore, risk of injury) from its course within the pterygomandibular space medial to the mandibular ramus, anteriorly into the IAC at the mandibular foramen, and terminally at its division into the mental and incisive nerves. Therefore, the surgeon must plan to access all these areas through a single surgical incision for the best visibility and for any and all possible surgical manipulations, including neurorrhaphy or reconstruction of a nerve gap (see Table 5-2). In some patients, the favored approach is through a submandibular skin incision, but this depends on individual patient requirements (adequacy of access; visualization and instrumentation; the desire to avoid a visible scar in the upper neck) and the surgeon's judgment and experience. In the current patient, because the horizontal osteotomy cuts were seen to traverse the anterior aspect of the inferior alveolar canals, surgical planning called for exposure of the MN/IAN junctions transorally (Figure 9-16, *A*). Further proximal (posterior) exposure of the IANs could be attempted through the same incisions in the mouth. If an injury to the IANs could not be adequately visualized and treated, a submandibular approach could then be used. The patient was advised of all these considerations, with their relative risks and benefits, and he consented to either of the two surgical approaches, depending on the surgeon's determination at the time of the operation.

The patient was taken to the hospital operating room, and general oral endotracheal anesthesia was administered. Alternate compression devices were applied to both lower extremities and activated, and the urinary bladder was catheterized. The face and perioral region were sterilely prepped and draped. A pharyngeal pack was inserted, and the mouth was thoroughly rinsed with chlorhexidine solution. Bilateral IAN blocks and infiltration of the mandibular labiobuccal vestibule were done with 0.5% bupivacaine/epinephrine 1:100,000. An incision was made from right to left in the mandibular vestibular mucosa, including the previous surgical scars. A full labiobuccal mucoperiosteal flap was raised, and both mental nerves were identified and protected. All osteotomy sites in the mandible were well healed and ossified. The genioplasty and right and left mandibular internal fixation plates and screws were removed. The entire right IAC was exposed by removal of overlying lateral mandibular bone with the

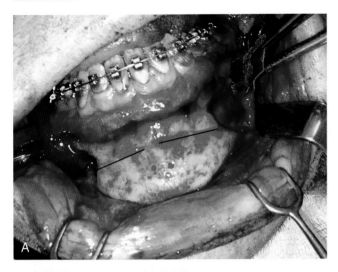

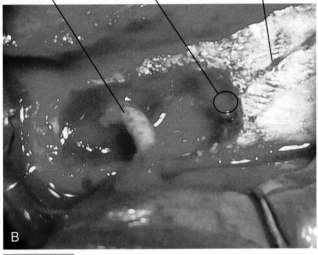

| Nerve graft and | Position of | Area of prior |
| repositioned IAN/MN | mental foramen | genioplasty osteotomy |

Figure 9-16 **A,** Exposure of the mandible, mental nerves, and IAN via a circumvestibular incision. The black lines outline the prior genioplasty osteotomy line that transects both IANs. The IANs can be further exposed posteriorly by extension of the incision. **B,** Reconstruction of the right IAN using an peripheral nerve allograft (AxoGen, Inc.; Alachua, Florida).

high-speed drill, fine osteotomes, and curettes. There was a complete discontinuity defect of the right IAN at its junction with the MN. The remainder of the IAN was intact proximally to where it entered the IAC at the mandibular foramen. Inspection under magnification (foot-controlled operating microscope with ports for surgeon, assistant and/or camera, or surgical loupes of ×2.5-×5.0, depending on surgical needs and the surgeon's preference) revealed that the proximal stump of the IAN ended in a neuroma-like bulb surrounded by considerable scar tissue. The IAN proximal to this area was intact, as was the MN with its three branches proceeding distally into the buccal mucosa. The stump ends of the IAN and MN were debrided and prepared for reconstruction with removal of the neuroma (later verified by the pathologist's report) and scar tissue and exposure of viable nerve fascicles. This left a significant nerve gap (2 cm). Microsurgical repair

was done using a processed heterogenous nerve graft sutured (interrupted 8-0 nylon ophthalmic sutures) to the epineurial layers of the IAN proximally and the MN distally (Figure 9-16, *B*). The reconstructed nerve was entubulated by a processed nerve cuff. (A nerve cuff enhances the healing process in the nerve by preventing percolation of blood and the ingrowth of scar tissue between the nerve stumps.)

Alternately, the nerve gap can be reconstructed using an autogenous nerve graft, commonly either the great auricular nerve (GAN) in the neck or the sural nerve (SN) in the lower extremity (Figure 9-17).

Next, the left IAC was unroofed similarly to the procedure in the right mandible. The left MN was found to be intact. In the midportion of the left IAN there was a neuroma-in-continuity of 0.6 cm in length. The neuroma and associated scar tissue were excised and the nerve stumps debrided to expose viable fascicles; this left a nerve gap of 1 cm. The left incisive nerve was transected, which allowed mobilization of the MN to bring it into tension-free approximation with the distal stump of the IAN. A microsurgical neurorrhaphy through the epineurial layers only was done using four interrupted 8-0 ophthalmic nylon sutures. The repaired left IAN was entubulated with a nerve cuff.

The entire operative site was thoroughly irrigated with sterile saline. There was good hemostasis. The incision was closed in two layers using 3-0 chromic sutures. The throat pack was removed, and the oral cavity and pharynx were irrigated and suctioned. A pressure dressing was applied externally to the chin and mandible. The urinary bladder catheter was removed. General anesthesia was concluded, the patient was extubated, and then he was taken to the postanesthesia care unit in good condition.

The patient did well after surgery. The next morning the pressure dressing was removed, and he was discharged from the hospital. The incision healed normally. The patient was maintained on clonazepam for 1 month. This was then tapered gradually until it was discontinued after the second postoperative month, without return of neuropathic pain. There was mild paresis of the right lower lip (marginal mandibular nerve weakness, most likely due to prolonged soft tissue flap retraction for the right IAN reconstruction), which resolved after about 3 months with the assistance of daily motor exercises performed at home by the patient. At 6 months after surgery, the patient began to experience spontaneous tingling in his left lower lip. Seven months postoperatively, the left lower lip, chin, and labial gingiva responded to painful stimuli and light touch. At 9 months after surgery, the right lower lip, chin, and gingiva began to respond to stimuli. There was no hyperesthesia. Sensory reeducation exercises for the lower lip, chin, and gingiva were begun and continued three times daily. One year after the operation, the left lower lip, chin, and labial gingiva responded to painful stimuli and static light touch at normal thresholds, and the two-point discrimination (2 pd) threshold in the left lower lip was 12 mm (Table 9-5). The patient continued sensory reeducation exercises for another 6 months. Eighteen months after the surgery, the right side had achieved a 2 pd threshold of 11 mm, and on the left side it

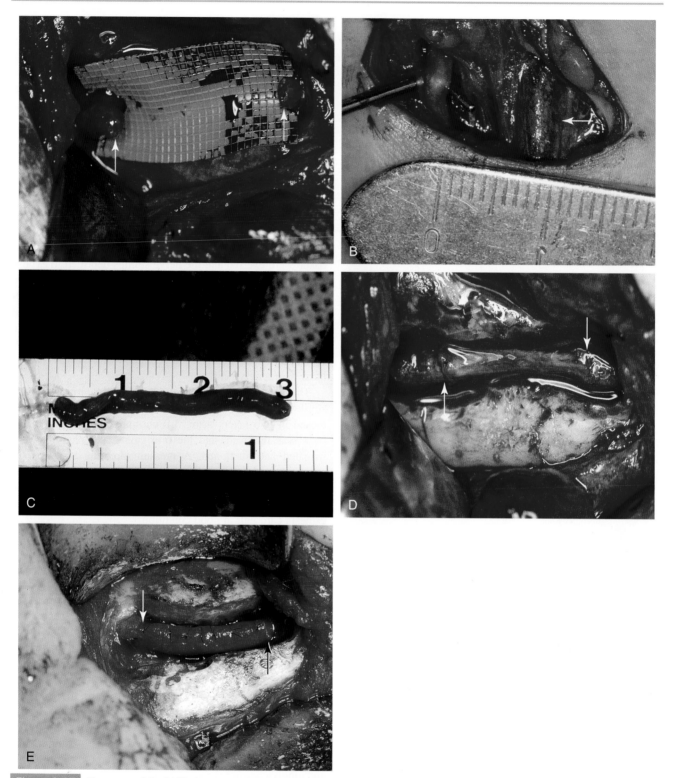

Figure 9-17 Exposure of the IAN via a transcutaneous approach. **A,** The damaged IAN segment has been removed. **B,** Exposure of the great auricular nerve (GAN) (cradled by a nerve hook) in the right side of the neck. The external jugular vein *(arrow)* is an important adjacent anterior landmark. **C,** A 3-cm graft has been harvested from the donor right GAN. **D,** The right IAN nerve gap has been reconstructed with the GAN autogenous graft *(arrows* indicate the suture lines). **E,** Reconstructed right IAN using the GAN graft. The reconstructed right IAN has been encircled by an absorbable collagen nerve cuff *(arrows* indicate the ends of the cuff).

Table 9-5	Medical Research Council Scale for Evaluation of Peripheral Nerve Function (Modified for the Trigeminal Nerve)

Score*	Assessment
S0	No recovery of sensation
S1	Recovery of deep cutaneous sensation
S2	Return of some superficial pain/tactile sensation
S2+	Same as S2 with hyperesthesia
S3	Same as S2 without hyperesthesia; static two-point discrimination (2 pd) > 15 mm
S3+	Same as S3 with good stimulus localization; 2 pd of 7-15 mm
S4	Same as S3+, except 2 pd is 2-6 mm

Modified from Meyer RA, Rath EM: Sensory rehabilitation after trigeminal injury or nerve repair, *Oral Maxillofac Surg Clin North Am* 13(2):365, 2001.
*S3 and S3+ indicate useful sensory function. S4 is complete recovery. Hyperesthesia is an exaggerated stimulus response (e.g., allodynia, hyperpathia, hyperalgesia).

was now 6 mm. The patient was free of pain. He was able to chew food, brush his teeth, wash and shave his face, speak and kiss without difficulty. He was encouraged to continue the daily sensory reeducation exercises until he felt that sensation was equal on both sides of his lower lip and chin. He was satisfied with his sensory function and ability to perform normal orofacial functions, and he was dismissed from care.

COMPLICATIONS

Whenever surgery is performed on a sensory nerve, four possible outcomes must be considered: (1) increased sensory loss (if it was incomplete before surgery) or worsening of neuropathic pain, (2) minimal, unacceptable, or no improvement, (3) acceptable improvement, or (4) return of normal, or nearly normal sensation and/or total relief of pain. None of these is assured, but maximal likelihood of a successful outcome (outcomes 3 and 4, or grades S3, S3+, and S4 on the Medical Research Council Scale [MRCS]; see Table 9-5]) is significantly related to the time from injury to surgical repair (best results are seen within 6 months; a large drop-off in the success rate occurs after 9 to 12 months), the age of the patient (the success rate decreases after age 45 for the lingual nerve [LN] and age 51 for the IAN), and the experience and technical skill of the microsurgeon. A patient in whom the major symptom or complaint is numbness or loss of sensation is at minimal risk of developing a neuropathic pain syndrome after microsurgical nerve repair. Preoperatively, if a patient's pain is relieved by a successful local anesthetic block of the suspected nerve, there is a reasonable chance that the pain is emanating from that nerve (rather than from the central nervous system or a collateral pathway, such as adjacent sympathetic fibers [so-called sympathetic-mediated pain], or reflex sympathetic dystrophy) and that microsurgical intervention might relieve some or all of the pain (often caused by a neuroma).

Microsurgical operations on the IAN pose risks that are considered in the informed consent process and in the planning of the operation. Because the IAN is subjected to surgical manipulation from the pterygomandibular space to the mental foramen, the surgeon must be prepared to expose the nerve in such a way that this entire area can be inspected and surgically accessed under direct vision. Therefore, an IAN injury resulting from an SSRO may, in some patients, require exposure through a submandibular skin incision. When a submandibular approach exposes the IAN, the adjacent marginal mandibular branch (MBr) of the facial nerve (cranial nerve [CN] VII) is at risk of injury. Most commonly, this is a temporary injury due to retraction of the superior soft tissue flap (which contains the MBr of CN VII), resulting in transient paresis (weakness) of the ipsilateral lower lip musculature with a "crooked smile" or deficient puckering. When the injury to the IAN is located beneath or anterior to the first molar tooth, it might be accessed via a transoral approach, which avoids an externally visible surgical scar. Although the MBr is not directly exposed transorally, it is still at risk of injury when prolonged retraction of the soft tissue flap is necessary for the microsurgical procedure (as occurred with the current patient).

Patient concerns regarding a visible skin scar are addressed by explaining the method of careful cosmetic skin closure performed, in addition to the injection of a corticosteroid (e.g., dilute triamcinolone) into the incision margins before closure in African American or other darkly pigmented patients, who have an increased tendency to form hypertrophic scars or keloids. Such injections can be repeated postoperatively as needed.

The harvesting of an autogenous nerve has its own risks, most commonly loss of sensation in the area supplied by the harvested donor nerve. When the GAN is the donor nerve, this causes anesthesia of the lower portion of the earlobe and a variable sized area of skin at the angle of the mandible. This is generally well tolerated by most patients. Harvesting of the SN leaves the patient with loss of sensation on the lateral aspect of the foot and sometimes the heel. Patients who depend on position sense and tactile accuracy in their feet (e.g. runners, climbers, and some professional athletes) may have difficulty with this sensory deficit. The most feared complication in the donor nerve surgical site is the development of pain, often but not always due to development of a proximal nerve stump neuroma. This is minimized, or in most cases eliminated, by a nerve redirection procedure in which the proximal stump of the donor nerve is sutured to adjacent muscle (the sternocleidomastoideus in the neck; the gastrocnemius in the lower extremity), or by epineurial capping (Figure 9-18). The donor nerve selected depends on the length of the nerve gap to be reconstructed. Generally, about 3 cm is the greatest length of GAN that is available for harvest. Therefore, when the nerve gap is greater than 2.5 cm (allowing for contracture of the graft after harvesting), the SN (which is available from the popliteal fossa to the lateral malleus of the ankle) is usually selected for grafting.

Recently, decellularized human cadaveric nerves (AxoGen, Inc.; Alachua, Florida) have become available for peripheral

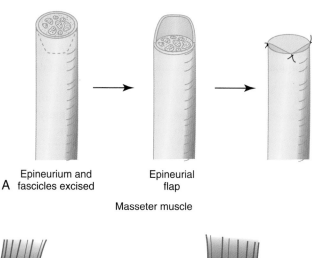

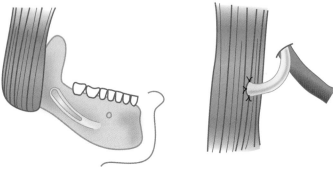

Figure 9-18 Management of the proximal stump of the donor nerve. **A,** Epineurial capping. Sufficient epineurium and fascicular material is excised to create an epineurial flap. The flap is folded over the exposed axons in the nerve stump and sutured under magnification with fine, nonreactive sutures (i.e., 8-0 or 10-0 nylon). **B,** Nerve redirection. The proximal stump of the donor nerve is mobilized and rotated into contact with adjacent muscle (i.e., the sternocleidomastoideus in the neck; the gastrocnemius in the lower extremity). Under magnification, the epineurial margins are carefully sutured to the muscle, leaving sufficient laxity in the proximal nerve to accommodate bodily movement. *(Redrawn from Bagheri SC, Meyer RA: Management of mandibular nerve injuries from dental implants,* Atlas Oral Maxillofac Surg Clin North Am *19[1]:47-61, 2011.)*

nerve reconstruction, not only in the oral and maxillofacial region, but also in other areas of the body (e.g., the hand) requiring peripheral nerve reconstruction. The use of this type of nerve graft eliminates the necessity of a donor site incision and the risks associated with nerve harvesting described previously. As yet, the success rate for nerves reconstructed with processed cadaveric grafts, compared to those using autogenous grafts, have not been established in well-controlled studies. However, our early experience and that of other surgeons has shown good results with the processed grafts.

Because microsurgical repair of the IAN often necessitates reconstruction of a nerve gap with a nerve graft, it is frequently a lengthy procedure requiring several hours. Good airway control and anesthetic management are important in reducing pulmonary atelectasis and the development of pneumonitis. The risk of urinary bladder distention requires

catheterization in most patients. Venous stasis in the lower extremities and the risk of deep vein thrombosis and embolism are minimized by the application of alternating compression devices on the lower extremities.

DISCUSSION

The most frequent causes of IAN injury in oral and maxillofacial surgery practice, from most common to least common, are (1) removal of mandibular third molars, (2) sagittal split mandibular ramus osteotomy (SSRO), (3) maxillofacial trauma, (4) dental implants, and (5) root canal treatment. Other causes seen less often are biopsies and excision of tumors or cysts, mandibular ridge augmentation procedures, and injection of a local anesthetic. Of all these, the treatment of a nerve injury associated with the SSRO is the most problematic, because it is often difficult to determine preoperatively the exact location of the IAN injury, even with the assistance of CBCT.

Proactive measures taken to avoid injuries to the IAN, MN, and LN have lessened the risk of such injuries during orthognathic surgery (i.e., SSRO and genioplasty) on the mandible in the authors' practice. Steps taken during the SSRO to reduce the risk of IAN injury include (1) determination of the exact location of the IAC with appropriate preoperative imaging studies; (2) protection of the IAN where it enters the medial surface of the mandibular ramus; (3) making the vertical anterior osteotomy cut just barely through the buccal cortical bone; (4) using anterior and superior border "spreaders" to initiate separation of the proximal and distal mandibular segments until the IAN is directly visualized; (5) removing irregular bone from the medial surface of the proximal mandibular segment, which might impinge on the IAN when the osteotomized segments are fixated; (6) inserting autogenous or bank bone grafts between the distal and proximal segments superior to the IAC before clamping the segments together for internal fixation; and (7) placing bicortical screws only along the superior border of the mandible, to minimize compression of the IAN, and using monocortical screws no longer than 5 mm, to avoid entering the IAC.

The risk of LN injury is reduced by (1) careful dissection and elevation of the medial mandibular periosteum in the retromolar area; (2) not allowing the drill to penetrate more than just barely through the mandibular lingual plate when preparing holes for internal fixation screws; and (3) selecting fixation screws of the correct length so that the lingual nerve is not impinged upon.

In performing the horizontal mandibular osteotomy for genioplasty, the most important steps for reducing the risk of injury to the MN are (1) good imaging studies that show clearly the position of the mental foramen and its relationship to the IAC and (2) making the osteotomy cuts sufficiently below the inferior border of the IAC.

Special considerations arise regarding diagnosis, selection of surgical procedures, and timing of treatment in patients who have sustained IAN injuries from removal of mandibular third molars (M3s), maxillofacial trauma, dental implants, root canal treatment, and ablative tumor surgery. For more information, the reader is directed to the pertinent references listed in the Bibliography: M3s—Kim et al., 2012; maxillofacial trauma—Bagheri et al., 2009; dental implants—Bagheri and Meyer, 2011; root canal treatment—Meyer, 1992; ablative tumor surgery—Meyer and Bagheri, 2013.

Because the IAN has a rather straight course within the IAC, there is often little to be gained by attempting mobilization of the proximal and distal nerve limbs, as can be done with the LN. Some surgeons section the incisive nerve (IN) to allow greater mobilization and lateralization of the IAN/MN and achieve closure of a small (i.e., less than 1 cm) nerve gap without grafting (as was done in the patient described previously). However, after debridement of all abnormal tissue and preparation of the nerve stumps for repair, nerve gaps in the IAC are often larger than 1 cm and, despite the additional mobilization created by IN transection, they may not be amenable to approximation without tension. Therefore, reconstruction with either an autogenous nerve graft (the GAN in the neck or the SN in the lower extremity), a processed allogeneic nerve graft, or guided regeneration through a nerve tube is often necessary. All of these have been successful in various situations, depending on the surgeon's judgment and experience.

Sensory reeducation is an essential aspect of the care and rehabilitation of the patient whose peripheral nerve injury has been repaired. As soon as the patient regains responses to painful stimuli and static light touch (which demonstrate that the nerve has reinnervated the target tissue end organs), a series of stimulating exercises on the affected area and the contralateral (or adjacent, in the patient with bilateral IAN injuries, such as the patient presented previously) normal side are performed three times daily, in front of a mirror with the eyes open and then with the eyes closed. Such exercises aid in the recovery of *graphesthesia* (the ability to identify objects by their "feel"), more closely localize a stimulus to its point of origin (loss of this skill is termed *synesthesia*), overcome new axonal connections and transmission to different areas of the central nervous system than existed before injury, adapt to differing speeds of impulse conduction, and decrease or resolve hypersensitivity (aided by control of hyperesthesia with neurotropic medications). Sensory reeducation exercises are performed by the patient on a daily basis until he or she is satisfied with the result or for at least 1 year, whichever is longer. The patient is monitored by NST at bimonthly visits with the surgeon during this time. (For an in-depth discussion of sensory rehabilitation, the reader is referred to the articles by Meyer and Rath, 2001, and by Phillips et al., 2011, listed in the Bibliography.)

The results of microsurgical repair of the IAN, as assessed by NST and graded on the MRCS, are successful in 80% to 90% of patients, depending upon the cause of the injury, the length of time from injury to repair, the age of the patient, and the experience and technical skill of the microsurgeon. Based on this information, microsurgical repair of peripheral trigeminal nerve injuries is an acceptable and recommended

treatment for patients who meet the diagnostic criteria discussed in this chapter.

Control of chronic neuropathic pain in the patient who is not a candidate for peripheral nerve surgery or in whom surgical intervention has failed to relieve pain is often a difficult problem. Neurotropic medications such as clonazepam, gabapentin, and pregabalin act directly on pain impulses in the central nervous system and are generally the initial choices for pharmacologic management of chronic neuropathic pain. Abolition of neuropathic pain soon after its onset reduces the risk of the development of an intractable pain syndrome. Once this problem has developed in susceptible patients, as early as a few months after pain onset in some cases, treatment becomes extremely problematic. The choice of medication and the optimal dose vary among patients. Once a satisfactory level of pain control with little or no sedation has been established, it is generally maintained, in the absence of surgical intervention, for 6 months before attempting to wean the patient off this medication. Cessation is done slowly, over a period of several weeks, after long-term administration to avoid the risk of a seizure. If neurotropic medications provide inadequate pain relief, some patients may be candidates for narcotics. However, strict dosage schedules and close patient monitoring are essential. Such patients are often best managed in a multispecialty pain clinic, where all aspects of their lives that are affected by chronic pain (e.g., activities of daily living, nutrition, interpersonal relationships, employment, psychological issues) can be addressed simultaneously and comprehensively by appropriate specialists.

Bibliography

Bagheri SC, Meyer RA, Ali Khan H, et al: Microsurgical repair of trigeminal nerve injuries from maxillofacial trauma, *J Oral Maxillofac Surg* 67:1791, 2009.

Bagheri SC, Meyer RA, Ali Khan H, et al: Microsurgical repair of the peripheral trigeminal nerve after mandibular sagittal split ramus osteotomy, *J Oral Maxillofac Surg* 68(11):2770, 2010.

Bagheri SC, Meyer RA: Management of mandibular nerve injuries from dental implants, *Atlas Oral Maxillofac Surg Clin North Am* 19(1):47, 2011.

Bagheri SC, Meyer RA: Management of trigeminal nerve injuries. In Bagheri SC, Bell RB, Khan HA (eds): *Current therapy in oral and maxillofacial surgery*, pp 224-237, St Louis, 2011, Saunders.

Essick GK: Comprehensive clinical evaluation of perioral sensory function, *Oral Maxillofac Surg Clin North Am* 4(2):503, 1992.

Gregg JM: Studies of traumatic neuralgias in the maxillofacial region: symptom complexes and responses to microsurgery, *J Oral Maxillofac Surg* 48:135, 1990.

Gregg JM: Medical management of traumatic neuropathies, *Oral Maxillofac Surg Clin North Am* 13(2):343, 2001.

Kim J-W, Cha I-H, Kim S-J, et al: Which risk factors are associated with neurosensory deficits of inferior alveolar nerve after mandibular third molar extraction? *J Oral Maxillofac Surg* 70(11):2508, 2012.

LaBanc JP: Classification of nerve injuries, *Oral Maxillofac Surg Clin North Am* 4(2):285, 1992.

Meyer RA: Applications of microneurosurgery to the repair of trigeminal nerve injuries, *Oral Maxillofac Clin North Am* 4(2):405, 1992.

Meyer RA: Nerve harvesting procedures, *Atlas Oral Maxillofac Surg Clin North Am* 9:77, 2001.

Meyer RA, Bagheri SC: Clinical evaluation of peripheral trigeminal nerve injuries, *Oral Maxillofac Surg Clin North Am* 19(1):15, 2011.

Meyer RA, Bagheri SC: Nerve injuries from mandibular third molar removal, *Oral Maxillofac Surg Clin North Am* 19(1):63, 2011.

Meyer RA, Bagheri SC: Etiology and prevention of nerve injuries. In Miloro M (ed): *Trigeminal nerve injuries*, Heidelberg, 2013, Springer (in press).

Meyer RA, Bagheri SC: Clinical evaluation of nerve injuries. In Miloro M (ed): *Trigeminal nerve injuries*, Heidelberg, 2013, Springer (in press).

Meyer RA, Bagheri SC: Microsurgical reconstruction of the trigeminal nerve, *Oral Maxillofac Surg Clin North Am* 25(2):287-302, 2013.

Meyer RA, Rath EM: Sensory rehabilitation after trigeminal injury or nerve repair, *Oral Maxillofac Surg Clin North Am* 13(2):365, 2001.

Miloro M, Kolokythas A: Inferior alveolar and lingual nerve imaging, *Oral Maxillofac Surg Clin North Am* 19(1):35, 2011.

Phillips C, Blakey G, Essick GK: Sensory retraining: a cognitive behavioral therapy for altered sensation, *Oral Maxillofac Surg Clin North Am* 19(1):109, 2011.

Schultz JD, Dodson TB, Meyer RA: Donor site morbidity of great auricular nerve harvesting, *J Oral Maxillofac Surg* 50:803, 1992.

Wolford LM, Rodrigues DB: Autogenous grafts/allografts/conduits for bridging peripheral trigeminal nerve gaps, *Atlas Oral Maxillofac Surg Clin North Am* 19(1):91, 2011.

Woods DD, LaBanc JP: Complications and morbidity associated with trigeminal nerve repairs, *Oral Maxillofac Surg Clin North Am* 4(2):473, 1992.

Ziccardi VB: Microsurgical techniques for repair of the inferior alveolar and lingual nerves, *Oral Maxillofac Surg Clin North Am* 19(1):79, 2011.

Zuniga JR, Meyer RA, Gregg JM, et al: The accuracy of clinical neurosensory testing for nerve injury diagnosis, *J Oral Maxillofac Surg* 56:2, 1998.

Computer-Assisted Surgical Simulation: Virtual Surgical Planning for Orthognathic Surgery

Nathan G. Adams and Kevin L. Rieck

CC

A 16-year-old male presents for combined surgical and orthodontic correction of his facial asymmetry and apertognathia. He describes his chief complaint as an inability to bring his anterior dentition into occlusion, which makes eating difficult. He is also concerned about his facial asymmetry and weak-appearing chin.

When orthognathic surgery is considered, it is important always to assess the patient's chief complaint as it relates to function and esthetics to ensure that any planned surgical intervention adequately addresses the patient's concerns and to fully inform the patient about any anticipated changes in facial appearance as a result of the surgery.

HPI

The patient has a significant past medical history of bilateral retinoblastoma, which was treated at 5 months of age by enucleation of the left globe and radiotherapy of the right orbit. Significant facial asymmetry due to radiotherapy-induced growth disturbance is readily evident. The patient had been in orthodontic therapy for 15 months prior to this consultation, and he is primarily concerned about masticatory dysfunction. His deformity consists of anterior open bite and facial asymmetry with diminished right periorbital volume and enophthalmos. His first premolar teeth have been removed in preparation for the surgery, and he is also missing teeth #1 and #32. Teeth #16 and #17 remain impacted.

PMHX/PSHS/MEDICATIONS/ALLERGIES/SH/FH

Bilateral retinoblastoma, with the left globe treated by enucleation and the right eye with radiotherapy at 5 months of age. No history of recurrence. At present the patient denies any regular use of medications or history of allergies.

EXAMINATION

General. No acute distress, well nourished, and appropriate mental capacity.

Head. Growth status complete. Orbital prosthesis present in left orbit. The right periorbital region is diminished in volume, with presence of enophthalmos and decreased projection of the right zygomatic buttress and arch.

Further maxillofacial examination proceeded as follows.

1. **Skeletal aspects**
   - Significant facial asymmetry is present.
   - Midpoints
     - Upper dental midline is 5 mm to patient's right.
     - Lower dental midline is 2 mm to patient's right.
     - Chin point is 4 mm to patient's right.
   - Vertical: Occlusal plane is canted upward to patient's right.
   - Profile: Convex
   - Chin: Retrusive, but signs of mentalis strain are evident (indicative of muscular activity to assist with lip competency).
   - Nose: Large
   - Nasolabial angle: Obtuse (normal is 100 degrees ± 10 degrees)
   - Throat length: Short
2. **Lips**
   - Upper lip is in normal anterior-posterior position.
   - Lower lip is protrusive.
   - Incompetent, open 11 mm.
   - Upper lip is thin.
   - Lower lip is thick and protrusive.
3. **Dental aspects**
   - Anterior open bite malocclusion with contact only on posterior first and second molars bilaterally. Complete orthodontic appliances are in place.
   - Upper incisor to lip line at repose is 5 mm.
   - Upper incisor to lip line smiling is 11 mm with 0 mm of gingival display.
   - Lower incisor show to lip line at repose is 3 mm of exposed.
   - Lower incisor show to lip line at smiling is 10 mm exposed.
   - No centric relation/centric occlusion (CR/CO) discrepancy noted.
   - No macroglossia noted.

IMAGING

Although this chapter focuses on the use of three-dimensional, computer-assisted surgical simulation software in conjunction with a preoperative computed tomography (CT) scan, panoramic and cephalometric radiographs continue to be used by clinicians to assist in preoperative surgical planning. Some practitioners choose to obtain these radiographs separately; however, they can also be easily generated from CT or cone-beam CT (CBCT) data set manipulation via a number of software programs.

For the current patient, recent panoramic and cephalometric radiographs (Figure 9-19, *A* and *B*) were present at the time of consultation and revealed impacted teeth #16 and #17, in addition to considerable facial asymmetry. The vertical height of the mandible was measured as 1 cm shorter on the right than on the left (disruption of the growth center of the mandible secondary to radiotherapy and/or to altered growth of the functional matrix of the face on the right side), and cephalometrics revealed obvious apertognathia, as noted on clinical exam (Figure 9-19, *C*). CT imaging was obtained after the initial consultation but correlated with the radiographic findings and provided additional information regarding the hypoplastic nature of the right facial skeleton and its contributions to the facial asymmetry. The CT imaging protocol used for computer-assisted surgical simulation is very important, and the surgeon must adhere to it closely for accuracy of procedures and splint fabrication.

LABS

The patient's current medical status and planned surgical interventions did not require preoperative laboratory assessment.

ASSESSMENT

Marked facial asymmetry secondary to radiation therapy for retinoblastoma; occlusal dysfunction as a result of underlying hypoplastic right mandibular body, anterior open bite, and significant occlusal cant.

Correction of this type of asymmetric deformity requires combined surgical and orthodontic treatments. Surgical intervention requires osteotomies of both the maxilla and mandible, preceded by precise preoperative planning, to achieve both functional and cosmetic correction.

Although surgical planning has historically used two-dimensional radiographs and model surgery, with documented

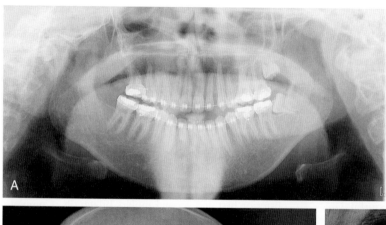

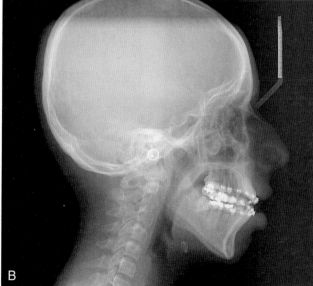

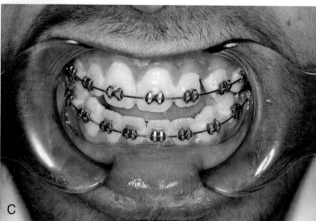

Figure 9-19 Preoperative panoramic **(A)** and cephalometric **(B)** radiographs show impaction of tooth #16 and tooth #17, along with extensive facial asymmetry. The vertical height of the mandible is 1 cm shorter on the right than on the left. Observable apertognathia can be seen on the clinical view **(C)** and on the cephalometric radiograph.

success, the use of computed tomography and virtual surgical planning software in a preoperative work-up provides precision and detail of movements and position not previously available. By evaluating maxillary and mandibular movements in relation to the entire facial skeleton in a virtual three-dimensional model, the surgeon can make more accurate decisions, and a more precise splint can be fabricated.

TREATMENT

Isolated cases of apertognathia historically have been treated with a LeFort I osteotomy involving posterior impaction and some maxillary advancement. Alternatively, isolated mandibular surgery consisting of bilateral sagittal split ramus osteotomies and counterclockwise rotation of the mandible to close the anterior open bite is possible, assuming rigid fixation is used. The current patient has a combination of apertognathia and significant facial asymmetry, which makes any attempts at isolated treatment of the maxilla and mandible futile. Facial asymmetry cases require a great deal of preoperative planning to ensure that the deformity is corrected appropriately.

Virtual surgical planning software, marketed and used by various modeling companies, can assist the surgeon in making important, complex decisions. To use such planning, the surgeon must obtain specific preliminary records. They include:

- Clinical assessment measurements (i.e., midline discrepancies, facial asymmetries)
- Clinical photographs
- Natural head position measurements (using a gyroscope or intraoral fiducial markers)
- Fabrication of a specialized CR bite jig registration, to be in place at the time of CT acquisition
- CT/CBCT scan with the CR bite jig registration attached to the radiographic fiducial marker device
- Stone models that are hand articulated into ideal occlusion and referenced accordingly for laser scanning and incorporation into the CT imaging data

After these records have been acquired and delivered to the modeling company, the surgeon is ready for the online Web meeting to initiate planning. This meeting allows the surgeon and the modeling team to make precise movements of the maxillomandibular complex by visualizing bony osteotomies, condylar position, and overlaps and gaps between bony segments. This type of visualization allows the surgeon to make changes in the roll, pitch, and yaw of the segments, thereby creating the most favorable and stable osseous position of all segments. Such capabilities are particularly invaluable in facial asymmetry cases.

In the current patient, a LeFort I osteotomy and bilateral sagittal split ramus osteotomy were used to correct the apertognathia and facial asymmetry (Figure 9-20, A). The LeFort procedure was performed first; an intermediate splint was used to level the maxillary occlusal plane and align dental midlines with facial midlines. The maxilla was impacted 7.3 mm posteriorly and 3.5 mm anteriorly, with 6.1 mm of impaction on the left and 0.9 mm on the right. After rigid fixation of the maxilla, bilateral sagittal split ramus osteotomy was performed, bringing the dentition into final occlusion. The unique aspect of this case is the quality and precision of the movements afforded by the use of preoperative planning software. As shown in Figure 9-20, B, the maxillary dental midline is coincident with facial midline; however, the maxillary yaw is shifted significantly to the patient's left. Figure 9-20, C, illustrates the yaw correction of the maxilla, which places the maxilla in the most ideal yaw, pitch, and roll position. Once the maxillary movements have been planned, the mandible is brought into the final occlusion based on the scanned, hand-articulated models provided to the modeling company. Visualization of the mandibular osteotomies, and the gaps naturally created by the asymmetric movements of the mandible, are easily reviewed and examined (Figure 9-20, D). As noted, the overlapping aspects of the proximal and distal segments are less than ideal (Figure 9-20, E), and fixation in this position would require a great deal of adjustment to the proximal segment or result in flaring of the right mandibular condyle. However, with the maxilla and mandible locked in final occlusion, mild adjustments are made to the yaw of the entire maxillomandibular complex, allowing for a more favorable overlap of the mandibular proximal and distal segments (Figure 9-20, F). Clearly, selected areas of bony reduction or modification and/or the placement of bone shims in certain areas may be necessary to allow for ideal positioning of the proximal and distal segments of the mandible in cases such as this. Postoperative panoramic and lateral cephalometric radiographs reveal the stable fixation and the correction of skeletal asymmetries, in addition to the enhancement of the chin position as predicted by the use of virtual surgical planning technology (Figure 9-21).

COMPLICATIONS

Orthognathic surgery requires attention to detail and an excellent knowledge of facial anatomy to minimize surgical complications. Failure to appreciate the patient's specific anatomy and poor surgical technique can lead to intraoperative complications; however, unforeseen complications also can occur in any orthognathic procedure. Such complications may include nerve injury, bleeding, unfavorable fractures, and technical difficulties in bony positioning and fixation. The goal of every orthognathic surgeon should be to minimize the risk of these complications by understanding the patient's specific anatomy and undertaking sound preoperative planning. The use of virtual surgical planning software provides the surgeon with additional means to better understand these case-specific details. Specific anatomic structures, such as the neurovascular bundles in the mandible, can be highlighted and referenced to the anticipated osteotomies for improved safety.

Complications of maxillary and mandibular orthognathic surgery are discussed in greater detail elsewhere in this text.

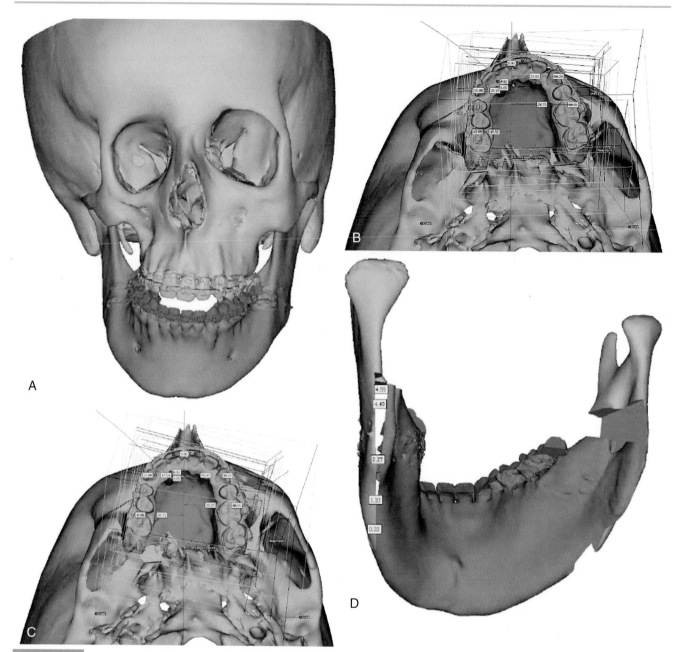

Figure 9-20 Computer-aided surgical simulation planning. **A,** Composite skull model showing original condition of apertognathia and facial asymmetry. **B,** Inferior view showing that the maxillary dental midline is coincident with the facial midline, whereas the maxillary yaw is shifted greatly to the left. **C,** Inferior view showing the maxilla in the ideal yaw, pitch, and roll position. **D,** Left posterior view showing the mandibular osteotomies and the gaps caused by the asymmetric movements of the mandible.

DISCUSSION

Facial asymmetry is ubiquitous among individuals to some degree. These asymmetries obviously vary in severity and may be perceived differently by different individuals. Recognition of asymmetry is crucial in examining a patient for potential orthognathic surgery, because some asymmetries are subtle, whereas others are more obvious. It is the responsibility of the clinician and surgeon to understand the patient's perception of his or her facial asymmetries, because the practitioners' perceptions may not coincide entirely with that of the patient. The patient may not perceive a need for correction or may have unrealistic expectations of what can truly be accomplished; both are important aspects of surgical planning.

Significant asymmetries require a great deal of surgical experience and skill, because they can involve a variety of tissues and occur in multiple planes, making correction complex. In the current patient, the asymmetry was caused by radiotherapy at a young age, secondarily altering the growth of a variety of tissues at a variety of levels. Orthognathic

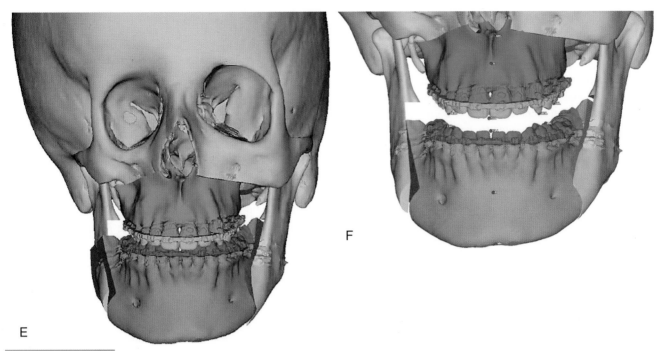

Figure 9-20, cont'd **E,** Frontal view demonstrating the overlapping aspects of the proximal and distal segments. **F,** Postoperative computer simulation after maxillary and mandibular surgery.

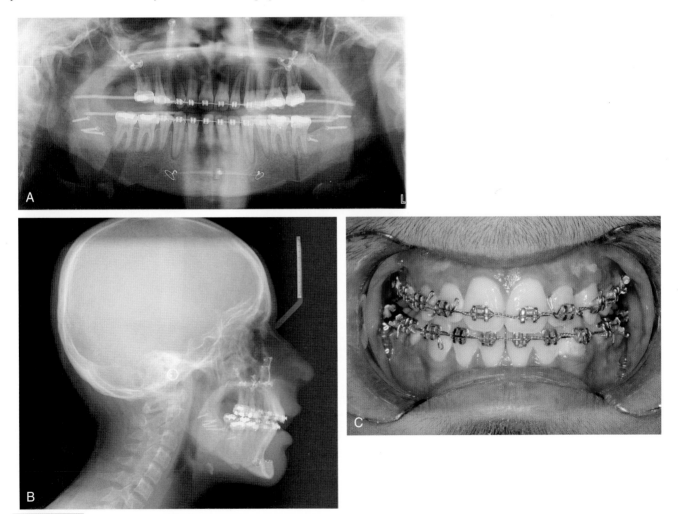

Figure 9-21 Postoperative panoramic **(A)** and cephalometric **(B)** radiographs showing stable fixation, correction of the skeletal asymmetries, and enhancement of the chin position. **C,** Postoperative clinical view no longer shows apertognathia.

surgery in this patient was the first phase of treatment in correcting his asymmetries, with future plans for facial augmentation by alloplastic or autogenous means, if necessary or if desired by the patient. Understanding the limits of orthognathic surgery in correction of asymmetries is also important, because additional procedures and methods may be required to achieve balance in facial esthetics.

Diagnosis of facial asymmetry begins with a thorough clinical evaluation. Although the methodologies by which a surgeon may clinically evaluate a patient may differ, a detailed, systematic, and comprehensive approach is required as the first step in the evaluation of potential orthognathic patients. As discussed previously, the adjunct information obtained from three-dimensional imaging techniques and the use of virtual surgical planning can enhance the surgeon's ability to properly diagnose and treat the details of facial asymmetry. However, as with generic model surgery, a firm understanding of this technology is paramount to using it properly in the treatment of our patients. As with all advancements in medical technology, the primary goal should be to enhance the clinician's ability to improve patient care.

Bibliography

Gateno J, Xia JJ, Teichgraeber JF, et al: Clinical feasibility of computer-aided surgical simulation (CASS) in the treatment of complex craniomaxillofacial deformities, *J Oral Maxillofac Surg* 65:728, 2007.

Guyuron B, Ross RJ: Computer generated model surgery, *J Craniomaxillofac Surg* 17:101, 1989.

Hassfeld S, Muhling J: Computer assisted oral and maxillofacial surgery: a review and an assessment of technology, *Int J Oral Maxillofac Surg* 30:2, 2001.

Hatcher DC, Aboudara CL: Diagnosis goes digital, *Am J Orthod Dentofacial Orthop* 125:512, 2004.

McCormick SU, Drew SJ: Virtual model surgery for efficient planning and surgical performance, *J Oral Maxillofac Surg* 69:638, 2011.

Orentlicher G, Goldsmith D, Horowitz A, et al: Applications of 3-dimensional virtual computerized tomography technology in oral and maxillofacial surgery: current therapy, *J Oral Maxillofac Surg* 68:1933, 2010.

Quevedo LA, Ruiz JV, Quevedo CA: Using a clinical protocol for orthognathic surgery and assessing a 3-dimendionsal virtual approach: current therapy, *J Oral Maxillofac Surg* 69:623, 2011.

Schendel S, Jacobson R: Three-dimensional imaging and computer simulation for office-based surgery, *J Oral Maxillofac Surg* 67:2107, 2009.

Wolford LM: Facial asymmetry: diagnosis and treatment considerations. In Fonseca RJ (ed): Oral and maxillofacial surgery, ed 2, vol III, St Louis, 2009, Saunders.

Xia JI, Gateno J, Teichgraeber JF: Computer-aided surgical simulation for orthognathic surgery. In Bagheri SC, Bell RB, Khan HA (eds): *Current therapy in oral and maxillofacial surgery*, St Louis, 2011, Saunders.

CHAPTER 10

Temporomandibular Joint Disorders

This chapter addresses:
- Myofascial Pain Dysfunction
- Internal Derangement of the Temporomandibular Joint
- Arthrocentesis and Arthroscopy
- Degenerative Joint Disease of the Temporomandibular Joint
- Ankylosis of the Temporomandibular Joint

Care of the patient with temporomandibular joint (TMJ) disorders is difficult. At present there is no formal TMJ specialty. There are TMJ interest groups, but many of the members of these groups are not surgeons. Although the majority of patients with temporomandibular joint dysfunction (TMD) are treated nonsurgically, it is clear that oral and maxillofacial surgeons are in a unique position to treat TMJ disorders; they can provide the full scope of treatments, ranging from occlusal guards to total TMJ replacement.

Disorders of the TMJ can result in debilitating pain and limited function. Although TMD includes a broad spectrum of disease states, it can be classified into two general categories: intracapsular disease (internal derangement or ankylosis) and extracapsular disease (myofascial pain dysfunction). Most cases of TMD can be managed nonsurgically with conservative therapy. Accurate diagnosis of the etiology of TMD is paramount for avoiding unwarranted invasive treatment.

The teaching cases in this chapter cover identification and management strategies for internal derangement, myofascial pain disorder, degenerative joint disease, and ankylosis of the temporomandibular joint. Arthrocentesis and arthroscopy also are discussed. The distinction between intracapsular and extracapsular TMD is emphasized. As in many complex disorders, the majority of information is obtained from the patient's presenting complaint and history of symptoms. In these cases the key features of the chief complaint (CC) and the history of the present illness (HPI) are emphasized. The significant findings in the physical examination are highlighted, along with explanations of these findings.

Although nonsurgical management strategies are more consistent between individual practitioners, various surgical strategies have been used based on surgeons' preferences and the clinical presentation. Some of the advantages and disadvantages of different treatment modalities are outlined. Surgical options are discussed, along with the rationale for treatment and the relative success rates. Reconstructive strategies for advanced disease states are also presented.

Myofascial Pain Dysfunction

Gary F. Bouloux, Ibrahim M. Haron, and Chris Jo

CC

A 43-year-old Caucasian woman presents with a 6-month history of daily bitemporal headaches that worsen as the day progresses.

Temporomandibular joint dysfunction is a heterogenous group of disorders that includes myofascial pain dysfunction (MPD), which predominantly affects females.

HPI

The patient reports that the pain is dull and, while often present upon awakening, it continues to worsen throughout the day (characteristic of MPD). When asked to point to the regions of pain, she readily identifies the areas over her temporalis and masseter muscles. She has difficulty falling asleep and wakes up frequently throughout the night. The pain is worse when eating food, especially when chewing tough foods, such as steak (increasing pain and muscle fatigue during mastication are typical findings in MPD). She has modified her diet by excluding hard and chewy foods to reduce the pain and discomfort associated with eating. She reports no history of migraines but admits to a high level of stress at work (work- or home-related stress can exacerbate MPD). She denies any prior history of temporomandibular joint dysfunction and is not aware of any parafunctional habits such as bruxism. (Bruxism is grinding of the teeth. Many patients may be unaware of nocturnal bruxism, unless reported by their bed partner. Also, patients with nocturnal bruxism are characteristically worse on waking and improve over the course of the day).

PMHX/PDHX/MEDICATIONS/ALLERGIES/SH/FH

The patient's medical and dental histories are unremarkable. She is happily married and has one child. She denies any history of depression (depression is a risk factor for MPD). She works at a regional bank and was recently promoted to vice president, a job that she finds quite stressful (stress is a risk factor for MPD).

EXAMINATION

General. The patient is a well-developed and well-nourished, anxious woman.

Maxillofacial. There is no facial swelling or asymmetry. On palpation, there is tenderness of the temporalis, masseter, and sternocleidomastoid muscles bilaterally (temporalis and masseter muscles are most commonly involved in MPD). There is no TMJ capsular tenderness and no clicks or crepitus (making an intracapsular source of pain less likely). The patient has a maximal incisal opening of 28 mm (less than normal) with a soft end feel, which can be stretched to 39 mm with pain (limited opening due to muscle guarding that can be slowly stretched to a normal opening is consistent with MPD). Her left and right lateral excursions are 9 and 8 mm, respectively (normal condylar translation makes TMJ internal derangement less likely). The remainder of her physical examination is noncontributory.

IMAGING

A panoramic radiograph is the initial screening examination of choice. Although it cannot diagnose MPD, it provides a general overview of the teeth and related bony structures to rule out other sources of pain. Magnetic resonance imaging (MRI) and computed tomography (CT) scans are ordered based on the clinical suspicions of pathology in conjunction with MPD (see the section on Internal Derangement of the Temporomandibular Joint). However, MRI and CT are not indicated when MPD is the sole clinical diagnosis.

The panoramic radiograph in the current patient reveals no odontogenic or osseous pathology.

LABS

Laboratory tests are not indicated in the work-up of MPD unless associated with other suspected or diagnosed medical conditions (e.g., rheumatoid arthritis or neuromuscular disorders). A suspicion of temporal arteritis would warrant further laboratory testing (erythrocyte sedimentation rate and C-reactive protein as markers of inflammation) and biopsy of the superficial temporal artery.

ASSESSMENT

Myofascial pain dysfunction (MPD) syndrome.

The diagnosis of MPD is largely based on the patient history, which is confirmed with a thorough clinical examination. MPD can occur alone (as in the current patient) or in association with internal derangement of the TMJ (see the section Internal Derangement of the Temporomandibular Joint, later in this chapter).

TREATMENT

The treatment of MPD begins with the correct diagnosis. The etiology of MPD is multifactorial; therefore, the management of MPD requires a multimodal approach. Initially, the patient should be reassured that the pain is purely myofascial and likely to be the result of increased muscle activity secondary to any of a number of entities. These may include stress, anxiety, bruxism, clenching, malocclusion, parafunctional oral habits, internal derangement of the TMJ, rheumatologic diseases (polymyalgia rheumatica), fibromyalgia, and vasculitis (e.g., temporal arteritis). Treatment must address the etiology; however, given the difficulty associated with correct diagnosis, the approach is often generic.

Conservative therapy is generally the first-line treatment unless other identifiable associated diagnoses (tumors, infection, severe internal derangements, degenerative joint disease) are present that are thought to exacerbate the symptoms of MPD. Treatment options include reassurance, stress management (relaxation exercises, biofeedback), occlusal splint therapy, physical therapy, application of heat to affected muscles, nonsteroidal antiinflammatory drugs (NSAIDs), muscle relaxants, and anxiolytics (anxiolytics should be prescribed with caution due to abuse potential). Conservative treatment often results in significant improvement in or resolution of the MPD.

Patients who do respond to conservative therapy with an occlusal splint and have a significant malocclusion may be considered for orthodontic treatment or orthognathic surgery (there is some evidence that malocclusion may be associated with MPD). These modalities may offer a long-term solution to MPD, but they are invasive and not without complications.

Trigger point injections may be beneficial in a select group of patients with MPD who are refractory to all conservative approaches. Typically, a local anesthetic (with or without a steroid) is injected directly into tender areas in the muscles. This can be repeated as often as necessary. It may also be possible to improve MPD with injection of botulinum toxin into the muscle to reduce muscle activity. This may need to be repeated every 3 to 6 months, due to the temporary effect of the botulinum toxin. Regeneration of the nerve endings at the motor end plate of the neuromuscular junction is responsible for cessation of the clinical effects. Excessive muscle activity alone may not explain the majority of cases of MPD, and the response to botulinum toxin is not predictable. Intraarticular procedures, including arthrocentesis, arthroscopy, and arthroplasty, have no place in the management of isolated MPD.

The current patient was encouraged to manage her life stressors more effectively by taking stress management classes and using biofeedback to reduce muscle tension. She was instructed to avoid hard-to-chew foods and to apply moist heat (using a warm, moist towel) to the affected muscles as often as necessary for symptomatic relief. A short course of ibuprofen 800 mg three times a day was prescribed (a muscle relaxant can be added to this regimen). A hard, flat-plane maxillary occlusal splint was constructed, and the patient wore this at all times, except while eating or brushing her teeth. The splint was adjusted weekly to ensure good contacts in centric relation and no interferences during lateral excursions. Splint adjustments became less frequent as the occlusion stabilized, and by 2 months the patient was wearing the splint only at night and was able to open to 44 mm, with complete resolution of her pain.

COMPLICATIONS

With conservative (nonsurgical) approaches to the treatment of MPD, complications are relatively uncommon and are mostly related to the failure of available treatments to alleviate pain, the side effects of medications, or difficulties with occlusal splint therapy.

NSAIDs are often helpful and carry no risk of physiologic dependence, although gastrointestinal irritation and/or bleeding, platelet dysfunction, and decreased renal function are potential complications. The use of some muscle relaxants and anxiolytics can be associated with dependence and abuse, which are compounded by the frequently chronic and recurrent nature of MPD.

Occlusal splint therapy is not without complications (especially when the splint is inappropriately designed). Several different types of splints are used by prescribing clinicians, and unfortunately, there are no clear evidence-based guidelines for splint therapy. Different splints include maxillary, mandibular, flat-plane, anterior repositioning, and pivotal splints. Flat-plane occlusal splints, whether maxillary or mandibular, are the most popular and technically the least demanding. Although complications related to conservative splint therapy are uncommon, an incorrectly adjusted splint can result in exacerbation of the preexisting TMJ dysfunction, tooth movement, and/or the development of new symptoms. Anterior repositioning splints are occasionally useful in patients with Class II malocclusions and function by holding the mandible in a forward position; this unloads the richly innervated retrodiscal tissue within the TMJ and helps to reestablish a more normal disk-condyle relationship. These splints are likely to be associated with permanent occlusal changes, and considerable clinician experience is required in their use. Pivotal splints are rarely used and are thought to function by decreasing masticatory muscle forces (via periodontally mediated biofeedback).

After splint therapy, changes in the occlusion are not uncommon. Before splint therapy, most patients have a centric occlusion–centric relation discrepancy. A flat-plane occlusal splint may eliminate this discrepancy over time, resulting in a less than ideal occlusion when the splint is removed or discontinued. This may necessitate continued splint therapy, occlusal adjustment, orthodontics, or orthognathic surgery.

DISCUSSION

Myofascial pain disorder of the masticatory muscle system is the most common of all temporomandibular joint disorders.

The main muscles of mastication are the temporalis, masseter, lateral pterygoid, and medial pterygoid muscles. They all function harmoniously during speech and deglutination. As with any group of muscles, they are susceptible to inflammation, which may in turn cause pain. This is commonly due to excessive activity of these muscles, but the exact pathophysiology has not been clearly defined. The causes of muscle hyperactivity are many and may include malocclusion, parafunctional habits, TMJ internal derangement, cervical pain, and psychological stressors. Management of the acute symptoms of MPD is generally similar, regardless of the etiology, but long-term treatment and success need to address any known precipitating or etiologic factors. As is often the case, no definitive factors can be identified; consequently, a generic approach using several modalities must be adopted.

Bibliography

Giannakopoulos NN, Keller L, Rammelsberg P, et al: Anxiety and depression in patients with chronic temporomandibular pain and in controls, *J Dent* 38:369-376, 2010.

Graff-Radford SB: Temporomandibular disorders and headache, *Dent Clin North Am* 51:129-144, 2007.

Hersh E, Balasubramaniam R, Pinto A: Pharmacologic management of temporomandibular disorders, *Oral Maxillofac Surg Clin North Am* 20:197-210, 2008.

Klasser G, Greene C: Oral appliances in the management of temporomandibular disorders, *Oral Surg Oral Med Oral Pathol Oral Radiol Endod* 107:212-223, 2009.

Kurtoglu C, Gur OH, Kurkcu M, et al: Effect of botulinum toxin-A in myofascial pain patients with or without functional disc displacement, *J Oral Maxillofac Surg* 66:1644-1651, 2008.

Okeson JP, Leeuw RD: Differential diagnosis of Temporomandibular disorders and other orofacial pain disorders, *Dent Clin North Am* 55:105-120, 2011.

Schmitter M, Kress B, Leckel M, et al: Validity of temporomandibular disorder examination procedures for assessment of temporomandibular joint status, *Am J Orthod Dentofacial Orthop* 133:796-803, 2008.

Scrivani SJ, Keith DA, Kaban LB: Temporomandibular disorders, *N Engl J Med* 359:2693-2705, 2008.

Vedolin G, Lobato V, Conti P, et al: The impact of stress and anxiety on the pressure pain threshold of myofascial pain patients, *J Oral Rehabil* 36;313-321, 2009.

Internal Derangement of the Temporomandibular Joint

Gary F. Bouloux, Ibrahim M. Haron, and Chris Jo

CC

A 24-year-old female college student presents with several months of a painless "pop" in front of her right ear while eating. (Temporomandibular joint dysfunction [TMD] is a heterogenous group of disorders, including temporomandibular joint [TMJ] internal derangement, and is more commonly diagnosed in females.)

HPI

The patient first noted a "popping" sound in her right temporomandibular joint soon after she had her annual visit to her dentist 4 months earlier. The sound is noticeable when she is chewing, yawning, and brushing her teeth. The click is not associated with pain. She denies any history of trauma (which may precipitate internal derangement), and she had never had any symptoms of temporomandibular joint dysfunction (e.g., popping, clicking, pain, open lock, closed lock, or limited range of motion) before her annual dental visit.

PMHX/PDHX/MEDICATIONS/ALLERGIES/SH/FH

The patient's past medical and dental histories are noncontributory. She is in her final year of college.

EXAMINATION

General. The patient is a well-developed and well-nourished woman in no apparent distress.

Maxillofacial. The right external auditory meatus is patent, without evidence of erythema or exudate. The tympanic membrane is normal. There is no TMJ capsular tenderness. An opening click (caused by the condyle translating and recapturing a normal position beneath the disk) and a reciprocal click (a second click that occurs during closure of the mandible with anterior displacement of the disk) are evident within the right TMJ to both lateral capsular and endaural palpation. Auscultation over the TMJ reveals a harsh opening click and a softer closing click. No crepitation is present (crepitus would be suggestive of disk perforation with degeneration of the condyle and glenoid fossa). The left TMJ clinical examination is within normal limits. There is no evidence of masticatory muscle tenderness (masseter and temporalis muscles). The patient has an initial interincisal opening of 22 mm with a right-sided deviation (due to restricted right condylar translation), followed by a right TMJ click and correction of the deviation (as the anteriorly displaced right disk is recaptured). The maximum interincisal opening is 44 mm. The Mahan test is bilaterally negative (biting on a tongue depressor on one side, eliciting pain in the contralateral TMJ, is a positive test result that suggests intracapsular pathology). The patient is noted to have a Class II division II malocclusion (may be associated with an increased incidence of TMD). The remainder of her clinical examination is unremarkable.

IMAGING

The panoramic radiograph is the initial screening study of choice for assessment of TMDs, especially when pain is present (to assess pain of odontogenic origin). It provides a general overview of the bony morphology of the mandible and condyle. Magnetic resonance imaging (MRI), in open and closed mouth positions, is considered the standard when evaluating for TMJ internal derangement. It provides the most information regarding the soft tissue structures and disk position. A TMJ arthrogram (fluoroscopy with dye injected into the superior joint space) is an invasive procedure that shows the disk in dynamic function and is the only study that can readily identify disk perforations. Arthrograms can also be used to evaluate disk position, but the study is technique sensitive and is not readily available in most institutions. Computed tomography (CT) scans are indicated when bony or fibrous ankylosis of the TMJ or other bony pathology is suspected.

In the current patient, no osseous or dental abnormalities were seen on the panoramic radiograph. Sagittal and coronal MRI scans showed an anteromedially displaced (most frequent location of a dislocated disk) right TMJ disk in the closed mouth position (Figure 10-1, *A*), which reduced to a normal anatomic relationship in the open mouth position (Figure 10-1, *B*). The disk demonstrated a normal morphology (anatomy is best seen with T1-weighted images). No joint effusion was seen (inflammation and effusions are best evaluated with T2-weighted images).

LABS

No routine laboratory tests are indicated for the work-up of anterior disk displacement (ADD) of the TMJ. Clinical suspicion of systemic arthropathy (e.g., rheumatoid arthritis, systemic lupus erythematosus, psoriatic arthritis, and gout) would dictate further laboratory testing.

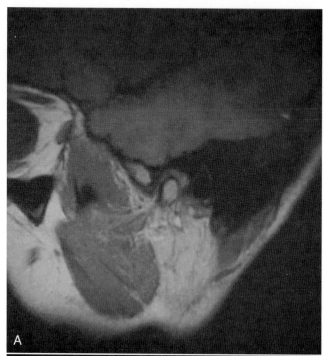

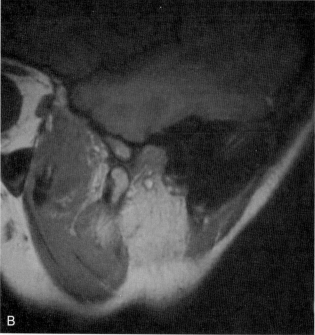

Figure 10-1 **A,** T1-weighted MRI scan in the closed mouth position showing anterior disk displacement. **B,** T1-weighted MRI scan in the open mouth position showing recapture or reduction of the disk.

ASSESSMENT

Internal derangement of the right TMJ; a nonpainful anterior disk displacement (ADD) with reduction of the right TMJ.

Patients with ADD with or without reduction may present with or without pain originating from the joint itself or from the muscles of mastication (i.e., myofascial pain dysfunction

[MPD]). ADD without reduction presents with different clinical findings, including no opening or closing click, and potentially with restricted condylar translation on the affected side (reduced lateral excursion to the contralateral side). The MRI scan would demonstrate anterior displacement of the disk with no evidence of disk recapture during opening. It is not uncommon for MPD to accompany a painful internal derangement of the TMJ. It is important to distinguish between internal derangement and MPD, because their treatment is very different. MPD may also present as the sole source of pain, which warrants proper diagnosis to avoid unnecessary and inappropriate surgical management (see the section Myofascial Pain Dysfunction earlier in this chapter).

The Wilkes classification system for internal derangement of the TMJ characterizes progression of the disease as having five stages, based on the clinical, radiographic, anatomic, and pathologic features (Table 10-1).

TREATMENT

Treatment of internal derangement is generally guided by the presence of pain and/or limited function. In the absence of symptoms, active treatment may be avoided or minimized, as long as adequate patient education and reassurance are provided.

Conservative (reversible or nonsurgical) treatment is generally the first line of therapy in symptomatic patients. Such treatment includes splint therapy; a soft, nonchewing diet; elimination of parafunctional habits (bruxism); warm, moist compresses; physical therapy; nonsteroidal antiinflammatory drugs (NSAIDs); and muscle relaxants. However, protocol-driven treatment should be avoided, and individualized patient assessment is necessary. Undue delay with conservative therapy, when an effective surgical solution is indicated, can be counterproductive, resulting in a delay in resolving the problem and further frustration for the patient and clinician.

Patients who are unresponsive to conservative therapy or who present with advanced disease are candidates for various invasive (surgical) interventions. Surgical options include arthrocentesis, arthroscopy, arthroplasty with disk plication, meniscectomy (with or without autogenous, allogeneic, or alloplastic graft/replacement), modified condylotomy, and total joint replacement.

Arthrocentesis is accomplished by irrigating and distending the superior joint space with lactated Ringer's solution, removing inflammatory mediators, and improving joint mobility by lysis of immature adhesions. A steroid or hyaluronic acid injection may follow, particularly if pain is a significant component of the patient's complaint.

Arthroscopy is a more invasive procedure, often requiring general anesthesia, but it enables the surgeon to visualize, irrigate, and lyse adhesions within the superior joint space. Arthroscopy is reported to have a success rate approaching 80%. Coblating instruments and the holmium:YAG laser can be used during arthroscopy for lysis of adhesions, discectomy, and partial synovectomy of the inflamed synovium. Arthroscopy may be expected to produce a similar reduction

Table 10-1	Wilkes Classification System for Internal Derangement of the TMJ		
Stage	Clinical Findings	Radiologic Findings	Surgical Findings
I	Painless clicking No locking No restricted motion	Slight anterior disk displacement that reduces on opening Normal osseous contours	Normal disk form Slight anterior disk displacement
II	Occasional painful clicking Intermittent locking Headaches	Slight anterior disk displacement that reduces on opening Early disk deformity Normal osseous contours	Thickened disk Anterior disk displacement
III	Frequent pain Joint tenderness Headaches Locking Restricted motion	Anterior disk displacement that does not reduce on opening Moderate disk deformity Normal osseous contours	Disk deformed and displaced Variable adhesions No bone changes
IV	Chronic pain Headaches Restricted motion with crepitus	Anterior disk displacement that does not recapture on opening Marked disk deformity Degenerative osseous changes	Disk perforation, displacement, and adhesions Degenerative changes in condyle and/or fossa
V	Variable pain Joint crepitus	Anterior disk displacement that does not recapture on opening Marked disk deformity Degenerative osseous changes	Disk perforation, displacement, and adhesions Degenerative changes in condyle and/or fossa

Modified from Wilkes CH: Internal derangement of the temporomandibular joint: pathological variations, *Arch Otolaryngol Head Neck Surg* 115:469-477, 1989.

in pain but a greater increase in the mean interincisal opening, compared with arthrocentesis.

Open joint arthroplasty with disk plication, the most conservative open technique, involves mobilizing the anteriorly displaced disk and plicating it posteriorly (with sutures or titanium anchors) to ensure that it rests in the correct anatomic position on the mandibular condyle. Success rates approaching 90% have been reported.

Meniscectomy involves removal of the disk, and although it readily eliminates the disk displacement, it may be associated with significant degenerative joint disease (DJD) unless it is replaced with some type of graft (cartilage, fat, and dermis grafts have been used) or flap (temporalis muscle–fascia flap).

The modified condylotomy is an extraarticular procedure that spares the TMJ itself but involves allowing the mandibular condyle to reposition inferiorly and anteriorly to facilitate a more normal relationship between the condyle and disk. This procedure is associated with significant postoperative occlusal changes that can be difficult to manage in the long term, especially when the procedure is performed bilaterally.

In total joint replacement (TJR), the condyle is removed and the condyle and fossa are replaced with a prosthesis. TJR is performed in certain circumstances, such as ankylosis, degenerative joint disease, aseptic necrosis of the condyle, and systemic arthritides (rheumatoid arthritis, ankylosing spondylitis). Success after total joint replacement, in terms of pain and range of motion, is strongly influenced by the number of prior open surgical procedures.

In the current patient, although anterior disk displacement with reduction was present within the right TMJ, no symptoms were present. The patient did not require any treatment; she was reassured that her clinical findings were not uncommon and, in the absence of pain or limited function, observation was all that was necessary.

COMPLICATIONS

Although not complications, the sequelae of observational treatment include progression to symptomatic disease and the development of ADD without reduction or DJD. Progression of disease may warrant further noninvasive and/or invasive surgical treatment (see Discussion), each with its associated potential complications.

Complications associated with arthrocentesis are rare and mostly related to traumatic needle placement. Arthroscopy is more invasive and therefore may be associated with several complications, including facial nerve injury; penetration into the middle cranial fossa; damage to the joint structures; laceration or edema of the external auditory canal; otologic injury, resulting in hearing loss; infection; and instrument failure. Increased joint noise is common after arthrocentesis or arthroscopy, especially in patients with ADD without reduction.

Open joint procedures are the most invasive and are associated with the most potential complications, which include those mentioned for arthroscopy. Preauricular or endaural incisions are most commonly used to access the joint, which may result in sensory and motor nerve injuries. Injury to the auriculotemporal nerve (most common sensory nerve injury) usually results in altered sensation to the skin overlying the preauricular region (although this is usually temporary). Frey's syndrome (auriculotemporal nerve syndrome or gustatory sweating) may result from injury to the auriculo-temporal nerve, which carries parasympathetic fibers to the parotid gland and sympathetic fibers to the sweat glands of the skin. Misdirected nerve regeneration may cross the sympathetic and parasympathetic pathways, causing ipsilateral facial sweating when tasting or smelling food. Gustatory neuralgia (much less common) is similar to Frey's syndrome but results in electric shock and/or pain in the preauricular region when tasting or smelling food. Injury to the temporal (frontal) branch (most common motor nerve injury) of the facial nerve (crosses the zygomatic arch 8 to 35 mm, 20 mm on average, anterior to the external auditory meatus) results in weakness or paralysis of the frontalis (resulting in eyebrow ptosis) or orbicularis oculi muscles (resulting in lagophthalmos). Other branches or the main trunk of the facial nerve may be injured when more complex reconstructive joint procedures are performed due to the need for wider access and multiple incisions. There is a higher incidence of motor nerve injury in patients who have undergone multiple TMJ operations.

Temporary postoperative malocclusion (ipsilateral posterior open bite) is common after many invasive joint procedures. This may result from anatomic changes and edema in the joint. Modified condylotomy (extracapsular procedure) is associated with temporary or permanent postoperative malocclusion (anterior open bite and increased overjet), especially when performed bilaterally. This may result from condylar sag and loss of posterior vertical height or from condylar dislocation. Most cases of malocclusion may be treated with elastics, but surgical correction may be required.

Progression to DJD may occur both in patients who have undergone surgery and those who have not. The literature is inconsistent concerning the need for disk replacement after discectomy. There is concern that discectomy without replacement has a higher incidence of progression to DJD or ankylosis. Heterotopic bone formation may occur after any open joint procedure and may result in bony ankylosis.

DISCUSSION

Asymptomatic ADD with reduction is present in a significant proportion of the general population. The criteria for treatment are based on the degree of pain and functional impairment. Surgical intervention should be reserved for those with significant impairment and/or those for whom conservative therapy has failed. Disk displacement with reduction, whether symptomatic or not, may progress to disk displacement without reduction. This is thought to be the natural progression of the disease toward a more complex pathologic process that is more difficult to treat. The natural progression of disk displacement has been classically described by Wilkes, although a simpler functional description with ADD with or without reduction is more frequently used.

For patients with disk displacement with reduction who are asymptomatic, reassurance is often all that is needed. The potential for progression to disk displacement without reduction should be discussed. For patients desiring treatment, conservative splint therapy should be offered. Although flat-plane occlusal splints are most popular, an anterior repositioning splint that holds the mandible in a protruded position may help recapture the anteriorly displaced disk. An anterior repositioning splint is much more likely to result in occlusal changes that will necessitate further treatment, including occlusal equilibration, orthodontics, or orthognathic surgery.

Bibliography

Abramawicz S, Dolwick M: Twenty-year follow-up study of disc repositioning surgery for temporomandibular joint internal derangement, *J Oral Maxillofac Surg* 68:239-242, 2010.
Bays R: Surgery for internal derangement. In Bays RA, Quinn P (eds): *Oral and maxillofacial surgery: temporomandibular disorders*, pp 275-300, Philadelphia, 2000, Saunders.
Klasser G, Greene C: Oral appliances in the management of temporomandibular disorders, *Oral Surg Oral Med Oral Pathol Oral Radiol Endod* 107:212-223, 2009.
Mercuri LG, Wolford LM, Sanders B, et al: Long-term follow-up of the CAD/CAM patient fitted with a total temporomandibular joint reconstruction system, *J Oral Maxillofac Surg* 60:1440-1448, 2002.
Sidebottom A: Current thinking in temporomandibular joint management, *Br J Oral Maxillofac Surg* 47:91-94, 2009.
Wilkes CH: Internal derangement of the temporomandibular joint: pathological variations, *Arch Otolaryngol Head Neck Surg* 115:469-477, 1989.
Wolf J, Weiss A, Dym H: Technological advances in minimally invasive TMJ surgery, *Dent Clin North Am* 55:635-640, 2011.
Zhang S, Yang C, Cai X, et al: Prevention and treatment for rare complications of arthroscopic surgery in the temporomandibular joint, *J Oral Maxillofac Surg* 69:e347-e353, 2011.

Arthrocentesis and Arthroscopy

Brian E. Kinard and Gary F. Bouloux

CC

A 38-year-old female reports moderate right temporomandibular joint pain that has not responded to 3 months of splint therapy.

HPI

The patient reports a 4-month history of right-sided jaw pain that is worse with biting, chewing, and yawning. The pain is worsening and is severe enough to limit her diet to soft foods. She also reports a previous asymptomatic right-sided jaw click, present for many years, which stopped about the time she developed the right-sided pain. She reports limited jaw opening. Three months ago she saw her dentist, who prescribed a course of conservative therapy, including an occlusal splint, nonsteroidal antiinflammatory drugs (NSAIDs), use of a heating pad, and diet modification; this has provided little relief of her pain and scant improvement in her jaw opening.

PMHX/PDHX/MEDICATIONS/ALLERGIES/SH/FH

The patient's past medical and dental histories are noncontributory.

EXAMINATION

General. The patient is a well-developed and well-nourished woman in no apparent distress.

Maxillofacial. There is no tenderness on palpation of the temporalis or masseter muscles (no myofascial pain dysfunction), and the patient has no limitation or pain with movement of her neck (no cervical pain). There is right capsular tenderness on preauricular and endaural palpation. There is no clicking or crepitus on either palpation or auscultation of the temporomandibular joints bilaterally. The patient has a maximal interincisal opening of 32 mm, with deviation to the right and moderate pain. Her lateral excursive movements are 9 mm to the right and 3 mm to the left (suggesting decreased right TMJ condylar translation). She reports pain in the right joint when biting on a tongue blade placed between the molar teeth on the left side (positive Mahan test result, suggesting a right intracapsular source of pain). The remainder of her clinical examination is unremarkable.

IMAGING

A panoramic radiograph reveals no osseous abnormalities. Magnetic resonance imaging (MRI) reveals a normal left temporomandibular disk shape and position (11 o'clock position of the posterior band) and an anteriorly displaced right disk with a small joint effusion (suggesting inflammation).

LABS

No routine laboratory tests are indicated for the work-up of internal derangement unless there is clinical suspicion of undiagnosed systemic arthropathy (e.g., rheumatoid arthritis, systemic lupus erythematosus, psoriatic arthritis, and gout), which would dictate further laboratory testing.

ASSESSMENT

Internal derangement of the right TMJ; painful anterior disk displacement (ADD) without reduction of the right TMJ with capsulitis; Wilkes stage III (see Wilkes staging in the section Internal Derangement of the Temporomandibular Joint, earlier in this chapter).

TREATMENT

The initial treatment of temporomandibular joint dysfunction (e.g., symptomatic ADD without reduction) is often conservative. This may include an occlusal splint, NSAIDs, heating pads, diet modification, physical therapy or muscle relaxants. If after a short period of conservative treatment the patient has failed to improve adequately, surgical procedures should be considered.

The two most conservative surgical treatments are arthrocentesis and arthroscopy. Failure of one or both of these procedures may necessitate an open joint procedure, such as arthroplasty (see the section Internal Derangement of the Temporomandibular Joint, earlier in this chapter). All surgical procedures should be reserved for intracapsular sources of pain or limited function.

Arthrocentesis

Arthrocentesis is the process of irrigating and distending the superior joint space (rarely the inferior joint space) with Lactated Ringer's solution (LR) to remove inflammatory mediators and degraded proteins and to disrupt immature adhesions or a stuck disk. Arthrocentesis is generally indicated for patients with acute closed lock and arthralgia (often due to synovitis, chondromalacia, osteoarthritis, stuck disk phenomenon, or internal derangement). The procedure may result in an improvement in pain and range of motion. It can be accomplished under local anesthesia or sedation. The surgical field is prepared, and landmarks are identified by drawing a line extending from the superior aspect of the tragus to the lateral canthus of the eye. A point 10 mm anterior and 2 mm inferior along the tragal-canthus line is marked and serves as the initial puncture site. A local anesthetic is injected into the joint space and superficial tissues. Next, a 21-gauge needle is inserted into the superior joint space, and irrigation tubing is connected to it. Minor pressure is applied using a 60-ml syringe filled with LR to distend the joint space. A second 21-gauge needle can then be inserted into the joint space at a puncture point 4 to 5 mm anterior to the initial puncture site. Successful placement of the two needles is confirmed by the egress of LR from the second needle. The joint space is then irrigated with 50 to 200 ml of Lactated Ringer's solution (Figure 10-2). On completion of the irrigation, one needle can be removed and an adjuvant medication (e.g., corticosteroid or hyaluronic acid) can be injected into the joint space through the remaining needle. The mandible is then manipulated by opening maximally. The remaining needle is then removed, and pressure is applied to the injection site for 2 to 3 minutes.

The anticipated mean reduction in pain with arthrocentesis approaches 50%, and the mean increase in maximum interincisal opening approaches 15% over baseline.

Arthroscopy

Arthroscopy can be performed under local anesthesia, sedation, or general anesthesia in an ambulatory setting. Arthroscopy can be broadly classified as single or dual puncture, depending on how many trocars are used to penetrate the superior joint space. Dual-puncture arthroscopy is technically more difficult but provides the opportunity to instrument the joint space with hand instruments, motorized shavers, lasers, and coblation devices. There is no evidence that dual-puncture

arthroscopy is superior to single-puncture arthroscopy. The following description refers to single-puncture arthroscopy.

The surgical field is prepared, landmarks are identified (as per arthrocentesis), and a local anesthetic is injected into the joint space and superficial tissues. A sharp obturator/trocar is inserted percutaneously into the superior joint space. The obturator is then removed, the trocar is covered with a thumb to prevent backflow of irrigant, and irrigation tubing is connected to the trocar. Minor pressure is applied on a 60-ml syringe filled with lactated Ringer's solution. While the superior joint space is distended with the solution, a 21-gauge needle is inserted 4 to 5 mm anteriorly into the superior joint space. Appropriate positioning is confirmed with immediate egress of the irrigating solution. The arthroscope can then be inserted through the trocar with clear visualization of the superior joint space. Once the arthroscope is inside the anterior-superior joint space, a methodical sweep of the joint space is undertaken so that the retrodiscal tissue, medial trough, anterior recess, disk, and eminence are visualized. Evidence of synovitis, chondromalacia, fibrous adhesions, pseudowalls (synovium-covered, fibrous walls), perforations, or other pathology is readily identified. The joint space is irrigated with 150 to 200 ml of lactated Ringer's solution under pulsatile digital pressure (Figure 10-3). Adhesions can be disrupted with the scope and a lateral capsular stretch performed (lateral capsular impingement syndrome). The 21-gauge needle is then removed, and an adjuvant medication (e.g., corticosteroid or hyaluronic acid) is injected through the trocar. The trocar is removed, and digital pressure is applied for 2 to 3 minutes.

The anticipated mean reduction in pain with arthroscopy approaches 70%, and the mean increase in maximum interincisal opening approaches 40%.

COMPLICATIONS

Complications associated with arthrocentesis are rare and mostly related to traumatic needle placement with perforation

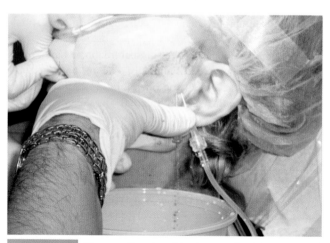

Figure 10-2 Two needles placed in the superior joint space and irrigation with lactated Ringer's solution.

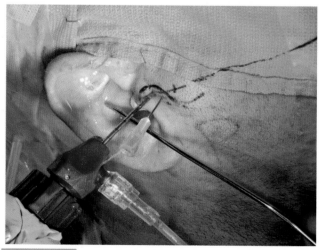

Figure 10-3 Arthroscope and outflow irrigating needle with egress of lactated Ringer's solution.

of the external auditory canal, middle ear, and middle cranial fossa. Complications with arthroscopy are also rare and include the previously described perforation injuries, in addition to injury to the facial nerve, iatrogenic injury to the joint, and instrument breakage, which may necessitate an open procedure.

DISCUSSION

The treatment for patients with symptomatic internal derangement is aimed at reducing pain and increasing range of motion. Many patients undergo a period of conservative treatment, which may fail to provide improvement. Ultimately the patient may benefit from arthrocentesis or arthroscopy. All surgical procedures must be used only for patients with intracapsular sources of pain or limited function (e.g., internal derangement). The choice between arthrocentesis and arthroscopy can be difficult to make and is often dictated by the surgeon's experience, the patient's preference, and the cost. The outcomes are comparable, although arthroscopy is more likely to result in a greater mean reduction in pain and improvement in maximum interincisal opening. Early arthroscopy (within 6 months of symptom development) has also been shown to be more successful than delayed arthroscopy. This may not be the case with arthrocentesis. For both procedures, a vigorous postprocedural jaw exercise regimen, which the patient performs at home for several weeks, is particularly important.

Controversy exists as to whether the injection of adjunct medication (e.g., corticosteroid or hyaluronic acid) is of additional benefit after either procedure. The choice of which medication to use is guided more by the surgeon's personal experience, although current literature provides equivocal support for both medications, depending on the pathology present and the joint involved. No clear guidelines exist specifically for the temporomandibular joint.

Bibliography

Basterzi Y, Sari A, Demirkan F, et al: Intraarticular hyaluronic acid injection for the treatment of reducing and nonreducing disc displacement of the temporomandibular joint, *Ann Plast Surg* 62:265-267, 2009.

Dolwick MF: Temporomandibular joint surgery for internal derangement, *Dent Clin North Am* 51:195-208, 2007.

Gonzalez-Garcia R, Rodriguez-Campo FJ, Monje F, et al: Operative versus simple arthroscopic surgery for chronic closed lock of the temporomandibular joint: a clinical study of 344 arthroscopic procedures, *Int J Oral Maxillofac Surg* 37:790-796, 2008.

Gonzalez-Garcia R, Rodriguez-Campo FJ, Monje F, et al: Influence of the upper joint surface and synovial lining in the outcome of chronic closed lock of the temporomandibular joint treated with arthroscopy, *J Oral Maxillofac Surg* 68:35-42, 2010.

Israel HA, Behrman DA, Friedman JM, et al: Rationale for early versus late intervention with arthroscopy for treatment of inflammatory/degenerative temporomandibular joint disorders, *J Oral Maxillofac Surg* 68:2661-2667, 2010.

Long X, Chen G, Cheng AH, et al: A randomized controlled trial of superior and inferior temporomandibular joint space injection with hyaluronic acid in treatment of anterior disc displacement without reduction, *J Oral Maxillofac Surg* 67:357-361, 2009.

Manfredini D, Bonnini S, Arboretti R, et al: Temporomandibular joint osteoarthritis: an open label trial of 76 patients treated with arthrocentesis plus hyaluronic acid injections, *Int J Oral Maxillofac Surg* 38:827-834, 2009.

McCain JP, de la Rua H: Principles and practice of operative arthroscopy of the human temporomandibular joint, *Oral Maxillofac Surg Clin North Am* 1:135-151, 1989.

Morey-Mas MA, Caubet-Biayna J, Varela-Sende L, et al: Sodium hyaluronate improves outcomes after arthroscopic lysis and lavage in patients with Wilkes stage III and IV disease, *J Oral Maxillofac Surg* 68:1069-1074, 2010.

Oliveras-Moreno JM, Hernandez-Pacheco E, Oliveras-Quintana T, et al: Efficacy and safety of sodium hyaluronate in the treatment of Wilkes stage II disease, *J Oral Maxillofac Surg* 66:2243-2246, 2008.

Onder ME, Tüz HH, Koçyiğit D, et al: Long-term results of arthrocentesis in degenerative temporomandibular disorders, *Oral Surg Oral Med Oral Pathol Oral Radiol Endod* 107:e1-e5, 2009.

Wilkes CH: Surgical treatment of internal derangements of the temporomandibular joint: a long-term study, *Arch Otolaryngol Head Neck Surg* 117:64-72, 1991.

Degenerative Joint Disease of the Temporomandibular Joint

Jason A. Jamali, Antonia Kolokythas, Chris Jo, and Michael Miloro

CC

A 55-year-old woman (DJD has a higher prevalence with advanced age and in female patients) presents to your office with a long history of temporomandibular joint dysfunction (TMD), complaining, "I've been through several TMJ surgeries, and now my right joint is very painful and makes grinding noises."

HPI

The patient reports several months of anxiety and stress that she relates to the pain centered around her right temporomandibular joint (TMJ); this pain is most pronounced upon mouth opening during mastication or speech. She has a long, progressive history of TMJ problems. In her late teens, she developed bilateral reciprocal TMJ clicking (suggestive of anterior disk displacement [ADD] with reduction, which was confirmed by an arthrogram (prior to the advent of MRI, arthrography was a commonly used modality for imaging the TMJ and diagnosing TMJ disorders). She also had intermittent right-sided preauricular pain and bilateral myofascial pain. She was managed nonsurgically with occlusal splint therapy and nonsteroidal antiinflammatory drugs (NSAIDs). She reported mild improvement and did not pursue further treatment, because she tolerated her discomfort by minimizing masticatory function. In her mid-20s, the right TMJ stopped clicking, and she developed an acute closed lock with severe right-sided pain and restricted left lateral excursive movements of the mandible without clicking (this is consistent with the progression of ADD with reduction to ADD without reduction on the right). She underwent right-sided TMJ arthrocentesis, which provided 8 months of symptomatic resolution. A second arthrocentesis procedure was performed, which provided only brief additional relief. Subsequent MRI studies showed evidence of ADD and degenerative joint disease (DJD) of the right TMJ (with a displaced, deformed, nonreducing disk and evidence of perforation of the posterior band of the disk, in addition to degenerative bony changes of the TMJ with decreased joint space, flattening of the condylar head, and osteophyte formation), in addition to ADD without reduction on the left side with associated degenerative bony changes. Her surgeon elected to perform a discectomy (removal of the disk) without disk replacement, which resulted in an excellent outcome for several years. She now presents with a 2-year history of loud, grinding noises or crepitus (crepitus is a pathognomonic sign of advanced osteoarthrosis) of the right TMJ with increasing levels of debilitating pain localized to the right TMJ.

PMHX/PDHX/MEDICATIONS/ALLERGIES/SH/FH

Noncontributory, except for arthritic changes diagnosed in the patient's cervical spine and the proximal interphalangeal joints of the hands. She has taken NSAIDs as needed for pain over the past several years. (Patients with arthritic degeneration of the TMJ frequently have involvement of other joints that precedes involvement of the TMJ. However, it is possible to have DJD of the TMJ with no evidence of arthritis in any other joints.)

EXAMINATION

General. The patient is a well-developed and well-nourished woman in moderate distress due to right-sided TMJ pain.

Maxillofacial. The patient has no facial swelling or asymmetry. The right TMJ is exquisitely tender to palpation (upon both preauricular and endaural palpation). The left TMJ is nontender. She has limited opening (20 mm) due to pain and a loud, bony crepitance of the right TMJ that is easily heard without a stethoscope. Lateral excursive movements are limited (3 mm to the left and 6 mm to the right). She has a Class I occlusion without an open bite (advanced condylar degeneration and loss of posterior mandibular height can lead to a contralateral posterior open bite or an anterior open bite). The external auditory canals are clear, and the tympanic membranes appear normal. Her preauricular surgical scar is well healed, and cranial nerve VII is intact (multiple open TMJ procedures increase the risk of cranial nerve VII injury, especially the frontal or temporal branch).

IMAGING

The panoramic radiograph is the initial imaging study of choice for evaluation of the TMJ. It provides a general overview of the bony morphology of the mandible and condyle. MRI scans, in the open and closed mouth positions, are considered the standard when evaluating for TMJ internal derangement to view the disk. MRI provides the most detailed information regarding the soft tissue structures (disk morphology) and disk position in the open and closed mouth positions (some patients may not be able to open sufficiently due to pain, ADD without reduction, or closed lock). A TMJ arthrogram (a fluoroscopic study in which contrast dye usually is injected into the inferior joint space), an invasive procedure that shows the disk in dynamic function, is an ideal study for detection of disk perforations (finding dye in the superior joint space indicates a perforation allowing contrast to exit the inferior joint space). A bony window computed tomography (CT) scan is indicated when bony or fibrous ankylosis of the TMJ, or other bony pathology, is suspected. A CT scan can be used to better delineate the bony anatomy of the TMJ, and demonstrate any degenerative changes.

For the current patient, the panoramic radiograph demonstrated evidence of bilateral osteoarthrosis (small condyles with arthritic remodeling, likely due to joint overloading), including flattening of the condylar head, subchondral eburnation (sclerosis), and osteophyte formation. The right condylar head (Figure 10-4, *A*) showed a greater loss of normal

anatomy, was significantly smaller than the left side, had sharp edges, and had lost its cortical definition (signs of advanced degeneration). Sagittal and coronal MRI scans showed an anteromedially displaced (most frequent location of a dislocated disk) left TMJ disk in the closed mouth position that did not reduce in the open mouth position, with moderate degenerative changes (TMJ soft tissue anatomy is best seen with T1-weighted images). T1-weighted MRI images of the right TMJ (Figure 10-4, *B*) revealed remnants of the anterior portion of the displaced disk (consistent with previous discectomy) and evidence of severe degenerative changes of the condylar head and inflammatory changes (TMJ inflammation and effusions are best seen with T2-weighted images, because they appear with increased signal intensity). A CT scan showed bilateral bony degenerative changes that

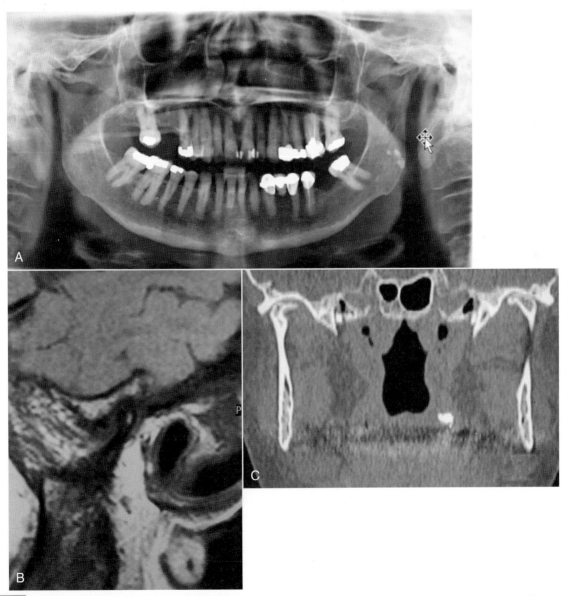

Figure 10-4   **A,** Panoramic radiograph revealing severe degenerative bony changes of the bilateral (right greater than left) condylar heads, including loss of normal architecture and loss of smooth cortical outline. **B,** T1-weighted MRI revealing remnants of the anterior portion of a displaced disk from a previous discectomy and significant degenerative changes of the condylar head. **C,** Direct coronal CT showing degenerative bony changes of the bilateral mandibular condylar heads (right greater than left).

were more severe on the right side, with decreased marrow space (Figure 10-4, *C*).

LABS

No routine laboratory testing is indicated for the work-up of DJD. Clinical suspicion of systemic arthropathies (e.g., rheumatoid arthritis, systemic lupus erythematosus, psoriatic arthritis, and gout) would dictate further laboratory testing. Other laboratory values are obtained based on the medical history, and the results of nonspecific laboratory studies of inflammation (e.g., C-reactive protein and erythrocyte sedimentation rate) may be elevated due to chronic inflammation. Baseline preoperative hemoglobin and hematocrit levels are recommended for patients undergoing an open joint procedure or total joint reconstruction.

ASSESSMENT

DJD of bilateral TMJs, with localized pain on the multiply operated right side.

TREATMENT

The goals of treatment for DJD of the TMJ are to decrease pain and swelling, improve joint function, and limit disease progression. Generally treatment follows a stepwise sequence, beginning with noninvasive or minimally invasive procedures and progressing to more advanced surgical treatment modalities when indicated.

Nonsurgical therapy includes a jaw rest regimen, occlusal appliances, physical therapy, warm compresses, and NSAIDs. Arthrocentesis is a minimally invasive treatment modality; however, the use of intra-articular adjunctive medications (e.g., corticosteroids and hyaluronic acid) is somewhat controversial. Arthroscopy does not offer additional outcome benefits over arthrocentesis, but it may provide a diagnostic advantage. The majority (about 80%) of patients respond, at least in the short term, to both noninvasive and minimally invasive treatments, perhaps as a result of the joint lavage and clearance of inflammatory mediators.

More invasive surgical modalities include open joint (arthrotomy) procedures, such as arthroplasty with osseous recontouring of the condyle and/or glenoid fossa and, if necessary, disk removal or repositioning. Discectomy may be performed in conjunction with placement of an interpositional material (e.g., autogenous fat graft, dermal graft, alloplastic graft, cadaveric graft, temporalis muscle–fascia flap, ear cartilage). With severe degeneration of the TMJ, reconstruction may be necessary using either autogenous options (e.g., free fibula flaps, costochondral/calvarial grafts) or an alloplastic prosthesis. Various alloplastic total joint implants are available either as one-stage or two-stage procedures (see the section Ankylosis of the Temporomandibular Joint, later in this chapter).

In the current patient, total joint replacement was performed using custom prefabricated condylar head and fossa alloplastic implants. This required a two-stage surgical approach. In the first stage, a gap arthroplasty was performed with a discectomy and condylectomy to provide adequate space (2 to 2.5 cm minimum distance) for the TMJ implant (a Silastic block can be left in situ to preserve the surgically created tissue space and prevent scarring). In the second stage, the TMJ fossa and condylar prosthesis were implanted via a preauricular approach with two stab incisions (in addition to the preauricular incision, a retromandibular approach can be used to facilitate fixation of the condylar component of the total joint replacement).

COMPLICATIONS

The possible complications of TMJ surgery for the treatment of DJD are similar to those of open arthrotomy surgery for internal derangement or TMJ ankylosis (see the sections on Internal Derangement of the Temporomandibular Joint and Ankylosis of the Temporomandibular Joint for a discussion of surgical complications). In addition, hardware failure, with screw loosening, may lead to prosthesis failure. With prosthetic joint replacement in ankylosis, the prosthetic components may act as osteoconductive scaffolds for heterotopic bone formation and reankylosis, especially if active physiotherapy is delayed or if the patient is noncompliant with postoperative rehabilitation. Also, these prosthetic components may have a limited life span (20 years) and may require replacement. However, clinical experience may show that replacement of a functional TMJ prosthesis, without any indication other than time in function, may be unnecessary.

DISCUSSION

Degenerative joint disease is a maladaptive response to mechanical joint loading, leading to destruction of hard tissue. During this process, the breakdown products lead to recruitment of inflammatory mediators, resulting in a secondary synovitis and capsulitis. The symptomatic inflammatory phase, known as *osteoarthritis,* may be distinguished from *osteoarthrosis,* which represents an end-stage phase of the spectrum.

TMD encompasses several related disorders of the TMJ. The Research Diagnostic Criteria for Temporomandibular Disorders (RDC/TMD) classification system organizes these disorders into three groups: group I (myofascial pain), group II (internal derangement), and group III (degenerative joint disease). Although these entities are interrelated, the data regarding a causative relationship between internal derangement and degenerative joint disease have not been definitive. The epidemiology reveals a bimodal distribution for the incidence of internal derangement (mean age, 38 years) and degenerative joint disease (mean age, 52 years). Studies have shown that degenerative joint changes may occur in elderly patients who show normal disk positioning. Establishing a causative relationship may have significant clinical implications for treatment planning, although it has been shown that pain does not correlate well with degenerative joint disease. Long-term studies have shown that the initial symptoms of DJD and internal derangement may follow a self-limiting course, with resolution by 30-year follow-up after nonsurgical therapy.

With regard to diagnosis, proper imaging analysis is an important adjunct to the clinical examination. In general, MRI is more helpful for delineating disk position, and CT scanning is most helpful for visualization of the bony changes associated with DJD. Crepitus is an important distinguishing finding on clinical examination, because it has a high correlation with DJD.

The Wilkes staging classification system for internal derangement of the TMJ (see Table 10-1) divides progression of the disease into five stages (early, early/intermediate, intermediate, intermediate/late, and late) based on the clinical, radiographic, and anatomic and pathologic features.

Bibliography

Auerbach SM, Laskin DM, Frantsve LME, et al: Depression, pain, exposure to stressful life events, and long-term outcomes in temporomandibular disorder patients, *J Oral Maxillofac Surg* 59:628-633, 2001.

Bays RA: Temporomandibular joint disc preservation, *Atlas Oral Maxillofac Surg Clin North Am* 4:33-50, 1996.

Bertolami CN, Gay T, Clark GT, et al: Use of sodium hyaluronate in treating temporomandibular joint disorders: a randomized, double-blind, placebo-controlled clinical trial, *J Oral Maxillofac Surg* 51:232-242, 1993.

Bjornland T, Larheim TA: Discectomy of the temporomandibular joint: 3-year follow-up as a predictor of the 10-year outcome, *J Oral Maxillofac Surg* 61:55-60, 2003.

Broussard J: Derangement, osteoarthritis, and rheumatoid arthritis of the temporomandibular joint: implications, diagnosis, and management, *Dent Clin North Am* 49:327-342, 2005.

Carvajal WA, Laskin DM: Long-term evaluation of arthrocentesis for the treatment of internal derangements of the temporomandibular joint, *J Oral Maxillofac Surg* 58:852-855, 2000.

de Souza RF, Lovato da Silva CH, Nasser M, et al: Interventions for the management of temporomandibular joint osteoarthritis, *Cochrane Libr* 4:1-38, 2012.

Dimitroulis G: A review of 56 cases of chronic closed lock treated with temporomandibular joint arthroscopy, *J Oral Maxillofac Surg* 60:519-524, 2002.

Dimitroulis G: The use of dermis grafts after discectomy for internal derangement of the temporomandibular joint, *J Oral Maxillofac Surg* 63:173-178, 2005.

Dolwick MF: Disc preservation surgery for the treatment of internal derangements of the temporomandibular joint, *J Oral Maxillofac Surg* 59:1047-1050, 2001.

Edwards SP, Feinber SE: The temporalis muscle flap in contemporary oral and maxillofacial surgery, *Oral Maxillofac Surg Clin North Am* 15:513-535, 2003.

Emschoff R, Rudisch A: Are internal derangement and osteoarthrosis linked to changes in clinical outcome measures of arthrocentesis of the temporomandibular joint? *J Oral Maxillofac Surg* 61:1162-1167, 2003.

Emschoff R, Rudisch A: Determining predictor variables for treatment outcomes of arthrocentesis and hydraulic distention of the temporomandibular joint, *J Oral Maxillofac Surg* 62:816-823, 2004.

Eriksson L, Westesson PL: Long-term evaluation of meniscectomy of the temporomandibular joint, *J Oral Maxillofac Surg* 43:263-269, 1985.

Eriksson L, Westesson PL: Discectomy as an effective treatment for painful temporomandibular joint internal derangement: a 5-year clinical and radiographic follow-up, *J Oral Maxillofac Surg* 59:750-758, 2001.

Feinberg SE: Use of local tissues for temporomandibular joint surgery disc replacement, *Atlas Oral Maxillofac Surg Clin North Am* 4:51-74, 1996.

Fricton JR, Look JO, Schiffman E, et al: Long-term study of temporomandibular joint surgery with alloplastic implants compared with nonimplant surgery and nonsurgical rehabilitation for painful temporomandibular joint disc displacement, *J Oral Maxillofac Surg* 60:1400-1411, 2002.

Guarda-Nardini L, Piccotti F, Mogno G, et al: Age-related differences in temporomandibular disorder diagnoses, *J Craniomandibular Pract* 30:103-109, 2012.

Hendler BH, Gateno J, Mooar P, et al: Holmium: YAG laser arthroscopy of the temporomandibular joint, *J Oral Maxillofac Surg* 50:931-934, 1992.

Indresano AT: Surgical arthroscopy as the preferred treatment for internal derangements of the temporomandibular joint, *J Oral Maxillofac Surg* 59:308-312, 2001.

Israel HA, Ward JD, Horrell B, et al: Oral and maxillofacial surgery in patients with chronic orofacial pain, *J Oral Maxillofac Surg* 61:662-667, 2003.

Iwase H, Sasaki T, Asakura S, et al: Characterization of patients with disc displacement without reduction unresponsive to nonsurgical treatment: a preliminary study, *J Oral Maxillofac Surg* 63:1115-1122, 2005.

Keith DA: Complications of temporomandibular joint surgery, *Oral Maxillofac Surg Clin North Am* 15:187-194, 2003.

Leeuw R, Boering G: Symptoms of temporomandibular joint and internal derangement 30 years after non-surgical treatment, *J Craniomandibular Pract* 13:81-88, 1995.

Mazzonetto R, Spagnoli DB: Long-term evaluation of arthroscopic discectomy of the temporomandibular joint using the holium YAG laser, *J Oral Maxillofac Surg* 59:1018-1023, 2001.

McKenna SJ: Discectomy for the treatment of internal derangements of the temporomandibular joint, *J Oral Maxillofac Surg* 59:1051-1056, 2001.

Milam SB: Chronic temporomandibular joint arthralgia, *Oral Maxillofac Surg Clin North Am* 12:5-26, 2000.

Nitzan DW, Price A: The use of arthrocentesis for the treatment of osteoarthritic temporomandibular joints, *J Oral Maxillofac Surg* 59:1154-1159, 2001.

Park J, Keller EE, Reid KI: Surgical management of advanced degenerative arthritis of temporomandibular joint with mental fossa-eminence hemijoint replacement prosthesis: an 8-year retrospective pilot study, *J Oral Maxillofac Surg* 62:320-328, 2004.

Reston JT, Turkelson CM: Meta-analysis of surgical treatments for temporomandibular articular disorders, *J Oral Maxillofac Surg* 61:3-10, 2003.

Stegenga B: Osteoarthritis of the temporomandibular joint organ and its relationship to disc displacement, *J Orofac Pain* 15:193-205, 2001.

Tucker MR, Spagnoli DB: Autogenous dermal and auricular cartilage grafts for temporomandibular joint repair, *Atlas Oral Maxillofac Surg Clin North Am* 4:75-92, 1996.

Umeda H, Kaban LB, Pogrel MA, et al: Long-term viability of the temporalis muscle/fascia flap used for temporomandibular joint reconstruction, *J Oral Maxillofac Surg* 51:530-533, 1993.

White RD: Arthroscopic lysis and lavage as the preferred treatment for internal derangement of the temporomandibular joint, *J Oral Maxillofac Surg* 59:313-316, 2001.

Yun PY, Kim YK: The role of facial trauma as a possible etiologic factor in temporomandibular joint disorder, *J Oral Maxillofac Surg* 63:1576-1583, 2005.

Zingg M, Iizuka T, Geering AH, et al: Degenerative temporomandibular joint disease: surgical treatment and long-term results, *J Oral Maxillofac Surg* 52:1149-1158, 1994.

Ankylosis of the Temporomandibular Joint

Vincent J. Perciaccante and Deepak G. Krishnan

CC

A 64-year-old woman presents to the oral and maxillofacial surgery (OMS) office complaining of a progressively worsening inability to open her mouth.

Although there is no gender predilection in ankylosis, there is a correlation with age and geographic distribution. Ankylosis in children is more common in developing countries. Ankylosis in most other populations is usually a result of end-stage joint disease, trauma, benign pathoses, or repeated TMJ operations in adults.

HPI

The patient has a protracted history of bilateral temporomandibular joint dysfunction (TMD) and multiple attempts at nonsurgical and surgical management (see the sections on Internal Derangement of the Temporomandibular Joint and Myofascial Pain Dysfunction) to alleviate the pain associated with her TMJs. The multimodality treatment she has undergone already includes splint therapy, physical therapy, nonsteroidal antiinflammatory drugs (NSAIDs), multiple arthrocentesis procedures (which resulted in transient relief of pain), and TMJ arthroplasties with bilateral disk plication, followed by bilateral discectomies and abdominal fat grafting (see the previous section on Degenerative Joint Disease of the Temporomandibular Joint). With unresolved symptoms, which included painful crepitus, and findings of atrophic failure of these grafts, she underwent bilateral temporalis muscle fascia interpositioning surgery 2 years earlier. She admits to being noncompliant with postoperative jaw opening exercises due to pain. However, since her last surgery, mouth opening has progressively decreased, and the associated TMJ pain has reduced considerably.

PMHX/PDHX/MEDICATIONS/ALLERGIES/SH/FH

The patient has chronic pain associated with the cervical spine and TMJ (osteoarthritis, chronic neck pain status post cervical spine fusion of C4-5).

Osteoarthritis can be an initiating factor in the cascade of events that leads to the ankylosis of an adult TMJ. Patients with chronic TMJ pain and associated myofascial pain dysfunction (MPD) may also present with significant chronic neck pain.

EXAMINATION

General. The patient is a well-developed and well-nourished woman in mild distress due to chronic neck pain and inability to open her mouth.

Maxillofacial. She has limited range of motion of her cervical spine, especially with flexion and extension (this increases the difficulty of intubation). Her maximal incisal opening is 2 mm, with a hard stop and no lateral excursive movements (consistent with mechanical obstruction). Palpation of the TMJs reveals a bony mass, and no condylar movement is palpable in any direction. The temporal (frontal) branch of the right facial nerve (cranial VII) is weak (the incidence of facial nerve injury increases with each open joint procedure in patients who have undergone multiple TMJ operations). Bilateral preauricular surgical scars are well healed. She is in Class I occlusion. There is tenderness of the masseter, temporalis, and sternocleidomastoid muscles upon palpation. There is mild masseteric hypertrophy. (The muscles of mastication constantly attempt to open an ankylosed joint; this effect is more profound in ankylosis in children, in whom masseteric hyperactivity also causes the formation of a prominent antegonial notch.)

IMAGING

A panoramic film is the initial screening study of choice when dealing with TMD, especially when pain is present (to evaluate for odontogenic causes of pain). It provides a general overview of the bony morphology of the mandible, the condyle, and the glenoid fossa. If a bony or fibrous ankylosis of the TMJ is suspected, bony window CT scans without contrast and with multiplanar views is the study of choice. These provide the most diagnostic information on the bony architecture (anatomic and pathologic) of the TMJ, including the presence of heterotopic bone formation. In addition, these images can be used for virtual treatment planning of the surgery and can aid construction of custom TMJ prosthetics, if indicated. MRI is indicated when internal derangement is suspected (see the section on internal derangement earlier in this chapter), but it has little diagnostic value in the case of ankylosis.

In the current patient, the panoramic radiograph showed normal adult dentition with multiple previous dental restorations. It also showed some evidence of heterotopic bone formation in the bilateral TMJ areas, with obliteration of normal joint space and distortion of the condylar articular anatomy.

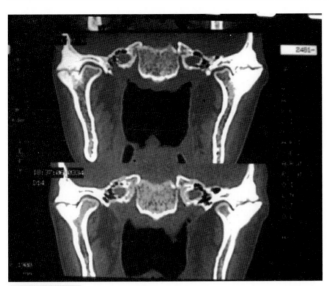

Figure 10-5 Bony window, direct coronal CT scans showing bilateral TMJ bony ankylosis.

Coronal bony CT scans (Figure 10-5) clearly demonstrated obliteration of the bilateral TMJ space. The heterotopic bone had a mushroom shape and appeared to distort the entire TMJ anatomy. No evidence of any remnants of normal disks or previously attempted grafts or flaps was visible.

LABS

For TMJ ankylosis, no laboratory values are needed in the initial work-up unless dictated by the patient's medical history. Preoperative hemoglobin and hematocrit levels are needed during the surgical phase of treatment because of potential intraoperative blood loss. Clinical suspicion of systemic arthropathy (e.g., rheumatoid arthritis, systemic lupus erythematosus, psoriatic arthritis, and gout) would dictate further laboratory work-up.

The current patient had a hemoglobin of 12 mg/dl and a hematocrit of 35.6%.

In addition to conventional lab testing, most patients with TMJ ankylosis benefit from a preanesthesia evaluation. This enables anesthetic risk stratification, which is important considering the patients' difficult airway access, altered anatomy, and chronic pain, in addition to other challenges in perioperative and postoperative management.

ASSESSMENT

Bony ankylosis of the bilateral TMJs and associated MPD.

Ankylosis of the TMJ has a variety of etiologies but eventually results in fusion of the mandibular condylar head to the glenoid fossa. The etiologies are all insults and invasions of the joint space in one form or another, such as trauma, surgery, or infection (an infectious etiology mostly is seen with direct spread from mastoiditis or otitis but rarely via the hematogenous route). Ankylosis can be bony or fibrous, complete or partial. Reference to fibrous ankylosis is made clinically and

radiographically when the limitation in motion of the joint is caused by fibrous adhesions or scar tissues rather than actual bone formation. Fibrous ankylosis often progresses to bony ankylosis.

TREATMENT

The goals of treatment for TMJ ankylosis are to release the ankylotic joint or joints and to reconstruct the diseased joint to function. This can be done as simultaneous procedures or as staged procedures, depending on the elected reconstructive modality (stock or custom-fabricated alloplastic TMJ prosthesis or autogenous costochondral, cranial, or vascularized bone grafts). Postoperative pain management, aggressive physical therapy, and prevention of reankylosis are paramount during the rehabilitation phase.

Release of ankylotic joint or joints. In the adult with TMJ ankylosis, the procedure of choice to release the ankylosis depends on the type and severity of the condition. In fibrous ankylosis, often detachment of the fibrous scars and a coronoidectomy (or coronoidotomy) provide good mouth opening. If there is bony ankylosis, a gap arthroplasty is warranted. Gap arthroplasty involves osseous recontouring of the deformed glenoid fossa and condylar head (condylectomy may be performed, depending on the reconstruction modality), removal of heterotopic bone, and creation of adequate space to accommodate the reconstructive plans. Ipsilateral coronoidectomy or coronoidotomy is indicated if mouth opening is restricted after release of the ankylotic joint, followed by contralateral coronoidectomy or coronoidotomy if opening is still restricted. The medial extent of large ankylotic joints often requires arthroplasty pursued in deeper recesses, where both access and visibility may be difficult. Recent advances in navigation-guided surgery allow careful access to the medial parts of the TMJ traditionally considered risky due to aberrant vasculature in the area. Navigation-guided surgery has also proven to be a reliable tool for preventing untoward perforations through the glenoid fossa into the middle cranium, made while preparing the site during gap arthroplasty.

Reconstruction of the TMJ. There is increasing evidence supporting the safety, utility, and longevity of alloplastic prosthetic reconstruction of the TMJ. Although this is not an option in the growing child, it may have a valuable role in the treatment of adults. Alloplastic TMJ prostheses may be custom-made or stock. If the joint is to be reconstructed with a custom CAD-CAM–generated prosthesis, the surgery sometimes (but not always) requires two stages. A custom-fabricated joint prosthesis uses patient-specific information obtained from the CT scan (Figures 10-6 and 10-7). Gap arthroplasty and setting of the occlusion to the desired position often are done preoperatively on a stereolithographic model, either manually or digitally. Stock prostheses rely on prefabricated fossa and condyle/ramus units that come in preset sizes. The clinician uses sizers and contouring drills to choose and then fit the appropriate-sized prosthesis for each patient.

Before the advent of total TMJ reconstruction systems, the costochondral graft was the workhorse of TMJ reconstruction.

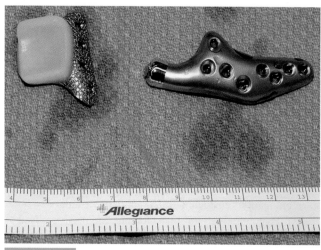

Figure 10-6 Example of a total TMJ prosthesis (the TMJ Concepts prosthesis [Ventura, California] is shown).

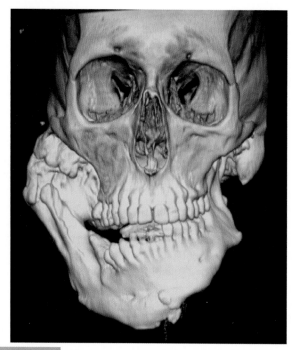

Figure 10-7 CT scan of another patient showing extensive right TMJ ankylosis caused by progressive fibrous dysplastic growth in the region. Although the more common etiology for ankylosis is end-stage joint disease, trauma, repeated TMJ operations or infections, the differential diagnosis should include benign pathology of the TMJ structures.

It is still the graft of choice for growing children. The most-cited disadvantage of the costochondral graft is its unreliable growth pattern, especially in children. Other autogenous bone grafts have been reported, including calvarial strips, metatarsal joints and sternoclavicular junction, and vascularized grafts from the fibula, second toe, and iliac crest. When autogenous grafting is used for reconstruction of the TMJ complex, the fossa is most often aligned and interpositioned by a pedicled temporalis muscle–fascia flap.

Rehabilitation and prevention of reankylosis. Postoperative pain management and physical therapy are critical to the success of TMJ ankylosis surgery. Reluctance and noncompliance by the patient in following a thorough physical therapy regimen are often cited as the most significant contributing factors in reankylosis or failure to achieve good mouth opening. There is also some evidence that low-dose radiation can prevent heterotopic bone formation after joint surgery (see Discussion). The current management algorithm in adult reconstruction of an ankylosed TMJ using a TMJ prosthesis virtually eliminates the chances of reankylosis. However, rehabilitation is necessary in these patients to maximize function after reconstruction.

COMPLICATIONS

TMJ ankylosis surgery carries all the potential complications associated with any open TMJ surgery, which may include scar formation, facial nerve damage, Frey's syndrome (gustatory sweating), external auditory meatus perforations, infection, and reankylosis (see the section on Internal Derangement of the Temporomandibular Joint earlier in this chapter).

Other potential complications include those associated with anesthesia related to hypomobility of the mandible, causing a difficult airway that may require advanced intubation techniques. Complications associated with concomitant procedures may be seen, including morbidities from a graft procurement (donor and recipient site), orthognathic surgery, or distraction osteogenesis procedures.

The greatest challenge for the surgeon is the probability of reankylosis. Sometimes despite aggressive resection, interpositioning, and aggressive physiotherapy, the intrinsic ability of a young adult to form heterotopic bone overcomes all obstacles, leading to reankylosis. The same low-dose radiation protocol used to prevent heterotopic bone formation after hip arthroplasties (i.e., 10 Gy fractionated in five doses) can be used to help prevent TMJ heterotopic bone formation. This has been suggested to be effective in preventing TMJ reankylosis after release and reconstruction. The chances of reankylosis are drastically lower in patients treated with a total joint prosthesis.

Complications associated with surgical techniques can include perforation into the middle cranial fossa from the gap arthroplasty. Dural exposure through the glenoid area should be carefully examined to ensure that the dura is intact. If a dural tear is seen or suspected, neurosurgical consultation is warranted.

Severe bleeding may be encountered from the medial infratemporal fossa. Peoples and associates reported management of an iatrogenic tear of the internal maxillary artery during TMJ arthroplasty via selective embolization. Their review of the literature showed that arguments against a carotid cutdown and ligation stemmed from the suspicion that continued bleeding could arise from the collateral vessels distal to the bleeding site. (Transantral ligation has also been documented as somewhat unreliable due to documented cases of continued postligation bleeding.) These researchers' choice of management is selective embolization to obtain proximal control. The locations of the middle meningeal artery, the internal jugular vein, and the main trunk of the third division of the trigeminal nerve can vary greatly, and this can make surgery more dangerous than may be anticipated. In resection of the medial aspect of the ankylosed TMJ, excessive bleeding can be attributed to the internal maxillary artery. This arterial bleeding can have the potential to cause serious morbidity. Navigation-aided resection of an ankylosis of the mandible has been reported as a safe technique that may become a routine part of craniomaxillofacial surgery.

DISCUSSION

Ankylosis alters the normal anatomy of the TMJ to varying degrees and can be classified according to the tissues involved and the extent of involvement. Classification can also be based on the location of the ankylosis. Consolidation and fibro-osseous restructuring of hemarthrosis form the basic pathogenic pattern of TMJ ankylosis. The destruction of a growing joint may directly affect the mandible and has secondary effects on the growing facial skeleton and soft tissues.

The objectives of TMJ ankylosis surgery can be summarized as follows:

- Restoring mouth opening and joint function
- Allowing for adequate condylar growth
- Correcting the facial profile
- Relieving any upper airway obstruction

The basic principles of ankylosis release should be followed, regardless of the patient's age or the type of ankylosis. These include:

- Gap arthroplasty for resection of the ankylotic mass
- Placement of an interpositional material to prevent the recurrence of ankylosis and to correct secondary deformities

The joint can be reconstructed in several ways. Advantages of autogenous grafting include:

- Ease of adaptation to the host site and remodeling over time
- Associated low morbidity from graft harvest
- Infrequent rate of infection
- Reduced relative cost and time for preparation compared to allografts

A disadvantage of costochondral grafts is the unpredictable growth pattern, which may lead to progressive dental midline shifts, occlusal changes, chin deviation, and modification of the graft itself.

Advantages of alloplastic grafting include:

- Ability to begin physical therapy immediately after surgery
- Avoidance of a secondary surgical site
- Ability to mimic normal anatomy

Contraindications to alloplastic grafting include:

- Growth requirements of the graft and a finite life span
- Uncontrolled systemic diseases
- Active infection at the implantation site
- Allergies to the materials used in the implant

Today's technology allows adult patients with severe TMJ ankylosis the option of complete TMJ prosthorehabilitation. However, no consensus has yet been reached on the optimum treatment options for children.

Bibliography

De Bont LGM, van Loon JP: The Groningen temporomandibular joint prosthesis, *Oral Maxillofac Surg Clin North Am* 12:125-132, 2000.

Dierks EJ, Buehler MJ: Complete replacement of the temporomandibular joint with a microvascular transfer of the second metatarsal-phalangeal joint, *Oral Maxillofac Surg Clin North Am* 12:139-147, 2000.

Donlon WC: Nonprosthetic reconstructive options, *Oral Maxillofac Surg Clin North Am* 12:133-137, 2000.

Edwards SP, Feinber SE: The temporalis muscle flap in contemporary oral and maxillofacial surgery, *Oral Maxillofac Surg Clin North Am* 15:513-535, 2003.

Gerard DA, Hudson JW: The Christensen temporomandibular joint prosthesis system, *Oral Maxillofac Surg Clin North Am* 12:61-72, 2000.

Guyuron B, Lasa CI: Unpredictable growth pattern of costochondral graft, *Plast Reconstr Surg* 90:880-889, 1991.

Hoffman DC, Pappas MJ: Hoffman-Pappas prosthesis, *Oral Maxillofac Surg Clin North Am* 12:105-124, 2000.

Kaban LB, Perrott DH, Fisher K: A protocol for management of temporomandibular joint ankylosis, *J Oral Maxillofac Surg* 48:1145-1151, 1990.

Mercuri LG: The TMJ Concepts patient fitted total temporomandibular joint reconstruction prosthesis, *Oral Maxillofac Surg Clin North Am* 12:73-91, 2000.

Milam SB: Chronic temporomandibular joint arthralgia, *Oral Maxillofac Surg Clin North Am* 12:5-26, 2000.

Pellegrini G: Preoperative irradiation for prevention of heterotopic ossification following total hip arthroplasty, *J Bone Joint Surg* 78A(6):870-881, 1996.

Peoples JR, Herbosa EG, Dion J: Management of internal maxillary artery hemorrhage from temporomandibular joint surgery via selective embolization, *J Oral Maxillofac Surg* 46:1005-1007, 1988.

Quinn PD: Lorenz prosthesis, *Oral Maxillofac Surg Clin North Am* 12:93-104, 2000.

Schmelzeisen R, Gellrich N, Schramm A, et al: Navigation guided resection of temporomandibular joint ankylosis promotes safety in skull base surgery, *J Oral Maxillofac Surg* 60:1275-1283, 2002.

Shah FR, Sharma RK, Hiloowalla RN, et al: Anesthetic considerations of temporomandibular joint ankylosis with obstructive sleep apnea: a case report, *J Indian Soc Pedod Prev Dent* 20(1):16-20, 2002.

Yu HB, Shen GF, Zhang SL, et al: Navigation guided gap arthroplasty in the treatment of temporomandibular joint ankylosis, *Int J Oral Maxillofac Surg* 38:1030-1035, 2009.

CHAPTER 11

Oral Cancer

Editors: Deepak Kademani and Shahrokh C. Bagheri

This chapter addresses:
- Squamous Cell Carcinoma
- Verrucous Carcinoma
- Malignant Salivary Gland Tumors
- Neck Dissections

Malignant diseases of the oral cavity include a spectrum of neoplastic disorders that can emerge from the cellular structures present in the oral cavity or, less frequently, from metastatic disease to the area. Primary oral squamous cell carcinoma accounts for more than 90% of all head and neck malignancies. Malignant diseases of the salivary glands, and ductal epithelium account for the majority of the remaining cases. A greater proportion of oral cancer is diagnosed and referred for treatment by dental professionals than by general medical practitioners. Therefore, recognition and knowledge of the diagnostic tools necessary to identify these disorders are the minimum requirements for general dental practitioners and oral and maxillofacial surgeons. Today an increasing number of oral and maxillofacial surgeons are additionally trained in the treatment of head and neck malignancies. Surgery remains the primary treatment modality for head and neck cancer.

Oral cancer poses a significant challenge to our specialty. As the future unfolds, advances in molecular biology, cell signaling, immunomodulation, and angiogenesis will result in novel targeted therapies that will allow patients with cancer to live longer and healthier lives. Therapies will be tailored to the biologic behavior of the tumor, whether benign or malignant, not just to the histologic diagnosis. This behavior, in turn, will be determined by pretreatment genetic, molecular, and proteomic assessment so that the prescribed cure matches the patient's disease.

In this chapter we present three cases representing the most commonly encountered oral cavity malignancies. One case discusses oral squamous cell carcinoma, and another case discusses verrucous carcinoma; these cancers originate from the epithelium. The third case discusses three salivary gland malignancies—acinic cell carcinoma, adenoid cystic carcinoma, and mucoepidermoid carcinoma. A new section discusses neck dissection, a procedure that is an important aspect of head and neck cancer treatment.

Box 11-1 outlines the TNM staging classification used for lip and oral cavity cancers; Box 11-2 looks at the staging of squamous cell carcinoma.

Box 11-1	TNM Staging for Lip and Oral Cavity Cancers*		
Designation	**Description**	**Designation**	**Description**
Primary Tumor (T)		**Regional Lymph Nodes (N)**	
TX	Primary tumor cannot be assessed.	NX	Regional lymph nodes cannot be assessed.
T0	No evidence of primary tumor	N0	No regional lymph node metastasis
Tis	Carcinoma in situ	N1	Metastasis in a single ipsilateral lymph node, 3 cm or less in greatest dimension
T1	Tumor 2 cm or less in greatest dimension		
T2	Tumor more than 2 cm but not more than 4 cm in greatest dimension	N2a	Metastasis in a single ipsilateral lymph node, more than 3 cm but not more than 6 cm in greatest dimension
T3	Tumor more than 4 cm in greatest dimension	N2b	Metastasis in multiple ipsilateral lymph nodes, none more than 6 cm in greatest dimension
T4 (lip)	Tumor invades through cortical bone, inferior alveolar nerve, floor of the mouth, or skin of the face (e.g., chin or nose).	N2c	Metastasis in bilateral or contralateral lymph nodes, none more than 6 cm in greatest dimension
T4a (oral cavity)	Tumor invades adjacent structures (e.g., through cortical bone into deep [extrinsic] muscle of the tongue [genioglossus, hyoglossus, palatoglossus, and styloglossus], maxillary sinus, or skin of the face).	N3	Metastasis in a lymph node more than 6 cm in greatest dimension
		Distant Metastasis (M)	
		MX	Distant metastasis cannot be assessed.
T4b	Tumor invades masticator space, pterygoid plates, or skull base and/or encases internal carotid canal.	M0	No distant metastasis
		M1	Distant metastasis
Note: Superficial erosion of bone/tooth socket by a gingival primary tumor is not sufficient to classify a tumor as T4.			

From Sobin L, Gospodarowicz M, Wittekind C: International Union Against Cancer (UICC) TNM classification of malignant tumors, ed 7, West Sussex UK, 2010, Wiley-Blackwell.
*Staging system of the American Joint Committee on Cancer.
M, Distant metastasis; *N,* regional lymph nodes; *T,* primary tumor; *Tis,* carcinoma in situ.

Box 11-2	Staging of Oral Squamous Cell Carcinoma
Stage	**TNM Findings**
0	Tis, N0, M0
I	T1, N0, M0
II	T2, N0, M0
III	T3, N0, M0
	T1, N1, M0
	T2, N1, M0
	T3, N1, M0
IVA	T4a, N0, M0
	T4a, N1, M0
	T1, N2, M0
	T2, N2, M0
	T3, N2, M0
	T4a, N2, M0
IVB	Any T, N3, M0
	T4b, any N, M0
IVC	Any T, any N, M1

From Sobin L, Gospodarowicz M, Wittekind C: International Union Against Cancer (UICC) TNM classification of malignant tumors, ed 7, West Sussex UK, 2010, Wiley-Blackwell.
M, Distant metastasis; *N,* regional lymph nodes; *T,* primary tumor; *Tis,* carcinoma in situ.

Squamous Cell Carcinoma*

Ketan Patel and Deepak Kademani

CC

A 55-year-old African-American man presents to your office and states, "There is something wrong with my tongue, and my dentist said I need to have it checked." (African Americans have a higher incidence of squamous cell carcinoma [SCCa] and double the mortality rates.)

HPI

The patient recently visited his general dentist for evaluation of his loose upper dentures. Upon examination, a red and white, fungating mass of the right lateral border of his tongue was noted (SCCa until proved otherwise). The patient was otherwise asymptomatic. (Early mucosal lesions of oral cancer are usually asymptomatic; painful ulcers would be more suggestive of an inflammatory or infectious etiology). Within 2 weeks he had an incisional biopsy of the lesion by a local oral surgeon, with a subsequent diagnosis of an invasive SCCa.

The biopsy report from the previous surgeon was requested and reviewed (it is important to confirm the diagnosis before definitive treatment). The histopathology report described a loss of normal maturation of the epithelial cells, with invasion of abnormal cells beyond the basement membrane into the underlying subcutaneous tissues and muscle layers (indicative of invasive tumor). Stranding and islands of keratin-like material are also noted (keratin is indicative of greater cellular differentiation). The abnormal cells appeared pleomorphic (having many different shapes) with an increased nuclear-to-cytoplasmic ratio and occasional mitotic figures (signs of cellular malignant transformation). Generalized inflammatory infiltration was noted at the deepest portion of the specimen. The diagnosis of a grade III (discussed later in this section) invasive SCCa was made.

PMHX/PDHX/MEDICATIONS/ALLERGIES/SH/FH

The patient has a 45 pack-year history of tobacco use. In addition, he regularly consumes alcoholic beverages on weekends and occasionally on weekdays (tobacco and alcohol are both risk factors for the development of oral SCCa; see Discussion). He does not receive routine medical or dental treatment.

The strong association between SCCa and tobacco use is well established. The risk of SCCa developing in a smoker is approximately five to nine times greater than in a nonsmoker. It is also postulated that smoking is responsible for approximately 90% of oral cavity tumors in men and 61% of those in women. Chewing tobacco is associated with an increased risk of oral SCCa. Alcohol use alone and in conjunction with tobacco use has been shown to pose an increased risk of oral SCCa. In studies controlled for smoking, those who consumed moderate to heavy amounts of alcohol were found to have a 3 to 9 times greater risk of the development of SCCa. When alcohol and smoking are combined, alcohol is considered to be a promoter and a possible co-carcinogen to tobacco, with some studies showing a 100-fold increased risk.

EXAMINATION

The examination of a patient with the diagnosis of SCCa should entail a complete head and neck examination to search for neck metastasis (the most common areas of distant metastasis are the lungs), synchronous primary tumors or, in cases of presenting neck disease, occult primary tumors. Particular attention is given to the status of the lymph nodes and the size of the presenting lesion. Previous studies have shown that on initial examination of a known primary tumor, there is a 3% to 7% incidence of a synchronous tumor in the upper aerodigestive tract. A nasopharyngoscopic examination is indicated to evaluate the subepiglottic and supraepiglottic regions, posterior oropharynx, and nasopharynx.

General. The patient is a well-developed and well-nourished African American man who appears his stated age, with no signs of cachexia (seen with advanced disease).

Maxillofacial. There is a 3.5-cm red and white, fungating mass on the right lateral border of tongue with central ulceration (a nonhealing ulcer in the oral cavity is considered to be SCCa until proved otherwise) (Figure 11-1). There is no pain or bleeding noted on palpation of the lesion (although ulcers from SCCa may occasionally bleed, they are usually painless). Some patients may also complain of ear pain if the lesions are deep and involve the lingual nerve. When ear pain is present, perineural invasion cannot be ruled out until final pathology. Examination of the remaining oral cavity, including the buccal mucosa, hard and soft palate, parotid and submandibular glands, oropharynx, and nasopharynx, reveals no other abnormalities. Nasopharyngoscopy reveals no abnormal tissues in the posterior oropharynx, subglottic or supraglottic regions, or nasopharynx (nasopharyngoscopy should

*The authors and publisher wish to acknowledge Dr. David C. Swiderski for his contribution on this topic to the previous edition.

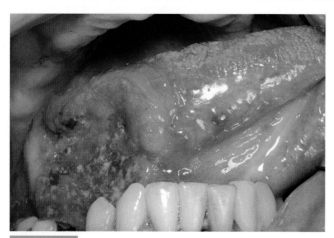

Figure 11-1 Ulcerating fungating mass of the right lateral border of the tongue, diagnosed as SCCa.

be performed as part of the head and neck evaluation of tongue SCCa).

Neck. No cervical or submandibular lymphadenopathy is noted (cancers of the tongue usually metastasize to the level I and II nodes). There is no pain on palpation of the neck (lymphadenopathy from cancer is usually painless).

The presence of occult neck disease in the N0 neck is related to the tumor's stage, size, and depth of invasion; perineural invasion; and histologic grade. Lesions greater than 4 mm in depth, along with a high-grade histology, have a greater than 20% risk of neck disease in the N0 neck.

IMAGING

The initial imaging modalities for the evaluation of patients with SCCa begin with a panoramic radiograph. This is a useful screening tool to evaluate for the presence of bony infiltration associated with the tumor. It also provides valuable information regarding the long-term prognosis of the remaining dentition, because some patients may require extraction of carious or periodontally involved teeth before radiotherapy.

A computed tomography (CT) scan of the head and neck is the commonly used imaging study of choice to delineate the lesion and assess the neck for cervical lymphadenopathy (nodes greater than 1.5 cm, with central necrosis, an ovoid shape, and fat stranding are indicative of nodal metastasis). Additional tests, such as magnetic resonance imaging (MRI) and ultrasonography, can be used to assess the status of the cervical nodes.

Anteroposterior and lateral chest radiographs are used to screen for underlying pulmonary disease and evaluate for pulmonary metastasis, because the lungs are the most common areas of metastasis for this tumor. Positron emission tomography (PET) scans are becoming a common modality for the evaluation of distant metastasis. This technology uses an 18F-fluorodeoxyglucose (FDG) marker to examine sites of increased glucose uptake, which are seen with metabolically active cancer cells. This imaging modality is commonly used

to rule out distant disease, and it is also helpful for clinically staging the tumor. Several studies have demonstrated that a standardized uptake valve (SUV) of greater than 3 correlates with hypermetabolism suggestive of a pathologic process. Clinical staging is helpful, because a treatment plan can be worked up for the patient and adjuvant modalities recommended.

In the current patient, axial and coronal CT images of the head and neck, with and without contrast, revealed a 3.5-cm, well-circumscribed lesion of the right lateral border of the tongue musculature. No evidence of cervical lymphadenopathy was noted. The PET scan performed with 18F-FDG showed a hypermetabolic area in the right tongue coinciding with the clinical lesion. No other abnormal uptake in the neck or chest was noted. The panoramic and chest radiographs revealed no abnormalities.

LABS

A complete metabolic panel (CMP), complete blood count (CBC), and coagulation profile (prothrombin time [PT], partial thromboplastin time [PTT], and international normalized ratio [INR]) are mandatory laboratory studies in the cancer patient because of metabolic, electrolyte, and nutritional derangements that may accompany malignant disease. Liver function tests are obtained as part of the complete metabolic panel and are important screening tests for liver metastasis or alcohol dependence. Other laboratory studies can be ordered based on the patient's medical history.

In the current patient, the CBC, CMP, liver function test results, and coagulation studies were within normal limits.

ASSESSMENT

T2, N0, M0 (tumor greater than 2 cm but less than 4 cm, with no positive nodes and no distant metastasis) stage II, oral SCCa of the right lateral border of the tongue with a Broders' histologic grade of III.

TREATMENT

Treatment of SCCa of the tongue begins with a complete history and physical examination, including nasopharyngoscopy. This is followed by appropriate tests, including CBC with differentials, electrolytes, liver function tests, chest radiographs, and CT with contrast. The role of PET scanning for occult metastasis continues to evolve.

The treatment of SCCa is site specific; surgical ablation with minimum 1 to 1.5-cm margins is the main modality of treatment. Most oral cavity tumors are approached intraorally; however, some tumors may need to be accessed extraorally via a transfacial approach. When the tumor is located in the mandible, the inferior border can be preserved (marginal mandibulectomy), depending on the degree of infiltration. However, when the cancellous portion of the mandible is invaded, segmental resection is required to maintain oncologic safety.

A common procedure that accompanies the removal of the tumor is the removal of the fibrofatty contents of the neck, for treatment of cervical lymphatic metastases and for complete staging of the cancerous process (see the section Neck Dissections later in this chapter).

Reconstruction and rehabilitation. Depending on the defect, the reconstructive surgery can be divided into soft tissue and/or bony reconstruction. Closing the defect primarily is ideal if it can be accomplished. Soft tissue surgical procedures include closure by secondary intention, skin grafts, local flaps, or microvascular free flaps. Simultaneous bony reconstruction can be accomplished using vascularized free flaps from the iliac crest, scapula, or fibula when needed. When large ablative and reconstructive procedures are performed, they can be performed simultaneously (see Chapter 12). Depending on the amount of healing and dysfunction anticipated, a percutaneous endoscopic gastrostomy tube and elective tracheostomy can be performed to secure the airway and aid in the nutritional support of the patient during the postoperative period.

Radiation therapy. Radiation therapy can be used as a primary or an adjuvant therapy. Primary radiotherapy is usually reserved for patients with significant comorbidities or when the primary tumor or the patient is not amenable to surgery. This is not a primary indication for early-stage SCCa because of the associated morbidity, including dysphagia and xerostomia. Another significant risk is the development of metachronous lesions after radiation therapy.

Postoperative radiation therapy is commonly used as a part of the comprehensive treatment. The indications for its use include positive or near margins, significant perineural or perivascular invasion, bone involvement, multiple nodal involvement, extracapsular spread, or stage III or stage IV disease. Typically, about 6,000 cGy in divided doses is administered, and treatment is initiated soon after healing from the initial surgery is complete. Surgery combined with radiation therapy and chemotherapy has increased the 5-year survival rates for stage III and stage IV cancers by 10%.

In the current patient, a right partial glossectomy via a transoral approach was performed with 1.5-cm margins. The status of the margins was evaluated using frozen section microscopy, which demonstrated negative margins. An ipsilateral supraomohyoid neck dissection (levels I through III) was completed for staging, which revealed no positive lymph nodes. The tongue defect was reconstructed with a radial forearm free flap, anastomosing with the facial artery and vein. An elective tracheostomy was performed.

After complete healing, the patient was followed closely for signs of recurrence (85% of recurrences occur in the first 3 years after initial treatment).

COMPLICATIONS

Complications are best categorized as intraoperative, postoperative (within 1 month), and long term (after 1 month).

Intraoperative complications. The main intraoperative concerns associated with oncologic ablative and reconstructive surgery include control of hemorrhage and anesthetic complications. Damage to adjacent structures, such as the lingual nerve and Wharton's duct, is possible with ablative procedures of the tongue and floor of the mouth. When simultaneous neck dissection is performed, additional complications may be seen, such as nerve palsies (facial and spinal accessory nerves),vascular injury to the carotid artery or internal jugular vein and, more rarely, pneumothorax, air embolism, and formation of a chylous fistula (especially on the left side).

Postoperative complications. Postoperative complications include wound infection, hematoma, skin necrosis, flap failure, orocutaneous fistula, poor speech, and swallowing dysfunction. Poor healing can also be noted in patients who are alcoholics, because their prealbumin status is usually low. Complications after bony reconstruction include malunion, nonunion, contour irregularities, resorption of bone, osteomyelitis, and hardware failure.

Long-term complications. The gravest long-term complications are recurrence of the primary tumor and death (85% of recurrences occur in the first 3 years). The lifetime risk of development of a second primary tumor is 2% to 3% per year, and the 5-year survival rate is 56% for all tumor stages. Routine diagnostic tests are performed based on the clinical suspicion of recurrence. Imaging studies can be difficult to assess in the postoperative setting due to the difficulty of separating recurrent tumors from postoperative anatomic changes. Recurrent disease usually occurs at the surgical wound margin. Other complications include lingual nerve hypoesthesia, duct obstruction, and flap failure. Dysphagia, xerostomia, mucositis, and the risk of osteoradionecrosis are associated with radiation therapy. The most common causes of death in patients with oral cancer are related to locoregional disease, distant metastasis, or cardiopulmonary failure. Metastases of SCCa tend to involve the lung, bones, liver, and brain.

DISCUSSION

SCCa accounts for roughly 90% of neoplastic cases in the head and neck. It has a 3:1 male predilection, and the median age of onset (diagnosis) is in the sixth decade of life (although recently there has been an increasing prevalence in the third decade). The overall 5-year survival rate for SCCa is over 50%. African Americans are reported to have significantly lower survival rates, approaching 35%. In 2005, an estimated 29,370 new cases were diagnosed, and 7,320 patients died of their disease. Roughly two thirds of these cases can be prevented with cessation of known risk factors (tobacco and alcohol).

From an epidemiologic and clinicopathologic standpoint, carcinomas in the head and neck region can be divided into three anatomic areas:

1. Carcinomas arising in the oral cavity, which includes the tongue, gingiva, floor of the mouth, hard palate, buccal mucosa, and retromolar area
2. Carcinomas of the lip vermilion
3. Carcinomas of the oropharynx, including the base of the tongue, lingual tonsil, soft palate, and uvula

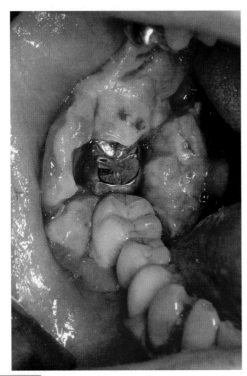

Figure 11-2 Squamous cell carcinoma of the right retromolar area in a different patient from the one shown in Figure 11-1.

Table 11-1	Oral Squamous Cell Carcinoma Survival Rates by Stage				
	Year 1	Year 2	Year 3	Year 4	Year 5
Stage I	93.9	84.4	77.5	73.0	68.1
Stage II	88.1	72.7	64.2	58.6	52.9
Stage III	77.5	60.9	52.5	46.0	41.3
Stage IV	60.3	40.6	33.5	29.3	26.5

Modified from the National Cancer Institute, US National Institutes of Health: Surveillance epidemiology and end results (SEER). Available at http://seer.cancer.gov/publicdata/access.html. Accessed December 2012.

Figure 11-2 shows a different patient with a large fungating SCCa of the right retromolar area.

In addition to alcohol and tobacco, the use of betel quid, or paan, which is popular in India and southeast Asia, has been associated with an increased risk for developing SCCa. The quid consists of a betel leaf wrapped around a mixture of areca nut and slaked lime, commonly in combination with tobacco. The slaked lime releases an alkaloid from the areca nut, causing a feeling of euphoria. Chronic use of the quid can lead to a debilitating condition known as *submucous fibrosis,* which is a premalignant condition.

Human papillomavirus (HPV) types 16 and 18 have been shown to increase the risk of SCCa. Data from recent studies show that HPV 16 and 18 increase the ratio of SCCa by approximately threefold to fivefold. Tonsillar SCCa has the highest rate of HPV infection, with approximately 50% testing positive. These HPV-positive oropharyngeal tumors are usually treated with chemoradiation.

Other known risks factors include chronic sun exposure leading to cutaneous SCCa of the lip. Several studies have suggested that oral lichen planus, particularly the erosive form, is associated with an increased risk for SCCa. Severe iron deficiency presenting as Plummer-Vinson syndrome is associated with an increased risk for pharyngeal and esophageal SCCa. Previous radiation exposure is linked to an increased risk for developing SCCa.

Premalignant conditions. There are several well-known entities pathologically that have a distinct association with SCCa: leukoplakia, erythroplakia, and lichen planus.

Leukoplakia is a white patch or plaque that cannot be characterized clinically or pathologically as any other disease. Erythroplakia is defined as a red lesion of the oral cavity that cannot be classified clinically or pathologically as any other lesion (see the section on Oral Leukoplakia in Chapter 7).

Oral lichen planus has been a subject of controversy in the literature concerning its possible role as a premalignant condition. Several recent studies have shown that the transformation rate of oral lichen planus to SCCa is approximately 0.04% to 1.74%.

Early oral SCCa usually presents as one of the premalignant conditions discussed: a white, red, or mixed red and white lesion. As the lesion matures, it can become centrally ulcerated, and the borders become less distinct. The surface can become exophytic with papillary projections or endophytic with raised, rolled borders.

The tongue is the most common site of SCCa (30%), followed closely by the floor of the mouth (28%). These sites are at the higher risk, probably due to carcinogens that pool with saliva in these areas, contributing to a greater exposure. The thin, nonkeratinized layer of epithelium in these areas may contribute to the greater susceptibility. The other areas of prevalence, in descending order, are the upper and lower alveolar ridges (including the hard palate), the retromolar trigone, buccal mucosa, and the lips.

Broders' classification system is an index of malignancy based on the fact that less differentiation (differentiation is defined as the degree of keratinization) is proportionally related to greater malignancy of the tumor. The classification is as follows:

Grade I: More than 75% differentiated cells
Grade II: 25% to 75% differentiated cells
Grade III: Fewer than 25% differentiated cells
Grade IV: Anaplastic with no cell differentiation

Histopathologic factors correlating with a poorer outcome include depth of invasion, perineural invasion, and extracapsular spread.

The 5-year survival rate remains about 50% and is related to the stage at diagnosis (Table 11-1). Unfortunately, there has been only a modest improvement in survival over the past several decades.

Bibliography

Braakhuis BJM, Tabor MP, Kummer JA, et al: A genetic explanation of Slaughter's concept of field cancerization: evidence and clinical implications, *Cancer Res* 63:1727-1730, 2003.

Broders AC: Carcinomas of the mouth: types and degrees of malignancy, *Am J Roentgenol Radium Ther Nucl Med* 17:90-93, 1927.

Funk FF, Karnell LH, Robinson RA, et al: Presentation, treatment, and outcome of oral cavity cancer: a national cancer data base report, *Head Neck* 24:165-180, 2002.

Hillbertz NS, Hirsch JM, Jalouli J, et al: Viral and molecular aspects of oral cancer, *Anticancer Res* 32:4201-4212, 2012.

Kademani D, Bell RB, Bagheri SC, et al: Prognostic factors for intraoral squamous cell carcinoma: the influence of histologic grade, *J Oral Maxillofac Surg* 63:1599-1605, 2005.

Marur S, D'Souza G, Westra WH, et al: HPV-associated head and neck cancer: a virus-related cancer epidemic, *Lancet Oncol* 11:781-789, 2010.

McClure SA, Mohaved R, Salama A, et al: Maxillofacial metastases: a retrospective review of one institution's 15-year experience, *J Oral Maxillofac Surg* 16(2):181-188, 2012.

Neville BW, Day TA: Oral cancer and precancerous lesions, *CA Cancer J Clin* 52:195-215, 2002.

Oliver AJ, Helfrick JF, Gard D: Primary oral squamous cell carcinoma, *J Oral Maxillofac Surg* 54:949-954, 1996.

Reichart PA, Philipsen HP: Oral erythroplakia: a review, *Oral Oncol* 41:551-561, 2005.

Schmidt BL, Dierks EJ, Homer L, et al: Tobacco smoking history and presentation of oral squamous cell carcinoma, *J Oral Maxillofac Surg* 62:1005-1058, 2004.

Schwartz LH, Ozsahin M, Zhang GN, et al: Synchronous and metachronous head and neck carcinomas, *Cancer* 74:1933-1938, 1994.

Shafer WG, Waldron CA: Erythroplakia of the oral cavity, *Cancer* 36:1021-1028, 1975.

Smith GI, O'Brien CJ, Clark J, et al: Management of the neck in patients with T1 and T2 cancer in the mouth, *Br J Oral Maxillofac Surg* 42:494-500, 2004.

Syrjanen S: Human papillomavirus (HPV) in head and neck cancer, *J Clin Virol* 32S:S59-S66, 2005.

Todd R, Donoff RB, Wong DTW: The molecular biology of oral carcinogenesis: toward a tumor progression model, *J Oral Maxillofac Surg* 55:613-623, 1997.

Van der Meij EHDDS, Schepman KP, Van der Waal I: The possible premalignant character of oral lichen planus and oral lichenoid lesions: a prospective study, *Oral Surg Oral Med Oral Pathol Oral Radiol Endod* 96:164-171, 2003.

Waldron CA, Shafer WG: Leukoplakia revisited: a clinicopathological study of 3,256 oral leukoplakias, *Cancer* 36:1386-1392, 1975.

Wooglar JA: Histological distribution of cervical lymph node metastases from intraoral/oropharyngeal squamous cell carcinomas, *Br J Oral Maxillofac Surg* 37:175-180, 1999.

Verrucous Carcinoma*

Ketan Patel and Deepak Kademani

CC

A 68-year-old Caucasian male farmer is referred to you. He complains, "I'm worried about this growth on my gums. It just won't seem to go away" (verrucous carcinoma is more commonly seen in the elderly male population, those over 60 years of age).

HPI

The patient reports a 6-month history of a rough, corrugated area on his anterior maxillary gingiva. He was seen by his dentist and was referred to you for evaluation of possible "oral cancer" (verrucous carcinoma cannot be distinguished clinically from squamous cell carcinoma [SCCa]). The area has not been painful but has recently become more irritated (pain is not characteristically seen with neoplastic processes). He has been inadvertently chewing on the area, with occasional bleeding. He denies any weight loss or constitutional symptoms (these may be seen with metastatic disease).

PMHX/PDHX/MEDICATIONS/ALLERGIES/SH/FH

The patient has a positive history of chronic obstructive pulmonary disease (secondary to chronic tobacco use). He sees his local dentist only when he develops a problem (he does not have routine oral cancer screening). He has used smokeless tobacco for 30 years and consumes three or four alcoholic beverages per week.

Many patients with verrucous carcinoma are reported to chew tobacco, but this association is not consistent. Both tobacco use and chronic alcohol consumption are risk factors for the development of SCCa. The association with verrucous carcinoma is uncertain.

EXAMINATION

General. The patient is a thin, elderly Caucasian man who appears older than his stated age; this is most apparent by his sun-damaged skin and extensive facial rhytids (chronic tobacco and sun exposure both contribute to early signs of aging secondary to changes in collagen synthesis).

Maxillofacial. The patient has deeply tanned skin with many rhytids (secondary to prolonged sun exposure). There

are no skin lesions in the sun-exposed areas (it is important to look for early signs of basal cell carcinoma and actinic keratosis), and there is no facial or cervical lymphadenopathy (enlarged lymph nodes would be suggestive of a malignant disease process).

Intraoral. The patient has multiple restored teeth, significant enamel staining (secondary to smokeless tobacco use), and moderate generalized periodontal disease. There is an exophytic grayish and white cauliflower-like growth involving the edentulous anterior maxillary ridge (the most common site of verrucous carcinoma is the buccal mucosa), measuring 2×3.5 cm (Figure 11-3). The lesion has areas of surrounding erythema with dispersed white patches that appear traumatized. It is firm to palpation and has rolled margins. The keratotic surface is covered with pink-red pebbly papules that do not rub off. The surrounding mucosa appears normal and does not feel indurated (ulceration is typically not seen with verrucous carcinoma).

IMAGING

A panoramic radiograph should be obtained to screen for any bony erosion or infiltration and to evaluate the dentition. Although verrucous carcinoma has a low tendency to metastasize, it does represent a malignancy; therefore, formal oncologic staging should be considered. A routine oncologic work-up includes an assessment of the extent of locoregional disease using clinical and radiographic modalities (panoramic radiograph, CT scan of the head and neck, nasopharyngeal laryngoscopy, and chest radiograph or CT). The likelihood of

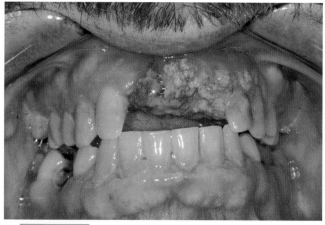

Figure 11-3   Verrucous carcinoma of the anterior maxilla.

*The authors and publisher wish to acknowledge Dr. Scott D. Van Dam for his contribution on this topic to the previous edition.

distant disease is remote and can be addressed based on system-driven findings.

In the current patient, a panoramic radiograph demonstrated normal bony anatomy of the jaws. The maxillary sinuses appear clear and have no evidence of widening of the periodontal ligaments or localized resorption of teeth (signs of infiltrative disease processes). A contrast-enhanced CT scan (contrast enhances visualization of soft tissue) of the head and neck was obtained. This showed focal thickening of the oral soft tissues in the area of the anterior maxilla. There was no evidence of infiltration or extension of the lesion, and no enlarged lymph nodes (signs of metastatic disease) were noted. Due to the risk of occult malignancy, a nasopharyngoscopy was performed. No abnormalities where detected.

An anteroposterior chest radiograph revealed mild cardiomegaly and lung hyperinflation (secondary to chronic obstructive pulmonary disease) but no focal lung lesions indicative of metastatic disease.

LABS

Routine laboratory tests are indicated in the routine workup of verrucous carcinoma as dictated by the medical history. A hemoglobin level may be obtained before the removal of larger lesions. Liver function tests are typically not required, because the risk of liver metastasis is extremely low.

DIFFERENTIAL DIAGNOSIS

Based on the history and clinical examination, verrucous carcinoma can be confused with a number of white lesions. These different lesions may represent a spectrum of similar diseases. Proliferative verrucous leukoplakia is a diagnosis for lesions that begin as simple hyperkeratosis and spread to other sites, become multifocal, and progress slowly through a spectrum of dysplasia to frank invasive carcinoma. Histologically, the associated dense inflammatory infiltrate may contribute to the occasional misdiagnosis as pseudoepitheliomatous hyperplasia or chronic hyperplastic candidiasis. Small lesions can resemble focal epithelial hyperplasia (Heck's disease).

BIOPSY

When a diagnosis of verrucous carcinoma is considered, a full-thickness biopsy sample, down to the periosteum or submucosa, must be taken to minimize the possibility of misdiagnosis. Appropriate treatment relies on a good biopsy technique, with attention to including the base of the lesion as part of the specimen. The key in differentiating between benign and malignant lesions is to take a biopsy sample that is both deep (full thickness) and large enough to allow examination of the relationship between the tumor and the underlying connective tissue. On occasion, multiple biopsies may be necessary to diagnose verrucous carcinoma.

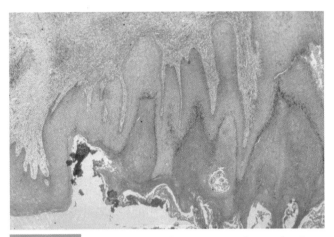

Figure 11-4 Histopathology of verrucous carcinoma showing a "pushing border" with a high degree of keratinization.

ASSESSMENT

Verrucous carcinoma and a low-grade SCCa.

For the current patient, under local anesthesia a full-thickness wedge biopsy sample, including normal tissue, was taken from the periphery of the lesion. The tissue was sent for permanent hematoxylin and eosin staining, which showed a thick surface layer of orthokeratinized squamous epithelium with occasional parakeratosis. There were exaggerated, blunt rete pegs extending into the lamina propria, with an intact, well-polarized basal layer and a "pushing border" appearance. The suprabasilar cells were well differentiated. Lymphocytic inflammation was seen throughout the lamina propria with a high degree of keratinization and minimal pleomorphism (Figure 11-4).

TREATMENT

Surgical resection is the mainstay of management of verrucous carcinoma of the oral cavity. For treatment planning purposes, preexisting comorbidities; the site, grade, and stage of the tumor; and the effectiveness of the particular therapy and its associated complications should be taken into account.

Due to the superficial, cohesive growth pattern and sharply demarcated margins of this lesion, a number of authors recommend surgical excision as the treatment of choice. Surgery involves wide excision of the primary lesion and surrounding tissues, including bone and muscle when invasion is suspected. Wide surgical excision with 0.5- to 1-cm margins is the recommended treatment for verrucous carcinoma. With adequately treated tumors, the recurrence rate is low. It should be noted that any oral cancer that invades beyond 4 mm carries an increased risk of cervical lymph node metastasis.

Radiation therapy can be used as an adjunctive procedure and offers the advantage of treating a wide field, especially in cases in which extensive surgery would cause significant morbidity. Patients should be aware of the risks of mucositis, xerostomia, radiation caries, and osteoradionecrosis of the jaws.

For the current patient, general anesthesia with nasal endotracheal intubation and local anesthetic injections were used. The lesion was excised with wide margins (0.5 to 1 cm) of uninvolved surrounding tissue. The specimen measured 2.5 × 4 cm. The depth of the specimen measured less than 2 mm relative to the surrounding normal mucosa, which included excision to the level of the buccinator fascia. After complete hemostasis was obtained, the wound bed was covered with a 0.015-inch, split-thickness skin graft harvested from the thigh.

COMPLICATIONS

The prognosis is excellent after adequate excision. Complications relate mainly to local destructive effects caused by the tumor itself and its surgical removal. Large lesions can be locally destructive, with invasion or erosion of adjacent tissue and bone. Metastasis is rare. Focal areas of invasive SCCa are sometimes found within an excised specimen. Those with hybrid features (verrucoid SCCa) should be treated similar to conventional SCCa.

DISCUSSION

The terms *verrucous carcinoma of Ackerman* and *oral florid papillomatosis* have been used to describe verrucous carcinomas occurring within the aerodigestive tract. This is an uncommon tumor; it is diagnosed in 1 to 3 individuals per 1 million people each year and accounts for 2% to 9% of oral cancers. Most patients with verrucous carcinoma are older than age 50 (the average age at the time of diagnosis is 65 years). Males are affected more often than females. Verrucous carcinoma is typically associated with a favorable prognosis, with 5-year survival rates up to 85% (compared to slightly greater than 50% for SCCa). Radiation can be used as adjuvant therapy for close margins or unresectable lesions; however, long-term survival rates drop to about 57.6%.

The most common site of verrucous carcinoma is the oral cavity. Verrucous carcinoma most commonly involves the buccal mucosa and the mandibular gingiva alveolar ridge, or palate. It typically presents as a nonulcerated, slow-growing, exophytic, "papulonodular" or "warty," fungating gray or white mass. Less frequently, the roughened, pebbly surface can be inconspicuous, and the tumor can present as a flattened white lesion. It can vary in size from a small patch to a confluent, extensive mass. Verrucous carcinoma can superficially invade the soft tissues and underlying bone structures, becoming fixed to the periosteum. Distant metastasis is exceedingly rare.

The etiology of verrucous carcinoma remains unclear, but tobacco is thought to play a significant role for lesions of the aerodigestive tract. Tobacco smoking and excess alcohol are known risk factors for the development of SCCa of the mouth, and they may play a role in the pathogenesis of verrucous carcinoma. Similarities between the morphologic features of verrucous carcinoma and virally infected epithelial lesions suggest a possible etiologic link with human papillomavirus (HPV) infection. HPV types 6, 11, 16, and 18 have been detected to varying degrees in verrucous carcinoma of the oral cavity.

The hallmark of this tumor is the discrepancy between the histologic pattern and the clinical behavior. Microscopically, verrucous carcinoma appears as a papillary or verrucous, low-grade (i.e., well-differentiated) SCCa. Verrucous carcinomas typically present clinically as exophytic lesions; they can also present with a mixed or an endophytic growth pattern. Squamous cells display minimal or no dysplasia, with infrequent mitoses localized to the invading (pushing) front. There is an overlying hyperorthokeratosis or parakeratosis, resulting in keratin-filled clefts of the surface epithelium with prominent, bulbous rete processes extending to a uniform distance into the underlying connective tissue; this creates a "pushing border" rather than an infiltrating quality at the base of this tumor. The basement membrane is intact, with little evidence of connective tissue invasion. An intense, mixed inflammatory infiltrate may surround and blend with the tumor, sometimes obscuring the epithelium–connective tissue interface.

As mentioned, verrucous carcinoma is an uncommon tumor that can be seen in the oral cavity. Excision of the tumor should be followed by frequent follow-up evaluations for recurrence and for new-onset squamous cell carcinomas of the upper aerodigestive tract.

Bibliography

Addante R, McKenna S: Verrucous carcinoma, *Oral Maxillofac Surg Clin North Am* 18:513-519, 2006.

Batsakis JG, Suarez P, El-Naggar AK: Proliferative verrucous leukoplakia and its related lesions, *Oral Oncol* 35:354-359, 1999.

Bouquot JE: Oral verrucous carcinoma: incidence in two US populations, *Oral Surg Oral Med Oral Pathol Oral Radiol Endod* 86(3):318-324, 1998.

Charles S: The man behind the eponym: Lauren V. Ackerman and verrucous carcinoma of Ackerman, *Am J Dermatopathol* 26(4):334-341, 2004.

Jordan RC: Verrucous carcinoma of the mouth, *J Can Dent Assoc* 61(9):797-801, 1995.

Jyothirmayi R, Sankaranarayanan R, Varghese C, et al: Radiotherapy in the treatment of verrucous carcinoma of the oral cavity, *Oral Oncol* 33(2):124-128, 1997.

Koch B, Trask D, Hoffman HT, et al: National survey of head and neck verrucous carcinoma: patterns of presentation, care and outcome, *Cancer* 92(1):110-120, 2001.

Mirbod S, Ahing S: Lesions of the oral cavity. II. Malignant lesions, *J Can Dent Assoc* 66:308-311, 2000.

Paleri V, Orvidas LJ, Wight RG, et al: Verrucous carcinoma of the paranasal sinuses: a case report and clinical update, *Head Neck* 26(2):184-189, 2004.

Schwartz RA: Verrucous carcinoma of the skin and mucosa, *J Am Acad Dermatol* 32(1):1-21, 1995.

Walvekar R, Chaukar DA, Deshpande MS, et al: Verrucous carcinoma of the oral cavity: a clinical and pathological study of 101 cases, *Oral Oncol* 45:47-51, 2009.

Malignant Salivary Gland Tumors*

Ketan Patel and Deepak Kademani

CC

The patient is a 64-year-old woman referred for evaluation of a mass on the right posterior hard palate. (Mucoepidermoid carcinoma occurs across a wide age range and has a slight female predilection. Adenoid cystic carcinoma [ACC] has a relatively equal male-to-female distribution and is most commonly seen in the elderly population.)

HPI

The patient first noticed a lump on her hard palate approximately 6 months earlier (the parotid gland is the most common site for mucoepidermoid carcinoma; minor salivary glands, especially from the palate, are the second most common). The patient is asymptomatic, although the mass has been slowly increasing in size (mucoepidermoid carcinoma usually presents as progressively enlarging, asymptomatic swelling). She denies pain, fever, chills, night sweats, nausea, vomiting, weight loss, or other constitutional symptoms. She also denies any history of dental pain or sinus congestion. (ACCs are more common in the submandibular gland and lower lips. Late-stage ACCs can present with progressive anesthesia on the lip due to the propensity for perineural invasion.)

PMHX/PDHX/MEDICATIONS/ALLERGIES/SH/FH

The patient denies tobacco or alcohol use.

Although exposure to ionizing radiation has been implicated as a cause of salivary gland cancer, the etiology of most salivary gland cancers cannot be determined. Occupations that may be associated with an increased risk for salivary gland cancers include rubber product manufacturing, asbestos mining, plumbing, and some types of woodworking. Tobacco and alcohol consumption do not seem to have a causal relationship with salivary gland tumors.

EXAMINATION

General. The patient is a well-developed and well-nourished Caucasian woman who appears her stated age and is in no apparent distress. She is noncachexic (cachexia may be a sign of advanced disease).

Maxillofacial. The face is symmetrical and without any extraoral swelling. The patient has no proptosis (maxillary sinus malignancies can invade both the palate and orbit). The infraorbital nerves are intact (low-grade mucoepidermoid carcinoma typically does not display perineural invasion).

Intraoral. A 2×2-cm submucosal swelling is present on the right posterior hard palate (Figure 11-5). The mass is firm, nonmobile, nonpulsatile, and nontender to palpation (highly suggestive of a neoplastic process). The overlying mucosa is pink (may present with a bluish or reddish color) and nonulcerated. The greater and lesser palatine nerves are intact. The dentition is in good repair, and all teeth are vital without pain on percussion. There are no other intraoral lesions or masses.

Neck. There is no lymphadenopathy (regional lymph node metastasis is uncommon, especially for low-grade lesions, but may occur with high-grade lesions or advanced disease).

IMAGING

The work-up for a biopsy-proved mucoepidermoid carcinoma involves a complete head and neck physical examination, CT scan of the head and neck (with intravenous contrast) for delineation of the primary tumors and regional metastasis, a panoramic radiograph (initial screening examination), and a chest radiograph for evaluation of pulmonary metastasis. Newer imaging modalities, such as positron emission tomography (PET) scanning, have become powerful tools

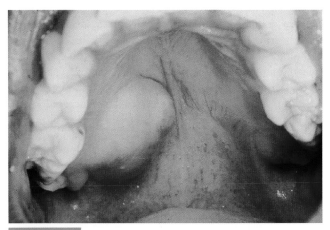

Figure 11-5 Submucosal swelling on the right posterior hard palate. *(From Ibsen OAC, Phelan JA:* Oral pathology for the dental hygienist, *ed 6, St Louis, 2014, Saunders.)*

*The authors and publisher wish to acknowledge Dr. David Rallis and Dr. David C. Swiderski for their contribution on this topic to the previous edition.

for delineation of local and distant disease. Most PET studies are performed using the glucose analog 18F-fluorodeoxyglucose (18F-FDG), which has been shown to accumulate in areas of higher metabolic activity. This is especially important in ACCs, because these tumors have a predilection for distant metastasis.

In the current patient, no abnormalities of the dentition or surrounding bony structures were identified on the panoramic radiograph. Axial and coronal views from the CT scan of the head and neck performed with intravenous contrast (for improved delineation of soft tissue) demonstrated a 2 × 1-cm enhancing soft tissue mass of the right posterior hard palate that did not appear to involve the underlying bone. No cervical lymphadenopathy was noted. The chest radiograph was normal.

LABS

For the biopsy procedure, routine laboratory studies are not indicated in an otherwise healthy patient. CBC, electrolyte studies, and coagulation studies may be performed to establish a baseline before the definitive surgery. Liver function tests are not routinely obtained, because liver metastasis is rare.

DIFFERENTIAL DIAGNOSIS

The differential diagnosis in the case of a submucosal mass of the posterior hard palate should include benign (pleomorphic adenoma, monomorphic adenoma, canicular adenoma) and malignant minor salivary gland tumors (mucoepidermoid carcinoma, adenoid cystic carcinoma, polymorphous low-grade adenocarcinoma, acinic cell carcinoma, and adenocarcinoma). Lesions of infectious etiology should be considered but are unlikely, given the presentation. Sarcomas can also occur on the palate and should be considered in the differential diagnosis. An incisional biopsy is indicated for the current patient.

BIOPSY

Mucoepidermoid carcinoma is graded on a scale of I to III (low, intermediate, and high grade, respectively); features of high-grade tumors include nuclear atypia, necrosis, perineural spread, mitoses, bony invasion, lymphatic and vascular invasion, intracystic component, and tumor front invading in small nests and islands. The grading system for mucoepidermoid carcinoma is subjectively assessed based on the degree of epidermoid versus mucinous cellular components. High-grade tumors have a relatively higher proportion of epidermoid cells (squamous and intermediate cells) and few mucus-producing cells, whereas low-grade tumors have a high proportion of mucus cells (Figure 11-6).

In adenoid cystic carcinoma, three major forms are recognized histopathologically: the cribriform, tubular, and solid variants (Figure 11-7). Microscopically, adenoid cystic carcinoma is composed of small cells arranged in groups that form

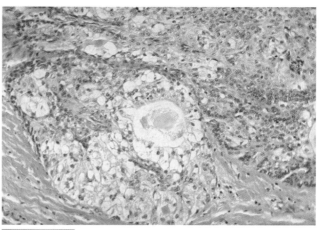

Figure 11-6 Histopathology image showing an abundance of mucus cells in a low-grade mucoepidermoid carcinoma.

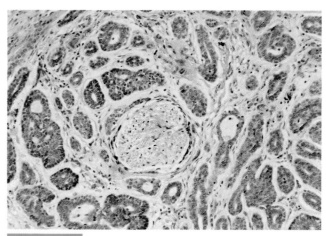

Figure 11-7 Adenoid cystic carcinoma showing perineural invasion.

glandular spaces filled with mucoid material or a hyaline plug. The cribriform variant is most common, and the solid variant has the worst prognosis.

In the current patient, an incisional biopsy of the central portion of the palatal mass was performed under local anesthesia. Histopathology of the specimen confirmed a low-grade mucoepidermoid carcinoma (high proportion of mucus cells with minimal cellular atypia). It is important to obtain a tissue sample from the center of the lesion in cases of suspected salivary gland neoplasms. A biopsy from the periphery may result in a nondiagnostic specimen due to inadequate depth.

ASSESSMENT

T1, N0, M0 (a tumor 2 cm or less in diameter, with no lymphadenopathy and no evidence of distant metastases) low-grade mucoepidermoid carcinoma of the right posterior hard palate.

TREATMENT

Once a biopsy-proven diagnosis of low-grade mucoepidermoid carcinoma has been made, the lesion is definitively treated by wide local excision with 1-cm margins. High-grade lesions may require more extensive resection, with surgical management of the neck, to limit the potential for locoregional recurrence.

For the current patient, the treatment of choice was a right partial maxillectomy with a split-thickness skin graft and immediate placement of a prosthetic obturator (see Discussion). Adjuvant radiation therapy is not indicated for low-grade lesions that are completely excised.

The patient was placed under general anesthesia and underwent a formal right partial maxillectomy, with 1-cm, tumor-free margins, via a transoral approach (a Weber-Ferguson incision may be indicated for larger tumors that require a more extensive ablative surgery). A split-thickness skin graft (0.015 inch) was harvested from the right thigh and used to line the ablative defect. This was bolstered using Xeroform gauze packing (Coe-Soft [GC America, Alsip, Illinois] denture liner can also be used) and a preformed surgical stent, which was secured to the maxilla with a midpalatal screw. The stent was removed after 2 weeks, and an impression was taken for fabrication of a temporary maxillary obturator.

COMPLICATIONS

Complications associated with a partial maxillectomy include bleeding due to vascular injury of the terminal branches of the internal maxillary artery (greater and lesser palatine vessels) or the internal maxillary artery itself.

Hemorrhage can be controlled with direct pressure, hemostatic agents, electrocautery, or vessel ligation. Uncontrollable arterial bleeding may require angiography and embolization of the feeding vessels to obtain proximal control. The use of a maxillary stent helps promote hemostasis and improve patient comfort and speech in the healing period.

Local recurrence or regional metastases, although uncommon, is a major concern (see Discussion). Complications associated with the rehabilitation and reconstruction of the defect can also have a significant impact on the patient's quality of life.

DISCUSSION

Salivary gland neoplasms exhibit an approximate distribution of 85% in the major salivary glands and 15% in the minor salivary glands. Of the major glands, the parotid accounts for 90% of these lesions, followed by the submandibular gland (5% to 10%); the lesions are rare in the sublingual gland. Of the minor salivary glands, the palate is involved in 60% of cases, followed by the lips (15%). In general, the size of the salivary gland is inversely related to the likelihood of tumor malignancy. Approximately 10% of parotid gland lesions, 30% of submandibular gland lesions, and 50% of intraoral salivary gland lesions are malignant.

Mucoepidermoid carcinoma is the most common malignancy originating from both the major and minor salivary glands; it is comprised of epidermoid, mucus-producing, and intermediate cells. It has been shown to account for approximately 3% to 15.5% of salivary gland tumors, and 12% to 34% are malignant. The parotid gland, followed by the palate and submandibular glands, are the most common sites of primary tumors (42%, 15%, and 10% of cases, respectively). The disease is seen most often in the third to fifth decades of life and has a slight female predilection. Tumor grade, stage, and negative margin status have correlated with disease-free survival. In studies involving mucoepidermoid carcinoma of both major and minor salivary glands, 5- and 10-year survival rates have ranged from 61% to 92% and 51% to 90%, respectively.

Low-grade mucoepidermoid carcinoma is a malignant process with a low risk of locoregional recurrence. Surgical extirpation is typically all that is required, along with long-term follow-up. High-grade mucoepidermoid carcinoma is an aggressive malignancy with affinity for regional lymphatic spread and has the potential for distant metastasis (the lungs are the most common site).

The primary goal in surgical treatment of mucoepidermoid carcinoma is to obtain widely negative margins at the primary location, but additional factors must be evaluated to determine the need for adjunctive therapy. Low-grade lesions (such as in the case presented) are typically resected with a 1-cm margin without adjunctive treatment. A recent study by Ord and Salama suggested that low-grade mucoepidermoid tumors do not necessarily need a bony resection if there is no evidence of bony invasion on imaging. High-grade lesions typically require more extensive resection, with additional management of the neck. When surgical margins are positive, radiotherapy with high-energy particles (protons and neutrons) has some efficacy in improving local control.

Mucoepidermoid carcinoma of the parotid gland (the most common site) typically presents with a unilateral, preauricular mass and facial swelling. These findings are nonspecific to parotid tumors. Although the majority of parotid tumors are benign and occur in the superficial pole of the gland, approximately 20% of parotid tumors may be malignant, and mucoepidermoid carcinoma is the most common type. When a lesion of the parotid is suspected and properly imaged with CT or MRI, fine-needle aspiration is performed to establish a preoperative diagnosis. Treatment consists of a parotidectomy with facial nerve dissection and preservation (the facial nerve is typically spared, except in high-grade lesions with direct involvement of the facial nerve). A margin of normal salivary gland tissue should be resected around the lesion. High-grade lesions may require multimodality treatments and a more extensive resection.

Adenoid cystic carcinoma is a salivary gland malignancy of myoepithelial and ductal cells. It is well known for its indolent course and propensity for perineural invasion, distant metastasis, and locoregional recurrence. Locoregional recurrence is thought to occur via "skip lesions" along nerve fibers. This implies that although the nerve may be without disease at the surgical margins, tumor cells may be present farther along the nerve sheath (i.e., skip lesions). For this reason, it is not uncommon during resection to sacrifice the nerve as far proximally as possible, often to the skull base.

Adenoid cystic carcinoma accounts for 35% of all submandibular malignancies. It usually occurs in the fourth through sixth decades of life. The peak incidence is in the fifth decade, although cases have been reported in the early third and the eighth decades. There is no gender predilection, although the reviewed literature is not entirely clear on this subject. Seventy percent of lesions appear in the minor salivary glands, with the most common locations being the hard and soft palates and the lip. The other 30% occur in the parotid and submandibular glands, in equal distribution. Differentiation between a minor gland tumor and that of the sublingual gland may be difficult.

There appears to be no predisposing factors for the development of adenoid cystic carcinoma. The tumor is very slow growing and takes many months to be noticed clinically. If treated at an early stage, there is a high 5-year survival rate. Unfortunately, there is a high rate of locoregional recurrence regardless of negative margin status. Adenoid cystic carcinoma also has a high rate of distant metastasis, with some studies reporting a rate as high as 50%. The lungs are the main organ of metastasis, followed by bone and liver. These lesions are classically described as "coin" lesions on chest radiographs. The survival rate continues to fall until the 20-year mark, when the survival rate is less than 5%.

Acinic cell carcinoma is another rare malignancy that accounts for about 6% of all salivary gland tumors. This tumor most commonly presents in females and is usually seen in the fifth and sixth decades of life. The parotid gland is the most common location; painful swelling is seen in 18% to 71% of patients, and facial paresis is reported in 11%. The survival rate has been reported as 76%, 63%, and 55% at 5, 10, and 15 years, respectively, although there is significant variation in the literature.

Acinic cell carcinoma is considered a low-risk tumor for regional and distant metastasis (12% and 16% metastatic rates, respectively). The lungs are the most common site of distant metastasis, followed by bone. Staging is the primary determinate of treatment, but the histologic grade, facial paralysis, age, pain, and extraglandular spread are prognostic factors that must be considered. A higher histologic grade and a lack of cellular differentiation have both been associated with a poorer prognosis. Postoperative radiotherapy may be used to improve local control.

As with any oncologic surgical procedure, the goal in treating acinic cell carcinoma is to obtain wide negative margins at the primary location. Equally important, the clinician must use diagnostic tools to accurately stage the malignancy and determine the need for adjunctive therapy.

Bibliography

Beckhardt RN, Weber RS, Zane R, et al: Minor salivary gland tumors of the palate: clinical and pathologic correlates of outcome, *Laryngoscope* 105:1155-1160, 1995.

Boahene DK, Olsen KD, Lewis JE, et al: Mucoepidermoid carcinoma of the parotid gland: the Mayo Clinic experience, *Arch Otolaryngol Head Neck Surg* 130(7):849-856, 2004.

Brandwein MS, Ivanov K, Wallace DI, et al: Mucoepidermoid carcinoma: a clinicopathologic study of 80 patients with special reference to histological grading, *Am J Surg Pathol* 25(7):835-845, 2001.

Carlson ER, Schimmele SR: The management of minor salivary gland tumors of the oral cavity, *Atlas Oral Maxillofacial Surg Clin North Am* 6:1, 1998.

Ellington CL, Goodman M, Kono SA, et al: Adenoid cystic carcinoma of the head and neck: incidence and survival trends based on 1973-2007 surveillance, epidemiology, and end results data, *Cancer* 15:118(18):4444-4451, 2012.

Goode R, Auclair P, Ellis G: Mucoepidermoid carcinoma of the major salivary glands: clinical and histopathological analysis of 234 cases with evaluation and grading criteria, *Cancer* 82:7, 1997.

Guzzo M, Andreola S, Sirizzotti G, et al: Mucoepidermoid carcinoma of the salivary glands: clinicopathologic review of 108 patients treated at the National Cancer Institute of Milan, *Ann Surg Oncol* 9(7):688-695, 2002.

Hosokawa Y, Shirato H, Kagei K, et al: Role of radiotherapy for mucoepidermoid carcinoma of the salivary gland, *Oral Oncol* 35:105-111, 1999.

Mullins JE, Ogle O, Cottrell DA, et al: Painless mass in the parotid region, *J Oral Maxillofac Surg* 58(3):316-319, 2000.

Ord R, Salama A: Is it necessary to resect bone for low-grade mucoepidermoid carcinoma of the palate? *Br J Oral Maxillofac Surg* 50(8):712-714, 2012.

Plambeck K, Friedrich RE, Schmelzle R: Mucoepidermoid carcinoma of salivary gland origin: classification, clinical-pathological correlation, treatment results and long-term follow-up in 55 patients, *J Craniomaxillofac Surg* 24:133-139, 1996.

Pogrel MA: The management of salivary gland tumors of the palate, *J Oral Maxillofac Surg* 52:454-459, 1994.

Li Quan, Zhang Xin-Rui, Liu Xue-Kui, et al: Long-term treatment outcome of minor salivary gland carcinoma of the hard palate, *Oral Oncol* 48:456-462, 2012.

Rapidis AD, Givolas N, Gakiopoulou H, et al: Adenoid cystic carcinoma of the head and neck: clinicopathological analysis of 23 patients and review of the literature, *Oral Oncol* 41:428-435, 2005.

Schramm VL, Imola MJ: Management of nasopharyngeal salivary gland malignancy, *Laryngoscope* 111(9):1533-1544, 2001.

Neck Dissections

Ketan Patel and Deepak Kademani

CC

A 60-year-old Caucasian man presents to your office. He states, "I have been told I have a squamous cell carcinoma on my tongue."

HPI

The patient noticed a spot on his tongue about a month ago. He reports that the lesion is painful, with radiating pain to the ear (this is a typical symptom of tongue carcinoma). He was initially seen by his general dentist and then referred to an oral and maxillofacial surgeon for a biopsy. The biopsy results described a squamous cell carcinoma (SCCa) (as described in the Section, Squamous Cell Carciroma).

PMHX/PDHX/MEDICATIONS/ALLERGIES/FH

The patient has a 45-year history of tobacco use. He also reports consumption of alcohol. (An association between tobacco and alcohol consumption and the development of SCCa has been well established.) The patient does not report any other significant medical problems.

EXAMINATION

The examination of the patient with a diagnosis of SCCa should include a complete head and neck exam. A neck examination is very important to evaluate for neck metastasis. Studies have shown that on initial examination of a known primary tumor, there is a 3% to 7% incidence of a synchronous tumor in the upper aerodigestive tract, especially in smokers. A nasopharyngoscopic examination is indicated to evaluate the subepiglottic and supraepiglottic regions, posterior oropharynx, and nasopharynx.

General. The patient is a well-developed and well-nourished male who appears his stated age, with no signs of cachexia.

Maxillofacial. The left tongue has a tumor, measuring approximately 4 × 2 cm, that feels endophytic and ulcerated. On palpation it seems to have possibly crossed the midline (Figure 11-8). The rest of the oral cavity is free of lesions. The patient also has multiple necrotic teeth that are grossly carious. (Some patients may also complain of ear pain if the lesions are deep and involve the lingual nerve. When ear pain is present, perineural invasion cannot be ruled out until a final pathology evaluation.) Examination of the rest of the oral cavity, including the buccal mucosa, hard and soft palate, parotid, oropharynx, and nasopharynx, reveals no other abnormalities. Adenopathy is palpable in the submental and the left submandibular regions of the neck. The nodes feel firm but not fixed (fixed nodes could be a sign of extracapsular spread).

Nasopharyngoscopy reveals no abnormal tissues in the posterior oropharynx, subglottic or supraglottic region, or nasopharynx (nasopharyngoscopy should be performed as part of the head and neck evaluation of tongue SCCa).

IMAGING

The initial imaging modality for evaluation of a patient with SCCa is a panoramic radiograph. This is a useful screening tool to evaluate for bony infiltration associated with the tumor. It also provides valuable information regarding the long-term prognosis of the remaining dentition, because some patients may require extraction of carious or periodontally involved teeth before radiotherapy.

A computed tomography (CT) scan of the head and neck is the commonly used imaging study of choice to delineate the lesion and assess the neck for cervical lymphadenopathy (nodes greater than 1.5 cm, with central necrosis, an ovoid shape, and fat stranding are indicative of nodal metastasis). Additional tests, such as magnetic resonance imaging (MRI)

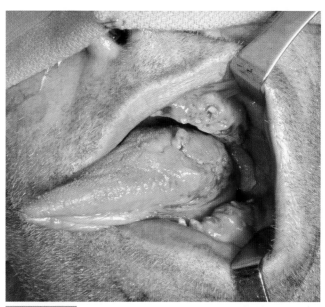

Figure 11-8 Clinical view showing a squamous cell carcinoma of the left lateral tongue and multiple necrotic teeth.

367

and ultrasonography, can be used to assess the status of the cervical nodes.

Positron emission tomography (PET) scans are becoming a common modality for the evaluation of distant metastasis. This technology uses a 18F-fluorodeoxyglucose (FDG) marker to examine sites of increased glucose uptake that are seen with metabolically active cancer cells. In addition to helping to rule out distant disease, PET aids in clinical staging of the cancer. Clinical staging is helpful, because a treatment plan can be worked up for the patient and adjuvant modalities recommended.

The current patient's axial and coronal CT scans of the head and neck, with and without contrast, revealed a 4-cm, well-circumscribed lesion of the left lateral border of the tongue musculature. Some adenopathy was noted in the submental region bilaterally and in the left submandibular region. (Usually nodes are oval in shape; however, in cancer patients with lymph node involvement, the nodes are more circular. Nodes greater than 1 cm in diameter should raise suspicion of metastatic disease. Central necrosis is another factor that correlates with a poorer outcome.) The PET scan performed with 18F-FDG showed a hypermetabolic area in the left tongue, coinciding with the clinical lesion, with an SUV of 17 (some studies suggest a correlation between a higher SUV and more aggressive tumors). Also noted were a single right level IB node, a single left level IB node, several left level IIA nodes, and a left level III node, all demonstrating associated FDG uptake. The largest node was a 1×1-cm level IIA lymph node demonstrating a maximum SUV of 5.4 (Figure 11-9). An SUV of greater than 3 has been shown to correlate with the increased metabolic activity associated with some pathologic conditions; however, clinical correlation must be completed.

In the current patient, the panoramic film showed that the condyles were seated on the fossa, with no bony invasion. In addition, several necrotic teeth with considerable periapical pathology were noted on the film.

LABS

A complete metabolic panel (CMP), complete blood count (CBC), and coagulation profile (prothrombin time [PT], partial thromboplastin time [PTT], and international normalized ratio [INR]) are mandatory laboratory studies in the cancer patient because of metabolic, electrolyte, and nutritional derangements that may accompany malignant disease. Liver function tests are obtained as part of the complete metabolic panel and are important screening tests for liver metastasis and alcoholism. Other laboratory studies can be ordered based on the patient's medical history.

In the current patient, the CBC, CMP, liver function test results, and coagulation studies were within normal limits.

ASSESSMENT

T2N2cM0 (tumor greater than 2 cm, with multiple bilateral nodes with no distant metastasis), stage IV, oral SCCa of the

left lateral border of the tongue with a Broders' histologic grade of III.

TREATMENT

The treatment of SCCa is site specific; surgical ablation with minimum 1- to 1.5-cm margins is the main modality of treatment. Most oral cavity tumors are approached intraorally; however, some tumors may need to be accessed extraorally

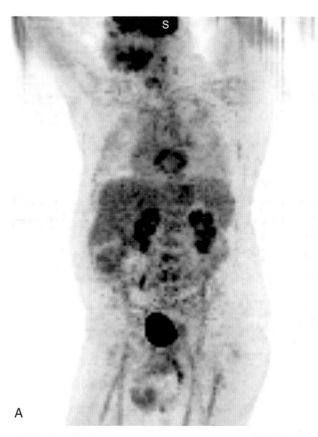

A

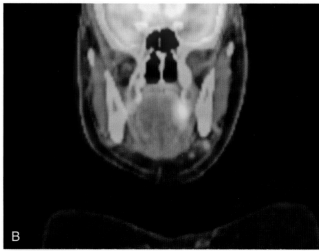

B

Figure 11-9   **A,** Full body PET scan shows some uptake in the nodes in the left neck in levels II and III. **B,** Head PET scan shows the primary tumor and an associated positive lymph node in level II.

via a transfacial approach. When the tumor is located in the mandible, the inferior border can be preserved (marginal mandibulectomy), depending on the degree of infiltration. However, when the cancellous portion of the mandible is invaded, segmental resection is required to maintain oncologic safety.

In the current case, several approaches were possible, including a transoral approach, a pull-through approach, a lip split mandibulotomy, and transoral robotic surgery (TORS), to obtain a cuff of normal tissue for the posterior tongue base margin. A transoral approach was used to excise the primary tumor. A common procedure that accompanies the removal of the tumor is neck dissection, or removal of the fibrofatty contents of the neck; this is done for treatment of cervical lymphatic metastases and also for complete staging of the cancerous process. In the current patient, selective neck dissection was performed on the right side (levels I through III) and on the left side (levels I through V). Bilateral neck dissection was performed because the tumor had crossed the midline and because the results of the PET scan were positive bilaterally. Vessel preservation was performed for a vascular free flap anastomosis (radial free forearm flap) to the facial artery and to the internal jugular vein.

The neck dissection procedure can be completed in many different ways. For the current patient, the following procedure was used, because it is the preferred method at our institution.

Selective neck dissection (levels I through III). After the patient had been prepped and draped, a surgical marker was used to delineate the incision site. Several variations of neck dissection incisions have been used historically (Figure 11-10). In this case a straight-line neck incision was used, with the incision situated in a resting skin tension line midway between the angle of the mandible and clavicle extending just slightly anterior to the auricle to the midline. (Any skin crease in the neck can be used, as long as it is approximately 2 cm below the inferior border of the mandible to avoid damage to the marginal mandibular branch of cranial nerve [CN] VII.) A no. 10 knife blade was used to create an incision through the skin and subcutaneous tissue to visualize the platysma; this was sharply dissected with a bovie electrocautery. Subplatysmal flaps were then raised to the level

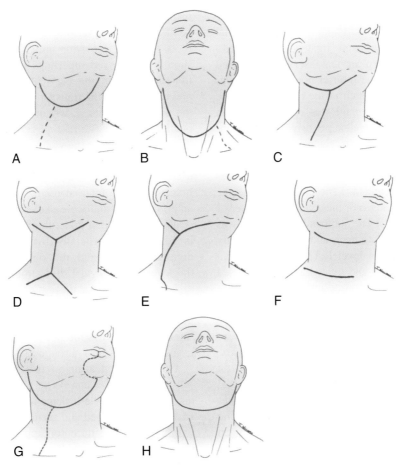

Figure 11-10 Variations of neck dissection incisions that have been used historically. **A,** Latyshevsky and Freund incision. **B,** Freund incision. **C,** Crile incision. **D,** Martin incision. **E,** Babcock and Conley incision. **F,** MacFee incision. **G,** Incision used for unilateral supraomohyoid neck dissection. **H,** Incision used for bilateral supraomohyoid neck dissection. *(From Rothrock JC: Alexander's care of the patient in surgery, ed 14, St Louis, 2011, Mosby.)*

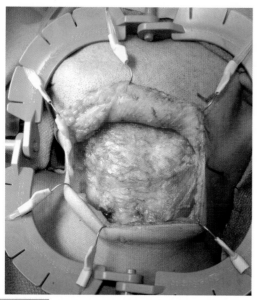

Figure 11-11 Clinical view showing the superior and inferior subplatysmal flaps.

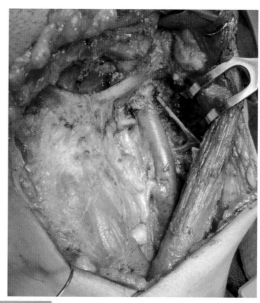

Figure 11-12 Clinical view showing the neck after removal of all the fibrofatty tissues from levels I through III.

of the inferior border of the mandible superiorly and the omohyoid muscle inferiorly (Figure 11-11). (This inferiorly based flap can be extended to just above the clavicle if further dissection to level IV is required. Care should be exercised to preserve the greater auricular nerve. The external jugular vein should be skeletonized, ligated, and divided.) The superficial layer of the deep cervical fascia was dissected approximately 1.5 cm below the inferior border of the mandible to protect the marginal branch of the facial nerve. The capsule of the submandibular gland was dissected, and a subcapsular dissection was initiated superiorly to the inferior border of the mandible. Bovie electrocauterization was used to dissect the fascia to the anterior belly of the digastric muscle in the submental triangle; this was continued posteriorly to the submandibular gland. (The lateral limit of the dissection is the midline diatheses or the contralateral anterior belly of the digastric muscle.) The submandibular gland was then retracted inferiorly into the neck and circumferentially dissected along the contents of level I. The common facial vein and artery were identified and ligated as they traversed the posterior aspects of the gland. Anteriorly they were once again identified and ligated (they are typically encountered on the medial side of the submandibular gland, thereby mobilizing the gland). An Army Navy retractor was placed beneath the myohyoid muscle to retract it superiorly. (The lingual nerve typically is visualized with the parasympathetic rami to the submandibular gland. The rami are transected with care to protect the lingual nerve.) The submandibular duct was then identified, skeletonized, and divided. (The entire contents of level I should be pedicled inferiorly on the digastric muscle. The fascia overlying the anterior border of the SCM superiorly from the level of the digastric muscle inferiorly to the omohyoid muscle is then separated from the muscle with bovie electrocauterization.) When the inferior surface of the SCM was dissected, the spinal accessory nerve

was identified approximately 1 cm below Erb's point and skeletonized. (When a clearance of level IIb is desired, the fascia above the CN XI is dissected deep to the level of the levator scapulae and splenius capitis. This fascia packet is then brought inferiorly beneath the nerve. The cervical roots form the posterior limit of the dissection, and fascia should be removed superficial to the nerve rootlets. Dissection deeper than the cervical roots should be avoided to prevent injury to the transverse cervical vessels and preserve the prevertebral fascia, which overlies the phrenic nerve and brachial plexus.) The fascia over the carotid sheath was then dissected over (once the white roll is identified on the anterior border of the internal jugular vein, a no. 15 blade can be used to skeletonize the fascia from the vein sharply). The branches of the internal jugular vein were identified on the anterior border and were skeletonized, ligated, and divided. (Once this has been done, the fascia from the jugular sheath is advanced superficially from the posterior belly of the digastric muscle and the omohyoid muscle inferiorly to the level of the level I dissection, which is pedicled on the digastric muscle. As the dissection continues, the anterior jugular veins are identified and ligated. The specimens can now be removed from the patient and orientated by level.) Figure 11-12 shows the neck after removal of the fibrofatty tissues from levels I through III.

Once the surgical field has been rendered hemostatic, the Valsalva maneuver can be performed to ensure that there is no evidence of chyle leakage or pneumothorax. A flat no. 10 Blake drain is placed and secured. Closure is then performed with 3-0 Vicryl suture for approximation of the platysma muscle. Skin closure can be completed with either 5-0 Prolene sutures or staples, and antibiotic ointment is applied. Extubation should be performed with minimal agitation while holding pressure to the surgical site to prevent the formation of a postoperative hematoma.

COMPLICATIONS

Complications of neck dissection are categorized as intraoperative, postoperative (within 1 month), and long term (after 1 month).

Intraoperative complications. The main intraoperative concerns associated with oncologic ablative and reconstructive surgery include the control of hemorrhage and anesthetic complications. When simultaneous neck dissection is performed, additional possible complications include nerve palsies (facial, lingual, spinal accessory nerves, and hypoglossal nerves); vascular injury to the carotid artery or internal jugular vein; and, rarely, pneumothorax, air embolism, and formation of a chylous fistula.

Postoperative complications. Postoperative complications include wound infection, hematoma, skin necrosis, orocutaneous fistula, poor speech, and swallowing dysfunction.

Long-term complications. The gravest long-term complications are recurrence of the primary tumor and death (85% of recurrences occur in the first 3 years). Other complications include lingual nerve hypoesthesia and duct obstruction. Dysphagia, xerostomia, mucositis, and the risk of osteoradionecrosis are associated with radiation therapy. The most common causes of death in patients with oral cancer are related to locoregional disease, distant metastasis, or cardiopulmonary failure. Metastases of SCCa tend to involve the lung, bones, liver, and brain.

DISCUSSION

Neck dissection was originally based on Halstead's principles of en bloc removal of lymph nodes in the neck for the management of patients with head and neck tumors. The term "neck dissection" has evolved to encompass several different operations that may be selected based on the nature of the disease. Neck dissection was first described in the late nineteenth century by von Langenbeck, Billroth, von Volkmann, and Kocher, who developed and reported the early cases of different types of neck dissection. The first report of a neck dissection published in the literature was by Crile in 1906, and several modifications were subsequently made.

The neck is divided into anatomic regions for purposes of neck dissection. The system most widely used today was adopted at the Memorial Sloan-Kettering Cancer Center. Researchers at that institution have defined seven regions, denoted as levels I through VII (Figure 11-13 and Box 11-3).

Several types of neck dissections have been described in the literature.

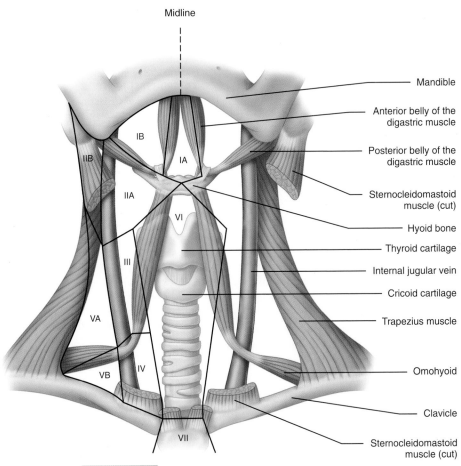

Figure 11-13 The levels of the neck for oncologic surgery.

Box 11-3   Seven Levels of the Neck

- **Level I: Submental and submandibular.** Contains the submental and submandibular triangles, which are bounded by the posterior belly of the digastric muscle, the midline, the body of the mandible superiorly, and the hyoid bone inferiorly. Level I can be further subdivided into Ia (submental triangle) and Ib (submandibular triangle).
- **Level II: Upper jugular.** Contains the upper jugular lymph nodes and extends from the skull base superiorly to the hyoid bone inferiorly. Anterior landmarks are the midline strap muscles; posteriorly, this level is bounded by the anterior border of the trapezius muscle. The spinal accessory nerve (XI) travels obliquely across this area and can be used to subdivide this area into IIa (anteriorly) and IIb (posteriorly).
- **Level III: Midjugular.** Contains the middle jugular lymph nodes from the hyoid bone superiorly to the level of the lower border of the cricoid cartilage inferiorly.
- **Level IV: Lower jugular.** Contains the lower jugular lymph nodes from the level of the cricoid cartilage superiorly to the clavicle inferiorly. Nodes that are deep to the sterna head of the sternocleidomastoid are categorized as IVa, and those deep to the clavicular are categorized as IVb.
- **Level V: Posterior triangle.** Contains the lymph nodes in the posterior triangle bounded by the anterior border of the trapezius muscle posteriorly, the posterior border of the sternocleidomastoid muscle anteriorly, and the clavicle inferiorly. This area may be further classified into the upper, middle, and lower levels, corresponding to the superior and inferior planes that define levels II, III, and IV.
- **Level VI: Prelaryngeal (delphian), pretracheal, and paratracheal.** Contains the lymph nodes of the anterior central compartment from the hyoid bone superiorly to the suprasternal notch inferiorly. On each side, the lateral boundary is formed by the medial border of the carotid sheath.
- **Level VII: Upper mediastinal.** Contains the lymph nodes inferior to the suprasternal notch in the superior mediastinum.

Radical neck dissection. This is the standard procedure for the removal of the entire cervical lymphatic chain from the unilateral neck, encompassing levels I through V, the spinal accessory nerve, the internal jugular vein, and the sternocleidomastoid muscle. Indications for this surgery include advanced neck disease with multiple-level positive lymph nodes with gross extracapsular spread and infiltration of the spinal accessory nerve, sternocleidomastoid muscle, or internal jugular vein.

Modified radical neck dissection. This procedure involves the removal of lymph nodes from levels I through V but requires the preservation of one or more of the nonlymphatic structures that are included in a radical neck dissection (e.g., spinal accessory nerve, internal jugular vein, or sternocleidomastoid muscle).

Selective neck dissection. This is an umbrella term encompassing several procedures in which neck nodes of certain ("selected") levels are removed and other areas are preserved.

Supraomohyoid neck dissection. This is the selective removal of levels I through III. Its main indication is for the N0 neck in cases of oral cavity SCCa with a 20% or greater chance of occult neck disease. The guiding parameters include an aggressive, high-grade tumor (characterized histopathologically): invasion of greater than 3 mm (if discussing oral SCCa); and perineural invasion. The procedure is performed on the ipsilateral side from the primary tumor, except in the case of primary tumors arising from midline structures such as the floor of the mouth, because such tumors are known to metastasize bilaterally.

Anterior compartment neck dissection. This is the selective removal of level VI nodes. The primary indications for this procedure are primary tumors of the thyroid gland, hypopharynx, cervical trachea, cervical esophagus, and subglottic larynx.

Posterolateral neck dissection. This is the removal of lymph nodes II through V. The procedure is indicated for scalp and auricular tumors.

Lateral neck dissection. This is the selective removal of levels II through IV. The main indication for this surgery is primary cancer of the oropharynx, hypopharynx, and larynx.

Extended neck dissection. This procedure includes removal of structures not routinely involved with radical neck dissection. Such structures can include retropharyngeal lymph nodes and the hypoglossal nerve, prevertebral musculature, or carotid artery. This surgery is indicated for advanced neck disease involving difficulty obtaining negative margins.

Bibliography

Crile G: Excision of cancer of the head and neck, with special reference to the plan of dissection based on 132 operations, *JAMA* 47:1780-1785, 1906.

Gavilan J, Gavilan C, Herranz J: Functional neck dissection: three decades of controversy, *Ann Otol Rhinol Laryngol* 101(4):339-341, 1992.

Kerawala CP, Heliotos M: Prevention of complications in neck dissection, *Head Neck Oncol* 1:35, 2009.

Lindberg, R: Distribution of cervical lymph node metastases from squamous cell carcinoma of the upper respiratory and digestive tracts, *Cancer* 29:1446-1449, 1972.

Martin H, Del Valle B, Ehrlich H, et al: Neck dissection, *Cancer* 4(3):441-499, 1951.

Medina JE: A rational classification of neck dissections, *Otolaryngol Head Neck Surg* 100:169-176, 1989.

Rinaldo A, Ferlito A, Silver CE: Early history of neck dissection, *Eur Arch Otorhinolaryngol* 265(12):1535-1538, 2008 (Epub: May 17, 2008.)

Shah JP: Patterns of lymph node metastases from squamous carcinomas of the upper aerodigestive tract, *Am J Surg* 160(4):405-409, 1990.

Smith GI, O'Brien CJ, Clark J, et al: Management of the neck in patients with T1 and T2 cancer in the mouth, *Br J Oral Maxillofac Surg* 42:494-500, 2004.

Wooglar JA: Histological distribution of cervical lymph node metastases from intraoral/oropharyngeal squamous cell carcinomas, *Br J Oral Maxillofac Surg* 37:175-180, 1999.

CHAPTER 12

Reconstructive Oral and Maxillofacial Surgery

Editors: Shahrokh C. Bagheri and R. Bryan Bell

This chapter addresses:
- Posterior Mandibular Augmentation
- Radial Forearm Free Flap
- Pectoralis Major Myocutaneous Flap
- Free Fibula Flap for Mandibular Reconstruction
- Mandibular Reconstruction with Iliac Crest Bone Graft

The term *reconstructive maxillofacial surgery* refers to the wide range of procedures designed to rebuild or enhance soft or hard tissue structures of the maxillofacial region. Ablative tumor surgery (benign or malignant) and traumatic injuries (especially avulsive) commonly demand reconstructive procedures to restore the functional and cosmetic deficit. Loss of soft or hard tissue secondary to infectious processes (e.g., osteomyelitis), or tissue injury due to irradiation (e.g., osteoradionecrosis) may also require reconstructive measures. In addition, the decrease in the quantity and quality of maxillomandibular structures with age (which may be accelerated by other processes, such as early loss of teeth) can be addressed with reconstructive measures to augment the tissue for restoration using dental implants.

In the past two decades, four developments have revolutionized the reconstruction of the maxillofacial structures. First, gains in our understanding of bone biology have allowed advanced bone grafting procedures in a variety of circumstances (e.g., sinus lift procedures, mandibular augmentation/reconstruction). Second, the advent of microvascular free flap techniques has enabled the transfer of tissue to reconstruct large soft and/or hard tissue defects (e.g., radial forearm fasciocutaneous or fibula osteocutaneous free flaps). Third, the development of and advances in dental implant techniques have allowed successful dental rehabilitation. Fourth, the introduction of computer-aided surgery, using CT-generated images and virtual surgery, has significantly changed the practice of reconstructive surgery. Future research may reveal improved methods of regenerating bone, neural, and muscle tissue. Future molecular biology techniques using gene therapy may provide knowledge that can be applied to maxillofacial reconstruction.

In this chapter, we present important teaching cases that describe some of the main issues in maxillofacial reconstruction. Mandibular reconstruction remains one of the greatest challenges in maxillofacial surgery. We present cases of mandibular reconstruction using corticocancellous bone grafts with implants and other cases using the free fibula osteocutaneous flap.

Posterior Mandibular Augmentation

William Stuart McKenzie and Patrick J. Louis

CC

A 69-year-old Caucasian male presents for evaluation for dental implants. He states, "I am interested in getting implants."

HPI

The patient was referred by his general dentist for extraction of periodontally involved teeth and evaluation for implant placement. He reports that he has difficulty chewing his food due to discomfort and mobility of several of his posterior teeth.

PMHX/PSHX/MEDICATIONS/ALLERGIES/SH/FH

The patient reports hypercholesterolemia, prostatic hypertrophy, gastroesophageal reflux disease (GERD), chronic neck pain, and chronic rhinitis/sinusitis. His current medications include aspirin 81 mg, fenofibrate, alfuzosin, and omeprazole. The past surgical history includes a hernia repair. The patient reports allergies to tramadol and hydrocodone. He also reports a history of cigarette smoking but quit 10 years ago. He denies alcohol and illicit drug use. The family history is negative for heart disease, diabetes, and head and neck malignancy.

EXAMINATION

General. The patient is a well-nourished, well-developed 69-year-old Caucasian male in no apparent distress.

Vital signs. Blood pressure is 156/87 mm Hg, heart rate 69 bpm, respiratory rate 16 per minute, and temperature 37°C.

Maxillofacial. Normocephalic. Skin is dry and intact, pupils equal, round, and reactive to light and accommodation (PERRLA), no scleral icterus, visual acuity grossly intact, external auditory canals clear bilaterally, tympanic membranes intact, nares patent, cranial nerves II through XII grossly intact bilaterally. Neck is supple and without lymphadenopathy.

Intraoral. Mucosa is moist and pink. No ulcers, masses, or discolorations of the oral cavity noted. Teeth #3, #11 through #15, #19, #20, and #30 are absent. Generalized periodontal disease is noted with root exposure on teeth #2, #4, #18, #21, #28, and #30. A buccal horizontal defect is present at teeth #19, #20, and #30.

IMAGING

Panoramic radiograph reveals no pathologic findings of the sinuses, maxilla, temporomandibular joints, or mandible. There is pneumatization of bilateral maxillary sinuses and generalized periodontal disease with periapical radiolucency at teeth #18, #28, and #31.

LABS

No labs are indicated at this time.

ASSESSMENT

Caucasian male, 69 years old, with a history of hypercholesterolemia, prostatic hypertrophy, GERD, chronic neck pain, and chronic rhinitis/sinusitis presents for an evaluation for dental implant placement after extraction of periodontally involved teeth. The physical exam reveals vertical insufficiency of the right mandibular and bilateral maxillary posterior alveolar ridges, in addition to a horizontal alveolar deficiency of the right mandibular posterior alveolar ridge (Figure 12-1).

TREATMENT

Alveolar deficiencies of the posterior mandible present unique surgical challenges. Defects must be accurately assessed for the horizontal and vertical deficiencies of bone and the amount of keratinized tissue available to support the final prosthesis. A host of reconstructive techniques and materials must be considered, and the most appropriate method selected to maximize the individual patient's outcome (Figure 12-2). The success of endosteal implant restorations and prostheses has made augmentation of the posterior mandible a necessary skill for oral and maxillofacial surgeons. The use of titanium mesh, autogenous bone, allogeneic/xenogeneic bone, and inlay bone grafting is discussed later.

Horizontal Defects

A horizontal defect is defined as an inadequate buccolingual dimension of bone with an adequate superoinferior dimension. Horizontal defects most commonly occur on the facial aspect of the mandible. Generally, implants 5 mm in diameter are placed in the molar region; this requires 7 to 8 mm of horizontal bone to ensure 1 to 1.5 mm of bone buccal and lingual to the implant.

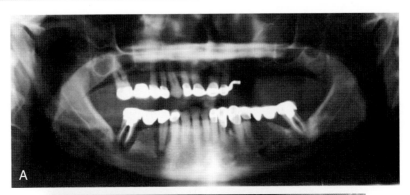

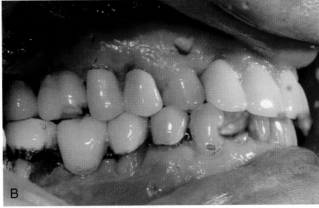

Figure 12-1   **A,** Initial panoramic radiograph showing generalized periodontal disease and insufficient height of bilateral maxillary and right mandibular posterior alveolar ridges for implant placement. **B,** Right posterior mandible showing severe periodontal disease and buccal horizontal defects at the posterior area.

Block Grafts

The autogenous block graft has been widely used for horizontal defects. The harvest site of the cortical bone depends largely on the length of bone required. For smaller defects, harvest from the mandibular symphysis or mandibular ramus allows for easy access with low long-term morbidity. However, temporary V3 paresthesia has been reported in 10% to 50% of symphysis grafts, and 0 to 5% of ramus grafts. For larger defects, distant harvest sites of bone are necessary. The calvarial graft, taken from the parietal bone, provides dense cortical bone that is resistant to resorption. Harvesting a split-thickness graft from this region provides an approximately 3-mm-thick segment of bone, and the harvest site has few complications. The ilium may also be used; however, the cortical bone is thinner and less resistant to resorption due to the endochondral origin of the ilium, compared with the intramembranous origin of the parietal bone. However, a large amount of bone may be harvested from the iliac crest. The main complications of iliac crest bone grafts include gait disturbances, paresthesia, hematoma/seroma, and fracture of the hip.

The use of block allografts has been presented in case series. Nissen and colleagues placed 29 cancellous block allografts in 21 patients with posterior mandibular atrophy; the graft failure rate was 20.7%, and the implant survival rate in the remaining grafts was 95.2% at 37-month follow-up. However, long-term outcomes for allogeneic block grafts from prospective, randomized clinical trials are lacking. A systematic review by Waasdorp and Reynolds found only nine articles that met inclusion criteria, and eight of the articles were case reports or case series. The authors concluded that, although the case reports demonstrated potential for allogeneic block grafts for alveolar ridge augmentation, there is insufficient evidence to establish treatment efficacy with regard to graft stability and long-term implant survival.

Procedure. The defect site is exposed using a crestal incision. The defect is then measured for the size of the graft needed. The appropriate-sized block graft is harvested from the donor site and is contoured to approximate the defect. The facial surface of the defect site also is contoured to allow for maximum surface area contact with the graft. Multiple sites of decortication are created on the defect site with a small round bur to promote neovascularization of the graft. The graft is secured with one or two resorbable or titanium screws. Particulate bone is packed into any gaps, and the site is covered with a resorbable or nonresorbable membrane. Tension-free closure is obtained using a periosteal releasing incision if necessary.

Particulate Bone

Particulate bone graft material is available from a wide array of sources, including autografts (from the patient), allografts (from a human donor), xenografts (from an animal donor),

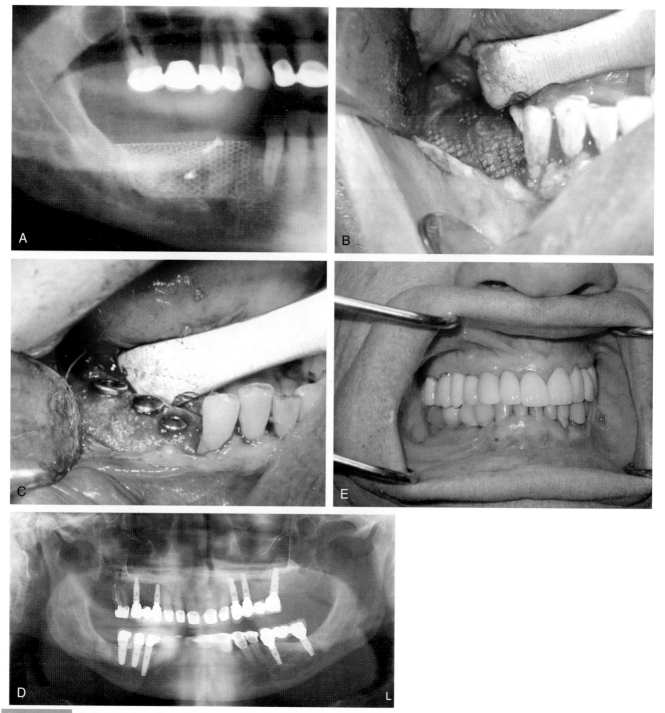

Figure 12-2 **A,** Panoramic radiograph showing titanium mesh placement for posterior ridge augmentation. A mixture of autogenous bone from a right mandibular torus, hydroxyapatite, and platelet-rich plasma was used under the mesh. **B,** Titanium mesh after 6 months of healing, with pseudomembrane intact. **C,** Implant placement at teeth #28, #29, and #30 after titanium mesh removal. **D,** Final panoramic radiograph showing right mandibular implants with restoration. The patient also underwent bilateral maxillary sinus lifts, right maxillary ridge split osteotomy, and implant placement at teeth #3, #5, #11, #12, #14, #18, and #20. **E,** Postoperative photograph showing restored posterior mandibular implants in function 8 years after placement.

and alloplastic material (synthetic material). Autogenous particulate bone may be harvested from intraoral sites, including cortical shaving from the symphysis, ramus, or zygoma, and cancellous bone can be harvested from the ilium or tibia. Autogenous bone is often combined with banked particulate bone; this increases the volume of graft material while maintaining the osteogenic and osteoinductive properties of the autogenous bone. The choice of graft material depends on the amount of particulate bone needed, osteoinductive versus osteoconductive properties, and the desires of the patient. Whether the graft is mineralized or demineralized determines the type of membrane required for graft stabilization. In general, mineralized particulate bone is able to better withstand the forces exerted on the surgical site during healing, requiring only a nonrigid membrane at the time of graft placement. Demineralized bone, however, requires a rigid membrane during the healing phase. Titanium mesh is well suited to protecting demineralized bone and can tolerate exposure to the oral cavity without a significant rate of graft failure. The titanium mesh is contoured and adapted to the alveolar ridge and secured with titanium screws.

Procedure. A crestal or vestibular incision is used to expose the defect. Decortication of the defect is performed using a small round bur. The particulate graft is placed. If a nonrigid membrane is used, the edges are trimmed and tucked underneath the flaps. If a rigid membrane is used, the membrane is contoured, packed with particulate bone, and then secured with screws to prevent movement. Tension-free closure is obtained using a periosteal releasing incision if necessary. The vestibular incision usually allows for tension-free closure without release of the periosteum.

Inlay Bone Graft

First described by Simion and colleagues in 1992, the alveolar split osteotomy technique for horizontal bone defects and subsequent implant placement has shown predictable results. The surgery is usually performed in a two-stage fashion in the mandible due to the dense cortical buccal plate. At least 3 mm of horizontal width is preferred for a controlled fracture; however, widths as narrow as 2 mm have been reported. The goal of the technique is to produce a vascularized bone flap through controlled fracture of the buccal plate. The gap produced by the fracture at the second stage can then be grafted with block or particulate bone, or implants can be placed along with a particulate graft. A membrane is generally used to protect the graft and implants during healing.

Procedure. The initial surgery requires a full-thickness flap to expose the buccal cortical plate. A crestal incision with releasing incisions away from the planned corticotomy sites is used. Crestal, apical, and two vertical corticotomies are performed and connected to create an outline of the intended bone flap. A piezoelectric drill is often used to preserve bone. The mucosal flap is then sutured. Stage 2 is performed after approximately 4 weeks; with this interval, the periosteal blood supply to the bone is restored, but callus is still present at the corticotomy sites. The crestal incision is made along the crestal corticotomy, with care taken to reflect as little periosteum as possible. Osteotomes are used to gently out-fracture the bone flap. The bone graft and/or implants can then be placed. Primary closure can be attempted using a periosteal releasing incision, but primary closure is often difficult, requiring the use of a membrane. If implants are not placed, 4 to 6 months of healing is allowed before implant placement.

Vertical Defects

Vertical defects of the posterior mandible refer to inadequate height of alveolar bone in relation to the inferior alveolar nerve. Vertical defects can be challenging to treat due to a small surface area of crestal mandibular bone for onlay grafting, difficulty with exposure of the graft due to tension of the soft tissue after augmentation, and resorption of graft material. Techniques described include onlay grafting, particulate bone grafts, inlay grafts, and distraction osteogenesis.

In 2009, Esposito and colleagues performed a Cochrane systematic review of randomized controlled trials (RCTs) for horizontal and vertical ridge augmentation. Of the 13 trials that met the inclusion criteria, 10, enrolling 218 patients, addressed vertical ridge augmentation. Analysis of the trials found that vertical augmentation resulted in a high complication rate (20% to 60%) and graft failure rates of 10% to 15%. Interestingly, two split-mouth trials compared alloplastic grafting (anorganic bovine bone and Regenaform, respectively) with autogenous bone grafting (iliac crest and particulate bone) and showed no statistical difference in outcomes. Although both studies had small sample sizes (10 and 5 patients), the reduction in operative time, cost, and patient discomfort certainly justify further investigation. The review also included a meta-analysis of two RCTs examining mandibular ridge augmentation (iliac crest inlay graft and anorganic bovine inlay) versus short implant placement without augmentation. The meta-analysis showed an increased implant failure rate (borderline significance; $p = 0.06$), and a statistically significant increase in the complication rate in the augmented group. The additional time, cost (e.g., general anesthesia, hospitalization), and patient discomfort are also important factors. However, the long-term outcomes of short implants in the posterior mandible have not been adequately evaluated to date.

Block Grafts

The use of onlay autogenous grafting for vertical augmentation has been widely described in the literature. One of the shortcomings of the onlay graft is resorption of the graft during healing. Studies using intraoral (symphysis and/or ramus) and posterior iliac crest have reported 17% to 41% resorption of the onlay graft at 4 to 6 months.

Procedure. Autogenous block grafts for vertical augmentation can be harvested in a fashion identical to that previously described. A crestal incision is made, and the block is adapted to the alveolar defect and secured with titanium screws. Gaps are packed with particulate bone, and a membrane is placed. The incision is sutured over the graft after periosteal release for tension-free closure.

Particulate Bone

Particulate bone grafting for vertical deficiency has been shown to be effective when used with a rigid membrane or titanium mesh. The use of titanium mesh has been shown to be effective in the reconstruction of alveolar ridge defects, regardless of the particulate bone source. The titanium mesh acts as a permanent, rigid barrier that is biocompatible and easily molded to the desired shape. Several studies have demonstrated successful vertical augmentation (maxilla and

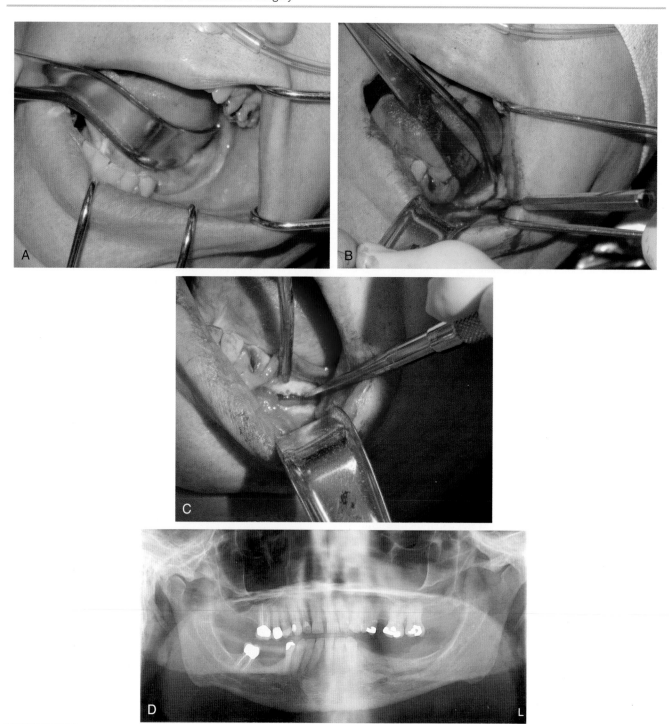

Figure 12-3   **A,** A 59-year-old Caucasian male with left posterior mandibular vertical deficiency. **B,** Completion of osteotomy for inlay graft (sandwich osteotomy technique). **C,** Mobilization of the mandibular alveolar segment. A block of allograft bone was used without fixation for the interpositional graft. **D,** Postoperative panoramic radiograph with block graft in place, showing adequate height for implant placement in left posterior mandible.

mandible) using titanium mesh, with average vertical gains of 3.71 to 14 mm and implant success rates in the grafted area of 93% to 100%. Exposure of the titanium mesh during the healing phase is commonly reported, with a rate ranging from 5% to 52%. However, the rates of infection and graft failure remain low compared to other nonresorbable barriers. Watzinger and colleagues demonstrated that the timing of the mesh exposure is critical to the final outcome. If exposure occurred within 4 to 6 weeks of the grafting procedure, graft take was poor. However, if exposure occurred after 4 to 6 weeks, these sites had outcomes similar to those for grafts that did not have exposure. Most areas of late exposure of titanium mesh (after 4 to 6 weeks) can be managed with local wound care; removal is required only if signs of infection are present.

Procedure. The technique for particulate bone grafting was described previously in the section on particulate bone grafting for horizontal deficiency.

Inlay Graft

Inlay grafting, or "sandwich" osteotomy, provides the advantage of having a pedicled segment of alveolar bone overlying the graft material. Felice and colleagues demonstrated significantly less bone resorption of the inlay graft, compared to onlay grafting of anterior iliac crest bone, in 20 patients. In another study by Felice, no statistical difference in outcomes was found for inlay grafts with anorganic bovine bone (Geistlich Bio-Oss [Geistlich Pharma North America, Inc., Princeton, N. J.]), compared with iliac crest bone, for vertical augmentation in the posterior mandible. The disadvantages of inlay grafting are the inability to address horizontal defects with the procedure and limitation of the amount of vertical augmentation by the lingual soft tissue pedicle to the mobilized alveolar segment. Additionally, there must be at least 4 mm of bone above the mandibular canal to preserve viability of the mobilized segment while avoiding damage to the nerve.

Procedure. A vestibular incision is made, and a subperiosteal flap is raised to expose the buccal surface of the alveolar ridge. The crestal and lingual tissue is not reflected. A reciprocating saw and/or piezoelectric handpiece is used to create the horizontal and two vertical oblique osteotomies, with care taken not to damage the lingual tissue. The horizontal osteotomy should be at least 2 mm superior to the mandibular canal, and the alveolar segment should ideally be at least 3 mm tall to tolerate the placement of titanium screws without fracturing. The bone graft is placed, and the transported and basal mandibular segments are plated with titanium miniplates and screws, thus stabilizing the graft. Gaps are filled with particulate bone, and the vestibular incision is closed. A healing period of 3 to 4 months is allowed before the hardware is removed and implants are placed.

DISCUSSION

With the growing popularity of implant restorations, mandibular ridge augmentation has become a necessary skill for oral and maxillofacial surgeons. The posterior mandible can be a particularly difficult area to successfully augment due to the unique anatomy of the area. A thorough understanding of surgical techniques and bone grafting options is vital to maximizing the final functional and esthetic outcomes for the patient (Figure 12-3).

Bibliography

Bell RB, Blakey GH, White RP, et al: Stages reconstruction of the severely atrophic mandible with autogenous bone graft and endosteal implants, *J Oral Maxillofac Surg* 60:1135, 2002.

Chiapasco M, Abati S, Romeo E, et al: Clinical outcome of autogenous bone blocks or guided bone regeneration with e-PTFE membranes for the reconstruction of narrow edentulous ridges, *Clin Oral Implants Res* 10(4):278-288, 1999.

Clavero J, Lundgren S: Ramus or chin grafts for maxillary sinus inlay and local onlay augmentation: comparison of donor site morbidity and complications, *Clin Implant Dent Relat Res* 5(3):154-160, 2003.

Cordaro L, Amade DS, Cordaro M: Clinical results of alveolar ridge augmentation with mandibular block bone grafts in partially edentulous patients prior to implant placement, *Clin Oral Implants Res* 13:103, 2002.

Corinaldesi G, Pieri F, Sapigni L, et al: Evaluation of survival and success rates of dental implants placed at the time of or after alveolar ridge augmentation with an autogenous mandibular bone graft and titanium mesh: a 3- to 8-year retrospective study, *Int J Oral Maxillofac Implants* 24:1119-1128, 2009.

Esposito M, Grusovin MG, Felice P, et al: The efficacy of horizontal and vertical bone augmentation procedures for dental implants: a Cochrane systematic review, *Eur J Oral Implantol* 2(3):167-184, 2009.

Felice P, Pistilli R, Lizio G, et al: Inlay versus onlay iliac bone grafting in atrophic posterior mandible: a prospective controlled clinical trial for the comparison of two techniques, *Clin Implant Dent Relat Res* 11(Suppl 1):e69-82, 2009.

Felice P, Marchetti C, Iezzi G, et al: Vertical ridge augmentation of the atrophic posterior mandible with interpositional bloc grafts: bone from the iliac crest vs bovine anorganic bone—clinical and histological results up to one year after loading from a randomized-controlled clinical trial, *Clin Oral Implants Res* 20:1386-1393, 2009.

Her S: Titanium mesh as an alternative to a membrane for ridge augmentation, *J Oral Maxillofac Surg* 70:803-810, 2012.

Louis P, Gutta R, Said-Al Naief N, et al: Reconstruction of the maxilla and mandible with particulate bone graft and titanium mesh for implant placement, *J Oral Maxillofac Surg* 66:235-245, 2008.

Louis P: Bone grafting the mandible, *Oral Maxillofac Surg Clin North Am* 23:209-227, 2011.

Mertens C, Decker C, Seeberger R, et al: Early bone resorption after vertical bone augmentation: a comparison of calvarial and iliac grafts, *Clin Oral Implants Res* 24(7):820-825, 2013.

Nissen J, Ghelfan O, Mardinger O, et al: Efficacy of cancellous block allograft augmentation prior to implant placement in the posterior atrophic mandible, *Clin Implant Dent Relat Res* 13(4):279-285, 2011.

Pieri F, Corinaldesi G, Fini M, et al: Alveolar ridge augmentation with titanium mesh and a combination of autogenous bone and anorganic bovine bone: a 2-year prospective study, *J Periodontol* 79:2093-2103, 2008.

Proussaefs P, Lozada J: The use of intraorally harvested autogenous block grafts for vertical alveolar ridge augmentation: a human study, *Int J Periodontics Restorative Dent* 25:351, 2005.

Proussaefs P, Lozada J, Kleinman A, et al: The use of ramus autogenous block grafts for vertical alveolar ridge augmentation and implant placement: a pilot study, *Int J Oral Maxillofac Implants* 17:238, 2002.

Roccuzzo M, Ramieri G, Spada MC, et al: Vertical alveolar ridge augmentation by means of a titanium mesh and autogenous bone grafts, *Clin Oral Implants Res* 15:73-81, 2004.

Roccuzzo M, Ramieri G, Bunino M, et al: Autogenous bone graft alone or associated with titanium mesh for vertical alveolar ridge augmentation: a controlled clinical trial, *Clin Oral Implants Res* 18:286-294, 2007.

Simion M, Baldoni M, Zaffe D. Jawbone enlargement using immediate implant placement associated with a split-crest technique and guided tissue regeneration, *Int J Periodontics Restorative Dent* 12:462–473, 1992.

Tolstunov L, Hicke B: Horizontal augmentation through the ridge-split procedure: a predictable surgical modality in implant reconstruction, *J Oral Implantol* 39(1):59-68, 2013.

Waasdorp J, Reynolds MA: Allogeneic bone onlay grafts for alveolar ridge augmentation: a systematic review, *Int J Oral Maxillofac Implants* 25(3):525-531, 2010.

Watzinger F, Luksch J, Millesi W, et al: Guided bone regeneration with titanium membranes: a clinical study, *Br J Oral Maxillofac Surg* 38:312-315, 2000.

Radial Forearm Free Flap

Jonathan Shum, Tuan G. Bui, Samuel Bobek, and R. Bryan Bell

CC

A 40-year-old edentulous man is referred by his general dentist for evaluation of a tongue mass. The patient states, "My tongue hurts."

HPI

The patient was referred to an oral and maxillofacial surgeon for evaluation of an ulcerative tongue lesion. The patient first noticed the lesion 8 months ago, and only for the past 2 months has the pain become worse. His general dentist had noted a large ulcerative lesion involving the left posterior lateral tongue. An incisional biopsy of the tongue mass was performed, resulting in the diagnosis of a poorly differentiated, invasive squamous cell carcinoma.

PMHX/PDHX/MEDICATIONS/ALLERGIES/SH/FH

The patient suffers from hypertension, gastroesophageal reflux disease (GERD), and high cholesterol. He is currently taking simvastatin, HCTZ, and Pepcid OTC. The patient also has a 60 pack-year history of cigarette smoking and has indulged in alcohol regularly for more than 20 years (risk factors for oral cancer). The family history is noncontributory.

EXAMINATION

General. The patient is a slim, pleasant white man who appears his stated age.

Intraoral. The patient is edentulous and has a prominent ulceration at the left posterior lateral tongue that measures 3 cm in length and 2 cm in width. The red and white lesion is tender and has a necrotic center with firm, everted edges along its periphery (Figure 12-4). The tongue is freely mobile. There appears to be no extension into the floor of the mouth.

Neck. There is no palpable lymphadenopathy.

Nasal fiber endoscopy. The lesion does not extend into the base of tongue; the bilateral tonsillar pillars, epiglottis, valleculae, arytenoids, piriform sinuses, and glottis are without obvious lesions.

Extremity. Peripheral pulses are 2+ for all extremities, and there is no cyanosis, clubbing, or edema. Bilateral Allen's tests revealed good collateral circulation to the hands.

Allen's test is used to assess the circulatory blood flow of the hand. The main blood supply to the hand is via the ulnar

and radial artery. The ulnar artery supplies the superficial palmer branch, and the radial artery supplies the deep palmer branch. (Communication between the superficial and deep systems allows perfusion of the hand if there is interruption of one of the two main arteries to the hand, such as with the radial forearm free flap harvest.) Allen's test determines the perfusion of the hand by simulating complete interruption of the radial artery. This is to ensure that the hand remains viable upon harvesting of the radial forearm free flap. Allen's test is performed by elevating the intended hand and digitally occluding both the ulnar and the radial arteries. The patient is asked to clench and release a fist to cause blanching of the hand. Next, the pressure over the ulnar artery is released, and the capillary refill of the hand is evaluated. A wide range of values for hand reperfusion have been noted, ranging from 3 to 15 seconds. Additional techniques to qualify hand perfusion include the use of finger oximetry and Doppler assessment in conjunction with the Allen's test. If hand perfusion is predominately based from the radial artery, use of the contralateral forearm or of an ulnar fasciocutaneous free flap should be considered.

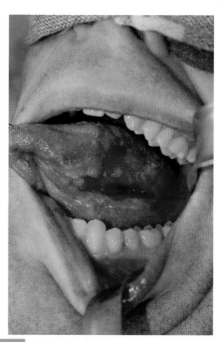

Figure 12-4 Squamous cell carcinoma of the left lateral and ventral tongue.

IMAGING

In general, if the patient has a normal result on Allen's test, no imaging is necessary prior to radial forearm free flap harvest.

The work-up of squamous cell carcinoma of the tongue includes CT scanning of the head and neck with intravenous contrast (for improved delineation of soft tissue) and a chest radiograph (see the section Squamous Cell Carcinoma in Chapter 11).

In the current patient, axial and coronal CT scans demonstrated a $3 \times 2 \times 1.5$-cm mass with poorly defined margins in the area of the tongue. No cervical lymphadenopathy was noted. The results of the chest radiograph were within normal limits.

Physical examination of the neck has variable reliability, with a sensitivity of 74%, specificity of 81%, and accuracy of 77%. As recommended by the National Comprehensive Cancer Network (NCCN) guidelines, the work-up for cancer of the oral cavity can include CT scans with contrast and/or MRI studies with contrast of the primary tumor location and the neck. CT imaging has a sensitivity of 83%, specificity of 83%, and accuracy of 83% for the detection of cervical metastasis. MRI, which has an effectiveness similar to that of CT, has been described as more sensitive in the identification of small metastatic cervical nodes. The combination of a physical examination with CT imaging increases the detection rate to 91%, whereas the detection rate for a physical examination alone is 75%.

LABS

Routine laboratory studies, such as a complete blood count (CBC), electrolyte studies, and coagulation studies, may be obtained to establish a baseline preoperatively. Liver function tests are obtained as part of the complete metabolic panel (CMP) and are important screening tests for liver metastasis. No specific laboratory tests are essential before radial forearm free flap harvest.

For the current patient, the results of all the laboratory studies mentioned were within normal limits.

ASSESSMENT

cT2N0M0, stage II (greatest clinical tumor dimension is between 2 and 4 cm, with no regional nodal metastasis and no distant metastasis on clinical or radiologic investigation) squamous cell carcinoma of the left lateral tongue.

TREATMENT

Surgery is the primary treatment modality for oral squamous cell carcinoma. Radiation therapy is an alternative with a comparable survival outcome; however, the treatment duration and likely complications of radiation-induced fibrosis and xerostomia make this option less appealing. Most patients opt for surgery, although medically compromised patients who are not suitable candidates for surgery may opt for radiation therapy.

Access to the lesion is considered first. In the current patient, the resection can be completed via a transoral approach. For larger oral squamous cell carcinomas of the oral cavity, it is not uncommon to gain access via a lip split mandibulotomy or "pull through" approach (Figure 12-5). Along with resection of the tumor, reconstruction of the defect is planned preoperatively. In general, reconstruction is based on the concept of the reconstructive ladder. The methods of reconstruction are ranked by complexity; most descriptions of the reconstructive ladder start with closure by secondary intention, primary closure, local flaps, regional pedicled flaps, and microvascular free flaps. In the current patient, the surgical defect after resection would result in a significant loss of tissue, because oncologic clearance generally incorporates 1 to 1.5 cm for the margins and, depending on frozen sections, may incorporate another 3 to 5 mm circumferentially.

With respect to tongue defects, reconstruction should consider preserving the patient's functions of speech and swallow. Resections incorporating the anterior tongue require the tongue tip for articulation and for propelling a food bolus posteriorly; the posterior tongue is largely involved with swallowing. Primary closure is an acceptable means of reconstruction if closure will not restrict tongue mobility. For the current patient, the radial forearm free flap was selected to provide bulk and to prevent restriction in tongue mobility that would affect speech and swallowing functions. Because tongue defects vary, a variety of free flaps can be used to restore form and function. When a glossectomy leaves more than 33% to 50% of the tongue, emphasis should be placed on maintaining mobility of the remaining tongue through the use of a thin, pliable flap, such as a radial or an ulnar fasciocutaneous free flap. When the defect leaves less than 33% of the original tongue, reconstruction shifts to the restoration of bulk to direct secretions toward the oropharynx and to provide contact of the neotongue with the palate for deglutition. For greater tissue bulk, the anterior lateral thigh free flap is an effective choice for reconstruction.

The radial forearm fasciocutaneous flap is the soft tissue flap of choice for reconstructing small to medium-sized oral and oropharyngeal defects. Based on the radial artery and cephalic vein and/or venae comitantes, it consists of thin, pliable skin and a very long pedicle, which make it well suited for use in the oral cavity. It can be designed to include tendons, muscle, or a segment of bone up to 12 cm in length, making it also useful for composite maxillary and mandibular defects.

The current patient was placed under general anesthesia and underwent a tracheostomy to secure his airway. A marking pen was used to delineate the planned resection edges, and a paper template was used to approximate the size and shape of the resection. A left hemiglossectomy was performed, and the margins of the resection were confirmed to be adequate with frozen sections (Figure 12-6, *A* and *B*).

A left selective neck dissection was performed to sample lymph nodes from levels I through III and to expose and preserve vessels for microvascular reconstruction

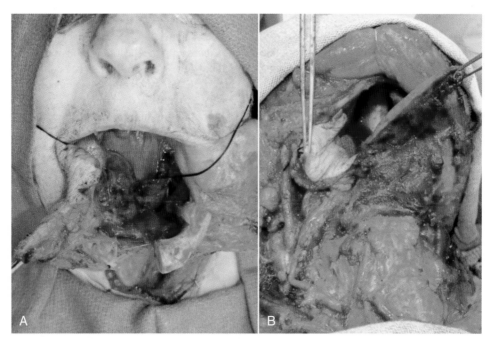

Figure 12-5 Access surgery for tongue resection. **A,** Lip split mandibulotomy approach. An osteotomy is completed through the symphysis of the mandible. A subtotal glossectomy was completed with the remaining base of the tongue identified by the attached black stitch. **B,** Pull-through approach. A subtotal glossectomy was completed by the release of the lingual attachments of the floor of the mouth and the tongue. The remaining tongue is demonstrated on the right side of the image; on the left side is the skin paddle of a radial forearm free flap that is secured to the remaining posterior right base of the tongue.

(Figure 12-6, *C*). These vessels included the internal jugular vein and the internal and external carotid arteries and their associated branches.

Simultaneous harvest of the radial forearm free flap was performed on the nondominant hand (Figure 12-6, *D*). The template was used to approximate the area of skin needed for the fasciocutaneous flap harvest. Generally, the skin of the entire volar forearm may be harvested, extending from the antecubital fossae to the flexor crease of the wrist. The skin and subcutaneous tissue are thinner in the distal forearm than in the proximal portion of the forearm. Also of note, the area of the distal forearm is thinner in males than in females.

Clinical landmarks that assist in the harvest of a radial forearm free flap include the distal extent of the flap within a flexor crease of the wrist, the antecubital fossae, and the brachioradialis, flexor carpi radialis, and palmaris longus, in addition to the outline of the planned flap. The flap is centered to overlap the region of the vascular pedicle located between the brachioradialis and flexor carpi radialis (Figure 12-6, *E*).

In the current patient, a tourniquet was placed proximal to the elbow and inflated to 250 mm Hg to facilitate dissection. An incision was made along the distal margin of the planned flap to expose and identify the vascular pedicle, cephalic vein, and superficial branch of the radial nerve. (After identification of the vascular pedicle, a confirmatory Allen's test can be performed with a bulldog clamp, the tourniquet let down and perfusion checked in the hand. A subfascial dissection is completed to the extent of the planned flap, with care taken to incorporate the vascular pedicle and to travel along the brachioradialis and flexor carpi radialis and to incorporate the

cephalic vein. At the proximal margin of the flap, the vascular pedicle is dissected free to the antebrachial fossae. Along the medial aspect of the skin flap, care is taken to avoid injury to the ulnar artery during dissection [deep between the flexor digitorum superficialis and flexor carpi ulnaris muscles.])

The radial artery was clamped and divided at its most proximal extent at the branching of the brachial artery to form the radial and ulnar arteries. (The cephalic vein is generally dissected free into the antebrachial fossae. The superficial branch of the radial nerve of the forearm runs with the radial artery beneath the distal belly of the brachioradialis. At approximately the midpoint of the brachioradialis, the nerve continues laterally and the radial artery courses medially. For this reason, it is often not included in the raised pedicle; therefore, the antebrachial cutaneous nerve is relied upon to supply the paddle.)

Once the radial forearm flap had been harvested, it was inset into the intraoral defect (Figure 12-6, *F*). Because of the vessel geometry, the pedicle was delivered medial to the left mandibular body and placed alongside the great vessels of the neck. Excess skin was removed to achieve the desired bulk, and the flap was secured to the resection wound edge prior to the microvascular vessel anastomosis. The term "ischemia time of the flap" refers to the time from harvesting of the flap to the moment the artery is reestablished. Free flap reconstructions require a period of tolerance to tissue ischemia. Studies have demonstrated that this period of tolerance varies with the tissue type. Most flaps incorporate skin, fascia, muscle, and bone tissue. Skin and fascia are the most resistant to ischemia; they have a tolerance period of 4 to 6 hours before

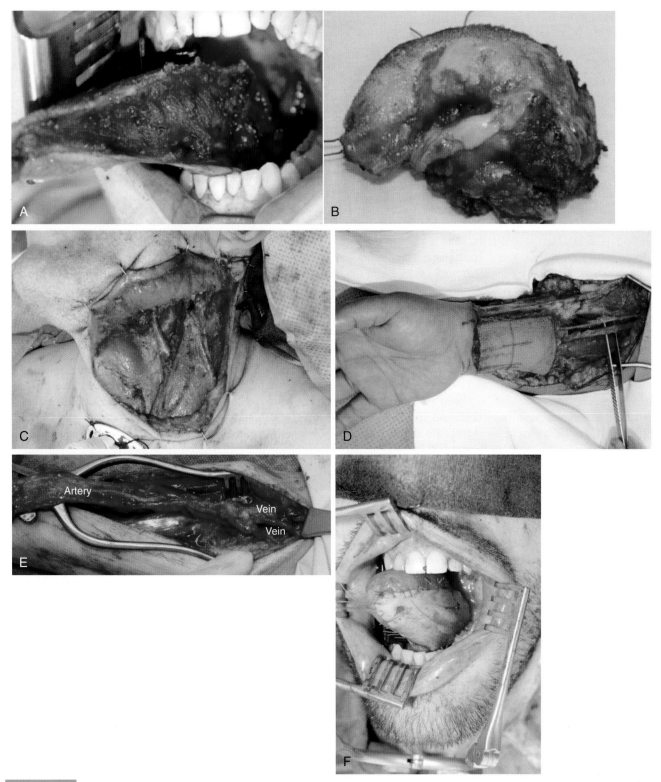

Figure 12-6 **A,** Left tongue defect after left hemiglossectomy. **B,** Left hemiglossectomy specimen. **C,** After completion of the supraomohyoid neck dissection. The sternocleidomastoid muscle, internal jugular vein, common facial vein, and external jugular vein are clearly exposed for the microvascular reconstructive phase. **D,** An 8 × 6-cm skin flap is raised on the distal volar surface of the forearm. Note the radial artery and the cephalic vein travelling toward the antecubital fossae. **E,** Radial forearm free flap vascular pedicle; also, artery and veins associated with the harvest of a radial forearm free flap with exposure to the antecubital fossae. **F,** Inset radial forearm fasciocutaneous free flap.

irreversible cellular injury occurs that could jeopardize the viability of the free flap. Muscle is generally the most sensitive to ischemia time; it has a tolerance period of less than 3 hours.

In the current patient, after flap harvest, the tourniquet was released, hemostasis was confirmed, and a split-thickness skin graft was harvested from the left thigh and grafted to the radial forearm free flap donor site. The arterial anastomosis was performed in an end-to-end fashion into the facial artery with 9-0 nylon sutures in an interrupted fashion, and the venous anastomosis was performed in an end-to-side fashion into the internal jugular vein. (During the microvascular anastomosis, heparinized saline [100 μ/ml] is used to mute the process of thrombosis in the lumen of the vessels. Inherent to the anatomy of blood vessels, arteries generally have a thicker media, whereas veins have thinner vessel walls; hence, anastomosis for the artery is commonly completed with sutures, and the veins are coupled together, because their thin walls make them amenable to coupling.) Adequate perfusion of the flap was confirmed clinically by assessment of color, texture, capillary refill, and temperature. (Doppler probes are also regularly used to assess blood flow through the free flap.)

Closure of the donor site was completed in a layered fashion, with dermal sutures followed by staples for the skin. The skin paddle donor site can be closed primarily if it is small, and techniques have been described for using local flaps (Z-plasty) to facilitate closure. Most defects are repaired with either a split-thickness or full-thickness skin graft. Unlike microvascular flaps, these grafts are dependent on nutrition from the recipient bed via plasmatic circulation or imbibition for 48 to 72 hours, until capillary in-growth occurs. During the initial wound healing phase, it is necessary to bolster the graft on the recipient bed to provide stability for the healing process. The split-thickness skin graft incorporates the layers of the epidermis and a portion of the dermis. Its advantages include the ability to cover large areas with a higher rate of successful graft take. On the other hand, split-thickness skin grafts are less esthetic, are susceptible to more contracture, and require an additional donor site. Full-thickness skin grafts incorporate layers of the epidermis and dermis and provide a more esthetic result with less late wound contracture. The donor site for the full-thickness skin graft can also be closed primarily, and the graft can be harvested from inconspicuous areas of the body, such as the supraclavicular area or, more commonly, the medial aspect of the upper arm.

In the current patient, the harvested split-thickness skin graft was bolstered with a wound vacuum-assisted closure system, and the wrist was immobilized for 5 to 7 days with a volar splint to prevent shearing of the skin graft. The flap remained viable at the recipient site and healed without complications.

COMPLICATIONS

The surgical complication rate among patients undergoing microvascular reconstruction after head and neck surgery is 19% to 22%. The majority of these surgical complications are related to the reconstructive effort and manifest as flap loss, partial loss, and wound healing complications at either the donor or recipient site. Preoperative risk factors that have been described to contribute to the incidence of surgical complications include American Society of Anesthesiologists (ASA) status of III or IV, low preoperative hemoglobin, prolonged operative time (longer than 10 hours), and prior radiation and/or surgery. Factors specific for free flap failure have been associated with the surgeon's experience, flap selection, and the patient's nutritional status. Free flap failure rates have improved significantly since this technique moved into mainstream use. Initial free flap survival rates, during the first decade of popularity in the 1980s, ranged from 85% to 89%; recent studies show that they have improved to more than 95%. A review of 248 consecutive microvascular free flap reconstructions at Legacy Emanuel Hospital in Portland, Oregon, found a 95.5% success rate. The radial forearm fasciocutaneous free flap was used in 52% of cases, reflecting its popularity for reconstruction of defects in the oral cavity. Specifically, the radial forearm free flap demonstrated excellent success, with flap survival rates of 96% to 100% in multiple studies.

The main disadvantage of the radial forearm fasciocutaneous free flap is the morbidity associated with the donor site. Inherent to the harvest of the graft is the manipulation of the superficial branch of the radial nerve, because this nerve is closely associated with the cephalic vein. The superficial branch of the radial nerve provides sensory input for the dorsal surface of the thumb and the second and third digits. Abnormal sensation (hypoesthesia, hypesthesia, or paresthesia) in the donor hand occurred in 82% of patients at 3 months after surgery; however, this improved to 26% during a mean follow-up period of 14 months.

Wound healing accounts for most of the complications associated with the donor site. Subfascial radial forearm fasciocutaneous free flap harvests demonstrated a higher incidence of skin graft loss, ranging from 16% to 28%; in this same subgroup, tendon exposure and delayed healing accounted for 13% to 28% and 22% to 28%, respectively. An alternative to harvesting of the radial forearm free flap involves suprafascial dissection, which tends to leave the exposed tendons of the forearm with investing fascia and some deep subcutaneous tissue to allow for a better foundation for the split-thickness or full-thickness graft. Skin graft losses in suprafascial donor sites are reported to be 4% to 6%. The incidence of skin graft loss has been associated with the likelihood of decreased grip strength. It is reported that subjective grip strength was significantly decreased in 5% to 10% of patients who demonstrated partial skin graft failure.

Use of the radial forearm flap as an osteocutaneous flap can be associated with the risk of radial fracture. A segment of vascularized bone can be harvested, and the length is limited by the attachments of the pronator teres muscle proximally and the brachioradialis muscle distally. On average, 10 to 12 cm in length and less than half of the radius can be harvested. Prophylactic plating of the radius is recommended to decrease the likelihood of radius fracture. Prior studies in which the radius was not plated after harvesting reported a fracture incidence of 15% to 67% in donor arms.

DISCUSSION

Since the original description of the radial forearm fasciocutaneous free flap, more than 30 years ago, this technique has evolved into a versatile and reliable flap for head and neck reconstruction. First described by Taylor in 1976 and publicized in oral cavity reconstruction by Soutar and colleagues in 1983, this flap continues to be a popular soft tissue flap despite the challenges with donor site morbidity. Alternative flaps, such as the cutaneous lateral arm flap, fasciocutaneous ulnar flap, and anterior lateral thigh perforator flap, have limited advantages, which focus on less donor site morbidity.

There are many applications for the radial forearm free flap in head and neck reconstruction. As demonstrated in this case presentation, tongue reconstruction with the radial forearm free flap is a common indication. Use of this type of flap has been described for reconstructing the ablative defects of the soft palate and mandible, restoring soft tissue deficiencies, and repairing tracheoesophageal fistulas. Dual skin flaps have been used to reconstruct through-and-through defects in the cheek and lip, and with two-stage procedures, prefabricated grafts can be prepared for reconstruction of complex structures such as the nose (Figure 12-7).

The surgical anatomy of the radial forearm flap is consistent and readily assessed. As previously mentioned, the viability of a donor site is based on the results of Allen's test. The blood supply is based on the radial artery, which is reliably found between the brachioradialis and flexor carpi radialis.

On average, the length of the radial artery, from the antecubital fossa to the wrist, is 18 to 20 cm, and the vessel has a diameter of 2 to 2.5 mm. It is relatively superficial, and dissection is completed within a subfascial plane guided by the brachioradialis and flexor carpi radialis. The radial artery is intimately associated with the overlying fascia and supplies perforating vessels that pass through to form subfascial, intrafascial, and suprafascial vascular plexuses. These networks establish the extensive subcutaneous vascular plexuses that supply the skin. The fascia provides a degree of additional protection to the pedicle and overall integrity of the flap.

Multiple variations of this flap can be developed from the incorporation of accessible anatomic resources. Additional bulk can be obtained from the brachioradialis, tendon and ligaments can be obtained from the palmaris longus when necessary, and innervation through the antebrachial cutaneous nerve and bone can be obtained through harvest of the radius.

Venous return for the free forearm flap is classified as a deep and superficial venous supply. The deep supply is composed of the venae comitantes, which run in the intermuscular septum along with the radial artery. The superficial venous supply consists chiefly of the cephalic vein. Both systems provide venous outflow for the tissue supplied by the radial artery. The harvest of both venous systems allows for anastomosis of two veins. A study of 492 head and neck free flap procedures performed at the University of Toronto compared two-vein anastomosis with single-vein anastomosis and demonstrated an improved success rate for the former (98.6% versus 93.6%). This finding was also illustrated in an evaluation of microvascular couplers in head and neck reconstruction; in this study, dual vein–coupled anastomosis showed a trend for improved success over single

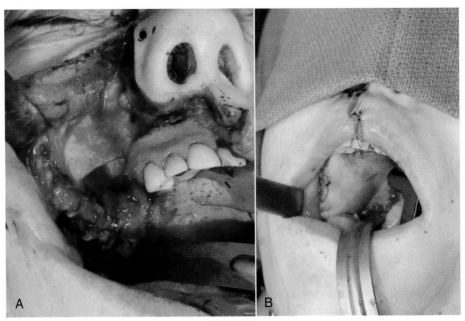

Figure 12-7   Example of maxillectomy defect reconstruction with radial forearm free flap. **A,** Access for ablation via the Weber-Ferguson approach. **B,** Obturation with radial forearm free flap.

vein–coupled anastomosis. When only a single vein is used for reconstruction, there are no differences in using the superficial over the deep venous system as the sole outflow for the flap.

In a vessel-depleted neck, a radial forearm hybrid flap can be used to compensate for the lack of vascular options. This scenario is most common in previously operated and irradiated fields. The radial forearm hybrid flap uses a single arterial anastomosis that is carried out between the radial artery of the flap and a recipient artery and the venous drainage (the cephalic vein), to remain in continuity with the systemic venous system. Technically, the cephalic vein is dissected up to the deltopectoral groove, pedicled over the clavicle, and delivered into the neck in the subcutaneous plane.

The radius is situated lateral to the ulna and articulates with the humerus and ulna proximally and with the ulna, scaphoid, and lunate bones distally. It averages 23 cm in length and in cross section the radial shaft appears triangular. Functionally the radius plays a minor role in the stability of the elbow; however, at the radiocarpal joint, it is an integral structure of the wrist. The proximal head of the radius allows the hand to pronate, and the distal head plays a role in hand flexion, extension, adduction, and abduction.

The brachioradialis functions to flex the arm at the elbow and for pronation and supination of the forearm. Its origin is at the lateral supracondylar ridge of the humerus, and it attaches to the distal styloid process of the radius by way of the brachioradialis tendon. It is located in the posterior compartment of the forearm and is innervated by the radial nerve. In reconstruction, the brachioradialis can be used to provide bulk, such as in a total glossectomy defect.

The skin available to be harvested on the forearm is defined by the radial artery angiosome. It extends from the flexor crease of the wrist to the antecubital fossa and from the medial third of the ventral surface of the forearm to the lateral third of the dorsal surface of the forearm. If an innervated flap is considered, the somatosome of the lateral antebrachial cutaneous nerve is used to guide the location of skin flap harvesting. The somatosome of the lateral antebrachial cutaneous nerve extends from the midline of the ventral forearm to the lateral third of the dorsal surface of the forearm.

Innervated tongue flaps are accomplished by neurorrhaphy of the lateral antebrachial cutaneous nerve to a recipient nerve. Sensation recovery of the innervated radial forearm flap was noted to be predictable in patients who did not receive postoperative radiotherapy and when neurorrhaphy was completed to the lingual or inferior alveolar nerve. Comparisons between reconstructed hemiglossectomy defects with innervated radial forearm free flaps and the nonoperated side revealed that the tongue tip, dorsum, ventral surface, and floor of mouth had comparable two-point discrimination at 18 months after surgery. Also, light touch sensation was similar at the tip and dorsum of the tongue; however, pain and light touch along the floor of the mouth were significantly decreased. Despite the sensation that is gained from reinnervation, these flaps do not offer a major functional advantage over noninnervated flaps.

In terms of function, when a glossectomy leaves more than 33% to 50 % of the original musculature, the emphasis for reconstruction is on the maintenance of mobility. A thin, pliable soft tissue flap, the radial forearm free flap is an ideal choice, because it can replace missing tissue without significantly restricting the mobility of the tongue. Studies that compared free flap reconstructions to prior methods for tongue reconstruction (e.g., the pectoralis major pedicled flap) showed that patients with free flaps had more intelligible speech. Furthermore, in a limited resection in which primary closure was performed, patients had equal or better function in terms of speech and swallowing functions. The reconstruction for a glossectomy defect that leaves less than 33% of the tongue base focuses on the replacement of bulk to direct secretions toward the oropharynx and to provide contact of the neotongue with the palate to facilitate swallowing.

Since its introduction three decades ago, the radial forearm fasciocutaneous free flap has become a staple of head and neck reconstruction. Variations on the originally described procedure have allowed it to become a solution for all aspects of microvascular reconstruction. Although donor site complications persist, it is difficult to discount the technique's proven success through its reliable and versatile characteristics, and it will undoubtedly continue as a "workhorse" of soft tissue reconstruction in head and neck surgery.

Bibliography

Asif M, Sarkar PK: Three-digit Allen's test, *Ann Thorac Surg* 84(2):686-687, 2007.

Avery C: Prospective study of the septocutaneous radial free flap and suprafascial donor site, *Br J Oral Maxillofac Surg* 45(8):611-616, 2007.

Avery CM, Pereira J, Brown AE: Suprafascial dissection of the radial forearm flap and donor site morbidity, *Int J Oral Maxillofac Surg* 30(1):37-41, 2001.

Bardsley AF, Soutar DS, Elliot D, et al: Reducing morbidity in the radial forearm flap donor site, *Plast Reconstr Surg* 86(2):287-292; discussion, 293-294; 1990.

Chen CM, Lin GT, Fu YC, et al: Complications of free radial forearm flap transfers for head and neck reconstruction, *Oral Surg Oral Med Oral Pathol Oral Radiol Endod* 99(6):671-676, 2005.

Engel H, Huang JJ, Lin CY, et al: A strategic approach for tongue reconstruction to achieve predictable and improved functional and aesthetic outcomes, *Plast Reconstr Surg* 126(6):1967-1977, 2010.

Janis JE, Kwon RK, Attinger CE: The new reconstructive ladder: modifications to the traditional model, *Plast Reconstr Surg* 127(Suppl 1):205S-212S, 2011.

Liu Y, Jiang X, Huang J, et al: Reliability of the superficial venous drainage of the radial forearm free flaps in oral and maxillofacial reconstruction, *Microsurgery* 28(4):243-247, 2008.

Lutz BS, Wei FC, Chang SC, et al: Donor site morbidity after suprafascial elevation of the radial forearm flap: a prospective study in 95 consecutive cases, *Plast Reconstr Surg* 103(1):132-137, 1999.

McConnel FM, Pauloski BR, Logemann JA, et al: Functional results of primary closure vs flaps in oropharyngeal reconstruction: a prospective study of speech and swallowing, *Arch Otolaryngol Head Neck Surg* 1998;124(6):625-630, 1998.

McGregor IA, MacDonald DG: Mandibular osteotomy in the surgical approach to the oral cavity, *Head Neck Surg* 5(5):457-462, 1983.

Merritt RM, Williams MF, James TH, et al: Detection of cervical metastasis: a meta-analysis comparing computed tomography with physical examination, *Arch Otolaryngol Head Neck Surg* 123(2):149-152, 1997.

Netscher D, Armenta AH, Meade RA, et al: Sensory recovery of innervated and non-innervated radial forearm free flaps: functional implications, *J Reconstr Microsurg* 16(3):179-185, 2000.

Quilichini J, Benjoar MD, Hivelin M, et al: Semi-free radial forearm flap for head and neck reconstruction in vessel-depleted neck after radiotherapy or radical neck dissection, *Microsurgery* 32(4):269-274, 2012.

Richardson D, Fisher SE, Vaughan ED, et al: Radial forearm flap donor-site complications and morbidity: a prospective study, *Plast Reconstr Surg* 99(1):109-115, 1997.

Ross GL, Ang ES, Golger A, et al: Which venous system to choose for anastomosis in head and neck reconstructions? *Ann Plast Surg* 61(4):396-398, 2008.

Ross GL, Ang ES, Lannon D, et al: Ten-year experience of free flaps in head and neck surgery: how necessary is a second venous anastomosis? *Head Neck* 30(8):1086-1089, 2008.

Santamaria E, Wei FC, Chen IH, et al: Sensation recovery on innervated radial forearm flap for hemiglossectomy reconstruction by using different recipient nerves, *Plast Reconstr Surg* 103(2):450-457, 1999.

Scheunemann H: Pull-through surgery in mouth floor: tongue neoplasms, *Acta Stomatol Belg* 72(2):229-230, 1975.

Shnayder Y, Tsue TT, Toby EB, et al: Safe osteocutaneous radial forearm flap harvest with prophylactic internal fixation, *Craniomaxillofac Trauma Reconstr* 4(3):129-136, 2011.

Soutar DS, Scheker LR, Tanner NS, et al: The radial forearm flap: a versatile method for intra-oral reconstruction, *Br J Plast Surg* 36(1):1-8, 1983.

Su WF, Hsia YJ, Chang YC, et al: Functional comparison after reconstruction with a radial forearm free flap or a pectoralis major flap for cancer of the tongue, *Otolaryngol Head Neck Surg* 128(3):412-418, 2003.

Sumi M, Kimura Y, Sumi T, et al: Diagnostic performance of MRI relative to CT for metastatic nodes of head and neck squamous cell carcinomas, *J Magn Reson Imaging* 26(6):1626-1633, 2007.

Timmons MJ: Landmarks in the anatomical study of the blood supply of the skin, *Br J Plast Surg* 38(2):197-207, 1985.

Timmons MJ: The vascular basis of the radial forearm flap, *Plast Reconstr Surg* 77(1):80-92, 1986.

To EW, Wang JC: Radial forearm free flap: hybrid version, *Plast Reconstr Surg* 104(4):1066-1069, 1999.

Villaret DB, Futran NA: The indications and outcomes in the use of osteocutaneous radial forearm free flap, *Head Neck* 25(6):475-481, 2003.

Zhang T, Lubek J, Salama A, et al: Venous anastomoses using microvascular coupler in free flap head and neck reconstruction, *J Oral Maxillofac Surg* 70(4):992-996, 2012.

Pectoralis Major Myocutaneous Flap

Allen Cheng, R. Bryan Bell, Saif Al Bustani, and Tuan G. Bui

CC

A 39-year-old man is referred to your office for evaluation of a large right parapharyngeal mass.

HPI

The patient reported having increasing pain in his throat. The pain began to extend to include his right posterior mandibular teeth. This prompted him to see his dentist, who noticed swelling in the right lateral oropharynx. A biopsy of this area demonstrated invasive squamous cell carcinoma (SCCa) of the right oropharynx, and the cancer was staged as cT3N1M0, stage III.

The patient underwent primary treatment with concurrent chemotherapy and radiation therapy (7,000 cGy of intensity-modulated radiation therapy [IMRT] with concurrent carboplatin and paclitaxel). Although he initially had a complete response and regression of the tumor, within 3 months of completion of treatment he began to complain of a return of his severe right throat pain. The clinical exam and imaging findings were consistent with local recurrence.

Head and neck SCCa is a heterogeneous disease that can behave differently, depending on the site involved. Therefore, the treatment of SCCa varies by site. Unlike oral cavity SCCa, which is treated primarily by surgery, with radiation and chemotherapy taking adjuvant roles, oropharyngeal SCCa often involves multimodality therapy. First-line treatment can be either surgical resection followed by radiation and/or chemotherapy or primary radiation therapy (with concurrent chemotherapy if indicated) followed by salvage surgery if necessary. Currently, surgery has mostly taken a secondary salvage role, because surgical ablation of oropharyngeal SCCa is morbid, often requiring a mandibulotomy to achieve sufficient access for an adequate oncologic resection.

Two recent developments have changed the way we understand oropharyngeal SCCa. First is the discovery of the role of high-risk human papillomavirus (HPV) infection in oropharyngeal SCCa. The clinical presentation of HPV-positive oropharyngeal SCCa is distinct. These tumors tend to present in a comparatively younger population with no typical risk factors (smoking, alcohol), with smaller primary tumors, and with more extensive nodal metastasis. However, despite more extensive regional metastasis, HPV-positive oropharyngeal SCCa has been found to have much better locoregional control and survival rates compared to HPV-negative tumors. The second development is the emerging role of transoral robotic surgery for the treatment of select early T-stage oropharyngeal SCCa. This technique allows for adequate surgical resection without an access mandibulotomy in select cases. The hope is that these tumors may then be treated primarily with a well-tolerated surgery, possibly obviating the need for radiation or allowing a reduction in the dose. Clinical trials are in progress to identify benefits from the use of this protocol.

PMHX/PDHX/MEDICATIONS/ALLERGIES/SH/FH

The patient has a 15 pack-year history of tobacco use and admits to drinking two to four cans of beer a day (both tobacco and alcohol are risk factors for intraoral squamous cell carcinoma).

There are no absolute contraindications to the pectoralis major myocutaneous flap. However, the flap is more likely to fail in a patient with severe systemic vascular disease, diabetes, or obesity. Additionally, some authors have described problems with skin paddle survival in females.

EXAMINATION

General. The patient is a well-appearing man in no acute distress.

Neck. No lymphadenopathy is appreciated. The skin shows evidence of postradiation changes.

Oropharynx. There is a large, exophytic mass that involves the right palatine tonsillar fossa and extends into and past the glossotonsillar sulcus into the floor of the mouth and base of the tongue (Figure 12-8). The mass is firm, indurated, and friable. It bleeds with manipulation. A fiberoptic exam demonstrates extension of the mass to include the lateral oropharynx and base of the tongue but not involving the hypopharynx or larynx.

Chest. The patient's lungs are clear on auscultation. His pectoralis major muscles are symmetric and of normal morphology and size.

The physical examination of patients with head and neck pathology should include an examination of the oropharynx, hypopharynx, and larynx. This can be performed in a number of ways. We typically perform a fiberoptic nasopharyngolaryngoscopy in the office setting. In patients who are difficult to examine or who have metastatic disease of an unknown primary, this is followed by direct laryngoscopy and biopsies in the operating room under general anesthesia.

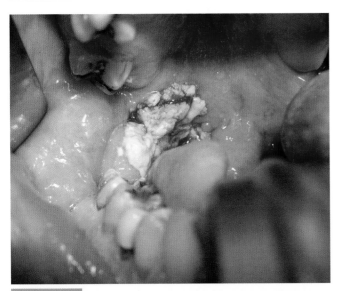

Figure 12-8 Intraoral photograph of right oropharyngeal lesion. This is an endophytic, verrucous lesion extending from the right retromolar trigone to involve the right palatine tonsillar fossa, the glossotonsillar sulcus, and the base of the tongue.

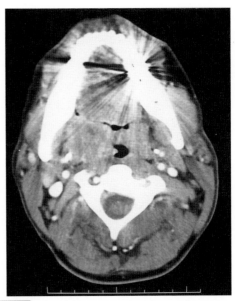

Figure 12-9 Computed tomography scan shows fluorodeoxyglucose (FDG)-avid lesion that corresponds to a large right oropharyngeal mass.

If a pectoralis flap is being considered as a reconstructive option, the chest should be examined to ensure that the muscle is adequately developed. Very rarely, the pectoralis major muscle can be completely absent in patients with Poland's syndrome.

IMAGING

A positron emission tomography/computed tomography (PET/CT) scan demonstrated a fluorodeoxyglucose (FDG)-avid focus, corresponding to soft tissue thickening in the area of the right tonsillar fossa. No FDG avidity or lymphadenopathy was identified in the neck.

There are many imaging modalities available and useful for evaluating patients with head and neck SCCa. PET/CT has the advantage of combining the ability to identify areas of high metabolic activity by PET with the anatomic detail of CT (Figure 12-9). This is often useful for patients with metastatic disease from an unknown primary, with indeterminate findings on CT or MRI, for patients at high risk for or suspected of having distant metastases, and for surveillance of patients after treatment. Patients, particularly smokers, should also have chest imaging, either by a plain chest film or chest CT, to screen for distant metastases or a second primary tumor.

LABS

Laboratory testing is dictated as much by the patient's past medical history and comorbidities as by the cancer itself. At a minimum, such tests include a complete blood count, metabolic panel, and coagulation panel. Many oncologic surgeons include liver function testing as a screen for distant metastases to the liver.

Direct Laryngoscopy and Biopsy

In the current patient, direct laryngoscopy under general anesthesia was performed. The exophytic, ulcerated lesion was seen to involve the right lateral oropharynx and the base of the tongue. The hypopharynx and larynx were not involved. Biopsy confirmed recurrent SCCa.

ASSESSMENT

Aggressive local recurrence of stage III cT3N1M0 oropharyngeal squamous cell carcinoma.

TREATMENT

Because concurrent chemoradiation therapy had failed, treatment planning focused on salvage surgery in the form of a right lateral pharyngectomy via a mandibulotomy approach and a right modified radical neck dissection (Figure 12-10), followed by reconstruction with a pectoralis major myocutaneous flap (Figure 12-11).

Unfortunately, the patient developed a local recurrence involving the supraglottic larynx. He was then treated with a second salvage surgery in the form of a total laryngectomy and reconstruction of the neopharynx with a second pectoralis major myocutaneous flap (Figure 12-12).

This type of ablative surgery leaves a sizeable soft tissue defect. Options to reconstruct soft tissue include microvascular free tissue transfer or regional flaps. Free tissue transfer is a critical component of the head and neck reconstructive surgeon's armamentarium; it is versatile and capable of filling large defects. Several free flaps are highly useful for soft tissue head and neck reconstruction, including the radial forearm free flap, the anterior lateral thigh flap, and the lateral arm flap. These are discussed elsewhere.

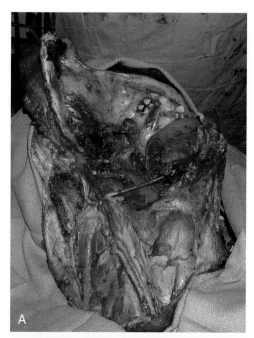

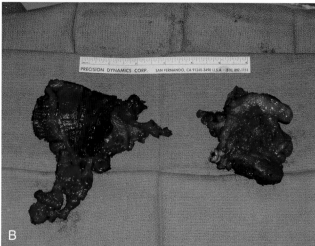

Figure 12-10 **A,** Large right oropharyngeal defect after wide resection and right radical neck dissection via a midline mandibulotomy approach. **B,** Specimens. *Left,* Right radical neck dissection. *Right,* Right oropharyngeal wide resection with marginal mandibulectomy.

Several regional flaps also can be used for reconstruction of oropharyngeal defects. These include the deltopectoral fascial flap, the pectoralis major flap, and the latissimus dorsi flap. Bakamjian initially described the deltopectoral fascial flap for head and neck construction, but it has several shortcomings, including lack of tissue bulk, unreliable distal perfusion when reconstruction is performed primarily, and the need for skin grafting at the donor site. As such, after Ariyan first described the use of the pectoralis major myocutaneous flap for head and neck reconstruction, it very quickly supplanted the deltopectoral fascial flap as the regional flap of choice.

Surgical Technique

In the current patient, we used a parasternal skin paddle. The procedure is performed as follows: Mark out a curvilinear incision from the clavicle, curving inferiorly into a parasternal limb, and then posteriorly into a horizontal inframammary limb. Draw out the planned skin paddle. Use a no. 10 blade to make the incision down to the pectoralis fascia, starting from the lateral edge of the skin paddle. Develop a skin flap laterally in this suprafascial plane, exposing the entire pectoralis major muscle. Complete the circumferential incision around the skin paddle. Suture the skin paddle down to the underlying muscle to prevent shearing between the skin and muscle and damage to the skin perforators. These sutures are removed prior to inset. Use blunt and sharp dissection to separate the sternocostal attachments. Ligate or cauterize the internal mammary artery perforators. Once the chest wall attachments have been divided, the dissection above the pectoralis minor can be done bluntly. As the flap is elevated, identify the pectoral branch of the thoracoacromial artery entering the deep aspect of the muscle. Identify and divide the attachment to the humerus. The clavicular head may also be divided, if necessary, to decrease bulkiness in the clavicular region. Similarly, the medial and lateral pectoral nerves can be divided to increase reach. Create a tunnel from the chest wall dissection into the neck dissection. This is done in a subplatysmal plane. The tunnel should be large enough to accommodate four fingers passing through comfortably. This is critical to prevent compression of the flap pedicle. The flap is then passed through into the neck for inset. Closed suction drains are placed under the skin flaps of the chest wall, and primary closure is performed.

Postoperative Care

The postoperative care of a patient with a flap focuses on eliminating factors that can lead to vascular thrombosis and then flap failure. It is critical to avoid compression of the pedicle underlying the neck skin flaps. It is helpful to mark the location of the pedicle so that the nursing staff knows to avoid pressure in these areas from dressings or tape; this includes tracheostomy ties if the patient has a surgical airway. The patient's neck movements should be restricted; excessive flexion or rotation of the neck should be avoided. Vasopressors should be avoided, if possible. Hypothermia should be avoided, because it may lead to vasoconstriction. Later in the postoperative period, surgical site infections are treated aggressively, because infections around the pedicle can lead to arterial thrombosis and flap failure. Physical therapy and occupational therapy are started as early as postoperative day 2.

COMPLICATIONS

Complications from the use of the pectoralis major flap, as reported in the literature, are shown in Box 12-1.

Total or partial flap necrosis occurs in a minority of cases. Higher rates in initial reports have been attributed to failure

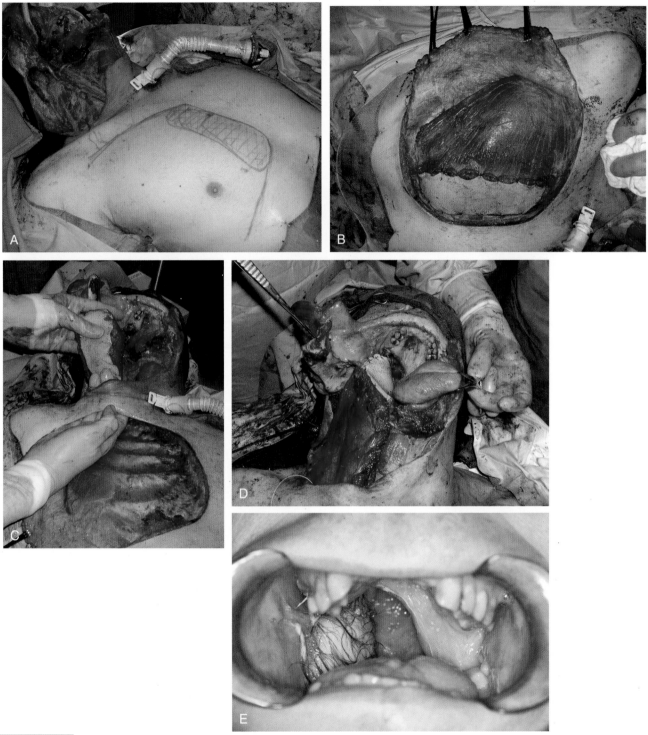

A, Right pectoralis major myocutaneous flap crescent incision marked out for a parasternal skin paddle. The location of the pedicle has been identified with a Doppler at the junction of the middle and lateral thirds of the clavicle. If a deltopectoral fascial flap is also to be used, the skin paddle is placed further inferiorly, and the superior horizontal limb is placed inferiorly to maintain the pedicle to the second flap. This superior incision would correspond with the inferior border of the deltopectoral fascial flap. **B,** Skin flap developed laterally in a plane superficial to the pectoralis fascia. The lateral extent of this dissection is taken to where the pectoralis major muscle narrows to its humeral attachment. The attachment is divided lateral to the pedicle, which is visualized on the underside of the flap. A gastrointestinal anastomosis (GIA) stapler can be used to divide the muscle. This provides good hemostasis and leaves a staple line that can be used for tacking sutures. The skin paddle is tacked down to the muscle prior to elevation of the flap to avoid shear injury to skin perforators. **C,** The flap is elevated off the chest wall and underlying pectoralis minor in a plane superficial to the clavicopectoralis fascia. The lateral aspect of this is done bluntly with finger dissection. Electrocautery is used to divide the sternal attachments of the pectoralis major muscle. The internal mammary artery perforators are identified and ligated to avoid vessel retraction and annoying bleeding. A subcutaneous tunnel is developed under the bridge of skin with blunt and/or sharp dissection. Enough room needs to be created to allow four fingers to pass easily; this prevents compression of the pedicle as it passes over the clavicle. Alternatively, the pedicle can be external and tubed (requiring a second-stage surgery to take down), a portion of clavicle can be removed, or the tunnel can be made subclavicular. **D,** The skin paddle is sewn into the oropharyngeal defect. The muscle provides excellent coverage to the exposed carotid, which is particularly important in patients who have or are to receive radiation therapy. **E,** Well-healed skin paddle. As is commonly seen, there is hair growth from the skin paddle.

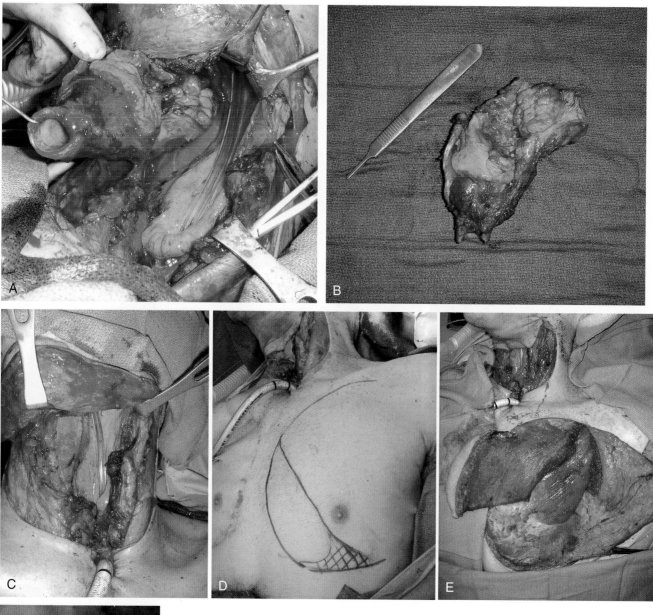

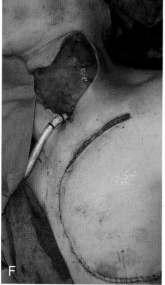

Figure 12-12   Total laryngectomy for local recurrence. **A,** The larynx is retracted laterally toward the patient's right after skeletonization of the left side of the larynx, division of the trachea, and resection along the left piriform recess. This gives a view looking at the posterior aspect of the supraglottic larynx. A large, endophytic, invasive mass involving the right oropharynx, hypopharynx, piriform recess, and supraglottic larynx can be seen. **B,** Total laryngectomy specimen viewed from posterior. The large right oropharyngeal mass can be seen extending to and involving the right aryepiglottic fold, arytenoid, piriform recess, and supraglottic larynx. **C,** Pharyngeal defect. A second pectoralis myocutaneous flap is used to reconstruct the pharynx to both increase the size of the lumen to prevent stricture and to decrease the risk of pharyngocutaneous fistulization. **D,** Left pectoralis major myocutaneous flap incision is marked out. In this case, a slight inframammary extension is included. Note the deformity on the right chest wall. **E,** The left pectoralis major myocutaneous flap is raised in the same fashion. **F,** The skin paddle is placed intraluminally to reconstruct the neopharynx. The muscle provides coverage over the reconstruction to prevent fistulization. The neck skin flaps are sutured to the muscle and not closed primarily to avoid compression. A split-thickness skin graft is placed over the exposed muscle.

Box 12-1	**Possible Complications with Use of a Pectoralis Major Flap**

- Total flap necrosis (1% to 7%)
- Partial flap necrosis (4% to 14%)
- Donor site hematomas or seromas
- Donor site wound dehiscence or skin necrosis
- Pulmonary complications
- Surgical site infection
- Osteochondronecrosis of the ribs
- Wound dehiscence and plate exposure
- Masking of recurrent malignancy
- Distortion of breast tissue
- Orocutaneous fistulas
- Hair growth
- Muscle atrophy

to include fasciocutaneous perforators, failure to include the rectus sheath when extending the flap caudally, and compression by the clavicle. Hematomas and seromas are rare. Donor site wound dehiscence can occur with closure of the wound under tension when larger skin paddles are used. Hair growth is an anticipated consequence of this flap in men. It is somewhat mitigated with radiation. The skin paddle can also be treated with electrolysis if the hair is annoying to the patient. As do all muscle flaps that have been denervated, the pectoralis major atrophies with time. This can be either problematic or beneficial, depending on the application, but should be expected. This atrophy is partially mitigated if the pectoral nerves are not divided.

DISCUSSION

The pectoralis major myocutaneous flap has been used in head and neck reconstruction since its initial description by Ariyan in 1979. Its reliability and versatility made it the workhorse flap of the 1980s until the widespread rise of microvascular surgeons and techniques relegated the pectoralis major flap to that of a salvage flap for failed microvascular reconstructions.

The pectoralis major is a broad, fan-shaped muscle that originates from the medial clavicle, sternum, and costal cartilages of the first through six ribs and the external oblique muscular aponeurosis. It inserts into the crest of the greater tubercle of the humerus. The pectoralis major muscle serves as an adductor, medial rotator, and extender of the arm.

The muscle is invested in the pectoralis fascia, which is distinct from the clavipectoral fascia that lies deep to it. The clavipectoral fascia is comprised of the pectoralis minor fascia, the subclavius fascia, the costocoracoid ligament, the costocoracoid membrane, and the suspensory ligament of the axilla. This is important, because the reconstructive surgeon uses the avascular plane between the clavipectoral fascia and pectoralis major fascia to raise the pectoralis major flap. The inferior free border of the pectoralis major forms the anterior axillary fold as it narrows to its insertion into the humerus.

The superior and lateral boundary is with the deltoid muscle. The plane between to the deltoid and pectoralis major forms the deltopectoral groove and is marked by the cephalic vein, which runs within it.

The vascular supply to the pectoralis major is based off branches of the axillary artery. The thoracoacromial artery is a branch off the middle portion of the axillary artery, deep to the pectoralis minor. This artery has four main branches: the pectoral, clavicular, acromial, and deltoid. The pectoral branch runs along and around the medial aspect of the pectoralis minor, pierces the clavipectoral fascia, along with the medial and lateral pectoral nerves, and runs inferiorly and obliquely along the deep aspect of the pectoralis major. It is the dominant pedicle of the pectoralis major muscle. However, the clavicular head has contributions from the deltoid branch; the medial portion of the pectoralis major is supplied by the internal mammary artery perforators, which are branches from the superior thoracic artery; and there can be important contributions by the lateral thoracic artery. The superior thoracic artery branches from the first portion of the axillary artery over the first intercostal space. The lateral thoracic artery branches from the middle portion of the axillary artery at the lateral edge of the pectoralis minor muscle.

The skin overlying the pectoralis major receives most of its blood supply from fasciocutaneous perforators that run along the lateral and inferior borders of the pectoralis major. To a lesser degree, the skin is also supplied by myocutaneous perforators.

Venous drainage is by the vena comitantes of the supplying arteries. Innervation is by the lateral and medial pectoral nerves off the brachial plexus.

The lateral pectoral nerve innervates the clavicular head, and the medial pectoral nerve innervates the sternocostal heads. The use of innervated pectoralis major flaps to improve swallowing in pharyngeal or esophageal reconstruction has not been shown to provide a measurable functional benefit.

Indications

- Soft tissue defects of the oral cavity, oropharynx, hypopharynx and skin of the head and neck
- Hypopharyngeal or pharyngoesophageal reconstruction
- Coverage of the carotid artery, especially after radical neck dissection with prior or anticipated radiotherapy
- Skull base coverage
- Alternative to free flaps in instances of free flap failure, lack of availability of free flap reconstruction, or patient inability to tolerate microvascular surgery

Although there are no specific contraindications to use of the pectoralis major myocutaneous flap, other than the absence of the pectoralis major muscle, the reconstructive surgeon should use caution in cases involving patients with significant restrictive lung disease, peripheral vascular disease affecting the thoracoacromial axis, or coverage of mandibular segmental defects without the ability to perform a bony reconstruction. For the latter, although adequate soft tissue coverage of mandibular hardware can be achieved, without a bony reconstruction, the pectoralis major flap has a high rate of wound dehiscence, which leads to plate exposure, fracture, and infection. This is particularly true in previously irradiated patients. Therefore, in this clinical scenario, the pectoralis major flap should be reserved for patients with a poor prognosis who cannot tolerate bony reconstruction. In addition, although this flap is useful for esophageal, pharyngeal, floor of the mouth, and even tongue reconstructions, when stretched to close maxillary or palatal defects, the skin paddle is prone to dehiscence from the pull of gravity.

Flap Design

The pectoralis major myocutaneous flap is a Mathes and Nahai type V muscle flap with one dominant pedicle (pectoral branch of the thoracoacromial) and secondary segmental pedicles (internal mammary perforators). It is an axial pattern flap, based off and following a named vessel. Several designs also incorporate random patterned extensions of the flap, based on the Taylor's angiosome concept, which theorizes the perfusion of adjacent angiosomes via choke vessels. Choke vessels are smaller, communicating, unnamed arteries that connect the vasculature of adjacent angiosomes, which are based on named arteries. In the case of the pectoralis major myocutaneous flap, the internal mammary and superior epigastric angiosomes are supplied by choke vessels communicating with the pectoral branch of the thoracoacromial artery.

The original flap design was a longitudinal skin paddle running along the axis of the pedicle (using a line drawn from the tip of the shoulder to the xiphoid) from the clavicle inferiorly and medially. The flap design included the skin, subcutaneous tissue, and pectoralis major muscle, elevated in a plane above the clavipectoral fascia with direct visualization and protection of the pedicle on the underside of the muscle. The intervening skin was tubed as part of a staged reconstruction. Ariyan later modified this to an island skin paddle over a muscle flap that is elevated and then tunneled under the skin. In this way, it could be used as a single-stage reconstruction. Several other variations have been described to optimize the flap for different reconstructive purposes, including the following:

- Inframammary skin paddle, which lengthens the arc of rotation, decreases cosmetic deformity of the donor site, and preserves the blood supply to the deltopectoral fascial flap for concurrent or later use
- Fasciocutaneous random pattern extension of flap inferior to the pectoralis major by including the rectus abdominis sheath
- Parasternal skin paddle, which reduces morbidity, provides a thinner skin paddle, and extends the arc of rotation
- Muscle flap only with skin graft (either two stage or single stage), which reduces the bulk of the flap
- Variety of tunneling techniques, including subcutaneous, underneath the clavicle, and removal of a segment of clavicle
- Bilobed "Gemini" skin paddle for reconstruction of two epithelial surfaces (intraluminal and cutaneous defects)
- Two separate flaps based off the thoracoacromial and lateral thoracic arteries
- Janus flap using an embedded skin graft in a two-stage fashion to create a flap with two epithelial surfaces
- Inclusion of the fifth rib for an osteomusculocutaneous flap for reconstruction of bony defects

Bibliography

Ariyan S: Further experiences with the pectoralis major myocutaneous flap for the immediate repair of defects from excisions of head and neck cancers, *Plast Reconstr Surg* 64(5):605-612, 1979.

Cohen MA, Weinstein GS, O'Malley BW Jr, et al: Transoral robotic surgery and human papillomavirus status: oncologic results, *Head Neck* 33:573-580, 2010.

Dennis D, Kashima H: Introduction of the Janus flap: a modified pectoralis major myocutaneous flap for cervical esophageal and pharyngeal reconstruction, *Arch Otolaryngol* 107:431-435, 1981.

Donegan JO, Gluckman JL: An unusual complication of the pectoralis major myocutaneous flap, *Head Neck Surg* 6:982-983, 1984.

Ferraro GA, Perrotta A, Rossano F, et al: Poland syndrome: description of an atypical variant, *Aesth Plast Surg* 29:32-33, 2005.

Freeman JL, Walker EP, Wilson JS, et al: The vascular anatomy of the pectoralis major myocutaneous flap, *Br J Plast Surg* 34:3-10, 1981.

Genden EM, O'Malley BW Jr, Weinstein GS, et al: Transoral robotic surgery: role in the management of upper aerodigestive tract tumors, *Head Neck* 34:886-893, 2011.

Hodgkinson DJ: The pectoralis major myocutaneous flap for intraoral reconstruction: a word of warning, *Br J Plast Surg* 35:80-81, 1982.

Moloy PJ, Gonzales FE: Vascular anatomy of the pectoralis major myocutaneous flap, *Arch Otolaryngol Head Neck Surg* 112:66-69, 1986.

Ossoff RH, Wurster CF, Berktold RE, et al: Complications after pectoralis major myocutaneous flap reconstruction of head and neck defects, *Arch Otolaryngol* 109:812-814, 1983.

Reid CD, Taylor GI: The vascular territory of the acromiothoracic axis, *Br J Plast Surg* 37:194-212, 1984.

Rikimaru H, Kiyokawa K, Inoue Y, et al: Three-dimensional anatomical vascular distribution in the pectoralis major myocutaneous flap, *Plast Reconstr Surg* 115:1342-1352, 2005.

Shah JP, Haribhakti V, Loree TR, et al: Complications of the pectoralis major myocutaneous flap in head and neck reconstruction, *Am J Surg* 160:352-355, 1990.

Shah GV, Wesolowski JR, Ansari SA, et al: New directions in head and neck imaging, *J Surg Oncol* 97:644-648, 2008.

Sharzer LA, Kalisman M, Silver CE, et al: The parasternal paddle: a modification of the pectoralis major myocutaneous flap, *Plast Reconstr Surg* 67:753-762, 1981.

Ueda M, Torii S, Nagayama M, et al: The pectoralis major myocutaneous flap for intraoral reconstruction: surgical complications and their treatment, *J Maxillofac Surg* 13:9-13, 1985.

Weaver AW, Vandenberg HJ, Atkinson DP, et al: Modified bilobular ("Gemini") pectoralis major myocutaneous flap, *Am J Surg* 144:482-488, 1982.

Weinstein GS, O'Malley BW, Magnuson JS, et al: Transoral robotic surgery: a multicenter study to assess feasibility, safety, and surgical margins, *Laryngoscope* 122:1701-1707, 2012.

Worden FP, Ha H: Controversies in the management of oropharynx cancer, *J Natl Compr Canc Netw* 6:707-714, 2008.

Free Fibula Flap for Mandibular Reconstruction*

Etern S. Park, Tuan G. Bui, and R. Bryan Bell

CC

A 66-year-old Caucasian woman presents to your office, stating, "I am having pain in my lower jaw, difficulty eating, and there is drainage from my face."

HPI

The patient sustained a mandibular fracture from a motor vehicle accident at age 20. Six years later she had her remaining teeth extracted, but she subsequently sustained a pathologic fracture of the mandible, which was treated with closed reduction using circummandibular wires fixated to her denture. In the following years, she underwent several preprosthetic procedures in an attempt to restore her dentition. Restoration eventually was accomplished with implants placed 15 years ago using a Hader bar and overdenture. The patient did well for 10 years; then she developed a pathologic fracture and was diagnosed with osteomyelitis. She was treated with intravenous antibiotics, decortication, open reduction and fixation using a reconstruction plate, and hyperbaric oxygen. Several years later, the reconstruction plate was removed after the screws loosened and became infected. She developed lower right facial swelling with a draining orocutaneous fistula over the right anterior mandible. The patient had excision of the orocutaneous fistula, multiple incision and drainage procedures, and debridements of the right mandible. However, the infection and exacerbating osteomyelitis did not respond to treatment. She eventually developed pathologic fractures of the right mandibular parasymphysis and left mandibular angle. The patient was referred to your office for definitive treatment.

PMHX/PDHX/MEDICATIONS/ALLERGIES/SH/FH

The patient has hypertension and non-insulin-dependent diabetes mellitus, both of which are well controlled.

Although hypertension and diabetes are not contraindications to microvascular surgery, it is important for both the blood pressure and glucose levels to be strictly controlled in the perioperative period. Severe peripheral vascular disease secondary to advanced atherosclerosis from diabetes may compromise microvascular treatment options.

---

*The authors and publisher wish to acknowledge Dr. Brian M. Woo for his contribution on this topic to the previous edition.

EXAMINATION

General. The patient is a well-developed and well-nourished, alert woman in no acute distress (morbid obesity and severe peripheral vascular disease would be contraindications to microvascular surgery).

Vital signs. Vital signs are stable and within normal limits. The patient is afebrile (an elevated temperature is not frequently seen with chronic osteomyelitis).

Maxillofacial. There is a draining orocutaneous fistula exiting the right submental region. The patient has severe mandibular atrophy with gross mobility and pathologic fractures of the mandible at the right parasymphysis and left mandibular angle. There is bilateral anesthesia of the third division (V3) of the trigeminal nerve at the mental nerve distribution.

Intraoral. The patient is completely edentulous and, in addition to the pathologic fractures, has a functional maxillary subperiosteal implant and a mobile Hader bar in the left anterior mandible.

Extremity. She has 2+ peripheral pulses without claudication or evidence of peripheral vascular insufficiency.

The lower extremities should be examined to evaluate for absent or diminished pulses in the anterior or posterior tibial arteries, because this may suggest atherosclerosis or vascular insufficiency. Absent or diminished anterior or posterior tibial pulses mandate a preoperative angiogram or magnetic resonance angiogram to define the vascular anatomy.

IMAGING

The panoramic radiograph and CT scan can be used to help determine the extent of the mandibular resection and to aid in predicting the size of the postresection mandibular defect. Stereolithographic models constructed from CT data can also be used to prebend a reconstruction plate before surgery.

In the current patient, the panoramic radiograph showed the fractures of the right parasymphysis and left mandibular angle, along with a maxillary subperiosteal implant and three mandibular endosteal implants with a Hader bar (Figure 12-13).

Preoperative imaging for the fibula transfer includes angiography/arteriography or magnetic resonance angiography of the lower extremities to evaluate the vascular anatomy for the possible absence or diminished size of the anterior and posterior tibial arteries and for narrowing or occlusion of the vessels secondary to atherosclerosis. However, some microvascular surgeons order these tests only when dictated

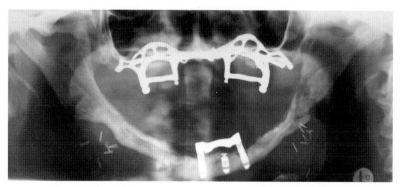

Figure 12-13   Preoperative panoramic radiograph showing fractures of the patient's right parasymphysis region and left mandibular angle, along with a maxillary subperiosteal implant and three mandibular endosteal implants with a Hader bar.

by physical examination findings. In about 10% to 20% of cases, the anterotibial or posterotibial artery may become attenuated. In these cases, a communicating branch from the peroneal artery supplies the attenuated vessel's territory; therefore, sacrifice of the peroneal artery could result in ischemia of the foot.

Routine use of preoperative angiography to evaluate lower extremity vasculatures remains controversial. Proponents claim that preoperative angiography results in surgical plan changes in 5% to 11% of patients. Opponents state that the normal clinical vascular examination is sufficient to ensure the adequacy of circulation in the lower extremity. We perform a clinical vascular exam, supplemented with a lower extremity CT angiogram, for most patients who are to have a fibula free flap. Angiography is reserved for patients with severe vascular disease.

LABS

Routine laboratory tests, such as a CBC and electrolyte and coagulation studies, may be performed to establish a baseline preoperatively.

ASSESSMENT

Chronic suppurative osteomyelitis with a draining orocutaneous fistula and nonunion of the mandibular right parasymphysis and left angle.

TREATMENT

The current patient presents a complex case demonstrating multiple attempts at reconstruction and management of an infected mandible. The goals of mandibular reconstruction include the following:

- Reestablishment of mandibular continuity and arch form and maintenance of the existing occlusion, with care taken to maintain the restored mandible's proper relationship to the maxilla to allow dental rehabilitation
- Provision of soft tissue closure and replacement of resected oral cavity soft tissue

- Dental rehabilitation
- Restoration of adequate function (speech, mastication, oral continence) and cosmesis, enabling the patient to enjoy a reasonable quality of life

Several treatment options are available, each associated with specific complications and limitations that reflect the difficulty of managing total mandibular reconstruction. These treatment options include:

- Reconstruction with only a mandibular reconstruction plate
- Reconstruction with a mandibular reconstruction plate and a pedicled myocutaneous flap (pectoralis major flap)
- Reconstruction with a mandibular reconstruction plate and a soft tissue free flap
- A nonvascularized bone graft (e.g., iliac crest, rib)
- A vascularized bone flap (e.g., fibula, ilium, radial forearm, scapula)
- Distraction osteogenesis (may be used alone or in combination with the other modalities)

The current patient was treated with segmental mandibulectomy, left neck dissection for vascular access, tracheostomy, and immediate reconstruction with an osseous fibula free flap (Figure 12-14).

COMPLICATIONS

The use of a mandibular reconstruction plate alone for mandibular reconstruction has been reported as having a failure rate ranging from 20% to 80%, with most of the failures resulting from plate extrusion. A higher percentage of failures also occurred in patients with segmental defects of the anterior mandible and in patients who received or were receiving radiation therapy, with or without chemotherapy Even with the use of pedicled myocutaneous flaps and soft tissue free flaps to provide coverage of the mandibular reconstruction plate, the failure rate has been reported to range from 7% to 44% (approaching the higher percentage with long-term follow-up). Most of these failures were also due to plate extrusion.

The use of vascularized bone grafts for mandibular reconstruction, however, has been reported to have a success rate

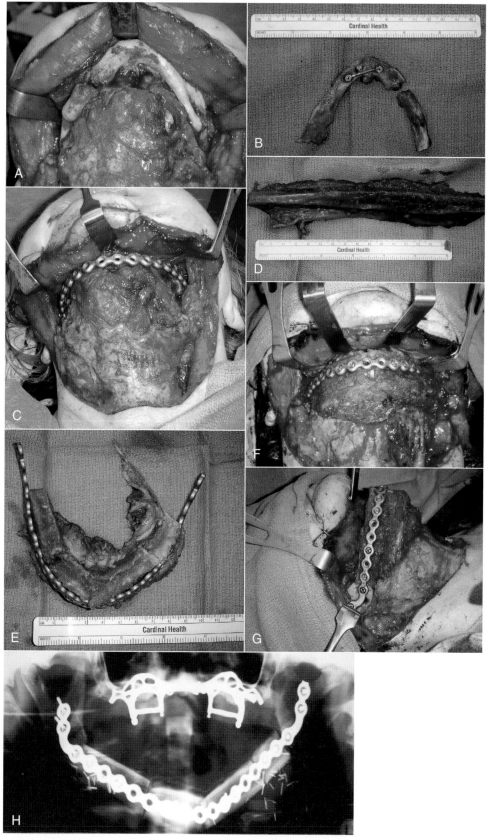

Figure 12-14   **A,** Intraoperative view showing surgical exposure of the mandible and fracture sites. **B,** Surgical specimen/resected mandible. **C,** Reconstruction plate contoured to the shape of the resected mandible. **D,** Free fibula graft. **E,** Fibula graft after it has been osteotomized and contoured to the shape of the resected mandible. **F,** Free fibula graft after it has been inset and secured in place. **G,** Lateral view of the inset free fibula graft. **H,** Postoperative panoramic radiograph of the free fibula graft in place.

greater than 90%, even in irradiated patients and in patients with segmental defects of the anterior mandible. Vascularized bone grafts also have the advantage of being able to accept endosteal implants for dental rehabilitation, which cannot be done if a mandibular reconstruction plate is used, with or without soft tissue coverage.

Despite the reported success rates, perioperative surgical and reconstructive complications and perioperative medical complications of the fibula free flap have been described in the literature (Box 12-2).

DISCUSSION

The application of the fibula free flap was first described by Taylor and colleagues. Hidalgo reported its first use in mandibular reconstruction in 1989. Since then, it has remained the method of choice for mandibular reconstruction after trauma and tumor ablation surgeries. The primary blood supply of the fibula free flap is from the peroneal artery and vein, which supply the fibula bone via endosteal and periosteal vessels. The peroneal artery is classically described as originating from the posterior tibial artery after the popliteal artery branches into the anterior and posterior tibial arteries. The peroneal artery and its two venae comitantes descend in the lower leg between the flexor hallucis longus and the tibialis posterior. The fibula can be transferred as a free osseous or free osteocutaneous flap. The skin is attached to the fibula by the posterolateral intermuscular septum and is supplied by the septocutaneous and musculocutaneous perforators arising from the peroneal artery and vein. An anatomic study by Schusterman and associates identified three types of perforators:

- Septocutaneous
- Musculocutaneous
- Septomuscular (which did not run within the muscle substance but is adherent to it)

These researchers also demonstrated that the musculocutaneous perforators were more numerous and proximal, whereas the septocutaneous perforators were less numerous and more distal. They found that the septocutaneous perforators were not present in 20% of their dissected specimens, and that in 6.25% of their dissected specimens there also were no muscular or septomuscular vessels. Eighteen of their clinical cases demonstrated a 33% skin paddle survival when dissected as a septocutaneous flap and a 93% skin paddle survival when dissected as a septomusculocutaneous flap. Based on these findings, it was recommended that a cuff of soleus and flexor hallucis longus be incorporated into the flap to help ensure flap viability. The lateral sural cutaneous nerve can be harvested and anastomosed to a recipient nerve to restore sensation to the skin component. Harvesting of the peroneal communicating branch as a vascularized nerve graft can be used to bridge the inferior alveolar and mental nerve to restore sensation to the lower lip.

The fibula free flap has several advantages. The fibula has thick cortical bone around its entire circumference, making it suitable to withstand the forces of mastication and for the placement of dental implants. Approximately 22 to 25 cm of bone can be harvested, leaving 6 to 7 cm proximally and distally to maintain adequate stability of the knee and ankle joints. Because of the length of bone that can be harvested, the fibula is suitable for restoration of subtotal and total mandibular defects. The length of the vascular pedicle that can be obtained is also an advantage. Additional length of the pedicle can be obtained by harvesting a more distal segment of bone and skin while discarding the proximal fibula. Hidalgo has described obtaining vascular pedicles as long as 12 cm through this technique. Another advantage is the ability to reconstruct soft tissue defects using the skin paddle (potential for sensory innervation) of the free fibula osteocutaneous flap. The width of the skin paddle is mainly limited only by the ability to achieve primary closure; however, a skin graft can be grafted to the donor site. Multiple osteotomies can be made in the bone for contouring the fibula to the shape of the mandible. These osteotomies are well tolerated if the osteotomized segments are at least 1 cm in length and the overlying periosteum is kept intact. Last, the donor site's distance from the head allows a two-team approach, if desired.

Criticism of the use of the fibula free flap in mandibular reconstruction has focused on the height discrepancy between the fibula bone and the native mandible and in the use of the flap for reconstruction of large oral cavity and through-and-through soft tissue defects. To decrease the discrepancy between the fibula bone and the native mandible, a "double barrel" technique has been described in which a 1-cm segment of the fibula bone is removed and the fibula is folded on itself lengthwise (Figure 12-15).

| Box 12-2 | **Possible Complications with Use of a Fibular Free Flap** |

Perioperative Surgical/Reconstructive Complications
- Venous thrombosis/arterial thrombosis
- Venous congestion
- Wound infection
- Salivary fistula
- Cervical hematoma
- Partial free flap necrosis
- Total free flap necrosis
- Hardware extrusion
- Carotid artery rupture
- Donor site complications (infection, skin graft failure, loss of knee and ankle strength, reduced ankle range of motion, damage to the peroneal nerve and its branches)

Perioperative Medical Complications
- Myocardial infarction
- Cerebrovascular accidents
- Deep venous thrombosis
- Congestive heart failure/pulmonary edema
- Pneumonia/atelectasis
- Acute respiratory distress syndrome
- Pneumothorax
- Cardiac arrhythmias
- Gastrointestinal hemorrhage/perforation
- Liver failure
- Mortality

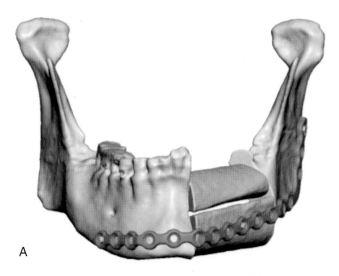

A

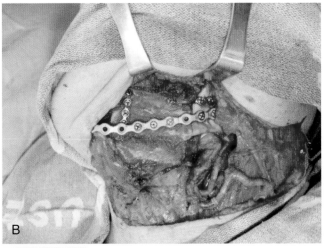

B

Figure 12-15 **A,** Preoperative planning for left mandibular reconstruction with fibula "double-barrel" technique. **B,** Intraoperative photograph of "double-barrel" technique.

Over the past decade, computer-assisted virtual surgery has been used for reconstruction of craniofacial defects. A cutting jig guides precise bony resection of mandibular pathology and of the fibula segment. Virtual surgery has eliminated much of the guesswork of mandibular and fibular osteotomies. A reduction in surgical time has been demonstrated with computer-assisted mandibular reconstruction. In addition, for selected cases of benign pathology, it allows the surgeon to place dental implants at the time of ablation to achieve a dental implant–supported prosthesis (Figure 12-16).

Use of a radial forearm flap in conjunction with the fibula flap has been described for the reconstruction of extensive soft tissue defects. The radial forearm flap can be used to reconstruct the oral cavity, and the free fibula osteocutaneous flap can be used to reconstruct the mandible and the cervical skin. This technique can also be used to reconstruct composite resections of the mandible, tongue, and floor of the mouth or composite resections of the mandible and lower lip. Combined ipsilateral maxillomandibular defects can also be reconstructed using the free fibula flap by removing a central 3-cm segment of the fibula and rotating the distal portion of the

fibula upward to reconstruct the maxilla and rotating the proximal portion downward to reconstruct the mandible.

Mandibular reconstruction with the use of nonvascularized bone grafts is well described in the literature. Before the availability of microvascular free tissue transfer, immediate bone grafting with nonvascularized grafts had a success rate of only 46%, as opposed to 91% in the delayed setting. Direct comparisons of nonvascularized versus vascularized bone grafts have shown a higher success of bony union with vascularized bone grafts. Pogrel and associates reported a 95% success rate of bony union using vascularized bone grafts and a 76% success rate using nonvascularized bone grafts for primary reconstruction of mandibular defects. Foster and colleagues reported similar results, with a 96% success rate using vascularized bone grafts and a 69% success rate using nonvascularized bone grafts. Pogrel and associates also found that the failure rate for nonvascularized grafts increased for segmental mandibular defects longer than 6 cm and that extreme caution should be used in using nonvascularized grafts for reconstructing segmental mandibular defects longer than 9 cm. The failure rate for nonvascularized grafts of 6 cm or shorter was 17%; this rate increased to 75% for grafts over 12 cm in length. This correlation of increasing failure rate with increased graft length was not seen with the use of vascularized bone grafts. Foster and colleagues also reported a higher success rate of osseointegration of endosteal implants in vascularized bone grafts (99%) over nonvascularized grafts (82%). In the studies by both groups, the predominant vascularized bone graft used was the fibula free flap.

Various vascularized osteocutaneous free flaps have been used for mandibular reconstruction; available choices include fibula, radius, ilium, scapula, rib, and metatarsal. Rib and metatarsal were among the first to be used for mandibular reconstruction but are rarely used today. The radial forearm flap provides a reliable, thin, and pliable skin flap and is excellent for reconstructing large intraoral defects. However, the radius bone provides only a short segment of unicortical bone (8 to 10 cm), is of poor quality for the reception of endosteal implants, and is easily devascularized with multiple osteotomies. There is also a risk of fracture with use of the radial forearm free flap. The scapula can provide a large and excellent skin paddle but with more soft tissue bulk than the radius. The bone of the scapula is thin, is of poor quality, and usually is able to provide only 10 to 14 cm of bone length. The scapula is also easily devascularized with multiple osteotomies and is not adequate for the placement of endosteal implants. Harvesting of the scapula also does not allow a two-team approach. The ilium, based on the deep circumflex iliac artery, can provide a large amount of bone, and its shape resembles that of the hemimandible. The number of osteotomies that can be made is also limited due to the risk of devascularization, making it more difficult to contour the ilium for anterior mandibular defects. The skin paddle of the ilium is also very bulky, and the donor site can be quite morbid and deforming. In addition, the vascular pedicle of the deep circumflex iliac artery flap is relatively short, making anastomosis into the recipient bed more challenging.

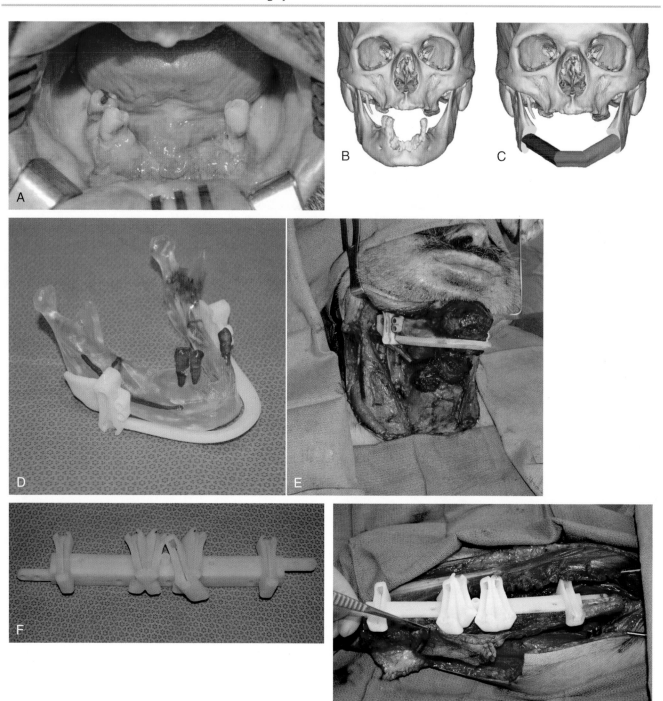

Figure 12-16 **A,** A 49-year-old male with squamous cell carcinoma, anterior mandible (pT4N0M0). **B** and **C,** Simulated mandible resection and reconstruction with fibula free flap, planned with patient-specific data. Mandibular cutting jig on stereolithic model **(D)** and applied to the patient's mandible to create the planned osteotomy **(E). F** and **G,** Fibula cutting guide designed from patient-specific data to create accurate closing wedge osteotomies, which were applied to the patient's left fibula. The skin paddle is shown with forceps.

Among the remaining choices, the fibula has been the most popular because of its numerous proven advantages: the length and quality of bone that can be harvested, a segmental blood supply that allows multiple osteotomies for shaping and contouring of the fibula, adequate bone height and width to receive endosteal implants, an intermediate-thickness skin paddle, a reliable vascular pedicle that can reach 8 to 12 cm in length, low donor site morbidity, and an ideal location for a two-team approach.

Bibliography

Anthony J, Rawnsley J, Benhaim P, et al: Donor leg morbidity and function after fibula free flap mandible reconstruction, *Plast Reconstr Surg* 96:146, 1995.

Bahr W: Blood supply of small fibula segments: an experimental study on human cadavers, *J Craniomaxillofac Surg* 26:148, 1998.

Blackwell K: Unsurpassed reliability of free flaps for head and neck reconstruction, *Arch Otolaryngol Head Neck Surg* 125:295, 1999.

Blackwell K, Buchbinder D, Urken M: Lateral mandibular reconstruction using soft-tissue free flaps and plates, *Arch Otolaryngol Head Neck Surg* 122:672, 1996.

Blanchaert R, Harris C: Microvascular free bone flaps, *Atlas Oral Maxillofac Surg Clin North Am* 13:151, 2005.

Boyd J, Mulholland RS, Davidson J, et al: The free flap and plate in oromandibular reconstruction: long-term review and indications, *Plast Reconstr Surg* 95:1018, 1995.

Buchbinder D: Discussion of "Analysis of reconstruction of mandibular defects using single stainless steel A-O reconstruction plates," *J Oral Maxillofac Surg* 54:862, 1996.

Choi S, Schwartz DL, Farwell DG, et al: Radiation therapy does not impact local complication rates after free flap reconstruction for head and neck cancer, *Arch Otolaryngol Head Neck Surg* 130:1308, 2004.

Cordeiro P, Disa J, Hidalgo D, et al: Reconstruction of the mandible with osseous free flaps: a 10 year experience with 150 consecutive patients, *Plast Reconstr Surg* 104:1314, 1999.

Cordeiro P, Hidalgo D: Soft tissue coverage of mandibular reconstruction plates, *Head Neck* 16:112, 1994.

Fong B, Funk G: Osseous free tissue transfer in head and neck reconstruction, *Facial Plast Surg* 15:45, 1999.

Foster R, Anthony J, Sharma A, et al: Vascularized bone flaps versus nonvascularized bone grafts for mandibular reconstruction: an outcome analysis of primary bony union and endosseous implant success, *Head Neck* 21:66, 1999.

Gilbert R, Dovion D: Near total mandibular reconstruction: the free vascularized fibular transfer, *Oper Tech Otolaryngol Head Neck Surg* 4:145, 1993.

Goodacre T, Walker C, Jawad A, et al: Donor site morbidity following osteocutaneous free fibula transfer, *Br J Plast Surg* 43:410, 1990.

Hayden R, O'Leary M: A neurosensory fibula flap: anatomical description and clinical applications. Presented at the Ninety-Fourth Annual Meeting of the American Academy of Facial Plastic and Reconstructive Surgery, Minneapolis, October 1, 1993.

He Y, Zhang ZY, Zhu HG, et al: Double-barrel fibula vascularized free flap with dental rehabilitation for mandibular reconstruction, *J Oral Maxillofac Surg* 69:2663-2669, 2011.

Hidalgo D: Fibula free flap: a new method of mandible reconstruction, *Plast Reconstr Surg* 84:71, 1989.

Hidalgo D: Discussion of "Fibula osteoseptocutaneous flap for reconstruction of composite mandibular defects," *Plast Reconstr Surg* 93:305, 1994.

Hidalgo D, Pusic A: Free-flap mandibular reconstruction: a 10 year follow-up study, *Plast Reconstr Surg* 110:438, 2002.

Hidalgo D, Rekow A: A review of 60 consecutive fibula free flap mandible reconstructions, *Plast Reconstr Surg* 96:585, 1995.

Horiuchi K, Hattori A, Inada I, et al: Mandibular reconstruction using the double barrel fibular graft, *Microsurgery* 16:450, 1995.

Jones N, Swartz W, Mears D, et al: The "double barrel" free vascularized fibular bone graft, *Plast Reconstr Surg* 81:378, 1998.

Khouri Cooley BC, Kunselman AR, et al: A prospective study of microvascular free-flap surgery and outcome, *Plast Reconstr Surg* 102(3):711-721, 1998.

Kim D, Orron DE, Skillman JJ: Surgical significance of popliteal artery variants: a unified angiographic classification, *Ann Surg* 210:776, 1989.

Kroll SS, Schusterman MA, Reece GP, et al: Choice of flap and incidence of free flap success, *Plast Reconstr Surg* 98:459, 1996.

Lee E, Goh J, Helm R, et al: Donor site morbidity following resection of the fibula, *J Bone Joint Surg* 72:129, 1990.

Levine JP, Patel A, Saadeh PB, et al: Computer-aided design and manufacturing in craniomaxillofacial surgery: the new state of the art, *J Craniofac Surg* 23:1, 288-293, 2012.

Markiewicz MR, Bell RB: Modern concepts in computer-assisted craniomaxillofacial reconstruction, *Curr Opin Otolaryngol Head Neck Surg* 19:295-301, 2011.

Myung-Rai K, Donoff RB: Critical analysis of mandibular reconstruction using AO reconstruction plates, *J Oral Maxillofac Surg* 50:1152, 1990.

Patel A, Levine JP, Brecht L, et al: Digital technologies in mandibular pathology and reconstruction, *Atlas Oral Maxillofac Surg Clin North Am* 20:95-106, 2012.

Pogrel MA, Podlesh S, Anthony J, et al: A comparison of vascularized and nonvascularized bone grafts for reconstruction of mandibular continuity defects, *J Oral Maxillofac Surg* 55:1200, 1997.

Sadove R, Powell L: Simultaneous maxillary and mandibular reconstruction with one free osteocutaneous flap, *Plast Reconstr Surg* 92:141, 1993.

Schusterman M, Reece G, Kroll S, et al: Use of the AO plate for immediate mandibular reconstruction in cancer patients, *Plast Reconstr Surg* 88:588, 1991.

Schusterman M, Reece G, Miller M, et al: The osteocutaneous free fibula flap: Is the skin paddle reliable? *Plast Reconstr Surg* 90:787, 1992.

Serletti J, Higgins JP, Moran S, et al: Factors affecting outcome in free-tissue transfer in the elderly, *Plast Reconstr Surg* 106:66, 2000.

Serlitti J, Coniglio J, Tavin E, et al: Simultaneous transfer of free fibula and radial forearm flaps for complex oromandibular reconstruction, *J Reconstr Microsurg* 14:297, 1998.

Shaari CM, Buchbinder D, Costantine PD, et al: Complications of microvascular head and neck surgery in the elderly, *Arch Otolaryngol Head Neck Surg* 124:407, 1998.

Singh B, Cordeiro PG, Santamaria E, et al: Factors associated with complications in microvascular reconstruction of head and neck defects, *Plast Reconstr Surg* 103:403, 1999.

Sphitzer T, Neligan PC, Gullane PJ, et al: Oromandibular reconstruction with the fibular free flap: analysis of 50 consecutive flaps, *Arch Otolaryngol Head Neck Surg* 123:939, 1997.

Sphitzer T, Gullane PJ, Neligan PC, et al: The free vascularized flap and the flap plate options: comparative results of reconstruction of lateral mandibular defects, *Laryngoscope* 110:2056, 2000.

Suh JD, Sercarz JA, Abemayor E, et al: Analysis of outcome and complications in 400 cases of microvascular head and neck reconstruction, *Arch Otolaryngol Head Neck Surg* 130:962, 2004.

Taylor GI, Miller GD, Ham FJ: The free vascularized bone graft: a clinical extension of microvascular techniques, *Plast Reconstr Surg* 55(5):533-544, 1975.

Ueyama Y, Naitoh R, Yamagata A, et al: Analysis of reconstruction of mandibular defects using single stainless steel A-O reconstruction plates, *J Oral Maxillofac Surg* 54:858, 1996.

Urken ML, Weinberg H, Buchbinl D, et al: Microvascular free flaps in and head and neck reconstruction. Report of Zoo cases and review of complications, *Arch Otolaryngol Head Neck Surg* 120:633, 1994.

Urken ML, Cheney ML, Sullivan MJ, et al: *Atlas of regional and free flaps for head and neck reconstruction*, Philadelphia, 1994, Lippincott Williams & Wilkins.

Wei FC, Seah CS, Tsai YC: Fibula osteoseptocutaneous flap for reconstruction of composite mandibular defects, *Plast Reconstr Surg* 93:294, 1994.

Young DM, Trabulsy PP, Anthony JP: The need for preoperative leg angiography in fibula free flap, *J Reconstr Microsurg* 10:283, 1994.

Mandibular Reconstruction with Iliac Crest Bone Graft

Solon Kao, Bradford Huffman, Rebecca Paquin, Chris Jo, and Shahrokh C. Bagheri

CC

A 28-year-old, otherwise healthy man is referred to your office for reconstruction of the left mandible. He states, "Now that the tumor is gone, I need my lower jaw reconstructed."

HPI

The patient is now 3 months status post resection of a large, expansile ameloblastoma of the left mandible (with 1.5-cm bony margins) and immediate placement of a locking reconstruction plate (a minimum of 3 months after ablative surgery is recommended to allow sufficient time for soft tissue healing before bone grafting). The tumor was resected via a transoral approach using a previously bent reconstruction plate that was placed to stabilize the mandible and the occlusion. (A custom-made, three-dimensional stereolithographic model [Figure 12-17], fabricated with the aid of a CT scan, was used to prebend the plate, reducing operating time and increasing the accuracy of the reconstruction). The inferior alveolar nerve was resected with the specimen (in select, benign cases, preservation of the nerve is possible using a nerve pull-out technique). There were no perioperative complications.

The patient is now ready for total mandibular reconstruction and functional rehabilitation.

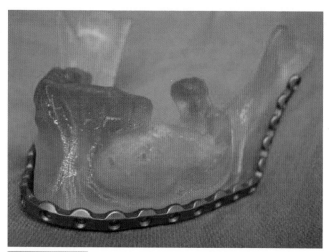

Figure 12-17 Stereolithographic model demonstrating an expanding mass of the left mandible and a well-adapted locking reconstruction plate to be used for surgical adaptation.

PMHX/PDHX/MEDICATIONS/ALLERGIES/SH/FH

Noncontributory. The patient has no history of cardiac or pulmonary conditions (increased intrathoracic pressure and hemodynamic changes associated with the prone position may not be tolerated well by patients with poor cardiac or respiratory reserves).

EXAMINATION

General. The patient is a well-developed and well-nourished man in no apparent distress.

Maxillofacial. Facial form and symmetry are good, with a slight loss of left lower lip support (secondary to the resection). There is anesthesia of the left mental nerve distribution. The marginal mandibular branch and the remaining branches of cranial nerve VII are intact.

Intraoral. The occlusion is as planned and reproducible, with a good range of motion. There are no traumatic occlusal or soft tissue interferences noted (traumatic occlusion, especially from a supraerupted maxillary third molar, can cause perforation of the soft tissue overlying the recipient bed). The remaining dentition is in good repair (compromised teeth, especially those adjacent to the recipient bed, should be restored or extracted before reconstruction to prevent graft infection). The soft tissue over the defect has healed well, with minimal scar contracture (a qualitative or quantitative soft tissue deficiency may require an alternative reconstructive plan, such as a myocutaneous flap [pectoralis major] or reconstruction with a vascularized free flap [free fibula or iliac bone]). There are no signs of infection, and there is no exposure of the reconstruction plate (bone grafting into a contaminated field is contraindicated).

IMAGING

A preoperative panoramic radiograph is the minimum radiographic study necessary to evaluate the size of the defect and to assess the integrity and stability of the hardware. In the current patient, the panoramic radiograph revealed an 8-cm continuity defect (10 ml of uncompressed cancellous marrow is needed for each centimeter of continuity defect). The dentition is in good repair, with no supraerupted maxillary teeth and no signs of residual or recurrent pathology.

LABS

The minimum preoperative laboratory studies necessary are hemoglobin and hematocrit levels. Tumor resection can be associated with an unpredictable amount of blood loss. Reconstructive procedures are usually more predictable, but a preoperative baseline measure of hemoglobin and hematocrit should be obtained. Other laboratory tests would be dictated by the past surgical and medical histories.

ASSESSMENT

Continuity defect (8 cm) of the left mandible, status post resection of a benign mandibular tumor (ameloblastoma).

TREATMENT

Reconstruction of the mandible has challenged surgeons for many years, and several techniques are available, all of which have their associated advantages and complications. Treatment is dictated by the surgeon's training, available resources, and the patient's preferences.

The current patient underwent reconstruction of a mandibular continuity defect, for which a transcutaneous approach (to minimize bacterial contamination of the graft) and a (posterior or anterior) iliac crest cancellous marrow graft were used. The surgical anatomy of the anterior and posterior ilium is shown in Figure 12-18.

Transcutaneous exposure and preparation of the recipient bed. The main advantage of a transoral resection of a

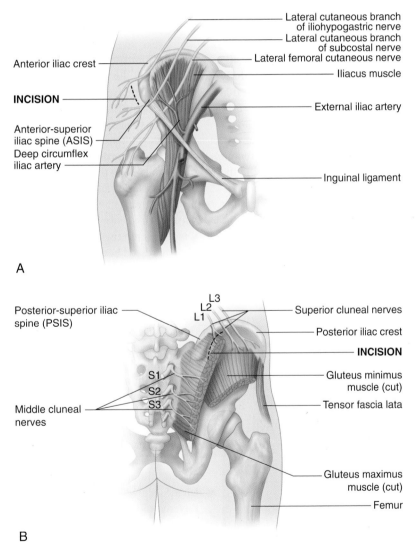

A

B

Figure 12-18 **A,** Anatomy of the anterior ilium. The anterior-superior iliac spine is seen along with the lateral cutaneous branches of the iliohypogastric nerve, subcostal nerve, and lateral femoral nerves (from posterior to anterior). The incision as shown is made 2 to 3 cm below the crest (to prevent wound dehiscence) and 1 to 2 cm posterior to the anterior superior iliac spine (to prevent injury to the subcostal nerve as it crosses over the anterior-superior iliac spine). **B,** Anatomy of the posterior ilium. Note that the posterior-superior iliac spine is the bony prominence adjacent to the sacroiliac (SI) joint where the gluteus maximus muscle originates. The cutaneous branches of the superior cluneal nerves (L1-L3) and middle cluneal nerves (S1-S3) are shown. The incision is made along the crest and centered over the posterior-superior iliac spine, avoiding injury to the superior and middle cluneal nerves.

benign tumor is the avoidance of a neck incision, and its associated scar tissue, upon making the transcutaneous exposure in preparation for the bony reconstruction phase. A curvilinear incision is marked at least 2 cm below the inferior border of the mandible with the head in a neutral position (to protect the marginal mandibular branch of the facial nerve) or further inferiorly in a neck crease. The exposure should be sufficient in length to fully expose the proximal and distal segments of the continuity defect. Nerve testing can be carried out to ensure that the dissection is below the marginal mandibular nerve. Dissection is then carried deep to the superficial layer of deep cervical fascia superiorly. The facial artery and vein are identified, ligated, and sectioned (carrying the dissection deep to these vessels ensures that the facial nerve is protected in the superior flap). The inferior borders of the mandible and reconstruction plate are identified. An incision is made through the periosteum (proximal and distal bony segments) and through the fibrous capsule of the plate. The surgeon must be careful not to perforate into the oral cavity with overzealous dissection (the most common area of mucosal perforation is at the line angles of the distal segment). The fibrous capsule surrounding the reconstruction plate should be carefully excised (excessive scar tissue surrounding the reconstruction plate prevents capillary diffusion into the graft). Figure 12-19 demonstrates exposure of the recipient site and adaptation of a resorbable crib in preparation for bone graft placement. Some surgeons recommend completely removing the reconstruction plate for recipient bed preparation, then placing the plate back using the same screw holes (placed with nontapping screws). The graft bed is further prepared with blunt dissection to create a pocket sufficient to accommodate the bone graft without tension. If an intraoral perforation is noted, the wound should be immediately irrigated and closed in a double-layer fashion, followed by copious irrigation of the bed with an antibiotic solution (to reduce the bacterial load)

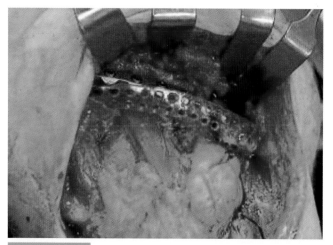

Figure 12-19 Complete exposure of the continuity defect, including the proximal and distal segments, via a transcutaneous approach. In this case, a resorbable, alloplastic crib was used to maintain the bone graft and prevent it from displacing inferiorly. It is important to avoid any intraoral perforations that would contaminate the graft with oral bacteria.

and redosing of the intravenous antibiotic if sufficient time has passed since the preoperative dose.

Posterior iliac crest bone graft harvesting technique. The main advantage of the posterior iliac crest bone graft is the quantity and quality of bone harvested. The main disadvantages are increased operating time, due to the change in position, and inability of two teams to work simultaneously. The patient is placed in the reverse flex prone position (decreases venous pressure and ooze) with hip and axillary/chest rolls. The posterior-superior iliac spine (a bony prominence where the gluteus maximus muscle originates) is palpated and marked (see Figure 12-18, *B*). A 10-cm, curvilinear incision (the length of the incision can vary, depending on the amount of bone to be harvested), 3 cm from the midline, is made along the crest. Dissection is carried through superficial fat and superficial fascia as the surgeon palpates the posterior iliac crest and posterior-superior iliac spine. The lumbodorsal fascia (deep fascia investing the deep muscles of the back and trunk) is identified and sharply incised to expose the posterior iliac crest and spine and its attachments (from medial to lateral: gluteus maximus, latissimus dorsi, and external oblique muscles). Bovie electrocautery can be used to make an incision through these attachments along the posterior crest down to bone. Subperiosteal dissection is carried out to reflect the gluteus maximus off the posterior superior iliac spine and part of the gluteus medius from the lateral aspect of the pelvis. A 5 × 5-cm corticotomy is made with a reciprocating saw (along the lateral third of the iliac crest and including a portion of the posterior-superior iliac spine). The sciatic notch and nerve are located 6 to 8 cm below the crest, which limits the vertical dissection and corticotomy. The corticocancellous window is removed (particulates into approximately 20 ml of uncompressed bone) with a curved osteotome. The cancellous marrow is removed with bone gouges and curettes and stored at room temperature in isotonic normal saline (95% cellular viability for up to 4 hours). The most abundant source of cancellous marrow is under the gluteus maximus insertion (posterior-superior iliac spine), which is a triangular bony prominence near the sacroiliac joint. Approximately 2 to 2.5 times more corticocancellous bone can be harvested from the posterior ilium than from the anterior ilium (an anterior iliac crest bone graft provides up to 50 ml of uncompressed bone). Hemostasis is achieved with electrocautery, judicious application of bone wax, and placement of Avitene (microfibrillar collagen) or platelet-poor plasma. Sharp bony edges should be rounded and smoothened. A drain with bulb suction can be placed, although it is not always necessary (Sasso and colleagues showed that there is no advantage to placing drains). Layered closure (periosteum, lumbodorsal fascia, subcutaneous, and skin) is performed, and a pressure dressing is applied.

The anterior iliac crest bone graft is an alternative to the posterior iliac crest bone graft when less volume of bone is needed. Its main advantage is the ability to simultaneously prepare the recipient bed and harvest the bone graft when working in two teams.

Anterior iliac crest bone graft (medial approach) harvesting technique (provides up to 50 ml of

corticocancellous bone). A hip and knee roll can be placed to externally rotate the hip and to flex the leg, respectively. The landmarks (anterior-superior iliac spine, crest, and tubercle) and incision site are carefully marked. The incision should be curvilinear, 4 to 6 cm in length, and 3 cm lateral to the crest (to prevent wound dehiscence); it should start 1 to 2 cm posterior and lateral to the anterior-superior iliac spine (to prevent injury to the lateral cutaneous branch of the subcostal nerve; see Figure 12-18, *A*). The incision should not extend beyond the tubercle (this can result in injury to the lateral cutaneous branch of the iliohypogastric nerve). The incision is carried through skin, superficial fat layer, and superficial fascia down to the deep fascia (fascia lata) and the iliotibial tract. The superficial and deep fat layers are bluntly swept superiorly to center the dissection over the anterior iliac crest. Sharp dissection to bone is performed, avoiding the musculature by keeping medial to the tensor fascia lata and gluteus medius muscles and lateral to iliacus and most of the external abdominal oblique muscles. Once the anterior iliac crest has been exposed, various corticotomy techniques can be used to access the cancellous marrow. Both medial and lateral approaches have been described in the literature, but the lateral approach is associated with greater morbidity due to stripping of muscles involved in ambulation and stance. The medial approach strips the iliacus muscle (when a corticocancellous block is needed), which is not a major contributor to gait. The "clamshell" approach (midcrestal greenstick split for small quantities of cancellous marrow), trapdoor approach (midcrestal pedicled osteotomy), Tschapp approach ("decapping" the crest), Tessier's approach (oblique osteotomies to maintain contour of crest), trephine techniques (for small bone grafts), or full-thickness grafts can be used, depending on surgeon preference. The authors prefer the technique described by Grillon and colleagues in 1984 (lateral decapping technique with attached superomedial pedicle to access the medial cortex), which allows for minimal dissection of the muscles attached to the anterior iliac crest. The iliacus muscle is dissected off the inner pelvis, and a 5 × 5-cm medial corticotomy can be made using a reciprocating saw and/or curved osteotomes. This block can be morselized with a bone mill (providing up to 20 ml of bone). Bone gouges and curettes are used to harvest the remainder of the cancellous marrow. The cancellous marrow is confined to the area anterior of the tubercle and 2 to 3 cm inferior to the iliac crest (medial and lateral cortices fuse or nearly fuse below this level). Up to 50 ml of uncompressed cancellous bone can be harvested and should be stored in an isotonic solution at room temperature. The anterior-superior iliac spine is vulnerable to fracture and avulsion because of muscle attachments (the seven attachments to the anterior-superior iliac spine are the fascia lata, inguinal ligament, tensor fascia lata, sartorius, iliacus, internal oblique, and external oblique muscles) and should not be undermined (this increases the risk of anterior-superior iliac spine fracture). The cap should be replaced and stabilized with a wire or suture (to prevent contour deformity). The wound is closed in layers, with or without drains.

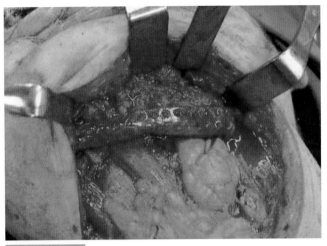

Figure 12-20   Morselized cancellous marrow graft compacted into the prepared recipient bed and alloplastic resorbable crib.

The harvested bone is milled and compressed into 10- or 12-ml syringes (compaction of the cancellous marrow increases the density of endosteal osteoblasts). The morselized bone is compacted into the prepared recipient bed (Figure 12-20). Various crib techniques can be used (resorbable or titanium mesh, cadaveric cribs, autogenous ribs) to stabilize the graft. The reconstruction plate itself serves as an excellent crib. The deep tissues are sutured to the plate, and the bone is packed from above, preventing inferior migration of the bone graft. The wound is closed in layers to further stabilize the graft. Some authors recommend 3 weeks of maxillomandibular fixation to prevent micromovement and shearing of budding capillaries penetrating the graft. Platelet-rich plasma, which has been shown to enhance bone grafting (earlier consolidation into lamellar bone and increased bony density) can be incorporated into the graft. Although there is some doubt regarding the efficacy of platelet-rich plasma in bone grafting, there are no well-controlled human studies to contradict its use.

Figure 12-21 is a panoramic radiograph demonstrating the bony reconstruction at 1 month. Dental implants can be placed into a mature graft (after 4 months) with a very high success rate. Animal studies have shown that implants placed into a cancellous marrow graft have a higher bone-to-metal contact and pull-out resistance than does native mandible.

COMPLICATIONS

Marginal mandibular nerve injury. This can be prevented by keeping the dissection inferior and deep to the nerve, retracting it in the superior flap. Dingman and Grabb studied 100 facial halves and found that the marginal mandibular branch is up to 1 cm below the inferior border of the mandible in 19% of cases. Anterior to the facial artery, it was found to be superior to the inferior border of the mandible. Ziarah and Atkinson studied 76 facial halves and found that 53% of the time the marginal mandibular branch was up to 1.2 cm below the inferior border of the mandible before reaching the facial

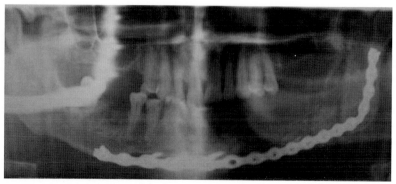

Figure 12-21   Postoperative panoramic radiograph showing an ideally placed reconstruction plate along the inferior and posterior borders of the mandible and a bone graft spanning the defect.

vessels. Six percent remained below the inferior border of the mandible, as far as 1.5 cm anterior to the facial artery.

Pain and gait disturbance. This is more frequently observed with an anterior iliac crest bone graft than with a posterior iliac crest bone graft (attributed to stripping of the tensor fascia lata muscle along the anterior iliac crest). A study by Marx and Morales (posterior group, N = 50; anterior group, N = 50) found that 6% of patients were limping after posterior iliac crest bone grafting at 10 days after surgery and no patients were limping at 60 days; however, for patients who underwent lateral-approach anterior iliac crest bone grafting, 42% and 15%, respectively, limped. These researchers also reported a higher pain score for the anterior group at postoperative days 1 and 10. When they compared the medial and lateral approaches for an anterior iliac crest bone graft, Grillon and associates found the lateral approach to be associated with greater morbidity (increased blood loss and number of days requiring a cane or crutch). Others have also found that a lateral approach is associated with more pain, prolonged gait disturbances, and wound hematoma. This is likely due to the stripping of the muscles attached to the lateral aspect of the anterior iliac crest (tensor fascia lata muscle), which is involved in gait and stance.

Infection and delayed wound healing at the donor site. This occurs in fewer than 4% of cases. Delayed wound healing has been reported mostly when the incision was directly over the bony prominence of the iliac crest.

Blood loss. This is directly related to the size of the corticocancellous graft harvested and the operative time. Brazaitis and colleagues reported a case of severe retroperitoneal hemorrhage (Grey-Turner sign, or ecchymosis on the flank, indicating retroperitoneal bleeding) that resulted in the patient's death after anterior iliac crest bone grafting.

Hematoma or seroma at the donor site. Some studies have suggested that the incidence of hematoma or seroma formation is lower when drains are used; however, this has not been consistently shown in the literature. Mazock and associates reported an 8.6% incidence of uncomplicated seromas. Marx and Morales reported a 12% incidence of seroma formation and a 2% incidence of hematoma formation for the anterolateral approach.

Adynamic ileus (decreased peristalsis due to the lack of smooth muscle contraction). This is a rarely reported complication; the signs and symptoms include abdominal pain and distention, nausea and vomiting, high-pitched or absent bowel sounds, a sentinel loop of gas per abdominal radiograph, and electrolyte abnormalities.

Orthopedic complications. The risk of fractures increases with graft size (2% to 13% incidence of anterior-superior iliac spine fracture, which can be prevented by limited undermining of the anterior-superior iliac spine). Acetabular fractures and iliac crest subluxations are rare. Pelvic instability in posterior iliac crest bone grafting is due to weakening of the sacroiliac joint and ligaments and should be avoided with careful dissection.

Contour defects of the anterior ilium. This is seen especially when the anterior iliac crest is removed and stripped from the periosteum. Hypertrophic scarring can also be seen at the incision site.

Sensory nerve injury. Laurie and associates reported a 10% temporary sensory loss after anterior iliac crest bone grafting (lateral cutaneous branches of the iliohypogastric and subcostal nerves). Nkenke and associates report 20% hypoesthesia after anterior iliac crest bone grafting, seen exclusively in the lateral femoral cutaneous nerve distribution (all resolved at 1 month). Others report that the lateral cutaneous branch of the iliohypogastric nerve is the most commonly injured nerve in anterior iliac crest bone grafting. Meralgia paresthetica (burning, stabbing pain along the lateral femoral cutaneous nerve distribution) has a reported incidence of 0% to 1.8% (86% of the time the lateral femoral cutaneous nerve runs deep to the inguinal ligament and is protected; however, in 2% of patients it runs over the anterior-superior iliac spine). The medial branch of the superior cluneal nerve is 6.5 cm from the posterior-superior iliac spine and 8 cm from the midline (Mazock and associates reported a less than 3% incidence of superior cluneal nerve injury that resolved at 6 months). Others have reported an incidence of 12% to 20% of temporary sensory loss to the cluneal nerves.

Pain and gait disturbances are rare after 6 months. Hernia, arteriovenous fistula formation, and ureteral injury have been reported but are rare complications.

DISCUSSION

Mandibular reconstruction using an iliac crest bone graft is a three-stage procedure:

- Stage I: Tumor resection
- Stage II: Bony reconstruction
- Stage III: Dental implants and rehabilitation

The main goal is to optimize the recipient bed (qualitatively and quantitatively) to improve bone graft survival. Stage I includes resection of the tumor (either malignant or benign) and stabilization of the mandibular segments and occlusion with a reconstruction plate. If there is a soft tissue deficiency at the time of ablative surgery, a soft tissue flap may be used (pectoralis major, latissimus dorsi, or free fibula, iliac crest, or radial forearm flaps). If postablative radiation therapy is used for the treatment of malignant tumors, a hyperbaric oxygen protocol can be used before and after stage II to optimize the quality of the recipient bed (some authors recommend bony reconstruction after 1 year of disease-free state, because 70% of recurrences occur within the first year). Bone grafting can be done 3 months after ablation of a benign tumor or 3 months after the last surgical procedure to optimize the recipient bed (including extractions, vestibuloplasties, scar excisions, or myocutaneous flaps).

Autogenous bone, in the form of a cancellous cellular marrow (formerly called "particulate bone" and "cancellous marrow"), is the gold standard for grafting in the maxillofacial region, because it has osteogenic (new bone formation from osteoprogenitor cells), osteoconductive (new bone formation from host-derived or transplanted osteoprogenitor cells along a biologic or alloplastic framework), and osteoinductive (formation of new bone by guided differentiation of stem cell precursors into secretory osteoblasts by bone inductive proteins) properties.

The ilium provides the highest cancellous cellular density (in descending order: posterior ilium, anterior ilium, tibial plateau, mandibular symphysis). Osteocompetent cells (endosteal osteoblasts and cancellous marrow stem cells) are transferred in a viable state to the recipient bed. The transplanted bone is hypoxic (oxygen tension of 3 to 10 mm Hg), acidotic (pH 4 to 6), and rich in lactate, which acts as chemotactic agent to recruit macrophages to secrete angiogenesis factors.

Bone grafting (first 3 to 5 days). Cells survive via diffusion of nutrients from the recipient bed. Vascularity of the recipient bed is important for graft survival. This can be optimized with hyperbaric oxygen, especially in previously irradiated patients (quality), added tissue bulk if needed (quantity), removal of scar tissue (to allow diffusion of nutrients into graft), and the absence of any infection. An oxygen gradient greater than 30 mm Hg stimulates macrophage chemotaxis and initiates angiogenesis.

Beginning on day 3, the capillary buds proliferate and begin to penetrate the graft (stimulated by multiple factors, including platelet-derived growth factors, macrophage-derived angiogenesis factors, and macrophage-derived growth factors). These new capillaries bring in nutrients to support mitogenesis and osteoid production.

Bone grafting (days 10 to 14). Completion of revascularization occurs at 2 weeks. An automated shut-off mechanism occurs when the oxygen gradient is obliterated. This is a critical period for bone graft survival, because small vessels can be easily sheared by micromovement. Two- to 3-week periods of maxillomandibular fixation and empiric antibiotic coverage are recommended during this revascularization phase.

Bone grafting (weeks 3 to 4). Phase I bone (woven bone) regeneration is dependent on the osteocompetent cellular density of the graft (which is increased by compacting the graft). Phase I bone is eventually replaced by phase II bone (mature lamellar bone) because of obligatory resorption of phase I bone by osteoclasts, releasing BMP and linking resorption with new bone formation (capable of self-renewal via the endosteum and periosteum). Ideally, phase II bone replaces phase I bone in a 1:1 ratio over the next several weeks.

Alternatives to a staged cancellous marrow bone graft for reconstructing a continuity defect of the mandible include the vascularized free fibula or deep circumflex iliac artery free flap. These can be used to reconstruct both the soft and hard tissues at the time of tumor ablation (see the section Free Fibula Flap for Mandibular Reconstruction in this chapter).

rhBMP can be used as adjunct therapy. rhBMP-soaked Gelfoam sponges can be placed into a defect using various cribs (allogeneic split rib is very versatile). rhBMP has been shown to be osteoinductive, creating bone de novo by recruiting circulating mesenchymal cells and initiating their differentiation into functional osteoblasts. Human studies have failed to identify any major local toxicity or adverse systemic effects related to rhBMP-2 or rhBMP-7, but several clinical studies and case reports have reported a greater amount of local edema at rhBMP sites during the postoperative period, most likely secondary to the influx of mesenchymal cells recruited by the rhBMP graft. The use of rhBMP is contraindicated in patients who are pregnant, are allergic to any materials contained in the graft, have an infection near the surgical incision, have had a tumor removed in the area of implantation, or are skeletally immature. In larger defects requiring bone grafting, it has been reported that the combination of rhBMP with platelet-rich plasma (PRP) and crushed cancellous freeze-dried allogeneic bone provides a composite cell signal and matrix for maximum bone regeneration.

Platelet-rich plasma, another adjunct, consists of concentrated blood plasma exceedingly rich in platelets. This highly concentrated source of platelets, once activated with the addition of thrombin and calcium chloride, causes degranulation from the alpha granules to release growth factors, making it ideally suited for augmenting wound healing. Growth factors, along with cytokines, coordinate cellular chemotaxis, proliferation, angiogenesis, provisional matrix formation, epithelialization, and maturation.

The acquisition of PRP causes very little donor morbidity. Blood is easily obtained via venipuncture 30 minutes before the surgery using a conventional sterile phlebotomy

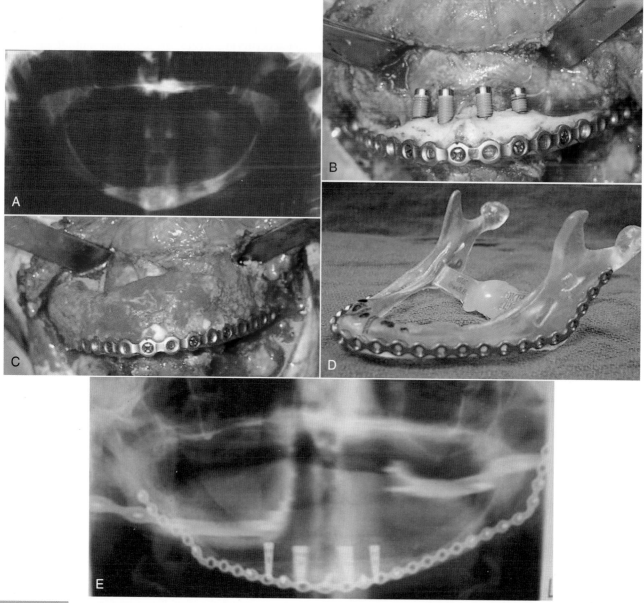

Figure 12-22 **A,** Panoramic radiograph of a severely resorbed edentulous mandible with bilateral body fractures, with severe telescoping on the left side. **B,** Four 15-mm dental implants are placed in the anterior mandible. **C,** A cancellous marrow bone graft from the posterior ilium and platelet-rich plasma are packed from ramus to ramus and around the implants. **D,** A stereolithographic model is used to prebend a low-profile, 2.3 locking reconstruction plate from angle to angle. The telescoped segment was sectioned on the model and glued together in a reduced position before the plate was bent. The position of the condyles was kept the same by fabricating glenoid fossae; the condylar heads were impressed into a plastic emesis basin filled with dental stone. **E,** Postoperative panoramic radiograph of the mandible, which was reconstructed using a modification of the tent pole technique.

technique. A small amount of whole blood is required (about 40 ml anticoagulated with citrate dextrose). Currently, two methods have been approved by the U.S. Food and Drug Administration (FDA) for preparation of PRP, essentially by gentle centrifugation separation. Pure PRP is an autologous preparation and as such avoids the risk of contagion or immunologic reaction.

The human platelet count ranges from 150,000 to 300,00/μL. The platelet count for optimal PRP is about 1 million/μL. The average platelet life span is 7 to 10 days. The complex cell signaling pathway that regulates cytokines and growth factors to promote soft tissue and bone healing is not fully understood at this time. Some studies indicate that short-term changes are beneficial for accelerating bone neoformation without producing cell cycle changes that might carry a risk of malignant transformation. Other studies show evidence of negative results from PRP, although opponents believe that these findings are based on improper preparation of or poor quality PRP. The research on PRP, in many different fields of medicine, is still in early clinical trials. Although there is much potential benefit in faster healing, it would be premature to state a definitive benefit without further clinical trials. The process of cell signaling is not fully understood, and more clinical trials are necessary

Bone marrow aspirate is another material that can be combined with rhBMP carriers or osteoconductive materials to use as a source of mesenchymal stem cells and osteoprogenitor cells. Bone marrow aspirate is most commonly harvested from the posterior-superior iliac spine; it can be harvested from the sternum, but this poses a higher risk of damaging the coronary vasculature. For harvesting of posterior iliac spine bone marrow aspirate, the patient is positioned in the prone lateral decubitus position and prepped and draped in sterile fashion. Local anesthesia is infiltrated into the area of the posterior iliac spine. The aspiration needle perforates the skin until it comes in contact with the bone, and the outer cortex then is penetrated. Bone marrow aspirate is withdrawn with a twisting motion to remove the semiliquid marrow. The contraindications to bone marrow aspiration are few; the primary contraindication is a severe bleeding disorder or skin breakdown or infection in the area of the posterior iliac spine. Bone marrow aspirate concentrate is another osteoinductive source that may have the ability to enhance early-phase bone regeneration. Further research and clinical trials are needed.

Reconstruction of a severely resorbed mandible is a unique challenge to all reconstructive surgeons (Figure 12-22, A). The severely resorbed mandible lacks sufficient bone height to accommodate dental implants 10 mm or longer, and wearing a non-implant-supported lower denture is nearly impossible (insufficient vestibular depth, mental nerve impingement, and lack of retention). These patients are also susceptible to mandibular body fractures (usually the thinnest and weakest area). The tent pole technique was introduced by Marx and has been found to be a predictable reconstructive modality for the severely resorbed mandible (height of bone 6 mm or less). With this technique, four to six 15-mm implants are placed in the anterior mandible (Figure 12-22, B), which act to "tent" up or expand the perimandibular soft tissue matrix, and immediate iliac crest bone grafting is performed from ramus to ramus around the implants via a transcutaneous approach (submental omega incision; Figure 12-22, C) to increase the bony dimensions of the mandibular body and reduce the risk of atrophic fractures. Marx presented 64 cases with a mean initial bone height of 4.8 mm. All patients maintained 15 mm of bone height and had an osseointegration rate of 99.5%, with functional rehabilitation of all patients at a mean follow-up of 4.9 years. This concept has been successfully applied to patients with a severely resorbed mandible and bilateral body fractures. In this situation, a visor incision is used, and a low-profile locking reconstruction plate is adapted from angle to angle (prebending the plate on a stereolithographic model is advantageous; Figure 12-22, D). The screws are placed in the anterior mandible (anterior to the mental nerve) in every other hole to allow placement of the implants and in the posterior body/ramus region (posterior to the inferior alveolar nerve). Autogenous bone is packed around the fractures and implants from ramus to ramus as

previously described. Figure 12-22, E, shows the postoperative panoramic radiograph.

Bibliography

Brazaitis MP, Mirvis SE, Greenberg J, et al: Severe retroperitoneal hemorrhage complicating anterior iliac bone graft acquisition, *J Oral Maxillofac Surg* 52:314-316, 1994.

Carlson ER: Mandibular bone grafts: techniques, placement, and evaluation, *Oral and Maxillofacial Surgery Knowledge Update* 1, 1994.

Carlson ER, Marx RE: Mandibular reconstruction using cancellous cellular bone grafts, *J Oral Maxillofac Surg* 54:889-897, 1996.

Catone GA, Reimer BL, McNeir D, et al: Tibial autogenous cancellous bone as an alternative donor site in maxillofacial surgery: a preliminary report, *J Oral Maxillofac Surg* 50:1258-1263, 1992.

Davies SD, Ochs MW: Bone morphogenetic proteins in craniomaxillofacial surgery, *Oral Maxillofac Surg Clin North Am* 22:17-31, 2010.

Dingman RO, Grabb WC: Surgical anatomy of the mandibular ramus of the facial nerve based on dissection of 100 facial halves, *Plast Reconstr Surg* 29:266-272, 1962.

Garcia-Martinez O, Vallecillo-Capilla MF, Ruiz C, et al: Effect of platelet-rich plasma on growth and antigenic profile of human osteoblasts and its clinical impact, *J Oral Maxillofac Surg* 70:1558-1564, 2012.

Grillon GL, Gunther SF, Connole PW: A new technique for obtaining iliac bone grafts, *J Oral Maxillofac Surg* 42:172-176, 1984.

Herford AS, King BJ, Audia F, et al: Medial approach for tibial bone graft: anatomic study and clinical technique, *J Oral Maxillofac Surg* 61:358-363, 2003.

Marx RE: Osteoradionecrosis: a new concept of its pathophysiology, *J Oral Maxillofac Surg* 41:283-288, 1983.

Marx RE: Mandibular reconstruction, *J Oral Maxillofac Surg* 51:466-479, 1993.

Marx RE: Philosophy and particulars of autogenous bone grafting, *Oral Maxillofac Surg Clin North Am* 5:599-612, 1993.

Marx RE: Biology of bone grafts, *Oral and Maxillofacial Surgery Knowledge Update* 1, 1994.

Marx RE: Clinical application of bone biology to mandibular and maxillary reconstruction, *Clin Plast Surg* 21:377-392, 1994.

Marx RE: Platelet-rich plasma: evidence to support its use, *J Oral Maxillofac Surg* 62:489-496, 2004.

Marx RE, Ames JR: The use of hyperbaric oxygen therapy in bony reconstruction of the irradiated and tissue-deficient patient, *J Oral Maxillofac Surg* 40:412-420, 1982.

Marx RE, Carlson ER, Eichstaedt RM, et al: Platelet-rich plasma: growth factor enhancement for bone grafts, *Oral Surg Oral Med Oral Pathol* 85:638-646, 1998.

Marx RE, Ehler WJ, Peleg M: Mandibular and facial reconstruction: rehabilitation of the head and neck cancer patient, *Bone* 19:(1 Suppl):59S-82S, 1996.

Marx RE, Ehler WJ, Tayapongsak P, et al: Relationship of oxygen dose to angiogenesis induction in irradiated tissue, *Am J Surg* 160:519-524, 1990.

Marx RE, Johnson RP: Studies in the radiobiology of ORN and their clinical significance, *J Oral Maxillofac Surg* 64:379-390, 1987.

Marx RE, Morales MJ: Morbidity from bone harvest in major jaw reconstruction: a randomized trial comparing the lateral anterior and posterior approaches to the ilium, *J Oral Maxillofac Surg* 48:196-203, 1988.

Marx RE, Shellenberger T, Wimsatt J, et al: Severely resorbed mandible: predictable reconstruction with soft tissue matrix expansion (tent pole) grafts, *J Oral Maxillofac Surg* 60:878-888, 2002.

Marx RE, Smith BR: An improved technique for the development of the pectoralis major myocutaneous flap, *J Oral Maxillofac Surg* 48:1168-1180, 1990.

Marx RE, Snyder RM, Kline SN: Cellular survival of human marrow during placement of marrow cancellous bone grafts, *J Oral Surg* 37:712-718, 1979.

Marx RE: Stevens MR: *Atlas of oral and extraoral bone harvesting*, Chicago, 2010, Quintessence.

Mazock JB, Schow SR, Triplett RG: Posterior iliac crest bone harvest: review of technique, complications, and use of an epidural catheter for postoperative pain control, *J Oral Maxillofac Surg* 61:1497-1503, 2003.

Nkenke E, Weisbach V, Winckler E, et al: Morbidity of harvesting of bone grafts from the iliac crest for preprosthetic augmentation procedures: a prospective study, *Int J Oral Maxillofac Surg* 33:157-163, 2004.

Sasso RC, Williams JL, Dimasi N, et al: Postoperative drains at the donor site of iliac crest bone grafts: a prospective, randomized study of morbidity at the donor site in patients who had a traumatic injury of the spine, *J Bone Joint Surg Am* 80:631-635, 1998.

Smith SE, Roukis TS: Bone and wound healing augmentation with platelet-rich plasma, *Clin Podiatr Med Surg* 26:559-588, 2009.

Stevens MR: Bone harvesting techniques, *Oral and Maxillofacial Surgery Knowledge Update* 1, 1994.

Ziarah HA, Atkinson ME: The surgical anatomy of the mandibular distribution of the facial nerve, *Br J Oral Surg* 19:159-170, 1981.

Zhong W, Sumita Y, Asahina I, et al: In vivo comparison of the bone regeneration capability of human bone marrow concentrates vs platelet-rich plasma, *PLoS One* 7(7):e40833; 2012.

CHAPTER 13

Facial Cosmetic Surgery

Editors: Shahrokh C. Bagheri and Husain Ali Khan

This chapter addresses:

- Botulinum Toxin A (Botox) Injection for Facial Rejuvenation
- Lip Augmentation
- Rhinoplasty
- Nasal Septoplasty
- Cervicofacial Rhytidectomy (Facelift)
- Upper and Lower Eyelid Blepharoplasty
- Genioplasty
- Endoscopic Browlift
- Facial Resurfacing

Facial cosmetic surgery in this section refers to soft tissue procedures of the face. In reality, modern facial cosmetic surgery includes procedures that enhance the appearance of the skeleton (orthognathic surgery), esthetic dental implantology and prosthetic rehabilitation, dermatologic procedures (skin resurfacing), hair restoration, and facial plastic surgery (Figure 13-1). Only oral and maxillofacial surgeons have the opportunity to provide all these services.

As in most cosmetic procedures, the vast majority of advances arise from the teaching of surgical skill sets to younger surgeons through operative training, textbooks, lectures, and symposia. The difficulty of developing randomized or prospective cohort studies and multicenter analysis for cosmetic procedures contributes to the progression via traditional (non-research-based) modes of teaching. Cosmetic surgery is unique among surgical specialties due to changing trends and racial and regional ethnic preferences that drive the patient's desires regarding what is considered an esthetic result.

Facial cosmetic surgery has gained tremendous popularity in the past decade. One reason for this rise in interest is the consumer's increased accessibility to information through television, the Internet, and other media sources. Also, the development of safe and effective surgical techniques, with reduced "downtime" and long-lasting, natural-appearing results, has popularized this field. Facial cosmetic surgeons must intimately understand facial anatomy, in addition to the anatomy and physiology of the aging process. Although some patients seek to rejuvenate their appearance to "turn back" the

hands of time, others are interested in altering their appearance to a more desirable social norm.

In each area of the face, several different surgical techniques have been developed to improve the appearance; each of these techniques has its own merits. It is the intent of this section to introduce readers to the concepts responsible for the evolution of facial cosmetic surgery techniques. Teaching cases involving facial cosmetic surgery include face-lift surgery, endoscopic brow lift, blepharoplasty, rhinoplasty, and genioplasty, in addition to injection of Botox and facial fillers. Each section is designed to emphasize the key points of the examination, contrasting the presenting deformity with the ideal, youthful norms. The rationale for surgical techniques to improve the outcome and achieve lasting results based on facial anatomy and the process of facial aging is described. Ultimately, the techniques used by facial cosmetic surgeons are based on the surgeon's preference and training and the clinical situation.

Both genetic and extrinsic factors contribute to the aging process. The genetic factors are fixed. Extrinsic factors can be altered and include excess sun damage, smoking, a healthy diet, and exercise. Rejuvenation of the face should be tailored to the individual by improving the patient's overall health, addressing the health of the skin, and possibly using adjunctive surgical procedures to enhance beauty. For smokers, the single most effective method of improving one's health (including the skin) is to stop smoking. For "sun lovers," it is old news: excessive sun exposure damages (burns and dries out) the skin. The goal of facial cosmetic surgery is to improve

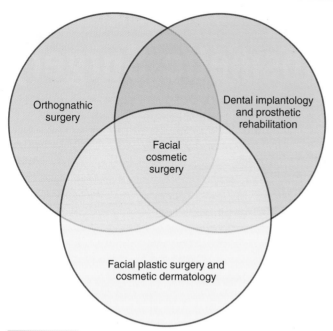

and refresh the appearance of the face without any signs of obvious surgical intervention after healing is complete.

Oral and maxillofacial surgeons are uniquely trained to recognize and manage facial deformities at all levels. Facial rejuvenation and cosmetic surgery has been described as analogous to building a house. First, the foundation must be established (skeletal surgery). Next, the framing and walls must be built (soft tissue surgery). Finally, the paint must be applied (skin resurfacing). With proper understanding and training, facial cosmetic surgery can be easily incorporated into the oral and maxillofacial surgery (OMFS) practice.

Botulinum Toxin A (Botox) Injection for Facial Rejuvenation

Eric P. Holmgren and Shahrokh C. Bagheri

CC

A 44-year-old Caucasian woman presents to your office for consultation regarding the wrinkles on her forehead. (The majority of patients seeking facial rejuvenation are females; however, interest in these procedures is growing in the male population.)

HPI

During an orthognathic surgery consultation for her daughter several months ago, the patient noticed the Botox pamphlets in the waiting room at your office (unlike other branches of OMFS, a busy cosmetic surgery practice is usually heavily dependent on marketing and advertisement). The patient states that "these lines" have recently appeared on her forehead and that she is tired of looking as if she is "scowling" or "frowning." Her husband has mentioned to her that the wrinkles make her appear "angry." Several of her friends have had satisfactory results with Botox injections for glabellar and periorbital lines. She has many questions regarding the safety and outcome of Botox injections for elimination of wrinkles.

PMHX/PDHX/MEDICATIONS/ALLERGIES/SH/FH

The patient does not have any known medical conditions. Specifically, she has no known history of neuromuscular diseases, including myasthenia gravis, amyotrophic lateral sclerosis, multiple sclerosis, Eaton-Lambert syndrome, or other motor neuron–related disorders (despite the absence of specific studies, Botox should be used cautiously in individuals with neuromuscular disorders due to potential exacerbation of any preexisting conditions). There is no significant family history of neuromuscular disorders.

The patient currently is not taking any aminoglycoside antibiotic or other medications that could interfere with neuromuscular transmission. (It is recommended that Botox injections be delayed or avoided in patients taking aminoglycosides.) She is not taking aspirin, a nonsteroidal antiinflammatory drug (NSAID), or other medication that can interfere with coagulation or platelet function (such drugs increase the risk of hematoma formation and bruising). She smokes one-half pack of cigarettes per day (smoking is not a contraindication to Botox injection).

There is no history of allergies to human albumin or of any previous adverse reactions to Botox. (Botox manufactured after 1997 has a lower albumin concentration and therefore a presumably lower risk of clinical antigenicity.) The patient currently is not pregnant or lactating. (Botox is contraindicated during nursing or pregnancy; it is classified by the U.S. Food and Drug Administration [FDA] as Pregnancy Category C, meaning that its safety profile during pregnancy has not been studied. It is unknown whether the toxin can cross the placenta or is excreted during lactation. However, the localized application of the drug would suggest the safety of application during pregnancy or nursing).

EXAMINATION

General. The patient is a thin, athletic, well-dressed female. She wears an extensive amount of makeup, which masks some of her facial features of aging. She wears her hair in a style that reduces the visibility of the forehead lines (subtle observations about appearance may be the key to successful patient rapport).

Maxillofacial exam. There are no pustules or signs of active dermatologic infections or pathology in the facial region (injections are contraindicated if an active infection exists at the injection site). There is no marked facial asymmetry or hypertrophic facial scarring (thick skin or a susceptibility to hypertrophic scars may be a relative contraindication to injections). No significant eyebrow ptosis is noted. (This is important for injection around the eyes or the forehead. Impairing the functioning of the frontalis can also lower the brow position from unopposed muscle action, resulting in an unappealing outcome. Similarly, large amounts of Botox injected around the eye can diffuse toward the levator palpebrae muscle, causing impaired eyelid closure. The degree of preoperative ptosis can be documented for postoperative comparison.)

Several prominent horizontal forehead wrinkles (due to frontalis muscle action) are present at rest (Figure 13-2, *A*) and are accentuated with animation (Figure 13-2, *B*). Multiple hyperdynamic rhytids (lines on the face) are seen lateral to the eye and are most pronounced on animation (orbicularis oculi region, also known as "crow's feet"; Figure 13-3, *C*). At rest, fine vertical glabellar furrows are present, and upon animation and frowning, the glabella muscle bulge becomes significantly prominent (the corrugator muscle is responsible for the vertical glabellar furrows, and the procerus muscle is responsible for the horizontal glabellar furrows). A glabellar spread test reveals that the glabellar lines are substantially decreased when physically manipulated or spread apart. (This

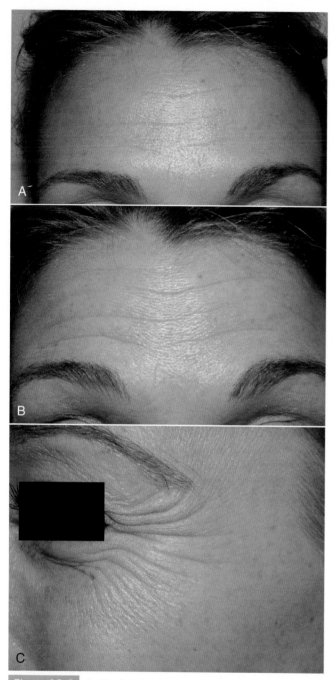

Figure 13-2 **A,** Forehead wrinkles secondary to frontalis muscle functioning. **B,** Forehead lines accentuated during frontalis function. **C,** Hyperdynamic periorbital lines (crow's feet) accentuated with animation.

is a good indication that the muscle and its overlying soft tissue are the etiology of the lines. During the physical exam, it is important to distinguish between dynamic and static wrinkles. Botox decreases dynamic wrinkles because of its effect on muscles. Static wrinkles may be treated using soft tissue fillers to decrease skin laxity at rest.)

No significant horizontal lines are present at the nasal root ("bunny lines"), and no prominent perioral vertical ("lipstick") rhytids are visible.

Intraoral exam. No abnormalities/lesions are noted (it is important to conduct an oral cancer screening exam, especially in a patient with a history of smoking).

Neck exam. No cervicomental lymphadenopathy is seen (enlarged lymph nodes are indicative of ongoing pathologic, inflammatory, or infectious processes).

IMAGING

Standard facial photographic documentation of the areas to be treated is recommended (but not essential) for Botox injection. Comparisons of preinjection and postinjection photographs may be important for future dosing and for surgeon education toward optimal results.

LABS

No routine laboratory tests are indicated. Patients taking large doses of anticoagulants are at risk for small hematoma formation at the injection site. The treating surgeon should inquire about any coagulation studies to assess the risk and to educate the patient about this potential temporary yet undesired effect.

ASSESSMENT

Multiple areas of hyperfunctioning facial muscles and signs of aging are present involving the periorbital, glabellar, and horizontal forehead regions. The patient desires injection of Botox for effacement of the wrinkles associated with the periorbital and forehead regions. (Although there may be many findings amendable to cosmetic surgery, the assessment and treatment are dictated by the patient's desires.)

TREATMENT

After a complete discussion of the procedure, risks, and alternatives, the patient signed the informed consent (which addressed all the complications listed later). One hundred units of Botulinum Toxin A was reconstituted with 3.3 ml of unpreserved normal saline. (According to a study by Alam and colleagues in 2002, the use of preservative-containing normal saline is less painful than preservative-free saline. However, this is not in accordance with the manufacturer's recommendations.) Botox is available in a sealed vacuum container that allows for easy reconstitution with saline. The resulting solution provides 3 units per 0.1 ml, or 15 units per 0.5 ml. Botox should be reconstituted gently (shaking and trauma to the toxin can diminish its potency) with a 21-gauge needle and then gently drawn into a tuberculin syringe. The syringe can be used with a short 30-gauge needle.

The patient was seated upright, close to a 60-degree position. After the injection sites had been prepared with alcohol, the patient was asked to frown (or lower the eyebrows) to highlight the regions of maximum muscular contraction. Six injection sites were identified to inject the frontalis muscle. To minimize the chance for blepharoptosis, the injections were performed at least 1 cm above both the central eyebrow and the supraorbital ridge. (It is important to avoid injections on the forehead lateral to the lateral canthus, to prevent inhibition of temporalis function. The goal of forehead injections is not to completely eliminate the frontalis muscle action, because this can cause undesirable brow ptosis.) Ice packs were applied immediately prior to injection to blunt the pain response from needle injection. The needle was inserted into the belly of the muscle, aspiration was performed, and Botox was then slowly injected. After the injections no manipulation was performed, and an ice pack was allowed to rest on the area (manipulation can enhance diffusion into other muscles, affecting the levator palpebrae superioris and causing blepharoptosis, especially with injections near the eyelid). Attention was then turned to the orbicularis oculi region. After the area had been prepared with alcohol, 9 units total was injected into three sites, on each side just below the skin (to minimize diffusion in this area). A total of 36 units was used for the forehead and crow's feet regions (18 units in the forehead and 18 units total for both eyes).

Ice was allowed to rest on the injection sites for as long as the patient tolerated. The patient was instructed to remain upright for at least 4 hours and was allowed to apply makeup 4 hours after injection (to minimize manipulation and thus diffusion of the toxin). She was allowed to resume exercise the next day. She was instructed to expect a noticeable effect in 3 to 4 days, with maximum benefit in 30 days (Figure 13-3). Follow-up was scheduled in 1 week. The areas can be reinjected after a minimum of 3 months has elapsed (earlier injections can increase the chance of antibodies developing).

COMPLICATIONS

Many patients have been safely treated with Botox since its introduction. The complications of treatment with Botox include:

- Undesired effect (can be related to the patient's expectations or rate of metabolism, dosing, anatomic variations, or inadequate site of injection).
- Short duration of the desired effect.
- Postinjection bruising: This is most common in the periorbital region and can be minimized by avoiding aspirin or NSAIDs for 7 to 14 days prior to injection.
- Blepharoptosis: The reported occurrence is 1% to 2% of periorbital injections. This can be treated with an α_2-adrenergic agonist (apraclonidine 0.5% eye drops, to be used 30 minutes before social situations), which stimulates Mueller's muscle, resulting in hours of transient lid opening.
- Transient headaches, pain, edema, and erythema at the injection site.
- Formation of neutralizing antibodies: This has been reported to occur with repeat injections within 1 month of the previous injections; it also was reported with doses greater than 100 units per treatment session. This has not been reported for the cosmetic use of Botox;

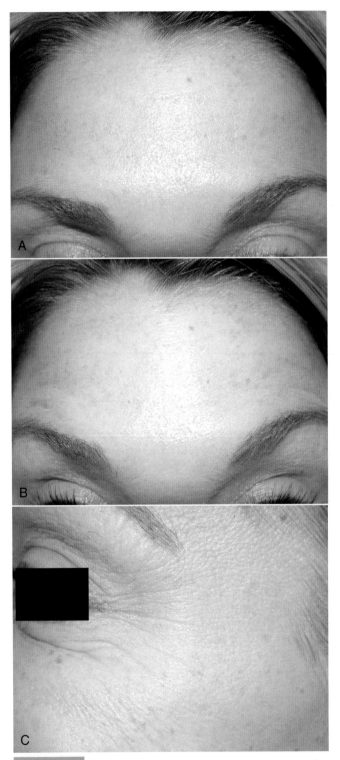

Figure 13-3 **A,** One month postoperative view at rest, showing significant reduction of horizontal forehead lines. **B,** One month postoperative view upon brow elevation, showing significant reduction of horizontal forehead lines with animation. **C,** One month postoperative view of the lateral periorbital lines (crow's feet) seen during animation.

however, it is recommended that a period of at least 3 months elapse between injections.

* Hematoma formation at the injection site.

DISCUSSION

Botox is a formulation of botulinum toxin A purified neurotoxin complex, produced from fermentation of the gram-positive spore-forming bacteria *Clostridium botulinum* type A. When injected into striated muscle, it produces a dose-dependent local muscle weakness by preventing the release of acetylcholine from the nerve terminal at the neuromuscular junction (chemical deinnervation). The action involves a four-step process that culminates with the cleavage of the 25kD synaptosome-associated protein (SNAP), which is essential for the exocytosis of acetylcholine. The paralytic effect is temporary, because there is a gradual recovery of the activity of the nerve terminal over 3 to 6 months. The unit of measurement for Botox is derived from work with mice. One unit of Botox is the lethal dose in 50% of mice (LD_{50}). The LD_{50} in humans is 2,500 to 3,000 units (40 units/kg). Dosing for the clinical effects of Botox can vary among individuals. Thicker muscles and male patients often require more Botox units to achieve the desired effect.

Unopened vials of Botox can be stored for 24 months in a refrigerator (2° to 8°C). Opinions vary regarding its shelf life, once reconstituted, beyond the manufacturer's recommendation of only 4 hours. Studies have suggested no clinical difference for up to 6 weeks after reconstitution, but others have noticed diminished potency beyond 48 hours.

As of this writing, FDA approval for the use of Botox includes treatments for dystonia, torticollis, blepharospasm, strabismus, wrinkles caused by the procerus and corrugator muscles (glabellar region), and severe primary axillary hyperhidrosis in patients younger than 65 years of age. However, common off-label uses are numerous and include hyperhidrosis for the palms, Frey's syndrome, migraine headaches, myofascial pain, bruxism, masseter hypertrophy, chronic temporomandibular dislocation, limb spasticity, and platysmal banding, among many others.

In the oral and maxillofacial surgery office, injections are commonly administered in the upper face region, such as the glabella, lateral canthal lines (crow's feet), and forehead (frontalis). Selective brow raising techniques can be done. By injecting the lateral orbicularis muscle without injecting the frontalis in select areas, the brow peak can rise as a result of unopposed frontalis muscle action. Noncosmetic injections for trigger pain regions of the temporalis and masseter muscle also can be performed. Lower face injections to treat "lipstick lines" should be reserved for experienced surgeons and may cause oral incompetence. Fillers, such as a non-animal-sourced hyaluronic acid (Restylane [Medicis Pharmaceutical Corporation, Bridgewater New Jersey]), can be used concomitantly with Botox to augment static wrinkles. Patient satisfaction has been shown to be increased with the use of these two techniques.

Bibliography

Alam M, Dover JS, Arndt KA: Pain associated with injection of botulinum A exotoxin reconstituted using isotonic sodium chloride with and without preservative: a double-blind, randomized controlled trial, *Arch Dermatol* 138(4):510-514, 2002.

Carruthers J, Carruthers A: A prospective, randomized, parallel group study analyzing the effect of BTX-A (Botox) and nonanimal sourced hyaluronic acid (NASHA, Restylane) in combination compared with NASHA (Restylane) alone in severe glabellar rhytides in adult female subjects: treatment of severe glabellar rhytides with a hyaluronic acid derivative compared with the derivative and BTX-A, *Dermatol Surg* 29:802-809, 2003.

Connor MS, Karlis V, Ghali GE: Management of the aging forehead: a review, *Oral Surg Oral Med Oral Pathol Oral Radiol Endod* 95(6):642-648, 2003.

Frampton J, Easthope S: Botulinum toxin A (Botox Cosmetic): a review of its use in the treatment of glabellar frown lines, *Am J Clin Dermatol* 4(10):709-725, 2003.

Freund B, Schwarz M, Symington JM: Botulinum toxin: new treatment for temporomandibular disorders, *Br J Oral Maxillofac Surg* 38:466-471, 2000.

Henriques Castro W, Santiago Gomez R, da Silva Oliveira J, et al: Botulinum toxin type A in the management of masseter muscle hypertrophy, *J Oral Maxillofac Surg* 63(1):20-24, 2005.

Hexsel DM, De Almeida AT, Rutowitsch M, et al: Multicenter, double-blind study of the efficacy of injections with botulinum toxin type A reconstituted up to six consecutive weeks before application, *Dermatol Surg* 29(5):523-529, 2003.

Kane M: Botox injections for lower facial rejuvenation, *Oral Maxillofac Surgery Clin North Am* 17(1):41-49, 2005.

Lorenc ZP, Kenkel JM, Fagien S, et al: A review of onabotulinumtoxin A (Botox), *Aesthet Surg J* 33(1 Suppl):9S-12S, 2013 (doi: 10.1177/1090820X12474629).

Niamtu J III: Botulinum toxin A: a review of 1,085 oral and maxillofacial patient treatments, *J Oral Maxillofac Surg* 61(3):317-324, 2003.

Rohrich R, Janis J: Botox for the treatment of dynamic and hyperkinetic facial lines and furrows: adjunctive use in facial aesthetic surgery, *Plast Reconstr Surg* 112(5 Suppl):53S-54S, 2003.

Solish N, Benohanian A, Kowalski JW: Canadian Dermatology Study Group on Health-Related Quality of Life in Primary Axillary Hyperhidrosis: prospective open-label study of botulinum toxin type A in patients with axillary hyperhidrosis—effects on functional impairment and quality of life, *Dermatol Surg* 31(4):405-413, 2005.

Trindade De Almeida AR, Kadunc BV, Di Chiacchio N, et al: Foam during reconstitution does not affect the potency of botulinum toxin type A, *Dermatol Surg* 29(5):530-531, 2003.

Vartanian AJ, Dayan SH: Facial rejuvenation using botulinum toxin A: review and updates, *Facial Plast Surg* 20(1):11-19, 2004.

Lip Augmentation

Shahrokh C. Bagheri and Chris Jo

CC

A 30-year-old, healthy Caucasian woman presents for consultation for upper lip augmentation. She complains that her upper lip is "thin" and does not match her lower lip. She desires a "mild" augmentation of her upper lip and specifically does not want to have an excessively "pouty" upper lip.

HPI

The patient has no previous history of facial filler for soft tissue augmentation. She has recently gone through a divorce and desires to improve her looks for the new year. She appears to have realistic expectations and is well educated, via the Internet, about the different products available on the market. She has had previous breast augmentation surgery, with satisfactory results.

PMHX/PDHX/MEDICATIONS/ALLERGIES/SH/FH

Noncontributory.

EXAMINATION

Maxillofacial. The patient does not have lymphadenopathy. Her facial skin is without any lesions, and her oral mucous membranes are moist. Oral hygiene is excellent. Nasal and maxillary dental midlines are aligned.

Evaluation of volume (height, fullness), projection, vermillion exposure, and definition of the lips is important in preparation for lip augmentation procedures.

Lips. The lips are symmetrical (Figure 13-4). The upper lip to lower lip height ratio is about 1:2 (in general, an

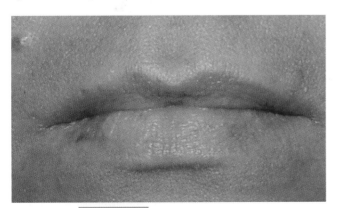

Figure 13-4   Lips before treatment.

aesthetic upper lip is one third of the total lip mass, and the lower lip represents two thirds of the total lip height). The upper lip is relatively deficient in volume compared with the lower lip. Cupid's bow and the vermillion border are well defined, with good profile projection. Four millimeters of central incisors is visible at rest (normal range is 3 to 4 mm for females and 2 to 3 mm for males), with no gingival show on smiling (no "gummy" smile). She does not exhibit lip incompetence. The nasolabial angle is within normal limits (100 degrees ± 10 degrees).

Normal esthetic parameters for the lips are differently defined among persons of different races and cultures; therefore, "normal" parameters are not well established. As in any cosmetic procedure, the patient's desires and expectations, along with fashionable trends emphasized by the media and celebrities, play a major role in the patient's and surgeon's decisions regarding cosmetic intervention.

IMAGING

Standard frontal facial photographs and close-up views of the lips are routine. Profile and oblique preoperative and postoperative close-up views of the lips may also be helpful.

LABS

Lab tests are not indicated unless there is a known history of coagulopathies (increased risk of hematoma, bruising, and erythema at the injection site). Unlike collagen, hyaluronic acid is identical among species, making it highly biocompatible and thus eliminating the need for allergy testing (see Complications).

ASSESSMENT

Patient desires upper lip augmentation to enhance both definition and volume.

TREATMENT

Restylane is a stabilized, lower-molecular-weight, partially cross-linked hyaluronic acid that has been approved by the U.S. Food and Drug Administration (FDA) for soft tissue augmentation. It is created via bacterial fermentation from streptococcal species. This material has been used in Europe and Canada since 1996 and received FDA approval for use in the United States in 2003. Hylaform

Gel is a hyaluronic acid extract derived from rooster combs.

Bilateral infraorbital nerve blocks are given to achieve upper lip anesthesia without local infiltration in the areas to be augmented to avoid temporary tissue distortion secondary to the injection. The white roll is augmented on the upper lip, starting at the midline and following the contour of Cupid's bow to enhance both definition and projection. The material is injected in a linear threading fashion as the needle is withdrawn away from the midline via two or three injection sites. The upper lips are intermittently massaged to achieve uniform distribution of the filler. The contralateral side is injected in a similar fashion. The body of the lip is also injected in a similar fashion to achieve volume enhancement of the lips. For the current patient, a total of one syringe was used for the upper lip (Figure 13-5).

Many surgeons actively involve the patient by allowing her to occasionally evaluate the lips in a mirror to achieve the desired effect and to give the patient a sense of participation in the treatment.

Other materials and techniques used for lip augmentation include AlloDerm (cadaveric acellular dermal collagen framework), polytetrafluoroethylene, autologous fat transfer/injection (harvested from periumbilical right medial thigh fat), injectable collagen, or a strip of superficial musculoaponeurotic system (SMAS) when concurrent facelift procedures are performed.

COMPLICATIONS

The ideal facial augmentation material should be inert, biocompatible, and safe and should remain stable over time. Bovine collagen has dominated the facial filler market until recently. The main concern associated with it is the risk of severe allergy, requiring allergy skin testing before injection. The use of autologous collagen harvested from the patient's own skin eliminated the need for allergy testing, but it needs to be harvested, which involves associated morbidity and limited supply. Autologous fat also eliminates the need for skin testing, but it also involves harvesting. This may be desirable if simultaneous liposuction is being performed. Dermalogen (Collagenesis; Beverly, Massachusetts) is human collagen prepared from human donor tissue processed from cadavers. This material undergoes extensive screening for infectious

agents and is irradiated before use. Skin testing is not required by the FDA.

Several formulations for hyaluronic acid are available for injection into soft tissue, but not all are FDA approved. Olenius conducted the first clinical study to evaluate biodegradable implants. He evaluated 113 subjects after injection with partially cross-linked hyaluronic acid and reported no allergic reactions and infrequent side effects; these were limited to localized erythema and swelling related to superficial placement of the material, small hematoma formation, and lumpiness secondary to uneven injection. In 2001, Lowe and associates studied 709 patients injected with hyaluronic acid preparations. They reported a 0.42% incidence of delayed inflammatory skin reactions that started about 8 weeks postinjection. A review of worldwide data on 144,000 patients treated in 1999 indicated that the major reaction to injectable hyaluronic acid was localized hypersensitivity, occurring in approximately 1 of every 1,400 patients treated. This study concluded that hypersensitivity to non-animal-source hyaluronic acid gel is the major adverse event and is most likely secondary to impurities of bacterial fermentation. More recent data indicate that the incidence of hypersensitivity appears to be declining after the introduction of a more purified hyaluronic acid raw material.

Knowledge of vascular anatomy is essential. Case reports have noted that intraarterial injection of hyaluronic acid can cause localized skin changes and autologous fat embolization, resulting in ocular and cerebral ischemia.

DISCUSSION

A common question asked by patients is the duration of the augmentation. In the study by Olenius, injection of partially cross-linked hyaluronic acid demonstrated the greatest degree of effectiveness at 2 weeks (98%), with subsequent decline at 3 months (82%), 6 months (69%), and 1 year (66%). Although the effects of this filler are not permanent, repeat injections may require smaller amounts of filler to achieve similar results.

It is essential that surgeons do not apply a single method of augmentation for every patient who presents to the office. Accurate diagnosis of the facial deformity or the desired effect is the key to satisfactory outcomes. A thorough knowledge of multiple techniques, in addition to the safety profiles of the existing materials and their clinical effects, is essential for successful soft tissue augmentation.

Bibliography

Danesh-Meyer HV, Savino PJ, Sergott RC: Case reports and small case series: ocular and cerebral ischemia following facial injection of autologous fat, *Arch Ophthalmol* 119(5):777-778, 2001.

Douglas RS, Donsoff I, Cook T, et al: Collagen fillers in facial aesthetic surgery, *Facial Plast Surg* 20(2):117-123, 2004.

Duranti F, Salti G, Bovani B, et al: Injectable hyaluronic acid gel for soft tissue augmentation: a clinical and histological study, *Dermatol Surg* 24(12):1317-1325, 1998.

Fagien S: Facial soft-tissue augmentation with injectable autologous and allogeneic human tissue collagen matrix (Autologen and

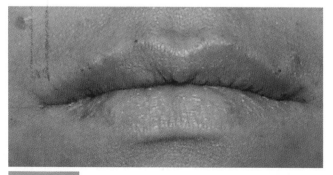

Figure 13-5   Lips after upper lip augmentation with Restylane.

Dermalogen), *Plast Reconstr Surg* 105(1):362-373, discussion, 374-375; 2000.

Friedman PM, Mafong EA, Kauvar AN, et al: Safety data of injectable nonanimal stabilized hyaluronic acid gel for soft tissue augmentation, *Dermatol Surg* 28(6):491-494, 2002.

Lowe NJ, Maxwell CA, Lowe P, et al: Hyaluronic acid skin fillers: adverse reactions and skin testing, *Am Acad Dermatol* 45(6):930-933, 2001.

Niamtu J: New lip and wrinkle fillers, *Oral Maxillofac Surg Clin North Am* 17(1):17-28, 2005.

Olenius M: The first clinical study using a new biodegradable implant for the treatment of lips, wrinkles, and folds, *Aesthetic Plast Surg* 22(2):97-101, 1998.

Schanz S, Schippert W, Ulmer A, et al: Arterial embolization caused by injection of hyaluronic acid (Restylane), *Br J Dermatol* 146(5):928-929, 2002.

Rhinoplasty

Shahrokh C. Bagheri and Chris Jo

CC

A 24-year-old woman presents for consultation regarding her nose. She explains that it is too bulky and that she does not like the "bump" on it.

HPI

The patient works in the beauty industry but has been aware of the shape of her nose since college. Several years ago, she noticed the prominence of her nasal dorsum and the bulky mid dorsal area when she looked in the mirror. In addition, she complains of difficulty breathing through her right nostril. She reports breathing better through the left nostril, and when she pulls her right cheek inferiorly and laterally, she experiences improved airflow through the right nostril (positive Cottle's sign).

PMHX/PDHX/MEDICATIONS/ALLERGIES/SH/FH

The patient has no previous history of septoplasty, cosmetic rhinoplasty, or nasal trauma. (Previous nasal surgery is particularly important, because the anatomy may be altered. If the septal cartilage has been previously harvested or adjusted and there is a need for cartilage grafting, ear or rib cartilage can be used). She denies any seasonal or drug allergies (it is important to note symptoms of allergic rhinitis or recent upper respiratory tract infections). There is no history of psychiatric disorders or treatment (patients with certain psychiatric disorders may not be candidates for elective cosmetic procedures). There is no history of smoking or cocaine or other drug use (cocaine-induced vasoconstriction compromises wound healing and increases the risk of septal perforation). She also has no history of granulomatous or autoimmune disorders (e.g., Wegener granulomatosis, which can affect the nasal mucosa) or of epistaxis (a prior history of unexplained epistaxis should be investigated for blood dyscrasias, such as von Willebrand disease).

EXAMINATION

Examination of the nose for cosmetic surgery has to include both cosmetic and functional factors. Cosmetic evaluation should encompass the entire face, but for planning purposes, the nose can be examined in five regions:

1. Skin
2. Radix
3. Dorsum
4. Tip
5. Nostrils and alar base

Each region is evaluated in three dimensions. The functional aspects of the nose (mainly breathing) require a careful endonasal speculum examination. Correction of cosmetic parameters may cause or exacerbate nasal function (e.g., narrowing the nose may compromise breathing).

General. The patient is a well-developed and well-nourished woman with realistic expectations and a knowledge of nasal cosmetic surgery.

Maxillofacial. There is no evidence of upper respiratory infection (no postnasal drip, discharge, or erythema of mucous membranes).

Examination of the Nose

Skin. The skin meets the criteria of Fitzpatrick type II with no evidence of acne or excessive sebaceous secretions. The skin and soft tissue envelope have adequate thickness over the dorsum and tip (Figure 13-6).

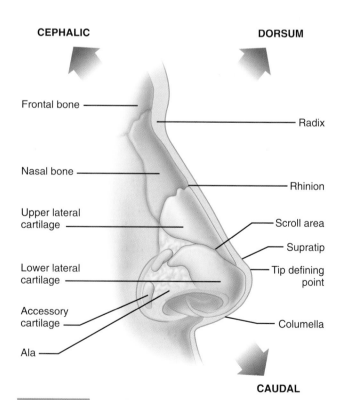

CEPHALIC · DORSUM

Frontal bone — Radix

Nasal bone — Rhinion

Upper lateral cartilage — Scroll area

— Supratip

Lower lateral cartilage — Tip defining point

Accessory cartilage —

Ala — Columella

CAUDAL

Figure 13-6 Anatomy of nasal structures as seen from profile.

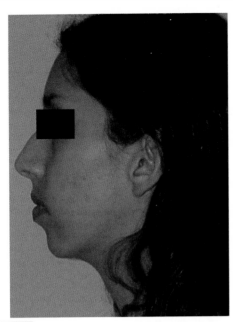

Preoperative facial profile before septorhinoplasty.

Table 13-1	Anatomic Regions of the Nose and Their Main Characteristics for Cosmetic and Functional Rhinoplasty
Anatomic Region	**Main Characteristics**
Radix	Location, size
Dorsum	Width, size, symmetry
Tip	Volume, projection, shape, definition, rotation, width
Nasal base	Alar base shape, nostril size, columellar anatomy, alar width, symmetry
Septum	Deviation, perforation
Turbinates	Size, obstruction of airflow, inflammation

From Bagheri SC, Bell RB, Khan HA (eds): *Current therapy in oral and maxillofacial surgery,* St Louis, 2012, Saunders.

Radix. The soft tissue nasion is between the lash and crease line of the upper lid (within normal limits). The nasofacial angle is 34 degrees (within normal limits).

Dorsum. There is a prominent dorsal hump on the profile view (Figure 13-7). The mid dorsum is rectangular in shape on the frontal view. The nasal dorsum is wide but symmetrical.

Tip. The tip is slightly bulbous with prominent lower lateral cartilages. The nasolabial angle is 100 degrees (normal is approximately 105 degrees).

Nasal base. There is adequate width (coincident with the medial canthus). The nostrils are symmetrical, with no significant nostril show or hanging columella.

Speculum exam. There is linear deviation of the quadrangular cartilage (nasal septum) to the right and partial blockage of the right internal nasal valve (the angle formed by the nasal septum and upper lateral cartilage). There is compensatory inferior turbinate hypertrophy on the left, with mild erythema of the nasal mucosa and turbinates.

The different anatomic regions of the nose and their main characteristics for cosmetic and functional rhinoplasty are shown in Table 13-1.

IMAGING

Preoperative and serial postoperative photoimaging is mandatory for cosmetic procedures. Standard photography for cosmetic rhinoplasty includes frontal, right and left lateral, right and left oblique, and basal ("worm's eye") views. Photographs should be standardized to allow optimal preoperative and postoperative comparisons.

Computed tomography (CT) is not necessary for cosmetic rhinoplasty, but it can be used in selected cases to delineate the severity of septal deviation and identify sinus pathology.

LABS

No routine laboratory testing is indicated for cosmetic rhinoplasty unless dictated by the medical history.

ASSESSMENT

Patient desires cosmetic rhinoplasty: prominent dorsal hump on profile; wide nasal dorsum on frontal view ("boxy dorsum"); bulbous tip as seen on the frontal view, with good projection; deviated septum with compromised right nasal valve function.

It is important to assess both the cosmetic and the functional aspects of the diagnosis.

TREATMENT

Treatment is dependent not only on the physical findings (diagnosis) but, more important, also on the patient's desires and expectations. Many of the fundamental principles of cosmetic rhinoplasty have evolved since the popularization of this procedure in the past 40 years. Initially rhinoplasty was primarily performed as a reductive procedure, focused on removal of the dorsum and cartilage excision. More recently cartilage grafting and advanced suturing techniques have caused a paradigm shift toward tissue preservation and anatomic form. The concept of "balanced" rhinoplasty refers to alterations of nasal anatomy by reduction, augmentation, or alteration to achieve the anatomic harmony between the radix, dorsum, tip, and alar base. The surgical access to the nasal structures has also seen the dramatic popularization of the open approach.

The current patient complains of a large nose and difficulty breathing through the right nostril. Treatment should address both the esthetic and functional disturbances. Cosmetic alterations frequently exacerbate functional parameters. The surgical plan must be developed preoperatively, based on the patient's function and cosmetic desires and needs.

The surgical approach (endonasal versus open rhinoplasty) depends on the complexity of the case and the experience and

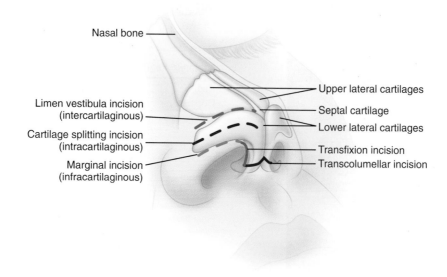

Nasal bone

Upper lateral cartilages

Limen vestibula incision
(intercartilaginous)

Septal cartilage

Lower lateral cartilages

Cartilage splitting incision
(intracartilaginous)

Transfixion incision

Marginal incision
(infracartilaginous)

Transcolumellar incision

Figure 13-8 Common sites of incisions for rhinoplasty.

preference of the surgeon. Incisions for endonasal rhinoplasty include the following (Figure 13-8):

- Intercartilaginous or limen vestibula incision (between the upper and lower lateral cartilages)
- Intracartilaginous or cartilage-splitting incision (through the upper aspect of the lateral crura of the lower lateral cartilage)
- Infracartilaginous or marginal incision (on the inferior aspect of the lower lateral cartilage)

Standard incisions for approaching the nasal septum include the transfixion incision (through the membranous septum) and the Killian incision (incision over the cartilaginous septum). Most simple rhinoplasties can be done via an endonasal approach. However, if complex tip work or spreader grafts are required, an open transcollumellar incision allows greater access and visibility than the cartilage delivery approach (Figure 13-9). The scar from this incision is usually not visible several months after the procedure.

For any rhinoplasty surgery, a treatment plan should be outlined to address the patient's desires within the confines of the surgeon's ability to achieve the outcome and without compromise of nasal function. The following surgical plan was created for the current patient.

Open Septorhinoplasty

1. Septoplasty and harvest of septal cartilage
2. Submucous resection and turbinate outfracture
3. Transcolumellar incision for access to the dorsum, septum, and nasal valve
4. Reduction of the nasal dorsum (rasp or osteotome reduction)
5. Nasal tip refinement (resection and/or suture techniques can be used, based on the surgeon's preference)
6. Bilateral spreader grafts (from septum) for opening of the nasal valves

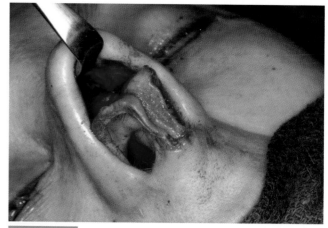

Figure 13-9 Exposure of nose with an open rhinoplasty incision. *(From Bagheri SC, Bell RB, Khan HA (eds): Current therapy in oral and maxillofacial surgery, St Louis, 2012, Saunders.)*

7. Bilateral low to high nasal osteotomies for narrowing of the dorsum and closure of the "open book" deformity

Under general anesthesia, lidocaine with epinephrine was injected along the nasal septum, columella, dorsum, and nostril areas, and adequate time was given for vasoconstriction (some surgeons limit the amount of subcutaneous local anesthetic injected to minimize tissue distortion, for improved intraoperative assessment). A septoplasty and septal cartilage harvest were performed via a left hemitransfixion incision (a minimum 1-cm strut of dorsal and caudal cartilage should be left intact for adequate support), followed by submucosal resection with lateral displacement of the right inferior turbinate. Careful attention was given to maintaining adequate dorsal and columellar cartilage, to avoid a saddle nose deformity. An open rhinoplasty (inverted V transcolumellar with infracartilaginous incisions) was performed, with subsequent resection of 4 mm of the cephalic margin of the lower lateral cartilages (cephalic trim or volumetric reduction). Domal equalization and creation sutures were used to provide tip definition (some surgeons may elect to split the domes). Reduction of the bony dorsum was performed using a rasp, followed by excision of the cartilaginous dorsum using fine scissors. Strut and shield grafts were not used in this patient (although some authors suggest that strut and shield grafts be used in most patients). The nasal tip was supported by suturing the medial crura of the lower lateral cartilages to the nasal septum (a columellar strut can be used to achieve greater tip projection). The septum was disarticulated from the upper lateral cartilages bilaterally, and a spreader graft was placed (to increase the internal nasal valve). Finally, low-to-high lateral nasal osteotomies were performed, and the nasal complex was fractured in to close the open "book deformity" and address the width of the dorsum. Figure 13-10 shows the postoperative patient profile.

COMPLICATIONS

Cosmetic rhinoplasty is a difficult procedure to master. It is imperative to recognize complications early and not to ignore a potentially correctable finding. Management of a dissatisfied patient can be challenging, but foresight, honesty, and a caring approach frequently aid in resolving an unsatisfactory outcome. These unsatisfactory outcomes may include a polly beak, saddle nose, open roof deformity, undercorrection, dorsal irregularities, nasal tip deformities, or asymmetrical dorsum/tip. An overall revision rhinoplasty rate of 5% to 15% has been reported. Other reported complications include hemorrhage (1% to 4%), infection (0% to 3%), septal perforation (0.1%), skin sloughing (rare), and nasal obstruction (1% to 10%).

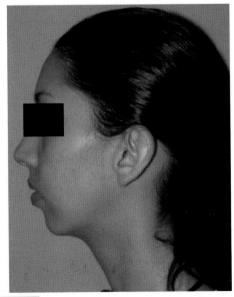

Figure 13-10   Postoperative facial profile after septorhinoplasty.

Patients undergoing open rhinoplasty should be informed about the postoperative anesthesia or profound hypoesthesia of the nasal tip. This is usually temporary but can take 6 months to 1 year to resolve.

DISCUSSION

Primary cosmetic rhinoplasty is the surgical manipulation of a previously unoperated nose for esthetic enhancement. A history of septoplasty in the absence of any cosmetic nasal alterations may change the treatment plan related to septal harvest, yet the procedure remains a primary cosmetic rhinoplasty. This is distinguished from revision and reconstructive rhinoplasty. In a revision procedure, the surgeon attempts to correct or further modify a previously operated nose. A revision procedure may be indicated if the patient and surgeon agree that the expected or planned results were not obtained from the primary procedure or if results are compromised due to complications. This is further distinguished from a repeat, or "re-do," rhinoplasty, in which a patient presents after a primary rhinoplasty requesting changes from a previously satisfactory result. Reconstructive rhinoplasty is the esthetic and/or functional enhancement of a nose that is altered by trauma, pathology, or ablative tumor surgery.

The most important factor in a successful cosmetic rhinoplasty is patient selection. Equally important is the surgeon's ability to recognize his or her limitations in meeting the patient's cosmetic demands. The nose needs to be examined in conjunction with the rest of the face, and considerable attention needs to be given to the patient's ethnic background. Most normal anatomic nasal measurements in the literature are for Caucasians; therefore, treatment planning must be done with caution. A systematic approach to analyzing the nose, both as a component of the face and as an independent entity, is essential. For example, a prominent nose may be accentuated by a hypoplastic mandible or chin, and the patient may benefit from an advancement genioplasty or alloplastic augmentation. Additionally, both cosmetic and functional aspects need to be addressed and anticipated. It is imperative for the surgeon to realize that an optimal cosmetic outcome may compromise nasal function. A good example is internal nasal valve compromise secondary to excessive nasal dorsum narrowing. Additional procedures may be considered, such as spreader grafts (cartilaginous graft between the nasal septum and upper lateral cartilage) to widen the nasal valve area.

Ultimately a successful cosmetic rhinoplasty requires that the patient clearly communicate his or her desires and expectations for surgery. The surgeon must take the time to understand and recognize unrealistic requests, ambiguity, and contradictions in the patient's desires. Subsequently, the surgeon must have a complete grasp of the surgical maneuvers at his or her disposal and be able to translate them into an custom operation that meets the patient's requests. It is essential that the surgeon recognize that each surgical intervention has a standard range of applications and an error margin that can cause deviations from the planned procedure. The more complex the set of interventions, the greater the margin of error. The current principles of rhinoplasty emphasize adherence to minor but key changes that result in more predictable and lasting outcomes. When possible, surgeons should evaluate their results beyond the first 6 to 12 months. Although to a lesser extent, the nose continues to change beyond this period. The stability of the cosmetic result depends on the degree of cartilaginous, ligamentous, bony, and soft tissue disruption and on surgically designed structural modifications. Long-term results can be difficult to decipher, not only due to difficulty in follow-up, but also because the nose continues to age, along with the other facial structures

Bibliography

Bagheri SC: Primary cosmetic rhinoplasty, *Oral Maxillofac Surg Clin North Am* 24(1):39-48, 2012.

Bagheri SC, Khan HA, Cuzalina A (eds): *Rhinoplasty; current therapy*: Oral Maxillofac Surg Clin North Am 24(1):ix-x, 2012.

Bagheri SC, Khan HA, Jahangirian A, et al: An analysis of 101 primary cosmetic rhinoplasties, *J Oral Maxillofac Surg* 70(4):902-909, 2012.

Beekhuis GH: Nasal obstruction after rhinoplasty: etiology and techniques for correction, *Laryngoscope* 86:540, 1976.

Bohlouli B, Bagheri SC: Revision rhinoplasty. In Bagheri SC, Bell RB, Khan HA (eds): *Current therapy in oral and maxillofacial surgery*, pp 901-910, St Louis, 2012, Saunders.

Daniel RK: *Rhinoplasty: an atlas of surgical techniques*, New York, 2002, Springer.

Gunter JP: The merits of the open approach in rhinoplasty, *Plast Reconstr Surg* 99(3):863-867, 1997.

Johnson CM, Toriumi DM: *Open structure rhinoplasty*, Philadelphia, 1990, Saunders.

Kamer FN, McQuown SA: Revision rhinoplasty, *Arch Otolaryngol Head Neck Surg* 114:257, 1988.

Maniglia AJ: Fatal and major complications secondary to nasal and sinus surgery, *Laryngoscope* 99:276, 1989.

Teichgraeber JF, Riley WB, Parks DH: Nasal surgery complications, *Plast Reconstr Surg* 85:527, 1990.

Teichgraeber JF, Russo RC: Treatment of nasal surgery complications, *Ann Plast Surg* 30:80, 1993.

Nasal Septoplasty

Shahrokh C. Bagheri and Roger A. Meyer

CC

A 28-year-old male presents for a consultation regarding his symptomatic third molars. There have been three episodes of pericoronitis requiring antiobiotic treatment in the past year. He also complains of difficulty breathing through the left side of his nose.

HPI

The patient reports no history of prior nasal surgery. However, his nose was forcefully struck in a sporting accident at age 24 (prior nasal injury is a risk factor for deviated septum). No surgical treatment was provided at that time. Subsequent to that injury, he has not been able to breathe through his left nostril. (Nasal obstruction due to septum deviation can occur due to birth trauma or, more likely, secondary to developmental changes or, as in the current patient, facial trauma).

PMHX/MEDICATIONS/ALLERGIES/SH/FH

No significant medical illness. The patient denies a history of abuse of cocaine or other nasally inhaled substances, such as nose drops or sprays (rhinitis medicamentosa can cause postoperative septal perforation due to chronic mucosal vasoconstriction). He does not have symptoms of nasal allergy (seasonal, due to pollens; perennial, due inhaled or ingested irritants, infectious agents or a combination of these) or vasomotor rhinitis (nasal congestion, hypersecretion, sneezing due to parasympathetic system instability). Such conditions should be diagnosed and controlled or resolved prior to nasal septal surgery. There is no history of Wegener granulomatosis (small and medial-sized vasculitis that can affect the nose, causing pain, epistaxis, and nasal deformities due to septal perforation). The patient denies tobacco use. (Tobacco smoke is irritating to the nasal mucosa, and nicotine causes generalized vasoconstriction. Smoking after a nasal—or any—operation seriously interferes with the healing process and may become a critical factor in wound breakdown and/or the development of an infection).

EXAMINATION

The nose is examined in conjunction with the other facial structures for both its functional and cosmetic aspects (see the section Rhinoplasty in this chapter). Physical examination should include inspection and direct visualization of the septum, turbinates, nasal mucosa, nasal passages, nasal valve, radix, dorsum, columella and anterior nasal spine. (Occasionally a tumor occurs in the nasal passages, and an area showing changes suspicious for neoplasia should be biopsied.) The examination of the current patient proceeded as follows.

External nasal examination. The nasal bones are stable and symmetric. The tip and septum are deviated to the left. The anterior nasal spine is palpated and appears coincident with the facial midline, but the cartilaginous caudal septum is deviated to the left. The bony radix and dorsum are in the midline. The external cartilaginous caudal nasal structures (dorsum, tip, columella) show only mild deviation to the left (significant septal deviation is not always associated with a cosmetic nasal deformity of the columella, dorsum, or tip).

Rhinoscopy (examination of the nose with a speculum). Nasal mucosa is nonerythematous with normal moisture and absence of polypoid tissue (erythema, excessive secretions and polyps would be indicative of allergic rhinitis). The quadrangular cartilage and bony septum are significantly deviated to the left, closing the nasal valve angle with nearly complete blockage of the airway, prominent midseptal bowing, and contact of the septum with the left inferior turbinate. The septum is also deviated inferiorly to the left. Both of the inferior turbinates are enlarged, with the right larger (compensatory turbinate hypertrophy) than the left. The left nasal valve is obstructed by this deviation.

Endoscopic nasal examination. After spraying the nose with oxymetazoline (α_1 agonist and partial α_2 agonist), endoscopic examination confirms the presence of right inferior turbinate hypertrophy and leftward deviation of the septum with no visible mucosal pathology. (Endoscopy is not necessary to diagnose and treat a deviated septum. However, it can be helpful in the evaluation of the posterior nasal structures; that is, the superior nasal passages, the paranasal sinus meatuses, and the posterior nasal choanae, especially in the absence of CT examination).

Cottle's test (negative). This test did not improve airflow in the current patient. The test is done to evaluate airflow due to nasal valve obstruction or compromise. The contralateral nostril is gently closed by the examiner, and the ipsilateral cheek is pulled laterally to open the nasal valve. If airflow is improved by this maneuver, the nasal valve deficiency is potentially contributing to airflow obstruction. (This is a very unreliable test that produces many false positives; that is, lateral retraction of the cheek improves the airway in many patients who only have temporary nasal mucosal ingestion, not collapse of the nasal valve. Therefore, the examiner should be wary of the validity of this test with regard to nasal valve integrity.)

IMAGING

Advanced imaging studies (CT scan) are not necessary to diagnose a deviated septum. However, CT or in-office cone-beam computed tomography (CBCT) are helpful in the evaluation of the location and extent of the deviation and in the assessment of the turbinates, paranasal sinuses, and other related structures for additional pathology. The panoramic radiograph is not used for definitive evaluation of the nasal septum. However, this routinely obtained plain film does afford basic two-dimensional anteroposterior visualization of the septal position and can be used as a screening tool.

In the current patient, axial and coronal CBCT imaging demonstrated significant leftward deviation of the septum with reduced air space and compensatory enlargement of the right inferior turbinate (Figure 13-11, *A* and *B*). The panoramic radiograph obtained for third molar evaluation in this patient, shows impaction of the mandibular third molars, and also demonstrates the deviated septum (Figure 13-11, *C*).

LABS

No routine laboratory tests are indicated for nasal septoplasty surgery in an otherwise healthy patient. However, patients with a family history of clotting disorders are screened for possible undiagnosed coagulopathies (e.g., von Willebrand disease, platelet deficits or dysfunction, liver pathology, and clotting factor deficiencies). Patients taking anticoagulant medications are at risk for hematoma formation and uncontrolled hemorrhage.

ASSESSMENT

Severely deviated nasal septum to the left involving the quadrangular cartilage and the bony septum, causing impaired left nostril airflow and compromised flow in the right due to compensatory inferior turbinate hypertrophy. Impacted symptomatic mandibular third molars.

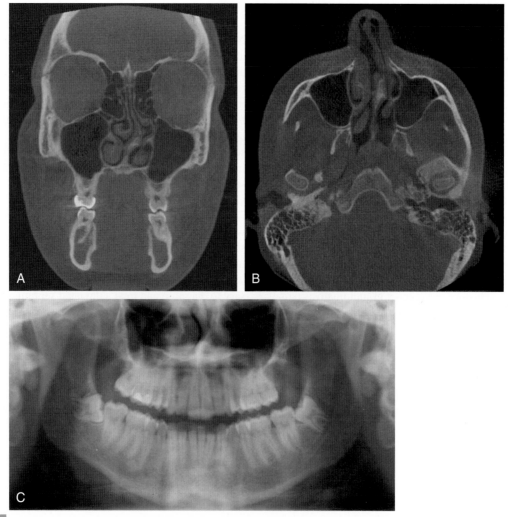

Figure 13-11   **A,** Coronal reconstruction CT scan showing significant midseptal deviation. **B,** Axial CT scan of septum showing deviated bony and cartilaginous septum with significant right inferior turbinate hypertrophy. **C,** Panoramic radiograph showing deviated septum.

TREATMENT

In the current patient, general anesthesia was induced and an oral endotracheal tube was placed for airway maintenance and administration of oxygen and anesthetic agents. Two main incisions are used to approach the septum, the Killian incision and the hemitransfixion incision (Figure 13-12). The Killian incision is the most common and is used to approach the septum without direct access to the caudal segment. It is the best incision for preserving tip support. The hemitransfixion incision allows exposure of the caudal septum and anterior nasal spine by placing the incision in the membranous septum just anterior to the cartilage. Critics of this incision argue that it can weaken tip support by affecting the foot plates of the lower lateral cartilage. The septum can also be approached via the open rhinoplasty incision (transcolumellar). This is usually done when nasal and septal surgery for both cosmetic and functional correction are planned. Access to the septum via the Le Fort I osteotomy is easily done in combination with orthognathic surgery. Correction of the deviated septum should be included in the orthognathic surgical plan. Special consideration is required with maxillary impaction, because the vertical height of the septum must be reduced adequately to allow the planned amount of maxillary superior intrusion and to avoid compression and postoperative nasal septum deviation.

In the current patient, 12 ml of 0.5% Marcaine with 1:100,000 epinephrine was injected into the septum and inferior turbinates for vasoconstriction and hydrodissection both anteriorly and posteriorly. Oxymetazoline (for vasoconstriction) was applied into both nasal passages using cotton pledgets. (Inferior turbinate removal is best performed prior to septoplasty surgery to avoid injury to the operated nasal septum during retraction. The inferior turbinate is removed [Figure 13-13, *A*], along with any prominent bony segment, to increase the airway space. A submucous resection combined with turbinate out-fracture was used, with careful attention to hemostasis. The inferior turbinates are resected using an angled scissors, with hemostasis achieved by electrocautery.)

A Killian incision was made in the right nasal mucosa (after adequate time for vasoconstriction [i.e., 5 to 7 minutes]), and a full mucoperichondrial flap was raised using a Cottle elevator. The deviated septum was exposed (Figure 13-13, *B*) and showed significant leftward deviation of the quadrangular cartilage. The dissection was carried out inferiorly to the floor of the nose, allowing reflection of the periosteum off the nasal crest of the maxilla inferiorly and laterally (this is the most common location of septal perforation, especially with

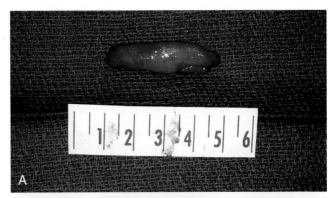

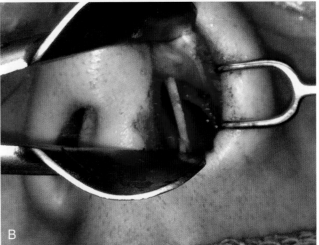

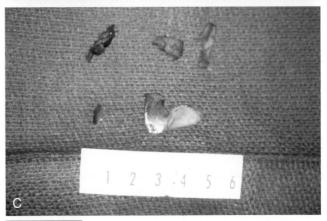

Figure 13-13   **A,** Resection of inferior turbinate. **B,** Exposure of the deviated septum via a Killian incision. **C,** Cartilage and bone removed via the Killian incision.

Figure 13-12   Sagittal view of septum showing the Killian and hemitransfixion incisions. *(From Azizzadeh B, et al: Master techniques in rhinoplasty, Philadelphia, 2011, Saunders.)*

Killian incision

Hemitransfixion incision

prominent bony deviations). After full exposure of the bone and cartilaginous septum, a segment of the cartilage was removed with preservation of approximately 1.5 cm at the dorsum and caudal strut (Figure 13-13, *C*). (Removal of the bony septum, including the perpendicular plate of the ethmoid bone, should be done with care, using double-action or through-cutting rongeur forceps, and with minimal lateral movement to avoid a cribriform plate fracture and possible cerebrospinal fluid [CSF] leak.) After irrigation, closure of the incision was done with 4-0 chromic gut suture. (A quilting suture is done with 4-0 chromic and a straight [Keith] needle to approximate the opposing mucoperichondrium, reduce the potential dead space, and prevent septal hematoma formation.) Bilateral internal Silastic nasal splints were inserted to prevent synechia formation and provide additional protection against septal hematoma. The splints were sutured to the caudal septum. (Nasal splints are removed 1 to 7 days postoperatively, depending on the surgeon's preference. Recent studies suggest that early removal [within 48 hours] is sufficient for synechia prevention.) The mandibular third molars were removed in a standard fashion with the oral endotracheal tube in place.

COMPLICATIONS

The risks and complications of nasal septoplasty can be divided into intraoperative, early, and late types.

Intraoperative. Intraoperative bleeding should be promptly recognized and treated. Posteriorly, bleeding from the posterior ethmoidal and sphenopalatine arteries can be brisk and its source difficult to visualize and staunch. Maintenance of a subperichondrial dissection can usually prevent injury to these vessels. Bleeding from Kiesselbach's plexus (formed by the confluence of the superior labial, anterior ethmoidal, and incisive arteries) in the anterior septum is more easily identified and controlled. Intraoperative control of hemorrhage can usually be achieved with reinjection of vasoconstrictor, electrocautery and/or applied pressure (anterior or posterior nasal packing). In rare circumstances, vessel ligation or arterial embolization might be required. Septal perforations (either preexisting or those created during the operation) should be repaired at that time and carefully evaluated postoperatively for maintenance of closure. CSF leakage is a rare occurrence and is usually associated with fracture of the cribriform plate during removal of the perpendicular (cribriform) plate of the ethmoid bone (PPEB). To avoid this complication, the PPEB should be removed with a crushing instrument (e.g., a side-cutting rongeurs). Attempts at lateral mobilization (rocking) and out-fracture of the PPEB that can lead to fracture of the skull base through the cribriform plate are to be avoided.

Early. A septal hematoma is a surgical emergency. It is the consequence of postoperative bleeding after septal manipulation (it can also be seen with nasal fractures). Bleeding occurs between the perichondrium and underlying/remaining cartilage (Figure 13-14). Because septal cartilage derives its blood supply from the perichondrium, a hematoma separates the

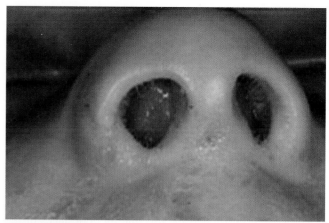

Figure 13-14 Nasal septal hematoma. *(From Nease CJ, Deal RC: Septoplasty in conjunction with cosmetic rhinoplasty,* Oral Maxillofac Surg Clin North Am *24[1]:49-58, 2012.)*

underlying cartilage from its nutrient vessels and causes ischemia or necrosis of both the cartilage and mucosa. The patient may present with pain, nasal deviation, nasal mass, ecchymosis, and possibly fever. Early recognition and drainage are important. Careful hemostasis, placement of a quilting suture to closely approximate the opposing perichondrium (using a straight Keith needle), and nasal packing are surgical steps that reduce the risk of this complication.

Because of the extensive blood supply of the nasal septum and mucosa, postoperative infections are rare, except when an allogenic or alloplastic material is used for concomitant nasal and/or septal reconstruction. In those isolated instances of infection, any foreign material should be removed, adequate drainage is created, and appropriate antibiotic cover is provided. A septal abscess is an emergency, because, similar to a septal hematoma, it can cause septal cartilage or mucosal necrosis. If the infection ascends via the angular veins to communicate with intercranial vessels, it might progress to cavernous sinus thrombosis. A single dose of preoperative intravenous antibiotics is thought to reduce the incidence of postoperative nasal infections.

CSF leakage is rare. Patients may present with headache and/or nasal pain or have no symptoms whatsoever. There may or may not be visible CSF rhinorrhea. An easy bedside clinical test can be performed to differentiate nasal secretions from CSF. A handkerchief is placed beneath the nose to collect nasal fluid, and this material is allowed to dry. Mucus starches (stiffens) the handkerchief, whereas CSF does not. Neurosurgical consultation is indicated. A CSF leak is usually treated expectantly with antibiotics and bed rest (with the head elevated). Occasionally surgical intervention is necessary to obliterate the communication between the intracranium and the superior nasal passage.

Late. Complications from nasal septoplasty can arise from days to several months after surgery. Assessment for internal valve collapse is done after several weeks of healing. This can be caused by scarring at the nasal valve angle due to the proximity of the incision, excessive cartilaginous reduction, or the development of adhesions. The selective use of spreader grafts in conjunction with septoplasty can improve the nasal valve angle.

Failure to improve airway patency and breathing can be related to undercorrection of the deviated septum or inadequate reduction of the turbinates. Posterior anatomic abnormalities that escaped preoperative diagnosis and went uncorrected can also compromise nasal airflow. Soft tissue edema or polyp formation from allergic phenomena or vasomotor effects that were not recognized and treated preoperatively can cause distressing postoperative nasal airway obstruction despite proper correction of bony and cartilaginous abnormalities in the nasal septum and turbinates.

A saddle nose deformity (collapse of the nasal dorsum) can result from excessive removal of cartilage. Maintaining at least 1.5-cm caudal and dorsal cartilaginous support prevents this complication.

When a nasal septal perforation develops postoperatively, it can be due to mucosal tears, (especially when bilateral), septal hematoma, septal infections, and abuse of recreational vasoconstrictor drugs, such as cocaine, nose drops, or sprays.

The development of nasal adhesions (synechiae) after septoplasty/turbinectomy is an undesirable complication that can be avoided. The use of internal nasal splints, although sometimes associated with discomfort, prevents synechiae. A short duration of intranasal splinting (5 to 7 days) is sufficient to preclude this complication.

DISCUSSION

A newborn infant usually has a straight nasal septum unless the nose is subjected to birth trauma. However, as the child grows and develops, the nasal septum commonly becomes curvilinear or otherwise deformed to various degrees, the form and size of the nasal turbinates change in response, and nasal breathing, except in cases of severe developmental or traumatic deformity, commonly adapts accordingly. Neither the mere presence of a deviated nasal septum nor the patient's complaint of "stuffy nose" or obstructed nasal breathing, in the absence of other findings, indicates that the nasal septum is the cause. As discussed previously, a thorough preoperative evaluation of the nasal airway includes attention to both the soft tissue components and the hard tissues elements (bone, cartilage).

Cosmetic rhinoplasty cannot be done without a full understanding of nasal septal surgery. There is an intimate relationship between "form and function" in nasal surgery. All surgeons who undertake cosmetic rhinoplasty must master septoplasty not only to harvest cartilage, but also to preserve or improve the shape and position of the nasal septum. Septoplasty for treatment of the deviated septum and nasal obstruction can make a dramatic change in the patient's quality of life by facilitating nasal airflow, allowing for better spontaneous drainage of the paranasal sinuses, possibly reducing mouth breathing and reducing or eliminating the symptoms of snoring, and perhaps by lessening the severity of obstructive sleep apnea syndrome.

Nasal septoplasty is indicated as an isolated procedure to improve the airway or for correction of a noticeable septal deviation. Frequently, however, it is done in combination with inferior turbinectomies and cosmetic rhinoplasty. A nasal septal cartilage graft is commonly used for nasal tip reconstruction (tip graft, struts, spreader grafts, shield grafts), correction of a crooked nose, or improvement of the nasal valve angle. In a recent review of 101 rhinoplasties, we found that most patients initially requested consultation solely regarding cosmetic nasal surgery (80%); only 20% desired correction of the nasal airway in addition to the appearance of the nose. However, the majority of the patients (63%) were treated with a septorhinoplasty, either for cartilage harvest or correction of septal deviation compromising nasal airway patency.

Among many who have contributed to advances in nasal septal surgery, three individuals cannot go without mention. In 1904, Killian described the incision that bears his name and the importance of cartilage preservation for support for the nasal dorsum and tip. He introduced the idea of preserving at least 1 cm of caudal and dorsal cartilaginous support, which to this day remains a fundamental concept of septal surgery. Freer, whose elevator is still widely used in nasal surgery, developed a similar operation at about the same time as and independently of Killian. Cottle (1898-1981), the designer of an eponymous surgical instrument (elevator), advocated the elevation of a mucoperichondrial flap on only one side of the nasal septum and promoted the hemitransfixion incision and the closed rhinoplasty approach.

Postoperative management for septoplasty should be focused on detecting a septal hematoma, infection, or perforation and verifying that the septum is correctly positioned. Nasal splints are removed 5 to 7 days after surgery. Moderate nasal mucosal edema is expected and gradually resolves within 2 to 4 weeks. Nasal irrigations with saline solution are used to prevent excessive dryness and crusting.

The patient who undergoes a successful nasal septoplasty operation experiences improved nasal breathing. Preoperative diagnosis and treatment of reactive nasal soft tissues (e.g., excessive secretions, edema or polyp formation due to allergic conditions, vasomotor rhinitis) improves airway conditions not correctable by surgical intervention. Surgical removal of those hard tissue (bone, cartilage) components (septum, turbinates) that interfere with nasal airflow should provide the patient with definitive relief of obstructed breathing. As a result of proper management of nasal soft tissue and hard tissue abnormalities, better spontaneous drainage of the paranasal sinuses is a frequent benefit to the patient. Retention of an adequate amount of septal cartilage ensures nasal support so that the external appearance of the nose is not adversely affected.

Bibliography

Aksoy E, Sering GM, Polat S, et al: Removing intranasal splints after septal surgery, *J Craniofac Surg* 22(3):1008-1009, 2011.
Bagheri SC: Primary cosmetic rhinoplasty. In Bagheri SC, Khan HA, Cuzalina A (eds): Rhinoplasty: current therapy, *Oral Maxillofac Surg Clin North Am* 24:49-58, 2012.

Bagheri SC: Rhinoplasty: current trends in rhinoplasty. In Bagheri SC, Bell RB, Khan HA (eds): *Current therapy in oral and maxillofacial surgery*, pp 891-900, St Louis, 2012, Saunders.

Bagheri SC, Khan HA, Jahangirian A, et al: An analysis of 101 primary cosmetic rhinoplasties, *J Oral Maxfac Surg* 70(4):902-909, 2012.

Behbrohm H, Tardy M: *Essentials of septoplasty*. New York, 2004, Thieme.

Cottle MH: Concepts of nasal physiology as related to corrective nasal surgery, *Arch Otolaryngol* 72:11, 1960.

Freer OT: The correction of deflections of the nasal septum with a minimum of traumatis, *JAMA* 16:362-75 1902.

Killian G:Die sumucose Fensterresektion der Nasenscheiwand, *Arch Laryngologie Rhinologie* 16:362-394 1904.

Nease CJ, Deal RC: Septoplasty in conjunction with cosmetic rhinoplasty. In Bagheri SC, Khan HA, Cuzalina A (eds): Rhinoplasty: current therapy, *Oral Maxillofac Surg Clin North Am* 24:49-58, 2012.

Newman MH: Surgery of the nasal septum, *Clin Plast Surg* 23:271, 1996.

Oneal RM, Beil RJ, Schlesinger J: Surgical anatomy of the nose, *Clin Plast Surg* 23:195, 1996.

Cervicofacial Rhytidectomy (Face-Lift)

Husain Ali Khan, Chris Jo, and Shahrokh C. Bagheri

CC

A 52-year-old Caucasian woman presents to your office for evaluation for possible facial cosmetic surgery. She complains of excessive skin laxity and wrinkling in her face and neck (Figure 13-15).

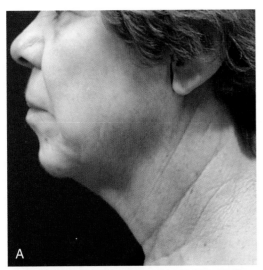

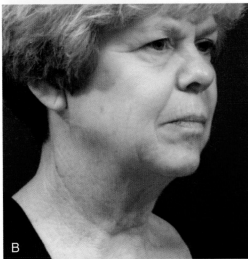

Figure 13-15 This patient exhibits the classic anatomy for which a lower face-lift and neck lift would be cosmetically beneficial. Major sagging in the jowls and neck usually requires a face-lift for correction. *(From Bagheri SC, Bell RB, Khan HA: Current therapy in oral and maxillofacial surgery, St Louis, 2012, Saunders; courtesy Dr. Angelo Cuzalina.)*

Although the majority of patients seeking facial cosmetic surgery are females, there is an increasing trend of male patients in recent years. Given the elective nature of facial cosmetic surgery, the chief complaint should strongly influence the selection of surgical procedures. It is our belief that for successful cosmetic surgery, the surgeon should focus on facilitating the patient's desires, as opposed to "selling" any procedure that falls within the surgeon's armamentarium.

HPI

The patient has no history of prior facial cosmetic surgery. She had recently attended a cosmetic seminar at your office, which sparked her interest in facial surgery (unlike other aspects of oral and maxillofacial surgery, a successful facial cosmetic practice requires adequate marketing and patient education). The patient specifically points to her jowls, cheeks, and submental regions, explaining that she has progressively noticed "sagging" of her face and neck over the past 3 years. She is constantly aware of her appearance, to the point that it consistently bothers her, and she desires a more youthful appearance of her face. She reports using sunscreen and tries to avoid sunlight exposure, because she does not tan and burns rather easily (Fitzpatrick type I skin).

The two most important factors related to the aging of skin are sunlight exposure and individual genetic characteristics. The later cannot be altered; therefore, exposure to sunlight is the single most important factor in skin care. Many skin care products are available on the market, most of which work by promoting hydration, protecting the skin from UV light, or facilitating exfoliation of superficial epithelium and dead cells.

PMHX/PSHX/MEDICATIONS/ALLERGIES/SH/FH

The patient has hypertension, which is well controlled with Lopressor HCT (a combination of a β-blocker and a thiazide diuretic). (Perioperative control of blood pressure is paramount for prevention of postoperative hematoma.)

She is also taking daily aspirin 81 mg for cardioprotective effects. (Aspirin or other nonsteroidal antiinflammatory drugs [NSAIDs] that interfere with platelet function should be stopped prior to face-lift procedures. Generally it is recommended that aspirin be discontinued 2 weeks prior to and for 1 week after the procedure to reduce the risk of hematoma formation.)

She denies smoking or illicit drugs use. (Smoking is associated with an increased risk of flap necrosis. Ideally, all nicotine-containing products should be stopped 4 to 6 weeks prior to cervicofacial rhytidectomy. Patients who are unable to quit smoking may be candidates for less invasive procedures such as the S-lift, or short flap rhytidectomy.)

There is no prior history of fever blisters (prophylaxis is required when concomitant laser or chemical resurfacing is performed). Face-lift procedures should be postponed in the presence of active herpes simplex virus [HSV] blisters).

EXAMINATION

General. The patient is a well-developed, well-nourished, pleasant female in no apparent distress.

Maxillofacial. The maxillofacial exam is divided into evaluations of the bony structure, soft tissue, and dermatologic factors.

- *Bony structure*
  - The facial structures are symmetric, with good malar projection and symmetric mandibular angles. There is no orbital dystopia (difference in position of the globe). The bony nasal pyramid and nasal tip are midline, with no dorsal hump. Examination of the nasal septum reveals no deviation. The hyoid bone is in good position (a low, anterior hyoid position compromises esthetic results in the neck).
  - The maxillary and mandibular dental midlines are coincident with the face. The occlusion is a Class I skeletal relationship. The chin is symmetric with good anteroposterior and vertical dimensions (recognition and subsequent correction of microgenia can significantly improve the facial contour of the chin and neck).
- *Soft tissue*
  - The eyebrows are in good position (in the female patient, the apex of eyebrow should be approximately 8 to 10 mm above the superior orbital rim and between the lateral limbus and canthus).
  - The upper eyelids show minimal dermatochalasis (excessive eyelid skin laxity).
  - There is no lateral hooding (excess skin of the lateral portion of the upper eyelid descending past the eyelid margin and obstructing vision in the lateral gaze).
  - There is no upper eyelid ptosis (the upper lid margin should cover 2 to 3 mm of the superior iris). The lower eyelids show good contour with no fat herniation. The snap test is normal (the lower lid should reapproximate the globe within 1 second when it is pulled inferiorly and released).
  - The nasolabial groove is deepened (formed by insertions of the zygomaticus muscles), and the nasolabial fold is full (caused by descent of the malar fat pad).
  - There is moderate jowling, most pronounced at the lower facial third and neck, causing blunting of the inferior border of the mandible.
  - Moderate submental lipomatosis and skin laxity are present, with a poorly defined cervicomental

(cervical-submental) angle and visible platysmal bands (an esthetically pleasing neck is defined as having a cervical-submental angle of 115 degrees ± 10 degrees, a distinct inferior border of the mandible, an anterior border of the sternocleidomastoid muscle, a depression posterior and inferior to the angle of the mandible, gentle contours without bands or folds, smooth skin, proportionate length, and, in men, a slight prominence of the thyroid cartilage).

- *Dermatologic factors*
  - Fair skin (Fitzpatrick skin type I: ivory white fair skin that never tans and always burns).
  - Glogau type II skin classification (early to moderate photoaging with wrinkles in motion, typically appearing in the fourth decade of life).
  - Fine dynamic cervicofacial rhytids in the periorbital region (crow's feet) and perioral region (marionette lines).

IMAGING

Standard preoperative and postoperative photodocumentation is mandatory for the face-lift patient. This should include a full frontal view in repose and with a full smile, right and left three-quarter obliques, and bilateral profile views.

LABS

In the absence of any significant medical problems, no routine laboratory testing is necessary for a cervicofacial rhytidectomy. Coagulation studies may be obtained if there is any suspicion of undiagnosed blood dyscrasias. An electrocardiogram is obtained based on the patient's age and risk factors for cardiovascular disease. A complete blood count and electrolyte panels can be obtained as needed.

ASSESSMENT

Patient desiring face-lift procedure secondary to cutis laxis, designated as type III cervical facial laxity (defined as moderate redundancy and jowling, platysmal banding, accentuated nasolabial folds, and variable degrees of cervical facial lipomatosis).

Dedo's classification of facial profiles categorizes the lower facial third into six distinct groups:
- Class I (normal)
- Class II (cervical skin laxity)
- Class III (submental lipomatosis)
- Class IV (platysmal banding)
- Class V (retrognathia or microgenia)
- Class VI (low hyoid bone)

TREATMENT

Cervicofacial rhytidectomy, submental lipectomy with platysmaplasty (commonly known as a "full face-lift") is the gold standard for treatment of type III cervical facial laxity. All modern face-lift techniques involve modifications of the superficial musculoaponeurotic system (SMAS) to achieve lasting cosmetic outcomes. The SMAS was first accurately described in 1976 by Mitz and Peyronie. Four basic approaches can be applied for correction of cervicofacial redundancy:

- Meloplication (e.g., barbed suture "thread-lift")
- S-lift (short flap rhytidectomy, described by Saylan; several modifications for incision designs and SMAS suspension suturing techniques have been described)
- Superficial plane face-lift
- Deep plane face-lift

For each of these techniques, various modifications have been described in the literature. The two most commonly used rhytidoplasty techniques are the S-lift and the superficial plane face-lift, with various incision designs for management of the SMAS, the platysma muscle, and suspension suturing techniques.

Superficial Rhytidectomy with Platysmaplasty

For the superficial rhytidectomy with platysmaplasty, the incision design must be carefully planned; it differs from surgeon to surgeon, based on the surgeon's preference and the technique (it must be modified for male patients to preserve the sideburns). First, the preauricular region is marked along the preauricular skin crease. Some surgeons prefer an endaural incision for improved scar camouflage, but this approach is often criticized as causing tragal deformities. The retroauricular incision is carried onto the posterior surface of the conchal bowl (in the crease for men) up to the level of the external auditory canal. It then makes a right-angle turn onto the mastoid skin and gently fades into the hairline. The temporal incision can extend superiorly from the preauricular incision as a temporal extension or can be made perpendicular to end at the anterior temporal tuft of hair (this incision should be beveled to allow regrowth of hair to hide the scar) (Figure 13-16). A 3-cm curvilinear horizontal incision is marked in the submental region 3 mm posterior to the submental crease; this incision is used for the submental lipectomy and platysmaplasty.

Next, tumescent solution is injected into the submental and submandibular triangles and the bilateral cheek areas in the superficial fat layer (tumescent solution has been shown to facilitate dissection and reduce postoperative complications). A local anesthetic with epinephrine can be injected into the incision sites.

Dissection begins in the submental region. A skin subcutaneous flap is elevated (leaving 3 to 5 mm of fat attached to the dermis). The boundaries of dissection should be the inferior border of the mandible, anterior border of the sternocleidomastoid, and 3 cm beyond the inferior border of the

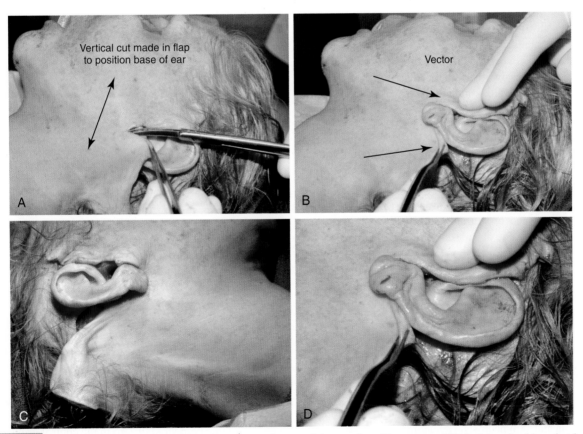

Figure 13-16 Setting the base of the ear is critical after the deep work is complete. The vector of lift is determined by what looks best and most natural on the table. The location of the base of the ear with respect to the flap is critical to allow normal redraping and for posterior hair alignment. Cutting too far one way or the other can cause major closure problems. *(From Bagheri SC, Bell RB, Khan HA:* Current therapy in oral and maxillofacial surgery, *St Louis, 2012, Saunders; courtesy Dr. Angelo Cuzalina.)*

area of neck ptosis. Excessive fat is sharply removed, and gentle open liposuction is performed. The central aponeurosis/ fascia-platysma muscle complex and deep fat are sharply excised to identify the anterior borders of the platysma muscle. A suture platysmaplasty is performed to close this decussation (platysma suspension sutures and "Giampapa sutures" can be placed here to engage the anterior platysma border at the depth of the new cervical-submental angle, which later is suspended to the contralateral mastoid fascia).

Next, the preauricular and postauricular incisions are made along the previous markings. A superficial flap is developed using face-lift scissors. This dissection joins the submental dissection that was previously carried out. Once the flap has been completely developed, the SMAS and platysma may be mobilized in a posterior-superior vector by a variety of techniques (e.g., imbrication, plication, lateral SMASectomy).

We prefer the lateral SMASectomy, as described by Baker in 2000, in which a 1.5 to 2-cm strip of SMAS parallel to the nasolabial fold (from the malar eminence to the angle of the mandible) is sharply excised and the margins reapproximated with 3-0 PDS sutures. This maneuver elevates the SMAS in a posterior-superior vector. Other surgeons prefer to fold the SMAS upon itself (plication) with sutures, and still others prefer to incise the posterior aspect of the SMAS and perform sub-SMAS dissection with imbrication of the SMAS. The posterior border of the plastyma/SMAS is identified and suspended to the mastoid fascia (if platysma suspension sutures were placed earlier, they are also sutured to the mastoid fascia).

The skin–subcutaneous tissue flap is then allowed to passively redrape by sweeping the flap in a posterior-superior vector without excessive tension. The flap beds are checked for hemostasis (meticulous attention to hemostasis reduces the incidence of postoperative hematoma). Platelet-rich plasma (PRP) or fibrin glue can be sprayed beneath the flaps (this is shown to decrease the incidence of seroma, edema, and ecchymoses). Key sutures are placed superiorly at the superior helix and at the lobule of the ear. Excess skin in the preauricular and postauricular regions is excised with face-lift scissors, and the areas are closed in layers (5-0 PDS in subcutaneous tissue and 6-0 Ethilon for skin); the sutures are removed in 7 days. The excess skin in the temporal (vertical or horizontal) and mastoid regions is excised, and the area is carefully closed. Finally, the submental incision is inspected for hemostasis and closed in layers. A pressure dressing is applied (some surgeons still prefer to use drains instead of PRP or fibrin sealant). Figure 13-17 shows the patient 18 months after surgery.

COMPLICATIONS

Hematoma is the most common postoperative complication (the incidence ranges from 0 to 9%) and can lead to prolonged facial edema and skin necrosis. Hematomas (most commonly occurring within the first 24 hours) can be classified as either large ("major" or "expanding") hematomas, which require immediate surgical intervention (evacuating the hematoma

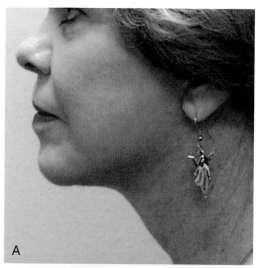

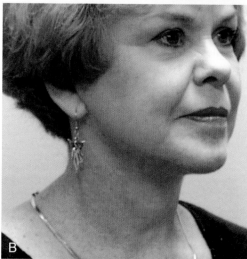

Figure 13-17   Eighteen months after surgery. The patient had additional age-related problems that were simultaneously corrected with other procedures: endoscopic forehead and brow lift, face-lift/ neck lift, submentoplasty and minor liposuction, upper and lower blepharoplasties, full-face laser skin resurfacing, chin implant, and injection of botulinum toxin. (*From Bagheri SC, Bell RB, Khan HA: Current therapy in oral and maxillofacial surgery, St Louis, 2012, Saunders; courtesy Dr. Angelo Cuzalina.*)

and achieving hemostasis) or minor hematomas ("microhematoma"), which can be treated with needle aspiration and/ or massage therapy. Signs include increased facial pain (especially when unilateral), swelling, tightening of the facial dressing, or ecchymosis of the buccal mucosa, lips, and neck.

In 2004 Jones and Grover reviewed 678 consecutive superficial face-lifts and found no significant difference in major hematoma rates between groups treated with pressure dressing, drains, fibrin glue, or tumescence (overall rate was 4.4%). When he compared tumescents with and without adrenaline, he found that the adrenaline-containing group had a 4.8% hematoma rate compared to zero in the control group. A separate study by the same authors showed that a tumescent technique significantly reduces the incidence of skin necrosis (14:1), alopecia (19:1), hypertrophic scarring (25:1), stretched scarring (21:1), and subsequent scar revision. Griffin and Jo in 2006 reviewed 178 consecutive face-lifts and reported a 2.8% incidence of major hematoma and a 1.7% incidence of minor hematoma after superficial rhytidectomy.

In 1976 Berner and colleagues found postoperative hypertension to be an etiologic factor in hematoma formation after rhytidectomy. In 1977 Straith and co-workers found that an admission blood pressure greater than 150/100 mm Hg had a 2.6 times greater incidence of hematoma formation. The next year, Rees and colleagues found that intraoperative hypotension increased the risk of hematoma; this was attributed to subsequent rebound hypertension. All three studies strongly suggest that blood pressure should be well controlled throughout the perioperative period. In 1995 Kamer and Kushnick found a twofold increase in expanding hematomas (2% versus 4.2%) when propofol was used for anesthesia; a 26% drop in systolic blood pressure was seen in the propofol group, compared with a 16% drop in the control group (no propofol).

Fibrin glue has been used to reduce the incidence of seroma. In 2001 Oliver and colleagues prospectively showed that fibrin glue reduces the amount of serosanguineous output, which obviated the need for drains to prevent seromas (no effect was seen on the incidence of major hematomas). In 1994 Marchac and Sandor reported a significant reduction in major hematomas and ecchymoses when fibrin sealant was used, without the need for drains or pressure dressings. However, a later study by Jones and co-workers did not find a difference in major hematoma rates when fibrin glue was used.

Platelet-rich plasma is used by some surgeons for its ability to enhance soft tissue healing and decrease the amount of edema and ecchymoses. Man and colleagues in 2000 and Powell and co-workers in 2001 reported the benefits of PRP when used in cervicofacial rhytidectomy. Neither fibrin glue, PRP, nor other adjunctive maneuvers were a good substitute for meticulous hemostasis in the prevention of major postoperative hematomas. In 2001 Palaia and colleagues found that DDAVP reduced the incidence of minor hematomas.

Seromas can also cause delayed wound healing and should therefore be aspirated. In 1997 Perkins and co-workers found that placing suction drains significantly decreases the incidence of seroma (37% without drains compared with 15% with drains). However, hematoma rates were similar in the two groups. The differential diagnosis of a fluctuant swelling beneath the flap must also include a parotid pseudocyst (resulting from damage to the parotid gland parenchyma). In 1996 McKinney and colleagues found that placing a suction drain, rather than repeated aspirations and pressure dressings, allowed more rapid resolution of parotid pseudocysts (within 1 week).

Postsurgical auricular deformities (e.g., downward and forward auricular displacement and rotation, increased auriculocephalic angle, hidden or buried tragus, pixie ear deformity) can be minimized by attention to suture anchoring of the soft tissue flaps.

Direct injury to branches of the facial nerve is a rare complication. Almost all motor nerve injuries are temporary. In 1983 Baker reviewed 7,000 cases of superficial rhytidectomy from multiple surgeons and reported 55 cases of motor nerve injury (the temporal and marginal mandibular branches were most commonly injured), seven of which were permanent. In 1992 Hamra found that deep plane dissection was most likely to cause temporary paresis of the upper lip and injury to the frontal branch. He also found a higher incidence of pseudoparesis of the lower lip due to platysmal transaction.

The greater auricular nerve (C2, C3) is the most common sensory nerve to be injured during a face-lift. It crosses the posterior border of the sternocleidomastoid muscle at Erb's point (along with three other cutaneous branches of the cervical plexus: the lesser occipital, transverse cervical, and supraclavicular nerves). It supplies the skin of the back of the ear, mastoid region, and angle of the mandible.

In 2003 Daane and Owsley reviewed 2,002 cases and found a 1.7% incidence of pseudoparalysis of the marginal mandibular nerve, in which the lower lip eversion was intact, but an asymmetrical "full denture-type smile" was caused by injury to the cervical branch of the facial nerve or direct platysmal injury. All cases fully recovered within 3 weeks to 6 months.

The most feared of all complications is flap necrosis and slough (incidence of 0 to 3%). This is the result of vascular compromise (decreased arterial perfusion, venous congestion, and small vessel disease seen with diabetes mellitus and smoking). Other causes include late hematoma evacuation and wide undermining with a wound closed under tension. Small areas of necrosis along the flap edge most commonly occur in the postauricular region (allow to heal by secondary intention). Smoking significantly increases the risk of skin slough because of its negative effect on wound healing and flap vascularity. In 1984 Rees and colleagues reported a 12 times greater risk for skin slough in smokers. In 1986 Webster and co-workers found that a conservative technique was safe in smokers and advocated use of the S-lift for noncompliant patients. It is recommended that the patient stop smoking 4 to 6 weeks before surgery and for 2 to 4 weeks after surgery. Wellbutrin is reported to be a good therapy for smoking cessation. Ice packs should be avoided, because they may cause decreased flap perfusion.

DISCUSSION

Facial aging is the result of a progressive gravitational descent of soft tissue that occurs in a predictable course based on anatomic and biologic certainties, which must be understood for facial rejuvenation surgery. The genetic differences between individuals give each patient his or her unique variations (timing and extent) of facial aging (skin laxity, soft tissue descent, fat atrophy and volume loss, orbital fat herniation, loss of facial volume, bony resorption of the anterior facial skeleton, and skin changes). Facial subcutaneous tissue, fascia, and overlying skin are supported or "anchored" by four true retaining ligaments (orbital, zygomatic, buccal-maxillary, and mandibular) and by three false retaining ligaments (platysma-auricular, buccal-maxillary, and masseteric-cutaneous). Areas of the face that have loosely adherent areolar tissue become preferentially ptotic. These loose areolar planes exist in the forehead and eyebrow region, the temporal region, the anterior and middle cheek, and in the lower face and neck, and they account for the characteristic pattern of facial aging in the upper face, midface, and lower face and neck.

The aging pattern of the upper face is characterized by horizontal forehead lines (frontalis muscle hypertrophy), oblique and transverse frown lines (corrugator and procerus muscles, respectively), soft tissue descent over the lower forehead (due to depressor muscle tone overwhelming the frontalis muscle), and soft tissue descent of the unsupported temporal tissue overlying the temporalis fascia (causing eyebrow ptosis and contributing to an aged upper eyelid appearance). (Rejuvenation of the upper face is discussed in a separate section.)

The aging pattern of the midface is characterized by attenuation and lengthening of the soft tissues, causing ptosis and pseudoherniation of the orbital fat pads and suborbicularis oculi fat pad (SOOF). Also, loss of support from the retaining ligaments of the midface causes descent of the malar fat pad, resulting in a deepened nasolabial groove, thickened nasolabial fold, and hollowing of the upper midface.

The aging pattern of the lower face and neck is characterized by ptosis of midfacial soft tissue and fat (the facial SMAS complex loses adherence and support from deep facial fascia and bone), which descend behind the mandibular retaining ligament and below the inferior border of the mandible (resulting in "jowling" and blunting of the inferior border of the mandible). The major plane of aging in the neck is the deep fat (areolar) layer (subfascia-platysma layer) due to the release of central adherence between the superficial cervical fascia and superficial layer of deep cervical fascia. This manifests as laxity in the submental region, blunting of the cervical-submental angle with lipomatosis or fat atrophy of the superficial fat layer, lipomatosis of the central deep fat layer, and platysma bands.

Most facial cosmetic surgeons prefer the superficial plane face-lift due to its technical simplicity, decreased operating time, decreased recovery time, decreased morbidity, and good patient satisfaction. Many other surgeons advocate the deep plane face-lift for its long-term stability and more natural rejuvenated appearance. Deep plane rhytidectomy was first introduced by Skoog in 1974 and has been popularized by the works of Owsley, Hamra, Barton, and others. The philosophy behind deep plane face-lifts is that the skin, subcutaneous tissue, platysma muscle, and SMAS should be elevated as one unit off the underlying facial muscles and repositioned to restore a more youthful appearance. This composite rhytidectomy technique is beyond the scope of this chapter.

Recently, minimally invasive techniques (Contour Thread Lifts) have been developed to rejuvenate the aging face. Although these are celebrated for their simplicity of technique, their short- and long-term stability is questionable.

Examination and treatment for facial cosmetic surgery should focus on the hard and soft tissues. Optimal cosmetic results are often obtained by combining surgical procedures that involve the underlying bony architecture and the soft tissue envelope. Recent trends in maxillofacial esthetics place greater emphasis on addressing the hard tissue deformities of the dentofacial region. A knowledge of orthognathic surgery, orthodontics, and dental esthetics can be beneficial to the facial cosmetic surgeon, allowing oral and maxillofacial surgeons to better serve the cosmetic needs of many patients.

Bibliography

Baker DC: Complications of cervicofacial rhytidectomy, *Clin Plast Surg* 10(3):543–562, 1983.

Baker D: Rhytidectomy with lateral SMASectomy, *Facial Plast Surg* 16:209-213, 2000.

Berner RE, Morain WD, Noe JM: Postoperative hypertension as an etiological factor in hematoma after rhytidectomy, *Plast Reconstr Surg* 57:314, 1976.

Brink RR: Auricular displacement with rhytidectomy, *Plast Reconstr Surg* 108(3):743-749, 2001.

Chisholm BB: Surgical facial rhytidectomy: the evolution of an esthetic concept, *Oral Maxillofac Surg Clin North Am* 12:719-728, 2000.

Cuzalina A, Copty TV, Khan HA: Rhytidectomy (face-lifting). In Bagheri SC, Bell RB, Khan HA (eds): *Current therapy in oral and maxillofacial surgery*, p 942, St Louis, 2012, Saunders.

Daane SP, Owsley JQ: Incidence of cervical branch injury with "marginal mandibular nerve pseudo-paralysis" in patients undergoing face lift, *Plast Reconstr Surg* 111(7):2414-2418, 2003.

Evans TW, Stepanyan M: Isolated cervicoplasty, *Am J Cosmetic Surg* 19:91-113, 2002.

Ghali GE, Smith BR: A case for superficial rhytidectomy, *J Oral Maxillofac Surg* 56:349-351, 1998.

Griffin JE, Epker BN: Correction of cervicofacial deformities, *Atlas Oral Maxillofac Surg Clin North Am* 12:179-197, 2004.

Griffin JE, Jo C: Complications after superficial plane cervicofacial rhytidectomy: a retrospective analysis of 175 consecutive face-lifts and review of the literature, *J Oral Maxillofac Surg* 65(11):2227-2234, 2007.

Hamra ST: Composite rhytidectomy, *Plast Resconstr Surg* 90:1-11, 1992.

Hamra ST: Prevention and correction of the "face-lifted" appearance, *Facial Plast Surg* 16:215-229, 2000.

Jones BM, Grover R: Avoiding hematoma in cervicofacial rhytidectomy: a personal 8-year quest—reviewing 910 patients, *Plast Reconstr Surg* 113(1):381-387, 2004.

Jones BM, Grover R: Reducing complications in cervicofacial rhytidectomy by tumescent infiltration: a comparative trial evaluating 678 consecutive face lifts, *Plast Reconstr Surg* 113(1):398-403, 2004.

Kamer F, Kushnick SD: The effect of propofol on hematoma formation in rhytidectomy, *Arch Otolaryngol Head Neck Surg* 121(6):658-661, 1995.

Man D, Plosker H, Wildland-Brown JE: The use of autologous platelet-rich plasma (platelet gel) and autologous platelet-poor plasma (fibrin glue) in cosmetic surgery, *Plast Reconstr Surg* 107(1):229-237, 2000.

Marchac D, Sandor G: Face lifts and sprayed fibrin glue: an outcome analysis of 200 patients, *Br J Plast Surg* 47(5):306-309, 1994.

McKinney P, Zuckerbraun BS, Smith JW, et al: Management of parotid leakage following rhytidectomy, *Plast Reconstr Surg* 98(5):795-797, 1996.

Mitz V, Peyronie M: The superficial musculo-aponeurotic system (SMAS) in the parotid and cheek area, *Plast Reconstr Surg* 38:80-88, 1976.

Newman JP, Koch RJ, Goode RL, et al: Distortion of the auriculo-cephalic angle following rhytidectomy: recognition and prevention, *Arch Otolaryngol Head Neck Surg* 123(8):818-820, 1997.

Obagi S, Bridenstine JB: Chemical skin resurfacing, *Oral Maxillofac Surg Clin North Am* 12:541-553, 2000.

Oliver DW, Hamilton SA, Figle AA, et al: A prospective, randomized, double-blind trial of the use of fibrin sealant for face lifts, *Plast Reconstr Surg* 108(7):2102-2105, 2001.

Palaia DA, Rosenberg MH, Bonanno PC: The use of DDAVP desmopressin reduces the incidence of microhematomas after facial plasty, *Ann Plast Surg* 46(5):163-166, 2001.

Perkins SW: Achieving the "natural look" in rhytidectomy, *Facial Plast Surg* 16:269-282, 2000.

Perkins SW, Williams JD, Macdonald K, et al: Prevention of seromas and hematomas after face-lift surgery with the use of postoperative vacuum drains, *Arch Otolaryngol Head Neck Surg* 123(7):743-745, 1997.

Powell DM, Chang E, Farrior EH: Recovery from deep-plane rhytidectomy following unilateral wound treatment with autologous platelet gel (a pilot study), *Arch Facial Plast Surg* 3:245-250, 2001.

Rees TD, Aston SJ: Complications of rhytidectomy, *Clin Plast Surg* 5:109-119, 1978.

Rees TD, Liverett DM, Guy CL: The effect of cigarette smoking on skin-flap survival in the face lift patient, *Plast Reconstr Surg* 73:911-915, 1984.

Rubin LR, Simpson RL: The new deep plane face lift dissections versus the old superficial techniques: a comparison of neurologic complications, *Plast Reconstr Surg* 97(7):1461-1465, 1996.

Saylan Z: The S-lift for facial rejuvenation, *International Journal of Cosmetic Surgery* 7:17-24, 1999.

Saylan Z: The S-lift: less is more, *Aesthet Surg J* 19:406-409, 1999.

Skoog T: *Plastic surgery: new methods and refinements*, Philadelphia, W.B. Saunders, 1974.

Straith RE, Raghava R, Hipps CJ: The study of hematomas in 500 consecutive face lifts, *Plast Reconstr Surg* 59:694-698, 1977.

Webster RC, Davidson TM, White MF, et al: Conservative face lift surgery, *Arch Otolaryngol* 102:657-662, 1976.

Webster RC, Kazda G, Hamden US: Cigarette smoking and face lift: conservative versus wide undermining, *Plast Reconstr Surg* 77:596-604, 1986.

Webster RC, Smith RC, Smith KF: Face lift. I. Extent of undermining of skin flaps, *Head Neck Surg* 5:525-534, 1983.

Webster RC, Smith RC, Smith KF. Face lift. II. Etiology of platysma cording and its relationship to treatment, *Head Neck Surg* 6:590-595, 1983.

Webster RC, Smith RC, Smith KF: Face lift. III. Plication of the superficial musculoaponeurotic system, *Head Neck Surg* 6:696-701, 1983.

Upper and Lower Eyelid Blepharoplasty

Shahrokh C. Bagheri and Chris Jo

CC

A 48-year-old female presents for consultation regarding excess skin on her upper and lower eyelids (dermatochalasis). Her co-workers constantly tell her that she "looks tired all the time."

HPI

The patient is able to point out areas of excess skin over both upper and lower eyelids in front of a mirror. In addition, she complains about the "dark circles and bags" under her eyes. She does not complain about any visual field restrictions (these can be caused by advanced dermatochalasis or lateral/temporal "hooding"). There is no history of dry eyes or other ocular problems, and she has not had any previous facial cosmetic surgery.

PMHX/PDHX/MEDICATIONS/ALLERGIES/SH/FH

There is no history of thyroid disease (Graves' ophthalmopathy may manifest as eyelid edema, lid retraction, or early proptosis and may mimic fat prolapse or aging). There is no history of coagulopathies or bleeding tendencies. The patient does not use aspirin, nonsteroidal antiinflammatory drugs (NSAIDs), vitamin E, herbal medications, or anticoagulants (medications that affect platelet or coagulation function and that may increase the risk of retrobulbar hemorrhage must be discontinued at least 10 to 14 days prior to the procedure).

EXAMINATION

General. The patient is a well-developed and well-nourished female in no apparent distress.

Ocular exams. Examination of the pupillary reactions, visual fields, visual acuity, and extraocular muscles reveals no abnormalities (Figure 13-18). Schirmer's test is normal (this test measures baseline tear production and can be used as needed to document preoperative lacrimal gland function).

Forehead–eyebrow–upper lid complex. This area is assessed first to evaluate for brow ptosis. For the current patient, the distance from the upper lid margin to the lower edge of the brow during primary gaze measures 10 mm (normal range). If this measurement is less than 10 mm, it is suggestive of brow ptosis, which can also contribute to the amount of temporal hooding (another reference is the distance from mid-pupil to the high point of the brow, which is about

25 mm). In cases of significant brow ptosis, consideration should be given to brow lift procedures (the eyebrows can be elevated to the ideal position with the thumb and index finger while examining the upper eyelid). There are no horizontal glabellar furrows (caused by the procerus muscle) or vertical furrows (caused by corrugator supercilii muscle) at rest.

Upper eyelid exam. The following elements are considered in the upper eyelid exam.

- *Skin* (examined with the eyebrows/forehead completely relaxed). In the current patient, excessive skin is centered over the mid-eyelid. The redundant eyelid skin is predominantly above the eyelid crease (smooth forceps can be used to pinch the excess tissue to demonstrate the amount of skin laxity). There is no ectropion (everted eyelid), entropion (inverted eyelid), or lagophthalmos (eyelid incompetence). Bell's phenomenon (a protective reflex to prevent corneal abrasion and erosion) is intact. The upper eyelid margin position is ideal (it should cover 2 to 3 mm of superior iris).
- *Herniated or prolapsed fat* (upper eyelid has two preaponeurotic fat pads). Areas of herniated/prolapsed orbital fat are noted nasally (most commonly noted in this area). (Gentle pressure on the globe while the eye is closed accentuates nasal fat herniation.)
- *Eyelid crease.* The eyelid crease is identified at 9 mm above the lid margin (within normal limits) at the level of the pupil.

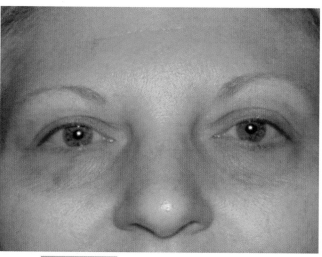

Figure 13-18 Preoperative frontal photograph.

- *Examination for blepharoptosis* (eyelid ptosis). The vertical interpalpebral fissure distance measures 10 mm (normal is 10 to 12 mm centrally). (This is the distance from the mid-upper to the mid-lower eyelid margin during primary gaze. A smaller distance is suggestive of blepharoptosis and levator disinsertion or dysfunction, in which the upper eyelid has decreased excursion upon superior gaze. This distance is increased with upper eyelid retraction, as is seen thyroid ophthalmopathy.)
- *Evaluation for prolapsed lacrimal gland.* No fullness in the temporal region is noted. (Fullness in this area would be suggestive of lacrimal gland prolapse or descent of the retroorbicularis oculi fat [ROOF]).

Lower eyelid exam. The lower eyelids should be examined in conjunction with the upper eyelid examination, even when the patient desires only upper eyelid surgery. The lower eyelids should be evaluated for excess skin, laxity, orbital fat herniation, and retraction.

- *Skin.* In the current patient, a moderate amount of excess skin is observed when the patient is looking upward.
- *Orbital fat.* The medial, central, and temporal areas (corresponding to the three lower orbital fat pads) are examined as the patient looks upward. In this patient, gentle pressure over the closed upper eyelid demonstrates accentuation of orbital fat herniation.
- *Lower eyelid retraction.* The lower eyelid is slightly above the level of the inferior limbus (no scleral show).
- *Lower eyelid laxity.* The snap test is normal (the lower lid reapproximates the globe within 1 second when it is pulled inferiorly and released).

Figure 13-19 shows the surface anatomy of the periocular region of a typical non-Asian patient in the youthful and aging states.

IMAGING

Preoperative and serial postoperative photo imaging is mandatory for cosmetic procedures. Close-up views of the eyelids in both the closed and open eyelid positions are recommended.

LABS

No routine laboratory studies are indicated for cosmetic eyelid surgery unless dictated by the medical history.

ASSESSMENT

The patient desires bilateral upper and lower eyelid blepharoplasties secondary to dermatochalasis (excess eyelid skin laxity) and prolapse of preaponeurotic fat.

TREATMENT

An understanding of the layers of the orbital anatomy is essential in performing eyelid surgery. The orbital septum is the extension of the periosteal envelope that covers the fat pads around the eye. Figure 13-20 illustrates some of the key anatomic landmarks.

For the current patient, bilateral upper eyelid blepharoplasty with resection of prolapsed fat is the treatment of choice to recreate an esthetically pleasing upper eyelid shelf. Because no eyebrow ptosis is present, a forehead/brow lift procedure would not be indicated. We emphasize that each patient presents with unique esthetic needs, mandating differences in the amount of skin, muscle, or fat that needs to be removed to achieve the optimal cosmetic result.

Blepharoplasties can be performed under local anesthesia in a cooperative patient, or general anesthesia can be used as needed. However, intravenous sedation is ideal for the patient's comfort. Prior to administration of any sedative-hypnotics or local anesthetic, the eyelids should be reexamined and marked in the upright position (after administration of topical tetracaine).

The eyelids are marked in the upright or semireclined position before the administration of sedation. The upper eyelid is elevated, and the inferior incision line is marked in the natural supratarsal lid crease, approximately 1 cm above the lid margin (the natural eyelid crease is 7 to 10 mm centrally in women and 6 to 8 mm centrally in men). Medially, the marking ends above the lacrimal punctum (extending the incision beyond the punctum increases the risk of webbing), with

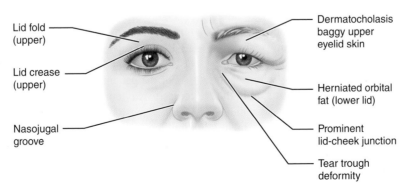

Lid fold (upper)

Lid crease (upper)

Nasojugal groove

Dermatocholasis baggy upper eyelid skin

Herniated orbital fat (lower lid)

Prominent lid-cheek junction

Tear trough deformity

Figure 13-19 Surface anatomy of the periocular region of a typical non-Asian patient in the youthful (*left*) and aging (*right*) states. (*From Bagheri SC, Bell RB, Khan HA:* Current therapy in oral and maxillofacial surgery, *St Louis, 2012, Saunders.*)

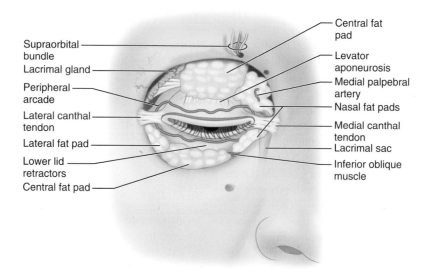

Supraorbital bundle

Lacrimal gland

Peripheral arcade

Lateral canthal tendon

Lateral fat pad

Lower lid retractors

Central fat pad

Central fat pad

Levator aponeurosis

Medial palpebral artery

Nasal fat pads

Medial canthal tendon

Lacrimal sac

Inferior oblique muscle

Figure 13-20 Anatomy of the anterior orbit. The surgeon often encounters the lacrimal gland and the inferior oblique muscle during upper and lower blepharoplasty. The former can be repositioned, and the latter should be left untouched. *(From Bagheri SC, Bell RB, Khan HA: Current therapy in oral and maxillofacial surgery, St Louis, 2012, Saunders.)*

a slight downward taper. Laterally, it is extended approximately 1 cm beyond the lateral canthus with a general upward slope (at the level of the lateral canthus, the incision should be approximately 5 mm above the level of the canthus). The superior incision line is marked as the excess skin is pinched with smooth forceps and the forehead/eyebrow is stabilized (slight eversion of the upper eyelid margin, with less than 1 mm of lagophthalmos, assures adequate but not an overly aggressive skin resection). A minimum of 20 mm of skin must remain between the upper eyelid margin and the lower eyebrow margin to prevent postoperative lagophthalmos. The superior incision is marked with the skin held by the forceps and curves into the inferior incision medially and laterally in an elliptical fashion (modifications to the incision design can be made at the medial and lateral junctions, depending on the clinical situation). The markings are again verified with smooth forceps to assure symmetry and lid competence. (When simultaneous lower eyelid blepharoplasty with a skin incision is planned, a minimum of 5 mm between the two incisions must be maintained laterally.)

After injection of local anesthetic with epinephrine, the incision can be made with various techniques (blade, radiofrequency, or CO_2 laser). The authors prefer to use a CO_2 laser (at 5 watts continuous wave) to make the skin incision along the previously marked incision line. The skin is sharply excised from the underlying muscle with the laser by using forceps to grasp the lateral point of the ellipse with gentle upward traction. Upper eyelid skin is the thinnest skin in the body and very mobile tissue, especially in the elderly patient. For these reasons, the CO_2 laser is ideal because of its precision. Some surgeons prefer to resect skin and muscle (orbicularis oculi) as a single unit, whereas others address the two separately.

A 3-mm strip of orbicularis oculi muscle, along the superior aspect of the wound, is excised from the lateral

pole to the medial pole with curved scissors (removal of redundant orbicularis muscle is necessary to obtain optimal results in most patients). After the muscle is excised, the orbital septum is exposed. The yellowish fat pads are visible through the septum. Gentle ballottement of the globe accentuates the prolapsed fat (the supine position can mask the excess fat, which is usually prolapsed when the patient is upright).

The orbital septum is incised, and the fat is allowed to herniate through, assisted by gentle traction (excessive traction can shear terminal branches of the ophthalmic artery and vein). The herniated fat can be clamped with a hemostat and then excised with electrocautery (which achieves hemostasis simultaneously) or simply excised with a laser as the fat is passively draped over a cotton swab (to avoid overresection). Not all patients require fat excision.

Hemostasis must be achieved prior to closure. The skin is closed using 6-0 nylon suture in a running fashion (some surgeons prefer to use absorbable sutures). An ophthalmic-grade antibiotic ointment is applied, and a cold compress (4 × 4 gauze soaked in ice water) is used to minimize edema (a preoperative dose of steroids can also be used).

Figure 13-21 shows the markings, the incision, skin removal, and (a different patient from the one shown in Figure 13-18) fat excision in a 46-year-old patient with dermatochalasis undergoing bilateral upper eyelid blepharoplasty.

For the patient in the case study, the lower eyelid blepharoplasty was conducted using a subciliary incision with a lateral extension within a natural skin crease, allowing for a minimum of 5 mm between the upper and lower eyelid incisions. A skin muscle flap was elevated, the orbital septum was incised and excess periorbital fat was gently removed in a similar fashion, with careful attention to hemostasis. A strip of skin and muscle was excised along the incision line to remove excess skin and restore the lower eyelid to a more

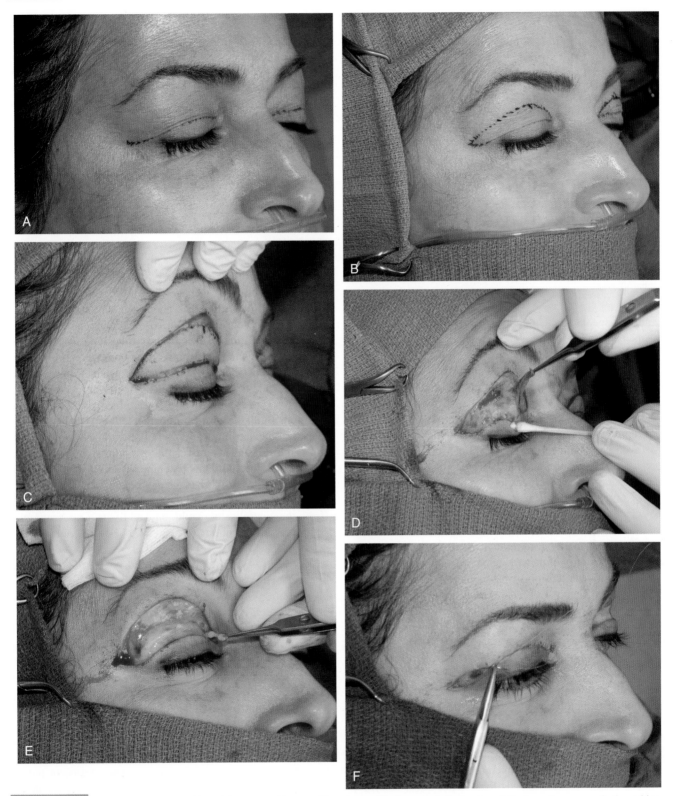

Figure 13-21 Bilateral upper eyelid excision on a 46-year-old patient with dermatochalasis. **A** and **B** show the presurgical markings. **C,** Skin incision. **D,** Removal of the skin. **E,** Fat excision. **F,** Closure (Note: this is a different patient from the one shown in Figure 13-18.)

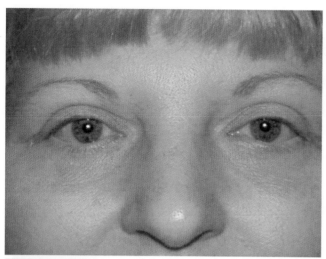

Figure 13-22 Six weeks after bilateral upper and lower blepharoplasties.

youthful appearance. Upon closure, attention is given to resuspension of the lateral aspect of the flap to the periosteum of the lateral orbital rim.

Alternatively, lower eyelid blepharoplasty can be performed via a transconjunctival approach for removal of fat only, or it can be combined with a skin pinch technique to remove excess skin without disrupting the orbicularis oculi muscle. Some surgeons advocate redistributing the fat instead of excising it. The ideal technique is determined by the surgeon's preference and the clinical presentation.

Postoperative care includes local wound care and application of antibiotic ointment. Overexertion must be avoided (especially during the first 48 hours after surgery), because it can increase postoperative edema and the risk of hematoma formation (especially a retrobulbar hematoma, a surgical emergency). Control of nausea and vomiting with antiemetics and control of hypertension are essential. Sutures are removed in 5 to 7 days. Figure 13-22 shows the postoperative photograph of the current patient at 6 weeks after upper and lower eyelid blepharoplasties.

COMPLICATIONS

Retrobulbar hematoma/bleeding, causing loss of vision. Retrobulbar hematoma after cosmetic blepharoplasty is the most feared complication, but it fortunately is rare (0.04%). It is more commonly reported in patients who failed to report the use of anticoagulation medications such as aspirin or herbal medications. A hematoma may be caused by shearing of small vessels in the fat pads located posteriorly or from uncontrolled hemostasis after excision of the fat. (The fat pads retract when released, making it difficult to control any small bleeders, so it is prudent to achieve hemostasis while the fat is being excised with electrocautery or laser.) The other theorized source of retrobulbar hematoma is hemorrhage from the cut edges of the orbicularis oculi muscle that gains retrobulbar access through the opened septum. The earliest sign is unilateral eye pain. This progresses to proptosis, ophthalmoplegia,

and decreased pupillary reflex with eventual visual disturbances (color discrimination is affected first, especially the color red). Sustained increased intraocular pressures (IOP) results in central retinal artery occlusion and optic nerve ischemia, resulting in irreversible damage. Treatment includes immediate removal of skin sutures and decompression of the orbit (this may require a lateral canthotomy and inferior cantholysis). Medical management includes high-dose steroids (dexamethasone 3 to 4 mg/kg, followed by a tapering dose), mannitol, acetazolamide, and papaverine (to decrease vascular spasm). Bed rest, elevation of the head, and avoidance of Valsalva maneuvers are important supportive measures.

Wound dehiscence. Due to the vascularity and quick healing time in the eyelids, wound dehiscence is uncommon. It can be seen after postoperative complications such as prolonged bleeding, hematoma, or infection. Patient noncompliance is another risk factor (e.g., early return to strenuous activity, eye rubbing). Management includes local wound care and allowing for healing by secondary intention, which generally occurs without scarring or cosmetic deformity.

Lagophthalmos and corneal abrasion. Transient lid incompetence is not uncommon after upper eyelid blepharoplasty. An intact Bell's phenomenon protects the cornea from abrasions and exposure keratitis when tear production is normal. Lagophthalmos with decreased tear production and/or a poor Bell's phenomenon increases the risk of exposure-related corneal complications. Lubrication ointment and an eye patch (plastic wrap over the eye works well) should be used during sleep until lagophthalmos resolves (as the lid skin stretches). Manual lid massage can be initiated 2 weeks after surgery to facilitate resolution. Full-thickness skin grafts (from the contralateral eyelid, banked tissue, or periauricular skin) may be required in cases of overly aggressive skin resection.

Eyelid ptosis. Postoperative eyelid ptosis may be caused by surgical injury or may result from an undiagnosed preexisting condition. Acquired senile ptosis (caused by dehiscence or disinsertion of the levator aponeurosis), accompanied by varying degrees of dermatochalasis of the upper eyelid, is common in the elderly population. Blepharoplasty performed in these patients without ptosis repair may result in postoperative exaggeration of the drooping eyelid. Therefore, it is prudent to identify such patients by properly examining levator function (normal excursion of 15 mm is considered excellent; greater than 8 mm is good; 5 to 7 mm is fair; and less than 4 mm is poor) and also the upper eyelid position at rest (normally covers 1 to 2 mm of the superior limbus). Periorbital edema and hematoma can cause transient ptosis. Otherwise, surgery for postoperative ptosis repair should be delayed 3 to 6 months to allow for resolution.

Keratoconjunctivitis sicca (dry eye syndrome). Tear production begins to decrease in the fifth decade of life. Blepharoplasty may produce subtle changes (increased width of the palpebral fissure, lower eyelid retraction, lagophthalmos), unmasking the borderline dry eye patient. Some authors recommend preoperative Schirmer's testing (a 5 × 35-mm strip of filter paper is placed on the lower conjunctiva for 5 minutes; less than 10 mm of wetting is considered abnormal). However, McKinney and Byun found that Schirmer's test was not a good predictor of post-blepharoplasty dry eye complication. Instead, the history (increased blinking, dryness, contact lens intolerance, grittiness, and pain) and anatomy (presence of scleral show, lagophthalmos, snap test, and negative vector) were found to be more important predictors of postoperative dry eye complications. Treatment options include topical ocular lubricants, wetting drops, ointments (night time), and punctal plugs.

Infection. Orbital cellulitis or abscess after blepharoplasty is extremely rare. Prevention includes identification and treatment of preexisting infectious diseases of the eyelid, conjunctiva, sinuses, and lacrimal sac. Appropriate surgical management may include opening a portion of the incision to allow drainage and systemic antibiotic coverage.

Cosmetic deformity (asymmetry, inappropriate fat resection, or lid malpositioning). Incomplete or overzealous resection of fat may cause residual fat bags or periorbital hollowing, respectively. Asymmetries of the lid arch, height and width of the palpebral fissure, residual fat, and lid crease are not uncommon. Photodocumentation of preexisting asymmetry and patient counseling are important. Careful surgical technique and attention to detail reduce the risk of asymmetry. Eyelid malpositioning (scleral show, ectropion, entropion, rounded eye) are mostly seen in lower eyelid blepharoplasty. Damage to the levator muscle, aponeurosis, or Mueller's muscle can result in upper lid malpositioning.

DISCUSSION

Examination of the blepharoplasty patient should encompass the whole face and should not be limited to the eyelids. Particular attention is given to the position of the upper lid (upper lid ptosis) and brow. Brow ptosis can cause excessive upper eyelid folds. This needs to be recognized and addressed in the treatment plan, for possible brow lift procedures.

Correct diagnosis is the first step to a successful outcome. The evaluation of the upper eyelid itself can be categorized into skin, muscle, and fat. Not all patients require surgical excision of all three components. Younger patients can demonstrate fat herniation/prolapse (especially the nasal/medial fat pad) without excess skin. A transconjunctival upper blepharoplasty (removal of excess medial upper eyelid fat) may be suitable for some patients. The aging patient may have excess eyelid skin and laxity (dermatochalasis), which requires skin excision only. However, most patients with varying degrees of dermatochalasis require resection of a small strip of orbicularis oculi muscle for a better-defined supratarsal crease and cosmetic outcome. Once the skin and muscle have been excised, the fat pads can be reevaluated under direct vision. Gentle ballottement of the globe accentuates the fat pads (which are normally prolapsed in the upright position but retracted in the supine position). If fat prolapses into the wound upon ballottement, the septum should be incised and the fat gently excised. It is important to keep in mind that the medial/nasal fat compartment is composed of two individual fat pads. It is also prudent to avoid excess traction on the fat pads, which can result in overresection of fat and shearing of the posterior vessels.

Management of the prolapsed lacrimal gland. A prolapsed lacrimal gland (superior lateral compartment of the orbit) should not be mistaken for a herniated fat pad. A prolapsed lacrimal gland can be repositioned using suture suspension techniques (the leading edge of the gland is sutured to the periosteum just posterior to the superior orbital rim); however, the gland should not be excised because of the increased risk of postoperative dry eye.

Adjunctive procedures during upper eyelid blepharoplasty. The corrugator supercilii muscle can be resected via the upper blepharoplasty incision, when indicated (to treat vertical glabellar rhytids). Some surgeons prefer to use this incision to facilitate subperiosteal dissection during an endoscopic-assisted forehead lift. If simultaneous forehead/eyebrow lifting is to be performed, the upper eyelid skin resection should be more conservative and should be marked with the eyebrow lifted to the ideal position (either procedure can be done first, depending on the surgeon's preference). Simultaneous laser resurfacing can also be performed.

Upper eyelid blepharoplasty in a male patient. An increasing number of male patients are seeking facial cosmetic surgery, particularly eyelid procedures. It is important to note the differences in anatomy and esthetic norms between the two genders. The male eyebrow should rest on the superior orbital rim (in females the apex of the brow should be 8 to 10 mm above); also, it is more flattened than the "arched" female brow. However, males can experience eyebrow ptosis and should be appropriately managed. The eyelid crease in men is typically lower, flatter, and less defined. In addition, the inferior skin incision is typically 6 to 8 mm above the upper eyelid margin centrally (in women it is 7 to 10 mm) and remains more flattened.

Special considerations for blepharoplasty in the Asian patient. The Asian patient requesting upper eyelid blepharoplasty deserves special attention. More than 50% of East Asians do not have a superior palpebral fold or supratarsal crease ("single eyelid"), and most of these patients requesting blepharoplasty seek surgical creation of a palpebral furrow or supratarsal crease ("double eyelid"). In the Asian "single eyelid," the superficial lamina of the levator aponeurosis/expansion does not penetrate the orbital septum and orbicularis oculi muscle to insert to the overlying dermis, as it does in the western "double eyelid." Instead, these fibers terminate on the tarsal plate (the height of the superior tarsal plate is 5 to 6 mm in Asians and 10 to 12 mm in Caucasians), and no palpebral fold is formed upon eyelid opening. The goal of Asian blepharoplasty is to create a well-defined supratarsal crease (the size and shape are dictated by the patient's desires) through various surgical techniques using supratarsal fixation sutures to adjoin the levator aponeurosis to the pretarsal skin. Several techniques can be used to create the "double eyelid" and manage the epicanthal fold, depending on the individual patient's anatomy and expectations.

Bibliography

Carraway JH: Surgical anatomy of the eyelids, *Clin Plast Surg* 14:693-701, 1987.

Cook BE, Lemke BN: Cosmetic blepharoplasty upper eyelid techniques, *Oral Maxillofac Surg Clin North Am* 12(4):673-687, 2000.

Fagien S: Discussion: the value of tear film breakup and Schirmer's tests in preoperative blepharoplasty evaluation, *Plast Reconstr Surg* 104:570-573, 1999.

Fagien S: Advanced rejuvenative upper blepharoplasty: enhancing aesthetics of the upper periorbita, *Plast Reconstr Surg* 110:278-289, 2002.

Ghali GE, Lustig JH: Complications associated with facial cosmetic surgery, *Oral Maxillofac Surg Clin North Am* 15:265-283, 2003.

Holt JE, Holt GR: Blepharoplasty: indications and preoperative assessment, *Arch Otolaryngol* 111:394-397, 1985.

Hughes SM: Evaluation of the cosmetic blepharoplasty patient, *Oral Maxillofac Surg Clin North Am* 12(4):649-670, 2000.

Januszkiewicz JS, Nahai F: Transconjunctival upper blepharoplasty, *Plast Reconstr Surg* 103:1015-1019, 1999.

Lisman RD, Hyde K, Smith B: Complications of blepharoplasty, *Clin Plast Surg* 15:309-335, 1988.

McCurdy JA: Upper Lid blepharoplasty: the double eyelid operation—external approach, *Facial Plast Surg Clin North Am* 4:7-23, 1996.

McCurdy JA: Upper blepharoplasty in the Asian patient: the "double eyelid" operation, *Facial Plast Surg Clin North Am* 10:351-368, 2002.

McKinney P, Byun M: The value of tear film breakup and Schirmer's tests in preoperative blepharoplasty evaluation, *Plast Reconstr Surg* 104:566-568, 1999.

Millay DJ, Larrabee WF: Ptosis and blepharoplasty surgery, *Arch Otolaryngol Head Neck Surg* 115:198-201, 1989.

Niamtu J: Cosmetic blepharoplasty, *Atlas Oral Maxillofac Surg Clin North Am* 12:91-130, 2004.

Seckel BR, Kovanda CJ, Cetrulo CL Jr, et al: Laser blepharoplasty with transconjunctival orbicularis muscle/septum tightening and periocular skin resurfacing: a safe and advantageous technique, *Plast Reconstr Surg* 106:1127-1145, 2000.

Seiff SR: Anatomy of the Asian eyelid, *Facial Plast Surg Clin North Am* 4:1-5, 1996.

Ullmann Y, Levi Y, Ben-Izhak O, et al: The surgical anatomy of the fat in the upper eyelid medial compartment, *Plast Reconstr Surg* 99:658, 1997.

Walrath JD, Hayek BR, Wojno T: Blepharoplasty. In Bagheri SC, Bell RB, Khan HA (eds): *Current therapy in oral and maxillofacial surgery*, p 986, St Louis, 2011, Mosby/Elsevier.

Zukowski ML: Endoscopic brow surgery, *Oral Maxillofac Surg Clin North Am* 12(4):701-708, 2000.

Genioplasty

Piyushkumar P. Patel and Shahrokh C. Bagheri

CC

A 25-year-old woman presents for consultation regarding chin augmentation. She explains, "I would like my chin to be bigger."

HPI

The patient states that she has been unhappy with the appearance of her lower face. In particular, she feels that her chin is small and that it influences her neck and facial profile. She has no prior history of facial cosmetic surgery or orthodontic treatment.

PMHX/PDHX/MEDICATIONS/ALLERGIES/SH/FH

Noncontributory.

EXAMINATION

General. The patient is a well-developed and well-nourished woman in no apparent distress.

Psychiatric evaluation. The patient's mood and affect are appropriate. Facial appearance is important to psychological well-being and social acceptance, and physical attractiveness may play a critical role in the development of an individual's self-concept or even career goals (e.g., modeling). It is important to assess the patient's motives and expectations for the surgery. Modern surgical interventions can safely enhance physical appearance, which in turn elevates self-confidence and personal well-being.

Maxillofacial. Chin deformities can manifest in any of the three dimensions (vertical, horizontal, and transverse) in isolation or in combination. The vast majority, however, are in the horizontal plane only. Careful scrutiny of the skeletal, dental, and soft tissue structures is required to obtain a good result.

On frontal view, the current patient exhibits good symmetry. The maxillary midline is coincident with the facial midline. The patient shows 2 to 3 mm of maxillary anteriors at rest (vertical maxillary excess can result in a clockwise rotation of the mandible, thus causing a retrognathic/microgenic appearance). The chin is symmetrical, with the soft tissue menton lying on the facial midline. Chin pad tissue thickness is approximately 10 mm (normal is 8 to 11 mm). On smiling, the lower lip is symmetrical. On elevation of the lower lip, no mentalis muscle hyperactivity or chin pad

fasciculations are seen (if alloplastic augmentation is to be used, muscle hyperactivity may place excessive force on the implant, leading to increased bone resorption or displacement of the implant).

On profile examination (Figure 13-23), the patient exhibits good nasal projection with a mild dorsal hump (a large nose makes the chin look small, and vice versa). The labiomental angle is obtuse at 160 degrees. (Ideally, the depth of the fold/sulcus should lie 4 mm posterior to a line drawn from the lower vermilion border to the pogonion. If the sulcus is shallow or high, augmentation results in enlargement of the lower face [chin and lip]; however, if the fold is deep and more inferiorly positioned, augmentation predominantly accentuates the chin.) The patient demonstrates a convex facial profile with a retrognathic appearance. The cervicomental angle is obtuse at 150 degrees (normal is 110 degrees to 120 degrees). On posturing of the mandible forward, there is significant improvement in the neck aesthetics (patients with microgenia can have altered neck aesthetics). There is a lack of the visible separation of the mandible and neck, giving the appearance that the face "flows" into

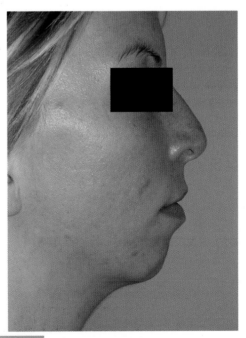

Preoperative profile view of the patient demonstrates a deficient chin in the horizontal plane.

the neck. To the untrained eye, this may appear to be secondary to tissue laxity or lipomatosis. Microgenia can further aggravate this condition. In such a case, the soft tissues of the neck should be examined with forward posturing of the mandible; if this produces less-than-optimal improvement in neck esthetics, cosmetic neck surgery may be indicated. In patients with macrogenia and a Class I relationship, an orthodontic history should be obtained to determine whether premolar extraction has been performed. In these patients, there usually is normal lip relationship with overprojection of the chin.

Intraoral. The patient's oral hygiene is excellent. (Some clinicians will not place an alloplastic implant in patients with active periodontal disease. Also, this may be an indicator of the patient's ability to keep the wound clean if an intraoral approach is to be used.) The patient has a Class I molar and canine relationship (a Class II malocclusion indicates that a skeletal abnormality exists; the patient should be informed of the option of orthodontic realignment and orthognathic surgery). The mandibular anterior teeth are in good position, neither retroclined nor proclined. Eversion of the lower lip results in deepening of the labiomental sulcus (this occurs with excess proclination of the anterior teeth).

IMAGING

Standard photographs of the frontal and profile views, both in repose and on smiling, are recommended. A panoramic radiograph and a lateral cephalogram are recommended for the work-up of patients requiring a genioplasty.

The panoramic radiograph is used to delineate the proximity of the mandibular canal/mental foramen, and the apices of the mandibular anterior dentition, in anticipation of a genial osteotomy. In addition, it provides a general overview of any mandibular osseous pathology.

Lateral cephalometric evaluations have been used to help determine the desired horizontal and vertical dimensions of the chin. Information gained from the cephalometric tracings includes the relationship of the maxilla and mandible to the skull base and to each other. It is important to identify any skeletal or occlusal disparities that can be corrected before or concomitant with a genioplasty procedure. Ideally, the chin (the soft tissue pogonion) should rest slightly posterior to the lower lip, and the lower lip should be posterior to the upper lip. Increasing sagittal projection beyond these relations may risk an unesthetic result.

The lateral cephalogram for the current patient shows the deficiency of the chin in the anteroposterior dimension and a Class I molar relationship (Figure 13-24).

Cone-beam CT facilitates appreciation of the three-dimensional anatomy of the mandible and also preoperative planning.

LABS

No routine laboratory testing is indicated for genioplasty procedures unless dictated by the medical history.

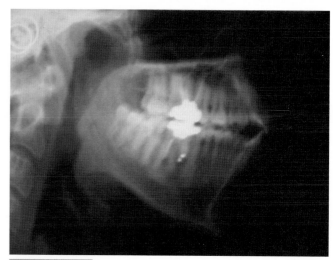

Figure 13-24 Preoperative lateral cephalogram showing the deficiency of the chin in the anteroposterior dimension and a Class I molar relationship.

Table 13-2	Comparison of the Two Currently Accepted Methods of Chin Augmentation
Osseous Genioplasty	**Alloplastic Augmentation**
Can correct deformities in vertical transverse and sagittal planes	Indicated only for correction of a mild to moderate sagittal deficiency
Useful in the correction of a failed alloplastic genioplasty	Relatively straightforward
More technically demanding	Can be performed via an intraoral or extraoral approach
No extraoral scarring	Precision increases with CAD/CAM-designed implants
Precision increases with computer-assisted surgery	

ASSESSMENT

Horizontal microgenia, in a patient who desires chin augmentation.

TREATMENT

Genioplasty refers to a horizontal osteotomy of the anterior mandible. *Chin implant* refers to either an alloplastic or autogenous implant. Alloplastic chin implants and sliding genioplasty are the two currently accepted methods of chin augmentation (Table 13-2). The anticipated soft tissue changes in response to hard tissue movements are shown in Table 13-3.

Careful treatment planning, meticulous surgical technique, and the surgeon's artistic sense are three important factors for successful and predictable chin surgery. For intraoral access,

Table 13-3 Soft Tissue Response to Hard Tissue Movements		
Procedure	**Soft Tissue Response (% of Hard Tissue Movement)**	**Comment**
Advancement		
Osteotomy (genioplasty)	90% to 100% horizontal	Labiomental fold deepens
Alloplast onlay	80% to 90% horizontal	Labiomental fold deepens
Bone onlay graft	60% to 70% horizontal	
Vertical Augmentation		
With interpositional graft	80% to 90 % of vertical augmentation	Labiomental fold flattens
Reduction Genioplasty		
Vertical reduction with wedge removal	90% of vertical reduction	
Vertical reduction with osteotomy of inferior border	25%	Highly unpredictable
Horizontal reduction (sliding)	90% to 100%	Labiomental fold flattens
Horizontal reduction (degloving with bur reduction)	25% to 30%	Overall flattening of chin

Modified from Peterson L, Indresano AT, Marciani RD, et al: *Principles of oral and maxillofacial surgery,* vol III, Philadelphia, 1992, Lippincott.

it is important to plan an incision that achieves the following goals:

- Ease of wound closure, ensuring that movable mucosa, rather than attached gingiva, forms the wound margin
- Avoidance of periodontal problems after wound contraction and scar formation
- Prevention of mental or inferior alveolar nerve severance
- Ability to resuspend the mentalis muscle to prevent chin (mentalis) droop

An incision in the depth of the vestibule results in excessive scar formation and should be avoided. A U-shaped incision extending from canine to canine that leaves 10 to 15 mm of mucosa anterior to the depth of the vestibule is ideal. The mentalis muscle is incised in an oblique fashion, leaving an ample amount superiorly to allow for closure. The mentalis muscle is stripped in a subperiosteal plane, exposing the symphysis. The mental nerves are identified bilaterally, and the periosteum is freed circumferentially around the foramen. Careful dissection in this area allows the surgeon to preserve all branches of this nerve. The planned osteotomy should lie a minimum of 5 mm below the longest tooth root (usually the canine) and a minimum of 10 to 15 mm superior to the inferior border. The osteotomy should also extend 4 to 5 mm below the lowest point of the mental foramen. It should be remembered that the angle of the osteotomy can influence vertical and horizontal changes. An osteotomy that is more parallel with the occlusal plane allows a greater vector of advancement in the horizontal dimension. If vertical shortening is desired, the angle should be more acute. The midline should be marked with a burr (fissure type) to prevent postoperative iatrogenic asymmetries. The osteotomy is completed with a reciprocating saw. The orientation of this saw should remain constant to ensure a symmetrical cut through the buccal and lingual cortices, to prevent interferences that may hamper the proposed movement. Once the osteotomy has been completed and the fragment repositioned, it can be secured through a variety of methods, including the use of wires, prebent chin plates, or lag screws. The wound should

be closed in layers; it is essential that the mentalis muscle be accurately repositioned. A dressing is applied to facilitate soft tissue reattachment and prevent hematoma formation.

Alloplastic augmentation can also be considered for the treatment of a genial deficiency. A wide range of materials can be used. Those most commonly used include high-density polyethylene (Medpor; Porex Surgical Products Group, Newnan, Georgia), hard tissue replacement polymer, polyamide mesh (Supramid; S. Jackson, Inc., Alexandria, Virginia), polydimethyl-siloxane (Silastic; Dow Corning, Midland, Michigan), and fibrillated ePTFE (Gore-Tex; W.L. Gore & Associates, Flagstaff, Arizona). Prior to the removal of Proplast from the American market, various forms of Proplast (Vitek; Houston, Texas) was used for genial augmentation, such as Proplast I (PTFE and graphite), Proplast II (PTFE and alumina), and Proplast hydroxyapatite. Many surgeons believe that polydimethyl-siloxane (Silastic) meets most of the criteria for an ideal alloplastic implant. The ideal characteristics of an alloplastic implant include the following:

- Anatomic configuration that has a posterior surface that contours to the external surface of the mandible and an external implant shape that imitates the desired outcome
- Readily implantable and nonpalpable
- Margins of the implant blend onto the bony surfaces
- Easily removable
- Malleable, comfortable, and inert
- Easily modifiable by the surgeon during the procedure

Placement of alloplastic implants via an extraoral submental incision can be combined with other procedures, such as submental liposuction or platysmal placation. The surgeon's experience is usually the deciding factor in whether an implant or an osteotomy is performed. It is generally accepted that mild to moderate abnormalities can be corrected with either alloplastic implantation or genioplasty (some clinicians recommend alloplastic augmentation for deficiencies up to 5 mm, because mandibular resorption beyond an augmentation of 5 mm is a concern). However, for severe abnormalities sliding genioplasty should be performed. Genioplasty is a more versatile procedure as it can address abnormalities in

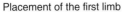

Placement of the first limb

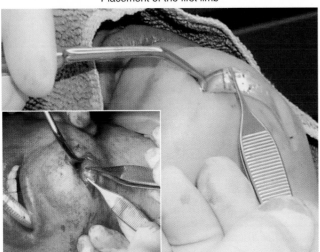

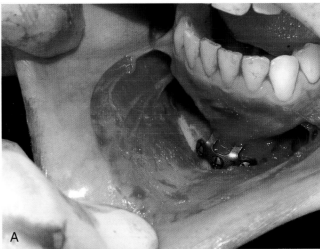

Figure 13-25   Insertion of a silicone chin implant via a submental incision. *(From Bagheri SC, Bell RB, Khan HA:* Current therapy in oral and maxillofacial surgery, *St Louis, 2012, Saunders.)*

any of the three dimensions. There is some debate on the superiority of either procedure for augmentation.

Computer-assisted osseous genioplasty involves performing the osteotomy virtually. From this a model can be fabricated and plates prebent. In addition, a surgical guide can be made to transfer the osteotomy line's screw positions and also a jig to accurately position the genial segment intraoperatively. Evaluation of the accuracy of this technique has shown that it is promising.

Three-dimensional computer-aided design (CAD) and computed-aided manufacture (CAM) of customized-designed implants reduce the need to carve or shape stock implants during surgery. Using established protocols, a CT is obtained, and a three-dimensional model is then fabricated. On this model the surgeon fabricates a template using silicone resin. An exact silicone elastomer implant is then fabricated (using the template) for insertion (Figure 13-25). In genioplasty patients, custom implants are usually used to correct contour irregularities from previous unsuccessful attempts.

The current patient underwent advancement of 7 mm with use of a prebent chin plate that was secured with six monocortical screws (Figure 13-26, *A*). Figure 13-26, *B,* shows the preservation of the branches of the mental nerve after careful dissection and plate stabilization. Figure 13-27 shows the postoperative lateral cephalogram and profile view at 4 weeks.

COMPLICATIONS

The most common complication after genioplasty surgery is a neurosensory disturbance, followed by hematoma and infection. Soft tissue changes, such as chin ptosis, excessive lower tooth display, devitalization of teeth, creation of mucogingival problems, asymmetry, and unesthetic results, are also known complications. Mandibular fracture, hemorrhage causing lingual hematoma and possible airway compromise, and

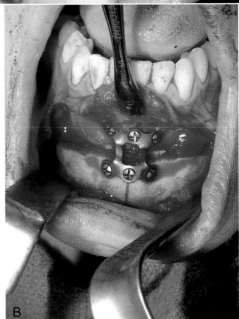

Figure 13-26   **A,** Intraoperative view showing the placement of a 7-mm prebent chin advancement plate. **B,** Intraoperative view showing the preservation of all branches of the mental nerve.

avascular necrosis of the mobilized segment are possible but rare complications of this procedure.

Injury rates to the mental nerve have been reported to range from 0 to 20% at 1 year after surgery. The etiologies of nerve injury include inadequate exposure, poorly designed flaps, inadequate protection during osteotomy, excessive stretching, and compression. The majority of patients undergoing genioplasty experience a transient neurosensory deficit, probably secondary to neuropraxia. However, most studies show resolution of any neurosensory deficit after several months. A reduction in the response to light touch (a sensitive marker for neurosensory deficit) has an incidence of 3.4%. This complication is associated with no adverse effect on the quality of life.

The inferior alveolar nerve travels inferiorly and anteriorly past the mental foramen before looping back and exiting the

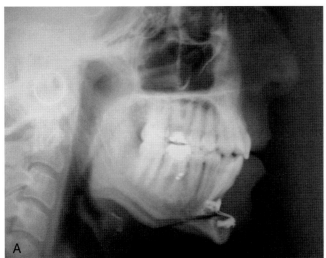

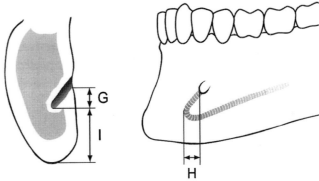

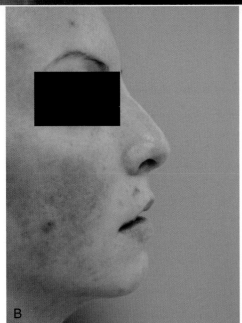

Figure 13-27 **A,** Postoperative lateral cephalogram showing the position of the chin after 7-mm advancement. **B,** Postoperative lateral view at 4 weeks after 7-mm advancement genioplasty.

Figure 13-28 Terminal mandibular canal in relationship to the mental foramen, demonstrating the looping of the nerve before exiting at the foramen. Looping terminal mandibular canal and mental foramen. G, Distance from terminal mandibular canal to mental foramen; H, Advanced anterior distance from terminal mandibular canal to mental foramen; I, Distance from terminal mandibular canal to inferior border of body near the mental foramen. The average distances of G, H, and I were 4.5 ± 1.9 mm, 5.0 ± 1.8 mm, and 9.2 ± 2.7 mm, respectively. *(From Hwang K: Vulnerability of the inferior alveolar nerve and mental nerve during genioplasty: an anatomic study, J Craniofac Surg 16:10-14, 2004.)*

mental foramen (Figure 13-28). It is recommend that the osteotomy line remain 5 mm (4.5 mm minimum) below the mental foramen to avoid injury to the inferior alveolar nerve.

Sensory innervation of the chin is divided into three territories: labial territory (the mental nerve supplies this area), mental territory (cutaneous branch of the mylohyoid nerve), and submental territory (cervical branches of the cervical plexus). Neurosensory deficits of the skin overlying the chin, without involvement of the mental nerve, can occur with injury to the mylohyoid nerve. When a horizontal osteotomy is performed using a reciprocating saw and sectioning involves not only bone but also some soft tissue of the floor of the mouth in this area, the potential for injury to the mylohyoid muscle exists, along with injury to the mylohyoid nerve. This can result in neurosensory deficits of the skin overlying the chin without involvement of the mental nerve. Other anatomic

structures at risk include the submental and sublingual arteries. Aggressive stripping of the soft tissue pedicle attached to the inferior and medial aspect of the mandibular symphysis can also involve the cutaneous branch of the mylohyoid nerve. Relapse in the immediate postoperative period is uncommon except in the case of fixation failure. There is generally good stability of the segment after genioplasty.

"Witch's chin deformity" is a term coined by Gonzales-Ulloa in 1971 to describe chin ptosis. Loss of mentalis muscle origination plays an important role in the pathogenesis of this problem. The mentalis muscle is the only muscle of significance when performing a genioplasty. It is the sole elevator of the lower lip, providing the majority of the lip's vertical support. If the muscle is not precisely reattached at the end of the surgery, chin ptosis and increased exposure of the lower incisors can occur. Advocates of alloplastic augmentation report that if the implant is placed through a submental approach, the mentalis muscle can be left attached.

The most common complications of alloplastic augmentation are infection, bone resorption under the implant (although some studies have shown that in the majority of patients, this has no clinical consequences, including esthetic changes in the soft tissue profile), extrusion, malpositioning or displacement of the implant, and improper sizing of the implant. The main theories on the cause of resorption under an alloplastic implant include the following:

- Pressure of the implant against bone. (Studies have shown that the implant's location with respect to the periosteum is irrelevant in the prevention of resorption; also, implants placed over alveolar bone tend to cause more resorption, and there is the risk of erosion into the roots of the mandibular anterior teeth. In addition, lower lip strain and an overactive mentalis may place additional pressure on an implant.)

- Loss of vascularity. (Preserving the lingual soft tissue has been shown to be beneficial in preventing resorption.)
- Micromotion. (A precise pocket, excellent contact between the implant and mandible, and consideration of the use of rigid fixation and porous implants that allow ingrowth have been shown to reduce micromotion.) Long-term follow-up of patients who have implants is recommended. In patients who demonstrate resorption, consideration can be given to removal of the implant and placement of a smaller implant or conversion to an osseous genioplasty.

DISCUSSION

Horizontal sectioning of the anterior mandible (genioplasty) was first described by Hofer in the German literature in 1957. This initial operation was performed on a cadaver, with preoperative and postoperative photographs demonstrating the results. Subsequently, Trauner and Obwegeser introduced the intraoral approach. Since then a number of technical variations have been described. Despite the versatility of the horizontal mandibular osteotomy, the biologic basis was not studied until the mid-1980s. Ellis and colleagues demonstrated that maintaining the soft tissue pedicle (the digastric musculature and the periosteum on the inferior and lingual border) is associated with less osseous resorption in the postoperative period. Storum demonstrated that close apposition of the margins of the osteotomy is important for vascular bridging and early osteogenesis. In patients with skeletal discrepancies who would benefit from conventional orthognathic surgery, Proffit and colleagues suggested three specific indications for an isolated genioplasty as a camouflage procedure:

- The borderline extraction patient with a good nasolabial angle, protruding mandibular incisors, and a deficient chin
- A patient with a short mandibular ramus in whom advancement may lead to an unstable result
- A patient with asymmetry that does not involve a significant malocclusion

Macrogenia can be seen in isolation or associated with mandibular hyperplasia. Some patients who are under the care of an orthodontist and would benefit from a mandibular setback are never referred to a surgeon, for a variety of reasons. In these cases the orthodontist extracts the lower premolars, followed by retroclining of the mandibular incisors. This results in normal occlusal and lip relationships; however, the patients usually exhibit macrogenia. Macrogenia can be classified into three subgroups, depending on the vectors of growth: anterior, vertical, or a combination. This can be corrected using either reduction of the mental protuberance with a bur or a horizontal sliding osteotomy. Removal of excess bone with a bur does not result in appreciable improvement of the soft tissue contour. The soft tissues drape poorly over the newly contoured bone, resulting in a double chin appearance. Lower lip ptosis can also be seen if the periosteum does not attach to the newly contoured bone. Lip

incompetence and a lack of cervicomandibular definition can also be associated with this technique. Submental ostectomy (burring down) of the prominence is acceptable when only a small amount of reduction is needed. Posterior repositioning with an osteotomy has been shown to produce a better result. However, this technique has the potential for mental nerve injury, not only from the procedure, but also because of the need to dissect around the inferior border to reduce the projecting wings. Submental ostectomy with soft tissue excision via an extraoral approach has been shown to prevent the negative sequelae of excessive submental tissue and chin ptosis.

Alantar and colleagues have shown that the mean number of branches of the mental nerve as it exits the foramen is two. However, the number of branches can range from one to four. The branches of the mental nerve are known to run in an oblique direction; the mean angle between the most medial branch and the long axis of the orbicularis oris muscle is 36 degrees. Based on this, it is recommended that an incision not be made parallel to the fibers of the orbicularis oris muscle. Damage can be avoided if the incision is made with an angle of 36 degrees to the long axis of the lip. Labial incisions should thus have a U shape. The two sides of the U should be as parallel as possible to the lower labial branches (36 degrees). Limiting the proximal extension of the incision to the canine region also reduces the incidence of neuronal injury.

Bibliography

Alantar A, Roche Y, Maman L, et al: The lower labial branches of the mental nerve: anatomic variation and surgical relevance, *J Oral Maxillofac Surg* 58:415-418, 2000.

Binder W: Custom-designed facial implants, *Facial Plast Surg Clin North Am* 16 (1):133-146, 2008.

Chang EW, Lam SM, Karen M, et al: Sliding genioplasty for correction of chin abnormalities, *Arch Facial Plast Surg* 3:8-14, 2001.

Chaushu G, Binder D, Taicher S, et al: The effect of precise reattachment of the mentalis muscle on the soft tissue response to genioplasty, *J Oral Maxillofac Surg* 59:510-516, 2001.

Ellis E, Dechow PC, McNamara JA, et al: Advancement genioplasty with and without soft tissue pedicle, *J Oral Maxillofac Surg* 42:637-645, 1984.

Frodel JL, Sykes JM, Johes JL, et al: Evaluation of vertical microgenia, *Arch Facial Plast Surg* 6:111-119, 2004.

Guyot L, Layoun W, Richard O, et al: Alteration of chin sensibility due to damage of the cutaneous branch of the mylohyoid nerve during genioplasty, *J Oral Maxillofac Surg* 60:1371-1373, 2002.

Hofer O: Die osteoplastiche verlaengerung des unterkiefers nach voneiselber bei mikrogenia, *Dtsh Zahn Mund Kieferheilkd* 27:81, 1957.

Hoffman GR, Moloney FB: The stability of facial osteotomies. Part 3. Chin advancement, *Aust Dent J* 40:289-295, 1995.

Hoffman GR, Moloney FB: The stability of facial osteotomies. Part 6. Chin setback, *Aust Dent J* 41:178-183, 1996.

Hwang K: Vulnerability of the inferior alveolar nerve and mental nerve during genioplasty: an anatomic study, *J Craniofac Surg* 16:10-14. 2004.

Hwang K, Han JY, Chung IH, et al: Anatomic studies: cutaneous sensory branch of the mylohyoid nerve, *J Craniofac Surg* 16:343-345, 2005.

Kim SG, Lee JG, Lee YC, et al: Unusual complication after genioplasty, *Plast Reconstr Surg* 109:2612-2613, 2002.

Lesavoy M, Creasman C, Schwartz RJ, et al: A technique for correcting witch's chin deformity, *Plast Reconstr Surg* 97:842-846, 1999.

Nishioka GJ, Zysset MK, Van Sickels JE, et al: Neurosensory disturbances associated with the anterior mandibular horizontal osteotomy, *J Oral Maxillofac Surg* 46:107-110, 1988.

Proffit WR, Turvey TA, Mariarty JD: Augmentation genioplasty as an adjunct to conservative orthodontic treatment, *Am J Orthod* 79:473-491, 1981.

Reed EH, Smith RG: Genioplasty: a case for alloplastic chin augmentation, *J Oral Maxillofac Surg* 58:788-793, 2000.

Storum KA: Microangiographic and histologic evaluation of revascularization and healing after genioplasty by osteotomy of the inferior border of the mandible, *J Oral Maxillofac Surg* 48:210-216, 1988.

Strauss RA, Abubaker AO: Genioplasty: a case for advancement osteotomy, *J Oral Maxillofac Surg* 58:783-787, 2000.

Trauner R, Obwegeser H: Surgical correction of mandibular prognathism and retrognathism with consideration of genioplasty, *Oral Surg* 10:677, 1957.

Varol A, Sencimen M, Kocabiyi K, et al: Clinical and anatomical aspects of possible mylohyoid nerve injury during genioplasties, *Int J Oral Maxillofac Surg* 38:1084-1087, 2009.

Ward J, Garri JI, Wolfe SA, et al: The osseous genioplasty, *Clin Plast Surg* 34:485-500, 2007.

White J: Management and avoidance of complications in chin augmentation, *Aesthet Surg J* 31:6, 634-642; 2011.

Zide BM, et al: Chin surgery. I. Augmentation: the allures and the alerts, *Plast Reconstr Surg* 104:1843-1853, 1999.

Zide BM, Pfeifer TM, Longaker MT: Chin surgery. II. Submental ostectomy and soft tissue excision, *Plast Reconstr Surg* 104:1854-1860, 1999.

Endoscopic Brow-Lift

Husain Ali Khan, Chris Jo, and Shahrokh C. Bagheri

CC

A 55-year-old female presents to your office with a chief complaint of, "My eyebrows have been drooping down slowly year after year, and I want them lifted back up."

HPI

The patient points to one eyebrow, lifts it superiorly with her fingers in front of a mirror, and states, "This is where my eyebrows used to be and should be, but now look how flat they are." (This maneuver may unmask pseudo upper eyelid dermatochalasis caused by the descended brow.) She also brings a picture of herself in her 30s to illustrate her desired surgical outcome. She denies any previous facial cosmetic surgery and appears to have reasonable expectations (surgeons should be cautious about patients with unreasonable expectations of cosmetic surgery).

PMHX/PDHX/MEDICATIONS/ALLERGIES/SH/FH

Noncontributory. The patient is not taking any medications that would affect platelet function (e.g., aspirin) or the coagulation cascade.

EXAMINATION

Forehead–eyebrow–upper lid complex. The forehead exhibits minimal horizontal rhytids (wrinkles) at rest and moderate dynamic horizontal furrows (caused by frontalis muscle hypertrophy/hyperactivity compensation for brow ptosis). The hairline (trichion) is 5 cm from the orbital ridge (within normal limits [WNL]). There are mild horizontal radix and vertical glabellar furrows at rest (caused by the procerus and corrugator supercilii muscles, respectively). The eyebrow (examined with the patient completely relaxed and in a neutral position) is relatively flat in shape (attractive female eyebrows are arched, as opposed to flattened in males). The position of the eyebrows is recorded (Figure 13-29); the inferior border of the eyebrow is measured from the superior orbital rim. Findings for the current patient are:

- *Medial brow region:* 1 mm below the superior orbital rim (ideally, the medial brow is 1 to 2 mm above the rim in females and males).
- *Brow apex* (halfway between the lateral limbus and lateral canthus): 3 mm above the superior orbital rim (ideally, the apex is 8 to 10 mm above the rim, or 25 mm diagonally from mid-pupil, in females and 1 to 2 mm above the rim in males).
- *Tail of brow* (lateral): 2 mm above the superolateral orbital rim (ideally, the tail is located 10 to 15 mm above the superolateral orbital rim in females and 1 to 2 mm above the rim in males) and ends just lateral to the line connecting the lateral canthus and nasal ala (WNL).
- **Upper eyelid** (also see the section Upper and Lower Eyelid Blepharoplasty). Exhibits pseudo dermatochalasis, or lateral hooding (Figure 13-30) secondary to brow fat pad and eyebrow ptosis (descent of the forehead–eyebrow–brow complex), which resolves when the forehead-eyebrow complex is manually raised into an ideal position by the surgeon's thumb.

IMAGING

Preoperative and serial postoperative photo imaging are mandatory for cosmetic procedures. A close-up view of the forehead–eyebrow–upper eyelid complex in frontal, three-quarter, and profile positions is recommended.

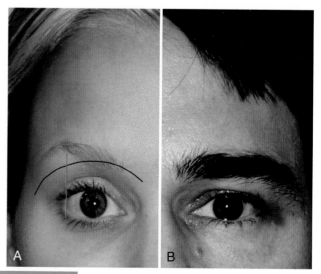

Figure 13-29　Ideal position of an esthetically pleasing, youthful eyebrow for a Caucasian female (**A**) and male (**B**). *(From Bagheri SC, Bell RB, Khan HA:* Current therapy in oral and maxillofacial surgery, *St Louis, 2012, Saunders.)*

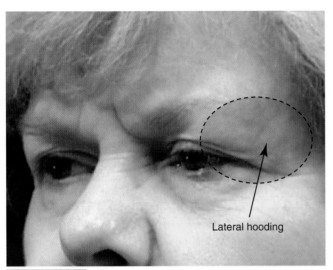

Figure 13-30 A 55-year-old patient with lateral hooding and heavy dynamic glabellar rhytids. *(From Bagheri SC, Bell RB, Khan HA: Current therapy in oral and maxillofacial surgery, St Louis, 2012, Saunders.)*

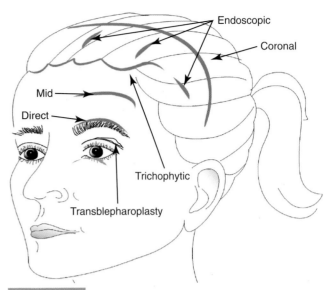

Figure 13-31 The different incisions and techniques used during forehead and eyebrow lifting. *(From Bagheri SC, Bell RB, Khan HA: Current therapy in oral and maxillofacial surgery, St Louis, 2012, Saunders.)*

LABS

Routine preoperative laboratory testing for outpatient brow lift procedures is not indicated unless dictated by the medical history.

ASSESSMENT

Patient desires brow lift procedure secondary to bilateral eyebrow ptosis caused by gravitational descent of the soft tissues of the upper facial third with age.

TREATMENT

For the current patient, upper facial rejuvenation with an endoscopic brow (forehead) lift is the treatment of choice to restore a youthful or esthetically pleasing eyebrow position. The most commonly used technique is described in this chapter, although there are multiple approaches to forehead and eyebrow lifting (Figure 13-31).

Incisions. Three 2-cm vertical incisions (one in the midline and two parasagittal incisions coincident with the lateral limbus) are made just behind the hairline down to bone, and two bilateral 3-cm vertical temporal incisions are made at 2 to 3 cm posterior to the hairline down to the deep temporal fascia (alternatively, some surgeons recommend two incisions coincident with the medial brow instead of one midline incision when more medial elevation is required).

Dissection. Subperiosteal dissection is initially carried out blindly, using the three frontal incisions, posteriorly toward the lambdoid suture, anteriorly to approximately 2 to 3 cm above the superior orbital rim, and laterally to the temporal crest. The endoscope is introduced into the midline incision and used to assist the subperiosteal dissection toward the superior orbital rim (there is strong periosteal adherence to

bone in this region) to avoid injury to the supraorbital and supratrochlear neurovascular bundles. It is important to release the periosteum down to the radix medially and past the orbital rims laterally.

The temporal incisions are then used to blindly dissect the initial 2 cm toward the lateral orbital rims. The endoscope is used to assist the remainder of the dissection. The temporal dissection should stay 1 cm above the zygomatic arch to prevent injury to the frontal branch of the facial nerve. The anterior extent of dissection is sufficient once the sentinel vein (zygomaticotemporal vein) is encountered. The temporal zone of fixation (conjoined tendon) is penetrated and released with a periosteal elevator, connecting the subperiosteal dissection in the forehead region and the subtemporoparietal dissection in the temporal region (connecting all three optical cavities). Some surgeons recommend removing a strip of deep temporal fascia to enhance scar formation and to improve long-term stability.

Prior to elevating the forehead and eyebrow, it is important to incise and release the periosteum just superior to the arcus marginalis from the lateral orbital rim, along the superior orbital rim, and across the radix of the nose. Several techniques can be used to release the periosteum. The authors prefer the technique described by Griffin and colleagues in which a 50-watt CO_2 laser is used (other surgeons prefer to use a long Colorado needle). The corrugator supercilii and/or procerus muscles can be disrupted if needed.

Elevation and fixation. Various methods can be used to elevate and fixate the forehead-eyebrow complex. Evans describes a very precise technique using two-hole miniplates; the forehead-eyebrow complex is secured to the miniplate with 2-0 Vicryl suture. Griffin describes a flap suspension suturing technique that secures the flap to the posterior scalp. It is important that the suture engage subcutaneous tissue,

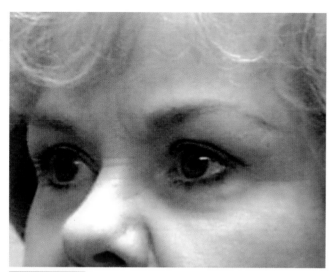

Figure 13-32   Patient 6 months after a brow lift and simultaneous upper and lower blepharoplasty. *(From Bagheri SC, Bell RB, Khan HA: Current therapy in oral and maxillofacial surgery, St Louis, 2012, Saunders.)*

galea, frontalis muscle, subgaleal areolar fascia, and periosteum (most important) at the anterior aspect of the incision. Resorbable endotines have been recently introduced; these are drilled into the frontal bone, and the spikes engage, holding the periosteum in place. The temporal tissues (superficial temporal fascia anteriorly to temporal fascia posteriorly) are suspended posteriorly by 2-0 Vicryl sutures through the temporal incision. The incisions are closed, and a head dressing is placed. Figure 13-32 shows the postoperative view of the current patient after simultaneous brow lift and upper and lower blepharoplast).

COMPLICATIONS

Endoscopic brow lift has minimal complications (infection, hematoma, nerve injury, alopecia, scarring, and brow malposition). As with all facial cosmetic procedures, relapse is the biggest concern for the surgeon, and long-term stability is one of the main goals of cosmetic surgery. Transient forehead paresthesia (anesthesia, hypoesthesia) is a consequence of surgery and is not considered a complication. Permanent nerve injury, although uncommon, may occur if the supraorbital or supratrochlear nerve is injured beyond a stretch injury (neuropraxia); this is usually avoided by performing careful dissection assisted by an endoscope. Despite correct technique and a thorough knowledge of the regional anatomy, nerve injuries can happen.

Evaluation of the brows should be done with particular attention to the upper eyelids. It is important to avoid performing an upper eyelid blepharoplasty on a patient who really requires a brow lift procedure. Lifting the brow to an ideal position may subsequently cause lagophthalmos due to excess upper eyelid skin excision.

DISCUSSION

Youthful or ideal appearance of the upper facial third. A youthful appearance of the upper third of the face includes smooth forehead skin without rhytids or furrows; arched, tapering eyebrows (for females); and a distinct supratarsal fold without excess skin or prolapsed fat. Males tend to have thicker and more horizontal eyebrows that are ideally 1 to 2 mm above and along the superior orbital rim. The goal of rejuvenation of the upper face is not only to restore the eyebrow to an esthetically pleasing form with a brow lift procedure, but also to restore the upper eyelid with a blepharoplasty as needed (see the section on upper and lower eyelid blepharoplasty) and to smoothen the forehead and glabellar rhytids or furrows with adjunctive procedures (see below). It is important to note that there are variations in what is considered a "normal" or esthetically pleasing eyebrow (see Figure 13-29) among different ethnic and racial groups.

Anatomy of aging of the upper facial third. The major plane of aging of the upper face is between the superficial fascia and deep fascia (gliding plane). This plane is called the *subtemporoparietal aerolar fascia* (in the temporal region) and the *subgaleal areolar fascia* (in the frontal region). The frontalis muscle inserts into the dermis of the medial two thirds of the eyebrow only, medial to the temporal fusion line. The lateral third of the eyebrow is unsupported by the frontalis muscle and begins to descend as the lateral support mechanism attenuates (temporal zone of fixation and orbital osteocutaneous ligament). The forehead-eyebrow-temporal soft tissues slide over the deep fascia-pericranium, which is loosely adherent; this causes ptosis of the eyebrows with a relatively greater effect on the lateral brow. Depressor action of the orbicularis oculi, depressor supercilii, corrugator supercilii, and procerus muscles and descent of the brow fat pad contribute to this aging process. Even though the changes in the sub–superficial musculoaponeurotic system (SMAS) plane are considered a main contributor to aging of the upper face, the long-term stability of forehead/eyebrow lift procedures depends on scarification of the periosteum to bone.

Alternative surgical procedures for forehead-eyebrow rejuvenation. Traditional approaches to the forehead and brow lift include a direct brow lift (incision/excision directly above the eyebrow), a mid-forehead lift (incision/excision along a horizontal forehead furrow), and a coronal lift (incision/excision along and/or within the hairline). The coronal lift (either coronal or pretrichial incisions) is still commonly used by some surgeons and is indicated in some cases. More recently, minimally invasive, barbed sutures (Contour Threads) have been introduced; however their long-term stability has come into question.

Adjunctive procedures. The endoscopic brow lift can be performed as an isolated procedure or can be combined with other facial cosmetic procedures (e.g., face-lift, upper or lower blepharoplasties, Botox injections), depending on the patient's needs and desires. It is important to realize that the positions of the upper eyelid and eyebrow are closely related, and the two must be examined together (refer to the section on Upper and Lower Eyelid Blepharoplasty). Botox is commonly used to treat vertical glabellar rhytids (corrugator supercilii muscle), horizontal forehead rhytids (frontalis muscle), and horizontal rhytids at the radix (procerus muscle). It can be used to achieve some elevation of the brow by reducing the downward force caused by the orbicularis oculi muscle.

Bibliography

Adamson PA, Johnson CM, Anderson JR, et al: The forehead lift, *Arch Otolaryngol* 111:325-329, 1985.

Beeson WH, McCollough EG: Complications of the forehead lift, *Ear Nose Throat J* 64:28-42, 1985.

Cook TA, Brownrigg PJ, Wang TD, et al: The versatile midforehead brow lift, *Arch Otolaryngol Head Neck Surg* 115:163-168, 1989.

Cuzalina A, Copty TV: Forehead, eyebrow and upper eyelid lifting. In Bagheri SC, Bell RB, Khan HA (eds): *Current therapy in oral and maxillofacial surgery*, St Louis, 2012, Saunders.

Cuzalina A: Endoscopic forehead and brow lift. In Fonseca RJ, Marciani R, Turvey TA (eds): *Oral and maxillofacial surgery*, ed 2, vol 3, St. Louis, 2009, Saunders.

Griffin JE, Frey BS, Max DP, et al: Laser-assisted endoscopic forehead lift, *J Oral Maxillofac Surg* 56:1040-1048, 1998.

Griffin JE, Owsley TG: Management of forehead and brow deformities, *Atlas Oral Maxillofac Surg Clin North Am* 12:235-251, 2004.

Knize DM: An anatomically based study of the mechanism of eyebrow ptosis, *Plast Reconstr Surg* 97:1321-1333, 1996.

Liebman EP, Webster RC, Berger AS, et al: The frontalis nerve in the temporal brow lift, *Arch Otolaryngol* 108:232-235, 1982.

Ramirez OM, Robertson KM: Update in endoscopic forehead rejuvenation, *Facial Plast Surg Clin North Am* 10:37-51, 2002.

Zukowski ML: Endoscopic brow surgery, *Oral Maxillofac Surg Clin North Am* 12(4):701-708, 2000.

CHAPTER 14

Syndromes of the Head and Neck

Editors: Shahrokh C. Bagheri

This chapter addresses:
- Cleft Lip and Palate
- Nonsyndromic Craniofacial Synostosis
- Syndromic Craniofacial Synostosis
- Hemifacial Microsomia
- Obstructive Sleep Apnea Syndrome

A multitude of anomalies and syndromes occur in the head and neck, most of which are beyond the scope of this book. The chapters in this section cover some of the most common anomalies or syndromes associated with the craniomaxillofacial region (Table 14-1). Congenital anomalies include nonsyndromic craniosynostosis, hemifacial microsomia, and cleft lip and palate; congenital syndromes include Apert and Crouzon. Obstructive sleep apnea syndrome, although not congenital in nature, is included in this section because its pathogenesis and manifestation are based on anatomic anomalies of the head and neck. Oral and maxillofacial surgeons are uniquely trained to play an integral role in the surgical management of these patients, syndromic or not.

The intent of these chapters is to familiarize the readers with the pathogenesis, presentation, and management of such anomalies. The chapters are structured so that key features of each syndrome or anomaly are emphasized. The reconstructive strategies and rationale for treatment are discussed. Because of the complexity of the craniofacial deformities involved in the growing child, the reconstructive efforts are generally staged. There is no consensus on the best timing of each stage; however, the general guidelines are presented. Various surgical strategies can be used, depending on the surgeon's preference and the clinical situation. These are presented in the various sections, along with the rationale for treatment.

Table 14-1	Characteristics of Some Craniofacial Syndromes				
Syndrome	Prevalence/ Inheritance	Genetic	Synostosis/Orbit	Limbs	CNS
Apert syndrome	15.5/million, AD or sporadic or new mutation M = F	Ser253Trp or Pro253 ARG on Ig II or III of FGFR2	Early fusion of coronal suture, widely patent midline calvarial defect	Fusion of digits 2, 3, and 4 Less common is fusion of digits 2, 3, 4, and 5 with digit 1 free	Patent sutures (except coronal) and open synchondroses, agenesis of septum pellucidum, agenesis of corpus callosum, cavum septum pellucidum, developmental delay
Crouzon syndrome	15-16/million, AD	15 mutations of Ig III FGFR2	Variable suture involvement and skull shape, exotropia, exposed conjunctiva and keratitis	None	Cerebellar tonsil herniation, jugular foramen stenosis, venous obstruction, increased intracranial pressure, headache (29%), seizure (10%), mental retardation (3%)
Pfeiffer syndrome	16-40/million, AD	FGFR1,2	Pronounced exorbitism, broad thumbs		Three types—type 1: normal life expectancy and intelligence; type 2: cloverleaf skull, exorbitism, elbow ankylosis, broad thumb and great toes; type 3: same as type 2 without cloverleaf skull. Types 2 and 3 have ventriculomegaly, progressive hydrocephalus, and cerebellar herniation
Saethre-Chotzen syndrome	Prevalence?	Twist gene 7P21	Low-set frontal hairline, deviated nasal septum		

AD, Autosomal dominant; *CNS*, central nervous system.

Cleft Lip and Palate

John M. Allen, Chris Jo, and Shahid R. Aziz

CC

As a member of the craniofacial multidisciplinary team, you are asked to evaluate a female infant born with a right complete cleft lip/palate (CLP).

There are both ethnic and racial variations in the incidence of CLP. It is most common in Asians (3.2 : 1,000), followed by Caucasians (1.4 : 1,000) and, least common, individuals of African descent (0.43 : 1,000). CLP occurs more often in males and on the left side. Isolated cleft palate (CP) is a different genetic entity with no racial predilection; it is more common in females.

HPI

The infant was born at a community hospital with no obstetric complications. She was subsequently diagnosed with a non-syndromic CLP and was referred for further evaluation and treatment. The pregnancy was uncomplicated, with no known environmental exposures.

Modern high-resolution ultrasonographic studies are able to diagnose complete CLP as early as 16 weeks in utero; therefore, prenatal diagnosis of CLP has become more common.

PMHX/PDHX/MEDICATIONS/ALLERGIES/SH/FH

Except for the CLP, the child has no other medical problems. She was born with Apgar scores of 8 and 9, at 1 and 5 minutes, respectively. There are no facial or systemic anomalies characteristic of any known syndromes (see Discussion later in this section), including any associated cardiac, respiratory, ophthalmologic, or musculoskeletal abnormalities. There is no family history of CLP or CP.

Pedigree analysis has demonstrated an increased incidence when a family member has CLP. In addition, if a couple has a child with CLP, the risk of having an affected second child is significantly increased (fortyfold).

Infants born with CLP are at increased risk for associated congenital syndromes, particularly congenital cardiac disease. As such, obtaining a screening echocardiogram should be considered to rule out congenital valvular heart disease or transposition of the great vessels. In addition, the presence of CLP interferes with appropriate feeding, which in turn can lead to failure to thrive in the infant. The use of special cleft nipples is recommended, in addition to consultation with a maxillofacial prosthodontist for obturator fabrication.

EXAMINATION

General. Female infant is in the 25th percentile for weight and height (likely due to difficulty with feeding).

Maxillofacial. The cleft lip (CL) is complete, penetrating the entire thickness of the lip, alveolus, nasal tip cartilages, and floor of the nose (Figure 14-1). The cleft is unilateral, right of midline (left side prevalence), and continuous with the palate (CLP is most commonly expressed unilaterally, with a 2 : 1 predilection for the left side).

Intraoral. The cleft continues through the hard palate and soft palate (structures anterior to the incisive foramen form the primary palate and posterior to the incisive foramen form the secondary palate). Throughout the cleft, the nasal cavity, nasal conchae, and posterior pharyngeal wall are readily visible. The nasal mucosa appears inflamed and ulcerated (due to irritation of the fragile tissue from feeding). Bidigital palpation identifies solid supportive bone along the palatal shelves bordering the cleft site (it is important to palpate the hard palate of any infant to detect the presence of a notch in the posterior border of the hard palate, suggesting the presence of a submucous cleft).

IMAGING

No imaging studies are indicated for the diagnosis and management of isolated CLP. When craniosynostosis or syndromic anomalies are suspected, craniofacial and head computed tomography (CT) scans are indicated.

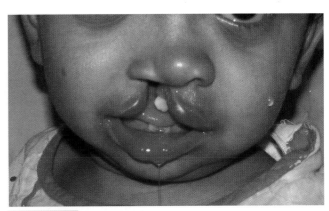

Figure 14-1 Preoperative photograph of patient showing unilateral cleft lip and palate. (Courtesy of Dr. Shahid Aziz.)

LABS

Baseline hemoglobin and hematocrit levels are indicated before surgical correction of any cleft. In general, a hemoglobin level of 10 mg/dl is deemed necessary before surgical intervention for lip repair (although there is no scientific rationale for this determination).

ASSESSMENT

Female infant with an isolated, complete, nonsyndromic CLP.

Although there are several classification systems for facial clefting, including one by Tessier, they are not routinely used at most centers.

CL is a unilateral or bilateral gap in the upper lip and jaw that forms during the third through seventh weeks of embryonic development. It develops from failure of fusion of the medial nasal process and the maxillary process. CLs are described as either complete or incomplete. A complete CL is a cleft of the entire lip and alveolar arch or premaxilla; an incomplete CL involves only the lip and often spares the soft tissue of the associated alar base. A CP is a gap in the hard and/or soft palate that forms during the fifth through twelfth weeks of development. CP forms as a result of failure of attachment and alignment of the levator veli, tensor veli palatini, uvular, palatopharyngeus, and palatoglossus muscles. The primary palate is formed by the lip, alveolar arch, and palate anterior to the incisive foramen (known as the *premaxilla*). The secondary palate is formed by the soft and hard palates posterior to the incisive foramen.

TREATMENT

There is no general consensus regarding the timing and techniques used for CLP surgery. Individual craniofacial centers and craniofacial surgeons follow various protocols according to their own experience, rationale, and preferences. The functional needs, esthetic concerns, and ongoing growth of affected individuals all create specific concerns that complicate the treatment process. Presurgical dentofacial orthopedics is increasingly used to optimize primary CL repair.

Table 14-2 outlines the sequence of management of patients with CLP. CL repair is usually addressed at 10 to 14 weeks of age. One advantage of waiting until this age is that it allows time for a thorough medical evaluation to determine whether

Table 14-2	Sequence of Management of the Cleft Palate	
Procedure	**Age or Timing**	**Comments**
Dentofacial orthopedics	First few weeks of life	Improves tension-free lip closure
Lip adhesion (two-stage repair)	After dentofacial orthopedics and before definitive nasolabial repair	Some centers prefer one-stage closure and do not perform lip adhesions
Definitive nasolabial repair	Traditionally done at 10 weeks (no scientific basis)	Timing may vary based on cleft type
	Centers now advocate lip closure at 3 to 6 months	
Cleft palate repair	Before 1 to 2 years	Earlier repair (before 1 year) is advocated to improve speech development
	Some centers advocate closure at 8 to 10 months	Maxillary growth should be monitored with earlier repairs
	Some centers advocate two-stage repair using an obturator to delay palate closure	
Correction of velopharyngeal insufficiency (pharyngeal flap or sphincter pharyngoplasty)	Speech assessment begins at 1½ to 2 years	Velopharyngeal insufficiency may occur after maxillary advancement and can be corrected 6 to 12 months later
Nasolabial revisions	Before 3 years	
Phase I orthodontics	Before alveolar cleft bone grafting	Differentially expands the anterior maxilla
Alveolar bone grafting	At 8 to 12 years (when maxillary canine root is one half to two thirds formed)	Bone graft from anterior ilium is usually preferred
Phase II orthodontics	Permanent dentition phase	
Correction of maxillary hypoplasia (orthognathic surgery and/or distraction osteogenesis)	After completion of growth	Distraction osteogenesis should be considered when maxillary advancement is greater than 10 mm
Rhinoplasty	At 6 to 12 months after maxillary advancement	

Modified from Kaban LB, Troulis MJ (eds): *Pediatric oral and maxillofacial surgery,* St Louis, 2004, Saunders.

the infant has any congenital defects. The surgical procedure is generally easier to perform when the child is slightly larger, because anatomic landmarks are more prominent and well defined. In addition, it has historically been accepted that the safest anesthesia time period for infants is based on the "rule of tens"—surgery can be performed when the child is at least 10 weeks of age, weighs at least 10 pounds, and has a minimum hemoglobin value of 10 mg/dl (however, there is no current scientific rationale to support this rule). With modern intraoperative pediatric monitoring techniques, general anesthesia can be performed safely at an earlier age as needed, although there is no documented benefit to performing lip repair before 3 months of age. In addition, excessive scarring and inferior esthetic results have been found to occur when surgery is performed earlier than age 3 months.

CP repair is usually performed between 9 and 18 months of age. It is intended to coincide with the progression of natural speech development and growth. In deciding upon the timing of repair, the surgeon must consider the delicate balance between facial growth restriction after early surgery and early speech development, which requires an intact palate. Most children require an intact palate to produce certain sounds by 18 months of age. If developmental delay is present and speech is not anticipated to develop until later, CP repair can be delayed. Coincident with CP repair is placement of myringotomy tubes, because CLP patients have a higher incidence of middle ear disease.

There is very little evidence to support palate repair before 9 months of age. Surgical repairs before this time are associated with a higher incidence of maxillary hypoplasia later in life and show no improvement in speech. After initial CP repair, 20% of the children develop inadequate closure of the velopharyngeal mechanism (velopharyngeal insufficiency). This is usually diagnosed at 3 to 5 years of age, when a detailed speech examination can be performed. Surgery is performed to correct the anatomic defect, with the goal of improving closure between the oral and nasal cavities and reducing nasal air escape during the production of certain sounds.

Approximately 75% of patients with any type of cleft present with clefting of the maxilla and alveolus. Bone graft reconstruction of the alveolus is performed during the mixed dentition period, before eruption of the permanent canine and/ or permanent lateral incisor. The timing of this procedure is based on dental development and not chronologic age. Reconstruction of the alveolus before the mixed dentition stage has been associated with a high degree of maxillary growth restriction, requiring orthognathic correction later in life. Autogenous bone grafted from the iliac crest has provided the best results for reconstruction of alveolar cleft defects. Although globally there are multiple recommendations with regard to the timing of the bone graft, most commonly in the United States the alveolar grafting is completed when the associated canine root is two thirds formed; that is, typically at 9 to 11 years of age. Prior to grafting, orthodontic expansion of the maxilla is indicated to maximize the amount of graft placed in the alveolus.

Orthognathic reconstruction of maxillary and mandibular discrepancies is generally performed from 14 to 18 years of age based on individual growth characteristics. This is performed in conjunction with orthodontics before and after surgery. Orthognathic surgery before this time frame is performed only for severe cases of dysmorphology.

Lip and nasal revision is best done once the majority of growth is complete, which generally occurs after 5 years of age; it is usually performed only for severe deformities. When orthognathic reconstruction is planned, rhinoplasty is best performed after orthognathic surgery, because maxillary advancement improves many characteristics of nasal form.

Treatment techniques for CL. Unilateral CL repair, as previously mentioned, is usually performed after 10 weeks of age. The technique most commonly used is the Millard rotation-advancement technique. The basic intent of the repair is to create a three-layer closure of skin, muscle, and mucosa that approximates the normal tissue and excises hypoplastic tissue at the cleft margins. The orbicularis oris muscle is adapted to form a continuous sphincter. The incision lines of the Millard technique also fall within the natural contours of the lip and nose on closure, which helps promote a natural form of symmetry. The C-flap can be used to lengthen the columella or create a nasal sill.

The Randall-Tennison technique is a Z-plasty technique used by some surgeons for unilateral CL repair. This technique does not achieve the same semblance of symmetry obtained with the Millard technique.

Primary nasal reconstruction may be performed at the time of lip repair to reposition the displaced lower lateral cartilages and alar tissues. Various techniques have been advocated, each with considerable variation. The repair essentially involves releasing the alar base, augmenting the area with allogenic subdermal grafts, or proceeding with open rhinoplasty with minimal dissection to avoid scar formation.

Bilateral lip repair is a very challenging technical procedure, primarily due to the lack of quality tissue present and the manner of separation of the tissues caused by the clefting. The typically shortened columella and rotation of the premaxillary segment make achieving acceptable aesthetic results difficult. Variations to surgical approaches range from aggressive lengthening of the columella with preservation of hypoplastic tissue to conservative primary nasal reconstruction as performed with McComb's unilateral CL technique. McComb's technique involves release and repositioning of the lower lateral cartilages and alar base on both sides without aggressive degloving of the entire nasal complex. Aggressive corrective techniques often produce initial results that are very good. Long-term results, however, are not so favorable due to the progression of natural growth processes. Excessive angulations and lengthened structures provide a less-than-optimal esthetic effect. Revision of these deformities is usually very difficult, and sometimes impossible. In general, if hypoplastic tissue is excised and incisions within the medial nasal base and columella are avoided, long-term esthetic results are excellent.

Treatment techniques for CP. Successful CP repair during infancy depends on two objectives. The first involves water-tight closure of the entire oronasal communication involving the hard and soft palate. The second involves anatomic repair of the musculature within the soft palate, which is critical for the creation of normal speech. The soft palate functions in coupling and decoupling of the oral and nasal cavities in the production of speech. The tensor and levator palatini and uvularis muscles, which usually join at the midline, forming a continuous sling, are separated and insert along the posterior edge of the hard palate. Surgical treatment of a CP is concerned with closing the palatal defect and releasing the abnormal muscle insertions. The timing for CP repair is correlated with the development of speech, which usually occurs around 18 months for a normally developing child. The velum, or soft palate, must be closed before the development of speech. If repair occurs after this time, compensatory speech articulations may result. The timing of surgery must also be balanced with the known biologic consequences of performing surgery during infancy, specifically during the growth phase, which could result in maxillary growth restriction. When repair of the palate is performed between 9 and 18 months of age, the incidence of maxillary restriction is approximately 25%. If repair is carried out earlier than 9 months of age, the incidence of severe growth restriction requiring future orthognathic surgery is greater. In addition, CP repair before 9 months of age is not associated with any increased benefit in terms of speech development. Performing CP repair between 9 and 18 months of age seems to best address the functional concerns of speech development and the potential negative impact surgery has on growth.

An approach used to address the speech issues with growth-related concerns involves staging the closure of the secondary palate with two procedures. This involves repair of the soft palate early in life, followed by closure of the hard palate later during infancy. The intent of this approach is to accomplish timely repair of the soft palate, which is critical for speech, while delaying hard palate repair until further growth has occurred. This technique offers the advantage of less growth restriction, easier repair of larger clefts, and less chance for fistula formation.

The basic premise of CP repair involves mobilization of multilayered flaps to close the defect created due to the failed fusion of the palatal shelves. The nasal mucosa is first closed, followed by reconstruction of the levator and tensor palatini muscles. The abnormal insertion of the levator and tensor palatini muscles on the hard palate must be removed and reconstructed to join in the midline. The musculature making up the velopharyngeal mechanisms are also reconstructed to allow the soft palate to close the space between the nasopharynx and oropharynx in order to create certain speech sounds. Closure of the oral mucosa completes the repair.

Many techniques have been devised for CP repair. The Bardach technique involves creation of two large, full-thickness flaps on each palatal shelf, which are layered and brought to the midline for closure (Figure 14-2, *A* and *B*). This technique allows for preservation of the palatal neurovascular

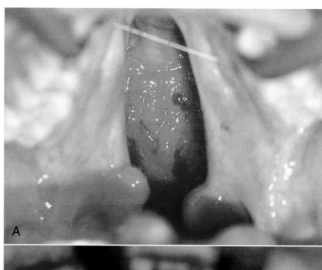

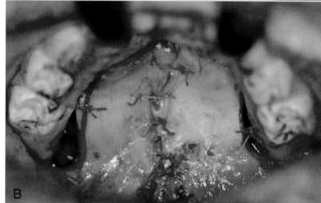

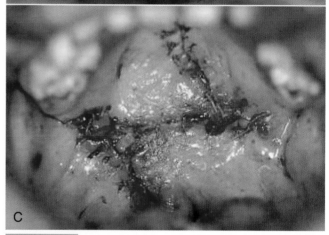

Figure 14-2 **A,** Complete cleft palate. **B,** Immediate postoperative photograph showing cleft palate closure using the Bardach technique. **C,** Immediate postoperative photograph showing cleft palate closure using the Furlow double-opposing Z-plasty technique.

bundle, which is contained within the pedicle of each flap. The Von Langenbeck technique is similar to the Bardach technique, but it preserves an anterior pedicle for increased blood supply to the flaps. It also involves elevation of large mucoperiosteal flaps from the palate with midline approximation of the cleft margins. Long lateral releasing incisions are made at the border of the palatal and alveolar bone to allow mobilization. The levator muscles are detached from their abnormal insertion along the hard palate. The Furlow double-opposing Z-plasty technique involves two Z-plasties, one on the oral mucosa and one in the reverse orientation on the nasal mucosa (Figure 14-2, *C*). The levator muscle on one side is included in the posteriorly based oral mucosa Z-plasty, whereas the levator muscle from the opposite side is included within the posteriorly based nasal mucosal Z-plasty flap. This procedure produces palatal lengthening and reorients and provides overlap of the malpositioned levator muscles. The Furlow Z-plasty has been reported to be associated with a higher rate of fistula formation at the junction of the soft and hard palates.

The Wardill-Kilmer-Veau technique is a V-Y advancement of the mucoperiosteum of the hard palate and is intended to lengthen the palate in the anteroposterior plane at the time of palatoplasty. Bone is left exposed in the area where the flaps were advanced. These areas granulate and epithelialize within 2 to 3 weeks but form excessive scat tissue that may contribute to maxillary growth disturbances. The vomer flap is used to achieve closure of the hard palate. A wide, superiorly based flap of nasal mucosa is elevated from the vomer and attached to the palatal shelf to close the defect. The vomer flap eliminates the need to elevate large mucoperiosteal flaps from the hard palate, thus avoiding possible maxillary growth disturbances.

For very wide clefts, a pharyngeal flap may be used. This technique allows the central portion of the cleft to be filled with posterior pharyngeal wall tissue, making the closure of the nasal and palatal mucosa easier. Patients with Pierre Robin sequence (malformation) or Treacher Collins syndrome have exceptionally wide clefts that are difficult to close without tension. The pharyngeal flap seems to address the concerns for CP repair with these patients. Pharyngeal flaps, however, pose an increased risk of bleeding, snoring, obstructive sleep apnea, and hyponasality.

Figure 14-3 shows the 1-year postoperative view of the patient seen in Figure 14-1.

COMPLICATIONS

The complications associated with cleft repair are essentially related to the technique used for treatment. The overall goals include nasal lining closure, adequate exposure, and release of soft tissue attachment along the bony borders of the cleft from the alveolar crest to the pyriform rim and closure of the oral mucosa with well-vascularized tissue that contains attached mucosa at the alveolar crest. Failure to address these concerns during treatment ultimately leads to complications that include wound infection with fistula formation, mucosal dehiscence, hypertrophic scar formation, and hemorrhage.

It is also important to note that many patients with CLP have coexisting systemic abnormalities that may negatively affect the outcome of the treatment provided. Patients who present with systemic abnormalities in general are expected to have a higher incidence of complications compared with healthy patients. With surgical correction of CLP, Lees and Pigott observed a high incidence of intraoperative and postoperative complications related to the respiratory system.

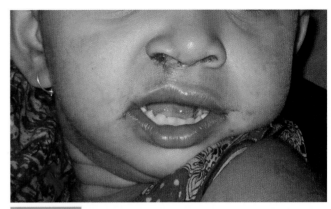

Figure 14-3 Postoperative photograph of patient in Figure 14-1 after lip and palate repair at 1 year of age. (Courtesy of Dr. Shahid Aziz.)

The most significant complication or unfavorable result of palate closure is the development of velopharyngeal insufficiency. This is manifested as a resonance problem, with creation of hypernasal or hyponasal speech. Velopharyngeal insufficiency can be secondary to maxillary orthognathic (advancement) surgery or the use of pharyngeal flaps. The resonance occurs from the modification of oronasal portals that are either too large or too narrow. Correction of this problem involves reconstructive surgery with revision or creation of a new pharyngeal flap, accompanied by aggressive speech therapy.

A common complication of lip repair is the "whistle" deformity, which occurs due to vertical retraction of the scar or from inadequate advancement and rotation of the skin flap. Various lip-lengthening procedures can be performed secondarily, such as the V-Y advancement, which corrects the deformity and creates a normal lip seal.

In cases of complete bilateral CLP, collapse of the alveolar segments posterior to the premaxilla is a common occurrence when orthodontic or palatal retention devices are not used. Correction of segment collapse is very complex, involving multiple surgeries over an extended period.

DISCUSSION

CL and/or CP malformations are the most common congenital abnormalities in the facial region. Worldwide, the incidence of CL is approximately 1:700 live births. The incidence of CP is approximately 1:2,000 live births. CLP patients routinely have impaired facial growth, dental anomalies, speech disorders, poor hearing, psychological difficulties, and poor social relationships. Due to the multiple factors associated with CLP, specialty multidisciplinary teams are involved in the overall care of these patients. The involvement of the team starts during the immediate neonatal period and continues through completion of growth and adolescence. The multidisciplinary team is composed of a craniofacial surgeon, an oral and maxillofacial surgeon, a pediatrician, an otolaryngologist, a pediatric dentist, an orthodontist, an audiologist, a speech and language therapist, a geneticist, a psychologist, and a social worker.

CP deficiencies commonly go undetected during infancy, only to be identified later during childhood when the resultant anomaly becomes very apparent with the emergence of speech, feeding, and growth complications. It is therefore very important to accurately assess the palatal anatomy of any infant before such deficiencies create significant problems. During the initial inspection and examination of the palatal anatomy of infants, the presence of a submucous cleft is quite frequently missed. With submucous clefts, on visual inspection the palate appears intact; however, the overlying oral and nasal mucous membranes are expanded against the cleft area, giving the illusion of an intact palate. Digital palpation identifies a notch or discontinuity along the posterior aspect of the bony hard palate. The submucous cleft represents a deficiency in the musculature of the palate due to failed midline fusion of the palatal muscles, namely, the levator veli palatini, tensor veli palatini, uvulus, palatoglossus, and palatopharyngeus muscles. A bluish midline streak is often present over the soft palate, which indicates the splitting of the muscle layers.

A number of concerns are associated with CLP.

- **Feeding.** Approximately 25% of CLP infants have early feeding difficulties, with poor weight gain for the first 2 to 3 months. Feeding sessions are prolonged due in part to ulceration of the nasal mucosa. Some infants also have increased metabolic needs due to congenital heart disease or airway obstruction. Initial poor weight gain usually resolves after cleft closure, and any deficiency in growth is corrected by 6 months of age. Height and weight progressions are routinely monitored.

- **Speech and language development.** Even after the palate has been repaired, children are still at risk for subsequent speech disorders. It is reported that 25% of children with CLP develop normal speech after primary surgery, whereas the remaining 75% require many surgical interventions throughout childhood and adolescence. Speech problems arise from velopalatal insufficiency, dental and occlusal problems, oronasal fistulas, and hearing problems. Approximately 15% to 20% of patients who have CP repair within the first 12 to 15 months of life have velopharyngeal insufficiency. As mentioned earlier, surgical intervention must be coordinated with the development of speech. Speech and language therapy must also be provided during this time. The monitoring of speech continues into adolescence and adulthood in conjunction with active orthodontic and surgical management.

- **Hearing.** Patients with CP are at increased risk of middle ear effusions and subsequent infections. The attachment of the levator veli palatini muscle around the eustachian tube is abnormal and leads to poor aeration and drainage of the middle ear. Regular assessment by the ear, nose, and throat (ENT) surgeon and audiologist is recommended to ensure that poor hearing is not a contributing factor to compromised speech.

- **General dental welfare.** Children with CLP are at great risk for developing malocclusion. When the cleft involves the alveolar process, odontogenic structures within this region are routinely absent or malformed. Orthodontic intervention is generally initiated during the preschool years. Active occlusal manipulation and correction should not be instituted until the permanent dentition has erupted.

- **Genetics.** There are three types of genetic risk groups for CLP: the syndromic group, identified by physical examination; the familial group, identified by history; and isolated defects, identified by exclusion of the first two groups. As mentioned earlier, the incidence of CL is approximately 1:700 live births, and the incidence of CP is approximately 1:2,000 live births. With one parent and one child affected, the chance of a second child having a cleft is 10%. When both parents are without clefts and two children have clefts, the chance of a third child having a cleft is 19%. When one parent has a cleft and two offspring are normal, the chance of the third child being born with a cleft is 2.5%.

- **Environment.** Epidemiologic studies have demonstrated a relationship between maternal exposure to environmental factors or teratogens during pregnancy and the development of CLP. These factors or teratogens include alcohol consumption, cigarette smoking, folic acid deficiency, corticosteroids, benzodiazepines, and anticonvulsants.

Bibliography

Bryne PJ, Sands NR: Secondary bone grafting of residual alveolar and palatal clefts, *J Oral Surg* 30:87-92, 1972.

Carici F: Recent developments in orofacial cleft genetics, *J Craniofac Surg* 142(2):130-143, 2003.

Chung K, Kowalski C, Kim HM, et al: Maternal cigarette smoking during pregnancy and the risk of having a child with cleft lip/palate, *Plast Reconstr Surg* 105(2):485-491, 2000.

Copeland M: The effect of very early palatal repair on speech, *Br J Surg* 43:676, 1990.

Costello BJ, Ruiz RL, Turvey T: Surgical management of velopharyngeal insufficiency in the cleft patient, *Oral Maxillofac Surg Clin North Am* 14:539-551, 2002.

Costello BJ, Shand J, Ruiz RL: Craniofacial and orthognathic surgery in the growing patient, *Select Readings Oral Maxillofac Surg* 11(5):1-20, 2003.

Dorf DS, Curtin JW: Early cleft repair and speech outcome: a ten year experience. In Bardach J, Morris HL (eds): *Multidisciplinary management of cleft lip and palate*, pp 341-348, Philadelphia, 1990, Saunders.

Glenny AM, Hooper L, Shaw WC, et al: Feeding interventions for growth and development in infants with cleft lip, cleft palate or cleft lip and palate, *Cochrane Database Syst Rev* 2, 2005.

Habel A, Sell D, Mars M: Management of cleft lip and palate, *Arch Dis Child* 74(4):360-366, 1996.

Lees VC, Pigott RW: Early postoperative complications in primary cleft lip and palate surgery: how soon may we discharge patients from hospital? *Br J Plast Surg* 45:232-234, 1992.

Marsh JL: Craniofacial surgery: the experiment on the experiment of nature, *Cleft Palate Craniofac J* 33:1, 1996.

McComb H: Primary correction of unilateral cleft lip nasal deformity: a ten year review, *Plast Reconstr Surg* 75:791-799, 1985.

Murray JC: Gene/environment causes of cleft lip and/or palate, *Clin Genet* 61:(4):248-256, 2002.

Padwa BL, Sonis A, Bagheri SC, et al: Children with repaired bilateral cleft lip/palate: effect of age at premaxillary osteotomy on facial growth, *Plast Reconstr Surg* 105:1261, 1999.

Posnick JC: Cleft orthognathic surgery: the unilateral cleft lip and palate deformity. In Posnick JC (ed): *Craniofacial and maxillofacial surgery in children and young adults*, pp 860-907, Philadelphia, 2000, Saunders.

Posnick JC: The staging of cleft lip and palate reconstruction: infancy adolescence. In Posnick JC (ed): *Craniofacial and maxillofacial surgery in children and young adults*, pp 785-826, Philadelphia, 2000, Saunders.

Ruiz RL, Costello BJ, Turvey T: Surgical correction of midface deficiency in cleft lip and palate malformation, *Oral Maxillofac Surg Clin North Am* 14(4):491-507, 2002.

Spritz RA: The genetics and epigenetics of orofacial clefts, *Curr Opin Pediatr* 13(6):556-600, 2001.

Takato T, Yonohara Y, Mori Y: Early correction of the nose in unilateral cleft lip patients using an open method: a ten year review, *J Oral Maxillofac Surg* 53A:28-33, 1995.

Nonsyndromic Craniosynostosis

Chris Jo, Shahrokh C. Bagheri, and Neil Agnihotri

CC

A 7-month-old male infant is referred by his pediatrician for evaluation of a craniofacial dysmorphology.

HPI

The mother of this 7-month-old, otherwise healthy male (craniosynostosis has a male predilection) has been concerned about the abnormal shape of his head, which was noticed immediately after birth. (Craniosynostosis is the premature fusion of the cranial sutures during intrauterine life. The deformity is often noticeable early [Figure 14-4].) The pediatrician has been closely observing this skull deformity for changes and resolution. It was initially assumed to be deformational plagiocephaly (skull deformity caused by vaginal delivery or early fetal decent into the pelvis) and later was thought to be secondary to a positional plagiocephaly, an acquired skull deformity caused by a repetitive head position during sleep (nonsynostotic posterior plagiocephaly has increased since the American Academy of Pediatrics issued a recommendation that infants be placed on their back during sleep to reduce the risk of sudden infant death syndrome [SIDS]). Despite conservative management, the child continued to exhibit the cranial deformity, which appeared to slightly worsen over time. He is otherwise in good health, and the mother denies any behavioral abnormalities. He is referred for craniofacial evaluation (the rate of detectable cranial abnormalities secondary to craniosynostosis has been reported to be as high as 1:1,700 to 1:1,900 births).

PMHX/PDHX/MEDICATIONS/ALLERGIES/SH/FH

Noncontributory. The patient is up-to-date with all childhood immunizations, and there is no previous surgical history. The patient had an otherwise uneventful vaginal delivery.

There is no significant family history. (Mendelian inheritance patterns are rare for nonsyndromic craniosynostosis and are usually associated with other abnormalities, except for metopic suture craniosynostosis, which has a 5% positive family history.)

With the exception of metopic craniosynostosis (which has a 43% incidence of associated malformations with no clear syndromic diagnosis), patients with nonsyndromic craniosynostosis are typically healthy and do not show other malformations commonly present in syndromic craniosynostosis.

EXAMINATION

General. The patient is a well-developed and well-nourished, pleasant child in no apparent distress.

Maxillofacial. Examination of the skull reveals a mild dysmorphology (the exact dysmorphology varies greatly and

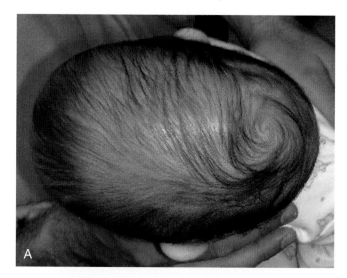

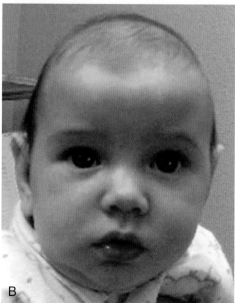

Figure 14-4 Sagittal synostosis. Top of head **(A)** and frontal view **(B)** before treatment. *(From Bagheri SC, Bell RB, Khan HA: Current therapy in oral and maxillofacial surgery, St Louis, 2012, Saunders.)*

depends on which portion or portions of the sagittal suture are involved) in which the cranial vault is narrow in the bitemporal and biparietal dimensions and abnormally elongated in the anteroposterior dimension (this is called *scaphocephaly,* meaning "long and narrow"). Frontal and occipital bossing is apparent (described as a "keel-like" appearance).

There is no midfacial or mandibular hypoplasia or asymmetry and no orbital dystopia (a relative discrepancy in globe position in the vertical and/or horizontal planes) or exophthalmos (anterior position of the globe relative to the orbital rims).

The fundoscopic examination is normal, with no evidence of papilledema (edema of the optic disc, which is indicative of elevated intracranial pressure).

Intraoral. The results of the examination are within normal limits (nonsyndromic craniosynostosis is not associated with an increased incidence of cleft lip/palate [CLP]).

Extremities. There are no deformities (nonsyndromic craniosynostosis does not have any associated abnormalities of the extremities).

IMAGING

Plain film complete skull series comprise the initial diagnostic radiographs of choice (the clinical diagnosis of craniosynostosis must be confirmed radiographically). In the current patient, the radiographs showed the absence of the entire sagittal suture. (Sagittal suture synostosis can involve the entire suture, the anterior portion only, or the posterior portion only. If the sutures appear patent on a radiographic study of diagnostic quality, craniosynostosis can be ruled out.)

Craniofacial axial and coronal (or reformatted) cut CT scans and three-dimensional reconstructions provide more detailed morphologic information, which is very useful during surgical planning (CT scans are also indicated when plain films are nondiagnostic). In the current patient, CT scans showed a scaphocephalic skull deformity, which is consistent with synostosis of the sagittal suture. CT scans of the head showed no masses (the possibility of an intracranial mass should be included in the differential diagnosis of cranial vault abnormalities) and no hydrocephalus (this is usually not encountered in single-suture craniosynostosis but may occur independently; hydrocephalus is seen in approximately 10% of cases in which multiple sutures are involved).

LABS

In an otherwise healthy, 7-month-old patient, the preoperative laboratory evaluation should include hemoglobin and hematocrit levels.

ASSESSMENT

Nonsyndromic craniosynostosis involving the entire sagittal suture.

TREATMENT

There are two primary goals in the surgical management of nonsyndromic craniosynostosis: (1) release of the fused suture or sutures to allow unrestricted growth of the brain and (2) reconstruction of all dysmorphic skeletal components to correct the anatomic form. The surgical team should be composed of a pediatric craniofacial surgeon and a pediatric neurosurgeon for optimal results ("strip craniectomy," previously performed by neurosurgeons working independently, did not address the dysmorphology of the craniofacial skeleton and resulted in residual deformities). Modern craniofacial management includes a formal craniotomy performed by a neurosurgeon and simultaneous skeletal reconstruction by the craniofacial surgeon. Reconstruction and reshaping include the removal, dismantling, and reassembly of all dysmorphic skeletal components into an anatomically desirable shape. The extent of the surgery depends on the suture or sutures involved and the resultant skeletal deformity.

Although craniosynostosis is surgically addressed during the first year of life, the exact timing of craniosynostosis repair is controversial. Some surgeons prefer early surgical correction, when the child is 3 to 6 months of age. In theory, early release of the suture or sutures allows the expanding brain to naturally reshape the cranial vault, minimizing the later-staged reconstructive efforts. Other surgeons prefer delaying the surgical correction until 9 to 11 months of age, permitting more growth of the cranial vault before reconstruction. The more stable cranial skeleton may result in fewer postsurgical deformities. Also, increased bony calcification allows for easier rigid fixation of the bony segments.

Surgical correction of nonsyndromic sagittal suture craniosynostosis involves a biparietal craniotomy for release of the fused suture and reshaping of the posterior and anterior cranial vault. The abnormal cranial components are dismantled and osteotomized into strips for reshaping of the cranial vault. The objectives are to increase the bitemporal and biparietal width and to decrease the anteroposterior length of the cranial vault (reduce frontal and occipital bossing). The bony segments are placed in the correct anatomic position and secured with rigid miniplates with monocortical screws. When the surgery is performed by age 2, most bony gaps, including full-thickness defects, completely fill with bone because of the osteogenic potential of the periosteum and dura mater. Complete healing of these defects is less predictable when surgery is performed between 2 and 4 years of age. After age 4, these defects may not heal without immediate reconstruction (with bone grafting or other alloplastic material).

If the entire sagittal suture is involved, reconstruction can be done in a single-stage procedure (associated with increased difficulty, surgical time, blood loss, and morbidity) or in a two-stage operation. The staged reconstruction involves addressing and reshaping the posterior two thirds of the cranial vault; this corrects the bitemporal and biparietal width and improves the anteroposterior cranial dimension. It does not correct the frontal bossing, which must be addressed during the second surgical phase, 6 to 12 weeks later. Others in the past have advocated strip craniectomy (at least 3 cm wide) from the anterior fontanelle to just beyond the lambdoidal suture as adequate treatment when the child is between 3 months and 1 year of age. However, this technique (along with its endoscopically assisted variation) has been criticized for its less-than-ideal cosmetic results.

When only the posterior portion of the sagittal suture is fused, surgical reshaping of the posterior two thirds of the cranial vault can be accomplished via a postauricular coronal scalp incision, with the patient in a prone position. Formal biparietal and occipital craniotomy is performed by the neurosurgeon. The bone flaps are removed, osteotomized, placed in the correct anatomic position, and secured with bone plates using monocortical screws. If only the anterior portion of the sagittal suture is involved, the resulting deformity is primarily frontal bossing. A coronal flap is elevated, and a bifrontal craniotomy is performed with the patient supine. The anterior cranial vault is reshaped and fixated as previously described.

COMPLICATIONS

Despite the very low complication rates associated with craniofacial surgery, both intraoperative and postoperative complications can occur. Massive blood loss and postoperative infection are the most common and most feared complications (Box 14-1). There is a high likelihood that homologous blood transfusion will be required during cranial vault reshaping. This is in part due to the low effective blood volume in infants and children. Acute normovolemic hemodilution (ANH) is a technique commonly performed intraoperatively to reduce the need for transfusion. Additional techniques include intraoperative blood salvage. Maintaining a "safe" hematocrit level, between 28% and 35%, has been recommended. However, the incidence of transfusion has been estimated to be as high as 90%.

Other complications include ocular complications (diplopia, temporary ptosis, strabismus, corneal abrasion and, rarely, visual loss), seizures (rare), cerebrospinal fluid leakage, elevated intracranial pressure, electrolyte disturbances (syndrome of inappropriate antidiuretic hormone secretion or cerebral salt-wasting syndrome, resulting in hyponatremia), airway embarrassment, fixation failure, translocation or migration, damage to the lacrimal drainage apparatus, and residual deformity, requiring secondary procedures.

DISCUSSION

Virchow coined the term "craniostenosis" in 1851. The word *craniosynostosis* describes the process of premature fusion of cranial sutures (six major suture areas and seven minor

---

Box 14-1   Intraoperative and Postoperative Complications in Craniofacial Surgery

Intraoperative Complications

Venous air embolism. Neonatal and pediatric calvaria have a large number of diploic and emissary channels that become exposed during a craniotomy procedure. Because the operative field is typically above the level of the heart, air could enter these exposed vascular channels and travel to the right atrium. A symptomatic air embolus could lead to profound hypotension and cardiovascular collapse. If venous air embolism is suspected, surgery should be stopped, the head of the bed lowered, and the surgical field irrigated and covered with a wet sponge; bone wax can be applied to the osteotomized bony edges. Nitrous oxide should be discontinued. Closed cardiac massage may be indicated in a severely compromised patient to force the air into the pulmonary circulation. A thoracotomy and direct massage with aspiration of intracardiac air are the last resort in failed attempts.

Oculocardiac reflex. Transcranial and fronto-orbital surgery can trigger the oculocardiac reflex in response to orbital manipulation and pressure, leading to bradycardia and hypotension. Care must be taken to prevent excessive orbital pressure and flap retraction. The anesthesia team should be notified during such maneuvers. Severe bradycardia and hypotension require the administration of atropine.

Dural lacerations. David and Cooter reported a 31% incidence of iatrogenic dural tears in a series of 53 patients. Others have reported an incidence of 5% to 60%. Direct repair usually has no detrimental sequelae.

Major blood loss. The continual oozing of blood from the vascular osteotomy sites over several hours of surgical time can amount to loss of a large portion of the patient's blood volume. The incidence of perioperative blood transfusions is variable and has been reported to be as high as 80% to 100% of patients undergoing cranial vault reconstruction. However, this is not universally accepted by all craniofacial surgeons. Major blood loss resulting in hypovolemic shock has a reported incidence of 0.3% to 4.6%. Appropriate fluid resuscitation with crystalloid, colloid, and blood and replacement of coagulation factors (fresh frozen plasma) should be anticipated.

Death. Reported mortality rates for craniofacial surgery range from 0% to 4.3%. Massive intraoperative bleeding, postoperative bleeding, intracranial bleeding, cerebral edema, infection, inadequate volume replacement, respiratory obstruction, and anesthetic complications are the most common causes.

Postoperative Complication

Infection. Infection can develop in the form of osteitis/osteomyelitis, meningitis, or intracranial abscess. It is the most common postoperative complication (infection rates range from 1% to 14%). Separation of the nasal and paranasal sinuses from the intracranial cavity is paramount in reducing the incidence of infection. The use of appropriate perioperative antibiotics, intraoperative antibiotic irrigation (or saline with dilute iodine), and reduction of surgical time also reduce infection rates. Monobloc advancement procedures have a higher rate of infection compared with other intracranial procedures.

Extradural and subdural hematomas. These are relatively rare occurrences. Poole reported less than a 1% incidence of hematoma. Suction drainage is not advocated because of concern that it can cause bleeding, cerebrospinal fluid leakage, or infection or draw nasal/sinus contamination intracranially. Close neurologic observation is needed to look for signs of an evolving intracranial hemorrhage.

sutures), which results in craniostenosis (outdated terminology). The craniofacial deformity is directly proportional to the area of sutures fused. Many classification systems have been developed to describe various subtypes of craniosynostosis. Three broad categories of craniosynostosis have been identified: simple (single suture) or compound (two or more sutures), primary or secondary (related to another disorder), and isolated (nonsyndromic) versus syndromic (Crouzon, Apert, Carpenter, Pfeiffer, Saethre-Chotzen, and other syndromes). In approximately 85% of patients, craniosynostosis is nonsyndromic in origin.

There are several different types of craniosynostosis. Sagittal suture craniosynostosis is the most common form of nonsyndromic single-suture synostosis, with a prevalence of approximately 1:5,000 live births and a 3:1 male predilection. It is characterized by a scaphocephalic deformity (long and narrow cranial vault) due to premature fusion of the entire sagittal suture or part of it. Absence or premature fusion of the sagittal suture results in no growth perpendicular to the suture and arrested development of the two parietal bone plates, causing bitemporal and biparietal narrowing. There is compensatory growth at the major sutures that remain patent (i.e., coronal, lambdoid, and metopic sutures) as the brain continues to expand, causing an abnormal, anteroposterior elongation of the cranial vault. This results in frontal and occipital bossing, often described as "keel-like." Portions of the sagittal suture (anterior or posterior portions) or the entire suture can be fused and determine the extent of the cranial deformity. The least common form is lambdoid suture synostosis.

Several theories have been proposed for the etiology of craniosynostosis. Virchow believed that the primary event was craniosynostosis and the associated cranial base deformity was secondary to that event. Moss theorized that the cranial base deformity was the primary malformation, resulting in premature fusion of the cranial sutures. Others theorized that mesenchymal defects resulted in both craniosynostosis and an abnormal cranial base. Growth of the midfacial skeleton also is restricted if sutures along the anterior cranial base are prematurely fused. A positive family history is a risk factor. This identifies the genetic relationship in craniosynostosis.

Maternal and environmental factors resulting in nonsyndromic craniosynostosis include advanced maternal age, maternal cigarette smoking, alcohol use, and use of clomiphene for infertility. However, these risk factors have been inconclusive because of the lack of large-scale studies.

Regardless of the pathogenesis, the prematurely fused suture or sutures inhibit growth of the neurocranium perpendicular to the fused suture or sutures. There is compensatory overgrowth at the normal (open) sutures to accommodate the growing brain (brain volume triples during the first year of life). Thus a unilateral synostosis results in a bilateral deformity. This phenomenon is known as *Virchow's law*. Despite this compensatory growth, an increase in intracranial pressure (greater than 15 mm Hg) may still be seen.

Neurologic impairment is rare with single-suture craniosynostosis (the single-suture type is most common, and the sagittal suture is most often affected), especially when the condition is treated before the age of 1 year (elevated intracranial pressure is seen in approximately 14% of children with untreated single-suture craniosynostosis and in 42% of those in whom two or more sutures are involved). However, if elevated intracranial pressure is left untreated, it may lead to irreversible neurologic and cognitive damage.

The major cranial sutures are the sagittal, metopic, coronal (right and left), and lambdoid (right and left) sutures. The minor sutures are the temporosquamosal, frontonasal, and frontosphenoidal sutures. In most patients with nonsyndromic craniosynostosis, only one suture is involved. Involvement of the sagittal suture is the most common type. Table 14-3 lists the major types of nonsyndromic craniosynostosis, along with their characteristic features and incidence.

Coronal suture craniosynostosis is the second most common type of nonsyndromic synostosis. Mutation of the fibroblast growth factor receptor 3 gene (FGFR3) has been

Table 14-3	**Types of Nonsyndromic Craniosynostosis**				
Sutures Affected	Head Shape	Name	Incidence	Elevated Intracranial Pressure	Central Nervous System (Mental Retardation)
Sagittal	Long and narrow	Scaphocephaly	1:5,000	Absent	Slight
Coronal	One hemicranium smaller than the other	Anterior plagiocephaly	1:10,000	Infrequent	Slight to moderate
Metopic	Triangular forehead	Trigonocephaly	1:15,000	Usually absent	Slight to moderate
Lambdoidal	One hemicranium smaller than the other	Posterior plagiocephaly	1:150,000	Infrequent	Slight to moderate
Bilateral coronal	Short, broad, and tall	Brachycephaly (acrobrachycephaly)	Rare	Infrequent	Slight to moderate
Sagittal and coronal	Short and narrow	Oxycephaly	Rare	Usually present	High

Modified from Dufresne CR: Classifications of craniofacial anomalies. In Dufresne CR, Carson BS, Zinreich SJ (eds): *Complex craniofacial problems,* pp 63-71, New York, 1992, Churchill Livingstone.

implicated in its pathogenesis. Due to early fusion of the coronal suture (either right or left), there is hypoplasia of the frontal and parietal bones on the affected side, resulting in flattening of the forehead (anterior plagiocephaly). Compensatory overgrowth of the unaffected sutures, including the contralateral coronal suture, results in frontal bossing of the unaffected side. Also, orbital dystopia (superior, posterior position of the affected orbit), ipsilateral zygomatic hypoplasia, and nasal asymmetry commonly occur. Midfacial hypoplasia and orbital dystopia are seen because of the involvement of the anterior cranial base along the frontoethmoidal, frontosphenoidal, and sphenoethmoidal sutures. This results in a "harlequin eye" deformity on an anteroposterior skull film. Surgical correction involves a bifrontal craniotomy, orbital osteotomies, fronto-orbital advancement, and anterior cranial vault reshaping.

Bibliography

AAP Task Force on Infant Positioning and SIDS: Positioning and SIDS, *Pediatrics* 89(6):1120-1126, 1992.

Ardalan M, Rafati A, Nejat F, et al: Risk factors associated with craniosynostosis: a case control study, *Pediatr Neurosurg* 48(3):152-156, 2012.

Carson BS, Dufresne CR: Craniosynostosis and neurocranial asymmetry. In Dufresne CR, Carson BS, Zinreich SJ (eds): *Complex craniofacial problems*, pp 167-194, New York, 1992, Churchill Livingstone.

David DJ, Cooter RD: Craniofacial infection in 10 years of transcranial surgery, *Plast Reconstr Surg* 80:213-223, 1987.

Dufresne CR: Classifications of craniofacial anomalies. In Dufresne CR, Carson BS, Zinreich SJ (eds): *Complex craniofacial problems*, pp 63-71, New York, 1992, Churchill Livingstone.

Eaton AC, Marsh JL, Pilgram TK: Transfusion requirements for craniosynostosis surgery in infants, *Plast Reconstr Surg* 95:277-283, 1995.

Faberowski LW, Black S, Mickle JP: Incidence of venous air embolism during craniectomy for craniosynostosis repair, *Anesthesiology* 92:20-23, 2000.

Fishman MA, Hogan GR, Dodge PR: The concurrence of hydrocephalus and craniosynostosis, *J Neurosurg* 36:621-629, 1971.

Fitzpatrick DR: Filling in the gaps in cranial suture biology, *Nat Genet* 45:231-232, 2013.

Gault DT, Renier D, Marchac D, et al: Intracranial pressure and intracranial volume in children with craniosynostosis, *Plast Reconstr Surg* 90:230-271, 1992.

Golabi M, Edwards MSB, Ousterhout DK: Craniosynostosis and hydrocephalus, *Neurosurgery* 21:63, 1987.

Greensmith AL, Meara JG, Holmes AD, et al: Complications related to cranial vault surgery, *Oral Maxillofac Surg Clin North Am* 16:465-473, 2004.

Jones BM, Jani P, Bingham RM, et al: Complications in paediatric craniofacial surgery: an initial four year experience, *Br J Plast Surg* 45:225-231, 1992.

Meyer P, Renier D, Arnaud E, et al: Blood loss during repair of craniosynostosis, *Br J Anaesth* 71:854-857, 1993.

Moss ML: The pathogenesis of premature craniosynostosis in man, *Acta Anat (Basel)* 37:351-370, 1959.

Phillips RJL, Mulliken JB: Venous air embolism during a craniofacial procedure, *Plast Reconstr Surg* 82:155-159, 1988.

Pietrini D: Intraoperative management of blood loss during craniosynostosis surgery, *Pediatr Anesth* 23:278-284, 2013.

Poole MD: Complications of craniofacial surgery, *Br J Plast Surg* 41:608-613, 1988.

Renier D, Sainte-Rose C, Marchac D, et al: Intracranial pressure in craniosynostosis, *J Neurosurg* 57:370, 1982.

Ruiz RL, Ritter AM, Turvey TA, et al: Nonsyndromic craniosynostosis: diagnosis and contemporary surgical management, *Oral Maxillofac Surg Clin North Am* 16:447-463, 2004.

Virchow R: Über den kretinismus, namentlich in Franken und über pathologische Schädelformen, Verhandlung der physikalischen-medizinischen Gesellschaft Würzburg, 2:231-284, 1851.

Syndromic Craniofacial Synostosis*

Mehran Mehrabi, Deepak G. Krishnan, and Shahrokh C. Bagheri

CC

A 14-year-old boy previously diagnosed with Apert syndrome presents to the craniofacial clinic for evaluation of his anterior open bite (apertognathia) with a chief complaint of "difficulty with chewing."

HPI

The patient was diagnosed with craniosynostosis (premature fusion of the cranial sutures) shortly after birth. Subsequently, he had fronto-orbital advancement at age 9 months. At age 2 years, he underwent craniofacial advancement to address the midface hypoplasia. Currently, the parents are unhappy with the child's appearance, because children at his school continually mock him about his appearance, particularly his open bite. The parents believe that this has affected their son's self-confidence and performance. The patient's mother indicates that the child has difficulty biting hard foods, such as steak or pizza, and has to use his posterior teeth for chewing. He is currently undergoing presurgical orthodontic treatment in preparation for combined surgical-orthodontic correction of the skeletal malocclusion. The parents are also concerned about their son's continued "sunken" face appearance (midface hypoplasia), which has persisted despite his corrective surgery at age 2 years (midface hypoplasia frequently persists despite early surgical advancement and often needs to be reoperated after completion of midfacial growth).

PMHX/PDHX/MEDICATIONS/ALLERGIES/SH/FH

The patient was also diagnosed with a heart murmur at birth and subsequently had corrective surgery, without complications (cardiovascular and valvular abnormalities, such as patent ductus arteriosus, are seen in 10% of patients with Apert syndrome). In addition, the patient had a history of hydronephrosis at birth, which resolved without surgery (genitourinary abnormalities are seen in about 10% of patients). At age 4 weeks he was diagnosed with pyloric stenosis, thickening of the pyloric valve that results in gastric obstruction (gastrointestinal abnormalities are seen in 1.5% of patients), and successfully underwent a laparoscopic pyloroplasty. The family history reveals that his two brothers and one sister are healthy (most cases of Apert syndrome are sporadic in nature, although autosomal dominance inheritance has been reported). Cognitive assessments at school have revealed that the patient is slightly developmentally delayed for his age (65% of patients have an intelligence quotient of less than 70, which is defined as mental retardation).

EXAMINATION

General. The patient is moderately cooperative. He has a poor attention span (secondary to developmental delay) but is able to follow simple commands. He has a short stature for his age and compared to his parents (megalocephaly [large head] results in the weight and height being above the 50th percentile early, but this decreases with age).

Maxillofacial. Examination of the skull reveals a steep frontal bone (Figure 14-5, *A*), flat occipital region, and bulging temporal region. He exhibits mild ocular esotropia (cross-eyed) and hypertelorism (diverging and widely spaced pupils, respectively). There is underdevelopment of the maxilla and zygomas bilaterally (midface hypoplasia; Figure 14-5, *B*). The fundoscopic examination is normal, with no evidence of papilledema (swelling of the optic disc, commonly seen in infants with Apert syndrome due to elevation in intracranial pressure).

Intraoral. The patient has an anterior open bite (apertognathia) with a narrow, high (V-shaped) maxillary arch (Figure 14-5, *C*) and a Class III molar relationship (Class III malocclusion with an anterior open bite is almost universal for Apert syndrome). Only two posterior molars are in contact on either side. There is no apparent hard or soft tissue clefting of the palate (this is seen in 30% of patients with Apert syndrome).

Extremities. The index, middle, and ring fingers are fused, and there is a common nail in both hands (symmetrical syndactyly) (Figure 14-5, *D*). The thumb and small fingers are not affected in either hand and show normal strength and mobility. The feet are normal and are not affected (lower extremities may be involved).

Skin. The child has yellow, raised papules on the dorsum of the hands (acne vulgaris involving the hands is seen in 70% of patients with Apert syndrome).

IMAGING

A panoramic radiograph and periapical radiographs are required to evaluate for supernumerary teeth, root crowding,

*The authors and publisher wish to acknowledge Dr. Chris Jo for his contribution on this topic to the previous edition.

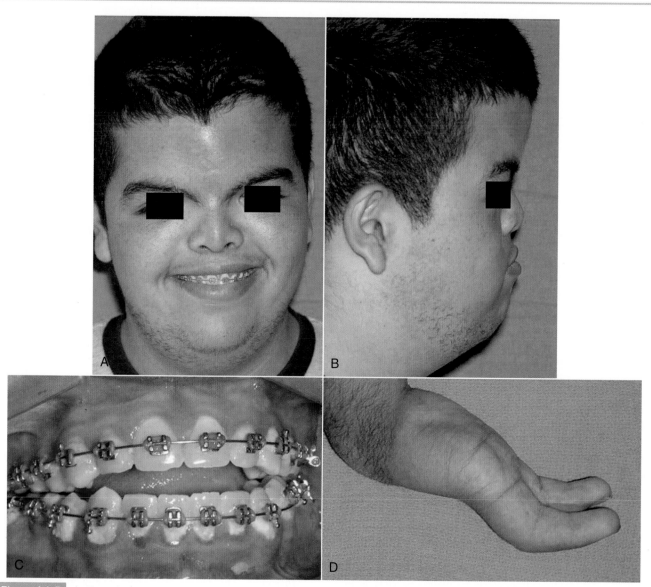

Figure 14-5 **A,** Frontal view showing general appearance of the patient. **B,** Profile view showing severe midfacial hypoplasia and frontal bossing. **C,** Intraoral view showing apertognathia. **D,** Syndactyly (seen in both hands).

and morphology and to detect caries. When impacted teeth are present (excluding third molars), periapical films from various angles can be obtained to evaluate the buccolingual position of the tooth (Clark's rule). A cone-beam CT could be beneficial for determining the spatial relationship and anatomic configuration of these impacted supernumerary teeth. A lateral cephalometric radiograph, along with cephalometric analysis, is used for evaluation and treatment of the dentofacial deformity. A conventional helical CT scan is not required but can be used for evaluation of opacified sinuses (which are not uncommon in maxillary hypoplasia) and for visualization of the three-dimensional anatomy as an aid in treatment planning. However, for more complex cases requiring orthognathic surgery, CT-guided treatment planning increasingly is being used. Often this does not necessarily require medical-grade CT; a cone-beam CT scan is more than adequate. Magnetic resonance imaging (MRI) also is not

required but can be useful in select cases for evaluation of soft tissue anatomy, such as brain parenchyma, orbital tissue, or pharyngeal structures. Obstructive sleep apnea (OSA) is commonly seen in patients with Apert syndrome, and the mentioned imaging modalities may be used to assess the posterior airway anatomy.

In the current patient, a panoramic radiograph and lateral cephalometric radiographs were obtained and used in treatment and cephalometric analysis. No teeth crowding, impactions, or supernumerary teeth were found; therefore, no periapical radiographs were obtained.

LABS

Preoperative laboratory testing includes a complete blood count (CBC) and a basic metabolic panel. For the current patient, neither of these demonstrated any abnormalities.

ASSESSMENT

Apert syndrome with maxillary hypoplasia and apertognathia requiring combined surgical orthognathic and orthodontic treatment.

TREATMENT

The initial evaluation of patients with Apert syndrome at birth focuses on the airway, central nervous system malformations, and feeding assessment. A retruded maxilla and limited nasopharyngeal airway increases the work of breathing and may require advanced airway interventions. Inability to pass a nasogastric tube may indicate nasopharyngeal obstruction. Most often these infants compensate with obligate mouth breathing and hence have an "open mouth" appearance. The central nervous system symptoms may manifest as seizures, hypotonia or hypertonia, and apnea. The high-arched palate, possible clefting, and obligate mouth breathing make feeding challenging. These patients may need a nasogastric or orogastric feeding tube or placement of a percutaneous endoscopic gastrostomy tube.

Surgical management of the craniosynostosis involves a staged reconstructive strategy. There is no clear consensus on the most appropriate timing and technique for each reconstructive stage (Box 14-2). Typically, there are three stages:
- Stage 1: Primary cranio-orbital decompression with reshaping and advancement
- Stage 2: Correction of midfacial deficiency and deformity with osteotomy and advancement (monobloc, facial bipartition, or extracranial Le Fort III osteotomies)
- Stage 3: Orthognathic surgery

Strip craniectomy, which allows for cranial decompression, has been performed in children younger than 3 months. However, due to unsatisfactory results, this procedure has been largely abandoned except for isolated sagittal synostosis. Fronto-orbital advancement is performed at age 6 to 9 months. In this procedure, the osteotomy is made across the nasofrontal junction, lateral orbital walls, and roof of the orbit. This increases the volume of the orbit, along with the anteroposterior cranial dimension, and decreases the bitemporal prominence. The fronto-orbital bar may be advanced up to 20 mm. Generally, there is no need for bone grafting (some surgeons use bone substitutes, such as demineralized bone, to fill in the defects), and the segments are commonly fixated using a resorbable plating system. A monobloc or craniofacial advancement is performed at age 9 months to 3 years. This procedure advances the cranium and midface simultaneously. This osteotomy consists of advancement of the frontal bone in two segments and a Le Fort III advancement. The retrofrontal dead space (the space created behind the frontal bone) makes this procedure dangerous, and it should be done only in patients with respiratory compromise. If midfacial distraction or advancement is used, it is best done between ages 3 and 5 years with a subcranial (extracranial) Le Fort III advancement.

> **Box 14-2** **Stages of Surgical Management of Dysmorphologies Associated with Crouzon Syndrome**
>
> **Stage 1.** Primary cranio-orbital decompression with reshaping and advancement is typically undertaken at 10 to 12 months of age. Some surgeons advocate earlier intervention, at 6 to 9 months. Elevation of intracranial pressures warrants earlier intervention. In stage 1, the coronal sutures are released bilaterally, and osteotomies are performed on the anterior cranial vault and upper orbits (across the nasofrontal junction, lateral orbital walls, and roof of the orbit), thereby advancing and decompressing both compartments. This increases the volume of the orbits, along with the anteroposterior cranial dimension, and decreases the bitemporal prominence. Repeat craniotomy may be required in later childhood in the presence of increased intracranial pressure.
>
> **Stage 2.** Correction of midfacial deficiency and deformity with osteotomy and advancement can be performed as early as 5 to 7 years of age (cranial vault and orbits are 85% to 90% of adult size at this age). The presenting deformity (in the vertical, horizontal, and transverse planes) dictates the osteotomy technique; monobloc, facial bipartition, or Le Fort III osteotomies can be used. An extracranial Le Fort III osteotomy is indicated when the supraorbital ridge is in good position and there is minimal ocular hypertelorism. If there is a residual deficiency in the supraorbital ridge and anterior cranial vault, along with midfacial deficiency, a monobloc osteotomy is indicated to advance the entire orbit and midface. If there is significant hypertelorism, a facial bipartition osteotomy (monobloc osteotomy with a vertical midline split and removal of a intraorbital wedge of bone) is indicated for orbital repositioning (this also widens the maxillary arch).
>
> **Stage 3.** Orthognathic surgery to correct residual jaw deformities and malocclusion should be performed after completion of facial growth in conjunction with other cosmetic procedures, such as malar or chin surgery.

The current patient was treated with a Le Fort III advancement. Mounted models with lateral cephalometric analysis were used to evaluate the extent of surgical movement. A custom-made, prefabricated occlusal splint was used to guide the position of the maxilla intraoperatively. Using a coronal, transconjunctival (or subtarsal), and circumvestibular maxillary incision, osteotomies were made along the roof on the orbit and lateral orbital wall, extending laterally and inferiorly to the pterygomaxillary fissure. The medial orbital wall osteotomy was connected to the inferior orbital fissure. This requires lifting the lacrimal sac without interruption of the medial canthal ligament. The nasofrontal osteotomy was extended laterally and inferiorly (behind the lacrimal groove) to meet the inferior cut. Then, a Rowe disimpaction forceps was used to mobilize and advance the midface. The position of the maxillary unit is dictated by the prefabricated splint. Bone grafts and/or distraction osteogenesis may be used in select patients. In patients with a normal occlusion, a Le Fort III with concurrent Le Fort I can be used. If the bizygomatic prominence is appropriate, Le Fort II osteotomy may be sufficient. Malar deficiencies may be addressed (often with augmentation bone grafts) at the same time, if indicated.

COMPLICATIONS

There are few reports in the literature on complications of Le Fort II and III orthognathic procedures. Complications of Le Fort I osteotomy have been extensively studied in the orthognathic surgery population and reported at a rate of about 6% to 9%. Most severe complications of Le Fort osteotomy (I, II, or III) result from an unwanted pterygomaxillary separation, with fractures extending to the skull base, orbital wall, and pterygoid plates. This is seen with a higher frequency in patients with craniosynostosis. Skull base fractures can result in a subarachnoid hemorrhage; there have been seven reported cases of skull base fracture in patients with craniosynostosis (Box 14-3). It is prudent to discuss this complication preoperatively. Other complications include increased frequency of intracranial aneurysms, seen in patients with Crouzon syndrome. Sporadic cases of blindness also have been reported after a Le Fort I osteotomy.

There are various modifications of maxillary osteotomies at the pterygomaxillary junction that can be done to prevent an unfavorable fracture. A straight osteotome can be used at the tuberosity rather than the pterygomaxillary fissure. Swann-shape osteotomes, which are designed to direct force anteriorly, and use of an oscillating saw and endoscopic techniques have also been discussed. However, most surgeons use a curved osteotome directed anteriorly, medially, and inferiorly as a measure to prevent an unwanted fracture and to avoid the internal maxillary artery.

Relapse of the surgical move and development of an anterior open bite are more frequently seen with larger moves. Overcorrection may be appropriate, especially in younger patients. Another strategy to address this complication is to plan the surgical procedure in two stages, with an initial monobloc advancement followed by a Le Fort I osteotomy to close the anterior open bite.

DISCUSSION

Craniosynostosis, or abnormal premature closure of cranial sutures, was first described by Hippocrates in 100 BC. It may present as an isolated finding (Table 14-4) or in combination with other physical findings; it the latter case, it is designated "syndromic craniosynostosis." Apert, Crouzon, Pfeiffer, and Saethre-Chotzen syndromes are the most commonly diagnosed syndromes that include craniosynostosis with midfacial hypoplasia. With involvement of the skull base with a hypoplastic midface, these are generally referred to as *dysostosis syndromes*.

Apert syndrome was first described in 1894 by S.W. Wheaton and later by Eugene Apert in 1906. This

---

Box 14-3 | Intraoperative and Postoperative Complications in Craniofacial Surgery

Intraoperative Complications

Venous air embolism. Neonatal and pediatric calvaria have a large number of diploic and emissary channels that become exposed during a craniotomy procedure. Because the operative field is typically above the level of the heart, air could enter these exposed vascular channels and travel to the right atrium. A symptomatic air embolus could lead to profound hypotension and cardiovascular collapse. If venous air embolism is suspected, surgery should be stopped, the head of the bed lowered, and the surgical field irrigated and covered with a wet sponge; bone wax can be applied to the osteotomized bony edges. Nitrous oxide should be discontinued. Closed cardiac massage may be indicated in a severely compromised patient to force the air into the pulmonary circulation. A thoracotomy and direct massage with aspiration of intracardiac air are the last resort in failed attempts.

Oculocardiac reflex. Transcranial and fronto-orbital surgery can trigger the oculocardiac reflex in response to orbital manipulation and pressure, leading to bradycardia and hypotension. Care must be taken to prevent excessive orbital pressure and flap retraction. The anesthesia team should be notified during such maneuvers. Severe bradycardia and hypotension require the administration of atropine.

Dural lacerations. David and Cooter reported a 31% incidence of iatrogenic dural tears in a series of 53 patients. Others have reported an incidence of 5% to 60%. Direct repair usually has no detrimental sequelae.

Major blood loss. The continual oozing of blood from the vascular osteotomy sites over several hours of surgical time can amount to loss of a large portion of the patient's blood volume. The incidence of perioperative blood transfusions is variable and has been reported to be as high as 80% to 100% of patients undergoing cranial vault reconstruction. However, this is not universally accepted by all craniofacial surgeons. Major blood loss resulting in hypovolemic shock has a reported incidence of 0.3% to 4.6%. Appropriate fluid resuscitation with crystalloid, colloid, and blood and replacement of coagulation factors (fresh frozen plasma) should be anticipated.

Death. Reported mortality rates for craniofacial surgery range from 0% to 4.3%. Massive intraoperative bleeding, postoperative bleeding, intracranial bleeding, cerebral edema, infection, inadequate volume replacement, respiratory obstruction, and anesthetic complications are the most common causes.

Postoperative Complication

Infection. Infection can develop in the form of osteitis/osteomyelitis, meningitis, or intracranial abscess. It is the most common postoperative complication (infection rates range from 1% to 14%). Separation of the nasal and paranasal sinuses from the intracranial cavity is paramount in reducing the incidence of infection. The use of appropriate perioperative antibiotics, intraoperative antibiotic irrigation (or saline with dilute iodine), and reduction of surgical time also reduce infection rates. Monobloc advancement procedures have a higher rate of infection compared with other intracranial procedures.

Extradural and subdural hematomas. These are relatively rare occurrences. Poole reported less than a 1% incidence of hematoma. Suction drainage is not advocated because of concern that it can cause bleeding, cerebrospinal fluid leakage, or infection or draw nasal/sinus contamination intracranially. Close neurologic observation is needed to look for signs of an evolving intracranial hemorrhage.

Table 14-4	Types of Nonsyndromic Craniosynostosis				
Sutures Affected	Head Shape	Name	Incidence	Elevated Intracranial Pressure	Central Nervous System (Mental Retardation)
Sagittal	Long and narrow	Scaphocephaly	1 : 5,000	Absent	Slight
Coronal	One hemicranium smaller than the other	Anterior plagiocephaly	1 : 10,000	Infrequent	Slight to moderate
Metopic	Triangular forehead	Trigonocephaly	1 : 15,000	Usually absent	Slight to moderate
Lambdoidal	One hemicranium smaller than the other	Posterior plagiocephaly	1 : 150,000	Infrequent	Slight to moderate
Bilateral coronal	Short, broad, and tall	Brachycephaly (acrobrachycephaly)	Rare	Infrequent	Slight to moderate
Sagittal and coronal	Short and narrow	Oxycephaly	Rare	Usually present	High

Modified from Dufresne CR: Classifications of craniofacial anomalies. In Dufresne CR, Carson BS, Zinreich SJ (eds): *Complex craniofacial problems,* New York, 1992, Churchill Livingstone.

acrocephalosyndactyly (deformity of the skull, face, and extremity) presents with a distinctive cranial vault shape, midface hypoplasia, and limb abnormalities, such as symmetrical syndactyly, acne vulgaris, and nail abnormalities. There have been more than 300 cases reported. Most cases are sporadic, but an autosomal dominance inheritance has also been observed. Advanced paternal age and parental consanguinity (seen in two patients) have been associated with an increased risk.

Early fusion of the coronal sutures, along with a widely patent sagittal suture (extending from the glabella to the posterior fontanelle), produces a short anterior cranial fossa and a steep, wide, flat forehead. This results in a bulging pterion and an obliquely contoured temporal bone. The occiput is also flat, which makes for a shorter anteroposterior dimension and increases the vertical dimension. The resulting skeletal deformity of craniosynostosis is caused by poor skeletal development perpendicular to the prematurely fused suture. The remaining sutures widen excessively, producing the final cranial form. This is referred to as *Virchow's law.*

The midface hypoplasia consists of an underdeveloped maxilla in all dimensions with a reduction in the nasopharyngeal airway space. Oral examination may show a high-arched palate, CP, dental crowding, and an anterior open bite. Ocular abnormalities present as orbital hypertelorism and exorbitism, which are generally not as severe as in Crouzon syndrome. Syndactyly consists of soft tissue fusion of the second, third, and fourth fingers or toes. This is seen with a variable extent of bony and fingernail fusion of the involved digits.

The effects of an abnormal skull shape on the brain include the development of progressive hydrocephalus (rare); distorted ventricle shape; agenesis of the septum pellucidum, corpus callosum, and cavum septum pellucidum; and possible developmental delay. Two cranial nerves can be affected, independent of cranial vault shape: cranial nerve I (9%), resulting in anosmia, and cranial nerve VIII, causing hearing impairment (10%).

Crouzon syndrome was first described in 1912 by O. Crouzon and later in a series of 86 cases published by Atkinson in 1937. The reported prevalence in the literature is 15 to 16 per 1 million births, accounting for 4.5% of all cases of craniosynostosis. The syndrome follows an autosomal dominant mode of distribution, although reports of sporadic cases from new mutations occur. Variability of expression characterizes this syndrome.

Abnormalities of the central nervous system may include progressive hydrocephalus, chronic cerebellar herniation, and stenosis of the jugular foramen with venous obstruction. An increased frequency of cerebellar herniation has been attributed to earlier patterns of suture closure in Crouzon syndrome compared with Apert syndrome. Differences in skull development between Apert and Crouzon syndromes have been suggested, including earlier closure of sutures, fontanelles, and synchondroses in Crouzon syndrome. This leads to marked differences in shape and the cranial volume of the skull in patients with Crouzon syndrome. Cranial malformation depends on the order and rate of progression of sutural synostosis. Brachycephaly is most common, but scaphocephaly, trigonocephaly, and cloverleaf skull may be observed.

Shallow orbits with ocular proptosis are an important diagnostic feature of Crouzon syndrome. Concomitant ocular findings include exotropia, poor vision or blindness, optic atrophy, nystagmus, exposure conjunctivitis, and keratitis, among others. Approximately 50% of patients with Crouzon syndrome have lateral palatal swellings that resemble a pseudocleft. CLP and a bifid uvula occur with less frequency.

Maxillary hypoplasia manifests as transverse and anteroposterior dental arch shortening. A high-arched palate and a unilateral or bilateral crossbite are seen. Crowding, ectopic eruption, and missing teeth are not uncommon. Conductive hearing loss deficit is found in 55% of patients, and atresia of the external auditory canals occurs in 13%. Crouzon syndrome should be distinguished from simple bilateral coronal synostosis and crouzonodermoskeletal syndrome.

Bibliography

Cohen MM, Kreiborg S: An updated pediatric perspective on the Apert syndrome, *Am J Dis Child* 147:989, 1993.

Cohen MM Jr, MacLean RE: *Craniosynostosis diagnosis, evaluation and management*, ed 2, New York, 2000, Oxford University Press.

David DJ, Cooter RD: Craniofacial infection in 10 years of transcranial surgery, *Plast Reconstr Surg* 80:213-223, 1987.

Fearon JA: The Le Fort III osteotomy: to distract or not to distract? *Plast Reconstr Surg* 107(5):1091-1103; discussion, 1104-1106; 2001.

Ferraro NF: Dental, orthodontic, and oral/maxillofacial evaluation and treatment in Apert syndrome, *Clin Plast Surg* 18:291-307, 1991.

Flores-Sarnat L: New insights into craniosynostosis, *Semin Pediatr Neurol* 9(4):274-291, 2002 [erratum: *Semin Pediatr Neurol* 10(2):159, 2003].

Girotto JA, Davidson J, Wheatly M, et al: Blindness as a complication of Le Fort osteotomies: role of atypical fracture patterns and distortion of the optic canal, *Plast Reconstr Surg* 102:1409-1421, 1998.

Iannetti G, Fadda T, Agrillo A, et al: Le Fort III advancement with and without osteogenesis distraction, *J Craniofac Surg* 17(3):536-543, 2006.

Juniper RP, Stajcic Z: Pterygoid plate separation using an oscillating saw in Le Fort I osteotomy, technical note, *J Craniomaxillofac Surg* 19:153-154, 1991.

Katzen JT, McCarthy JG: Syndromes involving craniosynostosis and midface hypoplasia, *Otolaryngol Clin North Am* 33:1257-1284, 2000.

Lanigan DT, Guest P: Alternative approaches to pterygomaxillary separation, *Int J Oral Maxillofac Surg* 22:131-138, 1993.

Lanigan DT, Romanchuk K, Olson CK: Ophthalmic complications associated with orthognathic surgery, *J Oral Maxillofac Surg* 51:480-494, 1993.

Lanigan DT, Tubman DE: Carotid-cavernous sinus fistula following Le Fort I osteotomy, *J Oral Maxillofac Surg* 45:969-975, 1987.

Lo LJ, Hung KF, Chen YR: Blindness as a complication of Le Fort I osteotomy for maxillary distraction, *Plast Reconstr Surg* 109:688-698, 2002.

Marsh J, Galic M, Vannier MW: The craniofacial anatomy of Apert syndrome, *Clin Plast Surg* 18:237-249, 1991.

Matsumoto K, Nakanishi H, Seike T, et al: Intracranial hemorrhage resulting from skull base fracture as a complication of Le Fort III osteotomy, *J Craniofac Surg* 14:545-548, 2003.

Newhouse RF, Schow SR, Kraut RA, et al: Life-threatening hemorrhage from a Le Fort I osteotomy, *J Oral Maxillofac Surg* 40:117-119, 1982.

Poole MD: Complications of craniofacial surgery, *Br J Plast Surg* 41:608-613, 1988.

Posnick JC: Craniofacial dysostosis, *Oral Maxillofac Surg Knowledge Update* 2, 1998.

Renier D, Arnaud E, Cinalli G, et al: Prognosis for mental function in Apert's syndrome, *J Neurosurg* 85:66-72, 1996.

Robinson PP, Hendy CW: Pterygoid plate fractures caused by the Le Fort I osteotomy, *Br J Oral Maxillofac Surg* 24:198-202, 1986.

Ruiz RL: Update in craniofacial surgery, *Oral Maxillofac Surg Clin North Am* 16(4):xi-xii, 2004.

Sakai Y, Kobayashi S, Sekiguchi J, et al: New method of endoscopic pterygomaxillary disjunction for a Le Fort I osteotomy, *J Craniofac Surg* 7:111-116, 1996.

Hemifacial Microsomia*

Jason A. Jamali and Michael Miloro

CC

A 21-year-old male patient with left-sided hemifacial microsomia (HFM) presents for treatment of a persistent facial asymmetry (HFM may have a male predilection, although some studies have shown an equal gender distribution).

HPI

The patient was diagnosed with hemifacial microsomia in early childhood. He was subsequently treated with distraction osteogenesis of the left mandible during childhood; however, his facial proportions have slowly but progressively worsened since the distraction procedure (asymmetry in HFM usually progresses with age). Additionally, the patient has had persistent malar hypoplasia and asymmetry of the left auricle. The patient denies any previous history of facial trauma (facial fractures in a growing child, especially to the mandibular condyle, can contribute to growth disturbances).

PMHX/PDHX/MEDICATIONS/ALLERGIES/SH/FH

Noncontributory. The patient is a student in good academic standing at a local college (mental and developmental retardation are unusually seen in patients with HFM).

EXAMINATION

General. The patient is a well-developed, well-nourished male in no apparent distress.

Neurologic. The cranial nerves are intact, specifically the facial (N_0), vestibulocochlear, and hypoglossal nerves bilaterally.

Maxillofacial. There are mild deficits in subcutaneous tissue and underlying muscle (S_1). No perioral or palatal clefting is present. There are no distortions in orbital size and no asymmetry in position/dystopia (O_0). The left malar eminence is hypoplastic. There is mild hypoplasia of the left ear with significant protrusion of the pinna (E_1).

There is hypoplasia of the left mandible; the left condyle is absent, along with a portion of the ramus. The TMJ articulation is absent, and the zygoma is hypoplastic (M_3).

There is no posterior stop to the mandible when upward force is directed at the angle. The left gonial angle is underprojected. There is canting of the mandible (upward on the left) with reciprocal canting of the maxilla. The maxillary midline is shifted left 3 mm, and the pogonion is deviated left 5 mm. (Malocclusion is prevalent in HFM, and the degree of malocclusion is proportional to the skeletal deformity. Dental crowding, inclination of the anterior teeth, and unilateral crossbite on the affected side are characteristic findings).

The patient is not missing any adult teeth, and there is no evidence of enamel hypoplasia. No caries or periodontal disease is evident. (However, patients with HFM are more likely to have missing teeth, compared to the general population, and frequently have delayed tooth development on the affected side. Dental agenesis and enamel hypoplasia are more likely to occur in severe skeletal deformities. Enamel hypoplasia of the primary incisors on the affected side is thought to be an additional early developmental marker for HFM.)

The lips and oral commissure are normal (macrostomia is seen in 35% of patients with HFM). The soft palate, hard palate, and alveolar processes appear normal (approximately 7% to 15% of HFM patients present with cleft lip and palate).

IMAGING

A panoramic radiograph is the initial radiograph obtained for evaluating the degree of deformity of the mandible and its articulation with the zygoma. Posteroanterior and lateral cephalometric radiographs may be obtained to evaluate the degree of deformity of the maxillomandibular complex in relation to the cranial base (Figure 14-6, *A*).

CT scans (with three-dimensional reformatting) provide the best understanding of the hard tissue abnormalities and relationships. Additionally, this information may be used for virtual surgical planning and fabrication of surgical splints.

For the current patient, the Panorex demonstrated significant hypoplasia of the left mandible with absence of the condyle-ramus unit (orbit, mandible, ear, nerve, soft tissues [OMENS] classification of M_3/Kaban type III).

The CT scan provided further information on the severity of the left zygomatic hypoplasia, in addition to the degree of occlusal plane canting and midline discrepancy in relation to the skull base (Figure 14-6, *B* and *C*).

*The authors and publisher wish to acknowledge Chris Jo, DMD, and Shahrokh C. Bagheri, DMD, MD, FACS, FICD, for their contribution on this topic to previous edition.

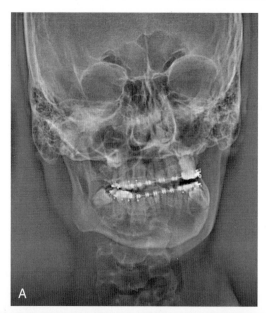

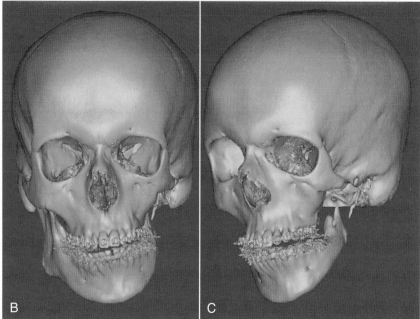

Figure 14-6   **A,** Posteroanterior cephalometric radiograph of a patient with left hemifacial microsomia. **B** and **C,** Three-dimensional CT scan showing the left HFM.

LABS

Preoperative hemoglobin and hematocrit levels were within normal range for this patient.

ASSESSMENT

A 21-year-old male with left-sided hemifacial microsomia; $O_0M_3E_1N_0S_1$ or Kaban type III (see OMENS classification system [Table 14-5]).

TREATMENT

The goals of treatment are both functional (restoration of occlusion/joint function) and esthetic (normalization of facial symmetry and contour). Other functional limitations (airway compromise, sleep disturbances, feeding difficulties, speech disorders, and hearing deficits) may require earlier or additional interventions.

Timing is an important consideration in the treatment of any craniofacial disorder, and this factor has generated the most controversy in the management of HFM. Growth

Table 14-5	OMENS Classification of Hemifacial Microsomia*

Classification	Description
O	Orbital distortion
O0	Normal orbital size and position
O1	Abnormal orbital size
O2	Abnormal orbital position
O3	Abnormal orbital size and position
M	Mandibular hypoplasia
M0	Normal mandible
M1	Small mandible and glenoid fossa with a short ramus
M2	Short and abnormal shaped ramus
M3	Complete absence of ramus, glenoid fossa, and temporomandibular joint
E	Ear anomaly
E0	Normal ear
E1	Mild ear hypoplasia and cupping with all the structures present
E2	Absence of external auditory canal with variable hypoplasia of the concha
E3	Malpositioned lobule with absent auricle
N	Nerve involvement
N0	Normal facial nerve
N1	Upper facial nerve involvement (temporal and zygomatic branches)
N2	Lower facial nerve involvement (buccal, mandibular, and cervical branches)
N3	All branches of the facial nerve affected
S	Soft tissue deficiency
S0	No apparent soft tissue and muscles deficiency
S1	Minimal muscle and subcutaneous deficiency
S2	Moderate deficiency
S3	Severe deficiency with muscles and subcutaneous tissue hypoplasia

Modified from Horgan JE, Padwa BL, LaBrie RA, et al: OMENS-plus: analysis of the craniofacial and extracraniofacial anomalies in hemifacial microsomia, *Cleft Palate Craniofac J* 32(5):405-412, 1995.

*Each subdivision is graded as 0 (normal), 1, 2, or 3 (most severe); these are added to obtain the OMENS score (e.g., $O_1M_2E_2N_3S_2$ = OMENS score of 10). If the OMENS score is greater than 6, there is an increased likelihood of extracranial comorbidities.

cessation and the progressive nature of the deformity are the key principles that govern the sequence of intervention. In general, treatment after growth cessation tends to produce the most stable results, with completion of growth following a cranial-caudal direction. Treatment for the different facial anatomic regions is discussed briefly.

Zygomatic and Orbital Reconstruction

Surgical intervention in the orbital/zygomatic area of the face may be undertaken earlier than surgery for the maxillomandibular deformity, typically after 5 to 7 years of age (growth of the orbital/zygomatic region is complete around age 7). Surgical access may require coronal flaps with the use of calvarial bone grafts for orbitozygomatic reconstruction. Orbital dystopia may be managed with facial bipartition, or orbital box, osteotomies.

Reconstruction of the Maxillomandibular Complex (MMC)

Treatment planning for restoration of the MMC must take into account the extent of deformities and the involvement of the TMJ. Type I and type IIA mandibular deformities will likely require ramus osteotomy in conjunction with a Le Fort osteotomy and genioplasty. Onlay grafts may be used to address hard tissue asymmetries that are not correctable with orthognathic surgery alone. Type IIB and type III mandibular deformities require reconstruction of the TMJ articulation. This may be done with a costochondral graft (for the ramus and/or zygoma) or total joint/prosthetic joint replacement in the adult.

Typically the changes in the maxilla occur secondary to limitation of growth imposed by the lack of growth of the mandible. In the past, early intervention prior to growth cessation was advocated to mitigate these reciprocal effects. Osteotomy and repositioning of the mandible during the mixed dentition phase (with or without a costochondral graft) were used to create an open bite on the side ipsilateral to the deformity. Closing the open bite slowly, over 18 to 24 months, allowed for normalization of the maxillary occlusal plane, primarily through dentoalveolar remodeling. Long-term stability in patients operated on prior to skeletal maturity has been a concern. Patients with type IIB and type III mandibles after costochondral reconstruction have less successful long-term stability, and this is worse when they are operated on early. Furthermore, long-term data on patients reconstructed with distraction osteogenesis in childhood and adolescence have shown that the benefits in facial symmetry initially gained from early intervention are completely lost after the patient achieves skeletal maturity. A literature review by Momaerts and Nagy has shown that there is no evidence to support early distraction osteogenesis in the HFM patient. Brusati compared the vertical ramus heights of the affected and nonaffected sides in patients with type I and IIA mandibles who underwent distraction osteogenesis between the ages of 5 and 7 years. By 1 year after surgery, 16% of the vertical correction in ramal height was lost. By 5 years, 75% of the correction was lost, and at the completion of growth, the ratio of the affected to nonaffected sides returned to the original preoperative proportion.

For nongrowing patients who require restoration of the TMJ articulation (e.g., failed costochondral grafts), combined total joint prosthesis placement, along with simultaneous orthognathic surgery, is an option.

Soft Tissue Reconstruction

Initial soft tissue abnormalities (e.g., skin tag removal, correction of macrostomia, eyelid deficiencies) may be addressed in early adulthood. After the osseous foundation has been addressed, final soft tissue modifications for restoration of symmetry are undertaken. Microvascular tissue transfer is commonly used (e.g., parascapular flap); however, serial fat grafts are a more conservative option for replacing or augmenting deficient facial soft tissues.

Auricular Reconstruction

Auricular reconstruction is performed using either autologous grafts or implant-retained prostheses. Both procedures are performed in a staged approach. The advantages of autologous grafting include increased long-term stability and success, less need for maintenance, and decreased long-term costs. Prosthetic reconstruction results in an improved symmetry with the contralateral ear; however, it often requires a lifetime of maintenance. Computer-aided design and manufacture (CAD/CAM) technology has improved the cosmetic outcome of the prosthetic options. Costal cartilage is usually grafted from the sixth or seventh rib. The timing of grafting is controversial; however, in the two-stage repair, delaying the rib harvest until age 10 years, as suggested by Nagata, has become increasingly common. Timing options include

grafting as early as 6 years of age, as recommended by Brent, or after 10 years of age, as recommended by Nagata. The timing of endosseous implant placement relates to the quality of the temporal bone; increased complications have resulted in children between 5 and 12 years of age secondary to thinner/softer temporal bone. The future of reconstruction will likely involve tissue engineering using chondrocyte cells seeded onto biodegradable polymer scaffolds (Figure 14-7).

COMPLICATIONS

Multiple interventions may be necessary for reconstruction and normalization of facial symmetry in the patient with HFM. Depending on the modalities used, multiple variable complications are possible. These include infection, hardware failure, relapse, nonunion, graft failure, donor site morbidity, damage to adjacent structures (neurovascular), scarring, and unfavorable cosmetic outcomes. Many of the complications depend on the treatment and are the same as those seen in

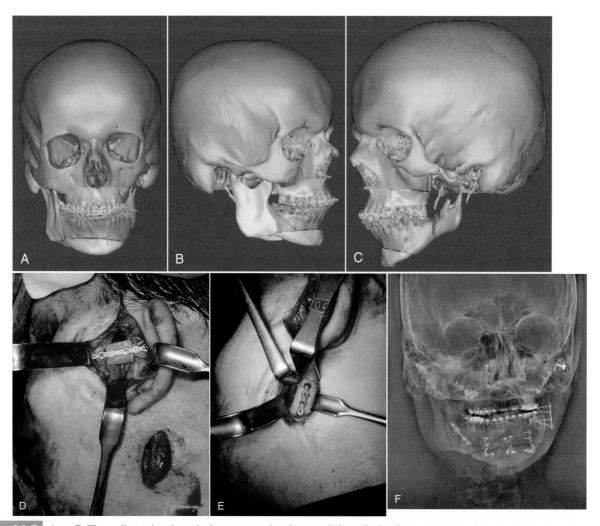

Figure 14-7 **A** to **C,** Three-dimensional surgical treatment planning consisting of a Le Fort osteotomy, right sagittal split osteotomy, and genioplasty, with plans for costochondral reconstruction of the left condyle-ramus unit. Intraoperative views of left zygomatic arch reconstruction (**D**) and left condyle-ramus unit reconstruction (**E**) with a costochondral graft. **F,** Posteroanterior cephalometric radiograph of the postoperative result showing restoration of facial symmetry.

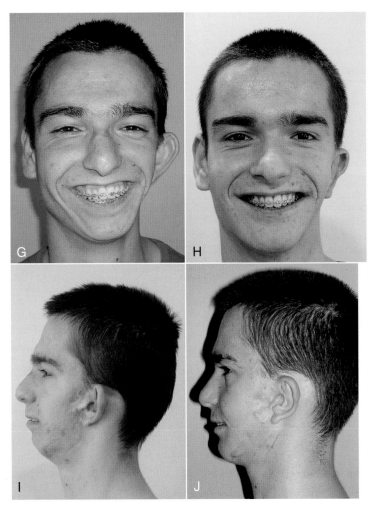

Figure 14-7, cont'd **G** and **H,** Comparison of preoperative and postoperative facial appearance on frontal view. **I** and **J,** Comparison of preoperative and postoperative facial appearance on profile view.

orthognathic surgery and distraction osteogenesis for non-HFM patients. These are discussed elsewhere in this book.

DISCUSSION

Hemifacial microsomia is a craniofacial disorder that results in varied malformation of the first and second branchial arch derivatives. Involvement of the mandible, TMJ, orbit, midface, ear, cranial nerves, and overlying soft tissue is common, in addition to extracranial abnormalities. The reported incidence ranges from 1:3,500 to 1:5,600 births, making HFM the second most common craniofacial abnormality after cleft lip and palate (CLP). There is a slight predilection for the right side of the face, and some studies have suggested a male predilection (3:2). Involvement is asymmetric and bilateral in 10% to 15% of cases.

The phenotypic expression is quite variable, and the disorder has been understood to exist along a spectrum known as ocular-auricular-vertebral spectrum, which includes Goldenhar syndrome. Additional nomenclature applied to HFM includes lateral facial dysplasia, craniofacial microsomia, otomandibular dysostosis, and first and second branchial arch syndrome. Treacher Collins syndrome may be confused with bilateral craniofacial microsomia, although Treacher Collins is symmetrical and has a well-defined inheritance pattern.

The mechanism of HFM is poorly understood; however, compromise of the branchial arches from vascular insult (hemorrhage and hematoma) to the stapedial artery has been proposed. Although a 2% to 3% recurrence rate has been seen in first-degree relatives, a well-defined inheritance pattern has not been demonstrated.

Given the extensive variability of HFM, several classification systems have been developed. The Kaban classification is a modification of the Pruzansky system, which characterizes the degree of mandibular involvement with particular attention to the ramus-condyle unit.

The Kaban type I mandible has mild hypoplasia of the ramus-condyle unit; however, the temporomandibular joint functions normally. A type IIA mandible is moderately hypoplastic with a deformed ramus-condyle unit but an intact articulation. A type IIB mandible has severe hypoplasia and

Table 14-6	Principal Maxillofacial Defects in Hemifacial Microsomia

Location	Principal Defects
Mandible	Mandibular hypoplasia (89% to100%)
	Malformed glenoid fossa (24% to 27%)
Ear	Microtia (66% to 99%)
	Preauricular tags (34% to 61%)
	Conductive hearing loss (50% to 66%)
Midface	Maxillary hypoplasia
	Zygomatic hypoplasia
	Occlusal canting
Soft tissue	Masticatory muscle hypoplasia (85% to 95%)
	Macrostomia (17% to 62%)
	Cranial VII nerve palsy (10% to 45%)

Table 14-7	Associated Defects in Hemifacial Microsomia

Craniofacial Defects	Other Defects
Velopharyngeal insufficiency (35% to 55%)	Vertebral/rib defects (16% to 60%)
Palatal deviation (39% to 50%)	Cervical spine anomalies (24% to 42%)
Orbital dystopia (15% to 43%)	Scoliosis (11% to 26%)
Ocular motility disorders (19% to 22%)	Cardiac anomalies (4% to 33%)
Epibulbar dermoids (4% to 35%)	Pigmentation change (13% to 14%)
Cranial base anomalies (9% to 30%)	Extremity defects (3% to 21%)
Eyelid defects (12% to 25%)	Central nervous system defects (5% to 18%)
Hypodontia/dental hypoplasia (8% to 25%)	Genitourinary defects (4% to 15%)
Lacrimal drainage anomalies (11% to 14%)	Pulmonary anomalies (1% to 15%)
Frontal plagiocephaly (10% to 12%)	Gastrointestinal defects (2% to 12%)
Sensorineural hearing loss (6% to 16%)	
Preauricular sinus (6% to 9%)	
Parotid gland hypoplasia	
Other cranial nerve defects (e.g., cranial nerves V, VII, IX, and XII)	

OMENS classification is used to score five anatomic structures based on severity (orbit, mandible, ear, nerve, soft tissues). A score is given for each category based on the degree of abnormality (Table 14-5), and the summation correlates with the severity of mandibular deformity. Several associated anomalies can exist in association with hemifacial microsomia (Tables 14-6 and 14-7). One study reported that more than half of patients with hemifacial microsomia had at least one extracranial anomaly.

Goldenhar syndrome (oculoauriculovertebral spectrum) has been described as a variant of hemifacial microsomia. However, it appears that hemifacial microsomia is within the broad range of expression of the oculoauriculovertebral spectrum, which is synonymous with Goldenhar syndrome.

Bibliography

Bauer BS: Reconstruction of microtia, *Plast Reconstr Surg* 124:14-26, 2009.

Brusati R: Comparison of mandibular vertical growth in hemifacial microsomia patients treated with early distraction or not treated: follow up till the completion of growth, *J Craniomaxillofac Surg* 40:105-111, 2012.

Kaban LB: Surgical correction of mandibular hypoplasia in hemifacial microsomia: the case for treatment in early childhood, *J Oral Maxillofac Surg* 56:628-638, 1998.

Mommaerts MY, Nagy K: Is early osteodistraction a solution for the ascending ramus compartment in hemifacial microsomia? A literature study, *J Craniomaxillofac Surg* 30(4):201-7, 2002.

Nagy K: No evidence for long-term effectiveness of early osteodistraction in hemifacial microsomia, *Plast Reconstr Surg* 124:2061-2071, 2009.

Padwa BL: Midfacial growth after costochondral graft construction of the mandibular ramus in hemifacial microsomia, *J Oral Maxillofac Surg* 56:122-127, 1998.

Posnick JC: Surgical correction of mandibular hypoplasia in hemifacial microsomia: a personal perspective, *J Oral Maxillofac Surg* 56:639-650, 1998.

Tanna N: Craniofacial microsomia soft tissue reconstruction comparison: inframammary extended circumflex scapular flap versus serial fat grafting, *Plast Reconstr Surg* 127:802-811, 2011.

Wang RR: Hemifacial microsomia and treatment options for auricular replacement: a review of the literature, *J Prosthet Dent* 82:197-204, 1999.

Wolford LM: Successful reconstruction of nongrowing hemifacial microsomia patients with unilateral temporomandibular joint total joint prosthesis and orthognathic surgery, *J Oral Maxillofac Surg* 70:2835-2853, 2012.

deformity of the ramus-condyle unit with a functional deficit. No articulation is present between the condyle and fossa, although a posterior stop may be present. The type III classification demonstrates aplasia of the ramus-condyle unit, lack of an articulation, and no posterior stop with palpation. The

Obstructive Sleep Apnea Syndrome

Martin Salgueiro, Chris Jo, and Shahrokh C. Bagheri

CC

A 46-year-old Caucasian man is referred to your office by his primary care physician for evaluation and management of obstructive sleep apnea syndrome (OSAS). (Four percent of middle-aged men and 2% of middle-aged women meet the criteria for a diagnosis of obstructive sleep apnea (OSA), making it more common in adults than asthma. The risk increases significantly after age 65 and in up to 50% of nursing home patients.)

HPI

The patient presents complaining of a long history of snoring and restless sleeping (sleep-disordered breathing includes hypopnea, apnea, and respiratory effort–related arousals). His wife of 20 years reports that he snores loudly, frequently stops breathing (apnea), and makes grunting, gasping, and choking sounds (bedroom partners are often the first to recognize the problem). The patient has noticed difficulty concentrating at work (OSAS decreases cognitive function) and difficulty staying awake during the day (daytime somnolence is a hallmark of OSAS). The patient scored above 10 on the Epworth Sleepiness Scale. (This scale is a questionnaire that subjectively assesses the level of daytime somnolence. Other screening tools include the Berlin questionnaire, the American Society of Anesthesiology checklist and the STOP-BANG questionnaire.) He also complains of morning dry mouth (nasal obstruction or congestion leads to mouth breathing, resulting in morning dry mouth), morning headaches, nocturia, and night sweats (common symptoms associated with OSAS). His primary care physician referred him to a sleep center for a polysomnogram (PSG) (the gold standard in diagnosis of OSAS); his respiratory disturbance index (RDI) score was 51 (see Discussion later in this section).

PMHX/PDHX/MEDICATIONS/ALLERGIES/SH/FH

The patient's past medical history is significant for hypertension (there is a direct relationship between OSAS and hypertension, resulting in cardiovascular morbidity), which is controlled with a β-blocker and a diuretic. His past surgical history is significant for tonsillectomy and adenoidectomy as a child (hypertrophic tonsils and adenoids increase the risk of OSAS in children, but this is more uncommon in adults).

He admits to drinking two or three beers a day (alcohol consumption can blunt the ventilatory response to hypercarbia and thereby worsen OSA) and occasional smoking (smoking can cause inflammation and edema of the upper airway mucosa, which increases airway resistance).

He is a sales manager and works more than 8 hours a day (overworking may contribute to lack of sleep, sleep-disordered breathing, and daytime somnolence). More recently, his co-workers have noticed that he is falling asleep at this desk (daytime somnolence also contributes to decreased productivity and can be particularly dangerous for individuals operating machinery or driving motor vehicles).

His father had similar signs and symptoms of OSAS that were untreated (a positive family history is commonly seen due to various genetic and environmental factors). He died at the age of 60 of a myocardial infarction (untreated OSAS significantly increases the risk of cardiovascular disease and cerebrovascular accident resulting in death).

EXAMINATION

Vital signs. Blood pressure is 150/95 mm Hg (stage I hypertension), heart rate 75 bpm, respirations 16, and temperature 37.6°C.

General. The patient is a moderately obese man in no apparent distress (obesity is an important risk factor for OSAS). His weight is 225 pounds, his body mass index is 32 kg/m² (class 1 obesity), and his waist-to-hip ratio is 1.2 (normal is 0.9 in males and 0.8 in females).

Maxillofacial. He displays mild retrognathia (retrognathia is a risk factor for OSAS). His neck measures 18 inches (a neck circumference of 17 inches or greater in men and 16 inches or greater in women increases the risk of OSAS and may be the best predictor of RDI in males).

Endonasal. The nares are equally patent bilaterally. There is no evidence of internal nasal valve collapse. A Cottle test is negative (a positive Cottle test may indicate internal nasal valve collapse). The nasal septum appears midline, and the inferior turbinates appear normal (a deviated nasal septum and/or turbinate hypertrophy may cause nasal obstruction). There are no nasal polyps.

Intraoral. His occlusion is Class II division II. The oral tongue is normal in size. The soft palate and uvula are long and not completely visible (Mallampati class III airway). The tonsils are not present. There are no tori. (Enlarged or redundant oral structures may cause oropharyngeal obstruction.)

Endoscopic nasopharyngoscopy in supine position (provides information on the presence and location of the obstruction, not evaluated with PSG). The nasopharynx is clear of any obstruction. The retropalatal airway space is narrow and has redundant soft tissue, and the space completely obliterates with Müller's maneuver (forced inspiratory effort against a closed mouth and nose). The retroglossal oropharynx and hypopharynx are narrow and partially obliterate (75%) with Müller's maneuver. Collapse of the lateral pharyngeal walls appears to contribute significantly to the airway collapse. There is no pathology of the endolarynx, and the vocal cords are functional.

IMAGING

The lateral cephalometric radiograph is the initial diagnostic study of choice, which can be taken in a relaxed position and with Müller's maneuver. Although it is a static, two-dimensional representation of a dynamic, three-dimensional space and is taken in an upright position on an awake patient, it is standardized, inexpensive, and readily available. It provides an excellent overview of the craniofacial skeleton for identifying and quantifying any skeletal deformities, including the position of the maxilla and mandible in relation to the cranial base, and also the soft tissue anatomy (see Chapter 9, on Orthognathic Surgery). Cone-beam computed tomography (CBCT) scanners are not uncommon in oral and maxillofacial surgery offices and are a valuable tool for obtaining a three-dimensional view of the airway. The distance from the hyoid bone to the mandibular plane (normal is 11 to 19 mm), the posterior airway space (normal is 10 to 16 mm), the length of the soft palate (normal is 34 to 40 mm), and the thickness of the soft palate (normal is 6 to 10 mm) are important measurements in the work-up of OSAS. Hospital-grade CT and magnetic resonance imaging (MRI) also provide three-dimensional and volumetric information on the upper airway and surrounding soft tissues, but they are not very practical or cost-efficient.

In the current patient, the lateral cephalometric radiograph showed a hypoplastic mandible causing a Class II skeletal discrepancy, a retropositioned pogonion, a posterior airway space of 6 mm, a long and thick soft palate, and a normal hyoid–to–mandibular plane distance.

LABS

No laboratory values are needed in the initial work-up of OSAS. Thyroid hormone or thyroid-stimulating hormone levels are routinely ordered at some sleep centers but may not be warranted. A preoperative CBC is required for patients undergoing surgical treatment (hemoglobin and hematocrit levels are commonly elevated in OSAS). A baseline arterial blood gas analysis is indicated in some individuals. Other laboratory values are ordered based on the patient's medical history.

An electrocardiogram is required for all patients with OSAS. OSAS is considered a cardiac risk factor. Hypertension and obesity are additional cardiac risk factors that are commonly seen in patients with OSAS.

In the current patient, the CBC and electrocardiogram were within normal limits.

POLYSOMNOGRAPHY

Polysomnography ("sleep study") is the gold standard for diagnosing sleep-related breathing disorders. The electroencephalogram, electrocardiogram, electro-oculogram, electromyogram, heart rate, oxygen saturation, airflow, and respiratory efforts are monitored and recorded during sleep. The number of apneas (cessation of airflow lasting 10 seconds or longer) and hypopneas (abnormal respirations lasting 10 seconds or longer, with a 30% or greater reduction in airflow and 4% or higher oxygen desaturation) are calculated. The episode of apnea is categorized as obstructive (no airflow despite inspiratory effort), central (no airflow and no inspiratory effort), or mixed (both central and obstructive component). The RDI, or apnea/hypopnea index (AHI), is the total number of apneic and hypopneic events divided by the total number of hours of sleep (i.e., the average number of apnea and hypopnea events per hour). The RDI is used to quantify the severity of OSA and to monitor the patient's response to treatment.

In the current patient, the PSG showed an RDI of 51. All episodes of apnea were obstructive in nature. The lowest oxygen saturation was 81%. There were no cardiac arrhythmias (prolonged hypoxemia can precipitate premature ventricular contractions or sinus bradycardia).

ASSESSMENT

A 46-year-old obese man with severe OSAS (also termed obstructive sleep apnea-hypopnea syndrome) *due to obstruction at the level of the oropharynx (retropalatal and retroglossal) and hypopharynx (Fujita type II obstruction).*

OSAS can be classified as mild, moderate, or severe based on the patient's RDI or AHI (a score of 5 to 15 is mild, 16 to 30 is moderate, and over 30 is severe); these are arbitrarily defined and therefore inconsistent in the literature. When OSA is associated with daytime somnolence, OSAS is diagnosed. Upper airway obstruction can occur at different levels (nasopharynx, oropharynx, and hypopharynx). The Fujita classification divides the airway in three categories, based on the anatomic location of the obstruction (Table 14-8).

Table 14-8	Fujita Classification: Airway Classification by Anatomic Location of the Obstruction	
Type	**Anatomic Location**	**Structures Involved**
I	Oropharynx	Palate, uvula, tonsils
II	Oropharynx and hypopharynx	
III	Hypopharynx	Base of the tongue, lingual tonsil, epiglottis

TREATMENT

The treatment of OSAS begins with a proper diagnosis, along with recognition of the level or levels of upper airway obstruction and severity of the disease. Nonsurgical management, namely lifestyle changes, should be initiated immediately, regardless of the severity of disease or anticipated surgical plan. This includes weight loss therapy and cessation of alcohol use. Obesity is seen in 60% to 70% of patients with OSAS. It has been shown that a 10% weight loss improves the RDI by 26%, whereas a 10% weight gain worsens the RDI by 32%. Alcohol or any other sedatives can worsen the RDI (longer and more frequent obstructions) in patients with OSAS or can cause snorers to develop OSAS. Thus alcohol avoidance is recommended in all susceptible patients.

Other nonsurgical treatments include nasal continuous positive airway pressure (nCPAP), oral appliances, and modified sleep positions (the RDI doubles when supine, compared with the lateral decubitus position). Upright posture during sleep, with the head of the bead elevated 60 degrees, has been shown to significantly reduce the RDI in some patients. nCPAP or bilevel CPAP (BiPAP) is titrated to pressures sufficient to eliminate upper airway obstruction by preventing soft tissue collapse. It is a highly effective treatment if the patient is able to tolerate the device (noncompliance is the major reason for failure of this modality). Autotitrating continuous positive airway pressure (APAP) can autoadjust the pressure from 5 to 20 cm of water while the patient sleeps, compensating for REM sleep and position changes. Despite these advantages, APAP has limitations and patient selection is important when prescribing this device. Some patients may elect to have a test trial of nCPAP before considering surgical options. True long-term compliance is much lower than the self-reported compliance, and the overall acceptance rate is near 50%. Several Food and Drug Administration–approved mandibular repositioning or advancement appliances are available (the Herbst appliance [Figure 14-8] and the Klearway appliance are the most popular). They work by positioning the mandible and tongue forward (50% to 100% of maximum protrusive movement as tolerated), which brings the attached soft tissue anteriorly, thereby opening the posterior airway space. On average, oral appliances reduce the RDI by 56%. The Herbst appliance has been reported to decrease the mean RDI from 48 to 12. The Klearway appliance was shown to improve the RDI to less than 15 in 80% of patients with moderate OSA and 61% of patients with severe OSA.

Tricyclic antidepressants and selective serotonin reuptake inhibitors have been tried as pharmacologic therapy for OSA; however, studies have failed to show significant success. The use of oxygen alone as the main therapy for OSA can result in blunting of the hypoxic drive.

If nCPAP or an oral appliance is not tolerated by the patient or if the oral appliance does not improve the patient's RDI to acceptable levels, surgical options should be considered.

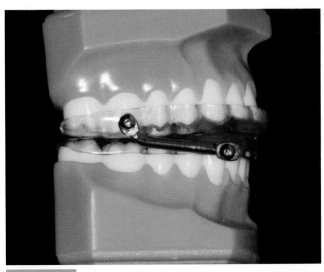

Figure 14-8 Herbst appliance. Bimaxillary appliance. Note that advancement of the mandible (Class III position) has advanced the genial tubercles and increased the airway space. *(Courtesy Dr. Daniel Levy, DDS. Department of Orthodontics, Georgia Health Sciences University, Augusta, Ga.)*

Tracheotomy was once considered the gold standard for OSA (100% effective), but it is no longer widely accepted except for very extreme cases. Site-specific or staged surgical reconstruction of the airway is now considered the standard of care. Nasal obstructions (deviated septum, inferior turbinate hypertrophy, internal nasal valve collapse, nasal polyps, or bony spurs) should be corrected in all patients, including those managed nonsurgically. Nasal reconstruction may include a septoplasty, radiofrequency inferior turbinate reduction (somnoplasty), spreader grafts, or polypectomy. A variety of staged-reconstruction protocols have been developed and studied. There is no conclusive evidence on which surgical protocol is most effective.

The soft palate (retropalatal oropharynx) is addressed by surgical ablation or radiofrequency volumetric reduction (somnoplasty). Uvulopalatopharyngoplasty (UPPP) was popularized by ear, nose, and throat (ENT) surgeons as an alternative to tracheotomy and was frequently and injudiciously recommended to almost all patients. When uvulopalatopharyngoplasty was the sole surgical modality, success rates were less than 50%. Failures were attributed to base of the tongue obstruction, which was not addressed with the uvulopalatopharyngoplasty. Others, who viewed the UPPP procedure as too radical, with an unacceptable incidence of velopharyngeal insufficiency and hypernasality, advocated the more conservative uvulopalatoplasty or uvulopalatal flap procedures. More recently, soft palate pillar implants have been introduced to stiffen the soft palate, reducing the amount of snoring and improving sleep apnea.

The retrolingual oropharyngeal and hypopharyngeal airway space can be improved with procedures that advance the genioglossus muscle and hyoid bone. The anterior mandibular osteotomy (genial window osteotomy, preferred when the pogonion is in normal position) or inferior sagittal osteotomy (sliding genioplasty, preferred when the pogonion is retropositioned) advances the genioglossus and geniohyoid muscles. The hyoid bone can be further positioned superiorly and anteriorly with a hyoid myotomy and suspension (the hyoid bone is suspended to the anterior mandible) or with a modified hyoid suspension technique (the hyoid bone is secured to the thyroid cartilage). When UPPP or uvulopalatoplasty is combined with a genial tubercle advancement with or without hyoid suspension, substantially higher success rates are reported.

Maxillomandibular advancement has been shown to improve posterior airway space and also to increase the stability of the lateral pharyngeal wall, countering its tendency to collapse. Maxillomandibular advancement may be performed in various stages of surgical treatment, depending on the surgeon's preference and the clinical indications. The maxillomandibular complex is typically advanced 10 mm. Adjunctive procedures (UPPP, genial advancement, hyoid suspension) can be performed based on site-specific principles. Success rates vary in the literature. Waite and colleagues reported a 65% success rate (RDI less than 10) when maxillomandibular advancement was the sole treatment. Prinsell reported 100% success (RDI less than 10) in 50 consecutive patients when maxillomandibular advancement was combined with genial advancement.

In the current patient, a trial of nCPAP was initiated, but the patient was unable to tolerate the device. He subsequently elected to undergo surgical management, consisting of an uvulopalatal flap procedure and advancement genioplasty (inferior sagittal osteotomy). A bilateral sagittal split osteotomy mandibular advancement, in conjunction with the uvulopalatoplasty and advancement genioplasty, would have been ideal, but the patient was not able to afford preoperative orthodontic therapy. His postoperative RDI was 20, with significant improvement in daytime somnolence. He was offered a modified hyoid suspension or maxillomandibular advancement as the second-stage surgery.

COMPLICATIONS

The morbidity and mortality of untreated OSAS far outweigh the individual complications of nonsurgical and surgical intervention. He and associates reported the 8-year survival rate of patients with an RDI greater than 20 to be 63%; an RDI of less than 20 corresponded to an 8-year survival rate of 96%. Hypertension is seen in one third to two thirds of all OSAS cases and is a major risk factor for coronary artery disease, congestive heart failure, and cerebrovascular accident. Untreated OSAS results in higher mortality rates from cardiovascular events. Untreated OSAS also increases the incidence of transient ischemic attacks and stroke, and this correlation may be stronger than that with coronary artery disease. Studies have also shown that daytime somnolence associated with OSAS is a major cause of traffic-related accidents and death.

Complications are specific for individual procedures, which are beyond the scope of this section. Velopharyngeal insufficiency is a well-documented postoperative complication of UPPP. The risk of velopharyngeal insufficiency is greater when UPPP is combined with maxillomandibular advancement. Li and colleagues reported a less than 10% incidence of "mild" velopharyngeal insufficiency with simultaneous maxillary advancement and UPPP.

DISCUSSION

Various staged surgical protocols have been developed that combine different site-specific surgeries into two or three stages. Because OSAS typically involves more than one anatomic level or area of obstruction, a combined surgical approach is warranted in most cases. This was recognized due to the low success rate when OSAS was treated with UPPP alone. Riley and associates described a two-stage process to treat type II obstruction. Stage 1 consisted of uvulopalatopharyngoplasty, genial advancement, and hyoid suspension. If stage 1 surgery was considered a failure, maxillomandibular advancement was performed as stage 2 surgery. In 1990 Riley and associates reviewed 40 patients undergoing stage 2 surgery (maxillomandibular advancement) and found a 97% success rate. In 1999 Lee and colleagues described a three-stage surgical treatment for type II obstruction:

- Stage 1: UPPP and genial advancement
- Stage 2: Maxillomandibular advancement
- Stage 3: Hyoid myotomy and suspension

In a review of 35 patients who had had the three-stage protocol, Lee and colleagues found a 69% success rate (RDI less than 20) after stage 1 treatment. The mean preoperative and postoperative RDIs were 53 and 19, respectively. Three patients underwent stage 2 surgery (maxillomandibular advancement), which resulted in a postoperative RDI of 10 or less in all three patients. Maxillomandibular advancement can also be used as an effective first line of treatment in moderate to severe cases of OSAS, as evidenced by Prinsell's review of 50 consecutive cases in 1999 with a reported 100% successful outcome.

Bibliography

Angelo J, De Dios A, Brass S: New and unconventional treatments for obstructive sleep apnea, *Neurotherapeutics* 9(4):702-709, 2012.

Chaples S, Rowley J, Prinsell J, et al: Surgical modifications of the airway for obstructive sleep apnea in adults: a systemic review and meta-analysis, *Sleep* 33:1396-1407, 2010.

Carvalho B, Hsia J, Capasso R: Surgical therapy of obstructive sleep apnea, *Neurotherapeutics* 9(4):710-716, 2012.

Chung F, Yegneswaran B, Liat P, et al: STOP questionnaire: a tool to screen patients for obstructive sleep apnea, *Anesthesiology* 108:812-821, 2008.

Chung F, Yegneswaran B, Liat P, et al: Validation of the Berlin questionnaire and American Society of Anesthesiology check list as screening tolls for obstructive sleep apnea in surgical patients, *Anesthesiology* 108:822-830, 2008.

Chung S, Hongbo Y, Chung F: A systemic review of obstructive sleep apnea and its implications for the anesthesiologist, *Anesth Analg* 107(5):1543-1563, 2008.

He J, Kryger MH, Zorick FJ, et al: Mortality and apnea index in obstructive sleep apnea. Experience in 385 male patients, *Chest* 94(1):9-14, 1988.

Lee NR, Givens CD Jr, Wilson J, et al: Staged surgical treatment of obstructive sleep apnea syndrome: a review of 35 patients, *J Oral Maxillofac Surg* 57(4):382-5, 1999.

Li KK, Troell RJ, Riley RW, et al: Uvulopalatopharyngoplasty, maxillomandibular advancement, and the velopharynx, *Laryngoscope* 111(6):1075-1078, 2001.

Mannarino M, Di Filippo F, Pirro M: Obstructive sleep apnea syndrome, *Eur J Intern Med* 23(7):506-593, 2012.

Morganthaler TI, Kapen S, Lee-Chiong T, et al: Practice parameters for the medical therapy of obstructive sleep apnea, *Sleep* 29(8):1031-1035, 2006.

Prinsell JR: Maxillomandibular advancement surgery in a site-specific treatment approach for obstructive sleep apnea in 50 consecutive patients, *Chest* 116(6):1519-29, 1999.

Riley RW, Powell NB, Guilleminault C: Maxillary, mandibular, and hyoid advancement for treatment of obstructive sleep apnea: a review of 40 patients, *J Oral Maxillofac Surg* 48(1):20-6, 1990.

Riley RW, Powell NB, Guilleminault C: Obstructive sleep apnea syndrome: a review of 306 consecutively treated surgical patients, *Otolaryngol Head Neck Surg* 108(2):117-125, 1993.

Shirin S: Perioperative management of obstructive sleep apnea: ready for prime time? *Cleve Clin J Med* 76(4):98-103, 2009.

Waite PD, Wooten V, Lachner J, et al: Maxillomandibular advancement surgery in 23 patients with obstructive sleep apnea syndrome, *J Oral Maxillofac Surg* 47(12):1256-1261, 1989.

Yaggi HK, Concato J, Kernana WN, et al: Obstructive sleep apnea as a risk factor for stroke and death, *N Eng J Med* 353:2034-2041, 2005.

Young T, Palta M, Dempsey J, et al: The occurrence of sleep-disorder breathing among middle-age adults, *N Engl J Med* 328:1230-1235, 1993.

Young T, Peppard PE, Gottlieb DJ: Epidemiology of obstructive sleep apnea: a population health perspective, *Am J Crit Care Med* 165:1217-1239, 2002.

CHAPTER 15

Medical Conditions

Editors: Shahrokh C. Bagheri

This chapter addresses:
- Congestive Heart Failure
- Acquired Immunodeficiency Syndrome
- Chronic Kidney Disease
- Liver Disease
- Von Willebrand Disease
- Oral Anticoagulation Therapy in Oral and Maxillofacial Surgery
- Alcohol Withdrawal Syndrome and Delirium Tremens
- Acute Asthmatic Attack
- Diabetes Mellitus
- Diabetic Ketoacidosis
- Acute Myocardial Infarction
- Hypertension

"Greater knowledge grants further humility."

Safe management of the oral and maxillofacial surgery patient requires an understanding of medial comorbidities that may complicate the perioperative or long-term outcome of procedures. Although it is not possible to describe the large array of medical conditions that may have surgical implications in oral and maxillofacial surgery, in this chapter we have elected 12 essential medical conditions that are encountered in the routine practice of any surgical subspecialty.

As the scope and depth of medicine and surgery expand, maintaining a command of all new developments becomes even more challenging. When necessary, consultation with practitioners in other medical or surgical subspecialties (e.g., cardiology, infectious diseases, ear/nose/throat) should be requested to obtain adequate information for safe surgical treatment.

Congestive Heart Failure

Michael R. Markiewicz, David Verschueren, Abdulrahman Doughan, and Shahrokh C. Bagheri

CC

A 71-year-old man who had been involved in a motor vehicle accident presents to the emergency department complaining of "shortness of breath, malocclusion, and broken bones in my face."

HPI

The patient had been involved in a motor vehicle accident in which he was an unrestrained driver in a low-velocity, head-on collision. He sustained injuries to the face, with no reported loss of consciousness. Upon presentation, he was also found to be in moderate respiratory distress. The patient is being admitted for multisystem trauma evaluation and possible acute congestive heart failure (CHF) exacerbation. The oral and maxillofacial surgery service was consulted to manage his facial injuries.

PMHX/PDHX/MEDICATIONS/ALLERGIES/SH/FH

The patient has a history of myocardial infarction 6 years earlier, with subsequent coronary artery bypass graft surgery without complications (documented previous coronary artery disease [CAD]). He also has a previous diagnosis of essential (idiopathic) hypertension, which is controlled by a single-drug regimen using hydrochlorothiazide (thiazide diuretic). He admits to poor compliance with his medications (risk factor for congestive heart failure [CHF] exacerbation) and had been previously diagnosed CHF, with a documented ejection fraction of 35% (the ejection fraction is the percentage of blood ejected forward into the systemic circulation by the left ventricle with each contraction; normal is greater than 55%). He is taking lovastatin (an HMG-CoA reductase inhibitor [cholesterol-lowering medication]) for hypercholesterolemia (risk factor for CAD). The patient has a 30 pack-year history of smoking (risk factor for CAD); he quit smoking after his myocardial infarction.

CAD involves varying degrees of impaired blood supply (oxygen) to the myocardium (causing ischemic heart disease), which puts the heart at risk for ischemic events (angina, myocardial infarction), with potential functional impairment of the myocardium and subsequent systolic dysfunction. This systolic dysfunction (heart failure) leads to the backup of blood (congestion); hence the term *congestive heart failure*. Risk factors for CHF include CAD (causes 50% to 75% of cases), uncontrolled systemic hypertension, valvular heart disease, cardiomyopathy (dilated or hypertrophic), stress (takotsubo), drugs (alcohol, cocaine, chemotherapy), and infections (viral myocarditis).

EXAMINATION

Advanced trauma life support (ATLS) primary survey. Negative except for moderate respiratory distress. The patient was immediately placed on supplemental oxygen via a nasal cannula and showed improvement of his work of breathing.

General. The patient is awake, alert, and oriented to person, time, and place. He shows an increase in respiratory effort, evidenced by use of accessory muscles of respiration.

Vital signs. Blood pressure is 110/75 mm Hg, heart rate 120 bpm (tachycardia), respirations 28 per minute (tachypnea), and temperature 37.1°C.

Maxillofacial. Findings consistent with a mildly displaced Le Fort I fracture (see the section Le Fort I Fracture in Chapter 8).

Cardiovascular. Fast but regular rhythm with normal S1 sound (closure of mitral and tricuspid valves) and S2 sound (closure of aortic and pulmonic valves). An S3 sound is auscultated at the left sternal border at the fifth intercostal space (an S3 sound is heard in early diastole and is secondary to rapid ventricular filling in a dilated cardiac chamber). The point of maximum impulse (generated by the left ventricle as it touches the inner chest wall during systole) is laterally displaced with a parasternal heave (elevation of the chest wall to the left of the sternum). The jugulovenous pressure is elevated at 15 cm (normal is less than 9 cm) with a positive hepatojugular reflex (distention of the jugular veins on application of pressure in the right upper abdominal quadrant). Hepatojugular reflex and elevated jugulovenous pressure are signs of venous congestion observed in association with heart failure and volume overload.

Pulmonary. Use of the accessory muscles of respiration (sternocleidomastoid, scalenes, pectoralis major and minor, and serratus anterior muscles). Dyspnea is exacerbated when patient assumes the supine position (orthopnea). Bilateral basilar rales (fluid in the alveolar spaces) with dullness to percussion (due to pleural effusions) in the lung bases (fluid accumulation in the lungs is secondary to left-sided heart failure).

Abdominal. Nontender and nondistended, with hepatomegaly. Liver was percussed at 10 cm below the costal margin (hepatic congestion due to right-sided heart failure).

Extremity. Lower extremities show 3+ pitting edema at the ankles (significant fluid in the extravascular compartments due to venous congestion, causing capillary leakage; this is usually first noted in the lower extremities due to the added effect of gravity; Figure 15-1).

IMAGING

A chest radiograph is the minimum imaging modality for the evaluation of CHF exacerbation. This is valuable for the evaluation of pulmonary edema and infiltration and for the approximation of the heart size. Echocardiography (transthoracic or transesophageal) is also useful for the evaluation of ventricular and valvular function and determination of the ejection fraction. The earliest finding of left-sided heart failure on the chest radiograph is cephalization of the pulmonary vessels. Normally, the vessels in the lung bases are larger and more numerous than those in the lung apices. This is secondary to the effects of gravity and the anatomically larger volume of the lungs at the base. With the progression of heart failure,

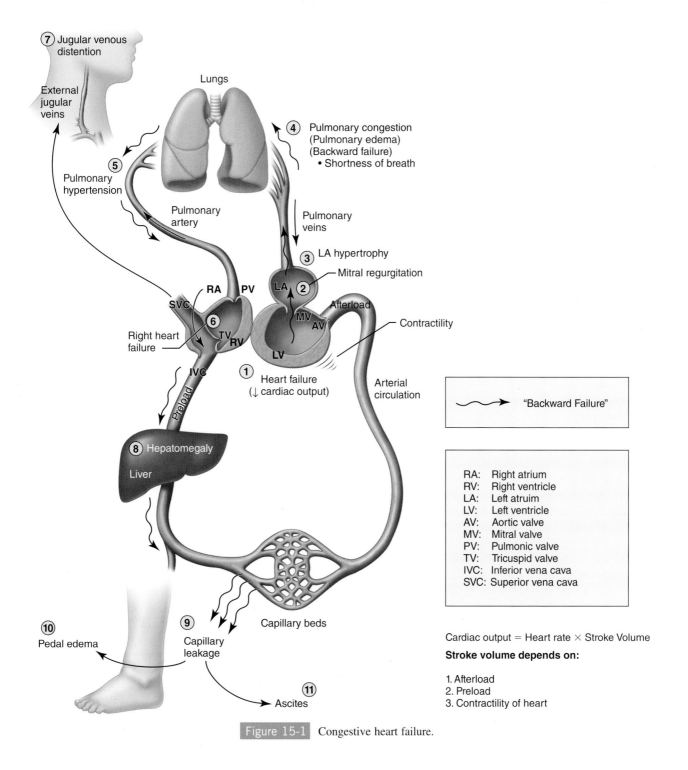

Figure 15-1 Congestive heart failure.

the increased pressure is transmitted "backward" to the pulmonary veins and capillaries (hence the term "backward failure"). The lung bases are affected first; therefore, blood is preferentially "shunted" to the upper, or more cephalad, lobes, giving the radiographic appearance of cephalization. If the pressure in the vessels continues to rise, the fluid in the interstitium becomes radiographically evident as interstitial edema, bronchial wall thickening, and interlobular septa. The most noticeable are the Kerley B lines. These are short, thin, perpendicular lines extending to the pleura at the lung bases on a chest radiograph. The following imaging findings were noted for the current patient.

Chest radiograph. Bilateral blunting of the costophrenic angles with pronounced infiltrates in the lower lobes (consistent with bilateral pleural effusions and pulmonary edema).

Cephalization of the pulmonary vessels bilaterally. Increased cardiac silhouette (an increased cardiac silhouette, spanning more than one third of the thoracic cavity on an anteroposterior film, is indicative of an enlarged heart or dilated cardiomyopathy).

Transthoracic echocardiography. Dilated left ventricle consistent with dilated cardiomyopathy with decreased wall motion (systolic dysfunction) and mild mitral regurgitation. The pulmonic, aortic, and tricuspid valves were without stenosis or regurgitation. The ejection fraction was estimated at 25% (compromised ventricular function). No pericardial fluid and normal wall thickness were seen in all four chambers. Moderate elevation of the pulmonary artery pressure was noted.

CT (maxillofacial). Mildly displaced fracture at the Le Fort I level. (A CT scan of the chest can also be used to further evaluate the pulmonary parenchyma and cardiac structures.)

LABS

Brain natriuretic peptide level was 2,000 pg/ml (normal is less than 100 pg/ml).

With CHF, increased pressure and workload on the heart trigger the myocardial cells to secrete natriuretic peptides. Atrial myocytes secrete increased amounts of atrial natriuretic peptide, and the ventricular myocytes secrete both atrial and brain natriuretic peptides in response to the high atrial and ventricular filling pressures. Both of these peptides work as natriuretic, diuretic, and vasodilator agents and help reduce both preload and afterload. The plasma concentrations of both hormones are increased in patients with asymptomatic and symptomatic CHF.

Electrocardiogram Findings

The electrocardiographic findings for the current patient were as follows:
- *Rate.* Tachycardic at 120 bpm
- *Rhythm.* Regular; each P wave followed by a QRS complex; each QRS complex preceded by a P wave; QRS complexes occurring at regular intervals
- *Axis.* Positive deflection in lead I; negative deflection in lead aVF (indicative of left-axis deviation secondary to left ventricular hypertrophy)

- *Intervals.* PR interval less than 0.20 second, or 5 small boxes on electrocardiograph paper (more than 5 small boxes is consistent with first-degree atrioventricular node block); QRS complex less than 0.12 second, or 3 small boxes (more than 3 small boxes indicates widened QRS complex); QT interval less than half the distance from QRS complex to QRS complex (normal)
- *Infarctions.* Q waves in leads V_1 through V_5 (hallmark of old anteroseptal myocardial infarction); no flipped T waves, and no ST-segment elevation or depression (signs of acute ischemic events)
- *Other.* Loss of precordial R wave progression in leads V_1 through V_6 (suggestive of old anteroseptal MI and loss of anterior electrical forces)

ASSESSMENT

A 71-year-old man status post motor vehicle accident with a previous history of heart disease now presenting with acute CHF exacerbation (class IV heart failure) and a mildly displaced Le Fort I fracture.

TREATMENT

The cardiology service was consulted, and the patient was treated with fluid and salt restriction, intravenous Lasix (loop diuretic), oral lisinopril (angiotensin-converting enzyme [ACE] inhibitor), and oral carvedilol (β-blocker). Inotropic support was not required due to preserved perfusion and absence of cardiogenic shock. The patient's cardiovascular symptoms and findings gradually improved within 36 hours (decreased shortness of breath, orthopnea, and paroxysmal nocturnal dyspnea; resolution of peripheral edema and pleural effusions; decrease in cardiac biomarker brain natriuretic peptide [BNP] level). He remained chest pain free and hemodynamically and electrically stable (no arrhythmias). After a careful perioperative cardiac risk assessment, the patient was taken to the operating room for fixation of the Le Fort fracture under general anesthesia.

DISCUSSION

Heart failure can result from any structural or functional cardiac disorder that impairs the ability of the heart to pump blood. It is characterized by several symptoms, such as dyspnea, fatigue, edema, and weight gain. There are several etiologies for heart failure, including myocarditis/endocarditis (viral/bacterial infections), ischemic heart disease, infiltrative disease (amyloidosis, sarcoidosis), peripartum cardiomyopathy, hypertension, human immunodeficiency virus (HIV) infection, connective tissue disorders, substance abuse, certain chemotherapy drugs, and idiopathic origin.

Fluid retention in heart failure is initiated by the fall in cardiac output, leading to edema and decreased effective arterial volume. The reduction of cardiac output sets into motion a cascade of hemodynamic and neurohormonal derangements that provoke activation of the renin-angiotensin-aldosterone and sympathetic nervous systems. Although initially beneficial in the early stages of heart failure, these compensatory mechanisms eventually lead to a vicious cycle of worsening heart failure, fluid retention, and volume overload.

The classification systems used for the management of CHF are based on the severity of the condition, systolic versus diastolic dysfunction, and left-sided versus right-sided failure. Heart failure is classified by severity of symptoms using the New York Heart Association (NYHA) classification (most commonly used). This categorizes patients into one of four functional classes, depending on the degree of effort needed to elicit symptoms:

- Class I: Symptoms of heart failure only at levels that would limit normal individuals
- Class II: Symptoms of heart failure with ordinary exertion
- Class III: Symptoms of heart failure on less than ordinary exertion
- Class IV: Symptoms of heart failure at rest

The American College of Cardiology/American Heart Association classification and guidelines for the treatment of heart failure can be found in Table 15-1.

When using the right-sided or left-sided designation as the etiology of heart failure, it is the symptomatology and physical and echocardiographic findings that determine the anatomic side of the failing heart. With right-sided heart failure, there is elevation of the jugulovenous pressure, peripheral edema, and hepatomegaly. In left-sided heart failure, fluid backs up in the lungs, causing dyspnea, cough, pleural effusions, and rales. Sustained left-sided heart failure eventually causes right-sided heart failure. After all, the most common cause of right-sided heart failure is left-sided failure.

The systolic versus diastolic designation of heart failure involves determining whether failure is the result of impaired contraction or inefficient relaxation. Systolic dysfunction is commonly defined as heart failure secondary to impaired ejection fraction, whereas diastolic dysfunction is characterized by heart failure in the setting of preserved ejection fraction. Causes of diastolic dysfunction include myocardial hypertrophy and infiltrative cardiomyopathy (cardiac amyloidosis).

The pharmacotherapy of heart failure (HF) is aimed at improving cardiac function (contractility and stroke volume) and reducing the workload of the heart (preload and afterload reduction). Most patients with HF should be routinely managed with a combination of three types of drugs: a diuretic, an ACE inhibitor (ACEI) or an angiotensin receptor blocker (ARB), and a β-blocker. The value of these drugs has been established by the results of numerous large-scale clinical trials. Patients with evidence of fluid retention should take a diuretic until a euvolemic state is achieved, and diuretic therapy should be continued to prevent the recurrence of fluid retention. Diuretics interfere with the sodium retention of HF by inhibiting the reabsorption of sodium or chloride at specific sites in the renal tubules.

Treatment with an ACEI or an ARB should be initiated and maintained in patients who can tolerate them. ACEIs are the best-studied class of agents in HF, with multiple mechanisms of benefit for both HF and coronary artery disease.

Table 15-1	Classification and Guidelines for the Treatment of Heart Failure	
Stage	**Characteristics**	**Treatment**
A	High risk for heart failure without structural heart disease or symptoms	ACEI or ARB
B	Structural heart disease without signs or symptoms	ACEI or ARB + β-blocker (devices such as defibrillators in appropriate patients)
C	Structural heart disease with prior/current symptoms of heart failure.	Routine use of diuretics, ACEI, or β-blockers, and aldosterone antagonist, ARB, digitalis, or hydralazine/nitrates, and devices such as biventricular pacing or implantable defibrillator in selected patients
D	Advanced heart disease	Medications from stages A through C, with optional use of palliative care, heart transplantation, chronic inotropes, permanent mechanical support, or experimental surgery or drugs

ACEI, Angiotensin-converting enzyme inhibitors; *ARB,* angiotensin receptor blocker.
Data from Hunt SA, Abraham WT, Chin MH, et al: ACC/AHA 2005 guideline update for the diagnosis and management of chronic heart failure in the adult: a report of the American College of Cardiology/American Heart Association Task Force on Practice Guidelines (Writing Committee to Update the 2001 Guidelines for the Evaluation and Management of Heart Failure). American College of Cardiology Web Site. Available at: http://www.acc.org/clinical/guidelines/failure//index.pdf.

They have been shown to favorably influence the long-term prognosis of HF.

β-blockers act principally to inhibit the adverse effects of the sympathetic nervous system in patients with HF. Sympathetic activation can increase ventricular volumes and pressure by causing peripheral vasoconstriction and by impairing sodium excretion by the kidneys. Long-term treatment with β-blockers can lessen the symptoms of HF, improve the clinical status of patients, and enhance the patient's overall sense of well-being. In addition, as do ACEIs, β-blockers can reduce the risk of death and the combined risk of death and hospitalization.

Therapy with digoxin as a fourth agent may be initiated at any time to reduce symptoms, prevent hospitalization, control rhythm, and enhance exercise tolerance. Digoxin is a digitalis glycoside that inhibits sodium-potassium (Na^+-K^+) adenosine triphosphatase. Inhibition of this enzyme in cardiac cells and vagal afferent fibers results in an increase in the contractile state of the myocardium and reduction in sympathetic outflow from the central nervous system, respectively.

Other treatments that can be initiated in heart failure patients include use of an aldosterone antagonist and use of a combination of hydralazine and isosorbide dinitrate. Spironolactone is the most widely used aldactone antagonist. It has been shown in long-term trials to reduce death and heart failure hospitalizations and to improve the functional class for patients with NYHA class III or class IV symptoms.

The combination of hydralazine and isosorbide dinitrate reduces mortality in patients with heart failure who remain symptomatic despite optimal medical therapy, particularly in the African American cohort of patients. Hydralazine and isosorbide are arterial and venodilators that act by lowering systemic vascular resistance (afterload). Other advanced therapies for heart failure include intraaortic balloon counterpulsation, cardiac resynchronization, and left ventricular assist devices.

CONCLUSION

Trauma patients commonly present with exacerbations of previous medical conditions due to the increased physiologic stress of trauma. Particular attention should be given to the overall status of the patient and not just to the maxillofacial region. Early recognition of an acute exacerbation of a preexisting medical condition, such as congestive heart failure, is critical. The unpredictable progression to multisystem failure can be devastating. A thorough physical examination and a high index of suspicion must be maintained to assess cardiac, pulmonary, and volume status.

Bibliography

Dickstein K, Cohen-Solal A, Filippatos G, et al: ESC guidelines for the diagnosis and treatment of acute and chronic heart failure 2008: the Task Force for the Diagnosis and Treatment of Acute and Chronic Heart Failure 2008 of the European Society of Cardiology. Developed in collaboration with the Heart Failure Association of the ESC (HFA) and endorsed by the European Society of Intensive Care Medicine (ESICM), *Eur J Heart Fail* 10(10):933-989, 2008.

Grady KL, Dracup K, Kennedy G, et al: Team management of patients with heart failure: a statement for healthcare professionals from the Cardiovascular Nursing Council of the American Heart Association, *Circulation* 102:2443, 2000.

Hunt SA, Abraham WT, Chin MH, et al: 2009 Focused update incorporated into the ACC/AHA 2005 guidelines for the diagnosis and management of heart failure in adults: a report of the American College of Cardiology Foundation/American Heart Association Task Force on Practice Guidelines developed in collaboration with the International Society for Heart and Lung Transplantation, *J Am Coll Cardiol* 53(15):e1-e90, 2009.

Knudsen CW, Omland T, Clopton P, et al: Diagnostic value of B-type natriuretic peptide and chest radiographic findings in patients with acute dyspnea, *Am J Med* 116:363, 2004.

Young JB, Gheorghiade M, Uretsky BF, et al: Superiority of "triple" drug therapy in heart failure: insights from the PROVED and RADIANCE trials—prospective randomized study of ventricular function and efficacy of digoxin; randomized assessment of digoxin and inhibitors of angiotensin-converting enzyme, *J Am Coll Cardiol* 32(3):686-692, 1998.

Acquired Immunodeficiency Syndrome

Mehran Mehrabi and Shahrokh C. Bagheri

CC

A 46-year-old man who is seropositive for the human immunodeficiency virus (HIV) is referred to your office. He complains, "I am having pain in my mouth, and I need my teeth out in order to get dentures."

HPI

The patient has been receiving routine dental care, but during a recent yearly checkup, he was found to have multiple mobile teeth (accelerated periodontal disease is seen with HIV infection). This sudden change in his oral health has coincided with a recent exacerbation of his HIV infection, as measured by an increase in his viral load, a decrease in his CD4 cell count, and the onset of gastrointestinal and constitutional symptoms. He has had several previous hospital admissions. Currently, he complains of a foul-smelling mouth odor (halitosis), gingival pain, loosening teeth, gingival bleeding, and exposed roots. The onset of pain has contributed to difficulty with hygiene and further accumulation of calculus.

PMHX/PDHX/MEDICATIONS/ALLERGIES/SH/FH

The patient tested positive for HIV 6 years ago. He believes he acquired the virus through unprotected sexual contact. On his most recent hospital admission, his CD4 count was 108 cells/μl; therefore, he was diagnosed with acquired immunodeficiency syndrome (AIDS). (An absolute CD4 count below 200 cells/μl is an AIDS-defining feature in adults; in pediatric patients, the CD4 cell percentage is more accurate.) The patient's internist indicated that the patient's recent episode of pneumonia was due to the recent decline in his CD4 count.

There are no particular preoperative criteria for maxillofacial surgery in patients with HIV infection or AIDS. However, each patient should be assessed for risks and benefits of surgery. Some of the common concerns in a surgical patient are the hemoglobin level and platelet count. Despite popular belief, neither the lymphocyte count nor the viral load alters maxillofacial surgical intervention. Nonetheless, a patient with a rapidly declining lymphocyte count or a rise in viral load should be reassessed before any surgical intervention.

EXAMINATION

General. The patient is a cooperative man with evidence of muscle wasting (cachexia) who appears anxious (generalized muscle wasting is seen with advancing AIDS).

Vital signs. Blood pressure is 121/79 mm Hg (hypotension), heart rate 90 bpm, respirations 14 per minute, temperature 37.8°C (with advanced AIDS, it is not uncommon to have a normal temperature despite the presence of an acute infection; this is due to the failure and/or deficiency of available white blood cells to mount an appropriate inflammatory response, which results in fever), and SaO$_2$ 92% on room air (a recent history of pneumonia can result in a decrease in baseline oxygen saturation on room air).

Maxillofacial. There is no evidence of hair loss or patchy ulceration on the scalp. (Scalp ulceration may be seen in patients with disseminated fungal diseases, such as cryptococcal infection. These ulcerations may also present in the oral cavity or on the peripheral extremities. A biopsy can be used to confirm the diagnosis. This finding can be used as a sign to evaluate other organs for fungal invasion.) Bilateral temporal wasting and prominent zygomatic arches are noted. Examination of the neck reveals a soft dorsal hump. (Lipodystrophy may result either directly from HIV or as a side effect of antiretroviral therapy, particularly protease inhibitors. Other physical signs to investigate are seborrheic dermatitis [dandruff], vesicular rash with central umbilication in the forehead [molluscum contagiosum], and enlargement of the parotid glands [differential diagnoses consist of lymphoepithelial cyst, lipodystrophy, and lymphoma].)

Intraoral. Oral hygiene is poor, and the breath is fetid. A generalized inflammation of the maxillary and mandibular gingivae, exposed buccal bone, and mobility of the teeth are noted. Gentle palpation of the gingival tissue results in bleeding and pain. There is no facial or intraoral fluctuance and no obvious swelling. (In addition to HIV gingivitis and HIV periodontitis, the oral examination should concentrate on the presence of warts [human papillomavirus]; oral neoplastic growths, such as Kaposi sarcoma [human herpes virus 8]; hairy leukoplakia [Epstein-Barr virus]; candidiasis; and other fungal infections. Aphthous ulcers, lymphoma, herpes, and cytomegalovirus ulcerations also may be seen in patients with AIDS.)

Chest. Chest is clear on auscultation (if the patient presents with crackles, a chest radiograph is indicated).

Cardiovascular. Regular rate and rhythm, S1 and S2, and no gallops, rubs, or murmurs (HIV may affect the heart, resulting in dilated cardiomyopathy, but this is not common).

IMAGING

A routine preoperative chest radiograph is not indicated unless the patient's history or clinical examination is suggestive of symptoms such as shortness of breath, a decrease in oxygen saturation on room air, or a productive cough. However, a chest radiograph, along with arterial blood gas analysis, may be valuable.

For the current patient, the panoramic radiograph demonstrates areas of moderate and severe vertical interproximal bone loss consistent with severe to moderate periodontal disease.

LABS

During the perioperative evaluation of a patient with HIV infection, a complete blood count is valuable but should be used with caution. A rise in the white blood cell count may not be seen in response to physiologic or inflammatory demands, as would be seen in immune-competent individuals. The lymphocyte subset can be used to assess the susceptibility to opportunistic infections. The neutrophil count may be elevated with bacterial infections. The hemoglobin and hematocrit levels may be used to assess volume status (hemoglobin would be falsely elevated). Hemoglobin and platelet levels may be depleted, and patients may require packed red blood cell or platelet transfusions before major surgery.

Additional tests may be helpful, depending on the extent of the surgical procedures or the presence of concurrent comorbidities associated with immune suppression. Arterial blood gas analysis is helpful for assessing the pulmonary status of a patient with active pneumonia. A basic metabolic panel may be used to evaluate intravascular fluid status in dehydrated and volume-depleted patients. A blood urea nitrogen to creatinine ratio greater than 20 is suggestive of volume depletion. The coagulation factors are rarely depleted in patients with HIV, but HIV or other infections may predispose a patient to disseminated intravascular coagulation (DIC). Coagulation studies should be obtained as needed. Evaluation of hepatic function is also important. Although HIV may affect liver function directly, of more concern is a concurrent infection with hepatitis B or C virus (note that the route of transmission is similar for HIV and the hepatitis B and C viruses).

ASSESSMENT

AIDS secondary to HIV infection, now complicated by acute necrotizing ulcerative periodontitis, requiring full mouth extraction.

TREATMENT

There is some controversy regarding the optimal time to initiate treatment for patients who are seropositive for HIV. Most infectious disease specialists start pharmacotherapy when the CD4 count drops below 50 cells/µl. Regardless of the CD4 count, treatment should be initiated as soon as possible in patients with HIV nephropathy, pregnant patients, and those coinfected with hepatitis B. Current recommendations consist of a combination of a nucleoside reverse transcriptase inhibitor (NRTI; Table 15-2), a non–nucleoside reverse transcriptase inhibitor (NNRTI; Table 15-3), protease inhibitors (Table 15-4), integrase inhibitors, fusion inhibitors, and CCR5 antagonists. A combination of these medications is commonly referred to as *highly active antiretroviral therapy* (HAART).

When a patient presents with a CD4 count below 200 cells/µl, they are started on trimethoprim-sulfamethoxazole for *Pneumocystis jirovecii* (formerly called *Pneumocystis carinii*) prophylaxis. At a CD4 count below 100 cells/µl, the patient is increasingly susceptible to toxoplasmosis infections. Because this is treated with the same medication, no additional prophylactic is needed. When the CD4 count drops below 50 cells/µl, there is a high risk of *Mycobacterium avium* complex infection. This is empirically treated with clarithromycin or azithromycin (macrolide antibiotics). Viral infections, such as herpes simplex virus, are treated with famciclovir

Table 15-2	Nucleoside Reverse Transcriptase Inhibitors	
Nucleotide Reverse Transcriptase Inhibitor	**Abbreviation**	**Side Effects**
Retrovir	AZT	Anemia, neutropenia
Videx	DDI	Pancreatitis, peripheral neuropathy (PN)
Hivid	DDC	Pancreatitis, PN
Zerit	D4T	Pancreatitis, PN
Epivir	3TC	Also used for hepatitis B virus (HBV) infection
Ziagen	ABC	Rash, death

Table 15-3	Nonnucleoside Reverse Transcriptase Inhibitors	
Nonnucleoside Reverse Transcriptase Inhibitor		**Side Effects**
Nevirapine (Viramune)		Hepatotoxicity, hepatic necrosis during the first 4 weeks
Delavirdine (Rescriptor)		Rash, headache
Efavirenz (Sustiva)		Teratogenic; Stevens-Johnson rash, hallucinations, nightmares

Table 15-4	Protease Inhibitors	
Protease Inhibitor	**Number of Pills Taken Daily**	**Common Side Effects**
Indinavir (Crixivan)	6	Nephrolithiasis
Ritonavir (Norvir)	12	Weakness, loss of appetite, nausea and vomiting
Invirase/Fortovase (Saquinavir)	9	Gastrointestinal disturbances
Nelfinavir (Viracept)	10	Gastrointestinal disturbances (most commonly diarrhea)
Amprenavir (Agenerase)	16	Severe rash
Lopinavir/ritonavir (Kaletra)	6	Hepatitis

or acyclovir (there is prophylactic treatment; patients are treated only in the face of infection). Some infections, such as *Candida* species, may present at a CD4 count below 500 cells/μl, but prophylactic treatment of fungal infections is not recommended.

The initial treatment of acute necrotizing ulcerative periodontitis consists of fluid resuscitation as needed, analgesics, and antibiotic therapy. With generalized severe periodontal disease, full mouth extraction is both definitive and curative. Patients with HIV infection are treated aggressively to prevent any odontogenic sources of infection, which may cause severe complications in a patient with a declining immune system.

The current patient underwent outpatient full mouth extraction under intravenous sedation. After surgical treatment, the alveolar ridges healed without complications.

Immune suppression can be due to defects in various aspects of the immune system. Concerns and cautions are not the same when dealing with different defects of the immune system. For example, a patient who is neutropenic is more susceptible to bacterial infection, whereas T-lymphocyte deficiency increases susceptibility to fungal, viral, and parasitic infections.

In oral surgical procedures, there are more complications associated with neutropenia (sepsis, oral ulceration, periodontal disease) than with lymphopenia. For the neutropenic patient, preoperative antibiotics are used to prevent sepsis. Postoperative antibiotics may also be used.

COMPLICATIONS

Patients affected by HIV infection may present with thrombocytopenia. This can be due to idiopathic thrombocytopenic purpura or thrombotic thrombocytopenic purpura. Idiopathic thrombocytopenic purpura is an autoimmune disorder, resulting from antibodies to glycoprotein platelet 2β3α-receptors. This may present as an acute condition (mostly in children) or a chronic condition (mostly in adult women). Treatment

consists of prednisone, intravenous immunoglobulin, splenectomy, azathioprine, or vincristine. Thrombotic thrombocytopenic purpura presents as a combination of five symptoms: renal failure, central nervous system abnormalities, fever, thrombocytopenia, and anemia. The exact etiology is not well understood. A similar syndrome, hemolytic uremic syndrome, is caused by *Escherichia coli* O157:H7. In the presence of neurologic symptoms, the diagnosis of thrombotic thrombocytopenic purpura is made; however, when renal failure is the prominent feature, it is usually due to hemolytic uremic syndrome. The treatment for thrombotic thrombocytopenic purpura is plasmapheresis.

There also are other causes of both idiopathic thrombocytopenic purpura and thrombotic thrombocytopenic purpura. Idiopathic thrombocytopenic purpura may be caused by any viral infection, leukemia, lupus erythematosus, cirrhosis, antiphospholipid syndrome, and medications (quinine, heparin). Thrombotic thrombocytopenic purpura can be caused by cancer, bone marrow transplantation, pregnancy, and medication (ticlopidine, clopidogrel, cyclosporine, mitomycin, tacrolimus/FK-506, interferon-α).

The risk of postoperative infection in a patient with HIV infection or AIDS who undergoes maxillofacial surgery is controversial at best. Although earlier studies showed an increased risk of infection in those with HIV, this has not been confirmed by more recent studies. Most studies were conducted before the advent of HAART. There is a need for prospective evaluation for the risk of infections after various maxillofacial surgeries. Currently there are no recommendations regarding the presurgical or postsurgical care of a patient with HIV infection compared with that of healthy control patients.

DISCUSSION

Immune deficiency may be an inherited, acquired, or iatrogenic disorder. Inherited defects may result from quantitative or qualitative defects of the cells or cellular pathways involved in immunity (neutrophil, macrophages, complement, lymphocytes). Immune suppression is also seen with organ transplantation for prevention of host-versus-graft or graft-versus-host disease and in chemotherapy. Acquired immune deficiency is seen with conditions such as diabetes, leukemia, and AIDS.

AIDS was recognized in 1981 after multiple homosexual male patients were diagnosed with *Pneumocystis* pneumonia and Kaposi sarcoma (more recently found to be also associated with human herpes virus 8). Before 1981, *Pneumocystis* pneumonia was commonly seen in cancer patients, and Kaposi sarcoma was endemic to Africa and the Mediterranean region. In 1984, HIV, a retrovirus belonging to the Lenti virus family, was discovered concurrently by French and American scientists. The virus can be transmitted via exposure of body fluids through sexual contact, sharing of needles or paraphernalia, blood transfusions (horizontal transmission), or from mother to fetus (vertical transmission). Once in the bloodstream, HIV targets the lymphocytes and macrophages, which are the only cells with CD4+ receptors. T cells with a CXCR4 chemokine coreceptor are called *T tropic,* and macrophages with CCR5 are called *M tropic.* The virus is unable to infect these cells in the absence of these coreceptors. Interaction of the CD4 receptor with the viral glycoprotein 120 changes its stereo-chemistry, exposing glycoprotein 41, which binds to heparin sulfate in the membrane of the host cells, fusing the viral envelope with the cell membrane. Once genetic material enters the cell, a complementary DNA or coda is made from the original RNA by the enzyme reverse transcriptase. This complementary DNA joins the host DNA by using the enzyme integrase, forcing the cell to make necessary proteins to replicate the virus. Finally, the packaged virus leaves the host cell, using the cell membrane as a viral envelope, and subsequently infecting other cells. CCR5 inhibitors, fusion inhibitors, integrase inhibitor, NRTIs and NNRTIs are respectively used to inhibit every step in this process.

After inoculation, a patient typically seroconverts in approximately 3 weeks, although the time period can range from 9 days to as long as 6 months. Routine laboratory testing for HIV before this date results in a negative test. The patient may be asymptomatic or may develop flulike symptoms. The viral load rapidly rises and then falls during this period, and the CD4 count rapidly drops before returning to nearly its original level. During the following years, if the infection goes untreated, there is a steady decrease in the CD4 cell count, along with an increase in the viral load. In general, the viral load is a reflection of the speed of progression of AIDS, whereas the CD4 cell count reflects the current immune status and is used to evaluate susceptibility to opportunistic infections.

More than 1 million Americans (1,106,400) had been infected with HIV by 2006, according to the Centers for Disease Control and Prevention (CDC). This population is increasing at the rate of 40,000 new infections each year. Among oral and maxillofacial surgery patients, the prevalence of HIV is estimated to be as high as 4.8% in certain demographic areas. Although HAART has resulted in a significant drop in opportunistic infections, such as those presenting with oral manifestation, it has not eradicated these complications.

Oral manifestation of HIV may aid in both the diagnosis and prognosis of the disease. These lesions are seen in up to 30% to 80% of patients who have tested positive for HIV, and they may be infectious (bacterial, viral, fungal, and parasitic), neoplastic, or idiopathic. A study published by Diz Dios and colleagues found a reduction in oral lesions from 74.2% to 28.5% after the use of HAART. However, in that study there was a significant drop in patient follow-up due to death or relocation. A study by Aguirre and associates evaluated 72 patients with various oral diseases. A significant improvement was seen in the prevalence of pseudomembranous candidiasis (from 80% to 32%) with the use of HAART. Only a small change was seen in acute necrotizing periodontitis. Tappuni and Flemming evaluated 284 patients infected with HIV and concluded that oral lesions are seen significantly less often in patients receiving monotherapy compared with patients

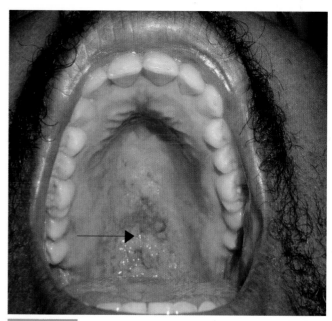

Figure 15-2 Cryptococcal infection of the palate in a patient with AIDS.

receiving no therapy. Furthermore, the use of HAART resulted in a statistically significant reduction in lesions compared with the use of monotherapy.

The differential diagnosis of oral lesions seen with HIV may be divided into bacterial, viral, fungal, neoplastic, and idiopathic categories. Bacterial infections may present as acute necrotizing gingivitis or periodontitis. Viral infections, such oral papillomas, are caused by the human papillomavirus and are commonly seen. Fungal infections, such as histoplasmosis or cryptococcosis (Figure 15-2), can cause oral ulcerations. An example of intraoral neoplastic disease is Kaposi sarcoma, caused by human herpes virus 8, which is most commonly seen in homosexual males. Idiopathic xerostomia is commonly seen, resulting in cervical caries.

The surgical management of patients with HIV infection or AIDS requires an understanding of the pathophysiology, medications, and associated disease processes.

Bibliography

Aguirre JM, Echebrria MA, Ocina E: Reduction of HIV-associated oral lesion after highly active antiretroviral therapy, *Oral Surg Oral Med Oral Pathol Oral Radiol Endod* 88:114-115, 1999.

Carey JW, Dodson TB: Hospital course of HIV-positive patients with odontogenic infections, *Oral Surg Oral Pathol Oral Med Oral Radiol Endod* 91:23-27, 2001.

Centers for Disease Control and Prevention: *HIV/AIDS surveillance report,* vol 18, Atlanta, 2008, the CDC.

Depoala LG: Human immunodeficiency virus disease: natural history and management, *Oral Surg Oral Med Oral Pathol Oral Radiol Endod* 90:266-270, 2000.

Diz Dios P, Ocampo A, Miralles C, et al: Changing prevalence of human immunodeficiency virus–associated oral lesion, *Oral Surg Oral Med Oral Pathol Oral Radiol Endod* 90:403-404, 2000.

Dodson TB: HIV status and the risk of post-extraction complications, *J Dent Res* 76:1644-1652, 1997.

Dodson TB: Predictors of postextraction complications in HIV-positive patients, *Oral Surg Oral Med Oral Pathol Oral Radiol Endod* 84:474-479, 1997.

Dodson TB, Nguyen T, Kaban LB: Prevalence of HIV infection oral and maxillofacial surgery patients, *Oral Surg Oral Med Oral Pathol Oral Radiol Endod* 76:272-275, 1993.

Dodson TB, Perrott DH, Gongloff RK, et al: Human immunodeficiency virus serostatus and the risk of postextraction complications, *Int J Oral Maxillofac Surg* 23:100-103, 1994.

Frame PT: HIV disease in primary care, *Prim Care* 30:205-237, 2003.

Mehrabi M, Bagheri S, Leonard MK Jr, et al: Mucocutaneous manifestation of cryptococcal infection: report of a case and review of the literature, *J Oral Maxillofac Surg* 63:1543-1549, 2005.

Miller EJ Jr, Dodson TB: The risk of serious odontogenic infection in HIV-positive patients: a pilot study, *Oral Surg Oral Med Oral Pathol Oral Radiol Endod* 86:406-409, 1998.

Panel on Antiretroviral Guidelines for adult and Adolescents: Guidelines for the use of antiretroviral agents in HIV-1 infected adults and adolescents. Department of Health and Human Services. Available at: http://aidsinfo.nih.gov/contentfiles/lvguidelines/adultandadolescentgl.pdf. Accessed August 26, 2012.

Patton LL: Hematologic abnormalities among HIV-infected patients: associations of significance for dentistry, *Oral Surg Oral Med Oral Pathol Oral Radiol Endod* 88:561-567, 1999.

Ray N, Doms RW: HIV-1 coreceptors and their inhibitors, *Curr Top Microbiol Immunol* 303:97-120, 2006.

Schmidt B, Kearns G, Perrott D, et al: Infection following treatment of mandibular fractures in human immunodeficiency virus seropositive patients, *J Oral Maxillofac Surg* 53:1134-1139, 1995.

Shanti RB, Aziz SR: HIV-associated salivary gland disease, *Oral Maxillofac Surg Clin North Am* 21:339-343, 2009.

Sleasman JW, Goodenow MM: HIV-1 infection, *J Allergy Clin Immunol* 111:S582-S592, 2003.

Tappuni AR, Flemming JP: The effect of antiretroviral therapy on the prevalence of oral manifestations in HIV-infected patients: a UK study, *Oral Surg Oral Med Oral Pathol Oral Radiol Endod* 92:623-628, 2001.

Chronic Kidney Disease

Gary F. Bouloux, Sung Hee Cho, and Shahrokh C. Bagheri

CC

A 68-year-old (age is a risk factor) African American (highest risk factor) woman with a history of chronic kidney disease presents with her third episode of acute pericoronitis in 18 months.

HPI

The patient has an impacted lower third molar that causes intermittent pain and has given rise to moderate right-sided facial swelling, fever, malaise, and anorexia.

PMHX/PDHX/MEDICATIONS/ALLERGIES/SH/FH

The patient's medical history is notable for poorly controlled diabetes mellitus, hypertension, hypercholesterolemia (all risk factors), and chronic kidney disease. Her dental history is significant for multiple extractions over the past 20 years. Medications include insulin, felodipine (calcium channel blocker), metoprolol (β-blocker), losartan (angiotensin receptor blocker), and furosemide (loop diuretic). She has a 28 pack-year smoking history (risk factor).

EXAMINATION

General. The patient is a mildly obese woman in mild distress secondary to pain.

Vital signs. Blood pressure is 162/98 mm Hg, heart rate 104 bpm, respirations 18 per minute, and temperature 38.8°C.

Neurologic. Patient is alert and oriented to place, time, and person.

Maxillofacial. There is fluctuant, tender, and erythematous right-sided facial swelling extending from the angle of the mandible to the right submandibular space. The floor of the mouth and the oropharyngeal airway are normal. The right mandibular third molar (tooth #32) is impacted, with swelling of the surrounding operculum. Right submandibular lymphadenopathy is noted.

Pulmonary. The chest is clear on auscultation bilaterally.

Cardiovascular. Regular rate and rhythm with no murmurs, rubs, or gallops.

Extremity. There is no swelling, edema, or muscle weakness.

IMAGING

A panoramic radiograph reveals a mesioangular impacted right mandibular third molar with a pericoronal radiolucency. Renal osteodystrophy (secondary hyperparathyroidism) is evident, as seen by a generalized "ground-glass" pattern of the bone, loss of lamina dura, and a maxillary unilocular radiolucency (osteitis fibrosa cystica). This is a result of decreased renal conversion of 25-hydroxycholecalciferol to 1,25-dihydroxycholecalciferol (active vitamin D). A decrease in active vitamin D results in reduced gastrointestinal adsorption of calcium, with a corresponding increase in parathyroid hormone to augment serum calcium levels by increasing bone resorption.

LABS

Laboratory tests are ordered based on the severity and acuity of symptoms related to chronic kidney disease in conjunction with the patient's nephrologist/internist. A baseline complete blood count, metabolic panels, liver function tests, and coagulation studies are usually obtained.

The following laboratory study results were obtained for the current patient:

- *Complete blood count:* White blood cells 14,000/μl, hemoglobin 9.2 g/dl, hematocrit 29.2%, platelets 265,000/μl
- *Chemistry:* Sodium 145 mEq/L, potassium 5.6 mEq/L, bicarbonate 22 mEq/L, blood urea nitrogen 48 mg/dl, creatinine 3.9 mg/dl, glucose 167 mg/dl, calcium 7 mg/dl, phosphate 5.2 mg/dl
- *Coagulation studies:* Prothrombin time 11 seconds, partial thromboplastin time 33 seconds, international normalized ratio 1.0
- *Liver function tests:* Aspartate aminotransferase 42 U/L, alanine aminotransferase 33 U/L, γ-glutamyl transpeptidase 43 U/L, alkaline phosphate 34 U/L
- *Urinalysis:* 300 mg/dL proteinuria; no red blood cells, white blood cells, or casts

The laboratory findings are characteristic of chronic renal disease. The hemoglobin and hematocrit are decreased secondary to the decreased production of erythropoietin by the kidneys. The elevated blood urea nitrogen and creatinine levels reflect the decreased glomerular filtration rate, which is also responsible for the elevated serum potassium. Proteinuria is a result of increased glomerular permeability. The decreased calcium is a result of decreased gastrointestinal absorption secondary to decreased renal production of active vitamin D.

ASSESSMENT

Chronic kidney disease complicating management of an odontogenic abscess.

TREATMENT

The management of a patient with chronic kidney disease is often complicated. Of particular concern is fluid status and electrolyte balance. Correction of metabolic and fluid abnormalities should be done in conjunction with the nephrologist before any surgical intervention. This may be accomplished by judicious hydration, careful electrolyte replacement, and medications. As chronic renal disease progresses to end-stage renal disease (ESRD), either peritoneal dialysis or hemodialysis becomes necessary. Hypertension is typically very difficult to adequately treat with medication alone and usually involves a salt restriction. In some cases, some degree of hypertension may need to be tolerated. Many medications, particularly antibiotics, need to be appropriately dosed for the reduced glomerular filtration rate or avoided altogether. All patients able to take oral nutrition should have a renal diet low in sodium, potassium, and protein. Patients requiring dialysis are best scheduled for surgery the day after their dialysis treatment (to optimize fluid and electrolyte balance) with a resumption of their usual dialysis the day after surgery. Because patients frequently are heparinized for dialysis, a minimum of 6 hours is prudent after cessation of heparin. In emergency cases in which surgery cannot wait, the dialysis treatment can be done without heparin. Patients with successful renal transplants may be considered to have adequate renal function but are commonly receiving immunosuppressive drugs, including corticosteroids, placing them at increased risk for infections and adrenal insufficiency in the perioperative period.

The initial management of the current febrile and anorexic patient included judicious fluid resuscitation. Normal saline (500 ml bolus) was given, followed by a maintenance rate of 50 ml/hr. Fluid resuscitation reduced the serum creatinine to 3.4 mg/dl, suggesting that some of the renal insufficiency was secondary to dehydration. In patients with end-stage renal disease who are dialysis dependent, fluid resuscitation may not be necessary. The patient's elevated temperature was treated with acetaminophen (avoid nonsteroidal antiinflammatory drugs in chronic kidney disease, because they decrease renal blood flow). Although the degree of hyperkalemia was only mild, an electrocardiogram was performed to evaluate for loss of P waves, widened QRS complex, and peaked T waves (none of which were present). Kayexalate was given orally to lower the serum potassium level. The patient was begun on intravenous clindamycin. No dosing adjustment was needed, because the clearance of this drug is largely hepatic.

Preoperative pain control was achieved primarily with a scheduled hydrocodone/acetaminophen combination, with morphine for breakthrough pain. Hydrocodone and morphine are metabolized hepatically via conjugation, but their metabolites are renally excreted. The half-lives, therefore, tend to increase in chronic kidney disease, and a reduction in the frequency of administration (every 8 hours) was needed to avoid toxicity and excessive sedation.

Hyperglycemia was initially treated with sliding scale insulin. On the second day after admission, incision and drainage of the right submandibular abscess and removal of the right mandibular third molar were performed under a general anesthetic. The postoperative course was uneventful. The patient was placed on a renal diet (low protein) with a caloric restriction as soon as she was able to eat, and at that time her usual insulin regimen was begun.

COMPLICATIONS

The development of uremic syndrome due to end-stage renal disease (often when the glomerular filtration rate is less than 10 ml/minute) is associated with a variety of symptoms (Table 15-5) and herald the urgent need for dialysis. This syndrome is due to the combined effects of the accumulation of various metabolites (not just urea). Other indications for dialysis include acidosis, electrolyte abnormalities, drug toxicity, and fluid overload. Thrombosis, hypotension, occlusion through blood pressure cuffs, and improper tucking of extremities may compromise the vascular access (arteriovenous fistulas, synthetic grafts, and central venous catheters) used to perform dialysis and should be avoided.

The single most feared complication of chronic renal disease is the development of acute renal failure (ARF) on top

Table 15-5	Symptoms of Uremic Syndrome Due to End-Stage Renal Disease
System	**Symptoms**
Central nervous	Irritability, insomnia, lethargy, seizures, coma
Musculoskeletal	Weakness, gout, pseudogout, renal osteodystrophy
Hematologic	Anemia, coagulopathy
Pulmonary	Noncardiogenic pulmonary edema, pneumonitis
Cerebrovascular	Pericarditis, arrhythmias, cardiomyopathy, atherosclerosis
Gastrointestinal	Nausea, vomiting, anorexia, gastrointestinal bleeding
Acid-base/volume	Hyperkalemia, volume overload (other electrolyte disturbances)
Endocrine	Hyperparathyroidism, hyperlipidemia, increased insulin resistance
Dermatologic	Pruritus, skin discoloration (yellow)

of the underlying chronic renal insufficiency. A quick assessment of kidney function can be determined by measuring the urine output. Normal urine output is 0.5 ml/kg/hr in adults; 1 ml/kg/hr in children; and 2 ml/kg/hr in infants. Causes of acute renal failure can be divided into prerenal, renal, and postrenal causes. The most likely cause of prerenal failure is hypovolemia secondary to blood loss or dehydration (as in the current patient). Laboratory indices that suggest a prerenal source include a blood urea nitrogen to creatinine ratio greater than 20 and a fractional excretion of sodium of less than 1%. Furthermore, rapid improvement in the serum creatinine level with fluid resuscitation is highly suggestive. Renal causes of acute renal failure include acute tubular necrosis, acute interstitial nephritis, and acute glomerulonephritis. Acute tubular necrosis may occur secondary to either hypoperfusion or toxic agents, such as myoglobinuria (rhabdomyolysis), contrast agents, drugs (aminoglycosides, amphotericin), crystals (acyclovir, sulfonamides), and uric acid (tumor lysis syndrome). The hallmark laboratory feature of acute tubular necrosis is muddy brown casts in the urine. Acute interstitial nephritis may occur with many drugs and is a potential concern in any patient with chronic kidney disease. Drugs that can cause acute interstitial nephritis include cephalosporins, β-lactams, penicillins, sulfamethoxazole-trimethoprim (Bactrim), diuretics, and nonsteroidal antiinflammatory drugs. The presence of eosinophils in the urine is highly suggestive. The last potential cause of acute renal failure is postrenal obstruction. This is usually secondary to urethral obstruction from calculi or prostatic hypertrophy. It can also occur temporarily after removal of a regular urethral Foley catheter in an otherwise healthy individual. Narcotics are another cause for acute renal retention. A postrenal cause of acute renal failure that is distal to the ureteral orifices can be diagnosed with measurement of the postvoid residual. This can be measured by having the patient void naturally and then placing a temporary catheter in the bladder or by using bladder ultrasound to record the volume of remaining urine. A volume of less than 50 ml is considered normal.

Drug toxicity, another common complication of chronic kidney disease, can occur when there is a failure to adjust medication doses for the degree of renal insufficiency. Most drugs are metabolized in the liver and ultimately excreted by the kidney. Many metabolites of hepatically metabolized drugs are themselves metabolically active to some degree. The net result is an increase in the half-life of many drugs. In the presence of chronic kidney disease, it is possible to develop drug toxicity from failing to adjust either the drug dose or, more important, the frequency of drug administration. Drugs that are primarily renally cleared are also likely to accumulate if not dosed appropriately and need to be adjusted accordingly. Although many drugs are relatively nontoxic, failure to renally dose a drug can result in significant morbidity and mortality.

DISCUSSION

There are many causes of chronic kidney disease. Diabetes mellitus is a common cause and, as in the current patient, may be complicated by uncontrolled hypertension and hypercholesterolemia. General management of the patient with chronic kidney disease includes a low-protein diet (less than 50 g/day), sodium restriction (less than 2 g/day), potassium restriction, fluid restriction, correction of hyperkalemia/hypokalemia, and either peritoneal or hemodialysis as required. The management of hyperkalemia requires an electrocardiogram (wide QRS, peaked T waves, loss of P waves), moderate intravenous hydration, Kayexalate and, in severe cases, intravenous calcium gluconate or chloride to stabilize the myocardium, combined with dextrose and insulin to lower the serum potassium. Hypokalemia is typically a result of excessive loop diuretic and requires judicious oral or parenteral replacement. Furthermore, perioperative care may complicated by impaired drug excretion, corticosteroids or immunosuppressive drugs, hypertension, anemia, and arrhythmias related to hyperkalemia. Bleeding may also complicate chronic kidney disease as a result of uremia. Bleeding time is typically elevated due to platelet dysfunction and von Willebrand factor abnormalities. Uremia is best controlled through dialysis, whereas von Willebrand factor levels may be increased with 1-deamino-8-D-arginine vasopressin (DDAVP), cryoprecipitate, or fresh frozen plasma.

Recent studies have shown that patients who experience ARF have a higher risk for chronic renal failure and ESRD. Although there is no consensus on a standardized risk stratification system, the adverse outcomes of ARF have significant morbidity and mortality if they are not recognized early and treated properly. Therefore, it is important to obtain an early nephrology consultation in patient management.

Bibliography

Carrasco LR, Chou JC: Perioperative management of patients with renal disease, *Oral Maxillofac Surg Clin North Am* 18:203-212, 2006.

Coca SG, Singanamala S, Parikh CR: Chronic kidney disease after acute kidney injury: a systematic review and meta-analysis, *Kidney Int* 81:442-448, 2012.

Susantitaphong P, Altamimi S, Ashkar M, et al: GFR at initiation of dialysis and mortality in CKD: a meta-analysis, *Am J Kidney Dis* 59(6):829-840, 2012.

Liver Disease

Gary F. Bouloux, Sung Cho, and Shahrokh C. Bagheri

CC

A 54-year-old Caucasian man presents to the emergency department, complaining, "I was hit in the face, and my teeth do not meet right. It has not stopped bleeding."

HPI

The patient was punched in the face the day before admission while intoxicated with alcohol. He denies loss of consciousness but reports the progressive development of left facial swelling, pain, difficulty eating (secondary to malocclusion), and numbness of his left lower lip. In addition, he describes persistent ooze from inside his mouth where he was hit (secondary to coagulopathy). He was subsequently diagnosed with a left mandibular angle fracture.

PMHX/PDHX/MEDICATIONS/ALLERGIES/SH/FH

The patient was diagnosed with alcoholic cirrhosis of the liver and associated portal hypertension 2 years ago. He has had several hospital admissions over the past year for worsening ascites (fluid in the abdomen) and one for upper gastrointestinal bleeding (secondary to esophageal varices). He has had no regular dental care. His current medications include furosemide (loop diuretic), spironolactone (potassium-sparing diuretic), propranolol (nonselective β-blocker), and omeprazole (proton pump inhibitor). He drinks 2 quarts of wine every other day.

EXAMINATION

General. Generalized muscle wasting (secondary to poor nutrition and protein catabolism) and lethargy (secondary to hepatic encephalopathy).

Vital signs. Blood pressure is 155/92 mm Hg (elevated blood pressure), heart rate 72 bpm, respirations 22 per minute (tachypnea), and temperature 36.2°C.

Neurologic. The patient is alert and orientated times three (person, place, and time) but intermittently confused, with asterixis (flapping of the hands with the arms and palms fully extended, a sign of hepatic encephalopathy).

Maxillofacial. Scleral icterus (due to hyperbilirubinemia), fetor hepaticus (due to elevated serum ammonia level), enlarged parotid glands (due to metabolic and nutritional derangements associated with chronic alcoholism), decreased

sensation to light touch and direction of left V3, and left mandibular angle swelling and ecchymosis.

Chest and pulmonary. Bilateral crackles in the lung bases (fluid in the alveolar spaces), bilateral gynecomastia (enlarged breasts secondary to increased levels of estrogen), and hair loss over the chest.

Cardiovascular. Regular rate and rhythm, with no murmurs, gallops (S3 or S4), or rubs.

Abdominal. The abdomen is nontender and distended, with shifting dullness (due to ascites) and splenomegaly (due to portal hypertension secondary to liver cirrhosis). Nodular hard hepatomegaly and caput medusa (tortuous periumbilical veins secondary to portal hypertension) are also noted.

Extremity. Bilateral lower extremity 1+ pitting edema (secondary to hypoalbuminemia), Dupuytren contracture in the right index and middle finger (flexion deformity of the fingers secondary to flexor tendon fibrosis), and palmar erythema.

Skin. Multiple small petechiae, spider angiomas, and testicular atrophy (all secondary to decreased hepatic metabolism of estrogen) are present.

LABS

The laboratory test in the work-up of liver disease can be complex and crucial to the evaluation of the extent of liver injury and the degree of dysfunction with associated systemic involvement. A complete metabolic panel includes hepatic transaminases. Elevated hepatic enzymes reflect hepatocellular dysfunction. In the current patient, both aspartate aminotransferase and alanine aminotransferase levels are elevated (the aspartate aminotransferase–alanine aminotransferase ratio usually is greater than 2:1 with alcoholic hepatic damage). Ordered separately, elevated alkaline phosphatase and γ-glutamyl transpeptidase levels are also seen (reflecting biliary system abnormalities). Elevated blood urea nitrogen and creatinine levels can be seen, especially if there is associated hepatorenal syndrome (HRS). Hypokalemia and hypomagnesemia are also common with malnutrition and need to be corrected.

A complete blood count generally shows a macrocytic anemia (mean corpuscular volume is greater than $100/\mu m^3$) (secondary to vitamin B_{12} and folate deficiency) with thrombocytopenia (secondary to hypersplenism, increased sequestration, and decreased hepatic production of thrombopoietin). An elevated prothrombin time, partial thromboplastin time, and international normalized ratio are secondary to decreased synthesis of coagulation factors. The prothrombin time is often elevated first because of the shorter half-life of the vitamin K–dependent factor VII that is part of the extrinsic pathway measured best by the prothrombin time (even small decreases in factor VII result in increased prothrombin time) or the international normalized ratio (INR). High blood ammonia levels reflect the inability of the liver to convert ammonia to urea for excretion by the kidneys. Hypoalbuminemia is reflective of decreased albumin production in the liver. Finally, unconjugated hyperbilirubinemia (causing scleral icterus) is seen because of decreased bilirubin conjugation by the liver.

For the current patient, the following laboratory tests were obtained:

- *Chemistry:* Sodium 133 mEq/L, potassium 3.1 mEq/L, blood urea nitrogen 48 mg/dl, creatinine 1.6 mg/dl, glucose 172 mg/dl, magnesium 1.0 mg/dl, bilirubin 1.3 mg/ dl, ammonia 67 mmol/L, albumin 2.2 mg/dl
- *Complete blood count:* White blood cells 4,500/μl, hemoglobin 9.5 g/dl, hematocrit 30.1%, platelets 62,000/μl
- *Coagulation studies:* Prothrombin time 17 seconds, partial thromboplastin time 43 seconds, international normalized ratio 1.5
- *Liver function tests:* Aspartate aminotransferase 141 U/L, alanine aminotransferase 84 U/L, γ-glutamyl transpeptidase 45 U/L, alkaline phosphatase 51 U/L.

IMAGING

A panoramic radiograph revealed a fracture of the left mandibular angle.

For evaluation and diagnosis of liver cirrhosis, a CT-guided liver biopsy can be done as needed to demonstrate destruction of normal hepatic architecture with fibrotic changes, confirming the diagnosis of liver cirrhosis.

ASSESSMENT

Mandibular fracture complicated by hepatic dysfunction secondary to alcoholic cirrhosis.

TREATMENT

Preoperative preparation of patients with severe liver disease is of paramount importance to prevent perioperative complications. Preoperative management includes administration of thiamine 100 mg (to prevent Wernicke encephalopathy, characterized by ophthalmoplegia, ataxia, and memory impairment), a nutritious diet, and multivitamins with folic acid and vitamin B*12* supplementation (excess alcohol consumption is often associated with nutritional deficiencies). Any coagulopathy needs to be addressed preoperatively (see Complications section).

In the current patient, hypokalemia and hypomagnesemia were corrected with potassium chloride and magnesium sulfate infusions. Librium, a benzodiazepine, was given as a

taper over 4 days to prevent life-threatening alcohol withdrawal (delirium tremens). Due to the risk of aspiration (increased in alcoholics), the patient was also continued on a proton pump inhibitor (decreases gastroesophageal reflux and the degree of chemical pneumonitis should aspiration occur). Due to the patient's obvious respiratory distress as a result of the ascites, paracentesis (removal of peritoneal fluid) was performed; the removal of 4 L of fluid (with care taken to prevent hypotension) brought an immediate reduction in the work of breathing and the respiratory rate. The patient was started on furosemide and spironolactone to reduce the severity and frequency of recurring ascites. The hepatic encephalopathy was treated with administration of lactulose (to decrease ammonia production by enteric bacteria). The coagulopathy was treated with 6 units of fresh frozen plasma (to overcome deficiencies of multiple coagulation factors) and 4 units of platelets (to increase the platelet numbers to greater than 100,000 cells/μl). Subsequently, the patient underwent open reduction with internal fixation of the fracture without complications.

COMPLICATIONS

Complications for patients with liver disease are inherently dependent on the degree of functional impairment of the liver and concomitant preoperative systemic conditions.

Patients tend to be protein depleted, fluid overloaded, vitamin deficient, and coagulopathic, with electrolyte abnormalities, and often have an impaired ability to metabolize medications.

Adjunctive enteral feeding (nasogastric or orogastric tube) may be necessary in the perioperative period to meet caloric needs, especially in the setting of oral and maxillofacial surgery, when chewing may be difficult (e.g., intermaxillary fixation, swelling, pain). Parenteral nutrition may also be considered, but only in the setting of compromised gastrointestinal function (if the gut works, use it). Caloric requirements should be calculated with consideration to reducing the protein/amino acid content to prevent exacerbation of any encephalopathy. The latter is thought to relate to the blood ammonia level, which can be further reduced with the use of lactulose. Malnutrition and impaired protein synthesis impair wound healing, which can present as increased wound breakdown and delayed healing.

Coagulopathy may be the result of decreased platelets from splenic sequestration (hypersplenism occurs secondary to portal hypertension, which is secondary to liver cirrhosis). Platelet transfusion is the only treatment for thrombocytopenia. Spontaneous bleeding is seen with platelet counts less than 30,000/μl; for most minor procedures, a count greater than 50,000/μl is appropriate. Ideally, the patient should be transfused to a platelet count greater than 100,000/μl for major surgeries and procedures.

Coagulopathy may also be the result of decreased hepatic synthesis of clotting proteins, as is often the case with end-stage liver disease, or it may be the result of decreased absorption of fat-soluble vitamins (vitamins A, D, E, and K) from the gastrointestinal tract. The latter is more common with cholestatic liver disease (decreased bile salts reduce the absorption of fat and fat-soluble vitamins). In this situation, vitamin K can be administered, with an appropriate increase in the synthesis of vitamin K–dependent coagulation factors (factors II, VII, IX, and X). The end point of management is a substantial improvement in or normalization of the prothrombin time or INR. When decreased hepatic synthesis of coagulation proteins is the result of intrinsic liver disease (as in the current patient), transfusion with fresh frozen plasma is the treatment of choice. Care must be taken to avoid worsening of the total body fluid overload, which is typical of ascites and may precipitate pulmonary edema.

Liver failure may also be associated with hepatopulmonary syndrome, hepatorenal syndrome (with electrolyte disturbances), upper gastrointestinal bleeding, nonalcoholic steatohepatitis, and subacute bacterial peritonitis. Most drugs are metabolized by the liver and as such may need to be dosed appropriately or avoided altogether. Drugs that are renally excreted are preferable to those that require hepatic metabolism.

End-stage liver disease (ESLD) can be treated with liver transplantation, although most patients die of liver disease or are not eligible for transplantation. In 2002, the Mayo Clinic began to stratify ESLD liver transplant recipients with an objective calculator to determine the severity of liver dysfunction. The Model for End-Stage Liver Disease (MELD) score can be used to predict morbidity and mortality in patients needing nonliver surgery. The MELD score is readily calculated using the patient's INR, bilirubin and creatinine. The formula is available at the website *www.mayoclinic.org/meld/mayomodel5.html*. Elective nonliver surgery is acceptable in a patient with a MELD score below 10; a score between 10 and 15 necessitates careful assessment of risks and benefit; and a score above 16 effectively eliminates elective procedures. Our patient, despite a MELD score of 16, was a candidate for open reduction and internal fixation of his fractured mandible, because this is not elective surgery. However, elevated MELD scores are associated with increased perioperative morbidity and mortality. Successful liver transplant recipients have a functionally normal liver but are immunosuppressed to prevent graft rejection. This may result in an increase in both opportunistic and perioperative infections.

DISCUSSION

Liver disease can be the result of many insults. The most common causes are alcohol consumption and viral hepatitis. Hepatitis C is more common than hepatitis B, with an estimated 4 million cases in the United States. As many as 90% of these cases are chronic. Viral hepatitis also poses a risk for transmission to the surgeon and operating room staff from needle stick injury. Particular care should be taken to reduce this risk. The causes of liver dysfunction are many, but the consequences are often similar. Cirrhosis is the final common pathway of chronic inflammation and is irreversible. Alcoholic cirrhosis may coexist with alcoholic hepatitis. Liver dysfunction is associated with malnutrition, protein catabolism, poor wound healing, coagulopathy, portal hypertension, splenomegaly, ascites, portosystemic venous shunts (esophageal, periumbilical, retroperitoneal and hemorrhoidal shunts), encephalopathy, and impaired drug metabolism and clearance. A proper history and physical examination, in addition to appropriate laboratory tests, are critical in the perioperative period for the surgeon. All these factors combine to make management of the patient with liver disease a challenging and difficult task.

Bibliography

Kamath PS, Wiesner RH, Malinchoc M, et al: A model to predict survival in patients with end-stage liver disease, *Hepatology* 33:464-470, 2001.

Muir AJ: Surgical clearance for the patient with chronic liver disease, *Clin Liver Dis* 16:421-433, 2012.

O'Leary JG, Yachimski PS, Friedman LS: Surgery in the patient with liver disease, *Clin Liver Dis* 13:211-231, 2009.

Von Willebrand Disease

Danielle Cunningham, Shahrokh C. Bagheri, and Kambiz Mohammadzadeh

CC

A 16-year-old Caucasian girl is referred to your office for evaluation of an asymptomatic, radiopaque mass of the maxilla consistent with a complex odontoma.

HPI

The lesion was identified on routine radiographic examination for an unerupted primary premolar. There was no history of pain, fever, swelling, or drainage from the area.

PMHX/PDHX/MEDICATIONS/ALLERGIES/SH/FH

The parents denied any significant PMHx. However, on further questioning, a history of prolonged bleeding, including heavy menstruation and several episodes of epistaxis without the need of hospitalization, were identified (positive history of abnormal bleeding). This was first noted after the loss of her mandibular primary incisors. Careful questioning also revealed a history of "easy" bruising on her extremities. The parents recall previous episodes of prolonged bleeding with other family members (von Willebrand disease [vWD] is an autosomal dominant disorder). The remaining history was negative.

EXAMINATION

General. The patient is a well-developed and well-nourished, cooperative girl in no apparent distress whose height and weight are above the 50th percentile.

Maxillofacial. There is no notable facial swelling. During intranasal examination with a nasal speculum, slight epistaxis was noted. Intraoral examination reveals bilateral buccal mucosa ecchymosis (skin discoloration caused by the escape of blood into the tissues from ruptured blood vessels).

Chest, abdominal, and extremities. Multiple petechiae (pinpoint-size hemorrhages of small capillaries, often seen with quantitative and qualitative platelet dysfunction) are seen on the upper and lower extremities, abdomen, and chest.

IMAGING

A panoramic radiograph reveals a well-defined radiopacity of the right anterior maxilla with multiple teethlike structures and an associated impacted first premolar (consistent with a compound odontoma). No routine imaging studies are necessary to evaluate vWD unless there is a suspicion of internal hemorrhage, especially in the setting of trauma.

LABS

The initial laboratory studies to evaluate for vWD should include routine coagulation studies (CBC with platelets, prothrombin time [PT], partial thromboplastin time [PTT], international normalized ratio [INR], bleeding time). These are good general screening tests that can be ordered at the discretion of the physician. The CBC is generally normal, except in vWD type 2B, in which the platelet count may be decreased. Bleeding time is a good screening test, although it is not sensitive or specific. Normal results do not rule out vWD. PT and INR are normal. However, the PTT, in addition to measuring factor VIII activity, may also measure concurrent deficiencies with other clotting factors. This may be prolonged in vWD type 2N, severe disease, and 25% of patients with vWD type 1.

Abnormal coagulation studies in addition to history and physical examination may trigger the specialist to order further diagnostic studies.

There are other laboratory tests used to screen for and diagnose vWD:

- *Plasma von Willebrand factor (vWF) levels* (vWF:RCo) (ristocetin cofactor activity assay, used to measure platelet aggregation). Plasma vWF levels may vary from day to day. They are influenced by stress, pregnancy, hormone replacement therapy, and blood type (individuals with type O have decreased levels); a single level within the reference range does not exclude the disease.
- *Plasma vWF antigen.* The total plasma concentration of vWF protein, depending on the assay, could be the total of vWF binding sites or the total vWF protein present in the plasma. It does not reflect molecular structure; therefore. this value could be normal in patients with abnormal multimers.
- *Factor VIII activity.* This is a measure of the cofactor function of the clotting factor (factor VIII) in plasma.

The ristocetin cofactor activity assay is the gold standard for diagnosis of vWD; however, it is difficult to obtain an accurate level. The levels of vWF rise during pregnancy and periods of stress and with hormone replacement therapy; therefore, patient anxiety may acutely elevate the vWF level despite a relative deficiency. A positive screening test and/or a high index of suspicion based on the clinical history may indicate further testing is necessary.

A vWF multimer and ristocetin-induced platelet aggregation can be used to confirm the diagnosis. These tests are also used to determine the vWD subtype. An additional test that is gaining acceptance is the platelet function test, which is dependent on vWF and platelet function. This is used as a screening test for vWD due to its high specificity and sensitivity.

ASSESSMENT

Compound odontoma of the maxilla requiring removal, complicated by vWD.

TREATMENT

There are five modalities of treatment for vWD:
1. Desmopressin (1-desamino-8-D-arginine-vasopressin [DDAVP])
2. vWF replacement therapy (using cryoprecipitate)
3. Antifibrinolytic agents
4. Topical agents (thrombin or fibrin sealants)
5. Estrogen therapy in women with no contraindications

DDAVP is a synthetic analog of antidiuretic hormone, without vasopressor activity. It acts by increasing vWF and factor VIII levels, by indirectly stimulating the release of vWF from endothelial cells. DDAVP may be administered intravenously, intramuscularly, or intranasally. If given intravenously or intramuscularly for acute bleeding, the dose is 0.3 μg/kg (maximum, 20 μg). Increases in vWF and factor VIII levels are seen within 30 to 60 minutes, with a duration of approximately 6 to 12 hours. Intranasal administration has gained popularity with patients who have less serious bleeding and for premedication before minor surgical procedures. The usual dose is 150 μg for children weighing less than 50 kg and 300 μg for larger children and adults. A test dose should be administered to observe the effects on vWF. DDAVP should not be administered to patients with type 2B vWD because it may worsen the disease (see the Discussion section). It also does not seem to be as efficacious in patients with severe bleeding disorders and type 3 disease, probably secondary to the lack of stored vWF.

Replacement therapy with vWF would appear to be the gold standard for treatment. However, for cryoprecipitate (which contains factor VIII) to contain viable vWF, it cannot be pasteurized, only screened. If possible, this should be avoided, because there is an increased risk of viral transmission. Most factor VIII concentrates do not contain sufficient high-molecular-weight vWF; however, the drugs Humate-P (human antihemophilic factor/vWF complex) and Alphanate (antihemolytic factor) do contain sufficient amounts. These drugs may be used with cryoprecipitate in patients with type 2B or type 3 vWD, because these patients cannot be treated with DDAVP. For significant bleeding, the goal of replacement therapy is to maintain the activity of factor VIII and vWF between 50% and 100% for 3 to 10 days.

Fibrinolytic therapy with tranexamic acid (Amicar) can also be used. This prevents the lysis of blood clots and can be especially useful for bleeding from the mucous membranes. This class of drugs may be given orally or intravenously. With oral administration, the drug must be given three or four times over a 24-hour period (because of the medication's short half-life) for 3 to 7 days. Topical agents such as Gelfoam (absorbable sponge made from gelatin) and Surgicel (oxidized regenerated cellulose) soaked in topical thrombin can also be used for local hemostasis.

In several studies, estrogen was found to increase the levels of vWF in women taking oral contraceptives and hormone replacement therapy. However, no long-term studies have looked at the risk/benefit ratio for hormone replacement therapy in vWD.

Treatment is determined by clinical findings and the extent of hemorrhage. There are no good laboratory tests that correspond with the severity of the disease. vWF is not a reliable marker of severity, because this value can be artificially elevated in certain physiologic states, such as stress or pregnancy; therefore, a past history of bleeding is an important clue to the severity of the disease and to determination of optimal therapy.

The current patient was referred to a hematologist for preoperative consultation and evaluation. Subsequently, the patient had normal ristocetin activity and platelet levels. The hematologist recommended premedication with 150 μg of DDAVP and four doses of Amicar postoperatively for 24 hours. The patient was subsequently sedated in the office, and the odontoma was removed. Surgicel was placed in the defect and sutured with resorbable sutures. Hemostasis was observed in the office before discharge. At 1-week follow-up, the patient denied any complications and was healing appropriately.

COMPLICATIONS

The most obvious complication of vWD is persistent hemorrhage. If hemorrhage is persistent after extractions, Surgicel, topical thrombin, direct pressure, and DDAVP may be used unless contraindicated. In the setting of acute bleeding, cryoprecipitate is the treatment of choice. Cryoprecipitate can be used to treat all types of vWD. (Cryoprecipitate contains factors VIII and XIII, vWF, fibrinogen, and fibronectin. It can be stored at −18°C for up to 1 year.)

Each treatment regimen has various side effects. DDAVP may cause vasodilation, headache, hypotension, or hypertension (which is usually mild). More serious complications of DDAVP include tachyphylaxis (rapid development of immunity to a drug) and significant hyponatremia and seizures secondary to water retention. Therefore, DDAVP is usually limited to once-daily dosing, along with water restriction and careful monitoring of serum sodium levels.

Replacement with cryoprecipitate carries an increased risk of transmission of blood-borne pathogens secondary to the inability to adequately pasteurize the extract. Fortunately, as a result of the improved sensitivity of blood testing, the risk of transmission is low.

Prolonged use of antifibrinolytic therapy carries the risk of thrombosis. Hypercoagulable patients need to be carefully evaluated. Topical agents are generally safe but are costly and can only be used as a local measure. Certain preparations of topical thrombin may contain bovine factor V; broad exposure could precipitate the formation of antibodies to this factor that cross-react with human factor V, aggravating hemorrhage.

DISCUSSION

vWD is the most common inherited bleeding disorder, affecting approximately 1% of the population. Most patients do not seek medical attention and are only diagnosed on the basis of unexplained heavy bleeding (e.g., during menstruation) or easy bruising. This disorder is characterized by a mutation in vWF itself or in the amount of vWF produced. This factor is responsible for primary hemostasis by aiding platelet aggregation and adherence to the endothelial lining and by serving as a carrier protein for factor VIII. Factor VIII has a significantly shortened half-life when it is not bound to vWF; this is the reason factor VIII levels are evaluated through laboratory tests.

There are three subtypes of inherited vWD. Types 1 and 2 are autosomal dominant, and type 1 is the most common form of the disease (approximately 70%). Type 1 is a quantitative deficiency in vWF itself. Symptoms range from mild to moderately severe (Figure 15-3). It is possible that the deficiency may be from abnormally fast clearance of the protein or inadequate production.

Type 2, which is usually autosomal dominant, is a qualitative abnormality of vWF. Type 2 is subdivided into four subtypes: 2A, 2B, 2M, and 2N. The classification is based on where the mutation occurs on the vWF itself.

- Type 2A is a qualitative defect in which the quantity levels are normal but the ability of the factor to bind to platelets is diminished. This type of vWF also does not coalesce well with other vWF, resulting in diminished large multimers, which in turn results in decreased platelet adhesiveness. Therefore, vWF antigen assay results are normal, but cofactor assays and large multimers are reduced or absent.
- Type 2B (approximately 5%) contains the defect on the platelet binding site itself, which actually increases binding of platelets to vWF. This takes platelets out of circulation, causing thrombocytopenia. It is imperative to determine whether the patient has this subtype, especially if treatment is to be instituted, because treatment with DDAVP may actually exacerbate the condition. DDAVP causes an increase in the release of vWF, subsequently causing increased binding of platelets to vWF and removing more platelets from circulation, worsening the thrombocytopenia.
- Type 2M is characterized by a qualitative defect and can form appropriate multimers; however, its ability to bind to platelets is diminished. Therefore, plasma antigen levels are normal, large multimers are present, but the cofactor assays are decreased.
- Type 2N (N is for Normandy, where this type was first described) is a rare autosomal recessive disorder. The

CLINICAL BLEEDING SYMPTOMS ASSOCIATED WITH TYPE 1 VON WILLEBRAND DISEASE

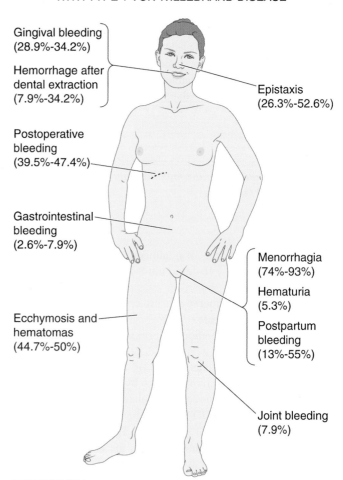

Gingival bleeding (28.9%-34.2%)

Hemorrhage after dental extraction (7.9%-34.2%)

Epistaxis (26.3%-52.6%)

Postoperative bleeding (39.5%-47.4%)

Gastrointestinal bleeding (2.6%-7.9%)

Menorrhagia (74%-93%)

Hematuria (5.3%)

Postpartum bleeding (13%-55%)

Ecchymosis and hematomas (44.7%-50%)

Joint bleeding (7.9%)

Figure 15-3 Clinical bleeding symptoms by type and frequency (%) in patients with type 1 von Willebrand disease. *(From Armstrong E, Konkle BA: von Willebrand disease. In Young NS, Gerson SL, High KA (eds): Clinical hematology, St Louis, 2006, Mosby.)*

defect affects the ability of vWF to bind to factor VIII, but the ability to bind with factor VII remains normal. Therefore, platelet function remains normal (as does the quantity of available vWF), but factor VIII levels are greatly reduced. Because this subtype is recessive, a second mutated allele must also be inherited for symptoms to develop. It can be difficult to distinguish this subtype from factor VIII deficiency (hemophilia), because in both conditions the patients have low levels of factor VIII. Type 2N vWD should be considered when a patient presents with a family history of autosomal penetrance (seen in both males and females, not gender-linked, mendelian genetics) rather than X-linked.

Type 3 is rare (approximately 1 in 1 million people) and is characterized by complete absence or very low levels of vWF; this results from different genetic defects, including nonsense, missense, and frameshift mutations. These patients have severe bleeding and at first may be diagnosed as having factor VIII deficiency, before vWF testing is obtained.

vWD may also be acquired with various disease states, usually autoimmune conditions such as systemic lupus erythematosus. Other mechanisms include decreased synthesis, proteolysis, binding to tumor cells, and increased clearance of vWF.

Bibliography

Aledort LM: Treatment of von Willebrand's disease, *Mayo Clin Proc* 66:841, 1991.

Batlle J, Torea J, Rendal E, et al: The problem of diagnosing von Willebrand's disease, *J Intern Med Suppl* 740:121-128, 1997.

Chang AC, Rick ME, Ross Pierce L, et al: Summary of a workshop on potency and dosage of von Willebrand factor concentrates, *Hemophilia* 4(Suppl 3):1, 1998.

Federici AB, Berntorp E, Lee CA, et al: A standard trial infusion with desmopressin is always required before factor VIII/von Willebrand factor concentrates in severe type 1 and 2 von Willebrand disease: results of a multicenter European study [abstract], *Thromb Haemost* (Suppl):795, 1999.

Lee CA, Brettler DB: Guidelines for the diagnosis and management of von Willebrand disease, *Haemophilia* 3:1-25, 1997.

Lethagen S, Harris AS, Sjorin E, et al: Intranasal and intravenous administration of desmopressin: effect on factor VIII/vWF, pharmacokinetics and reproducibility, *Thromb Haemost* 58:1033, 1987.

Mannucci PM: Treatment of von Willebrand's disease, *N Engl J Med* 351:683, 2004.

Mazurier C, Dieval J, Jorieux SK, et al: New von Willebrand factor (vWF) defect in a patient with factor VIII deficiency but with normal levels and multimeric patterns of both plasma and platelet vWF: characterization of abnormal vwF/ FVIII interaction, *Blood* 75:20, 1990.

McKeown LP, Connaghan G, Wilson O, et al: 1-Desamino-8-arginine-vasopressin corrects the hemostatic defects in type 2B von Willebrand's disease, *Am J Hematol* 51:158, 1996.

Moffat EH, Giddings JC, Bloom AL: The effect of desamino-D-arginine vasopressin (DDAVP) and naloxone infusions on factor VIII and possible endothelial cell (EC) related activities, *Br J Haematol* 57:651, 1984.

Posan E, McBane RD, Grill DE, et al: Comparison of PFA-100 testing and bleeding time for detecting platelet hypofunction and von Willebrand disease in clinical practice, *Throm Haemost* 90:483, 2003.

Ratnoff OD, Saito H: Bleeding in von Willebrand's disease, *N Engl J Med* 290:1089, 1974.

Rodeghiero F, Castaman G, Dini E: Epidemiological investigation of the prevalence of von Willebrand's disease, *Blood* 69:454, 1987.

Schneppenheim R: The pathophysiology of von Willebrand disease: therapeutic implications, *Thromb Res* 128(Suppl 1):S3-S7, 2011.

Shepherd LL, Hutchinson RJ, Worden EK, et al: Hyponatremia and seizures after intravenous administration of desmopressin acetate for surgical hemostasis, *J Pediatr* 114:470, 1989.

Sutor AH: DDAVP is not a panacea for children with bleeding disorders, *Br J Haematol* 108:217, 2000.

Wagner DD: Cell biology of von Willebrand factor, *Annu Rev Cell Biol* 6:217, 1990.

Oral Anticoagulation Therapy in Oral and Maxillofacial Surgery

Gary F. Bouloux, Damian R. Jimenez, and Shahrokh C. Bagheri

CC

A 54-year-old woman is referred to your clinic for removal of multiple teeth before partial denture construction.

HPI

The patient has multiple carious teeth that are nonrestorable. She is planning to have a new maxillary partial denture constructed after the removal of the teeth. She does not complain of any pain or swelling. She had not previously seen a dentist for 8 years. She has not had any extractions other than her wisdom teeth, which were removed 35 years earlier.

PMHX/PDHX/MEDICATIONS/ALLERGIES/SH/FH

The patient's past medical history is remarkable for paroxysmal atrial fibrillation and multiple transient ischemic attacks in her late 40s and a subsequent cerebrovascular accident at age 49. As a result of the cerebrovascular accident, she has significant left leg weakness. She has a 30 pack-year history of smoking, elevated serum cholesterol and triglycerides, and hypertension (all are additional risk factors for cerebrovascular accident). Her current medications include warfarin (Coumadin), atorvastatin (HMG CoA reductase inhibitor), hydrochlorothiazide (diuretic), and felodipine (calcium channel blocker). She has no known drug allergies.

EXAMINATION

General. The patient is a cooperative woman in no acute distress.

Vital signs. Blood pressure is 130/84 mm Hg, heart rate 66 bpm, respirations 12 per minute, and temperature 36.5°C.

Intraoral. There are multiple carious teeth and retained roots.

Neurologic. Weakness (3/5) of left lower extremity with brisk knee and ankle reflexes (sign of upper motor neuron injury secondary to cerebrovascular accident). There are no other focal neurologic signs.

Extremities. Mild atrophy of the left lower extremity (disuse atrophy) is seen.

Skin. Multiple bruises are noted on the upper and lower extremities (secondary to anticoagulation therapy).

LABS

The prothrombin time (PT) is used to measure the adequacy of the extrinsic and common pathway of the clotting cascade. Specifically, it measures the clotting ability of factors I (fibrinogen), II (prothrombin), V, VII, IX, and X. Deficiencies of these clotting factors prolong the prothrombin time (normal range, 11 to 13 seconds). However, most laboratories report PT results that have been adjusted to the international normalized ratio (INR), using the international sensitivity index for the particular thromboplastin and instrument combinations used to perform the test. The normal value is designated as 1.0. Coumadin therapy affects the function of factors II, VII, IX, and X. Factor VII has the shortest half-life and therefore is the most important factor in initially determining the functioning of the extrinsic pathway.

For the current patient, the following laboratory test results were observed:

- Complete blood count: White blood cells 4,000/µl, hemoglobin 12.4 g/dl, platelets 365,000/µl
- Coagulation studies: PT 48 seconds, partial thromboplastin time (PTT) 33 seconds, INR 3.2

Bleeding time, platelet aggregation studies, and platelet flow cytometry, which are tests of platelet function, were not indicated in this patient.

IMAGING

A panoramic radiograph revealed multiple maxillary carious teeth and several retained roots.

ASSESSMENT

Multiple carious teeth and retained roots requiring surgical extraction in a patient on anticoagulation therapy with Coumadin for prevention of thromboembolic disease.

TREATMENT

Given the potential for paroxysmal atrial fibrillation and therefore the risk of further thromboembolic events, it was decided to continue Coumadin in the current patient in the perioperative period. However, after consultation with the primary care physician, her regular dose of Coumadin was reduced to lower the INR below 2.5 (this reduced the likelihood of excessive perioperative bleeding, yet maintained a satisfactory level of anticoagulation). Under general anesthesia, multiple teeth were removed using small, atraumatic mucoperiosteal flaps and minimal bone removal. Any soft tissue bleeding was controlled with electrocautery. The extraction sockets were then packed with hemostatic bovine collagen (Avitene; Davol, Providence, Rhode Island), and the wounds were closed carefully with slowly resorbing polyglactin (Vicryl) horizontal mattress sutures. The wounds were carefully inspected before the procedure was terminated. The patient was given a 5% tranexamic acid mouthwash, to be used four times a day for 5 days. She continued to take her Coumadin throughout the hospital admission. A soft diet and avoidance of strenuous activity were recommended for the first postoperative week.

COMPLICATIONS

Postoperative bleeding can complicate any surgical procedure. Although this may occur secondary to inadequate wound hemostasis, postoperative wound breakdown, or infection, it may also be the result of systemic coagulopathy (the condition seen in the current patient). When postoperative bleeding occurs, rapid assessment of the severity of the bleeding must be made. If the bleeding is severe, the patient must be admitted to the hospital for fluid resuscitation; typed, screened, and cross-matched; and transfused if the hemoglobin and hematocrit levels are sufficiently low or the patient is symptomatic. After initial stabilization, attention must be directed toward stopping the bleeding. Local measures can aid in hemostasis. However, in coagulopathic patients (as in the current patient), local measures may not suffice, and a systemic approach to the control of hemorrhage may be necessary. Platelets, fresh frozen plasma, and cryoprecipitate all can be given, depending on the etiology of the bleeding.

Bleeding secondary to therapeutic Coumadin can be treated with vitamin K, although it usually takes 12 to 24 hours for any significant reversal of the anticoagulation to occur. Bleeding secondary to unfractionated heparin can be treated with protamine sulfate, with immediate reversal of the anticoagulation. Bleeding associated with the use of low-molecular-weight heparins (e.g., Lovenox) cannot be directly reversed due to a different mode of action (indirect inhibitor factor Xa); ultimately, treatment with fresh frozen plasma is required. Bleeding secondary to the use of dabigatran (Pradaxa), a direct thrombin inhibitor, cannot be directly reversed; reversal requires the administration of fresh frozen plasma, recombinant factor VIIa, or prothrombin complex concentrate. Dialysis may also be of benefit in any patient with life-threatening bleeding secondary to use of Pradaxa, because it can reduce plasma levels up to 60% in 2 to 3 hours. Bleeding secondary to use of Xarelto (rivaroxaban), a direct factor Xa inhibitor, also cannot be directly reversed and requires fresh frozen plasma. Bleeding secondary to thrombasthenia (dysfunctional platelets but normal numbers) may be hereditary (Glanzmann thrombasthenia or Bernard-Soulier syndrome) or, more commonly, may be due to the use of aspirin or Plavix (clopidogrel is a platelet adenosine diphosphate receptor inhibitor). The only immediate therapy available is platelet transfusion.

Bleeding may also occur secondary to von Willebrand disease (vWD), one of the more common hereditary hematologic disorders, in addition to hemophilia A. Deficiency of von Willebrand factor (vWF) may be treated with 1-deamino-8-D-arginine vasopressin (DDAVP) if mild or with fresh frozen plasma, cryoprecipitate, or factor VIII concentrate if severe (see the preceding section on vWD). Hemophilia A and hemophilia B are hematologic disorders characterized by deficiencies of factors VIII and IX, respectively; they can be readily treated with recombinant factor replacement. The need to replace these factors is largely dependent on the baseline factor level and the planned surgical procedure.

Necrosis of the skin is a rare complication of oral anticoagulation with Coumadin. The lesions can present as ecchymosis, followed by the development of large bullae containing a deep red fluid. The condition does not appear to be dose related. The etiology of Coumadin-related skin necrosis is unclear, although it presents histologically as vasculitis and thrombosis. It may be a result of a transient prothrombotic state that occurs with the initiation of Coumadin therapy. The necrosis is thought to be the result of reduced levels of functional proteins C and S, which are potent inhibitors of coagulation. Proteins C and S have shorter half-lives than do factors II, VII, IX, and X and therefore are theoretically the first proteins of the coagulation cascade to be affected by the initiation of Coumadin therapy. The diagnosis of skin necrosis mandates cessation of Coumadin therapy and replacement with unfractionated or low-molecular-weight heparin.

Coumadin also has a narrow therapeutic window and many important interactions with other medications. Many other drugs inadvertently increase the level of anticoagulation by displacing Coumadin from albumin (it is 99% bound to albumin). Furthermore, Coumadin is metabolized by the liver, and other drugs may either induce or suppress hepatic enzymes, with resultant alterations in the level of anticoagulation. All medications that are to be administered to a patient taking Coumadin should be reviewed for possible drug interactions.

Recently, additional options for oral anticoagulant therapy have become available. Dabigatran (Pradaxa) and rivaroxaban (Xarelto) were mentioned previously. Dabigatran, a direct thrombin inhibitor with fewer side effects and complications than current oral anticoagulants, is used to prevent blood clots in patients with atrial fibrillation and deep venous thrombosis (DVT). Although the management of patients on dabigatran anticoagulant therapy does not routinely require monitoring, the best way to monitor the level of anticoagulation is the Ecarin clotting time (ECT) or the thrombin time (TT). The indications for rivaroxaban are similar to those for dabigatran; however, rivaroxaban is a direct inhibitor of factor Xa, and factor Xa inhibition must be measured to monitor the adequacy of anticoagulation, if clinically desired.

DISCUSSION

Coumadin is a potent anticoagulant that inhibits the cofactor function of vitamin K. Factors II, VII, IX, and X and proteins

C and S are all dependent on vitamin K for their synthesis, which occurs in the liver. Coumadin treatment results in the inhibition of the enzyme vitamin K epoxide reductase, which is required to maintain vitamin K in the reduced state needed for functional coagulation protein synthesis. Proteins C and S are required for fibrinolysis, and the production of nonfunctional proteins usually results in a minimal and clinically insignificant prothrombotic state. Factors II, VII, IX, and X are required for thrombosis and clot formation, and the production of nonfunctional proteins results in a state of anticoagulation that is clinically significant.

When surgery is planned, the simplest way to manage patients on Coumadin is to continue therapy before the surgical procedure. Simple extractions and minor oral surgery can usually be completed in patients taking Coumadin without complication, using local measures, provided the INR is less than 2.5 to 3.0. Local measures include minimizing surgical trauma, primary closure, and the use of hemostatic material, such as bone wax, oxidized cellulose, or bovine collagen. Antifibrinolytics, such as γ-aminocaproic acid and tranexamic acid, stabilize the formed blood clot by helping to reduce the natural process of fibrinolysis. The advantages of 5% tranexamic acid mouthwash are that it can be used as a topical treatment and it has no systemic effect. More involved surgery requires the same local measures, but in addition the patient must be switched to another anticoagulant or anticoagulation must be discontinued. Bridging with low-molecular-weight-heparin (LMWH) is recommended, as an alternative to heparin, for patients taking Coumadin who are admitted for ambulatory or inpatient procedures. LMWH acts by and potentiating antithrombin III and its ability to inactivate factors Xa and II. Bridging with LMWH avoids hospitalization during the recovery period, because patients taking LMWH do not need laboratory monitoring while the INR returns to the therapeutic range. The risk of a hypercoagulable state that theoretically occurs when Coumadin is stopped and then restarted is avoided when bridging therapy is used. Initially, all patients should be stratified according to their risk of thromboembolism (Table 15-6).

In patients taking Pradaxa or Xarelto, minor surgical procedures (e.g., extractions) probably require no modification of dosing, as long as local measures are used to control bleeding; however, no literature currently exists to guide the approach. For patients requiring major surgical procedures, Pradaxa or Xarelto should be stopped 1 to 2 days before surgery if renal function is normal or 3 to 5 days if renal function is impaired.

Bibliography

Aldridge E, Cunningham L: Current thoughts on treatment of patients receiving anticoagulant therapy, *J Oral Maxillofac Surg* 68:2879-2887, 2010.

Brohi K, Cohen M, Davenport R: Acute coagulopathy of trauma: a mechanism, identification, and effect, *Curr Opin Crit Care* 13:680-685, 2007.

Dunn A, Turpie A: Perioperative management of patients receiving oral anticoagulants: a systematic review, *Arch Intern Med* 163(8):901-908, 2003.

Konkle B: Bleeding and thrombosis. In Longo DL, Fauci AS, Kasper DL, et al (eds): *Harrison's principles of internal medicine*, ed 18, New York, 2012, McGraw-Hill.

Levi M, Eerenberg E: Bleeding risk and reversal strategies for old and new anticoagulants and antiplatelet agents, *J Thromb Haemost* 9:1705-1712, 2011.

Nagarakanti R, Ellis C: Dabigatran in clinical practice, *Clin Ther* 34:2051-2060, 2012.

Syed J: Peri-procedural thromboprophylaxis in patients receiving chronic anticoagulation therapy, *Am Heart J* 147:3-15, 2004.

Tiede D, Nishimura RA, Gastineau DA, et al: Modern management of prosthetic valve anticoagulation, *Mayo Clin Proc* 73:665-680, 1998.

Table 15-6	Patients at Risk for Thromboembolism	
Risk Level	**Condition**	**Action**
Low	• Atrial fibrillation • Deep venous thrombosis (DVT) without high-risk features	Stop Coumadin several days before procedure; resume Coumadin on the day of surgery *or* Stop Pradaxa or Xarelto 1-2 days prior to procedure
Intermediate	• Atrial fibrillation and age > 65 years with diabetes mellitus • Coronary artery disease or hypertension • Prosthetic heart valves • DVT > 3 months without high-risk features	Stop Coumadin several days before surgery; use low-molecular-weight heparin (LMWH) perioperatively subcutaneously (hold LMWH on day of surgery); resume Coumadin on the day of surgery
High	• Atrial fibrillation with heart failure • Multiple prosthetic heart valves • DVT > 3 months with high-risk features (e.g., malignancy) • Known thrombophilic state	Stop Coumadin several days before surgery; use unfractionated heparin perioperatively intravenously (hold unfractionated heparin 6 hr before procedure); resume Coumadin on the day of surgery

Alcohol Withdrawal Syndrome and Delirium Tremens

Fariba Farhidvash and Chris Jo

CC

A 35-year-old Caucasian man presents to the emergency department, stating, "I was hit in the face, and I think that my jaw is broken." Alcoholism is 2.5 times more prevalent in males.

HPI

The patient was involved in a bar fight several hours earlier, and another man punched him in the face, causing a displaced left mandibular angle fracture (confirmed with a panoramic radiograph). On arrival at the emergency department, the patient appeared intoxicated and had a strong odor of alcohol on his breath. However, he was alert and oriented times three (person, place, and time) and denied any loss of consciousness. He was admitted to the oral and maxillofacial surgery service in preparation for open reduction with internal fixation of the mandibular fracture. The admitting resident did not include delirium tremens precautions in his admission orders, because the patient denied any history of excessive alcohol use or abuse or previous withdrawal symptoms (patients frequently describe the tremulousness, agitation, and/or anxiety of alcohol withdrawal as the "shakes"). The patient had an uneventful first night, but his operation was postponed due to problems with operating room availability. On the second hospital day, early symptoms of alcohol withdrawal were noted (agitation, anxiety, tremulousness, nausea, and vomiting). Later that evening, the patient wandered the halls of the ward, mumbling to himself and unable to sleep (insomnia). He became progressively more agitated, exhibiting aggressive behavior toward the nursing staff.

You are called to evaluate the patient in the middle of the night. You find him trembling in his bed, yelling incoherently at the television, claiming that there are spiders in the room (visual hallucinations). He will not cooperate with an examination and does not respond to questions. Detailed questioning of the available family members reveals that the patient has been a heavy drinker for several years and had been on a binge for the past several days.

PMHX/PDHX/MEDICATIONS/ALLERGIES/SH/FH

The patient drinks at least a six-pack of beer and half a pint of gin a day (alcohol dependence/addiction). His last drink was 2 nights ago, just before he was assaulted.

The diagnostic criteria for alcohol dependence and abuse listed in the *Diagnostic and Statistical Manual of Mental Disorders, Fourth Edition* (DSM-IV) is beyond the scope of this section. To summarize, alcohol dependence is based on tolerance to alcohol, the presence of withdrawal symptoms, and excessive time spent to obtain and use alcohol, along with persistent and increased use despite alcohol-related problems. Alcohol abuse manifests as the recurrent use of alcohol, despite disruptions at home or work, physical hazards, or legal problems, occurring over a 12-month period.

The CAGE questionnaire is a simple verbal test, composed of four questions, that can be quickly administered to identify patients at risk for alcoholism (Box 15-1). Patients with two affirmative answers are seven times more likely to be alcohol dependent. The sensitivity of the CAGE questionnaire is 75% to 90% in most studies. Other questionnaires used in the clinical setting are the AUDIT and TWEAK questionnaires.

EXAMINATION

General. The patient is extremely agitated, sweating, and shaking and is moving about restlessly in bed (signs of sympathetic overdrive).

Vital signs. Blood pressure is 180/90 mm Hg (hypertensive), heart rate 130 bpm (tachycardia), respirations 22 per minute (tachypnea), and temperature 37.8°C (rules out fever as the cause of altered mental status).

Neurologic. The patient is awake but extremely agitated and is not oriented to place, time, or situation. His speech is slurred; his pupils are dilated (mydriasis secondary to sympathetic overdrive) but equal and reactive to light (dilated pupils that are not reactive may indicate intracranial injury and elevated intracranial pressures); extraocular eye movements are intact; and the face is symmetric (facial asymmetry during

Box 15-1	CAGE Questionnaire

The **CAGE** questions are:

C   Have you ever felt the need to *cut down* on drinking?

A   Have you ever been *annoyed* with criticism about your drinking?

G   Have you ever felt *guilty* about something you did while drinking?

E   Have you ever had a morning *eye-opener* to get you going or to treat withdrawal symptoms?

From Ewing JA: Detecting alcoholism: the CAGE questionnaire, *JAMA* 252:1905-1907, 1984.

animation may indicate an upper or lower motor neuron lesion of cranial nerve VII). He is uncooperative with the motor and sensory examination but is moving all extremities well and is very tremulous (the grossly normal strength examination of the extremities and symmetric facial movement make a focal cerebral lesion unlikely).

Reflexes. Findings reveal +2/4 in all extremities, and the toes are downgoing bilaterally (upgoing toes is an abnormal finding in the adult patient and is termed a *Babinski sign*). (A nonfocal motor examination with downgoing toes is supportive of the absence of a focal upper motor neuron lesion.)

Maxillofacial. The examination is consistent with a left mandibular angle fracture.

Cardiovascular. The patient is tachycardic with no murmurs, gallops, or rubs (chronic alcoholics may have significant cardiac comorbidities).

Abdominal. The patient has a soft, nontender, slightly enlarged liver (hepatomegaly due to chronic alcohol consumption) and no ascites (intraperitoneal serous fluid or ascites would be seen in advanced hepatic dysfunction).

IMAGING

Imaging studies for evaluating the trauma patient with altered mental status should include a noncontrast head CT scan. Altered mental status can be due to acute drug or alcohol intoxication or withdrawal, electrolyte disturbances, hypoxia, infection/sepsis, or metabolic derangements. Altered mental status can also be a manifestation of a closed head injury, particularly intracranial bleeding in the current trauma patient. Any acute changes in mental status warrant a head CT scan to rule out an undetected or blossoming intracranial injury.

For the current patient, an initial head CT scan was not ordered upon admission due to the absence of focal neurologic signs or loss of consciousness. Although this patient is most likely experiencing alcohol withdrawal syndrome and delirium tremens, a head CT scan was ordered after the onset of his altered mental status to evaluate for closed head injury; the scan was normal.

Plain radiographic studies of the mandible confirmed the diagnosis of a left mandibular angle fracture.

LABS

During the initial evaluation of an intoxicated trauma patient with maxillofacial injuries, a blood alcohol level and urine drug screen, in conjunction with a head CT scan, are recommended to account for altered or decreased mental status. Liver function tests (including aspartate aminotransferase, alanine aminotransferase, albumin, bilirubin, prothrombin time, partial thromboplastin time, and international normalized ratio) are indicated for patients with liver cirrhosis to evaluate for possible coagulopathies, if the patient will or may undergo surgery. A complete blood count (including platelets) is warranted, because anemia (particularly macrocytic) and thrombocytopenia (due to liver dysfunction) are common in alcoholics. A complete metabolic panel is mandatory to rule

out electrolyte derangements as the source of altered mental status and to monitor the electrolyte abnormalities associated with chronic alcohol abuse and malnutrition (e.g., hypomagnesemia). A baseline electrocardiogram is recommended, especially in older patients, because cardiac disorders are commonly associated with alcohol consumption.

The current patient presented with an initial blood alcohol level of 250 mg/dl (the legal intoxication level is 0.08%, or 80 mg/dl, in most states) and a negative urine drug screen. Aspartate aminotransferase and alanine aminotransferase levels were 110 U/L and 50 U/L, respectively (aspartate aminotransferase and alanine aminotransferase are typically double or triple the normal values in patients who are chronic alcoholics). His hemoglobin was 11 g/dl, hematocrit 34%, and mean corpuscular volume 110 μm^3 (macrocytic anemia due to malnutrition and likely vitamin B_{12} deficiency). The electrocardiogram showed sinus tachycardia. The remainder of the laboratory values were within normal limits.

ASSESSMENT

A 35-year-old man with a left mandibular fracture, now complicated by alcohol withdrawal syndrome and delirium tremens, presenting with altered mental status and agitation (hyperexcitable state).

Alcohol withdrawal syndrome and delirium tremens describe a spectrum of symptoms observed after a relative or absolute withdrawal from alcohol in susceptible individuals (especially those who are chronic consumers of large amounts of alcohol). The physiologic mechanisms of alcohol withdrawal are based on the inhibitory γ-aminobutyric acid (GABA) and excitatory (glutamate) neurotransmitters of the brain. Alcohol increases the effects of GABA on the GABAA receptor, thus increasing its inhibitory effects. Also, it inhibits the excitatory effects of glutamate at the N-methyl-D-aspartate (NMDA) receptor, thereby decreasing neuronal excitability. During alcohol withdrawal, a state of hyperexcitability and autonomic dysfunction becomes apparent (hypermetabolic state).

TREATMENT

Identification of patients who are at risk for developing alcohol withdrawal syndrome or delirium tremens is the most important step for prevention of these two conditions. Patients with a recent history of significant alcohol consumption (chronic or binge drinkers) and those with a history of alcohol withdrawal and/or delirium tremens are at risk for alcohol withdrawal syndrome and delirium tremens. Older patients with other medical comorbidities are at greater risk. With hospitalization, patients do not have access to alcohol and may develop a range of signs and symptoms consistent with alcohol withdrawal syndrome, withdrawal seizures, and delirium tremens (some hospital facilities have alcoholic beverages available for delirium tremens prevention).

Preventive measures should be taken to reduce the risk of the development of alcohol withdrawal syndrome and delirium tremens. Benzodiazepines are the first-line agents for treatment and prevention; they are used either as needed or on a fixed schedule to prevent the development of the symptoms, based on the patient's history and the severity of symptoms. Scheduled dosing is recommended for patients considered to be at moderate or high risk; this also allows for a smoother withdrawal. With scheduled dosing of medications, doses high enough to relieve symptoms are given over the first 24 to 48 hours, and the patient is slowly weaned (by about 20% a day) over the next 3 to 5 days. Longer acting benzodiazepines, such as diazepam (Valium), starting at 5 to 10 mg PO/IV/IM every 6 to 8 hours, or chlordiazepoxide (Librium), starting at 25 to 100 mg PO/IV/IM every 4 to 6 hours, may be used to reduce rebound effects and significantly decrease withdrawal symptoms. In patients with significant comorbidities (e.g., liver failure, with associated decreased hepatic metabolism), shorter acting benzodiazepines may be used, such as lorazepam (Ativan), 1 to 4 mg PO/IV/IM every 4 to 8 hours, or oxazepam (Serax), starting with 15 to 30 mg PO every 6 to 8 hours. Nonpharmacologic measures include maintaining a calm, tranquil environment and a nonconfrontational interaction to help reduce the patient's anxiety. Patients presenting with symptoms of anxiety, tremulousness, and agitation after recent cessation of alcohol use should be treated promptly (with longer acting benzodiazepines).

Intravenous fluids, replacement of electrolytes (e.g., magnesium), folic acid, and intravenous thiamine (given before administration of glucose to prevent the development of Wernicke's encephalopathy) are essential to rehydrate the patient and correct any possible vitamin deficiencies. Standard "delirium tremens precautions/prophylaxis" orders include thiamine 100 mg IM/IV daily, folate 1 mg PO/IV daily, multivitamins PO/IV, magnesium sulfate 1 g IM/IV daily, and benzodiazepines as needed or scheduled, as discussed earlier.

With the onset of full-blown delirium tremens, the patient should be admitted to the intensive care unit, with administration of scheduled benzodiazepines to ameliorate delirium symptoms and reduce the incidence of seizures. For the autonomic symptoms (e.g., tachycardia and hypertension), antihypertensive medications may become necessary. β-Blockers may be used to treat tachycardia and hypertension, but caution should be used, because these drugs may precipitate delirium. Clonidine (a central α-agonist) may also be used to treat autonomic symptoms without any adverse effects on mental status. If withdrawal symptoms are severe and refractory despite benzodiazepine therapy, the patient may require endotracheal intubation for airway protection and administration of a general anesthetic, such as a propofol (propofol has been shown to be effective in refractory delirium tremens). Usual supportive care is included throughout delirium tremens (this may include four-point restraints).

The differential diagnosis of altered mental status can be extensive, particularly in the absence of an appropriate history and examination. Broad categories include toxic (drug overdose or toxicity), metabolic (hypoglycemia, hepatic encephalopathy, or uremia), infectious (systemic or central nervous system), inflammatory (demyelinating disease or central nervous system vasculitis), vascular (large vessel infarction or intracranial hemorrhage), and traumatic etiologies (increased intracranial pressure secondary to closed head injury); hypoxemia and/or hypercarbia; and acute psychotic episodes secondary to underlying psychiatric disorders. The differential diagnosis should be categorically narrowed to the most likely etiology given the clinical setting. Head imaging to rule out traumatic brain injuries, vascular accidents (e.g., intracranial hemorrhage), infectious processes (e.g., cerebral abscesses), or other cerebral lesions should be obtained early. If an infectious etiology involving the central nervous system is suspected, a lumbar puncture (after checking the prothrombin time, partial thromboplastin time, and international normalized ratio) is essential to rule out meningitis or encephalitis. Urine and/or serum toxicology screens can rule out drug or alcohol abuse. A complete metabolic panel, including liver function tests, calcium, magnesium, ammonia, vitamin B_{12} level, and thyroid function tests, can help identify certain metabolic derangements. Urinalysis and blood cultures should be obtained in cases of suspected urinary or hematogenous infectious processes contributing to mental status changes. In the obtunded patient, subclinical seizure activity should be considered. This can be evaluated using an electroencephalogram.

For the current patient, failure to identify the patient's risk factors and poor communication among staff members contributed to the lack of preventive measures for alcohol withdrawal syndrome and delirium tremens. At the onset of symptoms of delirium tremens, scheduled lorazepam 2 mg IV and chlordiazepoxide 50 mg IV every 4 hours were initiated, followed by replacement of fluids, electrolytes, and multivitamins. The patient's condition progressively improved over the course of the day, with resolution of the tachycardia and normalization of the blood pressure. Librium was continued on a scheduled basis for the next 2 days and subsequently slowly tapered (25 mg PO every 4 hours on day 3, followed by 10 mg PO every 4 hours on day 4) to prevent benzodiazepine withdrawal. Clonidine was not used, because the patient's autonomic dysfunction normalized. The patient underwent open reduction with internal fixation of the mandibular fracture without complications (closed reduction is frequently not well tolerated by patients who are poorly compliant). The patient was counseled about the importance of drinking cessation and the long-term effects of heavy alcohol use and was assisted to obtain help via support groups such as Alcoholics Anonymous or from professional counselors (psychiatrists or psychologists), with the help of the hospital social worker.

COMPLICATIONS

Inherent to the diagnosis of delirium tremens is the autonomic instability (fluctuating blood pressure, heart, and respiratory rates) that is life-threatening if not appropriately managed. Withdrawal seizures rarely require aggressive antiepileptic pharmacologic interventions (benzodiazepines are usually sufficient). Rarely, the seizure may become prolonged, leading to status epilepticus, a neurologic emergency characterized by continuous seizures (clinical or subclinical) lasting longer than 5 minutes or multiple seizures with a 30-minute period in which the patient does not return to baseline between seizures. This may lead to permanent cerebral damage or death if not managed aggressively. The mortality rate for untreated alcohol withdrawal syndrome and delirium tremens is about 15%, mostly secondary to cardiovascular and respiratory collapse.

DISCUSSION

Alcohol withdrawal syndrome and delirium tremens characterize the spectrum of symptoms observed after a relative or absolute withdrawal from alcohol, especially with chronic use. Delirium primarily involves alterations of attention and is characterized by a fluctuating course, difficulty with concentration, and altered mental status. Tremens refers to the tremors seen in patients with delirium tremens. Most patients who stop alcohol use acutely do not develop withdrawal symptoms, or they simply experience minor symptoms that do not require medical attention. Clinically significant alcohol withdrawal symptoms occur in up to 20% of patients. If the symptoms go untreated, 10% to 15% of these patients progress to withdrawal seizures. Delirium tremens is the last stage of alcohol withdrawal; it occurs in 5% to 10% of alcohol-dependent individuals, with a mortality rate of 5% to 15% when left untreated.

The physiologic mechanism of alcohol withdrawal is based on the inhibitory and excitatory neurotransmitters of the brain. Alcohol increases the effects of the GABAA receptor by increasing its inhibitory effects. In contrast, glutamate (excitatory neurotransmitter that acts on the NMDA receptor) is inhibited, thereby decreasing neuronal excitability. The presence of alcohol has an inhibitory effect by enhancing GABAA and depressing the NMDA receptor. On withdrawal of alcohol, there is an abrupt cessation of the neuronal inhibition and a subsequent state of hyperexcitability.

There are multiple stages of withdrawal based on the chronology of symptoms occurring after the cessation of alcohol use. These stages, from least to most severe, include acute intoxication, alcohol withdrawal, withdrawal seizures, and delirium tremens. Withdrawal may be apparent as early as 6 hours after the last drink but may last up to 12 to 24 hours; symptoms include depression, anxiety, tremulousness, and insomnia. Withdrawal seizures, which have a 2% to 5% incidence in alcohol withdrawal syndrome and delirium tremens, typically occur approximately 48 hours after cessation of alcohol use and present as generalized tonic-clonic seizures. Delirium tremens peaks at 48 to 72 hours after the last drink. The patient may present with delirium, hallucinations (visual, auditory, or tactile, with awareness that he or she is hallucinating), diaphoresis, or fever, but the key feature of delirium tremens is autonomic instability. Scales such as the Clinical Institute Withdrawal Assessment for Alcohol (CIWA-Ar) may help determine the severity of alcohol withdrawal symptoms.

Wernicke-Korsakoff syndrome encompasses two different syndromes associated with chronic alcohol use and severe malnutrition. Wernicke's encephalopathy is primarily a clinical diagnosis involving the classic triad of encephalopathy, ophthalmoplegia, and ataxia. Confusion is usually of a subacute to chronic nature and is characterized by inattention, memory loss, and apathy. Ophthalmoplegia (weakness or paralysis of one or more of the extraocular muscles) mostly involves the lateral recti but may also involve any of the extraocular muscles. Nystagmus (rhythmic oscillation of the eyes) is commonly present in the lateral and/or vertical gaze. Ataxia is the unsteady, clumsy motion of the extremities and, more commonly, the trunk. Left untreated, Wernicke's encephalopathy has a mortality rate of 10% to 20%. It is treated with the administration of thiamine 50 to 100 mg IV once a day (this should be given before glucose, because glucose further depletes thiamine and accelerates the development of Wernicke's encephalopathy). Korsakoff syndrome primarily involves memory impairment without significant deficits of other cognitive functions, such as attention or social behavior. It is also characterized by both anterograde and retrograde amnesia, along with confabulation, in which the patient's recall is distorted in relation to reality (a prominent feature). This condition also is treated with thiamine, but the prognosis is less favorable.

Bibliography

Aisa D, Lebrun G, Coursing D, et al: Alcohol withdrawal and delirium tremens in the critically ill: a systemic review and commentary, *Intensive Care Med* 39:16-30, 2012.

Al-Sanouri I, Dikin M, Subani AO: Critical care aspects of alcohol abuse, *South Med J* 98:372-381, 2005.

Bayard M, McIntyre J, Hill K, et al: Alcohol withdrawal syndrome, *Am Fam Physician* 69:1443-1450, 2004.

Eyre F, Schuster T, Felgenhauer N, et al: Risk assessment of moderate to severe alcohol withdrawal-predictors for seizures and delirium tremens in the course of withdrawal, *Alcohol Alcohol* 46:427-433, 2011.

Maimon WN, Davis LF: Management of acute alcohol withdrawal, *J Oral Maxillofac Surg* 40:361-366, 1982.

Morris PR, Mosby EL, Ferguson BL: Alcohol withdrawal syndrome: current management strategies for the surgery patient, *J Oral Maxillofac Surg* 55:1452-1455, 1997.

Acute Asthmatic Attack

Joyce T. Lee, Shahrokh C. Bagheri, and Ali R. Rahimi

CC

A 17-year-old male with a history of asthma is referred to your office for evaluation of symptomatic partially impacted third molars.

Asthma is seen in about 3% to 5% of the population and can occur in any age group; however, it is particularly common in children and young adults and is the most common chronic disease in this age group.

HPI

The patient is a high school student with a history of pain and recurrent episodes of pericoronitis of the mandibular third molars. He was referred by his general dentist for evaluation and treatment.

PMHX/PDHX/MEDICATIONS/ALLERGIES/SH/FH

The patient has a history of asthma, diagnosed at age 8. He states that his asthmatic episodes are usually exacerbated by exercise and seasonal allergies (other common triggers of asthma exacerbation include cold weather, tobacco smoke, recent upper respiratory infection, and certain medications, including nonsteroidal antiinflammatory drugs [NSAIDs]). He has had two previous visits to the local emergency department (ED) secondary to acute episodes that did not readily respond to his albuterol (β_2 agonist) inhaler; he required intravenous methylprednisolone (systemic corticosteroid), nebulized albuterol, and ipratropium (anticholinergic bronchodilator). The episodes resolved without the need for endotracheal intubation (ED visits and endotracheal intubation both correlate with the severity of the asthma). The patient does not have a history of status asthmaticus (asthmatic episode refractory to treatment). His last asthma attack was approximately a month ago (the frequency of attacks is an indicator of the control of this patient's asthma).

His current medications include an albuterol metered-dose inhaler, used as needed, and Montelukast (leukotriene receptor antagonist) 10 mg daily. He routinely monitors his status with a peak flow meter (patients use this device to monitor changes in the forced expiratory volume in 1 second [FEV_1]; Figure 15-4).

The patient states that he smokes occasionally (cigarette smoke is an airway irritant that may precipitate bronchospasm). He also has a history of allergic rhinitis (hay fever) and eczema. There is a positive history of asthma in several of his family members. (In patients with an allergic component to their asthma, there frequently is a strong family history of asthma or other allergies. Genetic factors may play a role in the pathogenesis of asthma. However, it is important to mention that not all asthmatic patients have allergies and that the association between asthma and allergies is not entirely clear.)

EXAMINATION

General. The patient is a well-developed, well-nourished male in no apparent distress.

Vitals. Stable with normotensive blood pressure.

Oral and maxillofacial. Partially erupted, impacted third molars are noted. The tongue is normal in size. The patient has a Class I skeletal and dental relationship. The maximal interincisal opening is 45 mm. The uvula and soft and hard palates are easily visualized; bilateral tonsils are within normal limits in size and recessed within the tonsillar crypts (Mallampati Class I). The thyromental distance is greater than four finger widths (evaluation of the airway is important, especially in patients who may require advanced airway interventions).

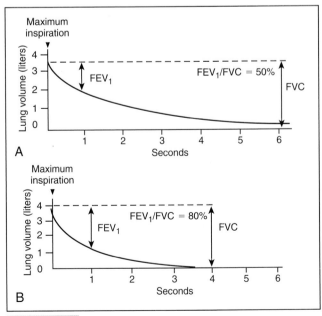

Figure 15-4 Forced vital capacity in a patient with an airway obstruction **(A)** and in an individual with an unobstructed airway **(B)**.

Cardiovascular. Regular rate and rhythm with no murmurs, gallops (S3 or S4), or rubs (patients with asthma can have other comorbidities, such as chronic obstructive pulmonary disease (COPD), which may produce "splitting" of the second heart sound with an accentuated pulmonic component).

Chest. Bilaterally clear on auscultation. (The major symptoms during an acute asthmatic attack are cough, dyspnea, expiratory wheezing, and chest tightness. Wheezing is not pathognomonic for asthma and reflects airflow obstruction through a narrow airway).

LABS

None are indicated in the routine care of a patient with well-controlled asthma. However, patients whose asthma is poorly controlled are often referred for pulmonary function testing. The most objective and relevant tests for measuring the degree of airway obstruction in asthmatic patients are the FEV_1 and the peak expiratory flow (PEF). In patients with well-controlled asthma, the FEV_1 should be 80% of the forced vital capacity (FVC). (Comparison of obstructive with restrictive pulmonary diseases reveals that the vital capacity [VC] and FEV_1 are decreased in both; however, in obstructive diseases, both the functional residual capacity [FRC] and the residual volume [RV] are increased, whereas in restrictive lung diseases, both the FRC and RV are decreased.)

IMAGING

In the current patient, the panoramic radiograph is significant for partial bony impacted third molars.

Chest radiographs are not indicated in asymptomatic patients with a history of asthma and are not particularly helpful except for ruling out other diseases. During acute asthmatic exacerbations, the chest radiograph may reveal hyperinflation of the lung fields (flattened diaphragm) and decreased vascular markings.

ASSESSMENT

ASA II patient with four impacted third molars, planned for extraction under intravenous sedation anesthesia.

The American Society of Anesthesiologists classification ASA II is defined as a patient with a mild systemic disease that is well-controlled, and poses no limitations for daily activities.

TREATMENT

After reviewing the risks, benefits, and alternatives, the patient elected to have his third molars removed under intravenous general anesthesia the next day. The patient was instructed to record his peak flow the morning of the surgery and to bring his albuterol metered-dose inhaler with spacer to the office (spacers are devices used to increase the effectiveness of medication delivery).

The day of surgery, the patient's lungs were clear on auscultation bilaterally (due to the episodic nature of asthma, pulmonary auscultation should be conducted routinely prior to surgery). After the patient had been prepared for surgery, he self-administered three puffs of albuterol (90 µg per puff) using his spacer. Intravenous general anesthesia was achieved with midazolam 5 mg, fentanyl 50 µg, and propofol titrated to effect (propofol is the preferred general anesthetic for the asthmatic patient, because there is a higher incidence of wheezing during anesthesia induction with intravenous methohexital [Brevital] compared to propofol).

Upon removal of the last third molar, the patient became diaphoretic, agitated, tachycardic (140 bpm), and tachypneic, with shallow breaths (25 per minute) (tracheal tugging, use of accessory muscles of respiration, and intercostal retractions are other signs of severe asthmatic exacerbation). The surgical sites were packed, the oropharynx was suctioned, and the tongue was retracted as the airway was repositioned and supported. The patient's condition continued to deteriorate, with a progressive decline in oxygen saturation as measured by the pulse oximeter. Inspiratory suprasternal retractions revealed the obstructive nature of the patient's condition. The diagnosis of an acute asthmatic attack was made. Two puffs of albuterol were given, in addition to two puffs of ipratropium bromide, while the vital signs were monitored closely. Supplemental 100% oxygen was delivered via a full face mask. Minutes later, the patient began to show worsening signs of respiratory distress, with a further drop in the pulse oximeter reading to below 85%. Emergency medical services (EMS) was activated. Meanwhile, 0.5 mg of a 1:1,000 solution of epinephrine was injected subcutaneously. An attempt to mask ventilate with 100% O_2 revealed airway resistance and chest tightness. Positive pressure ventilation using the bag-mask technique was unsuccessful despite airway repositioning. A 10-mg dose of IV succinylcholine was given, and the patient's anesthesia was deepened with 50 mg IV ketamine. (Ketamine is a dissociative agent with potent bronchodilatory effects. Causes of bronchospasm often are attributed to light anesthesia; therefore, ketamine is a valuable drug to consider.) The patient's airway soon became easier to ventilate with the bag-mask technique with 100% oxygen at a flow rate of 12 L/minute. (Consideration should be given to administration of diphenhydramine 50 mg IV in cases of suspected allergic response; 20 mg of dexamethasone IV can also be used to reduce the inflammatory response.) The patient responded to these measures, showing a gradual rise in the pulse oximeter reading, diminished chest wall rigidity, and improved air exchange and compliance. His vital signs normalized, except for a persistent tachycardia (a residual side effect of repeated doses of sympathomimetics is tachycardia). Upon arrival of EMS, the patient was transported to the hospital for further observation of his acute asthmatic event.

COMPLICATIONS

Complications arising in patients with asthma range from mild wheezing and dyspnea to severe bronchospasm, hypoxia, and death. Bronchospasm is a life-threatening emergency that must be treated as soon as it is recognized. In the office setting, it is important to alert EMS as soon as possible, because the patient's condition may deteriorate rapidly. The incidence of bronchospasm is low in patients with well-controlled asthma who are undergoing outpatient intravenous general anesthesia.

Bronchospasm is the acute manifestation of asthma. It results in increased airway resistance, which causes a decrease in the ratio of FEV_1 to FVC (see Figure 15-4). Signs and symptoms of bronchospasm include dyspnea, stridor, wheezing, mucus secretion, and hypoxia. Initial treatment should include 100% oxygen and an inhaled β_2 agonist. β_2 agonists relax the smooth muscle in bronchial walls and produce bronchodilation.

The clinician should also look for causes of the asthma exacerbation, such as undiagnosed latex allergies or medication allergies. Urticaria, pruritus, and facial edema are findings consistent with allergic reactions that may produce bronchospasm. If an allergic reaction is suspected, diphenhydramine and corticosteroids should be administered intravenously. Administration of epinephrine may be indicated in patients experiencing bronchospasm refractory to inhaled β_2 agonists; the most common dose and route of administration are 1 mg injected subcutaneously.

Theophylline and aminophylline (a phosphodiesterase inhibitor) produce bronchodilation and traditionally were used in the management of bronchospasm. (Aminophylline was used with caution, because it has a narrow therapeutic index and may produce arrhythmias.) However, in recent years multiple clinical trials have shown that aminophylline and theophylline not only result in no further bronchodilation, but also increase toxicity; consequently, this category of drugs has fallen out of the treatment protocol.

If bronchospasm persists and the patient is hypoxic, intubation is indicated. It is important to realize that intubation does not protect against or treat the bronchospasm. However, it facilitates ventilation of the narrowed airways and allows effective delivery of nebulized medications. If mechanical ventilation is used after intubation, it is important to be mindful that asthma is an obstructive airway disease and that overzealous high pressure or flow on inspiration can cause barotrauma, resulting in either a pneumothorax or tension pneumothorax.

DISCUSSION

Asthma is a common chronic respiratory condition that can present with acute exacerbations. It affects both children and adults and is highly variable in severity, response to treatment, and clinical presentation. Asthma is a form of obstructive airway disease characterized by an acute and reversible increase in airway resistance. Recent evidence suggests that asthma causes changes in the respiratory epithelium. The prevalence of asthma is 5% in adults and 10% in the pediatric population. There is evidence that this is increasing in the United States, especially in urban pediatric populations.

The various types of asthma are categorized according to the underlying etiology of the exacerbation. These types may include atopic or IgE-mediated, exercise-induced, occupational, infectious, or aspirin-induced asthma. Although the mediators that produce an acute asthmatic attack vary, the resulting physiologic responses are similar for all types of asthma. Because airway resistance is inversely related to the diameter of the bronchial lumen, pediatric patients are predisposed to rapid decompensation during bronchospasm (Figure 15-5).

Perioperative management of patients with asthma is primarily based on risk stratification. Successful management of asthma requires an active patient-physician partnership. Patients must understand the pathophysiology of their disease and the need for medication compliance, and they must be able to monitor the current status of the disease state. Many emergency visits by individuals with asthma are attributed to

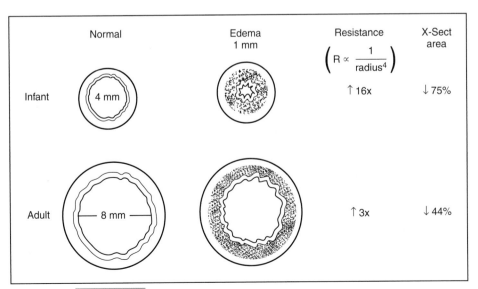

Figure 15-5 Airway resistance in the infant and in an adult patient.

the patients' lack of understanding about their disease. Elective surgery is contraindicated in asthmatic patients whose disease is not well controlled. Patients should be asked about their medication regimens, their understanding of medication delivery, and the use of peak flow meters. Patients whose understanding and medication compliance are not optimal should be referred to their primary care physician for evaluation prior to elective surgery.

Intraoperative management of asthmatic patients should emphasize adequate oxygenation, avoiding excessive airway stimulation by use of throat packs, and suctioning. A pretracheal stethoscope is recommended for auscultation monitoring. In patients who are intubated, decreased tidal volumes and increased end-tidal carbon dioxide levels may indicate bronchospasm. During extubation, minimal stimulation of the airway is advised. "Deep" extubation may be prudent to avoid excessive excitement in the emerging patient, because extubation may generate enormous negative pressure, resulting in acute pulmonary edema. Administering a dose of intravenous lidocaine prior to extubation also decreases airway stimulation. Despite these precautions, some patients with asthma experience bronchospasm during the course of surgery. Management of an acute asthmatic exacerbation should consist of early detection and intervention. Bronchospasm is a potentially life-threatening emergency that must be treated. Treatment should consist of assessment of vital signs, supplemental oxygen, inhaled β_2 agonists, injectable sympathomimetics, corticosteroids, and ventilatory support if indicated.

Bibliography

Bone RC: Goals of asthma management: a step-care approach, *Chest* 109:1056, 1996.

Currie GP: Recent developments in asthma management, *Br Med J* 330:585, 2005.

DiGiulio GA, Kercsmar CM, Krug SE, et al: Hospital treatment of asthma: lack of benefit from theophylline given in addition to nebulized albuterol and intravenously administered corticosteroid, *J Pediatr* 122:464, 1993.

Ezekiel MR: *Handbook of anesthesiology*, Laguna Hills, Calif, 2004, CCS Publishing.

Fanta CH, Rossing TH, McFadden ER Jr: Glucocorticoids in acute asthma: a critical controlled trial, *Am J Med* 74:845, 1983.

Hurford WE: *Clinical anesthesia procedures of the Massachusetts General Hospital*, ed 5, Philadelphia, 1998, Lippincott-Raven.

Newman KB, Milne S, Hamilton C, et al: A comparison of albuterol administered by metered-dose inhaler and spacer with albuterol by nebulizer in adults presenting to an urban emergency department with acute asthma, *Chest* 121:1036, 2002.

Ogle OE: *Management of medical problems*, Philadelphia, 1998, Saunders.

Owen CL: New directions in asthma management, *Am J Nurs* 3:99, 1999.

Pizov R, Brown RH, Weiss YS, et al: Wheezing during induction of general anesthesia in patients with and without asthma, *Anesthesiology* 82(5):1111, 1995.

Rea HH, Cragg R, Jackson R, et al: A case-controlled study of deaths from asthma, *Thorax* 41:833, 1986.

Rodrigo GJ, Rodrigo C: The role anticholinergics in acute asthma treatment: an evidence based evaluation, *Chest* 121:1977, 2002.

Rodrigo GJ, Rodrigo C, Hall JB: Acute asthma in adults: a review, *Chest* 125:1081, 2004.

Rossing TH, Fanta CH, Goldstein DH, et al: Emergency therapy of asthma: comparison of the acute effects of parenteral and inhaled sympathomimetics and infused theophylline, *Am Rev Resp Dis* 122:365, 1980.

Diabetes Mellitus

Mehran Mehrabi and Shahrokh C. Bagheri

CC

A 18-year-old man with a history of type 1 diabetes mellitus presents to the oral and maxillofacial surgery clinic, complaining, "My wisdom teeth are hurting."

HPI

For the past week, the patient has had mild, progressively exacerbating lower jaw pain that is worse with function. He denies any history of fever, swelling, or facial erythema. There is no history of trauma. He explains that his blood sugar has been well controlled (poorly controlled blood glucose decreases the ability to fight an infection).

PMHX/PDHX/MEDICATIONS/ALLERGIES/SH/FH

The patient was diagnosed with type 1 diabetes mellitus at age 10 and has been taking insulin for the past 8 years. He is currently being followed by his family practitioner. His medications include glargine (Lantus, a long-acting synthetic insulin that provides a steady concentration of insulin) once a day and preprandial lispro (Humalog, a rapidly acting insulin) three times a day. He has had no prior surgeries but was hospitalized for hypoglycemia twice during the previous year (previous episodes of hypoglycemia are a risk factor for future episodes). He reports that his blood glucose has been between 80 and 160 mg/dl during the prior week, as measured with his home Accu-Chek device (the ideal preprandial blood glucose level is 90 to 130 mg/dl).

There is no family history of diabetes mellitus. (Type 1 diabetes mellitus has a strong association with HLA-DR3, DR4, and DQ alleles; however, a family history is often lacking. A positive family history is often seen with type 2 diabetes mellitus.)

EXAMINATION

General. The patient is a thin, calm, and cooperative man (unlike patients with type 2 diabetes, those with type 1 are frequently thin and/or cachexic).

Vital signs. His vital signs are stable, and he is afebrile.

Maxillofacial. There is no facial edema, erythema, or induration. The patient is able to open his mouth without restriction.

Intraoral. Examination is consistent with bilateral pericoronitis of the left and right mandibular third molars (teeth #17 and #32, respectively). The right and left maxillary third molars (teeth #1 and #16, respectively) are in traumatic occlusion with the associated operculum of the mandibular third molars. The remainder of the dentition is free of caries or periodontal disease.

IMAGING

For the surgical management of patients with diabetes mellitus, the need for adjunctive imaging studies is dictated by the clinical findings and suspicion of sources of infection or pathology. Nonodontogenic sources of infection should be considered in all patients.

In the current patient, the panoramic radiograph showed partial bony impacted left and right mandibular third molars. The right and left maxillary third molars were supraerupted, with no other radiographic signs of pathology.

LABS

For the routine work-up of a patient with well-controlled diabetes mellitus, no routine preoperative laboratory testing is necessary for minor oral surgical procedures, except for a preoperative blood glucose level (especially important in a patient with poorly controlled diabetes). Hypoglycemia should be treated with oral or intravenous glucose (dextrose) or intramuscular glucagon as needed, and hyperglycemia may need to be treated with an insulin preparation. Elective surgical procedures should be delayed in the face of excessively abnormal blood glucose readings. Patients with infectious processes that require surgical intervention should be treated promptly, because infections are frequently the precipitating cause of the glycemic abnormality.

An effective, objective tool for assessing patient compliance and long-term hyperglycemic status is measurement of the glycosylated hemoglobin (HbA$_{1c}$) level. Prolonged elevation of serum blood glucose causes nonenzymatic, irreversible glycosylation of hemoglobin in red blood cells. Because the life expectancy of red blood cells is 120 days, the HbA$_{1c}$ gives an estimate of glycemic control during the past 90 to 120 days. An HbA$_{1c}$ greater than 6% is consistent with diabetes, and a value greater than 7% is indicative of poor glycemic control. Therefore, the HbA$_{1c}$ directly correlates with poor glycemic control for the previous 3 to 4 months. For patients undergoing major surgery, a complete metabolic panel and blood count should also be obtained.

For the current patient, the serum HbA$_{1c}$ was 6.5%, and the serum blood glucose level was 135 mg/dl.

ASSESSMENT

Pericoronitis of partially impacted left and right mandibular third molars, exacerbated by traumatic occlusion of right and left maxillary third molars, in a patient with well-controlled type 1 diabetes mellitus.

TREATMENT

Management of diabetes consists of a group effort by health-care providers concentrating on setting a goal, diet and exercise modification, smoking session, medications, self glucose monitoring, monitoring for complications of diabetes, and intermittent laboratory assessment and feedback. Although glycemic control is important, blood pressure and cholesterol monitoring should not be overlooked.

Pharmacologic management of diabetes mellitus (DM) consists of oral hypoglycemic agents (type 2 DM), insulin and insulin analogs (types 1, 2, and 4 DM), and insulin pumps (type 1 DM). Oral hypoglycemic agents decrease plasma glucose by various mechanisms. Sulfonylureas (glipizide, Glyburide) and meglitinides (repaglinide, nateglinide) stimulate the production of insulin by the pancreas. Glucophage (metformin, biguanides) decreases hepatic glucose production by inhibiting gluconeogenesis and glycogenolysis. α-Glycosidase inhibitors (acarbose), which are rarely used due to the high incidence of flatulence and abdominal discomfort, prevent carbohydrate absorption from the intestinal tract. Thiazolidinediones (TZDs) (pioglitazone [Actos] and rosiglitazone [Avandia]) stimulate target cells' response to insulin. There might be a higher risk of bladder cancer in patients taking pioglitazone (Actos) and of myocardial infarction in patients taking rosiglitazone (Avandia). Glucagon-like peptide (GLP-1) agonists (exenatide, liraglutide) stimulate glucose-dependent insulin secretion, decrease glucagon secretion, slow gastric motility, and induce early satiety. Dipeptidyl peptidase-4 inhibitors (DPP-4; sitagliptin, saxagliptin, linagliptin) slow degradation of GLP-1.

Current insulin formulations in the United States are biosynthetic, generated from human DNA since 1983. The traditional method of producing insulin by mashing pork or beef pancreas was introduced in the 1920s. In July 2005, the manufacturing company announced discontinuation of animal-based insulin production. However, it continues to be available in other countries.

For patients with type 2 DM, those with an HbA$_{1C}$ of 6.5 to 7.5 should be on monotherapy; those whose HbA$_{1c}$ is 7.6 to 9 should be on dual therapy; and those whose HbA$_{1c}$ is above 9 and who are symptomatic should be treated with insulin (asymptomatic could be treated with triple therapy). The insulin preparation may be rapid acting (e.g., lispro, glulisine, aspart insulin), short acting (regular insulin), intermediate acting (NPH), long acting (glargine, insulin detemir), or ultra long acting (degludec [awaiting approval by the FDA]).

Table 15-7	Some Commonly Available Insulin Preparations		
Preparation	**Onset**	**Peak Effect**	**Duration of Action**
Lispro (Humalog)	5 min to 0.25 hr	0.5-1 hr	2-4 hr
NovoLog	5 min to 0.25 hr	0.5-1 hr	2-4 hr
Regular insulin (Humulin R, Novolin R)	0.5 hr	2-5 hr	8-12 hr
NPH (Humulin N, Novolin N)	1-2.5 hr	8-14 hr	16-24 hr
Lente	1-2.5 hr	8-12 hr	16-24 hr
Protamine zinc (Ultralente)	4-6 hr	10-18 hr	>32 hr
Glargine (Lantus)	2-3 hr	7-12 hr	24-48 hr

Short-acting and rapid-acting insulin also may be prescribed for administration by the intravenous route. Table 15-7 provides a summary of some currently available insulin preparations.

The perioperative management of patients with diabetes is variable, depending on the type of diabetes, underlying pathologies, and the severity and extent of the anticipated procedure. An understanding of the acute and chronic complications of diabetes, along with a preemptive strategy, produces a successful outcome. The operation should be scheduled early in the morning. Generally, oral hypoglycemic agents are stopped the day before surgery. Short-acting insulin medications should be avoided on the morning of surgery to prevent dangerous hypoglycemia. For short ambulatory procedures, long-acting insulin preparations (e.g., glargine) may be continued. For major procedures requiring hospital admission, cessation of the long-acting insulin 1 to 2 days before surgery and administration of a short-acting insulin may be advocated.

Traditionally, when diabetes was discussed, the term "treatment" was not advocated, because the underlying disease was not altered with any of these medications. In 2000, clinical trials on islet cell transplantation showed promising results. Multiple cadaveric islets were prepared and transplanted into the recipient's liver. In the same year, Shapiro and associates studied seven patients who had received islet cell transplants; they found a success rate of 100%, with total independence from exogenous insulin.

The current patient was scheduled for extraction of the left and right mandibular and maxillary third molars using intravenous sedation. He was instructed to take nothing by mouth after midnight and was scheduled for an early morning appointment. He was instructed to continue taking glargine but to withhold lispro insulin in the morning.

On the morning of surgery, the patient appeared to be jittery and nervous. His skin was slightly clammy, and his palms were sweaty (sympathetic response to hypoglycemia).

He was found to be tachycardic (heart rate 120 bpm), and his blood pressure was 120/80 mm Hg. On placement of the intravenous catheter, the patient became less responsive (neurologic effect of hypoglycemia). Based on the patient's history and the clinical observations, a diagnosis of hypoglycemia was made and 1 ampule of 50% (25 g) dextrose was administered. A simultaneous Accu-Chek reading confirmed a blood glucose level of 55 mg/dl (hypoglycemia). Within minutes, the patient became more responsive and the heart rate decreased to 80 bpm. Retrospectively, it was found that the patient had misunderstood the preoperative instructions and, although he had refrained from breakfast in the morning, he had continued his routine insulin injections just before arriving at the office. The surgery was completed without any perioperative complications.

COMPLICATIONS

The complications of diabetes mellitus can be divided into acute and chronic categories. Acute complications primarily include diabetic ketoacidosis (discussed in the section, Diabetic Ketoacidosis), nonketotic hyperosmolar syndrome, and hypoglycemia. Chronic complications are predominantly related to the long-term effects of hyperglycemia on the vasculature and can be divided into microvascular retinopathy (nonproliferative, also known as *preproliferative,* and proliferative), nephropathy, neuropathy (peripheral distal symmetric polyneuropathy, autonomic neuropathy, proximal painful motor neuropathy, and cranial mononeuropathy), and macrovascular disease (accelerated atherosclerosis, coronary artery disease, myocardial infarction, and peripheral vascular disease). Although tight glycemic control has been shown to improve microvascular disease (Diabetic Clinical Control Trial), its role in macrovascular disease remains controversial. The United Kingdom Prospective Diabetes Study (UKPDS) indicated no benefits, but a follow-up study showed some improvement. There is no doubt that macrovascular disease may be improved with control of lipid levels and blood pressure, smoking cessation, and aspirin therapy.

The symptoms of hypoglycemia may be confused with those of cerebrovascular events, vasovagal syndrome, or a variety of disorders considered in the differential diagnosis of a delirious patient (hypoxia, infection, metabolic abnormalities, myocardial infarction, and medication overdose and withdrawal). Hypoglycemia is defined as a blood glucose level below 60 mg/dl. The symptoms may be divided into those that are neurologic and those that are secondary to increased adrenergic (sympathetic) outflow. Neurologic symptoms consist of visual disturbances, paresthesias, lethargy, irritability, delirium, confusion, seizures, and coma. Adrenergic symptoms consist of nausea, anxiety, weakness, sweating, and tremors. In a previously undiagnosed patient, the differential diagnosis should include primary or secondary hyperinsulinemia (insulinoma). Other important considerations include sepsis, malnutrition, and liver failure. The most common reason for hypoglycemia in a diabetic patient is insulin mismanagement. Patients with renal failure are more prone to hypoglycemia, because a small fraction of gluconeogenesis is conducted by the kidneys. Treatment of hypoglycemia in an awake patient consists of oral glucose administration (e.g., orange juice). If intravenous access is available, dextrose 10% or 50% in water (D10W or D50W) is acceptable. In the unconscious patient with no intravenous access, 1 mg of glucagon IM/SC can be administered. Diazoxide, octreotide, and hydrocortisone are other alternatives. Diabetic ketoacidosis and nonketotic hyperosmolar coma are discussed elsewhere in this book. It is important to treat any suspicion of hypoglycemia rapidly, because hyperglycemia in a misdiagnosed patient does not have any immediate emergent complications; however, untreated undiagnosed hypoglycemia may be devastating.

It is commonly known that patients with diabetes mellitus are more susceptible to infections. It is thought that various steps in neutrophil function are altered, including leukocyte adherence, chemotaxis, and phagocytosis. The antioxidants, which are involved in the bactericidal activity, may also be altered. The defects in neutrophil function are at least partially reversible by strict glycemic control (blood glucose between 80 and 110 mg/dl). However, it is hypothesized that the pathophysiology of the immunologic defects in diabetes mellitus is not exclusively related to glycemic control.

DISCUSSION

Diabetes mellitus is a prevalent and destructive endocrine disorder that may affect any organ in the body. More than 366 million people are affected worldwide. In the United States, approximately 26 million people have diabetes, and 79 million are prediabetic, according to the Centers for Disease Control and Prevention (CDC). Diabetes is the leading cause of blindness, nontraumatic leg amputation, and end-stage renal disease. It is also implicated as a risk factor in cardiac, cerebral, and vascular disease processes. The most common type, non-ketone-induced diabetes mellitus, is on the rise, correlating with the increased incidence of obesity in the United States. In 2001 Mokdad and colleagues randomly selected a cohort of 200,000 adult patients; they observed the prevalence of diabetes to be 7.9%, an increase from 7.3% in 2000. The prevalence of obesity, defined as a body mass index greater than 30 kg/m^2, was 20.9%, an increase of 5.6% from the previous year.

Insulin is an anabolic hormone produced by the β-cells of the pancreas. Its production is stimulated by elevated blood glucose, causing the subsequent effects of glucose uptake by cells, promotion of triglyceride synthesis and storage, inhibition of ketogenesis, activation of various enzymes (e.g., glycogen synthase, HMG-CoA reductase, lipid lipases), and inhibition of catabolic pathways, such as gluconeogenesis and ketogenesis (Figure 15-6). The counterregulatory hormones are cortisol, epinephrine, growth hormone, and glycogen. The hyperglycemia seen in diabetes is not only due to the lack of insulin, but also to the imbalance between insulin and its counterregulatory hormones.

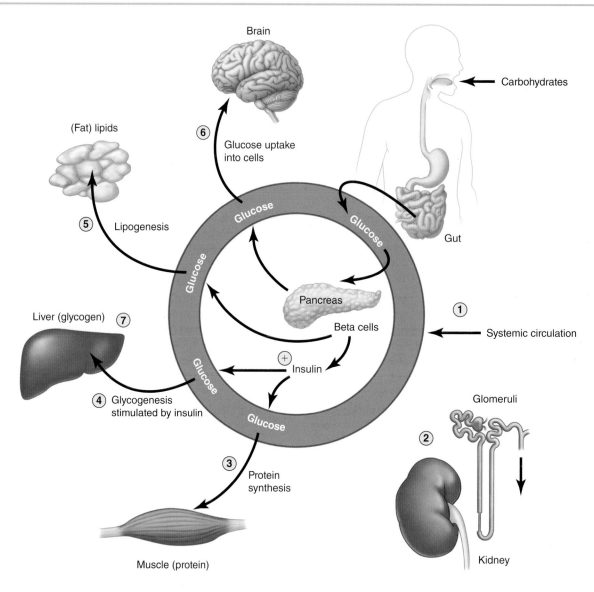

In the absence of insulin:

1. Blood glucose increases
2. Glucose spills out into the urine
   (osmotic diuresis causing dehydration)
3. Decreased protein synthesis (catabolism)
4. Increased gluconeogenesis and decreased glycogenesis
   further increasing plasma glucose

5. Lipid breakdown (lipolysis)
6. The brain cells cannot uptake glucose, and instead
   use ketones
7. Increased ketones (ketogenesis) causes ketoacidosis

Figure 15-6 The actions of insulin.

Diabetes is a disorder resulting from deficiency or defects in insulin action. The pathophysiology is related to four main etiologies: (1) defects in production (type 1 diabetes, juvenile-onset diabetes, ketoacidosis-prone diabetics), (2) defects at the site of action (type 2 diabetes, adult-onset diabetes, non-ketoacidosis-prone diabetics), (3) a consequence of another disease (type 3, or secondary, diabetes, including a wide variety of diseases such as Cushing's disease, hemochromatosis, and cystic fibrosis), and (4) gestational diabetes (type 4). The distinction among classifications has been blurred recently, because the pediatric population with type 2 diabetes is increasing, and patients with type 2 diabetes are being treated with exogenous insulin. A serum insulin or C-peptide level below 0.6 ng/ml suggests type 1 DM, whereas a level above 1 ng/ml suggests type 2 DM.

Symptoms of diabetes, although unique, are variable in onset of presentation, based on the type of diabetes. Type 1 diabetes mellitus commonly presents with acute symptoms, whereas type 2 diabetes mellitus may go undiagnosed for many years. Presenting symptoms of type 3 diabetes are variable, based on the primary disease. Women with type 4 diabetes usually present at 24 to 28 weeks of gestation due to elevation of prolactin-related peptide. Regardless of the diabetic subtype, symptoms consist of polyuria, weight loss, increased appetite, fatigue, blurred vision, and thirst. Postprandial hyperglycemia develops early, and the fasting blood glucose level eventually rises. The initial diagnosis is often made due to symptoms arising from oral or vaginal candidiasis and diabetic ketoacidosis.

Patients with impaired fasting glucose are more prone to develop type 2 diabetes than is the general population. Other risk factors for developing type 2 diabetes consist of age over 45 years, a family history of type 2 diabetes, racial predisposition (Hispanic, Native American, African American), hypertension and dyslipidemia, and a history of gestational diabetes or polycystic ovarian disease. Type 1 diabetes is more common in Caucasian and least common in Asian populations. Diabetes is diagnosed when the fasting blood glucose level exceeds 126 mg/dl; a random blood glucose level is greater than 200 mg/dl with polydipsia, polyuria (when serum the blood glucose level exceeds the threshold of 240 mg/dl), polyphagia, weight loss, and hyperglycemic crisis; a 2-hour postprandial blood glucose level is greater than 200 mg/dl after consumption of an oral glucose load of 75 g; or when the HbA_{1C} is 6.5% or higher. Prediabetic patients have a 2-hour postprandial glucose tolerance of 140 to 200 mg/dl or a fasting blood glucose level of 100 to 125 mg/dl. An individual has metabolic syndrome if he or she has three of the following conditions:

- Elevated triglycerides
- Low high-density lipoprotein
- Abdominal obesity
- Fasting glucose level of 100 mg/dl or higher
- Hypertension

Diabetes is a costly disease, and until recently only symptomatic treatment was available. A patient's compliance with daily injections and diabetic diets is frequently difficult to control, especially in an unmotivated patient. Islet cell transplantation for type 1 diabetes shows promise, providing an alternative with the potential for more definitive treatment.

Bibliography

Diabetes Control and Complications Trial Research Group: The effect of intensive treatment of diabetes on the development and progression of long-term complications in insulin-dependent diabetes mellitus, *N Engl J Med* 329(14):977-986, 1993.

International Diabetes Foundation: One adult in ten will have diabetes by 2030. Available at: http://www.idf.org/media-events/press-releases/2011/diabetes. Accessed February 27, 2013.

Joshi N, Caputo GM, Weitekamp MR, et al: Infections in patients with diabetes mellitus, *N Engl J Med* 341:1906-1912, 1999.

Marks JB: Perioperative management of diabetes, *Am Fam Physician* 67:93-100, 2003.

Mayfield J: Diagnosis and classification of diabetes mellitus: new criteria, *Am Fam Physician* 58:1355-1362, 1998.

Mokdad AH, Ford ES, Bowman BA, et al: Prevalence of obesity, diabetes and obesity related health risk factors, *JAMA* 298:76-79, 2003.

Rehman J, Mohammed K: Perioperative management of diabetic patients, *Curr Surg* 60:607-611, 2003.

Robertson PR: Islet transplantation as a treatment for diabetes: a work in progress, *N Engl J Med* 350:694-705, 2004.

Shapiro AMJ, Lakey JRT, Ryan EA, et al: Islet transplantation in seven patients with type 1 diabetes mellitus using a glucocorticoid-free immunosuppressive regimen, *N Engl J Med* 343:230-238, 2000.

UK Prospective Diabetes Study (UKPDS) Group: Intensive blood-glucose control with sulphonylureas or insulin compared with conventional treatment and risk of complications in patients with type 2 diabetes (UKPDS 33), *Lancet* 352(9131):837-853, 1998.

US Department of Health and Human Services/Centers for Disease Control and Prevention: National diabetes fact sheet: national estimates and general information on diabetes and prediabetes in the United States, 2011. Available at: http://www.cdc.gov/diabetes/pubs/pdf/ndfs_2011.pdf. Accessed February 27, 2013.

Diabetic Ketoacidosis

Mehran Mehrabi and Shahrokh C. Bagheri

CC

A 17-year-old diabetic female presents to the oral and maxillofacial surgery clinic 5 days after extraction of her four third molars. She complains of "nausea and vomiting."

HPI

The patient reports a history of poor oral intake and frequent emesis (vomiting) for the past 3 days. She has been feeling progressively more fatigued, with general malaise (secondary to dehydration). Because she has not been able to eat or drink regularly, she decided to discontinue all her insulin injections (lack of insulin is the key etiology in the development of diabetic ketoacidosis).

She also complains of blurry vision (secondary to volume depletion), vague abdominal pain (metabolic acidosis results in gastric distention and blockage, and β-hydroxybutyrate induces vomiting), cramping in her extremities (secondary to hypokalemia and dehydration commonly associated with diabetic ketoacidosis), an elevated temperature (secondary to development of infection and dehydration), and swelling of the left mandible that has progressively exacerbated over the past 48 hours. She reported an increase in the frequency of urination (polyuria) in the first few postoperative days but has not voided for the past day (initial osmotic diuresis causing dehydration). At first her mother was not concerned about a developing infection, because the patient's breath actually smelled "fruity" (acetone breath odor secondary to elevated plasma ketones). However, she became anxious when her daughter appeared progressively sleepy (stupor and coma can be caused by rapid increases in blood osmolarity, which cause water to be drawn out of the central nervous system, resulting in cellular dehydration and changes in consciousness). The on-call surgeon was contacted the night before and attributed the nausea and vomiting to excessive narcotic intake. The swelling was assessed via telephone to appropriately correspond to postsurgical edema. The patient was prescribed promethazine and advised to see the treating surgeon the next day. (Any suspicion of diabetic ketoacidosis should prompt evaluation in the emergency department as soon as possible. Unrecognized diabetic ketoacidosis can be deleterious.)

PMHX/PDHX/MEDICATIONS/ALLERGIES/SH/FH

The patient was diagnosed with diabetes mellitus type 1 at age 14. She takes regular insulin (short-acting insulin) and NPH (intermediate-acting insulin) twice a day under the care of an endocrinologist. She denies the use of alcohol, tobacco, or recreational drugs.

EXAMINATION

General. The patient is an intermittently nonresponsive girl who does not follow commands (altered mental status). She is breathing without obstruction, but it is deep and slow (Kussmaul breathing, partial respiratory compensation for metabolic acidosis).

Vital signs. Blood pressure is 101/50 mm Hg (hypotension), heart rate 114 bpm (tachycardia), respirations 8 per minute, and temperature 38.8°C (febrile).

Orthostatic. When the patient rises from a supine to a standing position, the heart rate increases to 140 bpm and the blood pressure decreases to 80/40 mm Hg (a rise in heart rate greater than 30 bpm and/or a decrease in systolic blood pressure by more than 20 mg/dl or in diastolic blood pressure by more than 10 mg/dl is an indication of severe volume depletion).

Maxillofacial. The patient has significant tenderness (dolor), edema (tumor), and erythema (rubor) of the left lower face, and her face is warm (calor) to the touch (these are the cardinal signs of inflammation). Fluctuance is palpated over the angle of the mandible. She is unable to open her mouth more than 10 mm (trismus, suggestive of masticator space infection). The patient is able to maintain her secretions (drooling would be indicative of significant oropharyngeal swelling or dysphagia).

Intraoral. Purulence is noted around the extraction socket of the left mandibular third molar, with surrounding gingival edema and erythema. The floor of the mouth is soft and is not raised. There is moderate swelling of the left lateral pharyngeal wall, with slight deviation of the uvula (indicative of left lateral pharyngeal spread of infection).

Cardiovascular. The patient has sinus tachycardia with intermittent pause, which correlates with premature ventricular contractions (electrolyte abnormalities, such as hyperkalemia, result in abnormal heart rhythms).

Pulmonary. Chest is bilaterally clear on auscultation with deep breathing.

Abdominal. Generalized pain on palpation, but otherwise nontender and nondistended.

IMAGING

A panoramic radiograph and a CT scan of the head and neck may be indicated to evaluate the spread of infection in the parapharyngeal and masticator spaces and for evaluation of the airway. In patients with compromised renal function, as determined by an elevated creatinine level, contrast CT is contraindicated. Noncontrast CT, although less useful for demonstrating soft tissue spread of infection, can still be of value.

CT/MRI

There should be a low threshold for ordering CT or MRI scans to search for brain edema, particularly in pediatric patients with altered mental status.

LABS

A full set of laboratory studies (complete blood count, electrolytes, and urinalysis) is essential in the management of diabetic ketoacidosis (DKA). DKA patients have a serum ketone concentration greater than 5 mEq/L. Ketones consist of acetoacetate, β-hydroxybutyrate, and acetone. The following laboratory study results also were obtained for the current patient:

- *Hemogram:* White blood cell count of 18.2 cells/μl with a differential of 70% neutrophils, 20% bands, 8% lymphocytes, 1% monocytes, and 1% eosinophils (elevated neutrophil count is indicative of acute inflammation); hemoglobin and hematocrit of 15 mg/dl and 45%, respectively (volume depletion results in overestimation of the hemoglobin and hematocrit); platelet count within normal limits
- *Basic metabolic panel:* Na^+ 130 mEq/dl (hyperglycemia induces an intracellular movement of sodium); K^+ 6.5 mEq/dl (elevated secondary to acidosis causing transcellular shift of K^+ into the extracellular space in exchange for H^+ ions); Cl^- 95 mEq/dl (normal chloride is consistent with an anion gap metabolic acidosis), bicarbonate 10 mEq/dl (a low bicarbonate level is indicative of metabolic acidosis), blood urea nitrogen 60 mEq/dl, creatinine 3 mEq/dl (blood urea nitrogen and creatinine are both elevated secondary to decreased intravascular volume [prerenal azotemia]), glucose 550 mg/dl (primarily secondary to the lack of insulin)
- *Arterial blood gas analysis:* pH 7.1, Pco_2 25 mm Hg, Po_2 90 mm Hg on Fio_2 of 40%. (A pH of 7.1 is a strong acidemia. These findings, along with a low Pco_2, are indicative of metabolic acidosis with respiratory compensation.)
- *Urine analysis:* Positive ketones, +3 glucosuria (the proximal convoluted tubules' ability to reabsorb glucose is maximized at a blood glucose of 180 to 200 mg/dl, after which glucose is spilled into the urine, causing osmotic diuresis); +2 proteinuria (glomeruli damage in diabetic nephropathy results in protein wasting and nephrotic syndrome; microproteinuria is indicative of

diabetic nephropathy and may be avoided or delayed by daily intake of angiotensin-converting enzyme [ACE] inhibitors)
- *Urine dip stick test:* +4 for nitroprusside (indicative of acetoacetate and acetone [ketones] in the urine). Rarely, urine ketone is negative. Although the predominant ketone in severe DKA is β-hydroxybutyrate, a urine dip stick cannot test for it. As the clinical condition improves, the urine dip stick may change from negative to positive as acetoacetate predominates.

Electrocardiogram

The electrocardiogram shows widened QRS complexes and peaked T waves (secondary to hyperkalemia) and occasional premature ventricular contractions.

ASSESSMENT

Diabetic ketoacidosis secondary to parapharyngeal and masticator space infection (infection is the leading cause of diabetic ketoacidosis).

TREATMENT

Treatment generally begins with assessment of the ABCs—airway, breathing, and circulation. Intravenous fluid is the first line of treatment; start with normal saline and subsequently switch to D5½NS (5% dextrose in 0.45% normal saline). This addresses dehydration and decreases the plasma glucose level by dilution. Any indication of cardiac instability (peaked T waves, wide QRS complexes, and premature ventricular contractions) due to hyperkalemia should be treated first with calcium gluconate. This is followed by an intravenous insulin drip to gradually decrease serum glucose and osmolarity (osmoles of solute per liter of solution). The difference between the measured osmolarity and calculated osmolarity (2Na + Glucose/18 + Blood urea nitrogen/2.8 + Ethanol/4.6) is called the *osmolal gap;* this would be elevated due to the high ketones or other anions (which are unmeasured anions and therefore the cause of an anion gap metabolic acidosis). A rapid reduction in osmolarity results in cerebral edema and should be avoided. Glucose is decreased at about 100 mg/dl/ per hour. A rapid reduction in glucose stimulates the counter-regulatory hormones and hence ketone production. The combination of hydration and insulin decreases potassium. Urine output is carefully monitored for evaluation of fluid status. With correction of acidosis, the serum potassium may precipitously decrease, requiring careful monitoring and supplementation (insulin causes transfer of hydrogen ions from the extracellular space to the intracellular space). Other electrolytes to consider are magnesium and phosphate, both of which may need to be replenished. Patients commonly have deficiencies of the B-complex vitamins (due to malnutrition), particularly thiamine, which should be corrected. Bicarbonate is rarely recommended for the treatment of acidosis (high risk for development of cerebral edema). It is generally reserved for patients with a pH below 7.0.

The current patient was admitted to the hospital and started on intravenous normal saline. Calcium gluconate was administered to maintain cardiac stability. The patient was started on a regular insulin drip, with frequent blood glucose checks to adjust the dose. The potassium level was evaluated intermittently and supplemented as needed. When the blood glucose level dropped below 200 mg/dl, dextrose supplementation was used to prevent dangerous hypoglycemia. The insulin drip was continued until resolution of the metabolic acidosis. Diagnostically, venous blood gas analysis may be just as valuable as arterial blood gas analysis and may be used to reduce arterial complications. The patient was empirically started on ampicillin-sulbactam (combination of β-lactam and β-lactamase inhibitor) and was taken to the operating room for surgical drainage of the lesion. The intravenous fluid was changed to D5½NS when the patient was deemed hemodynamically stable. Urine output improved, metabolic acidosis and pseudohyperkalemia (elevated plasma potassium despite total body depletion secondary to shift of potassium from the intracellular space due to high H^+ concentration) resolved, and the patient was transferred to the ward. An American Diabetic Association 1,800-kcal diet was initiated. The patient remained afebrile, with normalization of her white blood cell count, electrolytes, and urine analysis. She was subsequently discharged to home care on a 10-day regimen of amoxicillin with clavulanic acid.

COMPLICATIONS

Complications of diabetes can be divided into acute and chronic. The acute complications include hypoglycemia (see the Diabetes Mellitus section), diabetic ketoacidosis, and hyperosmolar hyperglycemic syndrome. Chronic complications include microvascular and macrovascular disease (see the Diabetes Mellitus section). Patients with diabetic ketoacidosis generally present with metabolic acidosis and a blood glucose level below 500 mg/dl, whereas patients with nonketotic hyperglycemia coma present with a blood glucose level above 1,000 mg/dl with no acidosis. The pathophysiology of both disorders is related to the physiologic response to stress. Acute insulin deficiency (due to lack of compliance, pump blockage, brittle diabetes), infection (the most common cause of diabetic ketoacidosis), trauma, ischemia (cerebrovascular accident, myocardial infarction), or volume depletion can induce signals to increase catecholamines, cortisol, growth hormone, and glucagon (insulin counterregulatory hormones that increase gluconeogenesis), resulting in an imbalance of glucose metabolism. These stress hormones increase blood glucose and osmolarity while decreasing cellular insulin. The lack of insulin results in ketone production by the liver and the development of an anion gap metabolic acidosis. Diabetic ketoacidosis also presents with nausea, vomiting, abdominal pain, polyuria, polydipsia, weight loss, diplopia, delirium, or coma. Objective laboratory studies reveal a metabolic acidosis, pseudohyperkalemia, glucosuria, and both serum and urine β-hydroxybutyrate and acetoacetate (ketones). Due to the rapid onset of acidosis and good renal clearance in younger patients with type 1 diabetes, the blood glucose level rarely exceeds 800 mg/dl.

Diabetic ketoacidosis is the most commonly observed acute complication of type 1 diabetes. Patients with type 2 diabetes may also develop diabetic ketoacidosis, but it is not common. The second most common cause of diabetic ketoacidosis is patient noncompliance with insulin.

DISCUSSION

The diagnosis of diabetic ketoacidosis is based on the history, clinical examination, and laboratory findings. This disease arises from a relative or an absolute deficiency of insulin and an increase in the counterregulatory hormones, resulting in gluconeogenesis, glycogenolysis, and lipolysis. The work-up should included the serum glucose and electrolyte levels; anion gap; blood urea nitrogen; creatinine; urinalysis, including ketones; electrocardiogram; complete blood count; arterial blood gas analysis; HbA_{1c} levels; and any tests required to determine the underlying cause.

The differential diagnosis of a patient with ketosis also includes alcoholism and starvation, but only diabetic ketoacidosis presents with hyperglycemia. The excess anions (ketones) in diabetic ketoacidosis cause an anion gap metabolic acidosis (gap acidosis) (see the Diabetes Mellitus section). The differential diagnosis includes methanol toxicity, uremia, diabetic ketoacidosis, paraldehyde ingestion, isoniazid toxicity, isopropyl alcohol toxicity, lactic acidosis, ethylene glycol toxicity, and salicylate toxicity. However, only diabetic ketoacidosis produces hyperglycemia. The symptoms of diabetic ketoacidosis can arise rapidly (within 24 hours), manifesting as polyuria, polyphagia, polydipsia, weakness, and fatigue, in addition to nausea, vomiting, and vague abdominal pain. Mental status may range from normal to profound coma. As dehydration becomes pronounced, the hypovolemic polyuria is not as prominent.

The differential diagnosis for hyperglycemia should include dawn and Somogyi phenomena. Dawn phenomenon results from a natural nocturnal rise in counterregulatory hormones (cortisol and growth hormone). The Somogyi effect results from a rise in nocturnal counterregulatory hormones due to midsleep hypoglycemia. Therefore, both the dawn and Somogyi phenomena result in hyperglycemia due to a rise in counterregulatory hormones. The difference is that the dawn phenomenon is a natural nocturnal rise in hormones, whereas the Somogyi effect is due to a rebound from hypoglycemia.

Acidosis results in a shift of potassium ions from the intracellular to the extracellular compartments. This causes elevation of the plasma potassium concentration. However, with the glucose-driven osmotic diuresis, potassium is excreted by the kidneys, causing depletion of total body potassium despite elevated plasma levels; hence the term *pseudohyperkalemia* (seen in more than one third of patients with diabetic ketoacidosis). With the correction of acidosis, the extracellular potassium shifts back to the intracellular space, causing significant lowering of plasma potassium. The plasma potassium needs to be replaced as the acidosis is corrected to avoid life-threatening hypokalemia.

Another acute complication of diabetes is hyperosmolar hyperglycemic syndrome, which has a less insidious onset than diabetic ketoacidosis. It generally begins with mild hyperglycemia, which is compensated by glycosuria. As hyperglycemia worsens, osmotic diuresis wastes more glucose through urine. If the patient maintains adequate hydration, the kidneys continue to excrete the excess glucose. As the patient becomes confused or incapacitated, oral hydration decreases, and the kidneys' ability to excrete glucose is diminished, exacerbating the hyperglycemia and causing mental status changes. During treatment, the plasma glucose level should be reduced no faster than 75 to 100 mg/dl/hour. A more rapid decline could cause brain edema.

Bibliography

Abramson E, Arky R: Diabetic acidosis with initial hypokalemia, *JAMA* 196:401-403, 1966.

Adrogue HJ, Lederer ED, Suski WN, et al: Determinants of plasma potassium levels in diabetic ketoacidosis, *Medicine* 65:163-172, 1986.

Adrogue HJ, Madias N: Management of life-threatening acid-base disorder. I, *N Engl J Med* 338:26-34, 1998.

Arora S, Henderson SO, Long T, et al: Diagnostic accuracy of point-of-care testing for diabetic ketoacidosis at emergency-department triage: β-hydroxybutyrate versus the urine dipstick, *Diabetes Care* 34(4):852-854, 2011.

Chiasson J, Aris-jilwan N, Belanger R, et al: Diagnosis and treatment of diabetic ketoacidosis and hyperglycemic hyperosmolar state, *CMAJ* 168:859-866, 2003.

Fulop M, Tannenbaum H, Dreyer N: Ketotic hyperosmolar coma, *Lancet* 2:635-639, 1973.

Herrington WG, Nye HJ, Hammersley MS, et al: Are arterial and venous samples clinically equivalent for the estimation of pH, serum bicarbonate and potassium concentration in critically ill patients? *Diabet Med* 29(1):32-35, 2012.

Jerums G, MacIsaac RJ: Treatment of microalbuminuria in patients with type 2 diabetes mellitus, *Treat Endocrinol* 1:163-173, 2002.

Joint British Diabetes Societies Inpatient Care Group: The management of diabetic ketoacidosis in adults. March 2010. Available at: http://www.diabetes.nhs.uk. Accessed October 17, 2012.

Kitabchi AE, Umpierrez GE, Murphy MB, et al: Hyperglycemic crises in patients with diabetes mellitus, *Diabetes Care* 26(Suppl 1):S109-S117, 2003.

Kreisberg RA: Diabetic ketoacidosis: new concepts and trends in pathogenesis and treatment, *Ann Intern Med* 88:681-695, 1978.

Matz R: Management of the hyperosmolar hyperglycemic syndrome, *Am Fam Physician* 60:1468-1476, 1999.

Narins RG, Cohen JJ: Bicarbonate therapy for organic acidosis: the case for its continued use, *Ann Intern Med* 106:615, 1987.

Page MM, Alberti KG, Greenwood R, et al: Treatment of diabetic coma with continuous low-dose insulin infusion, *Br Med J* 2:687-690, 1974.

Trachtenbarg DE: Diabetic ketoacidosis, *Am Fam Physician* 71:1705-1714, 2005.

Umpierrez G, Greire AX: Abdominal pain in patients with hyperglycemic crisis, *J Crit Care* 17:63-67, 2002.

Acute Myocardial Infarction

Ali R. Rahimi, Joyce T. Lee, and Shahrokh C. Bagheri

CC

A 57-year-old man with a history of hypertension, coronary artery disease, and hypercholesterolemia is referred to your office for evaluation of a biopsy-proved mandibular dentigerous cyst.

The perioperative cardiovascular risk assessment includes recognition of risk factors such as a history of ischemic heart disease, a history of compensated or prior heart failure, a history of cerebrovascular disease, diabetes mellitus, and renal insufficiency (preoperative serum creatinine level greater than 2 mg/dl).

HPI

The patient is diagnosed with a small dentigerous cyst of the posterior mandible.

The preoperative assessment includes inquiry into the patient's cardiovascular system review. This includes any history of chest pain, dyspnea, orthopnea (inability to sleep or lie prone without becoming short of breath), paroxysmal nocturnal dyspnea (spontaneous shortness of breath during sleep periods), pedal edema, palpitations, presyncope, or syncope. Positive symptoms or recent significant health events are indicators for additional preoperative questioning and testing. In addition, the patient's metabolic equivalent of task levels (METs) in performing daily activities is necessary to ascertain functional capacity. Typically, METs of 4 or higher (climbing a flight of stairs or walking up a hill), in the absence of cardiac complaints, precludes the need for cardiac stress testing for non-high-risk surgeries.

Risk assessment is not exclusively for patients with known cardiac disease, because a significant number of patients have undiagnosed heart disease. The guidelines published by the American College of Cardiology/American Heart Association outline the algorithm for cardiovascular risk assessment in individuals undergoing noncardiac surgery.

The current patient denies any cardiovascular complaints, including chest pain, shortness of breath, and dyspnea on exertion. He reports that he is able to climb a flight of stairs without difficulty (MET greater than 4).

PMHX/PDHX/MEDICATIONS/ALLERGIES/SH/FH

The patient has a history of hypertension, coronary artery disease, and hypercholesterolemia, for which he has been taking medications for the past 15 years (the two major types of angina are stable angina, which occurs with exertion, and unstable angina, which occurs at rest). He denies any history of previous myocardial infarction, cerebrovascular accident, or recent hospitalization (with a history of coronary artery disease, formal recommendations should be sought from the patient's cardiologist regarding the holding of any antiplatelet therapy during the perioperative period). The patient's last physical examination was several months ago, when a number of minor adjustments were made to his medications. His past surgical history includes an appendectomy and cholecystectomy under general anesthesia without any perioperative complications (a positive history of adverse events with anesthesia is significant in assessing the future risk of surgery under general anesthesia). His medications include atenolol (β-blocker), lisinopril (angiotensin-converting enzyme [ACE] inhibitor), atorvastatin (HMG-CoA reductase inhibitor, a cholesterol-lowering medication), and aspirin. He has smoked one pack of cigarettes per day for the past 20 years and admits to a sedentary lifestyle. He has no symptoms of depression (depression is a common comorbid condition in patients with CAD and a well-documented risk factor for recurrent cardiac events and mortality). His family history is significant for the death of his father at age 50 from a massive acute myocardial infarction (AMI).

EXAMINATION

General. The patient is a moderately obese man in no distress.

Vitals. Normal except for a baseline blood pressure of 155/88 mm Hg (stage I hypertension).

Maxillofacial. Minimal expansion of the buccal cortex of the left posterior mandible is noted.

Cardiovascular

- *Inspection:* The chest wall appears normal. The point of maximum impulse is located at the normal position along the midclavicular line at the fifth intercostal space.
- *Auscultation:* No audible bruits are heard using the bell of the stethoscope. This portion of the examination includes auscultation for bruits at the neck (carotid), mid-abdomen (aorta), and lateral flanks (renal). (Audible bruits would be indicative of significant atherosclerotic plaques, suggestive of systemic atherosclerosis.)
- Auscultation of the heart reveals a regular rate and rhythm, no murmurs, normal S1 and S2 with no S3

or S4 noted (S3 is caused by left ventricular volume overloading or dilation, as is present in heart failure; S4 is caused by poor compliance and stiffness of the left ventricles).

- *Jugular venous pressure:* Within normal limits at 3 cm above the sternal angle. (Jugular venous distention is a sign of venous hypertension, most commonly secondary to right-sided heart failure.)
- *Peripheral pulses and extremities:* No edema of the extremities (a sign of heart failure) or clubbing of the nail beds (seen with chronic pulmonary disease). (The peripheral pulses are inspected for symmetry and strength [pulsus alternans denotes an alternating strong and weak pulse and may signify left ventricular heart failure]).
- *Fundoscopic exam:* Bilateral retinal plaques (secondary to atherosclerosis) and arteriovenous nicking (secondary to hypertension). (Examination of the retina is an important part of a complete cardiovascular examination, because it allows direct visualization of the microvasculature.)

Pulmonary. The chest is bilaterally clear on auscultation. (With left-sided heart failure, blood backs into the pulmonary circulation, causing "congestion" and the leakage of fluid from the pulmonary capillaries into the interstitium; this leads to pulmonary edema ["wet lung"], which is detected as rales or crackles on auscultation of the lungs.)

IMAGING

Other than a panoramic radiograph, no other routine radiographic imaging studies are indicated for excision of a cyst under intravenous sedation. A preoperative chest radiograph may be obtained in select patients based on the history and physical examination findings.

In the current patient, the panoramic radiograph demonstrated a 2×2-cm unilocular radiolucency of the posterior mandible, consistent with a dentigerous cyst.

LABS/TESTS

The preoperative laboratory tests for the evaluation of a patient with significant cardiovascular disease should be done in conjunction with the treating primary care doctor and/or cardiologist.

A variety of stress tests, in conjunction with electrocardiographic monitoring, may be performed to further risk-stratify higher risk patients undergoing intermediate to high-risk surgery. The cardiovascular system is tested, or "stressed," either with physical activity (walking on a treadmill) or pharmacologically using sympathomimetic agents (e.g., Persantine or dobutamine), to test for any significant myocardial ischemia. Determination of cardiac function and risk stratification are based on the duration of exercise, any symptoms that develop, and the presence of electrocardiographic (ECG) findings such as flipped T waves or ST-segment depression or elevation. In addition to the ECG portion, stress testing may

include imaging with echocardiography or myocardial perfusion with labeled radioisotopes.

Echocardiography is a diagnostic test performed to assess cardiac structure and function. Several parameters can be estimated from echocardiography, such as the degree of valvular insufficiency or stenosis, wall motion abnormalities, and the ejection fraction. The ejection fraction is the percentage of the stroke volume that is expelled from the left ventricle with systole; the normal range is 55% to 70%. An echocardiogram is not routinely ordered unless the patient is having active or new cardiac complaints.

Cardiac catheterization is the gold standard for evaluating the coronary anatomy and assessing for the presence of significant atherosclerosis. However, it is not routinely recommended for preoperative assessment, given the invasive nature of the procedure, unless the patient has a significant abnormality on cardiac stress testing and it is recommended by the consulting cardiologist.

Evaluation of blood cholesterol levels is also important for assessment of future risks of cardiovascular events. The American College of Cardiology recommends targeting the low-density lipoprotein (LDL) level at below 100 mg/dl in individuals with coronary artery disease or diabetes mellitus. However, the target LDL level may be below 70 mg/dl, depending on the patient's comorbidities. The target high-density lipoprotein (HDL) level is above 40 mg/dl for males and above 50 mg/dl for females.

The current patient's most recent testing was done at his last physical examination several months ago. His total cholesterol was 190 mg/dl, LDL 125 mg/dl, and HDL 37 mg/dl. The basic metabolic profile was within normal limits (levels of potassium must be monitored in the hypertensive person on diuretics). A treadmill cardiac stress test done within the past year did not reveal any signs of myocardial ischemia.

A 12-lead electrocardiogram revealed no abnormalities. (Electrocardiography is an invaluable tool for obtaining information on cardiac conduction, chamber enlargement, electrolyte disturbances, drug toxicities, myocardial ischemia, and infarction. Elevation of the ST segment is strongly suspicious of myocardial injury, whereas ST depression is suggestive of myocardial ischemia.)

ASSESSMENT

A 57-year-old man with a history of coronary artery disease, hypertension, and hypercholesterolemia, requiring outpatient removal of a dentigerous cyst under intravenous sedation anesthesia.

The treating cardiologist was contacted for perioperative risk assessment for an elective low-risk surgery. He stratified the patient as intermediate risk for surgery with a recommendation to continue the existing atenolol regimen without interruption. He noted that the aspirin could be held preoperatively, if necessary, to minimize potential bleeding complications and then resumed after surgery. (A preoperative medical evaluation serves to assess the patient's risk of morbidity and mortality in the perioperative period. There is insufficient evidence to support the use of β-blockers in patients undergoing low-risk procedures; however, they are continued during the perioperative period in patients already on a β-blocker regimen.)

TREATMENT

After discussion of the risks, benefits, and alternatives, the patient elected to proceed with the procedure. He was instructed to withhold all his morning medications with the exception of his blood pressure pills, which were to be taken with a small sip of water. The patient was also counseled on the benefits of tobacco cessation and improved dietary and exercise habits.

Surgery was carried out with the patient monitored using the ASA I standards for outpatient procedures (ASA I monitoring includes electrocardiogram, blood pressure, heart rate, and pulse oximeter monitoring). Intravenous anesthesia was planned using a combination of Versed and fentanyl. Five minutes into the procedure, the electrocardiogram showed multiple unifocal premature ventricular contractions at the rate of about 10 per minute. The patient's oxygen saturation declined from 98% on room air to 92% with 4 L/min oxygen flow via a nasal cannula. His oxygen flow was increased to 8 L/min, resulting in improvement of the oxygen saturation to 97%. The patient then suddenly became noticeably agitated, tachypneic with shallow breaths, and tachycardic, with a heart rate of 135 bpm (agitation can be a sign of hypoxia). The procedure was aborted, and all intravenous anesthetics were halted. His blood pressure now measured 90/45 mm Hg (hypotension). His condition continued to deteriorate, with ST-segment elevation and multifocal premature ventricular contractions showing on the electrocardiogram. He remained tachycardic with persistent hypotension. The patient emerged from anesthesia and complained of chest tightness while putting his fist over this chest (a positive Levine sign; the patient places his or her hand over the sternal region due to the dull, aching, squeezing discomfort of an AMI). A diagnosis of AMI was suspected, and emergency medical services (EMS) was immediately activated. EMS personnel arrived within minutes and transported the patient to a local hospital.

A suspected AMI should be managed with use of the American Heart Association's adult advanced cardiovascular life support (ACLS) algorithm for ischemic chest pain. Immediate treatment should include administration of supplemental oxygen (to increase oxygen delivery), along with 325 mg of aspirin (to inhibit platelet function and clot propagation). Sublingual nitroglycerin (vasodilator) is administered to increase coronary blood flow, which reduces cardiac ischemia and therefore pain. If chest pain is not resolved, morphine should be administered intravenously. The mnemonic MONA (morphine, oxygen, nitroglycerin, and aspirin) outlines this treatment. Vital signs and oxygen saturation should be monitored during these interventions. Intravenous access should to be initiated immediately for drug delivery. A 12-lead electrocardiogram, serum cardiac markers, serum electrolytes and coagulation studies, and a portable chest radiograph should be obtained as soon as possible. The decision whether to treat the patient with pharmacologic agents, including intravenous heparin, glycoprotein IIb/IIIa receptor inhibitors, direct thrombin inhibitors, and nitroglycerin, is based on the electrocardiogram findings and continuous clinical assessment. In the setting of an ST-elevation myocardial infarction, rapid assessment and transport to a cardiac catheterization lab is essential; the goal is a door-to-balloon time under 90 minutes for revascularization of the affected vessel or vessels.

COMPLICATIONS

The most feared complication of an AMI is sudden death (most commonly due to ventricular fibrillation or myocardial rupture). The immediate- and long-term sequelae of an AMI are related to the extent and location of the necrotic myocardial tissue. Subsequent inflammatory and electrical conduction abnormalities that lead to mechanical dysfunction of the heart can be variable in both chronology and severity.

Cardiac arrhythmias are commonly seen during an AMI. Infarction of specialized myocardial tissue, such as the sinoatrial node, atrioventricular node, or bundle branches, can lead to a variety of arrhythmias and conduction blocks. Ventricular fibrillation is a nonperfusing rhythm that needs to be rapidly identified and treated via the ACLS protocol.

Impaired myocardial function can cause failure of the heart to adequately pump blood into the systemic circulation, with subsequent congestion of blood into the pulmonary circulation, resulting in congestive heart failure (CHF) (see the Congestive Heart Failure section earlier in this chapter). AMI may also lead to cardiogenic shock, which is defined as tissue hypoperfusion secondary to heart failure, resulting in decreased cardiac output and hypotension.

Ischemia or necrosis of specific anatomic locations may result in mechanical dysfunctions such as rupture of the papillary muscles, ventricular septal perforation, or rupture of the ventricular free wall and subsequent cardiac tamponade (usually resulting in death). Other long-term complications include pericarditis (inflammation of the pericardium) and thromboembolic events originating within the cardiac chamber secondary to endothelial injury, stasis of blood, and turbulent flow.

DISCUSSION

The prevalence of cardiovascular diseases in the United States is 20% to 25%; these diseases account for nearly 40% of fatalities from all causes. It is estimated that cardiac deaths and myocardial infarction occur in 0.2% (50,000 deaths) of all cases of surgery under general anesthesia annually. As the baby boomer population ages and the number of patients undergoing elective surgery increases, perioperative cardiovascular evaluation should be performed meticulously in patients at risk.

The etiologies of myocardial infarction span a broad range of pathologic processes, including atherosclerosis with thromboembolic events, vascular syndromes, coronary aneurysms, primary and drug-induced coronary spasms (cocaine), severe conditions of oxygen demand with hypotension (aortic stenosis, sepsis), and hyperviscosity states (polycythemia vera). Signs and symptoms of AMI are not always evident. Approximately 20% of patients who sustain an AMI are asymptomatic and have retrospective positive electrocardiographic findings. This is particularly significant in the diabetic patient, who may not experience painful symptoms due to underlying peripheral neuropathy.

Studies have provided evidence that the use of β-blockers reduces morbidity and mortality in patients with an AMI and those in heart failure due to left ventricular systolic dysfunction. By reducing the sympathetic drive to the myocardium (and hence workload), β-blockers have been shown to reduce the rate of reinfarction and recurrent ischemia. In addition, ACE inhibitors have been proven to increase survival in patients with AMI.

With progressive ischemia and subsequent myocardial infarction, the electrocardiographic findings include T-wave inversions (ischemia), ST-segment elevation (suggestive of acute myocardial infarct), ST-segment depression (nontransmural infarct or ischemia), and the development of Q waves (indicative of myocardial infarction). The leads in which an ST-segment elevation occur correspond to the area of cardiac injury. On a 12-lead electrocardiogram, leads V1 through V6 are designated as the precordial chest leads and leads I, II, III, aVL, aVR, and aVF are the limb leads. An inferior infarct commonly presents with abnormalities in leads II, II, and aVF, while findings on leads V1 through V6 represent injury to the anterior wall.

Cardiac enzymes are plasma diagnostic markers released during myocardial necrosis. Based on the onset of injury, concentration, and metabolic half-life of the enzymes released, myocardial cell necrosis can be confirmed. In addition, the approximate time of infarction can be predicted. Several enzymes are used, including creatine kinase, creatine kinase–myocardial band, and troponin I or T. Creatine kinase and myoglobin are not specific to myocardial tissue and can be elevated from other etiologies. The creatine kinase–myocardial band enzymes can also be found in skeletal muscles and are not as cardiac specific for myocardial tissue. Troponins T and I are currently the markers of choice for determining acute cardiac injury, because they have higher cardiac specificity and are much more sensitive than the creatine kinase–myocardial band enzyme. Troponin levels can be detected as soon as 4 to 8 hours postinjury and may remain elevated until 5 to 9 days later. Myocardial muscle creatinine kinase isoenzymes typically peak at 24 hours, with a return to the normal range in 48 to 72 hours.

In summary, a thorough patient history and physical examination are essential in determining the general health and preoperative risk of the patient. This should be done in cooperation with the patient's primary care physician and cardiologist when indicated. In the event of an AMI in the office setting, early detection of symptoms is critical. Management should follow ACLS guidelines, including defibrillation for indicated arrhythmias, symptomatic management with morphine, oxygen, nitroglycerin, and aspirin, and timely transfer to the hospital setting, where continued medical therapy and cardiac catheterization can significantly increase the likelihood of patient survival.

Bibliography

Andreoli TE, Benjamin I, Griggs RC, et al: *Andreoli and Carpenter's Cecil essentials of medicine*, ed 8, St Louis, 2011, Saunders.

Crawford MH: *Current diagnosis and treatment in cardiology*, ed 2, New York, 2006, McGraw-Hill.

Cummins RO: *ACLS provider manual*, Dallas, 2004, American Heart Association.

Farrell MH, Foody JM, Krumholz HM: Beta-blockers in heart failure: clinical applications, *JAMA* 287:890-897, 2002.

Fleisher LA, Beckman JA, Brown KA, et al: ACC/AHA 2007 guidelines on perioperative cardiovascular evaluation and care for noncardiac surgery: a report of the American College of Cardiology/American Heart Association Task Force on Practice Guidelines (Writing Committee to Revise the 2002 Guidelines on Perioperative Cardiovascular Evaluation for Noncardiac Surgery), *J Am Coll Cardiol* 50:e159-e241, 2007.

Fleisher LA, Beckman JA, Brown KA, et al: 2009 ACCF/AHA focused update on perioperative beta blockade incorporated into the ACC/AHA 2007 guidelines on perioperative cardiovascular evaluation and care for noncardiac surgery: a report of the American College of Cardiology Foundation/American Heart Association Task Force on Practice Guidelines, *J Am Coll Cardiol* 54:e13-e118, 2009.

Fuster V, Alexander RW, O'Rourke RA, et al: *Hurst's the heart*, ed 11, Philadelphia, 2006, McGraw-Hill.

Huffman JC, Smith FA, Blais MA, et al: Recognition and treatment of depression and anxiety in patients with acute myocardial infarction, *Am J Cardiol* 98:319-324, 2006.

Lilly LS: *Pathophysiology of heart disease*, ed 3, Philadelphia, 2002, Lippincott Williams & Wilkins.

Hypertension*

Mehran Mehrabi

CC

A 40-year-old African American man presents to the office with a referral for extraction of third molars due to periodontal disease (essential hypertension is most commonly diagnosed during the third to fifth decades of life, has a higher prevalence in African American males, and is more resistant to therapy in African Americans).

HPI

The patient complains of a 2-week history of bilateral posterior mandibular third molar looseness. Triage of the patient reveals that his blood pressure is elevated, which he attributes to anxiety. He states that he has never seen a primary care physician and denies any history of hypertension. He denies headache, dizziness, blurred vision, chest pain, lower extremity edema, and shortness of breath (signs of potential end organ damage, commonly seen hypertensive emergency).

PMHX/PDHX/MEDICATIONS/ALLERGIES/SH/FH

The patient describes himself as "healthy as a horse" (hypertension is an asymptomatic disease) but physically out of shape due to lack of exercise. He does not take any medications at this time. He smokes one pack of cigarettes daily and has consumed four alcoholic beverages daily for the past 10 years (smoking, consumption of alcohol, and a sedentary lifestyle increase the risk of hypertension and coronary artery disease [CAD]). He is single, and his typical diet consists of fast foods (a diet high in sodium, saturated fat, and simple sugars). His family history is significant for the sudden death of his father at age 44 from a heart attack (a family history of myocardial infarction is significant when the paternal age is less than 45 and the maternal age is less than 55). His father also was known to be a diabetic for the last 6 years (a family history of diabetes and CAD are nonpreventable risk factors, whereas obesity, smoking, and excessive alcohol consumption are preventable risk factors for cardiovascular disease).

EXAMINATION

General. The patient is alert and oriented, calm, and cooperative and follows commands well. He appears to be in no apparent distress. He weighs 240 pounds and is 5 feet 7 inches tall (a body mass index of 37.6 kg/m², consistent with class II obesity).

Vital signs. Blood pressure is 185/104 mm Hg in the right arm sitting and 181/101 mm Hg in the left arm sitting (although an interarm blood pressure difference of about 10 mm Hg may be normal, a greater difference may be consistent with aortic dissection or subclavian stenosis), heart rate 80 bpm, respirations 16 per minute, temperature 37.4°C, and visual analog scale for pain at 0 of 10 (severe pain may cause an acute increase in blood pressure).

Maxillofacial. No facial edema, erythema, or induration. Neck examination is benign, with no evidence of masses or lymphadenopathy. The jugular venous distention is undetectable. (A jugular venous pressure greater than 3 cm or a measured central venous pressure greater than 8 is consistent with right ventricular failure. The most common cause of right ventricular failure is left ventricular failure.)

Intraoral. Examination is consistent with mobile lower third molars with 8 mm periodontal probing depth.

Fundoscopic. Arteriovenous nicking and an arteriolar light reflex ("copper wiring"), with no evidence of retinal necrosis or disc edema. (Fundoscopic examination allows direct examination of the vasculature. The pathophysiology of the retinal vessels is similar to that of the cerebral and coronary blood vessels. The initial changes seen with hypertension include vasoconstriction followed by hyaline degeneration. As blood pressure increases, arterial narrowing [arteriovenous nicking] and arteriolar light reflex [copper wiring] may be seen. In uncontrolled hypertension, there is a breakdown of the blood-retina barrier and presentation of hemorrhage and areas of infarction [cotton-wool spots]).

Cardiovascular. No carotid, femoral, or renal bruits are present (these are indicative of peripheral vascular disease). On palpation of the heart, the apical impulse is palpated at the fifth intercostal space and the midclavicular line (normal position). It is enlarged at 4 cm (normal is 2 to 3 cm), sustained, and strong in intensity (indicative of ventricular hypertrophy). On auscultation, there is an S1 (first heart sound) and S2 (second heart sound), in addition to S4 gallop (a pathologic heart sound during the late diastolic period produced by the atrium pushing on an inelastic myocardium) just before S1 (S3, which may be present in patients with CHF, may be secondary to uncontrolled hypertension and is heard shortly after an S2). The rhythm is regular (irregularly irregular rhythm can be due to atrial fibrillation caused by hypertension). There is no murmur or rub on auscultation. Peripheral

*The authors and publisher wish to acknowledge Dr. Chris Jo for his contribution on this topic to previous edition.

pulses are bounding, with rapid upstroke and 2+ intensity, and synchronous with appropriate amplitude (a delayed femoral pulse, compared to the radial pulse, is consistent with coarctation, a congenital cause of hypertension).

Pulmonary. The chest is clear on auscultation bilaterally. There are no crackles or wheezing (cardiogenic wheeze is produced by pulmonary edema in acute CHF).

Abdomen. The patient is obese and has no evidence of surgical scars or striae (present in hypercortisolism secondary to adrenal tumor, pituitary tumor, or paraneoplastic syndromes). Bowel sounds are present on auscultation. The abdomen is soft and nontender to palpation. The kidneys are nonpalpable (individuals with enlarged kidneys, as are seen in polycystic kidney disease, may present with hypertension). The liver is 10 cm at the midclavicular line (normal is 10 to 12 cm). The aorta is not palpable and is not enlarged (if it were enlarged, this would be suggestive of an acute abdominal aneurysm).

IMAGING

The panoramic radiograph is the study of choice when evaluating third molars. In the current patient, there is evidence of bone loss surrounding the roots of mandibular third molars. In the setting of controlled hypertension, no additional radiographs are required for minor surgical procedures. On evaluation of hypertensive urgency or emergency in the emergency department, additional studies are required and may include a chest radiograph (to evaluate for cardiogenic pulmonary edema and cardiomegaly), electrocardiogram (to rule out AMI), and/or head CT (to rule out intracerebral hemorrhage). Depending on the clinical history and findings, a preoperative electrocardiogram may be warranted for patients undergoing general anesthesia who have risk factors for cardiovascular disease (hypertension, diabetes, smoking, hypercholesterolemia, and age over 45 in males and over 55 in females).

LABS

Laboratory studies are obtained based on the patient's medical history. For the patient with essential hypertension who presents for minor surgical procedures, no laboratory studies are indicated. Several laboratory parameters may be measured by the primary care physician or measured preoperatively to detect secondary causes of hypertension; these include plasma sodium (rennin-producing tumors, renal disease), potassium (renal or adrenal disease), creatinine (renal disease), urine vanillylmandelic acid (pheochromocytoma), serum cortisol, and thyroid-stimulating hormone, which are all markers of

potential causes of secondary hypertension. An astute clinician uses the patient's history and physical examination to develop a differential diagnosis. Radiographic, laboratory, and other tests are used to assess the validity of specific diagnoses.

ASSESSMENT

Chronic severe localized periodontitis complicated by elevated blood pressure.

The diagnosis of hypertension requires additional blood pressure readings. If these readings are confirmed in subsequent evaluations, the patient is classified as having stage II hypertension.

According to the seventh report of the Joint National Committee on Prevention, Detection, Evaluation, and Treatment of High Blood Pressure (JNC-7), a normal systolic blood pressure is below 120 mm Hg and a normal diastolic blood pressure is below 80 mm Hg. The blood pressure may be considered normal, prehypertensive, stage I hypertension, or stage II hypertension (Table 15-8). The effects on the end organs, such as the heart, brain, kidney, and eyes, are in a linear relationship.

TREATMENT

Management of the hypertensive patient begins with an accurate diagnosis. Blood pressure is determined by cardiac output (stroke volume multiplied by heart rate) and total peripheral resistance. It is measured with the patient in a sitting position with the arm at the level of the heart. Patients should avoid smoking and caffeine 30 minutes and 1 hour, respectively, before a blood pressure reading is taken. Note that a large cuff produces an erroneously low reading, and a small cuff produces an erroneously high reading. The blood pressure can be measured in both arms. A difference greater than 10 mm Hg may be suggestive of aortic dissection. The most common site for measurement of blood pressure is the brachial artery. The cuff is applied to the arm. It is tightened as the radial pulse is palpated, and the pressure is raised until it is 30 mm Hg above where the radial pulse disappears. This technique ensures that an auscultatory gap (a period of silence as the blood pressure cuff pressure decreases) does not result in an erroneously low reading. Measurements are repeated two or three times in different settings before the diagnosis of hypertension is made.

A blood pressure reading should be obtained before surgical procedures, even in the absence of symptoms or a positive medical history. Contraindications to surgery in a

Table 15-8	Classification of Blood Pressure in Adults			
Blood Pressure	**Normal (mm Hg)**	**Prehypertension (mm Hg)**	**Stage I Hypertension (mm Hg)**	**Stage II Hypertension (mm Hg)**
Systolic	<120	120-139	140-159	>160
Diastolic	<80	80-89	90-99	>100

hypertensive patient are not based on the actual blood pressure, but rather on clinical judgment in assessing the risks and benefits of surgical or nonsurgical interventions. Elective procedures should be deferred with a sudden, unexplained rise in blood pressure. When a hypertensive patient presents with symptoms of hypertensive emergency (diplopia, dizziness, headaches, shortness of breath, sudden leg swelling, chest pain), elective surgery is deferred and the patient is referred to the emergency department for further work-up and management.

Consultation with the primary care physician is valuable when possible but may not always be feasible. If there is no surgical emergency, temporary analgesia may be achieved with a long-acting local anesthetic and analgesic medications. When treating an urgent surgical problem in a hypertensive patient, the clinician may choose local anesthesia office sedation or hospital-based general anesthesia, depending on the clinician's training and comfort, location of practice, and the facility's monitoring capability.

When patients with a history of hypertension present for office intravenous sedation, they should continue with their daily antihypertensive medications. Abrupt withdrawal of certain antihypertensive medications, such as clonidine or β-blockers, may result in hypertensive urgencies (rebound hypertension). General anesthetic medications that may result in hypertension, such as ketamine (sympathomimetic effects), should be avoided or used cautiously. Local anesthetics with vasoconstrictors should be used cautiously and sparingly. Most dental literature recommends limiting epinephrine to 0.04 mg in patients with cardiovascular disease; however, this is a subject of controversy. A recent report, published by the Agency for Healthcare Research and Quality, evaluated the use of local anesthesia for dental extractions with and without epinephrine in hypertensive and normotensive individuals. The difference in systolic blood pressure and heart rate for epinephrine versus no epinephrine was 4 mm Hg and 6 bpm, respectively, in hypertensive patients when up to 2 carpules (1.8 ml each) of anesthetic agents were used.

The cause of intraoperative hypertensive episodes needs to be rapidly assessed and appropriately managed. Hypertension may be due to hypoxia, hypercarbia, anxiety, pain, full bladder, or prior medications, or it may be idiopathic (primary hypertension). Common intravenous antihypertensives used in ambulatory surgery are β-blockers and hydralazine. β-Blockers, such as esmolol (short acting) and labetalol (longer acting), reduce the blood pressure and heart rate; hydralazine reduces blood pressure with concurrent reflex tachycardia. It is extremely important not to treat numbers, but rather to evaluate the patient as a whole. Factors that must be considered include the patient's age, past medical history, family history (age, race, family history of hypertension), and social history (cocaine, methamphetamine, methoxymethyl methamphetamine abuse); initial blood pressure (baseline); type of procedure; medications used (ketamine); respiratory rate (pain); heart rate; and temperature (malignant hyperthermia).

During general anesthesia, patients on hypertensive medications may also be susceptible to episodes of hypotension. Propofol administered as a bolus can lower the systolic blood pressure up to 30 mm Hg, which can be exaggerated in patients with hypertension. Inhalation general anesthetics may also precipitously lower mean arterial pressures (due to vasodilation). Hypotension most commonly responds well to bolus fluid administration. If the patient is not responsive to conservative fluid treatment, a vasopressor agent may be required. The choice of vasopressor agent depends on both the blood pressure and heart rate. In the hypotensive and bradycardic patient, vasogenic stimulators that cause a reflex bradycardia should be avoided (phenylephrine). Ephedrine should be used for the hypotensive and bradycardic patient unresponsive to intravenous fluid bolus and a decreased the level of anesthesia. Phenylephrine is ideal for hypotensive and tachycardic patients.

Patients (particularly the elderly) admitted to the hospital are at greater risk of hypotension than hypertension. This may be due to a low-sodium diet, concurrent medications, narcotic use, or lack of physical activity. Therefore, hypertensive medications, such as diuretics, angiotensin-converting enzyme (ACE) inhibitors, angiotensin receptor blockers (ARBs), α-blockers, or calcium channel blockers, should be prescribed when the blood pressure is elevated. β-Blockers should be continued not only for their cardioprotective effect, but also for possible rebound tachycardia (perioperative administration of β-blockers has been shown to decrease anesthetic complications). Rebound hypertension also is common with the use of clonidine, but this medication is now rarely used. When patients are discharged from the hospital or office, they should continue their prior antihypertensive medication regimen.

The current patient was referred to his primary care physician for evaluation and management of his blood pressure. Three subsequent blood pressure readings in the physician's office, in addition to those from an automatic blood pressure monitor at the local pharmacy, reflected a systolic blood pressure of 175 to 185 mm Hg and a diastolic blood pressure of 95 to 105 mm Hg. The patient was instructed to restrict sodium and alcohol intake, to quit smoking, and to start aerobic exercise. However, the patient remained hypertensive at 150/90 mm Hg. He was subsequently placed on hydrochlorothiazide (diuretics are considered first-line therapy). At follow-up, his blood pressure was 130/82 mm Hg.

After his blood pressure had stabilized, the patient was scheduled for surgical extraction of the lower third molars using intravenous sedation. He was instructed to continue the hydrochlorothiazide (antihypertensive medications should be continued in the perioperative period). His blood pressure remained stable throughout the procedure.

COMPLICATIONS

Hypertensive urgency is hypertension with a blood pressure above 180/120 mm Hg in an asymptomatic patient. Patients are admitted to the emergency department, and the blood pressure is gradually lowered with oral medications. The blood pressure should not be abruptly reduced to less than 160/110 mm Hg due to the risk of cerebral and myocardial hypoperfusion. Hypertensive emergency is hypertension with evidence of end organ damage (brain, heart, kidneys, eyes), such as retinal hemorrhages and exudates, papilledema, renal failure (malignant nephrosclerosis), neurologic symptoms (headache, weakness, or neurosensory deficit), and cardiac symptoms, such as chest pain. Intravenous medications, such as nitroprusside (0.25 to 0.5 µg/kg/min, up to 8 to 10 µg/kg/min), nicardipine (5 to 15 mg/hour), or labetalol (0.5 to 2 mg/min), may be used to control blood pressure. Note that nitroprusside may result in cyanide toxicity, which can be treated with sodium thiosulfate. Nonintravenous routes (e.g., oral, nasal, or transcutaneous route) can be used, but they are not as titratable. A rapid decline in blood pressure can be as harmful as a rapid rise. Close monitoring of vital signs is more important than the route of administration.

Chronic complications of hypertension include CAD, CHF, cerebrovascular accident, renal disease, ophthalmologic disease, and others. Treatment of hypertension significantly reduces the risk of CAD, myocardial infarction, heart failure, and cerebrovascular accidents.

Antihypertensive medications can cause various side effects or complications, including orthostatic hypotension (especially in the elderly), resulting in syncope and ground-level falls.

DISCUSSION

Hypertension is frequently referred to as a "silent killer" and is a common disorder. In the United States, it is most prevalent among African Americans, followed by Hispanics and Caucasians. The incidence of hypertension increases with age and excess body weight. Other risk factors include genetics (hypertension is twice as common when one or both parents have hypertension), alcohol consumption, tobacco use, and male gender. Other factors, such as salt intake and type A personality, have not been shown to be risk factors for the development of hypertension. However, a low-salt diet decreases blood pressure in hypertensive patients, whereas a high-salt diet makes hypertension more resistant to therapy.

Hypertension may be divided into primary, or essential, (95%) and secondary (5%) categories. Although secondary hypertension is less common, diagnosis is important, because frequently a cure rather than treatment is possible. Essential (idiopathic) hypertension is generally diagnosed between the ages of 30 and 50, whereas secondary hypertension is most commonly identified prior to age 30 or after age 50. Secondary hypertension tends to be more severe and less susceptible to the routine treatment used for essential hypertension.

Secondary hypertension includes a variety of hormonal or structural defects. Elevation of steroid levels (primary adrenal tumor, secondary pituitary tumor, or tertiary paraneoplastic syndrome), calcium (hyperparathyroidism), and hypothyroidism (and hyperthyroid crisis) are common hormonal etiologies. A structural defect, such as coarctation of the aorta or renal artery stenosis and intracranial hypertension, may also cause systemic hypertension.

Treatment should be considered when two or three consecutive blood pressure readings are found to be above 140/80 mm Hg. Conservative treatment, such as weight reduction, a low-salt (sodium) diet, aerobic exercise, and cessation of alcohol and tobacco products, can be beneficial in preventing medical therapy.

Two landmark studies evaluated the effect of diet on hypertension. In the Treatment of Mild Hypertension Study (TOMHS), 902 patients with a diastolic blood pressure of 90 to 100 mm Hg participated in a regimen of sodium and alcohol restriction, weight reduction, and increased physical activity; they showed an improvement in the systolic and diastolic blood pressures of 8.6 mm Hg compared with the placebo group. The Dietary Approach to Stop Hypertension (DASH) study consisted of 459 hypertensive patients with blood pressures less than 160/90 mg Hg who were placed on a diet consisting of fruits and vegetables that was low in saturated fats. Blood pressure was reduced by 5.5/3 mm Hg in normotensive patients and by 11.4/5.5 mm Hg in hypertensive patients. This was followed by the DASH/low-sodium trial, which showed an additive effect. Blood pressure reduction with a low-sodium diet works independently of a healthy diet low in saturated fats and high in fruits and vegetables.

A variety of studies have examined various initial therapies for hypertension; these include the Medical Research Council (MRC) trial (showing the cardioprotective effect of β-blockers over thiazide diuretics in patients with CAD), Captopril Prevention Project (CAPPP study, showing the benefits of ACE inhibitors in diabetics), UK Prospective Diabetes Study, STOP Hypertension Trial, Heart Outcomes Prevention Evaluation (HOPE), Losartan Intervention for Endpoint Reduction (LIFE), and Australian National Blood Pressure (ANBP) studies.

The JNC-7 recommendations are based on the Antihypertensive and Lipid-Lowering Treatment to Prevent Heart Attack Trial (ALL-HAT). This study was a randomized examination of 45,000 patients with hypertension and one other risk factor (e.g., left ventricular hypertrophy, diabetes, cerebrovascular accident). The current recommendation is initiation of a low-dose hydrochlorothiazide (a sodium potassium channel blocker at the distal tubule of kidneys) as first-line antihypertensive therapy (higher doses may produce hypokalemia, hypertriglyceridemia, hyperglycemia, and gout).

A β-blocker may be a better choice in patients with CAD due to its post–myocardial infarction cardioprotective effect. Also, it may be the drug of choice in patients with migraine-type headaches, glaucoma, angina pectoris, essential tremor, and resting tachycardia. Sudden cessation of this medication can produce a withdrawal reaction and should be avoided. ACE inhibitors prevent the formation of angiotensin II and aldosterone. They are commonly considered the initial therapy in diabetic patients with microproteinuria, and they may be beneficial for post–myocardial infarction cardioprotection, comparable to that of β-blockers. ACE inhibitors are contraindicated in patients who develop angioneurotic edema or hyperkalemia, and in rare cases they can cause neutropenia. A dry cough is a side effect of ACE inhibitors, most likely due to the buildup of bradykinins; this is best treated by changing to another class of medication. ARBs are an alternative to ACE inhibitors in certain patients.

Calcium channel blockers are potent vasodilators; in general, they are not recommended for initial therapy. Their use in patients with CHF increases mortality. They also exacerbate reflux in patients known to have gastroesophageal reflux disorder (GERD). However, they are beneficial in patients with peripheral vascular disease or vasospasm, such as in Raynaud's disease. The α-blockers (e.g., prazosin, doxazosin, and terazosin) are not first-line medications. They produce syncope, headache, and weakness. They may be indicated in patients with benign prostatic hypertrophy. Antihypertensive medications considered safe during pregnancy include methyldopa and hydralazine, which generally are not considered in nonpregnant patients.

Other antihypertensive medications, such as clonidine (a central α_2-agonist), trimethaphan (a ganglionic blocker), and phentolamine and phenoxybenzamine (competitive and noncompetitive α_1- and α_2-blockers, respectively) are rarely used except for specific indications.

Hypertension is a common, asymptomatic disease; if left treated, it may result in various end organ injuries. CAD, CHF, cerebrovascular accidents, end-stage renal disease, retinal disease, and peripheral vascular disease are examples of complications. A dental office is more frequently visited than a primary care physician's office for "otherwise healthy" individuals and may be the first place a patient's blood pressure is evaluated. Nonpharmacologic therapy, such as weight reduction, diet modification, exercise, and alcohol and tobacco cessation, is an inexpensive and effective means of reducing blood pressure with few side effects. When pharmacologic therapy is indicated, a compromise should be made, focusing on the drug with the least problematic side effects that can prevent complications and achieve patient compliance.

Bibliography

Bursztyn M: Blood pressure difference between arms, *Arch Intern Med* 157:818, 1997.

Chobanian AV, Bakris GL, Black HR, et al: The seventh report of the Joint National Committee on Prevention, Detection, Evaluation, and Treatment of High Blood Pressure: the JNC 7 report, *JAMA* 289:2560-2572, 2003.

Dahlof B, Devereux RB, Kjeldsen SE, et al: Cardiovascular morbidity and mortality in the Losartan Intervention For Endpoint Reduction in Hypertension study (LIFE): a randomized trial against atenolol, *Lancet* 359:995-1003, 2002.

Hansson L, Lindholm LH, Niskanen L, et al: Effect of angiotensin-converting-enzyme inhibition compared with conventional therapy on cardiovascular morbidity and mortality in hypertension: the Captopril Prevention Project (CAPPP) randomized trial, *Lancet* 353:611-616, 1999.

Heart Outcomes Prevention Evaluation Study Investigators: Effects of ramipril on cardiovascular and microvascular outcomes in people with diabetes mellitus: results of the HOPE study and MICRO-HOPE substudy, *Lancet* 355:253-259, 2000.

Miall WE: Beta-blockers vs thiazides in the treatment of hypertension: a review of the experience of the large national trials, *J Cardiovasc Pharmacol* 16(Suppl 5):S58-S63, 1990.

Neaton JD, Grimm RH Jr, Prineas RJ, et al: Treatment of mild hypertension study: final results. Treatment of Mild Hypertension Study Research Group, *JAMA* 270:713-724, 1993.

Neutel JM, Smith DH, Wallin D, et al: A comparison of intravenous nicardipine and sodium nitroprusside in the immediate treatment of severe hypertension, *Am J Hypertens* 7:623, 1994.

Sacks FM, Svetkey LP, Vollmer WM, et al: Effects on blood pressure of reduced dietary sodium and the Dietary Approaches to Stop Hypertension (DASH) diet. DASH-Sodium Collaborative Research Group, *N Engl J Med* 344:3-10, 2001.

Schulz V: Clinical pharmacokinetics of nitroprusside, cyanide, thiosulphate and thiocyanate, *Clin Pharmacokinet* 9:239, 1984.

Vaughan CJ, Delanty N: Hypertensive emergencies, *Lancet* 356:411, 2000.

Index

Page numbers followed by "f" indicate figures, "t" indicate tables, and "b" indicate boxes.